EVERYONE'S GUIDE TO
Cancer Therapy

Other Books in the Series

Everyone's Guide to Cancer Supportive Care
Everyone's Guide to Cancer Survivorship

EVERYONE'S GUIDE TO

Cancer Therapy

*How Cancer Is Diagnosed,
Treated, and Managed Day to Day*

■ REVISED FIFTH EDITION

Andrew H. Ko, M.D.

Malin Dollinger, M.D.

Ernest H. Rosenbaum, M.D.

**Andrews McMeel
Publishing, LLC**
Kansas City

Everyone's Guide to Cancer Therapy, Revised Fifth Edition, copyright © 2008 by Andrew H. Ko, M.D., Malin Dollinger, M.D., and Ernest H. Rosenbaum, M.D. All rights reserved. Printed in the United States of America. No part of this book may be used or reproduced in any manner whatsoever without written permission except in the case of reprints in the context of reviews. For information, write Andrews McMeel Publishing, LLC, an Andrews McMeel Universal company, 4520 Main Street, Kansas City, Missouri 64111.

First edition, 1991. Second edition, 1994. Third edition, 1997. Fourth edition, 2002.

08 09 10 11 12   SHD   10 9 8 7 6 5 4 3 2 1

ISBN-13: 978-0-7407-6857-6

ISBN-10: 0-7407-6857-3

Library of Congress Cataloging-in-Publication Data

Ko, Andrew.
   Everyone's guide to cancer therapy : how cancer is diagnosed, treated, and managed day to day / Andrew Ko, Ernest Rosenbaum, Malin Dollinger. —Rev. 5th ed.
      p. cm.
   Rev. ed. of: Everyone's guide to cancer therapy / Malin Dollinger . . . [et al.], 2002.
   Includes index.
   ISBN-13: 978-0-7407-6857-6
   ISBN-10: 0-7407-6857-3
   1. cancer—Popular works. I. Rosenbaum, Ernest H. II. Dollinger, Malin. III. Everyone's guide to cancer therapy. IV. Title.

   RC263.D59 2008
   616.99'406—dc22

                                                                        2007021127

www.andrewsmcmeel.com

Contents

■ ■ ■ ■

PART THREE
Quality of Life

PART FOUR
New Advances in Research, Risk Assessment, Diagnosis, and Treatment

PART FIVE
Treating the Common Cancers

Foreword

■ ■ ■ ■

In 1978, I was diagnosed with terminal lung cancer. I was given three months to live and told there were no treatments that could help me. The following week, I went to a major cancer center in another state, where the doctor told me I could be cured.

Over the next three years, I learned a great deal about cancer. It is an extremely complex disease. There are hundreds of types and stages, with numerous treatment methods available. Progress in finding more effective treatments is being made at a staggering rate, and I soon came to realize there is no conceivable way any single human being could know the latest and most appropriate treatment for every kind of cancer. It is difficult to keep up with every current treatment for even one kind of cancer. Yet if cancer is to be beaten, it must be treated promptly, properly, and thoroughly. There is often no second chance.

I also came to realize that if a doctor is unaware of the latest and best treatment for an individual patient, all the research—all the work done and all the money spent—is wasted as far as that patient is concerned. Many lives can be lost not because treatments to cure or control a cancer haven't been discovered, but because the physician may be unaware of them.

In 1981, I was chairman of the board of H&R Block, Inc., my family's income tax firm. We had acquired a computer service company in Columbus, Ohio, named CompuServe. One of its services was a network whereby anyone with a computer could call a local telephone number, be connected with the huge mainframes in Columbus, and get all kinds of information instantly. One kind of information service offered was news.

When a newspaper is set today, it is done on a computer, and CompuServe had arrangements with eleven major newspapers in the United States to have their articles fed into the company's mainframes as they were set. At night, I could contact CompuServe with my home computer and read the next morning's *New York Times, Los Angeles Times, Washington Post,* or *Chicago Tribune.* I could read the front page, the editorial page, the sports or financial columns, or whatever I selected. And I could read it before the people in those cities could get their paper locally.

It seemed obvious that, in the same way, a continually updated computer database of the latest cancer treatments could instantly deliver state-of-the-art information to any practicing physician in his or her own office.

The National Cancer Institute (NCI) had been working along similar lines. The institute had the task of developing effective methods to prevent, diagnose, and treat cancer and was given additional resources by Congress to develop a program to disseminate cancer information.

First, since an international research data bank had already been established, in 1974, NCI began developing specialized systems to aid in collecting information to be made available to the scientific community. Mary Lasker, a member of the National Cancer Advisory Board at that time, requested that NCI publish a book of treatment protocols to help practicing physicians find out about promising investigational therapies. She also asked that the book be updated every six months, but it wasn't feasible to prepare the equivalent of a textbook on clinical cancer research and change it semiannually.

In response, Dr. Vincent T. DeVita Jr., then the director of NCI's Division of Cancer Treatment, decided to develop a computerized database called CLINPROT (Clinical Protocols) containing information on protocols supported by the institute. By 1980, Dr. DeVita had established a working group to expand the database with state-of-the-art treatment information and to make it available to the growing number of physicians with personal computers.

In 1981, I communicated to Dr. DeVita my idea of having an easily accessible database of cancer therapies. He heartily agreed about how important it was to communicate fresh information directly to physicians and explained that NCI was developing such a database in two stages. The first stage involved adding a geographic matrix to CLINPROT, allowing physicians to identify investigational studies by area and other factors. This new file would be called PDQ1. The second stage involved adding state-of-the-art treatment information to PDQ1 and developing a comprehensive directory of physicians and treatment facilities that could be contacted for cancer care. This expanded database was named the Physician Data Query system but came to be known simply as PDQ.

I was so enthusiastic about this project that I assembled a group of donors to purchase a building just off the National Institutes of Health (NIH) campus to house these activities. And in 1982, I became a member of the National Cancer Advisory Board. Throughout my six-year term on the board, I continued to support the development and refinement of the system.

PDQ is now available instantly to physicians in the United States as well as in many other parts of the world through their personal computers, their hospital computers, or the facilities of any medical library. And it is available absolutely free to any individual by calling 1-800-4-CANCER.

Everyone's Guide to Cancer Therapy continues this important work in making the most up-to-date cancer information as widely available as possible. In its tumor treatment sections, it expands on the PDQ database and translates the information into clear, easily understood terms. It is hoped that the guide will serve as a critical resource for cancer patients, their families, and anyone else whose life has been or might be affected by this disease. It is also hoped that it will serve health professionals who want additional information about cancer and supportive care techniques for themselves and for their patients.

The National Cancer Institute has stated that if physicians used the latest recommended therapy, cancer mortality would be reduced by 10 percent, saving some 40,000 lives annually.

Considering that the proper information can now be had so rapidly and easily, can there be any excuse to lose lives by failing to get it for every patient?

■ Richard Bloch

Kansas City, 1991

Editors' Note: Richard Bloch, a tireless and effective advocate for cancer patients, passed on in 2004. His message, so eloquently stated here, is still as valid today as it was when it was originally written—perhaps even more so. We will all remember him for his vital contribution to cancer care.

Preface to the Fifth Edition

Margaret A. Tempero, M.D., Deputy Director, UCSF Comprehensive Cancer Center, and Past President, American Society of Clinical Oncology

■ ■ ■ ■

Cancer is a common disease that will affect almost 1.5 million Americans in 2008. But for the first time, the news on the battlefront is extremely encouraging. We have finally come to the fruition of our hard work in cancer research, and what we are seeing is greater prevention and improved early detection and therapy, proving that the investment in NCI- and NIH-funded research is paying off.

For example, thanks to state initiatives, tobacco control is increasingly in force, a factor that undoubtedly has contributed to the declining death rate from lung cancer. The latest statistics show a precipitous decrease in lung cancer deaths in men and, finally, a plateau in what was previously an inexorable rise in lung cancer deaths in women. Wider use of screening has improved early detection in breast, colorectal, and prostate cancers; deaths attributable to these diseases continue to decline. Preventive strategies such as these, coupled with improved treatment, are increasing cure rates and prolonging lives. In the past fifteen years, the median survival for patients with metastatic colorectal cancer has quadrupled, and metastatic breast and prostate cancers can now often be viewed as chronic diseases.

Recent advances in our war against cancer include a new cancer vaccine that was borne out of our understanding of the importance of cancer causation by certain subtypes of human papillomavirus. In addition to cervical cancer, this vaccine has the potential to reduce the burden of anal cancer as well as certain types of head and neck cancers. In the therapeutic arena, our understanding of cancer biology has identified pathways that are critical for the maintenance of tumor cells and has allowed us to design drugs that can interrupt these critical circuits. The classic example of this is imatinib mesylate (Gleevec), a drug that targets an enzyme called BCR/ABL in chronic myelogenous leukemia cells. The adoption of this treatment has transformed the lives of patients with this chronic form of leukemia. Moreover, in the past five years (a short time in drug development!), drug resistance to imatinib has been addressed by understanding the structural biology of the enzyme, leading to the subsequent design of other drugs as well.

Cancer cells do not exist in a vacuum and it is now understood that the microenvironment plays an important role in tumor invasion and metastasis. Tumors need new blood vessels to grow; agents that interfere with molecules essential to new blood vessel formation (antiangiogenesis drugs) are now approved by the FDA and in widespread use. Bevacizumab (Avastin), a neutralizing antibody against an angiogenic molecule called vascular endothelial growth factor (VEGF), is improving survival in patients with colorectal, breast, and lung cancers. Small molecules such as sorafenib (Nexavar) and sunitinib (Sutent) that target the receptor of VEGF are prolonging the lives of patients with metastatic kidney cancer and liver cancer, diseases that previously had no established treatment.

Just as we are gaining a better understanding of the molecular targets to treat cancer, we are also beginning to understand better the molecular determinants that affect a patients' prognosis and response to treatment. Our previous approach to cancer medicine was a "one size fits all" strategy. We developed treatments that helped general groups of patients, but we could not always identify which specific drug could help any one particular individual. Now, by understanding the gene expression in breast cancer cells and correlating this with outcome, it is possible to identify genetic patterns that can identify women at low, intermediate, and high risk of recurrence. Armed with this information, women and their physicians can make decisions about whether or not additional therapy after surgery would increase their chance for cure. Once treatment is selected, choices of treatment can be more strategic. One example is the use of trastuzumab (Herceptin), an antibody against a growth factor (HER-2) expressed on a subtype of breast cancer. In the future, it is probable that most treatments will be selected based on either the tumor, the host genotype, or a combination of the two.

Reaching this level of individualized management for early detection or therapy requires team science. Cancer centers around the country have long understood the important contributions of different disciplines and the synergy that occurs when diverse talents collaborate to tackle the issues inherent in serious diseases. Team science allows discovery to be propelled to clinical application at the fastest possible pace and, similarly, allows clinical observations to inform basic research. Critical to this team approach are our patients, who are full partners in the progress that is being made.

That is why this book is such an important resource for people at risk for cancer and for patients and their families. Equipped with knowledge, we can all participate more effectively in this discovery process. *Everyone's Guide to Cancer Therapy* is a blueprint for health. This book gives readers the tools they need to adopt a healthier lifestyle, to enroll in early-detection programs when appropriate, and to identify and participate in the highest-quality cancer care. The future is bright and cancer patients have every reason for hope. *Everyone's Guide to Cancer Therapy* is an important resource that can help every patient navigate their way to the growing ranks of cancer survivors.

Editors' Preface

■ ■ ■ ■

For the fourth edition of this book, we titled our preface "2002—a Cancer Odyssey," a perhaps not-so-subtle allusion to the influential science-fiction narrative of a similar name. Of course, the major difference between that masterpiece by Stanley Kubrick and Arthur C. Clarke and *Everyone's Guide to Cancer Therapy* was (and is) that the content of our book was far from fictional. However, perhaps if scientists and clinicians living in decades past were transported to the present day, some of oncology might almost seem the stuff of science fiction, given the dizzying array of medical advances that have been made in cancer diagnosis, treatment, and prevention. Even over the past five years—the length of time that has elapsed between publication of the previous edition and this current one—we have been witness to a continued revolution in cancer biology and cancer medicine. To be more specific, our growing knowledge of the molecular bases by which a normal cell becomes cancerous, survives, multiplies, and spreads has improved our ability to treat patients with cancer with greater and more frequent success than anytime in the past.

We have been extremely pleased with the public acceptance and high regard for this book and wish to have it continue to serve its purpose of effective communication for many years to come. The past reviews of this book have been most heartwarming and inspire us to work even harder to fulfill the trust you have placed in us. We now have editions in Canada, Greece, India, Serbo-Croatia, and Poland, and on CD-ROM as well as on recordings for the blind. With this edition, we take great pleasure in announcing the addition of a new editor, Andrew H. Ko, M.D., a medical oncologist and an assistant professor of medicine at the University of California, San Francisco (UCSF), Comprehensive Cancer Center, who assumed a primary role in the compilation of this book. Again we have added a number of contributing authors, well-known and experienced physicians and scientists who have provided updates on key advances in cancer medicine that have occurred in the twenty-first century. We continue to be grateful to our faithful and devoted authors, who now number over 140.

As has been done in previous editions, the book is divided into five major parts. Part I, "Diagnosis and Treatment," offers an overview of what cancer is and why it often requires the input of multiple different specialists, and provides specifics about the various modalities that can be used to treat it. In particular, we welcome the new perspectives brought by John Park on biological therapy and immunotherapy; Raman Muthusamy on laser therapy; and Stanley Rogers on radiofrequency-generated heat treatment.

Parts II and III of this book focus on the supportive care aspects and quality-of-life issues surrounding cancer and its treatment—topics that have frequently received too little attention, even in a comprehensive book such as this. These have long been areas of intense interest and commitment by one of this book's senior editors in particular, Ernest Rosenbaum, who has dedicated much of his life's work to developing programs that improve the quality of life for patients and their families affected by cancer. We are pleased to have several new authors contribute to these sections, including Natalie Ledesma, a nutritionist whose work focuses on the unique nutritional and dietary needs of patients with cancer; Mitch Golant, who writes a thoughtful chapter on how to handle the distress that can come with a cancer diagnosis; and Mitch Rosen, who adds an important new chapter on fertility issues that patients with cancer often face. Moreover, we point readers' attention to the chapters on the health care system and paying for cancer care; these are especially timely and relevant issues given the increasing financial complexities—and the increasing costs—associated with cancer therapy as new medical breakthroughs in diagnosis and treatment are made.

Part IV of this book tackles many of the exciting new advances taking place in cancer medicine. As in previous editions, Vincent DeVita Jr.—one of the true giants in the field of oncology—together with his coauthor Amanda Psyrri, offers an insightful look at where we've been, where we are currently, and where we're going, in the chapter entitled "The Impact of Research on the Cancer Problem: Looking Back, Moving Forward." Major updates are provided in the chapters dealing with cancer biology, gene therapy, and investigational new agents. Of equal importance, we emphasize that cancer screening and prevention have the potential to save countless lives, more so than even the most exciting and innovative new anticancer drugs; thus, pay close attention to the chapters in this section dealing with these important topics. In another chapter, Beth Crawford and Amie Blanco, two genetic counselors at the UCSF Comprehensive Cancer Center, provide fresh insight in a reader-friendly way on

genetic risk assessment and counseling. Finally, this section closes with what we believe is an extremely useful chapter written by our cancer center librarians, Gail Sorrough and Gloria Won, pertaining to cancer Web sites on the Internet. We hope this chapter provides readers with a good starting point to help them navigate the dizzying array of options that can be found on the Web, and to do so in a way that preserves their sanity.

The fifth and final part of this book takes a site-based approach to explain each specific type of cancer, from A to Z. While this certainly represents the most user-friendly way of presenting information, in the future other classification schemes may be used more frequently, as cancers become more accurately categorized according to their molecular profiles rather than simply by the organ from which they originated. We welcome a number of new contributors to this section, too numerous to mention here, who provide fresh insight in chapters on cancers of the anus, bladder, brain, head and neck, lung, skin (including separate chapters on melanoma and Kaposi's sarcoma), pancreas, prostate, testis, penis, and thymus, as well as AIDS-associated lymphomas, soft-tissue sarcomas of both children and adults, and gastrointestinal stromal tumors. Of course, extensive updates have also been made in chapters addressing the most common cancers seen in the United States and worldwide, including cancers of the breast, colon, liver, and cervix, to name just a few in which significant medical advances have been made since the fourth edition.

In addition to a lot of facts, pathways, diagrams, and statistics, we wish above all that readers with cancer, and their families and friends, find hope and encouragement here. When we look back on the state of cancer medicine when the first edition of this book was published (1991), compared to where we are today, there is much reason to be optimistic. While we may not yet have found the cure for all types of cancer, we are getting closer to making this disease one that people can live with, rather than die from, and, better yet, one that they are more and more often able to look at in their rearview mirror.

Andrew H. Ko, M.D.
Malin Dollinger, M.D.
Ernest H. Rosenbaum, M.D.

To the Reader

■ ■ ■ ■

When your life has been touched, or rather grabbed, by cancer, many things change. Whether it has happened to you, a member of your family, or a friend, the impact of a cancer diagnosis is always the same. It's like being hit by a truck.

New emotions suddenly crop up, the greatest being the fear and anxiety associated with having a new and unknown disease. Cancer comes with its own vast vocabulary, much of it probably unfamiliar, that you have to learn in a short span of time. Many new words and complicated descriptions will become part of your everyday thinking. Furthermore, countless questions arise. What can be done to cure me? What medical and psychosocial help is available? Will I suffer? Will there be pain? How can I live with this disease? Do I have to die?

It is our wish and our purpose in this book to give you as thorough and as careful an understanding as possible of what you are facing, what can be done, and what you can expect. Our aim is to describe in easily comprehensible language the details and consequences of the particular cancer you or someone close to you may be confronting, what therapies are available, and what kinds of questions you should ask.

We have attempted to present the most current and the most accurate information available, but we recognize that it is not possible to convey every possible approach to cancer diagnosis and therapy that is out there. Although we have tried to reflect the treatment guidelines listed by the information services of the National Cancer Institute, the American Society of Clinical Oncology, and other key cancer organizations, there may occasionally be alternative, experimental, and/or newer methods of diagnosis and treatment that your physician may wish to present to you. If you have any questions or issues that you need clarification about, or even doubts—raise them. Sometimes a second opinion can be useful and important. Remember, your physician has the responsibility of discussing your various options with you, explaining why he or she is recommending a particular treatment given your particular circumstances and based on solid evidence and sound medical reasoning, and devising together with you the most appropriate treatment plan.

This book was created to help you get more out of these discussions by allowing you to understand the complex problems of cancer diagnosis and treatment, to ask the right questions, and to search for and obtain the best medical care. The more you equip yourself with knowledge, the more you can think of yourself as a full partner in the decision-making process, and the more comfortable and confident you will feel as you move forward with hope in your treatment and, ideally, your recovery.

Acknowledgments

■ ■ ■ ■

The successful completion of such a complex and comprehensive book depends upon the support, assistance, and help of a great number of people. In each of the first four editions, you will find a long list of contributors, friends, and colleagues without whom this project would not have been possible. Rather than repeat the names of each one here, we will simply offer a heartfelt thanks for each individual's previous and in many instances ongoing support. We feel both humbled and deeply appreciative when we think of how many people were vital to the success of this book, from its first edition back in 1991 all the way to the present day with this fifth edition. We have had the additional benefit of two editions in Canada, as well as the publication of editions in four other countries. It has been quite a journey.

I, Andrew Ko, would personally like to thank Ernest Rosenbaum for giving me the opportunity to join him and Malin Dollinger in working on this newest edition. Ever since I joined the faculty at the University of California, San Francisco (UCSF), Dr. Rosenbaum has been a tremendous support and source of encouragement to me and has gone out of his way to help further my career. His and his wife Isadora's generosity of spirit both to myself and to countless others has never ceased to touch and inspire me. It has been a privilege to work side by side at UCSF with, and to learn from, someone such as Ernie, as well as others at the forefront of their fields, including Margaret Tempero (a coeditor of the fourth edition of this book) and Alan P.

Venook. To them, as well as to all of my previous mentors in Baltimore, Boston, and Palo Alto during each phase of my medical training, I extend my sincerest appreciation.

Little did I know what a tremendous undertaking a book such as this would be—communicating with dozens of contributing authors, struggling to meet deadlines, reading and rereading text to make sure it flowed smoothly and was readable to the general public. It made me only further appreciate the efforts of Drs. Dollinger and Rosenbaum, and the other editors from earlier editions, to ensure the successful and timely completion of such a project. Thankfully, for this fifth edition, we were able to enlist the help of Julie A. Uy, whose organizational skills, keen attention to detail, and sharp eyes and mind were vital in ensuring everything was done smoothly and in a timely fashion. Her ability to juggle responsibilities in assisting with the book while simultaneously coordinating clinical trials at the UCSF Comprehensive Cancer Center and helping with the care of patients is a testimony to her myriad talents.

We owe our special thanks to many other members of the UCSF Comprehensive Cancer Center staff for their help with this fifth edition, including Paula Chung and Pamela Gonzales. Moreover, we wish to express our gratitude to the Board of Directors of the Mt. Zion Health Fund for their generous support of this project; to the Lillian and Stephen Stewart Fund; and to Robert T. Mendle, M.D., who remained committed to the success of the book even in the midst of his own courageous battle with cancer.

Obviously, none of these five editions would have been possible without the commitment and dedication of the talented team at Andrews McMeel Publishing. Special thanks are due the leadership of Andrews McMeel, including John P. McMeel (chairman), Hugh T. Andrews (president and CEO), and Christine Schillig (vice president and editorial director, book division). Christine, in particular, has been invaluable in making sure this reference work got done, and got done the right way. We also wish to acknowledge Tom Thornton, past president of Andrews McMeel, whose participation in the publication of prior editions was absolutely essential. An additional word of gratitude goes to our editor and cowriter of the first three editions, Greg Cable. We wish to acknowledge the hard work, dedication, and enormous effort he put into those previous editions to make highly complex medical information comprehensible to the general public.

Thanks are warmly extended as well to Lane Butler at Andrews McMeel for overseeing the entire editorial process of this fifth edition with such skill, attention, and kindness; Annette Corkey and Michelle Daniel for their matchless copyediting; David Shaw for his thorough proofreading; Peter Lippincott and John Carroll for their production assistance. We are also grateful for the artistic talent of medical illustrator Kam Yu.

Our contributing authors generously gave to this project the extremely important gifts of their time and energy, sharing with us their expertise in their particular fields. Their contributions were critical to ensuring that the information presented here would be as complete, comprehensive, and up-to-date as possible. We enlisted the help of a number of new authors for this fifth edition based on their expertise and reputations for excellence, and to each of them we offer both a note of welcome and a heartfelt thanks.

A very special acknowledgment is due the National Cancer Institute Information Center for originally providing the Physician Data Query (PDQ) database and literature updates. This book has served as a valuable knowledge link to PDQ. We want to express our appreciation to the National Cancer Institute for the concept of carrying the message of modern comprehensive cancer care to the practicing physician and the public, and to the staff of the institute's PDQ section for their cooperation in making the database available.

We, Malin Dollinger and Ernest Rosenbaum, would like to express our gratitude for inspiration and guidance early in our careers to Thomas Chiffelle, M.D., Laurance V. Foye Jr., M.D., Arthur Furst, Ph.D., Arthur C. Giese, Ph.D., and Norman J. Sweet, M.D. We also owe a tremendous personal debt to our teachers, Joseph Burchenal, M.D., William Dameshek, M.D., Harris Fishbon, M.D., David Karnofsky, M.D., Irwin Krakoff, M.D., Sidney Levin, M.D., John J. Sampson, M.D., and Russell Tat, M.D., who cared about the advance of knowledge, about their patients, and about us.

We also now understand why authors thank their spouses. Their acceptance and tolerance of the many hours, days, weeks, and months of time devoted to this book is an all-important ingredient in any manuscript's completion. Our spouses, Christine Ko, Lenore Dollinger, and Isadora Rosenbaum, have understood and accepted the many demands created by our professional relationships, and they have freely given us the support, the time, and the inspiration to continue.

Finally, we are grateful to our patients who have shared with us some of the most important and difficult struggles of their lives. They have allowed us to play a part in their struggle and in many cases to feel like one of the family. We have learned much from them over the years, not only about cancer and its treatment, but about hope, courage, and the indomitable human spirit. Many of them have also consented to participate in clinical trials, the basis on which most of the current advances on cancer treatment have been obtained. We, and society, owe all cancer patients a great debt and thanks.

Andrew H. Ko, M.D.
Malin Dollinger, M.D.
Ernest H. Rosenbaum, M.D.

Contributors

■ ■ ■ ■

Andrew H. Ko, M.D.
Assistant Clinical Professor of Medicine, University of California, San Francisco, Comprehensive Cancer Center.

Andrew H. Ko is the newest editor for this current edition of *Everyone's Guide to Cancer Therapy*. He did his undergraduate studies at Brown University, where he graduated magna cum laude and with honors in applied mathematics and biology. This was followed by medical training at the Johns Hopkins School of Medicine in Baltimore, Maryland, and an internship and residency at Boston's Beth Israel Hospital (a teaching hospital of Harvard Medical School). After completing a fellowship in medical oncology at Stanford University in 2001, he joined the faculty of UCSF and has built his academic career developing and leading clinical trials focusing on pancreatic cancer and other gastrointestinal malignancies. In 2003, he received a career development award from the American Society of Clinical Oncology (ASCO) to help support his research efforts. He currently serves on the Scientific Program Committee and as a specialty editor on the editorial board for ASCO, sits on the UCSF Comprehensive Cancer Center scientific Protocol Review Committee, and is an ad hoc reviewer for numerous scientific journals. He is the coauthor of more than thirty-five peer-reviewed articles, reviews, book chapters, editorials, and abstracts.

Malin R. Dollinger, M.D.
Clinical Professor of Medicine, University of Southern California, Los Angeles.

Malin R. Dollinger's lifelong dedication to the field of oncology and patient education has included a patient care and research position at the Memorial Sloan-Kettering Cancer Center in New York and a post as Director of Oncology at Harbor General Hospital/UCLA Medical Center in Los Angeles. He has been in the private practice of cancer medicine (medical oncology) for over thirty years. He is the author of over 100 articles and book chapters, has contributed to a number of books about cancer, and is a member of the peer-review editorial advisory boards of the *Medical Letter* (New York), of the *Annals of Internal Medicine,* and for the American Cancer Society.

He is a consultant to various scientific and medical organizations and now conducts a medical oncology practice devoted to second opinions for cancer patients (*TheCancerAnswer.org*). He teaches at the University of Southern California School of Medicine, has lectured extensively to medical professionals and the public, and has helped to educate the public about cancer in radio and TV appearances. He served as Vice President of Medical Affairs at the John Wayne Cancer Institute in Santa Monica, California, and was President of the local branch of the American Cancer Society, where he won awards for his public education programs. Additional training and experience have been in the fields of medical quality assurance, risk assessment, and managed care. He is especially interested in improving communication with cancer patients and their families and in the emotional issues associated with cancer.

Ernest H. Rosenbaum, M.D.
Clinical Professor of Medicine, University of California, San Francisco, Comprehensive Cancer Center; Adjunct Clinical Professor, Department of Medicine, Stanford University Medical Center; Director,

Stanford Cancer Supportive Care Programs National/International, Stanford Complementary Medicine Clinic, Stanford University Medical Center, Stanford, California.

Ernest H. Rosenbaum's career has included a fellowship at the Blood Research Laboratory of Tufts University School of Medicine (New England Center Hospital) and MIT. He teaches at the University of California, San Francisco, Comprehensive Cancer Center, was the cofounder of the Northern California Academy of Clinical Oncology, and founded the Better Health Foundation and the Cancer Supportive Care Program at the Stanford Complementary Medicine Clinic, Stanford University Medical Center.

His passionate interest in clinical research and developing ways to improve patient care and communication with patients and colleagues has resulted in over fifty articles on cancer and hematology in various medical journals. He has also participated in many radio and television programs and frequently lectures to medical and public groups.

He has written numerous books, including *Living with Cancer: A Home Care Training Program for Cancer Patients; Decisions for Life: You Can Live Ten Years Longer with Better Health; Cancer Supportive Care: A Comprehensive Guide for Cancer Patients and Their Families; Nutrition for the Cancer Patient; Everyone's Guide to Cancer Therapy;* and *Everyone's Guide to Cancer Survivorship.* For *Everyone's Guide to Cancer Therapy,* Ernest Rosenbaum, M.D., Malin Dollinger, M.D., and Greg Cable received an Honorable Mention in 1991 from the American Medical Writers Association for Excellence in Medical Publications. Ernest and Isadora Rosenbaum received the same award in 1982 for their book, *A Comprehensive Guide for Cancer Patients and Their Families.*

Arthur R. Ablin, M.D.
Professor Emeritus Clinical Pediatrics, University of California, San Francisco.

David S. Alberts, M.D.
Regents Professor of Medicine, Pharmacology, Nutritional Science, and Public Health and Director, Arizona Cancer Center and the College of Medicine, University of Arizona, Tucson.

James O. Armitage, M.D.
Professor of Internal Medicine and Joe Shapiro Distinguished Chair of Oncology, Section of Hematology/Oncology, University of Nebraska Medical Center, Omaha; past President (1996–1997) of American Society of Clinical Oncology.

Kenneth A. Arndt, M.D.
Clinical Professor of Dermatology, Yale University School of Medicine; Adjunct Professor of Medicine (Dermatology), Dartmouth Medical School; Clinical Professor of Dermatology, Beth Israel Deaconess Medical Center, Harvard Medical School; SkinCare Physicians, Chestnut Hill, Massachusetts.

Josefa Azcueta, R.N., O.C.N.
Administrator, Roze Room Hospice of the Valley, Sherman Oaks, California.

Joseph S. Bailes, M.D.
Past President (1999–2000), past Interim Executive Vice President and Chief Executive Officer (2005–2006), and current Cochairman of Government-Relations Council, American Society of Clinical Oncology; Founding Member and past President, Physician Reliance Network, Dallas, Texas; Executive Vice President for Clinical Affairs, US Oncology, Houston, Texas.

Emily K. Bergsland, M.D.
Associate Professor of Clinical Medicine, Division of Hematology/Oncology, University of California, San Francisco, Comprehensive Cancer Center.

J. Michael Berry, M.D.
Associate Clinical Professor of Medicine, Division of Hematology/Oncology, University of California, San Francisco, Comprehensive Cancer Center.

Kevin G. Billingsley, M.D.
Assistant Professor, Department of Surgery, University of Washington School of Medicine, Seattle.

Amie M. Blanco, M.S., C.G.C.
Genetic Counselor, Colorectal Cancer Prevention Program, Cancer Risk Program, University of California, San Francisco, Comprehensive Cancer Center.

Richard and Annette Bloch
(Richard Bloch deceased.) Founders of the Cancer Hot Line in Kansas City, Missouri; Founders of the R. A. Bloch Cancer Support Center at the University of Missouri; Founder (Richard Bloch), H&R Block, Kansas City, Missouri.

Stanley A. Brosman, M.D.
Urologist, Pacific Urology Institute, Santa Monica, California; Clinical Professor of Urology, UCLA David Geffen School of Medicine, Los Angeles, California.

Barbara J. Buckley, M.S.W., L.C.S.W.
Clinical Social Worker and Director (retired), Cancer Resource Center, University of California, San Francisco, Comprehensive Cancer Center.

David G. Bullard, Ph.D.
Clinical Professor of Psychiatry and Medicine, University of California, San Francisco, School of Medicine.

Nicholas A. Butowski, M.D.
Assistant Clinical Professor of Neurological Surgery, Neuro-Oncology Service, University of California, San Francisco.

David R. Byrd, M.D.
Professor of Surgery, University of Washington School of Medicine, Director of Melanoma Center, University of Washington Medical Center, Seattle.

Peter R. Carroll, M.D.
Associate Dean, University of California, San Francisco, School of Medicine; Ken and Donna Derr–Chevron Distinguished Professorship in Prostate Cancer; Professor and Chair, Department of Urology, University of California, San Francisco; Director of Strategic Planning and Clinical Services, Surgeon-in-Chief, and Leader of Urologic Oncology Program, University of California, San Francisco, Comprehensive Cancer Center.

Barrie R. Cassileth, Ph.D.
Chief, Integrative Medicine Service, and Laurance S. Rockefeller Chair in Integrative Medicine, Memorial Sloan-Kettering Cancer Center, New York, New York.

Susan M. Chang, M.D.
Director of Clinical Services, Neuro-Oncology Service, and Associate Member of the Brain Tumor Research Center, Department of Neurological Surgery, University of California, San Francisco, School of Medicine; Lai Wan Kan Endowed Chair of Neurological Surgery and Professor in Residence, University of California, San Francisco, Comprehensive Cancer Center.

David Claman, M.D.
Associate Clinical Professor of Medicine, Pulmonary and Critical Care Division, and Director of Sleep Disorders Center, University of California, San Francisco.

Orlo H. Clark, M.D.
Professor of Surgery and Chief of Surgery (Mt. Zion Medical Center), University of California, San Francisco, Comprehensive Cancer Center.

John P. Cooke, M.D., Ph.D.
Professor of Medicine, Division of Cardiovascular Medicine, Stanford University School of Medicine, Stanford, California.

Beth B. Crawford, M.S.
Genetic Counselor, Cancer Risk Program, Carol Franc Buck Breast Care Center, University of California, San Francisco, Comprehensive Cancer Center.

Lloyd E. Damon, M.D.
Clinical Professor of Medicine and Director of Apheresis and Stem Cell Collection Unit, University of California, San Francisco, Comprehensive Cancer Center.

Christine M. Derzko, M.D.
Associate Professor of Obstetrics and Gynecology and Internal Medicine (Endocrinology), University of Toronto, Ontario, Canada.

Marcel P. Devetten Jr., M.D.
Assistant Professor of Internal Medicine, Section of Hematology/Oncology, University of Nebraska Medical Center, Omaha.

Vincent T. DeVita Jr., M.D.
Amy and Joseph Perella Professor of Medicine, Yale Cancer Center, Yale University School of Medicine, New Haven, Connecticut.

Lenore Dollinger, R.N., Ph.D.
Certified Health Consultant, Rancho Palos Verdes, California.

W. Lawrence Drew, M.D., Ph.D.
Professor in Residence of Laboratory Medicine and Director of Clinical Virology, University of California, San Francisco, School of Medicine and University of California, San Francisco, Comprehensive Cancer Center.

Sarita Dubey, M.D.
Assistant Clinical Professor of Medicine, Division of Hematology/Oncology, University of California, San Francisco, Comprehensive Cancer Center.

Bernard Dubrow, M.S.
(Deceased.) Formerly, Scientist and Technical Manager, Redondo Beach, California.

Frederick Eilber, M.D.
Professor of Surgery and former Chief, Division of Surgical Oncology, UCLA David Geffen School of Medicine, Los Angeles, California.

Tony Y. Eng, M.D.
Associate Clinical Professor and Vice Chair, Department of Radiation Oncology, University of Texas Health Science Center, San Antonio.

Loren B. Eskenazi, M.D.
Founder, Women's Plastic Surgery Society, San Francisco, California; Member, American Society of Plastic Surgeons; Author, *Reconstructing Aphrodite* and *More Than Skin Deep: Exploring the Real Reasons Why Women Go Under the Knife.*

Jerry Z. Finklestein, M.D.
Clinical Professor of Pediatrics and Hematology/Oncology, UCLA David Geffen School of Medicine, Los Angeles, California; Pediatric Oncologist, Jonathan Jacques Children's Cancer Center, Long Beach, California.

Margaret I. Fitch, R.N., Ph.D.
Head, Oncology Nursing and Supportive Care, Toronto-Sunnybrook Regional Cancer Centre; Associate Professor, Faculty of Nursing, University of Toronto, Ontario, Canada.

Patricia Fobair, L.M.S.W., M.Ph.
Clinical Social Worker (retired), Department of Radiation Oncology, Stanford Cancer Center, Stanford, California;

Editor, *Surviving* (quarterly newsletter); Author, *Learning to Live Again.*

Leland J. Foshag, M.D.
Director of Pancreatic Research Program, John Wayne Cancer Institute, Santa Monica, California.

David A. Foster, Ph.D.
Professor of Biological Sciences, Hunter College of the City University of New York, New York, New York.

Nancy M. Gardner, Ph.D., A.R.N.P.
Nurse Practitioner, Gastrointestinal Oncology Program, H. Lee Moffitt Cancer Center and Research Institute, Tampa, Florida.

Mitch Golant, Ph.D.
Vice President, Research and Development, The Wellness Community, Los Angeles, California.

Robert E. Goldsby, M.D.
Assistant Professor of Clinical Pediatrics, Department of Pediatrics, University of California, San Francisco, Comprehensive Cancer Center.

William H. Goodson III, M.D.
Breast Surgeon and Senior Clinical Research Scientist, Department of Surgery, California Pacific Medical Center Research Institute, San Francisco, California.

Alexander R. Gottschalk, M.D., Ph.D.
Assistant Professor, Department of Radiation Oncology, University of California, San Francisco.

F. Anthony Greco, M.D.
Medical Director, Sarah Cannon Cancer Center, Nashville, Tennessee.

Mark L. Greenberg, M.B., Ch.B.
Senior Staff, Division of Pediatric Oncology, The Hospital for Sick Children, and Professor of Pediatrics and Surgery, University of Toronto, Ontario, Canada.

Daphne A. Haas-Kogan, M.D.
Associate Professor and Vice Chair for Research, Department of Radiation Oncology, University of California, San Francisco, Comprehensive Cancer Center.

John D. Hainsworth, M.D.
Director of Clinical Research, Sarah Cannon Cancer Center, Nashville, Tennessee.

Omid Hamid, M.D.
Medical Oncologist, The Angeles Clinic and Research Institute, Santa Monica, California.

Deborah Hamolsky, R.N., M.S., O.C.N., A.O.C.N.S.
Advanced Practice Nurse, Breast Care Clinic, University of California, San Francisco, Comprehensive Cancer Center; Assistant Professor, Department of Physiological Nursing, University of California, San Francisco.

Margaret Hawn, R.N.
Nurse Coordinator, Cancer Supportive Care Program, Infusion Treatment Area (ITA), Stanford Cancer Center, Stanford, California.

James T. Helsper, M.D.
(Deceased.) Formerly, Professor of Clinical Surgery, Norris Comprehensive Cancer Center, Keck School of Medicine, University of Southern California, Los Angeles, California.

Nora V. Hirschler, M.D.
President, CEO, and Medical Director, Blood Centers of the Pacific, San Francisco, California.

Sandra J. Horning, M.D.
Professor of Medical Oncology and Bone Marrow Transplantation, Stanford University Medical Center, Stanford, California.

Steven M. Horwitz, M.D.
Assistant Attending, Lymphoma Service, Department of Medicine, Memorial Sloan-Kettering Cancer Center, New York, New York.

I-Chow Joe Hsu, M.D.
Associate Professor, Department of Radiation Oncology, University of California, San Francisco.

Robert J. Ignoffo, Pharm.D.
Clinical Professor Emeritus, Department of Clinical Pharmacy, University of California, San Francisco.

David M. Jablons, M.D.
Ada Distinguished Professor of Thoracic Oncology and Associate Professor of Surgery, University of California, San Francisco at Mt. Zion; Leader of Thoracic Oncology Program, University of California, San Francisco, Comprehensive Cancer Center.

Thierry M. Jahan, M.D.
Associate Clinical Professor of Medicine and Director of Clinical Services, Division of Hematology/Oncology, University of California, San Francisco, Comprehensive Cancer Center.

Joanne M. Jeter, M.D.
Assistant Professor of Clinical Medicine, Arizona Cancer Center, Tucson.

Lawrence D. Kaplan, M.D.
Clinical Professor of Medicine and Director of Adult Lymphoma Program, University of California, San Francisco, Comprehensive Cancer Center; Director, AIDS-Malignancies Program, San Francisco General Hospital, San Francisco, California.

Mohammed Kashani-Sabet, M.D.
Herschel and Diana Zackheim Endowed Chair in Cutaneous Oncology, University of California, San Francisco; Co-Leader of Cutaneous Oncology Program and Director of Melanoma Center, University of California, San Francisco, Comprehensive Cancer Center; Associate Professor of Dermatology, University of California, San Francisco.

Patricia T. Kelly, Ph.D.
Medical Geneticist, Cancer Risk Assessment Program, Saint Francis Memorial Hospital, San Francisco, California.

Barbara Klencke, M.D.
Associate Medical Director, Medical Affairs, Genentech; Assistant Clinical Professor of Medicine, Division of Hematology/Oncology (past appointment), University of California, San Francisco, Comprehensive Cancer Center.

Boris Kobrinsky, M.D.
Fellow in Hematology/Oncology, New York University School of Medicine, New York, New York.

Badrinath Konety, M.D., M.B.A.
Associate Professor, Departments of Urology and Epidemiology/Biostatistics, University of California, San Francisco, Comprehensive Cancer Center.

Pat Kramer, M.S.N., R.N., A.O.C.N.
Oncology Nurse Educator and Consultant, Fatigue Management Program, Cancer Supportive Care Program, Stanford Cancer Center, Stanford, California.

Susan E. Krown, M.D.
Chair, AIDS Malignancy Consortium and Attending Physician, Memorial Sloan-Kettering Cancer Center, New York, New York.

Jasleen Kukreja, M.D.
Assistant Professor in Residence, Department of Cardiothoracic Surgery, University of California, San Francisco.

Larry K. Kvols, M.D.
Section Head of Neuroendocrine Oncology and Professor of Medicine, H. Lee Moffitt Cancer Center and Research Institute, Tampa, Florida.

Robert A. Kyle, M.D.
Professor of Medicine and Laboratory Medicine, Mayo Medical School, Mayo Clinic, Rochester, Minnesota.

Jack LaLanne
Author, lecturer, and fitness expert; Recipient of State of California Governor's Council on Physical Fitness Lifetime Achievement Award and Dwight D. Eisenhower Fitness Award.

Natalie L. Ledesma, M.S., R.D.
Oncology Dietitian, Cancer Resource Center, University of California, San Francisco, Comprehensive Cancer Center.

Alexandra M. Levine, M.D.
Chief Medical Officer, City of Hope Cancer Center, Duarte, California; past Medical Director, USC/Norris Comprehensive Cancer Center, and Distinguished Professor of Medicine and Chair, Division of Hematology, Keck School of Medicine, University of Southern California, Los Angeles.

Charles A. Linker, M.D.
Clinical Professor of Medicine, Division of Hematology/Oncology, Director of Adult Leukemia and Bone Marrow Transplant Program, and Co-Leader of Hematopoietic Malignancies Program, University of California, San Francisco, Comprehensive Cancer Center.

Britt-Marie Ljung, M.D.
Professor of Clinical Pathology and Director of Tissue Core Facility and Cytopathology Fellowship Program, University of California, San Francisco, Comprehensive Cancer Center.

Wendy Sara Long, M.D.
Assistant Clinical Professor, Department of Dermatology, New York University School of Medicine, New York, New York.

Francine Manuel, R.P.T.
Rehabilitation Specialist, past appointment with Exercise Program and Cancer Supportive Care Program, Stanford Center for Integrative Medicine, Stanford, California.

Lawrence W. Margolis, M.D.
Clinical Professor Emeritus, Department of Radiation Oncology, University of California, San Francisco.

Michael W. McDermott, M.D.
Robert M. and Ruth L. Halperin Endowed Chair in Meningioma Research, University of California, San Francisco.

Kerry Anne McGinn, R.N., N.P., M.S.N.
Nurse Practitioner and Ostomy Specialist; Author, *The Informed Woman's Guide to Breast Health.*

Anna T. Meadows, M.D.
Professor Emeritus, Department of Pediatrics, Division of Oncology, University of Pennsylvania School of Medicine; Medical Director, Cancer Survivorship and Living Well After Cancer Program, The Children's Hospital of Philadelphia, Pennsylvania.

Maxwell V. Meng, M.D.
Associate Professor in Residence, Department of Urology, University of California, San Francisco.

T. Stanley Meyler, M.D.
Clinical Professor of Radiation Oncology (retired), University of California, San Francisco, Comprehensive Cancer Center.

Lawrence Mintz, M.D.
Clinical Professor of Medicine/Infectious Disease (past appointment), University of California, San Francisco.

Malcolm S. Mitchell, M.D.
Special Assistant to the President, University of Texas at El Paso; Former Head of Program in Biological Therapy and Professor of Medicine, Immunology, and Microbiology, Karmanos Cancer Institute, Wayne State University, Detroit, Michigan.

Eugene T. Morita, M.D.
Clinical Professor of Nuclear Medicine and Radiology, University of California, San Francisco.

Franco M. Muggia, M.D.
Anne Murnick Cogan and David H. Cogan Professor of Oncology, Director of Division of Medical Oncology, and Associate Director for Clinical Research, Kaplan Comprehensive Cancer Center, New York University School of Medicine, New York, New York.

Sean J. Mulvihill, M.D.
Senior Director of Clinical Affairs, Huntsman Cancer Institute, and Professor and Chair, Department of Surgery, University of Utah, Salt Lake City.

V. Raman Muthusamy, M.D.
Assistant Clinical Professor of Medicine/Gastroenterology, University of California, Irvine.

Eric K. Nakakura, M.D., Ph.D.
Assistant Professor in Residence, Department of Surgery, University of California, San Francisco.

Kim-Anh Nguyen, M.D.
Associate Medical Director, Blood Centers of the Pacific, San Francisco, California.

Richard J. O'Donnell, M.D.
Associate Professor of Clinical Orthopaedic Surgery and Chief, Orthopaedic Oncology Service, University of California, San Francisco.

Bert O'Neil, M.D.
Assistant Professor of Medicine, Division of Hematology and Oncology, University of North Carolina School of Medicine, Chapel Hill.

John W. Park, M.D.
Associate Clinical Professor of Medicine and Neurosurgery and Director of Novel Therapeutics, Breast Oncology, University of California, San Francisco, Comprehensive Cancer Center.

Ramesh Patel, M.D.
Vice Chief of Staff, Gibson General Hospital, Princeton, Indiana.

Carlos A. Pellegrini, M.D.
Henry N. Harkins Professor and Chairman; Chair, Board of Directors, Institute for Surgical and Interventional Simulation (ISIS); Co-Director, Center for Videoendoscopic Surgery; and Co-Director, Swallowing Center, Department of Surgery, University of Washington Medical Center, Seattle.

Herbert A. Perkins, M.D.
Clinical Professor of Medicine, University of California, San Francisco; Senior Medical Scientist, Blood Centers of the Pacific, San Francisco, California.

Barbara F. Piper, D.N.Sc., R.N., A.O.C.N., F.A.A.N.
Associate Clinical Professor, Department of Physiological Nursing, University of California, San Francisco.

Joel M. Pollack, C.P.A.
Administrative Director, President's Office, John Wayne Cancer Institute, Saint

John's Health Center, Santa Monica, California.

Michael D. Prados, M.D.
Charles B. Wilson Endowed Chair in Neurological Surgery and Professor and Chief, Neuro-Oncology Service, University of California, San Francisco; Co-Leader, Neurologic Oncology Program, Univerisity of California, San Francisco, Comprehensive Cancer Center.

Amanda Psyrri, M.D.
Assistant Professor of Medical Oncology, Yale Cancer Center, New Haven, Connecticut.

Barbara Quinn
Manager and Billing and Collection Supervisor, John Wayne Cancer Institute, Saint John's Health Center, Santa Monica, California.

S. Vincent Rajkumar, M.D.
Professor of Medicine, Hematology, Laboratory Medicine, and Pathology, Mayo Clinic, Rochester, Minnesota.

James A. Recabaren, M.D.
Associate Professor of Clinical Surgery, Keck School of Medicine, University of Southern California, Los Angeles.

Elizabeth C. Reed, M.D.
Associate Professor of Internal Medicine, Hematology/Oncology, and Medical Director of Breast Cancer Program, University of Nebraska Medical Center, Omaha.

Brian I. Rini, M.D.
Associate Professor of Medicine, Departments of Solid Tumor Oncology and Urology, Cleveland Clinic Taussig Cancer Center, Ohio.

Mack Roach III, M.D.
Professor and Chair, Radiation Oncology, and Professor of Urology, University

of California, San Francisco; Investigator, Comprehensive Minority Institution/Cancer Center Partnership, San Francisco State University and University of California, San Francisco, Comprehensive Cancer Center.

Wendye R. Robbins, M.D.
CEO and President, Limerick NeuroSciences, Inc., San Francisco, California; Assistant Clinical Professor, Pain Management Center, Stanford University School of Medicine, Stanford, California.

Stanley J. Rogers, M.D.
Associate Clinical Professor, Department of Surgery, University of California, San Francisco.

Mitchell P. Rosen, M.D.
Infertility Specialist, University of California, San Francisco, Center for Reproductive Health; Adjunct Professor, Department of Obstetrics, Gynecology, and Reproductive Sciences, University of California, San Francisco.

Isadora R. Rosenbaum, M.A.
Medical Assistant (retired), Medical Oncology, University of California, San Francisco, Comprehensive Cancer Center.

Jonathan E. Rosenberg, M.D.
Assistant Clinical Professor of Medicine, Division of Hematology/Oncology, University of California, San Francisco, Comprehensive Cancer Center.

Phillip L. Ross, M.D.
Urologic Oncology Fellow, Department of Urology, University of California, San Francisco.

Hope S. Rugo, M.D.
Clinical Professor of Medicine, Division of Hematology/Oncology and Director of Breast Oncology Clinical Trials Program, University of California, San Francisco, Comprehensive Cancer Center.

Charles J. Ryan, M.D.
Assistant Clinical Professor of Medicine, Division of Hematology/Oncology, University of California, San Francisco, Comprehensive Cancer Center.

Terry Sarantou, M.D.
Oncologic Surgeon and Medical Director, Cancer Center, Frye Regional Medical Center, Hickory, North Carolina; Associate Member, Hickory Surgical Clinic, North Carolina.

Katsuto Shinohara, M.D.
Adjunct Professor, Department of Urology, University of California, San Francisco, Comprehensive Cancer Center; Staff Surgeon, Urology Section, Veterans Administration Hospital, San Francisco, California.

Edward A. Sickles, M.D.
Professor of Radiology and Section Chief of Breast Imaging Services, University of California, San Francisco, Comprehensive Cancer Center.

Allan E. Siperstein, M.D.
Vice Chairman, Surgical Division Office, Department of General Surgery, Cleveland Clinic, Cleveland, Ohio.

Eric J. Small, M.D.
Stanford W. Ascherman and Norman R. Ascherman Endowed Chair in Hematology/Oncology, University of California, San Francisco; Professor in Residence of Medicine and Urology, University of California, San Francisco; Director of Investigational Therapeutics and Co-Leader of the Prostate Cancer Program, University of California, San Francisco, Comprehensive Cancer Center.

Patricia (Penny) K. Sneed, M.D.
Professor in Residence, Department of Radiation Oncology, University of California, San Francisco.

Gail Sorrough, M.L.I.S.
Director, Medical Library Services, H. M. Fishbon Memorial Library, University of California, San Francisco.

Joycelyn L. Speight, M.D., Ph.D.
Assistant Clinical Professor, Department of Radiation Oncology, University of California, San Francisco.

David Spiegel, M.D.
Professor and Associate Chair of Psychiatry and Behavioral Sciences, Medical Director of Cancer Supportive Care Program, and Director of Center on Stress and Health, Stanford University Medical Center, Stanford, California.

Jeffrey L. Stern, M.D.
Gynecologic Oncologist, Women's Cancer Center, Berkeley, California; past Director, Division of Gynecologic Oncology, University of California, San Francisco.

Susan Sweeney, R.N., Ph.N.
Medical Social Worker, University of California, San Francisco (previous appointment).

Andrzej Szuba, M.D., Ph.D.
Clinical Assistant Professor of Medicine, Division of Cardiovascular Medicine, Stanford University School of Medicine, Stanford, California.

Margaret A. Tempero, M.D.
Doris and Donald Fisher Distinguished Professor of Clinical Cancer Research, University of California, San Francisco; Deputy Director and Director of Clinical Sciences, University of California, San Francisco, Comprehensive Cancer Center; past president (2003–2004), American Society of Clinical Oncology.

Jonathan P. Terdiman, M.D.
Associate Clinical Professor of Medicine/ Gastroenterology, Director of Colorectal Cancer Prevention Program, and Clini-

cal Director of Center for Inflammatory Bowel Disease, University of California, San Francisco, Comprehensive Cancer Center.

Pierre Theodore, M.D.
Assistant Professor in Residence, Department of Cardiothoracic Surgery, University of California, San Francisco.

Debu Tripathy, M.D.
Professor of Internal Medicine and Director of Komen/UTSW Breast Cancer Research Program, University of Texas Southwestern Medical Center, Dallas.

Alan P. Venook, M.D.
Professor of Clinical Medicine and Associate Chief, Division of Medical Oncology, University of California, San Francisco, Comprehensive Cancer Center.

Steven J. Wang, M.D.
Assistant Professor in Residence, Department of Otolaryngology–Head and Neck Surgery, University of California, San Francisco; Chief, Otolaryngology Section, Veterans Affairs Medical Center, San Francisco.

Robert S. Warren, M.D.
Professor, Department of Surgery of and Chief of Surgical Oncology Program, University of California, San Francisco, Comprehensive Cancer Center.

The Washington, D.C. Cosmetic, Toiletry, and Fragrance Association Foundation

Jeffrey S. Weber, M.D., Ph.D.
Chief, Division of Oncology, Bearle and Lucy Adams Chair in Cancer Research, and Chief of Medicine, University of Southern California Norris Cancer Hospital, Los Angeles.

Mark Welton, M.D.
Associate Professor and Chief, Colorectal Surgery, Stanford Cancer Center, Stanford, California.

Gloria Won, M.L.I.S.
Librarian, H. M. Fishbon Memorial Library, University of California, San Francisco.

Derrick Wong, M.D.
Clinical Fellow in Hematology/Oncology, University of California, San Francisco, Comprehensive Cancer Center.

K. Simon Yeung, Pharm.D., M.B.A.
Research Pharmacist and Manager, Herb/ Drug Information Center, Integrative Medicine Service, Memorial Sloan-Kettering Cancer Center, New York, New York.

Norman R. Zinner, M.D., M.S.
Medical Director, Western Clinical Research, Inc., Torrance, California.

PART ONE

Diagnosis and Treatment

— 1 —

Understanding Cancer

*Malin Dollinger, M.D., Andrew H. Ko, M.D.,
Ernest H. Rosenbaum, M.D., and David A. Foster, Ph.D.*

■ ■ ■ ■

Cancer is a general term for the abnormal growth of cells. Cells are the building blocks of our bodies. Every normal cell contains twenty-three pairs of chromosomes. Winding through each pair is the double helix of the DNA molecule, the genetic blueprint for life. DNA is the controller and transmitter of the genetic characteristics in the chromosomes we inherit from our parents and pass on to our children.

Our chromosomes contain millions of different genes—pieces of DNA containing information on how the body should grow, function, and behave. Genes determine the color of our eyes, tell injured tissues how to repair themselves, tell our stomachs how to make gastric juice, and direct the female breasts to make milk after a baby is born. Most of the time, these genes function properly and send the right messages. We remain in good health, with everything working as it should.

But there are an incredible number of genes and an unimaginable number of messages. And since the chromosomes reproduce themselves every time a cell divides, there are lots of opportunities for something to go wrong. Although the vast majority of "mistakes" that occur during chromosome reproduction or from damage by external factors are repaired by the body, sometimes something does go wrong in the process of cell division—a mutation that alters one or more of the genes.

Cancer results from genetic change or damage to a chromosome within a cell.

The altered gene sends the wrong message or a different message from the one it should give. A cell begins to grow rapidly. It multiplies again and again until it forms a lump that's called a malignant tumor, or cancer.

Uncontrolled Growth Rapid cell growth is not the same as malignancy. We all experience two normal situations in which our body tissues grow much more rapidly than they usually do. We grow from a single cell to a perfectly formed human being in nine months. Then we grow into a normal-sized adult human being over the next sixteen years or so. In addition, when we are injured and need rapid repair, restoration, and replacement of damaged tissues, our bodies can produce many new cells in a very short time.

When either of these processes— growth or healing—is completed, a set of genes tells the body that it is time to "switch off." We don't continue growing throughout our lives, and the scar we have after a cut has healed remains just that—a scar. Those are the rules.

But a cancer cell doesn't obey the rules. The change in its genetic code makes it "forget" to stop growing. Once growth is turned on, cancer cells continue to divide in an uncontrolled way. It's as though you set the thermostat in your house for a certain temperature, but no matter how hot your house gets, the furnace keeps running. No matter what you do to turn

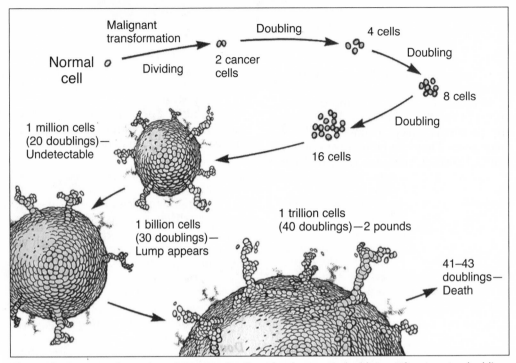

Normal cell

Dividing → Malignant transformation → 2 cancer cells → Doubling → 4 cells → Doubling → 8 cells → Doubling → 16 cells

1 million cells (20 doublings)—Undetectable

1 billion cells (30 doublings)—Lump appears

1 trillion cells (40 doublings)—2 pounds

41–43 doublings—Death

The malignant transformation of a normal cell and subsequent doublings. After twenty doublings (1 million cancer cells), the cancer is still too small to detect.

it off, it produces heat as if it had a mind of its own.

Doubling Times Cancer starts with one abnormal cell. That cell becomes two abnormal cells that become four abnormal cells and so on. Cells divide at various rates, called doubling times. Fast-growing cancers may double over one to four weeks; slower-growing cancers may double over two to six months. It may take up to five years for the duplication process to happen twenty times. By then, the tumor may contain a million cells yet still be only the size of a pinhead.

So there is a "silent" period after the cancer has started to grow. There is no lump or mass. It's too small to be detected by any means now known. What is not commonly appreciated is that the silent period is considerably longer than the period when we do know a tumor is present.

After many months, usually years, the doubling process has occurred thirty times or so. By then, the lump may have reached a size that can be felt, seen on an X-ray, or cause pressure symptoms such as pain or bleeding. To be able to see a tumor on an X-ray, it usually has to be about half an inch (1 cm) in diameter. At that stage, it will contain about 1 billion cells. When it is smaller, X-ray imaging techniques are not usually sensitive enough to detect it, although some newer imaging methods—especially computerized tomography (CT) and magnetic resonance imaging (MRI)—may sometimes detect such small tumors. Blood tests called tumor markers may be able to detect tiny cancers that are not visible on X-ray or MRI examination, for example,

PSA for prostate cancer (see chapter 2, "How Cancer Is Diagnosed").

Benign and Malignant Tumors Tumors are not always malignant. Benign tumors can appear in any part of the body. Many of us have them—freckles, moles, fatty lumps in the skin—but they don't cause any problems except (sometimes) cosmetic ones. They can be removed or left alone. However they are treated, they stay in one place. They do not invade or destroy surrounding tissues.

Malignant tumors, on the other hand, have two significant characteristics:

• They have no "wall" or clear-cut border. They put down roots and directly invade surrounding tissues.
• They have the ability to spread to other parts of the body. Bits of malignant cells fall off the tumor, then travel like seeds to other tissues, where they land and start similar growths. Fortunately, not all the many thousands of cancer cells that break off a tumor find a place to take root. Most die like seeds that go unplanted.

This spreading of cancer is called metastasis. And doctors are always concerned about whether the cancer has metastasized during the silent period. If it has, then the migrating cancer cells have begun to go through their own silent period. They, too, are too small to detect for many months or years.

Almost all cancers share these two properties, although cancers arising in various organs tend to behave differently. They spread to different parts of the body. They grow in very specific ways that are characteristic of that cancer. The consequence is that there is a specific method of diagnosis, staging, and treatment for each kind of cancer. One set of principles governs diagnosis and treatment of breast cancer, for example, while the rules for lung or colon cancer are just as complex but somewhat different.

What Causes Cancer

Although cancer is usually thought of as one disease, it is in fact more than 200 different diseases. For many of these cancers, no definite cause is known. There is no one single cause. In fact, cancer remains something of a mystery. But the clues we have discovered from research are greatly increasing our understanding.

The Roles of Oncogenes and Tumor Suppressor Genes One of the most exciting and important developments has been the discovery that some normal genes may be transformed into genes that promote the growth of cancer. These have been called oncogenes, the prefix *onco-* meaning tumor. This discovery has led to much research, better understanding of how cancer develops, and insights into methods of prevention, detection, and treatment.

Conversely, there is another set of genes called tumor suppressor genes, whose normal function is to help control cell growth. If tumor suppressor genes don't do their job properly or are missing altogether, the cancer-producing action of an oncogene may not be suppressed and cells may turn cancerous as a result (see chapter 44, "Investigational Anticancer Drugs").

The Implications for Screening All this new information raises the possibility that we may soon be able to test individuals— for example, with a blood test—to discover whether a specific oncogene is present and if the suppressor gene is defective or absent. The presence of certain oncogenes may even give us information about how likely it is that a cancer will spread. We may soon be able to identify people with a higher risk for cancer and possibly carry out other intensive detection and screening methods. Techniques for testing for oncogenes have recently been developed and are beginning to be available for general use. This new knowledge is already used in the study of

Cancer Risk Factors, with Percentages

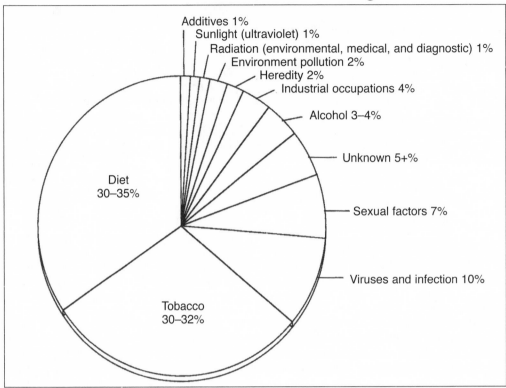

Additives 1%
Sunlight (ultraviolet) 1%
Radiation (environmental, medical, and diagnostic) 1%
Environment pollution 2%
Heredity 2%
Industrial occupations 4%

Alcohol 3–4%

Unknown 5+%

Sexual factors 7%

Viruses and infection 10%

Diet
30–35%

Tobacco
30–32%

familial (inherited) polyps of the colon and for familial breast cancer (see chapter 42, "The Impact of Research on the Cancer Problem: Looking Back, Moving Forward" and chapter 46, "Genetic Risk Assessment and Counseling," for additional screening information).

How the Process Works There are approximately 20,000 to 25,000 genes within a human cell, only a small fraction of which regulate cell growth or division. It is now also thought that we all carry normal cells that contain oncogenes in the chromosomes, but that these oncogenes are never activated. They simply lie dormant throughout our lives.

In other cases, a mutation may occur because of some assault on the cell structure.

Some stimulus or chemical agent turns on a "switch," several oncogenes are activated, and they set to work together to transform a normal cell into a cancer cell. This is thought to be at least a two-step process. First, the DNA must go through an initial change that makes the cell receptive. Then a subsequent change or set of changes in the DNA transforms the receptive cell into a tumor cell.

The big question is, what causes these changes in cellular DNA in the first place? There are several theories. One focuses on viruses, which can insert their own DNA into a cell's DNA and make the cell produce more virus-containing cells. Viruses may insert a viral oncogene or they might simply act as a random mutating agent.

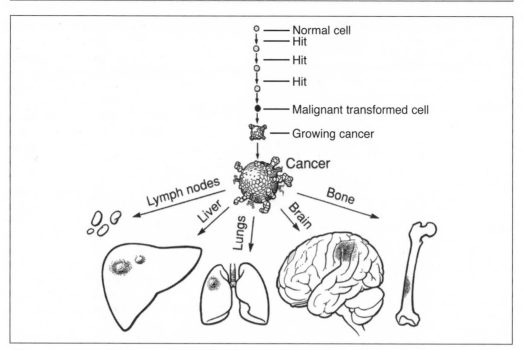

After two or more "hits," a transformed malignant cell grows into a lump we call cancer. Cells may eventually break off and spread (metastasize) via lymph vessels or blood vessels.

There is also some evidence that an assault by a "single carcinogenic bullet" hitting the cell at just the right spot can make a cell become cancerous. But the alternate theory that has gained a lot of support focuses on multiple "hits."

The Multiple Hit Theory According to this theory, all cancers arise from at least two changes or "hits" to the genes in the cell. Alfred G. Knudson, a cancer geneticist, developed his "two-hit" hypothesis in 1971 using hereditary retinoblastoma as a model. He postulated that patients who inherited one copy of a damaged gene (eventually discovered to be a tumor suppressor gene called RB) were at risk for developing this rare type of eye tumor, occurring mostly in children. That one bad copy alone was not enough to cause cancer; however, if a second hit to (or loss of) the good copy in the gene pair

occurred sometime after birth, retinoblastoma would result.

Most cancers do not fall into this direct hereditary pattern and require multiple "hits" to various genes that build up and interact over time. These "hits" may come from chemical or foreign substances that cause cancer, called carcinogens. These initiate the cancer process. Or the hits may be promoters that accelerate the growth of abnormal cells. Critical factors are the number and types of hits, their frequency, and their intensity. Eventually, a breaking point is reached and cancerous growth is switched on.

Initiators include

• Tobacco and tobacco smoke carcinogens. Lung cancer was a rare disease before cigarette smoking became widespread.
• X-rays and exposure to ionizing radiation. It is well known that there is an

increased incidence of leukemia among atomic bomb survivors. This same increase was noted in radiologists, the doctors who specialize in the use of X-rays, years ago. It should be pointed out that the average diagnostic use of X-rays does not increase the chance of getting cancer enough to rule out their use as a valuable health care tool. The risk of not having an X-ray may far outweigh the risk of cancer being caused by the use of X-rays for diagnosis. Used properly, X-rays are of great benefit in finding cancer at an early, curable stage.

- Certain hormones and drugs, such as DES (diethylstilbestrol), some estrogens (female hormones), and some immuno-suppressive drugs.
- Excessive exposure to sunlight.
- Industrial agents or toxic substances in the environment, such as asbestos, coal tar products, benzene, cadmium, uranium, and nickel.
- Dietary factors, such as high-fat and low-fiber diets, or carcinogens within food products or those created by the cooking process (see chapter 23, "Maintaining Good Nutrition").
- Obesity.
- Sexual practices, including the age of a woman when she first has intercourse and first becomes pregnant. Certain sexually transmitted viruses can cause cancers, and the risk of catching one of these viruses increases with unprotected sexual contact and with the number of sexual partners. This is particularly true for AIDS-related cancers such as Kaposi's sarcoma.

Promoters include

- Alcohol, which is a factor in 4 percent of cancers, mainly in cancers of the head and neck and the liver.
- Stress, which may weaken the immune system. Stress unfortunately relieved all too often with cigarettes, alcohol, rich food, and drugs.

Miscellaneous factors include

- Heredity.
- Weaknesses of the immune system, such as in transplant patients.

When two or more hits are combined—tobacco smoke and asbestos exposure, or cigarette smoking and alcohol, for example—the chance of getting cancer is not the sum of the individual risks. Rather, the chances are multiplied. Cancer is an additive process with many different hits occurring and interacting over many, many years.

What it comes down to is that the risk of developing cancer depends on

- who you are (genetic makeup),
- where you live (environmental and occupational exposures to carcinogens), and
- how you live (personal lifestyle).

Now that so many factors in our daily lives that affect the risk of getting cancer can be identified, cancer risk assessment has become increasingly vital to our continued good health. Risk assessment screening of apparently healthy people is now used in many cancer centers (see chapter 46, "Genetic Risk Assessment and Counseling").

How Cancer Spreads

It is possible for tumors to start to grow in several places simultaneously, though this is unusual. They usually start to grow at a single site, called the primary site. So if cancer spreads, it is usually because small bits of cancer cells are cast off the original, or primary, tumor and travel to other parts of the body. There are three ways for the cancer to spread.

Direct Extension As the tumor mass grows, it invades the organs and tissues immediately next to it. It tends to form roots, growing into the layers of surrounding tissue like carrots growing into the earth.

Through the Blood (Hematogenous Spread) Tumors have a blood supply. Arteries pump blood into the malignant cells and veins take it away. Pieces of the tumor can grow through the walls of these blood vessels, enter the bloodstream, and circulate around the body until they land in various organs. Fortunately, very few of these circulating cells actually find a place to grow.

Through the Lymphatic System There are two vascular systems in the body. One, the cardiovascular system, consists of arteries that move blood to all parts of the body, veins that return the blood to the heart, and small capillaries inside the organs and tissues that allow oxygen to be transferred.

The other, the lymphatic system, is a separate system of tiny vessels—called lymphatics—under the skin and throughout the body. These vessels carry a liquid called lymph. The purpose of lymph is to drain waste products such as infectious, foreign, and otherwise toxic materials.

Lymph Nodes Stations along these vessels, called lymph nodes, trap these materials. Tonsils, for example, are lymph nodes. When you have tonsillitis, you have a high temperature, you have trouble swallowing, and you generally feel awful. But you feel that way because the tonsils are doing their job by trapping bacteria and preventing them from getting into your body. If they weren't doing their job, you might develop a bloodstream infection.

The lymph system begins with very small tubes that drain into lymph nodes at different levels of the body. The system eventually feeds into the thoracic duct in the left side of the neck. That duct drains into the venous system, which returns the lymph fluid to the heart. From there, it is pumped through the body.

Tumor cells can easily spread into the lymphatic system. Breast cancer, for example, often spreads initially via lymphatic vessels to the lymph nodes in the armpit (axillary nodes). The cancer cells may continue traveling in the lymphatics to other locations in the body. In this situation, a doctor can sometimes feel the axillary nodes during a physical examination. But just to be sure, the nodes have to be examined under a microscope after they are surgically removed.

When breast cancer has spread to the lymph glands under the armpit, we hope the glands have done their job and prevented the cells from spreading any farther. You might visualize these lymph glands as train stations and the lymph vessels as tracks. We hope the cells behave like a local train, stopping at the next lymph node station, and don't behave like an express, scooting past several nodes and getting directly into the body.

Tumor Classification in Cancer Treatment

Treating cancer properly depends on defining each and every tumor precisely. All kinds of characteristics are taken into account when coming up with this definition, but all these characteristics essentially fit into three broad categories. The three key questions that have to be answered are, where is the tumor growing, how fast is it growing, and how big has it already grown?

The Different Kinds of Tumors The first of these questions is critical because, again, cancers that develop in different tissues tend to behave differently. There are generally three types of malignant tumors, which develop in the three kinds of tissues.

Carcinomas These develop in the tissues that cover the surface or line internal organs and passageways (epithelium). Most epithelial cancers—carcinomas—develop in an organ that secretes something. For example, lung tissue secretes mucus, breast tissue secretes milk, and the pancreas secretes digestive juices.

Sarcomas These are soft-tissue or bone tumors. They develop in any supporting or connective tissues—muscles, bones, nerves, tendons, or blood vessels. Since supporting or connective tissue is found throughout the body, sarcomas can be found anywhere.

The same organ that develops a carcinoma can also develop a sarcoma, since the organ has both epithelial cells and connective tissue in it. For example, most cancers that arise in the uterus are carcinomas, but, less commonly, uterine sarcomas can also be found.

Lymphomas and Leukemias These tumors develop in the lymph glands or arise from the blood-forming cells in the bone marrow.

Lymphomas (lymphosarcomas) are the tumors that develop in the lymph glands, the small round or bean-shaped structures found throughout the body. These tumors are almost always malignant. One specific kind of tumor in this broad class is called Hodgkin's disease, and all the other ones have come to be referred to as non-Hodgkin's lymphomas. To make things more complicated, there are many subvarieties of both Hodgkin's disease and non-Hodgkin's lymphomas.

The leukemias are cancers of the white blood cells and are named after the type of white blood cell affected. Plasma cell myeloma (multiple myeloma) is a cancer of the plasma cells in the bone marrow.

Understanding Tumor Names There are many different names for the various cancers, and it's easy to get confused. There are tumors in each of the three tumor categories that are named after the doctors who discovered them—Hodgkin's disease, Ewing's sarcoma of the bone, Kaposi's sarcoma, and Wilms' tumor of the kidney. Tumors may also be named after the

tissue of origin, such as a schwannoma, which is a tumor that develops in the Schwann cells surrounding nerves.

For the most part, there is a method to this confusing terminology. Every tissue or body part has a specific name. We all know these names in English. Bone is bone and fat is fat. But scientific medicine usually uses the Greek or Latin name for a body part and then adds a helpful tag onto the end of it. The rule for naming sarcomas, for example, is that if the tumor is benign, *oma* is usually added to the Greek or Latin name. If the tumor is malignant, *sarcoma* is added. The term for bone, for example, is *osteo*, so a benign tumor in the bone is an osteoma and a malignant tumor is an osteosarcoma. The term for fat is *lipo*, so there are lipomas and liposarcomas.

There are also different names for some organs, so a carcinoma of the stomach may be called a gastric carcinoma and a carcinoma of the kidney may be referred to as renal cell carcinoma. There are also alternative designations. For example, since the glands in the lung usually line the air passage (bronchus), carcinomas of the lung are sometimes called bronchogenic carcinomas (*genic* being the Latin way of saying "formed from").

Measuring the Rate of Growth The second way to classify tumors is according to how fast they are growing. It would be nice if there were a simple way of doing this, like pointing a radar gun at the tumor and getting a readout of the speed. But what usually has to happen is that a piece of the tumor is surgically removed and examined under a microscope, a process known as a biopsy. Its appearance and behavior can reveal a lot of information.

Well-Differentiated Tumors Under the microscope, some tumor cells look very much like the normal tissue they came from. If they do, they are called well differentiated. A normal pancreas has a characteristic look, for example. A pathologist can look at a slide of tissue and see that it's pancreas tissue, even if it is cancerous. Similarly, a follicular carcinoma of the thyroid resembles normal thyroid tissue rather well, so it is not difficult for a pathologist to know where that tumor comes from. Well-differentiated tumors tend to grow more slowly and are less aggressive.

Undifferentiated Tumors Other tumors don't particularly look like the normal tissues they come from. They resemble the tissue of origin only slightly or not at all. They look more primitive or immature. Sometimes they don't really look like any specific tissue. These are called undifferentiated or poorly differentiated.

Looking at a piece of undifferentiated tissue under the microscope, a pathologist will probably not be able to tell where the tissue was taken from. An undifferentiated tumor of the pancreas may look the same as an undifferentiated tumor of the lung, so the pathologist has to rely on the surgeon to say what area the tissue is from.

Undifferentiated or poorly differentiated tumors tend to be more aggressive in their behavior. They grow faster, spread earlier, and have a worse prognosis than well-differentiated tumors. But there are exceptions for both types of tumors. Some poorly differentiated tumors grow no faster than well-differentiated ones.

Moderately Differentiated Tumors As their name suggests, these tumors fall somewhere between well-differentiated and poorly differentiated tumors in their degree of differentiation and rate of growth.

High-Grade and Low-Grade Tumors There is another classification system that sometimes overlaps with the system based on differentiation. This system refers to tumors as "high grade" or "low grade." A high-grade tumor is immature, poorly differentiated, fast growing, and aggressive. A low-grade tumor is usually mature, well differentiated, slow growing, and less aggressive. The grading of tumors is used to help determine cancer prognosis.

Defining the Stages of Cancer The third classification used in cancer treatment is called the staging system. Staging has a number of purposes:

• It is a useful way of identifying the "extent" of the tumor—its size, the degree of growth, and the degree of spread. Obviously, if a tumor is found in only one place, it is in an early stage. If it has spread to some distant part of the body or is found in several places, it is in an advanced stage.

• It provides an estimate of the prognosis, since the chance of cure decreases as you move across the categories into more advanced or extensive stages.

• It provides a common and uniformly agreed upon set of criteria against which doctors around the world can compare treatments for a specific stage of tumor. They can then know that if one treatment has better results than another, the difference is really due to the treatment and not to differences between patients or the stages of the disease.

• It is generally the most important factor in deciding on the appropriate treatment.

The TNM System Several staging systems have been developed for different kinds of cancer. But in the past few years, a lot of thought and effort has been going on around the world to develop a relatively uniform classification system.

This system is known as TNM. T stands for the size of the tumor or the depth of penetration of the tumor through the wall of the organ, N for the degree of spread to lymph nodes, and M for the presence or absence of metastasis. A number is added to each of these letters to indicate degrees of size and spread.

Greatly simplified:

- T0 means there is no evidence of the primary tumor (typically because it was completely removed by the biopsy used to establish the diagnosis). T1 indicates the smallest tumor. T2, T3, and T4 indicate larger tumors or increasing depth through the wall of the organ and into surrounding tissues. TX means the tumor cannot be adequately assessed. This means the tumor is "in situ" (very early stage, not yet invasive).
- N0 means that the nearby lymph nodes are free of tumor. N1, N2, and N3 signify increasing degrees of involvement of these regional nodes. An N2 tumor is more serious than an N1 tumor.
- M0 means that no distant metastases (cancer cells) have been found. If there are metastases, the classification is M1.

This seems simple enough. But the system is actually quite complex. The classifications are defined differently for each kind of cancer, and each stage can include variations to the basic TNM classification. Following are the staging categories and stage grouping for breast carcinoma:

A breast cancer might be classified as a T2, N1, M0 lesion. This could represent a tumor 1 inch (2.5 cm) in diameter removed from the breast with some involvement of lymph nodes in the armpit but with no evidence of metastasis.

The TNM system has two overlapping classifications, the second having to do with the stage of cancer that represents a composite of the TNM classification. You will see in the tumor section that each tumor is grouped usually in one of four stages. Since there are many possible further TNM subdivisions, these are lumped together. You have to refer to the specific table for each cancer to be sure of the specific stage. For example, the T2, N1, M0

breast cancer described above is a Stage IIB cancer. A T3, N2, M0 cancer is Stage IIIA.

Staging and Treatment The significance of this classification is that treatment depends on the stage of the disease as defined by the TNM system. Your doctor has to know the stage to decide on appropriate therapy and to interpret the always evolving guidelines for treatment produced by major cancer centers and research groups.

This system has to be understood precisely so that very critical decisions can be made. Some stages of cancer are best treated surgically, others with radiotherapy, still others with chemotherapy. It is also becoming more and more common to use two of these treatment methods together and sometimes all three. Occasionally, they are given in sequence.

All these decisions are closely correlated with the stage of the tumor. In treating colon cancer, for example, chemotherapy is typically given following an operation for Stage III cancer, but not routinely for earlier stages of the cancer. Similarly, Stage I prostate cancer may be treated surgically. But surgery is not usually an option by Stage III, when the tumor has extended beyond the prostate.

Although the TNM system is not applicable to all cancers—it is not used with lymphomas, for example—it has now replaced earlier classification systems for tumors in the colon and rectum and is used to stage many other kinds of cancer. Since 1997, it has been the recommended staging system for most cancers.

Molecular Genetic Pathways to Cancer

Cancer is a complex disease caused by the uncontrolled proliferation of a single cell that has lost the ability to respond to the negative controls that restrict cell division.

American Joint Committee on Cancer Staging for Breast Carcinoma

T = Primary Tumor   **N** = Regional Tumor   **M** = Distant Metastasis

Primary Tumor (T)

TX   Primary tumor cannot be assessed

T0   No evidence of primary tumor

Tis*   Carcinoma in situ: Intraductal carcinoma, lobular carcinoma in situ, or Paget's disease of the nipple with no tumor

T1   Tumor 2 cm or less in greatest dimension

T2   Tumor more than 2 cm but not more than 5 cm in greatest dimension

T3   Tumor more than 5 cm in greatest dimension

T4†   Tumor of any size with direct extension to chest wall or skin

*Paget's disease associated with a tumor is classified according to the size of the tumor.
†Chest wall includes ribs, intercostal muscles, and serratus anterior muscle but not pectoral muscle.

Regional Lymph Nodes (N) (Clinical)

NX   Regional lymph nodes cannot be assessed (e.g., previously removed)

N0   No regional lymph node metastasis

N1   Metastasis to movable ipsilateral axillary lymph node(s)

N2   Metastasis to ipsilateral axillary lymph node(s) fixed to one another or to other structures

N3   Metastasis to ipsilateral internal mammary lymph node(s)

Distant Metastasis (M)

MX   Presence of distant metastasis cannot be assessed

M0   No distant metastasis

M1   Distant metastasis (includes metastasis to ipsilateral supraclavicular lymph node[s])

© 1989, American Cancer Society, Inc.

Stage Grouping			
Stage 0	Tis	N0	M0
Stage I	T1	N0	M0
Stage IIA	T0	N1	M0
	T1	N1*	M0
	T2	N0	M0
Stage IIB	T2	N1	M0
	T3	N0	M0
Stage IIIA	T0	N2	M0
	T1	N2	M0
	T2	N2	M0
	T3	N1, N2	M0
Stage IIIB	T4	Any N	M0
	Any T	N3	M0
Stage IV	Any T	Any N	M1

*The prognosis of patients with pN1a is similar to that of patients with pN0.

Natural selection has made sure that cancer is unlikely to occur during a normal life span, which varies substantially for different species. However, when life expectancy is increased, cancer incidence increases. Animals in the wild rarely get cancer, whereas cancer becomes common in animals maintained in zoos, where life span is frequently extended. Prior to the twentieth century, cancer was a relatively rare disease in humans; however, during the twentieth century, life expectancy for most human populations nearly doubled. With increased longevity, there has been a corresponding increase in cancer incidence.

Cancer occurs when a single cell acquires a set of mutations to genes that encode the proteins that control cell proliferation. These mutations make it possible for a cell to divide in an environment where cell proliferation is highly restricted. We all acquire mutations in our genes during our lifetime, and with the increasing life span of humans there has been a corresponding increase in the number of mutations that we acquire. As a result of increased longevity and genetic mutation, cancer has become responsible for 20 percent of all deaths in long-lived populations such as those in the United States.

During the past two decades, enormous strides have been made in characterizing the genes that are mutated as a normal cell progresses to a cancer cell. There are several discrete steps that a cell must take in order to proliferate uncontrollably and migrate to other sites where the dividing cancer cell ultimately becomes lethal. Each of these steps involves a genetic mutation that overcomes a strict control that keeps cell proliferation under control. A brief description of the control steps that must be overcome during tumor progression follows (these are adapted from an influential 2000 article in the scientific journal *Cell*, written by Doug Hanahan and Robert Weinberg, titled "The Hallmarks of Cancer"):

Cell Division Signals A cell divides only when instructed. The instructions come from other cells usually in the form of small molecules known as ligands, also commonly termed growth factors. These ligands function by binding to receptors on the surface of a cell, which induces changes on the inside of the cell such that the cell responds in some specific way. For example, the response might involve the assembly of a "signaling machine" within the cell. This signaling machinery consists of enzymes that become activated as a consequence of the ligand-receptor binding. The best character-ized mutations in cancer cells are in the genes that encode the receptors or various downstream components of this signaling machine. These mutations result in a constant signal to divide even in the absence of the signaling ligand, leading to unchecked cell growth and division.

Numerous genes have been identified that, when appropriately mutated, cause a signal to be sent that instructs the cell to divide.

Tumor Suppressor Genes Mutations that cause cell division signals to be sent, in general, are not sufficient to stimulate cell division. Just prior to replicating the genetic material (DNA), there is a criti-cal checkpoint that is guarded by a set of genes that are known as tumor suppres-sor genes. The tumor suppressor genes encode proteins that prevent DNA repli-cation and cell division unless the cell is supposed to divide. For reasons that are not yet clear, tumor suppressor genes have the capability to recognize when inappro-priate cell division signals are being sent and prevent inappropriate cell division. The tumor suppressor genes must there-fore be neutralized in order for cell divi-sion to occur. Inactivating mutations to tumor suppressor genes are essential for progression to a cancer cell.

Programmed Cell Suicide (Apoptosis) In order to maintain a constant cell number in the body, cell division must be matched by cell death. Our bodies have evolved efficient means for ridding the body of unwanted cells. Unwanted cells commit a genetically programmed cell suicide; this suicide mechanism is emerging as a major defense against cancer. Introduction of a mutated gene from the signaling machin-ery to a normal cell will generally lead to cell suicide, unless another genetic change is present that suppresses a default cell-suicide pathway. In order for a cell to become cancerous, therefore, it must overcome the cell's ability to commit suicide.

Immortality Most of the cells in our body have a limited number of times they can divide. This is because each time a cell divides, it incompletely replicates the ends of the chromosome. Successive rounds of replication ultimately lead to a shortening of the chromosome, and genes near the ends of the chromosome are lost. Ultimately, chromosomal degradation results in a cell that is unable to function, and cell death occurs. In this way, cells have a limited number of times that they can divide and are therefore protected from becoming cancerous. However, there is an enzyme known as telomerase that is able to replicate the ends of the chromosomes and prevent shortening and the loss of needed genes. The presence of this enzyme is generally restricted to the germ cells (sperm and egg), where it is critical that the entire complement of genetic material be protected for passage to succeeding generations. Cancer cells are somehow able to stimulate the telomerase gene to maintain the ends of the chromosomes, achieving the immortality needed to divide indefinitely and become fully cancerous.

Invasion and Angiogenesis Once a cell has attained the ability to divide in the absence of cell division signals, it still must gain the ability to migrate to foreign sites in the body and then stimulate the formation of blood vessels—a process called angiogenesis—that will provide the nourishment needed for developing a large tumor mass. A primary tumor must gain access to the bloodstream in order to migrate or metastasize. This process involves digging through connective tissue and blood vessel walls. Cancer cells accomplish this by secreting enzymes that break down tissue barriers, which then allows them to gain access to the circulatory system. Once a cancer cell has migrated to another site in the body and has begun to proliferate, it must stimulate the formation of blood vessels if it is to grow to a size that will be harmful to the invaded organ. Angiogenesis is initiated by secreting factors that stimulate the proliferation of cells that form blood vessel walls. Cancer cells must either secrete

these factors themselves or stimulate other cells to do so.

Caretakers Genetic mutations occur naturally during the replication of DNA during cell division. DNA can become chemically damaged by exposure to many compounds from diet and other sources. The ability to repair damaged DNA prior to replication is critical to preventing the mutations that contribute to cancer. DNA repair mechanisms are more efficient in species with longer life spans, indicating that DNA repair mechanisms have evolved in order to prevent cancer. Consistent with this hypothesis, individuals with inherited defects in DNA repair mechanisms have a greater risk for cancer. While defects in DNA repair do not contribute directly to uncontrolled cell proliferation, or cancer, the inability to repair chemically damaged DNA dramatically accelerates the accumulation of genetic alterations in genes that control cell proliferation. Genetic mutation in genes necessary for DNA repair is one of the most common reasons for a genetic predisposition to cancer.

Tumor Promotion A cell that has acquired some, but not all, of the genetic changes to become fully cancerous can sometimes be stimulated to divide by an external stimulus. Compounds that stimulate the proliferation of partially cancerous cells are known as tumor promoters. A well-known example of tumor promotion occurs in human breast cancer, where estrogen stimulates the proliferation of partially cancerous breast cells. In this situation, estrogen is acting as a tumor promoter to stimulate cell division. Cell division requires replication of DNA, which results in additional mutations. And these additional mutations will ultimately lead to a more malignant cell capable of dividing in the absence of the promoter. Compounds in diet and tobacco products that stimulate cell division and the replication of DNA, and, as a consequence, additional mutations, are likely the most significant causes of human cancer.

Understanding the genetic changes that occur as a normal cell progresses to a cancerous one reveals that there are many hurdles a cell must overcome to become a fully malignant tumor. These hurdles are overcome by the acquisition of several genetic mutations that (1) activate a signaling machine, (2) inactivate tumor suppressor genes, (3) overcome cell suicide programs, (4) attain immortality, (5) penetrate blood vessel walls, and (6) stimulate the production of blood vessels to provide nutrients. The genetic mutations that do all of the above can be accelerated by inherited defects in the ability to repair DNA or by tumor-promoting agents that stimulate excess cell proliferation.

In light of all the obstacles in the progression to cancer, it is somewhat surprising that as many as 40 percent of people in the United States will get the disease, and as many as 20 percent will die of cancer. However, if you consider that this number could be cut in half through avoidance of tobacco and changes in diet, the picture is not as bleak. During an average human life span, there are approximately 10^{16} (10 million billion) cell divisions that take place where the DNA is replicated and genetic changes are possible. In this regard, it is actually quite remarkable that as little as one in ten of us will acquire the set of genetic changes necessary for the formation of a fatal malignant cancer.

Cell proliferation leads to genetic changes and this is the basis for biological evolution. Natural selection has made sure that it is difficult for a cell to become cancerous in species with long life spans, where so much cell proliferation occurs. The process of progression to a malignant cancer is now beginning to be understood at the molecular and genetic levels and this understanding has provided many new targets for therapeutic intervention. The several steps that a cell must take to become a cancer provide an equally large number of places to therapeutically intervene. The next generation of cancer research promises to be one whereby the understanding of the molecular pathways to cancer are exploited to treat and eradicate this disease that has exposed itself with the increased longevity of human beings during the twentieth century.

— 2 —

How Cancer Is Diagnosed

Malin Dollinger, M.D., Britt-Marie Ljung, M.D.,
Eugene T. Morita, M.D., and Ernest H. Rosenbaum, M.D.

Cancer can be treated. But if it is going to be treated fully, it must be detected in its early stages. This isn't always easy because of the silent period of tumor growth—the months or years when the malignant cells are quietly doubling again and again—before the cancer is big enough to detect. For a long time, there may be absolutely no indication that this process is going on.

So how do we discover that the tumor is there? Your own complaint may be the tip-off. Or your doctor might pick up on some clue that appears during a physical. Whatever sets off the search for cancer, the investigative process that leads to a definitive diagnosis follows a standard pattern. Suspicions are aroused. Questions are asked. Answers are found through examinations, tests, images of body organs, and analyses of tissues under a microscope.

Symptoms

When a lump has grown to a certain size, its presence is signaled in a number of ways:

- It presses on nearby tissues, which sometimes produces pain.
- It grows into nearby blood vessels, which may produce bleeding.
- It gets so large that it can be seen or felt.
- It causes a change in the way some organ works. Trouble swallowing (dysphagia), for example, might be the sign of a tumor partially obstructing the esophagus, the passage between the throat and stomach. Hoarseness or change of voice might indicate a tumor in the larynx, or voice box. These symptoms—pressure, bleeding, a mass, or interference with function—are reflected in the American Cancer Society's list of *seven early warning signals:*

1. **C**hange in bowel or bladder habits.
2. **A** sore that does not heal.
3. **U**nusual bleeding or discharge.
4. **T**hickening or lump in breast or elsewhere.
5. **I**ndigestion or difficulty in swallowing.
6. **O**bvious change in wart or mole.
7. **N**agging cough or hoarseness.

Recognizing a symptom is the first critical step in the search for cancer. Unfortunately, many people don't pay any attention to these warning signals. They wait and wait, sometimes for months, before getting the medical attention that could save their lives.

The best chance of diagnosing cancer early depends on someone's thoughtful and perceptive awareness that something new has happened to his or her body—especially the appearance of one of these symptoms. Despite this, some cancers are silent until they grow to an advanced size, pointing out the need for sensitive tests for the early diagnosis of cancer.

The Physical Examination

The suspicion that a cancer is growing is often aroused during a routine physical examination, the major part of what should be a yearly checkup of your general health. The physical examination is a thorough, systematic, and progressive search throughout your body for signs of disease or abnormal function. To make sure that no significant area is missed, each physician generally develops his or her own standard pattern or sequence. Some start with the head and work down the body; others examine each organ system as a unit.

Whatever the pattern, a good physical examination with a view to detecting cancer involves a search of the entire body with a special emphasis on the parts that are most prone to malignancy.

• The nose and throat are examined. There is a quick and painless mirror examination of the larynx.
• The lymph-node-bearing areas—such as the neck above the collarbone, under the arms, and in the groin—are checked.
• Specific attention is paid to the breasts in women and the prostate gland in men.
• The abdomen is carefully pushed and probed to detect enlargement of any of the abdominal organs, especially the liver and spleen.
• Examination of the pelvic area in women, including a Pap smear, is essential to detect cancers of the cervix, uterus, and ovaries.
• A probing of the rectum with a gloved finger is an essential part of the physical for both men and women.

During the examination, your doctor will ask you many questions about various body functions. There will be specific questions about hoarseness, signs of gastrointestinal bleeding, constipation, swallowing problems, coughing up blood, and so on. A "yes" answer to any of these questions leads to more detailed questions, to more specific physical examinations, and possibly to blood tests, X-rays, or other studies.

You might also be asked questions about any family history of cancer, particularly among close relatives—parents, grandparents, aunts, uncles, brothers, and sisters. Detailed answers to these questions will help in the search for any cancers with a genetic basis, such as some breast and colon cancers.

Suspicious findings in any part of the physical examination will lead to further tests. An enlarged lymph node in the neck, for example, might indicate a cancer that has spread from somewhere else. This will set off a vigorous search for the primary site. Persistent coughing, especially with blood, might lead the doctor to look directly inside your lungs with a special instrument (a bronchoscope) to detect tumors (see "Endoscopy," in this chapter).

Blood Tests

The next level of the diagnostic process involves a laboratory analysis of blood samples. Two categories of blood tests are used to help in the diagnosis of cancer:

Nonspecific Tests Most blood tests are nonspecific. This means they can reveal an abnormality in the blood that indicates some illness but not which one.

A blood count, for example, may show anemia. Why would you be anemic? There are many reasons, including cancer. But the anemia may not be related to a tumor unless you have a history of bleeding in the bowel and X-rays show a cancer of the colon. Similarly, there are tests for liver function that indicate abnormalities in that organ. But the problem might be caused by gallstones, hepatitis, tumors, or drug toxicity. Certain patterns in the test results will suggest tumors or some other cause of bile obstruction. Other

Blood Tests Useful in Cancer Diagnosis

Nonspecific Tests

Alkaline phosphatase	Elevated in bone and liver disease
SGOT and SGPT	Elevated if there is liver damage
Bilirubin	Elevated in liver disease, especially with bile duct obstruction
LDH	Elevated in many diseases, including cancer
Uric acid	Elevated in gout, cancers of the blood and lymph nodes, and after cancer treatment
Creatinine and BUN	Elevated in kidney disease
Calcium	Elevated in cancer that has spread to the bone, with tumors that produce parathyroid hormone-like protein, and in multiple myeloma, as well as in some nonmalignant diseases
Electrolytes (sodium, potassium, carbon dioxide, chloride)	These levels are useful in metabolic and endocrine disease, and for monitoring both nutritional status and the effects of treatment
Amylase	Used to assess pancreatic disease

Specific Tests and Markers

Not all cancers produce these markers.

CEA (carcino-embryonic antigen)	Elevated in cancers of the colon, rectum, lung, breast, and pancreas
CA-125	Elevated in cancers of the ovary and uterus
CA 19-9	Elevated in cancers of the colon, pancreas, stomach, and liver
CA 15-3/CA 27-29	Elevated in breast cancer
Alpha-fetoprotein (AFP)	Elevated in primary liver cancer and some cancers of the testis
HCG (human chorionic gonadotropin)	Elevated in some cancers of the testis and ovary and some lung cancers; also elevated in pregnancy
Prostatic acid phosphatase (PAP)	Markedly elevated in some cases of prostate cancer
Prostate-specific antigen (PSA)	Helpful in diagnosing prostate cancer, in detecting recurrent disease, and in guiding treatment
Serum protein electrophoresis	Abnormal gamma globulin (monoclonal "spike") is found in myeloma
Serum protein immuno-electrophoresis (IgG, IgA, IgM)	Similar to above, but can classify the type of abnormal gamma globulin present

patterns will suggest hepatitis. But essentially these patterns are only important clues. They are not solutions to diagnostic questions.

There are so many tests used to detect abnormalities in different organ systems that physicians usually obtain a whole panel of them—blood counts, tests of metabolism (including levels of minerals such as calcium), and tests for the liver, kidneys, or thyroid. The test results may suggest certain types of tumors, but no specific diagnosis can be made on the basis of these tests alone.

Specific Tests Other blood tests are fairly specific for particular kinds of cancer, often several kinds. These tests will be ordered if your doctor strongly suspects one of these cancers.

Tumor Markers The most important are tests for chemicals called tumor markers. These are produced by various types of tumors. Breast, lung, and bowel tumors, for example, produce a protein called the carcinoembryonic antigen (CEA). Some inflammatory diseases may produce low levels of this chemical, but some tumors in these areas produce very high levels. If a very high CEA level is found, then a tumor is assumed to be present until proved otherwise. Similarly, prostate cancers and many cancers of the testicles and ovaries produce known chemicals.

Some very exciting research is now being done to find more and more accurate markers for different types of cancer. We can now envision the day in the not-too-distant future when specific blood tests will identify most human cancers. But at the moment, the few tests we do have are invaluable. They not only help make the diagnosis but are especially useful for keeping track of the cancer after treatment. If the marker is elevated at the time of diagnosis, then successful treatment should result in the level falling or disappearing altogether. The reappearance of the marker

often signals a relapse. If that happens, even if no other sign or symptom appears, there would be a search for a new tumor and consideration would be given to re-treatment. A problem with these tests, however, is that they can sometimes be elevated in the absence of cancer. Your doctor will need to evaluate these test results in the context of your individual condition.

Other Blood Tests When a cancer is in the blood cells themselves, tests of the blood and the blood-forming organs may be all that's needed to make the diagnosis. Cancer of the white blood cells—leukemia—can often be diagnosed by looking at a sample of blood taken from the finger or arm. The diagnosis can be confirmed by examining cells from the bone marrow, where these cells are made. Bone marrow analysis will also diagnose multiple myeloma, which is basically a malignancy of plasma cells in the marrow.

Tests of Fluids and Stools

Our bodies produce wastes—urine and stool—that can reveal clues about disease. But there are also other fluids that can be analyzed to detect cancer cells.

• The most familiar test of body fluids is the urinalysis that is part of a regular checkup. Analyzing the urine's composition can reveal all kinds of abnormalities. The presence of protein might indicate kidney disease. The level of sugar might indicate diabetes. Too many white blood cells can indicate an infection. Too many red blood cells could indicate bleeding, maybe because of a tumor, maybe from some other cause. If tumor cells are found, other tests will be done.

• A physical or X-ray examination may reveal the presence of fluid in the chest cavity, abdomen, or joints. A needle can be inserted into these areas and the fluid drawn out for examination.

• A lumbar puncture, also known as a spinal tap, is a special procedure to remove fluid from the spinal canal. It involves the insertion of a needle between the vertebrae, after you've been given a local anesthetic. Tests can identify any infection, inflammation, or cancer.

The Hidden Blood Stool Test Blood in the stool is always a sign of something going wrong in the digestive tract. Sometimes this blood can easily be seen in a bowel movement; most of the time, it's all but invisible. One simple procedure to find out whether there is blood in the stool is called the occult (hidden) blood test. A small amount of stool is smeared on specially treated paper and then chemicals that reveal the presence of blood are added. If blood is found, the upper and/or lower bowel will be examined with scopes or barium X-rays.

Blood in the stool is often caused by hemorrhoids, but a benign or premalignant tumor (a polyp) or a hidden cancer is always a possibility.

Imaging Techniques

Any suspicious findings in the physical exam or the lab test results will make your doctor want to find out what is going on inside your body. He or she could just look inside directly, either with special instruments or by opening up some area. But the first step usually involves the use of one or more devices that produce images of suspicious areas.

These "imaging studies" may show a tumor in a specific organ, and the image will help your doctor assess its size and whether it has involved surrounding tissues.

If you complain of indigestion, for example, your doctor may suspect stomach cancer. This would lead to an X-ray or endoscopy of the upper gastrointestinal tract. Lower digestive tract complaints such as constipation or bleeding might lead to an X-ray or endoscopy to diagnose a possible carcinoma of the colon. Blood in the urine may lead to an X-ray of the kidneys to confirm a suspected tumor in the kidneys or bladder. And complaints of severe headaches, together with other symptoms of increased pressure in the head, may result in a CT scan of the head in search of a brain tumor.

In the past, radiography (X-ray) was the only imaging technique available. If X-rays couldn't answer critical questions in the diagnostic investigation, then a surgeon would have to open up the body to take a direct look. But new techniques have revolutionized the art and science of diagnosis. Some of the new techniques involve the use of X-rays; others do not.

X-Rays This familiar imaging technique involves passing a small dose of ionizing radiation through a specific area of the body and onto a film. This produces a two-dimensional picture of the structures inside.

Bones and some other dense substances absorb more X-rays than other tissues, so they show up on the film as shadows that your doctor can interpret. But soft tissues can't be seen very well on X-rays. It is impossible to see the inside of a stomach, for example, without adding a substance that will prevent the X-rays from penetrating.

If your stomach is going to be X-rayed, you will be asked to swallow a barium "meal." The barium will improve the contrast and so produce a better picture. If your large bowel is going to be seen, you will be given a barium enema. If your kidneys are going to be examined, another type of contrast agent may be injected into a vein to fill the kidneys, which will allow them to be seen.

A fluoroscope might also be used. This lets the doctor see a continuous, moving image. In this procedure, the X-ray beam strikes a small fluorescent screen and the image is amplified through a video system.

Nuclear Scans Radioactive isotopes that emit gamma rays can produce an image on photographic film or on a scintillation detector. Some of these isotopes, generally given by injection, are organ specific, which means that they concentrate in that part of the body suspected of harboring cancer.

Different organs react to the isotopes in different ways. The isotopes used for liver scanning concentrate in normal tissues but are not taken up by cancer cells. So the image shows "cold spots" that may be cancerous areas. The isotopes used for bone scans, however, work in the opposite way. Cancer cells make the bone react to the isotope to a greater degree than normal bone, so "hot spots" light up the image of the skeleton. Hot spots can be produced by diseases other than cancer, however, such as bone injury or arthritis, and can represent healing bone.

Angiography This is a useful way to study the blood vessels in a specific area of the body. Angiography is sometimes used to diagnose and precisely locate tumors in the pancreas, liver, and brain, especially when surgery is being considered.

Angiography is also used in some chemotherapy treatments, when a small plastic tube (catheter) is placed in an artery to deliver anticancer drugs to the tumor. It is especially important in those cases to know the exact size of the tumor to make sure all of it is treated. It makes no sense to insert the catheter and then miss a portion of the tumor not supplied by the blood vessel being used. Angiograms safeguard against this problem by defining the blood vessels within the tumor, which have a different quality and appearance from the arteries next to the tumor.

CT Scans Computerized tomography (CT) scans are highly sensitive examinations that use small amounts of X-rays to see parts of the body that are difficult or impossible to view any other way. The images produced are far superior to those obtained by traditional X-rays. And the images are even clearer if you drink a contrast agent or get an injection before the scan is done.

The CT machine scans the area being investigated—chest, brain, abdomen, or any other part of the body—by taking X-rays of one thin layer of tissue after another. A computer puts the images together to create a cross section of the area. Looking at a set of CT images is the same idea as looking at a loaf of bread, with each slice laid out side by side in a row.

Although there is higher X-ray exposure with CT scans than with some conventional X-rays, such as chest X-rays, not undergoing the procedure is much riskier if cancer is strongly suspected. For example, the information from the scan is not only useful for diagnosis but very helpful in planning treatment. Today, some CT scans can be reconstructed with three-dimensional images. In some cases, these images can replace more invasive tests, such as colonoscopy.

Magnetic Resonance Imaging (MRI) The MRI scan can complement or even replace the CT scan in some cases. The images look similar to CT scan images, but there are no X-rays involved. The MRI scanner uses a powerful magnetic field to make certain particles in the body vibrate. Extremely sophisticated computer equipment measures the reaction and produces the images. Cross sections can be obtained not only across the body, as in CT scanning, but also from front to back and from left to right. This lets your doctor see your body from all three directions. In some cases, the images are superior to and provide more information than those obtained by CT scans. This is especially true for images of the central

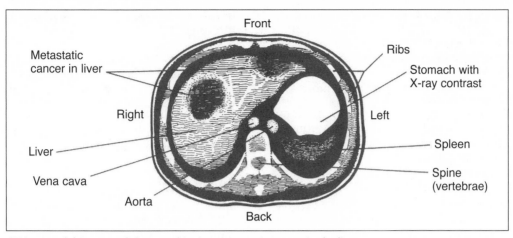

Front

Metastatic
cancer in liver

Ribs

Stomach with
X-ray contrast

Right

Left

Liver

Spleen

Vena cava

Spine
(vertebrae)

Aorta

Back

CT image of the upper abdomen, showing metastatic cancer in the liver.

nervous system and the spine. In some other cases, CT scanning is more useful than MRI scanning.

MRI is not suitable under certain conditions. An implanted metallic device such as a pacemaker, clip, or pump can be affected by the strong magnetic field.

Ultrasound This is a harmless and painless imaging technique. It is noninvasive, meaning that nothing enters your body except sound waves.

The technique involves spreading a thin coating of jelly over a particular area of the skin, then bouncing high-frequency sound waves through the skin onto internal organs. It works basically on the same principle as the sonar used by the navy to detect submarines, where sound waves are sent through the water and the "ping" of the sound bouncing back is analyzed. In a similar way, the complex ultrasound scanning apparatus draws a picture of whatever organ the sound waves are bouncing off. This picture can reveal a lot of information.

Many people are aware of ultrasound as a safe way to examine a fetus to search for abnormalities. But it is also useful for detecting possibly malignant masses or lumps without the need for X-rays.

Ultrasound is used to examine the neck for tumors of the thyroid gland or of the parathyroids. It is the standard method to diagnose gallstones, since the sound waves bounce quite nicely off the stones. And it is often used in the pelvis to study possible enlargement of the prostate or an ovary. Benign ovarian cysts are common, and other ways of examining this part of the body are not very precise. It has also been adapted to be used with endoscopes to help stage rectal and esophageal cancers. Ultrasound is helpful to distinguish cysts from solid breast tumors.

Positron-Emission Tomography (PET) This noninvasive scanning technique is becoming a valuable aid in finding hidden cancers. In contrast to other types of scans (CT, MRI) that show that "something is taking up space" in a certain area, PET scans "light up" areas of growing tissue. These scans depend on differences in metabolic activity (rate of growth), since tumors grow faster than normal tissue. Thus, this scan might distinguish living cancer from dead cancer tissue or blood clots or scar tissue. For those who appreciate details, PET is an accurate way to detect cancer invasion and help stage cancer. This comprehensive assessment is helpful both in initial staging of newly diagnosed patients and for follow-up staging after treatment for the extent of disease. PET has thus helped physicians in making more accurate and rational decisions, and will likely be used more and more in the future.

PET uses an imaging agent, radioactive tracer F-18 fluorodeoxyglucose (FDG). It was developed in the late 1960s, and with greater availability of FDG and new technology, it provides an improved imaging technique by being able to image active cancer processes. Images are in three dimensions. Most malignant tumors use a lot of glucose and will "light up" on a PET scan. Then the PET scan can be compared or integrated with a CAT or MRI scan. PET scans can be viewed in three dimensions on a computer screen, and the image can be "rotated" to see the mass from any angle. Both cancer and some benign processes can be seen on PET scans but cannot be distinguished. Tissue biopsies are sometimes required for a cancer diagnosis.

It is now common to use PET scans for staging of lung cancer and melanoma. For example, in lung cancer, the PET has 85 percent accuracy versus 52 percent for CT scans. PET detects accurately 83 to 94 percent of metastatic lymph nodes versus 63 to 73 percent accuracy for CT scans. PET detects metastases outside the chest in up to 30 percent of patients with lung cancer. In one study, 41 percent of patients had a change in treatment management based on PET scans.

Three technologies are required for PET scanning to be possible:

1. A source for the FDG radioisotope. FDG is produced in a cyclotron and can be purchased from a radiopharmacy.

2. A scanner that can record the location of the FDG in the body, to localize tissue with active metabolism—especially cancer.

3. A powerful computer to reconstruct the signals into the three-dimensional images of the body, for the radiologist to interpret.

Newer techniques merging CT/MRI and PET have improved the efficiency of our ability to diagnose cancer and assess the effectiveness of its therapy. PET scanning is likely to become even more useful, and in fact frequently necessary, in the diagnosis and management of cancer.

Endoscopy

Sometimes images are not enough. The use of direct visualization has become more and more important in recent years, not only for diagnosing malignancies but in some cases as an aid in treatment (see chapter 10, "Laser Therapy").

Rigid, thin telescopes have been used for years to look inside body cavities with natural openings. A bronchoscope inserted into the mouth or nose and through the windpipe (trachea) can be used to look inside the lungs. A cystoscope inserted into the urethra can be used to examine the bladder. Sometimes mirrors are used with these rigid scopes to examine, for example, the nasal passage and the back of the mouth (nasopharyngoscope) and the larynx (laryngoscope).

Flexible Scopes Flexible fiber-optic "telescopes" have come into widespread use, as they are more versatile and comfortable than rigid telescopes. These scopes use bundles of glass fibers that can bend around corners and form perfect pictures of the tissues at their far ends. Doctors looking through one end of the scope can look into many areas of the body safely, often with a minimum of sedation or local anesthetic. Not only can your doctor see exactly what's going on in these areas, but he or she can also take photographs or remove cell samples.

The inside of the lung passages can be examined easily and quickly with the fiber-optic bronchoscope. A diagnosis of lung cancer can often be made by this method alone, without resorting to the surgical procedures that used to be necessary.

Usually as an outpatient procedure, the nose and throat are sprayed with a local anesthetic and a thin flexible tube is passed into the lung area. Specialized fiber optics allow the doctor to "see" inside the lungs, look for areas that appear abnormal, and do small biopsies to see if cancer is present.

Similar instruments have revolutionized the diagnosis of tumors in the stomach and bowel. With a flexible gastroscope or colonoscope, the entire stomach or colon can clearly be seen and pieces of tissue can be collected. Similar specialized instruments for other body cavities have made diagnostic procedures much safer. And the procedures can be repeated after treatment to see how effective the treatment has been.

Endoscopic-Ultrasound-Guided Fine Needle Aspiration An ultrasound probe can be integrated into an endoscope, allowing images of masses close to the esophagus, stomach, or bowel to be visualized and sampled with a thin needle. The ultrasound device makes it possible to watch the needle tip moving into the mass and collect a small sample for microscopic analysis and diagnosis. A general description of fine needle aspiration can be found below under "Cytological Studies." Masses in the pancreas, the esophagus, the stomach and the bowel walls as well as a subset of lymph nodes and other structures in the abdomen and the mediastinum can be visualized, reached, and sampled with this technique.

ERCP Clever adaptations of these endoscopic methods and tools are sometimes used for specialized diagnosis and therapy. In a procedure called endoscopic retrograde cholangiopancreatography (ERCP), for example, a doctor can pass a flexible fiber-optic telescope into your stomach, visualize the opening of the ducts draining bile from the liver, and insert a tube (stem) into these ducts from inside the

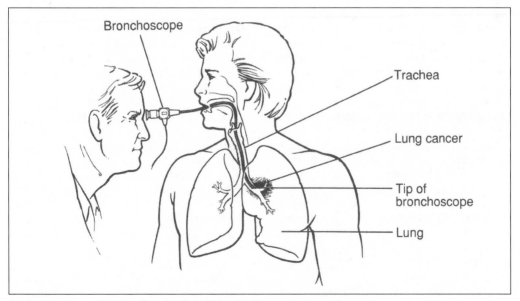

Lung cancer can often be diagnosed and biopsied through a bronchoscope.

stomach either to provide drainage or to take pictures showing the exact location of tumors in the bile ducts and exactly how involved the ducts are.

Cytological Studies

Cytology is simply the study of cells. In cancer diagnosis, the term *cytological studies* means the examination of cellular material removed from the body. The cells might be removed by natural means, such as coughing up sputum (phlegm). They might also be removed by washing a body cavity with a salt solution—the inside of the abdomen after abdominal surgery, for example—or by scraping the surface of an organ or a suspected cancer.

The best-known cytology test is the one developed by George Papanicolaou—the Pap smear. The cervix is scraped and brushed to remove for analysis cells that could be abnormal or cancerous. In the same way, the tongue, the esophagus, the stomach, or the lung's air passages can easily be scraped using a small brush through a scope.

Fine Needle Aspiration (FNA) Biopsy. This is another type of cytological test, used primarily to find out if a lump (for example, in the breast, thyroid, lung, lymph node, etc.) is benign or malignant. In most cases, it is also possible to find out exactly what type of benign or malignant process is causing the lump. In order to collect the cell sample for analysis, a very thin needle (thinner than a needle that is used to draw blood) is placed inside the lump, and over a duration of ten to twenty seconds, a small amount of cellular material is withdrawn for analysis. Usually at least two samples are collected. The discomfort experienced is usually comparable to a blood test, and the only common side effect is a limited local bruise with accompanying soreness lasting a few days.

The removed cells are put on slides, stained with dyes, and examined under a microscope. The cytotechnologist will screen the slide for the characteristic appearance of malignant or premalignant cells. A pathologist will subsequently examine the slides and may either diagnose cancer or report a strong suspicion of cancer. In some cases, a conventional surgical biopsy may be done to confirm the diagnosis.

FNA, when performed by well-trained practitioners, is suitable for definitive diagnosis of most types of cancer, including the majority of cancers involving lymph glands. For the latter, conventional microscopic interpretation is complemented by analysis of specialized stains highlighting markers on the surface of the tumor cells. This may be done by the flow cytometry method and/or by examination of the stained cells using a microscope.

Generally, specialized physicians who perform a large number of FNAs are more likely to provide a definitive diagnosis and a high rate of diagnostic accuracy. All diagnostic procedures carry a slight possibility of error (in the range of 1 to a few percent). If you are facing extensive treatment for cancer, you may want to consider obtaining a second opinion to confirm the diagnosis. Many institutions provide this by presentation at regularly scheduled multidisciplinary conferences, often called tumor boards, where experts from all aspects of cancer diagnosis and care come together to review diagnosis and treatment options for patients.

Tumor Tests Several other techniques for cell analysis, in addition to the usual examination under a microscope, are available. These techniques improve doctors' ability to diagnose cancer, help determine the likely clinical course, and help guide the choice of treatment options.

• *Special Stains* There are now a large number of special ways to stain cancer tissue in the laboratory. These stains are often of great help in determining the type of cancer when there is some uncertainty. They also provide helpful information about prognosis and treatment. Examples are hormone receptor analysis in breast cancer, Her-2/*neu* (c-*erb* B2), various cytokeratins, etc.

• *Flow Cytometry* This technique can analyze a tumor's DNA content to find out whether the cancer cells contain the normal number of chromosomes (diploid) or an abnormal amount (aneuploid). Aneuploid tumors tend to be poorly differentiated and aggressive.

• *S-Phase Testing* This technique measures how fast a tumor is growing. In the S-phase of a cell's growth cycle, new DNA is synthesized to prepare for the division of one cell into two. A tumor that is growing slowly may have less than 7 percent of cells in the S-phase. A more rapidly growing tumor has 8 percent or more. Tumors with higher rates of growth have a poorer prognosis and may need more aggressive treatment.

Biopsies

Ultimately the diagnosis of cancer depends on examining a small bit of tissue to see if

it has the characteristic patterns and cell types defined as cancer. The definitive way to diagnose a suspicious area may be by cytology, by core biopsy, or by performing a surgical biopsy. Sometimes this is done even before doing other tests.

This microscopic examination is carried out by a pathologist who is an expert in distinguishing the very exact criteria that separate malignant cells from normal or benign ones. It is essential to obtain a specimen of tissue to do this examination. The biopsy is the procedure for obtaining the tissue.

There are two types:

• An incisional biopsy involves cutting into a portion of the tumor, then stitching the area closed.
• An excisional biopsy involves removing the entire tumor.

The excisional biopsy is often done with small tumors that are easily accessible and relatively small, such as those involving the skin, the mouth or nasal cavity, lymph nodes, or a woman's reproductive system.

Biopsies are often done during the surgery that may be needed to expose the tumor. In such cases, it's customary to take tissue samples not only from the apparent

Types of Biopsy for Cancer Diagnosis

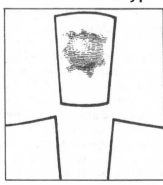
Excisional biopsy
Complete removal of tumor

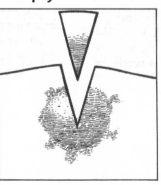
Incisional biopsy
Partial removal of tumor

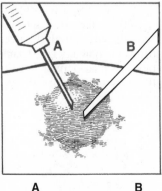
A
Fine needle
aspiration

B
Cutting needle
(core) biopsy

site of the tumor but also from the lymph nodes or other tissues in the neighborhood. This will help measure the tumor's potential or actual spread. This defines the stage of the cancer, so the staging process may be carried out at the same time as the diagnostic process. Of course, the surgeon may also try to carry out the most appropriate therapy at the same time by removing all the visible tumor.

Core Needle Biopsies These may be used to collect a slender piece of tissue from a palpable mass or an abnormal area seen on a radiological imaging study. If the mass is not palpable, then imaging guidance is necessary in order to correctly position the needle for sampling. Depending on the nature of the mass and the location in the body, ultrasound, CT (computerized tomography), or MRI (magnetic resonance imaging) may be used to guide the needle into the mass. The diameter of the needle varies from $\frac{1}{10}$ to $\frac{1}{6}$ of an inch.

Fine Needle Aspiration (FNA) Described earlier under the heading "Cytological Studies," fine needle aspiration can be utilized in a manner similar to core needle biopsies. The FNA needles are considerably smaller in diameter (25 to 22 gauge—smaller than a venipuncture needle). When FNA is utilized for deep-seated masses, requiring image guidance of the needle, it is common to have a cytologist present during sampling to examine a part of the material during the procedure in order to judge when enough material suitable for diagnosis has been collected.

What to Expect Local anesthetic is routinely used for all core needle biopsies and for deep-seated fine needle aspiration biopsies. Sedation is typically not needed. Local bruising is an expected side effect following both core needle biopsies and fine needle aspiration biopsies. The

thinner needles usually cause less bleeding and accompanying soreness after the procedure.

When sampling deep-seated masses in the abdomen and chest, bleeding can be more severe and very rarely life-threatening. Therefore a blood test, checking factors important for normal coagulation (clotting), is carried out before deep-seated sampling. In addition, patients are usually asked to temporarily stop taking "blood-thinning" medicines (aspirin, a variety of nonsteroidal anti-inflammatory drugs, heparin, Coumadin, etc.). If you are being scheduled for a procedure, make sure your provider knows what drugs you are on. Also ask when you should stop taking a particular drug. Several blood-thinning drugs take a number of days to clear from your body.

Very rare complications from needle biopsy include nerve damage and leakage of bile fluid or pancreatic juice that may cause serious peritonitis (inflammation in your abdomen). The risk of leakage is less with thinner needles and nerve damage has not been reported after using fine needle aspiration biopsy.

In order to limit bleeding after sampling of superficial masses, local pressure is applied for a few minutes (similar to a blood test). After deep-seated biopsies, patients are usually observed in the clinic/hospital for a few hours before release.

The Next Step Once the biopsy is performed and the diagnosis confirmed, the medical evaluation should rapidly be completed. At this point, treatment planning can begin.

Bone Marrow Examination

Bone marrow is analyzed to diagnose blood or bone marrow cancers and to find out if a malignancy from somewhere else has spread to the bone marrow.

The procedure is simple and brief. It can be done in a doctor's office using a local anesthetic similar to the one used by your dentist. In much the same way as blood is taken from your arm, a needle is inserted into either the breastbone or the pelvic bone, both of which are just under the skin and are easily entered. A small amount of liquid bone marrow is drawn into a syringe, placed on slides, and examined under a microscope for evidence of leukemia, lymphoma, or any other cancer cells. Sometimes a bone marrow biopsy may be done. A special cutting needle can be put into an anesthetized area of the pelvic bone and tiny bone chips (like pencil lead) can be removed. This procedure may be necessary for several reasons—to diagnose certain types of blood and bone marrow malignancies, to see if other cancers involve the marrow, or as part of the staging process.

Red marrow, which constitutes about 50 percent of an adult's marrow, actively produces red blood cells, white cells, and platelets. Yellow marrow contains fat cells and connective tissue and is inactive, but it can become active in response to the body's needs.

Bone marrow biopsies are helpful in staging using immunocytochemistry (cytokeratin) to detect micrometastases. One-third of women with breast cancer with negative lymph nodes had micrometastases. This ultrasensitive test is an independent prognostic predictor for relapse or death.

The Most Important Questions You Can Ask

Why is this test done?

A bone marrow biopsy may be done for the following reasons:

- To help the doctor diagnose blood diseases and anemias
- To diagnose primary and cancerous tumors
- To determine the cause of infection
- To help the doctor evaluate the stage of a cancer such as Hodgkin's disease

- To evaluate the effectiveness of chemotherapy and other treatments

What should you know before the test?

- The biopsy usually takes only five to ten minutes. Test results are generally available in one week.
- More than one bone marrow specimen may be required and a blood sample will be collected before biopsy for lab testing.
- The nurse will ask you to sign a consent form.
- You'll be told which biopsy site will be used (usually the breastbone [sternum] or the hip [iliac crest], but sometimes other places are used).
- You'll be given a local anesthetic but will feel pressure on insertion of the biopsy needle and a brief, pulling pain on removal of the marrow.

What happens during the test?

- The nurse or doctor has you lie down and urges you to remain as still as possible.
- The nurse or doctor may talk quietly to you during the procedure, describing what's being done and answering any questions.
- After the skin over the biopsy site is prepared and the area is draped, the doctor will inject the local anesthetic.
- After allowing time for the anesthetic to work, the doctor will then insert a needle into the bone and withdraw a bone marrow sample and then may do a needle biopsy.
- Immediate analysis is done on the sample taken from the bone marrow cavity by a hematologist, oncologist, or pathologist.

In a needle biopsy, a specimen is taken from the marrow cavity and sent to the lab.

What happens after the test?

- The nurse will apply pressure to the site for five minutes or so, then put on a bandage.

• If an adequate marrow specimen hasn't been obtained on the first attempt at aspiration, while your skin is still numb, the needle may be repositioned within the marrow cavity or may be removed and reinserted in another site within the anesthetized area. A needle biopsy may follow the aspiration biopsy.

Does the test have risks?

• Bone marrow biopsy isn't used in people with severe bleeding disorders, but bone marrow aspiration is still possible.

• Very rarely, bleeding and infection may be caused by bone marrow biopsy, which is why the nurse applies pressure to the site at the end of the procedure and why you are instructed to refrain from showering for twenty-four hours following the procedure and to leave the original dressing on for that duration. Problems or complications are very unusual, however.

What are the normal results?

Yellow marrow contains the fat cells and connective tissue. Red marrow contains various types of blood-making cells, fat cells, and connective tissue. An adult has a large blood-making capacity. An infant's marrow is mainly red, reflecting a small capacity.

What do abnormal results mean?

Microscopic examination of a bone marrow specimen can be used to detect scar tissue (myelofibrosis), inflammation (granulomas), or cancer, such as lymphoma and leukemias. Blood analysis, including cell counts, can alert the doctor to a wide range of blood disorders. Examples are iron deficiency, anemias of various types, infectious mononucleosis, and various kinds of leukemias and lymphomas. Rarely, cancer cells have spread to the bone marrow.

Bone marrow examinations are also sometimes done to check for infections, follow up the effectiveness of treatment, or discover how well the bone marrow could produce blood cells if really aggressive chemotherapy were to be given, which would require the bone marrow to work "extra hard" to produce new blood cells.

Bone marrow examinations, if needed, can greatly assist your physician in his or her search for the most complete and helpful information to use for diagnosis and treatment planning.

— 3 —

Working with the Health Care Team

Ernest H. Rosenbaum, M.D., Andrew H. Ko, M.D., Malin Dollinger, M.D.,
Lenore Dollinger, R.N., Ph.D., and Isadora R. Rosenbaum, M.A.

■ ■ ■ ■

After you've been diagnosed with cancer, you enter a world that is probably unfamiliar to you. The cancer treatment system is large and complex. Many different kinds of health care facilities and institutions are involved, and the system is populated by a bewildering array of professionals.

You may feel like you are being processed, sent from one place to another for tests or other procedures for reasons you don't quite understand. And at every turn, you meet new people who seem to speak a different language. It's easy to feel lost and disoriented in such a large system.

But it doesn't have to be that way. You simply have to remember that *you* are the one fighting for your life. And all the people and facilities are there to help you in your battle. Fighting cancer is fighting a war, and the more highly trained forces you can gather to attack the invader, the more successful you are likely to be.

Who Does What in the Cancer Treatment System

Cancer treatment today is very much a team effort that emphasizes total care. A wide range of medical specialists, therapists, technologists, counselors, social workers, and others become involved in your treatment and your rehabilitation.

Diagnosis By the time you are diagnosed as having cancer, you have already come in contact with several members of the health care team, even if you haven't met them all personally.

• Your cancer symptom may have been detected by your internist or primary physician—whoever it is you call when you have a fever or a pain you think should be looked at or when you're just feeling generally sick. If you are a woman, the primary physician may have been a gynecologist. If your child has the cancer, the primary physician may have been a pediatrician. Or it may have been a specialist in family practice, still fondly remembered by some as a GP, or general practitioner.

• A laboratory technician may have drawn your blood for tests.

• A radiologist may have interpreted your X-rays, CT scans, or other diagnostic imaging studies that provided information on the stage of your cancer.

• The tissue for a biopsy may have been taken by your primary physician, by a general surgeon, or possibly by a radiologist or medical oncologist doing a fine needle aspiration.

• Your tissue sample was then examined under the microscope by a pathologist, an expert in the analysis of tissue to identify disease.

Treatment Planning Once the diagnosis is made, the treatment team is assembled. Depending on the most appropriate kind of treatment for your particular tumor, you may deal with surgeons, medical or radiation oncologists, and/or internal medicine subspecialists.

• Medical oncologists—internists with additional training in the treatment of cancer—prescribe chemotherapy drugs as well as hormones and other biological agents.

• Surgeons—who remove as much cancerous tissue as possible, ideally before it has a chance to spread—also often specialize, operating only on specific areas of the body. But you should be aware that medical practices aren't always the same in all communities. Most general surgeons, for example, will operate on organs such as the colon and rectum. However, in larger cities, there are usually surgeons who specialize in this area of the body (proctologists). Some general surgeons do chest surgery; others do not. Some back operations will be done by neurosurgeons in some communities but by bone and joint (orthopedic) surgeons in others.

• Radiation oncologists are specialists in the use of high-energy X-rays to cause tumors to shrink. Within the radiation department, the radiation oncologist is supported by diagnostic radiologists, who interpret X-ray studies, and radiotherapy technologists and radiation physicists, who plan treatment and check the radiation dosage to make it as safe as possible.

• Internal medicine subspecialists include physicians who specialize in the endocrine system (endocrinologists), the gastrointestinal tract (gastroenterologists), the kidneys (nephrologists), the heart (cardiologists), and the lungs (pulmonologists). Depending on the type of cancer you have, one or more of these may be important players on your health care team.

Support Many other health care professionals work as a united team to help you through your cancer treatment and recovery.

• Oncology nurses play an essential role on the health care team. They have specialized knowledge and skill in giving chemotherapy and in meeting the special needs of cancer patients. They may specialize even further, as radiation oncology nurses, for example (see chapter 18, "Oncology Nursing").

• Nutritionists evaluate any deficiencies in your diet and prepare individualized plans that take your condition into account and make sure you get enough nutrients.

• Physical therapists can make sure you maintain proper muscle tone and adapt to any changes to your body that result from treatment.

• Occupational therapists help teach activities of daily living—how to eat, swallow, and use your body efficiently.

• Pharmacists prepare complicated medications and ensure correct dosages.

• Enterostomal therapists specialize in the care of ostomies (an ostomy is an opening from an area inside the body to the outside. For example, a colostomy allows passage of waste material out of the body if there is a blockage that does not permit bowel movements by usual means).

• Respiratory therapists help you keep your lungs and breathing passages clear.

• Speech therapists work with people who have lost their voice box (larynx) and have to learn to speak in a new way.

• Psychologists, psychotherapists, and other emotional counselors such as clergy and social workers help you through depression, fear, or other emotional problems you may have because of your cancer or its treatment.

• Dentists evaluate the state of your mouth before treatment and help you deal with treatment side effects such as mouth sores.

• Cosmeticians ensure proper skin care during treatment and help you cope with physical changes.

• Laboratory technologists perform specialized blood tests.

• Technologists make sure that breathing machines, chemotherapy pumps, home oxygen equipment, and other mechanical devices work properly at all times.

Direction As with any effective team, one person usually takes charge of the overall direction of the team's efforts. He or she is essentially the commander of the forces brought to bear on your cancer. He or she decides what "intelligence" information is needed, delegates specific tasks to the people best able to perform them, analyzes all the options, and makes the key decisions.

Most important, he or she is the one who reports to you on your situation. How do things look? What can be done? What are the risks? What are the odds? What are the alternatives?

Occasionally, the overall direction will be the responsibility of your primary physician. But since cancer treatment is so complex and so many specialists may be called in at various times, direction is now more often in the hands of an oncologist. And because medical oncologists are also specialists in internal medicine, they often assume overall responsibility.

There are many advantages to this chain of command. Medical oncologists see many cancer patients and are knowledgeable about the effects and likely results of the most up-to-date treatments. Oncologists also tend to do a lot of talking with you because cancer is serious business. Drugs are serious, radiation and surgery are serious, side effects are serious, and so is the prognosis. Nothing is trivial.

Choosing an Oncologist

There are several straightforward ways that an oncologist can become involved in your care. The most common is through a referral from your primary physician, who may recommend a specialist he or she has worked with before and has confidence in, who is an expert in the specific kind of cancer care you need. Sometimes you may know a specialist yourself, because of either your own experience or the experience of a family member or friend.

It is unusual these days that you have to choose a specialist without any help from family, friends, or general physicians. But if you do have to start from scratch, the American Cancer Society or other local medical societies in your area can supply you with names of several qualified physicians.

When you are choosing an oncologist, you can look into his or her credentials in a number of ways, the easiest being to check the *American Medical Directory* or the *Directory of American Specialists* at your local library. The latter lists doctors who have had special training and have demonstrated their competence to a recognized medical certification board (such as the American Board of Surgery or the American Board of Internal Medicine). You can also go to PDQ (Physician Data Query), a National Cancer Institute resource, at *www.cancer. gov.cancertopics/pdq/cancerdatabase* or call, from within the United States, 1-800-4-CANCER for a list of specialists. There are excellent oncology specialists who have had full training and are competent and up-to-date yet are not board certified. But if you are starting from scratch, the board certification may give you a little extra reassurance that you are in good hands.

Understanding What Your Doctor Is Saying

Right from the time you hear the cancer diagnosis, the medical team has to get a lot of new information across to you and your family. This isn't always an easy process, either for you or for your doctor. Each stage of cancer care involves a tremendous amount of information that is generally unknown to the lay public. And all too often doctors use technical terms that any nonmedical person has trouble understanding. Yet open and clear communication has become an essential part of a good medical relationship.

Cancer is a family affair. One member gets the disease, but the whole family goes through the experience. So it is very important that both you and your family know and understand all aspects of your disease. You should know how it is treated, what side effects there might be, and how you can best cope. Trying to learn how to deal with your new life situation may improve how you cope with your treatment program.

The Initial Visit Exactly where and how you find out about the diagnosis isn't always up to you. Yet this first confrontation with the fact that you have cancer can affect your relationship with the disease, your doctor, and the medical system.

Most doctors realize that difficult problems come up when someone is told he or she has cancer right in the recovery room after biopsy surgery. No one can fully appreciate what's going on in those circumstances. Most doctors also dislike telling someone he or she has cancer over the phone. It's very traumatic and it doesn't help the relationship. So doctors often try to make sure you are in a proper emotional state and have time to ask questions and discuss various aspects of treatment.

The proper emotional state is often hard to achieve. Your initial visit to an oncologist's office can be a very trying experience. Fear and anxiety about cancer, no matter how controllable or curable it might be, often limit the effectiveness of the visit. Often, after the diagnosis is made, it affects your ability to concentrate on the information being given. Faced with a serious, life-threatening illness, it becomes difficult to express feelings, ask questions, or assimilate all the new information.

When you are under such emotional stress, you often cannot think clearly. In our experience, after a one-hour consultation, one cancer patient, herself a medical social worker, walked from the doctor's office to the office waiting room. When her sister asked, "What did the doctor say?" she said, "I forgot." She had not even made it to the reception area.

Sharing the Information For this reason, many doctors encourage family members or close friends to come to the consultation. Some doctors record the initial consultation and dictate the letter to the referring physician in front of the patient during the office visit. A separate tape used to "translate" the technical letter and to explain the disease, treatment, and side effects, along with pertinent questions and answers, can also be very helpful. In a study at Minnesota's renowned Mayo Clinic, it was found that patients had to listen to an audiotaped discharge explanation at least three times before understanding the whole consultative message.

If your doctor audiotapes your initial consultation, it can be very beneficial to take the tape home and listen to it as often as you need to. You may wish to review it with your family and friends in a calm, relaxed atmosphere or even send copies to family members in other cities who wish to be informed. Tapes usually provide more comprehensive explanations for the patient, family, and friends.

Ignorance, confusion, and unspoken fears can isolate people from one another. In a situation filled with anxiety, the isolation can be especially severe and painful. When family and friends share information about treatment plans, medications, and side effects, cancer becomes more understandable and bearable for everyone concerned.

Besides reducing misunderstandings and improving communication, the use of audiotapes has the advantage of making the doctor's explanations more organized and concise. For the doctor, it will also mean fewer unanswered questions and fewer calls from family members trying to find out what's going on.

Getting More Information Besides the discussion and the audiotapes, your doctor may provide you with information in the form of handouts, pamphlets, or recommended reading. These are available free from the National Cancer Institute, the American Cancer Society, and many support organizations. Cancer resource centers also can provide books, literature, and computer analyses.

Pamphlets and books have their place in giving you both general and detailed information about your cancer and its treatment. Videos and DVDs can also accelerate the learning process. Videotapes may be especially important in the period just after your diagnosis because the emotional adjustment you need to make to having cancer can interfere with the concentration necessary for reading. It is common to experience a decrease in attention span and comprehension—or a feeling of emotional or mental paralysis. Videos and DVDs to explain CT scans, radiation therapy, good nutrition, exercise, or any other aspects of cancer and cancer therapy can be very helpful. They may be available from the National Cancer Institute or the American Cancer Society (see also "Useful Readings and Resources" in the appendix).

Videos and DVDs also bring the family together to watch and learn and talk about the procedures shown. They can present helpful ideas on how to cope and how to solve a simple problem such as how to set up a bedroom or tackle more serious problems. This can become a "quickie course" for family members to learn their role in supportive and home care.

The Doctor's Responsibility Doctors are well aware of the problems you and your family go through when you get the diagnosis of cancer. And your doctor does have a responsibility to reduce fears and confusion and to make it as easy as possible for you to understand what he or she is saying.

But not all doctors have learned to communicate effectively. If your doctor does not use such aids as audio- and videotapes and DVDs, ask about them. With your doctor's permission, perhaps you could take your own tape recorder into your consultations. Experience has shown that this technique promotes a more active discussion and does not intimidate physicians, patients, or families.

Communicating with Your Doctor

When you have cancer, the worry, fears, and concerns never stop, even after treatment. If your cancer is cured or permanently controlled, you always have that nagging fear that it might recur with a vengeance sometime in the years ahead. If it is not completely controlled, you worry that the treatment won't work, that you'll be a burden to your family or friends, or that you'll suffer pain and disability. No matter how hard you try to put these fears to rest, they reawaken and rise back up with each visit to the doctor.

You don't know whether you should be reassured by having extra tests or reassured by not having extra tests. You are always waiting for clear, definite answers to all the questions bombarding your brain. Am I really in remission? Is the cancer really gone? Will the pain go away? Can I go back to work? Will I ever feel safe? How long will I live?

While you are trying to understand everything your doctor is telling you, you may feel at a loss about how to get your concerns across. After all, you've had no training in how to deal effectively with specialists or even to deal with that nagging voice in your head that keeps whispering all the questions and fears.

What Helps and What Blocks Communication Two main factors affect the way you communicate with your doctor. Both can either help the process along or block effective communication.

• Your attitudes and feelings about yourself and about your illness
• Your need to be realistic, to understand your expectations, and to express your needs clearly

The attitudes and feelings that help communication are easy to list—openness, honesty, respect, clarity, responsibility, accountability, and a willingness to listen and to learn. What block effective communication are anger, resentment, dishonesty, intimidation, holding back information, and fear. And unless you do something to remove these blocks, you won't be receiving the best care your doctor can offer you.

Anger Sometimes the anger you might feel about having cancer or anger over a test result can hinder communication. Some people feel a generalized anger toward doctors, an anger that says, "They earn too much, they never listen, they're insensitive, they don't really care, they think they're God."

You may have good reason to feel angry. Your doctor may keep you waiting for an hour and then spend only five minutes with you. It may take forever for your calls to be returned. Whether your anger is justified or not, communicate how you feel. If you don't say it openly, the anger will be communicated anyway and will always be a barrier to openness and honesty.

You can express your anger and still be respectful. Make a list or compose a letter to the doctor. Write down how you feel clearly and concisely. If you write it down, it will be easier to speak without resentment. Then respect your doctor's time. Let the appointment desk know you want extra time during the next visit to talk about things that are bothering you and interfering with your ability to have a good working relationship.

When you tell your doctor how you feel, give him or her reasonable suggestions for resolving the problem, such as getting the first appointment of the day so you won't have to wait. Ask him or her what time calls are usually returned and say that you will call only at those times unless there's an emergency. Then stick to it.

Doctors know that anger is a secondary feeling rising up in response to fear, anxiety, or frustration. But doctors are also human and under a lot of pressure. So it might be difficult for your doctor to respond to you in a supportive way if you confront him or her only with anger. Ask yourself what lies beneath the anger—fear? rejection? disappointment?—and express those feelings. If it's emotional support you want and your doctor doesn't seem to have the time or compassion to meet your needs, ask if there is someone else who can. You have to be willing to accept your doctor's limitations, but be unwilling to accept less than *you* need.

Intimidation This is a two-way street. Many patients feel intimidated by their doctors. Patients can be afraid that doctors will think they're stupid if they ask too many questions or will not like them for taking up so much time. This is fear, pure and simple. Make it work for you. Simply say, "I'm afraid to take up your time, but I'm more afraid for myself." You'll be amazed how that kind of honesty can work for you.

The other side to intimidation is when the patient intimidates the doctor. If you think to yourself—or say right out (in a joking way, of course)—"I know as much as you do, so don't try to talk down to me," again recognize the fear at the source of this need to intimidate. Express this fear openly and honestly. If you really think your doctor is doing less than he or she should, talk about it and listen to how the doctor responds. Only then can you make a rational decision about what action you should take.

Withholding Information Holding back or not being completely honest and clear about how you feel not only blocks good communication, but also puts your doctor at a terrible disadvantage and doesn't serve your best interests at all.

If you have a lot of new symptoms, you may be afraid of sounding like a hypochondriac or appearing to be too emotional. So when the doctor asks you how you are, you reply, "Just fine." When you say that, you lose a golden opportunity to communicate your needs. These new symptoms may be causing you all kinds of worry and distress, but by your two little words, you've made sure that your doctor will not be able to put your mind at ease. You can only hope your doctor doesn't believe you.

And when your doctor explains a procedure, treatment, or test result and asks if you understand, don't just automatically say, "Sure. Got it." If you don't really understand, say so. All pretending can do is add to your confusion and increase your anxiety.

Dealing with Fear It should be clear by now that the feeling of fear can block communication. If fear stops you from asking perfectly reasonable questions or accepting needed treatment, or if it comes out as anger, it can badly damage your relationship with someone who is doing his or her best to make you well again.

But fear can also work for you in communicating with your doctor. Fear can make you stop and think for yourself. It can make you think seriously about all the alternatives before you and ask for explanations and support. Only then can you realistically evaluate the risks you have to take.

Talking About "What If . . . ?" There is one subject that many cancer patients don't want to talk about. Sometimes this is called the "What if . . . ?" scenario. What if the treatment doesn't help? What if everything that might help has already been done? What if the only goal now is to try to stay comfortable, physically and mentally?

It is hard to talk about all the aggressive treatments that might be used, the side effects, and your critical need to always have hope, and at the same time discuss "What if . . . ?" You may not want to talk about it at all. You don't always need to. And your doctor will respect your wishes. But if you do want to discuss it, let your doctor know.

There is one aspect of "What if . . . ?" that really should be discussed. If your situation does become grave, your doctor will need some guidance on how you want things handled. How heroic do you want your doctor to be, especially if the end seems near? If the situation does reach that stage, you may not be in any condition to discuss the question rationally. Your doctor may be able to talk it over with your family, but it is *your* wishes that are most important. There are now legal pathways (advance directives) to be sure your wishes are carried out (see chapter 41, "Planning for the Future").

How You Can Help Yourself Get an Effective Review

Fifteen minutes may not seem like a lot of time to cover critical information that may be important to your very survival. But a lot can happen during a fifteen-minute office visit. Unfortunately, relatively trivial matters can also use up a lot of time.

From the doctor's point of view, it sometimes may take three to five minutes to cover the strictly medical procedures. A schedule for a chemotherapy program, the dosage, and the side effects can be covered quickly. But a doctor has to deal with what happened last week, how you felt about things, what your hopes and fears are—all the secret things going on beneath the surface that might be important. So the other ten to twelve minutes are often given to psychological evaluation and counseling, rather than purely technical matters. Remember that the office staff can be very helpful in providing additional support.

All questions and problems are in some way important, but some are more important than others. To help yourself get the most from your medical review, there are certain rules or guidelines to keep in mind.

• *Focus on the matter at hand* Doctors try to take care of the most pertinent issues first. The doctor's most important questions will be about what's happening with you right now. Do you have a sore mouth? Are you losing weight? Do you have any major complaints? Do you have diarrhea? What's new since your last visit? The doctor then has to try to analyze and make sense of what's changing. Doctors are always trying to anticipate changes so they don't have to play catch-up. Until you have a problem, your doctor can't solve it. So give the clearest, most detailed answers you can without holding anything back. It might help if you kept notes of significant symptoms or events that you noticed between visits.

• *Be cooperative* Every doctor has seen patients who, because of anxieties—the fear of illness or death—simply aren't cooperative. They object to having extra blood tests or doing things that are sometimes necessary but that they simply don't want to do. When they come into the office, they should undress for an examination, yet some say, "I don't want to get undressed today." That's not the best way to get help. You have to follow certain patterns and be cooperative if you expect results.

• *Avoid raising irrelevant problems* Your doctor is always ready to deal with important problems like weight loss or nausea or a swollen arm or leg. With all that has to be covered during the office visit, it's hard to deal with problems such as a stubbed toe and other minor problems best treated by a primary doctor. Talking about half a dozen minor problems can use up half the appointment. Of course, the doctor realizes that what you are really saying is, "I'm scared. I'm frightened for my life." But, still, discussing extraneous problems is not the most effective use of office time.

• *Ask the pertinent questions* Unless you try to limit your questions to the most essential problems, you lose both focus and the chance for better explanations. All questions are relevant, but if you take a long list of questions, you are going to defeat yourself before you begin. As a patient, you have an obligation to be practical and to do your best to work with your physician. You may need to prioritize your questions if time is limited or leave them with your doctor to get back to you at a later time.

— 4 —

Deciding on the Appropriate Treatment

Malin Dollinger, M.D., Andrew H. Ko, M.D., and Ernest H. Rosenbaum, M.D.

■ ■ ■ ■

"Cancer is one of the most curable chronic diseases in this country today."
—Vincent T. DeVita Jr., M.D.

Medicine has now reached the stage where about half of all diagnosed cancers are cured. Of course, this statistic is an average. The cure rate for some cancers is much higher than for others. And some cancers can come back even after the five-years cancer-free interval that is often used to define "cure."

But even with cancers still considered incurable, proper therapy often yields tremendous benefits. Treatment can add months or years to a reasonably normal life. It can also greatly improve the quality of your life by relieving pain or ensuring the relatively normal functioning of your body processes. Many people live a normal life span with chronic cancer before succumbing to some other disease.

Unfortunately, far too many people still think a cancer diagnosis is a death sentence. Far too many take the attitude that if it can't be cured, there's no point in undergoing treatment. What is even more unfortunate is that this attitude is found not only among people with cancer and the lay public but within the medical community.

In many cases, cancer truly is an incurable disease. But it's not the only one. Diabetes and heart disease can't be cured, but they can be treated on an ongoing basis. They're treated all the time. Few people take the "Why

bother?" attitude with either of them. Why? Because they know both can be managed day by day and that people with either disease can lead long, active, and productive lives. The same can be true for cancer patients.

The key to getting the chance for cure or successful management is getting the best treatment as soon as possible after your diagnosis. What that treatment is, you will have to help decide. Yes, you should rely on experts with training and experience in fighting cancer. But it's your life on the line, and ultimately, the decisions must be yours. And you will have to base those decisions on a detailed analysis of your disease and the recommendations of your primary physician or cancer specialist.

What Are the Options?
A Treatment Overview

The three mainstays of cancer therapy over the years have been surgery, radiation, and chemotherapy. These have now been joined by biological therapy, which uses the body's immune system to combat growing cancer cells. The goals, procedures, risks, and side effects of each of these kinds of therapy (sometimes referred to as modalities) are detailed in chapters 6 to 9. Here, the treatment options are briefly reviewed.

Surgery This is the oldest and most successful approach to cancer treatment. If it is possible to cut it out safely and there is no residual disease, you may be cured. Two key questions have to be answered when deciding if surgery is the right thing to do:

• Is the tumor just in one place (localized)? Once the cancer has spread, surgery may or may not be appropriate.
• Can the tumor be removed without damaging vital organs or causing major functional problems? A cancerous lung or kidney can be removed because everyone has a spare. But a surgeon can't cut out the whole liver or vital parts of the brain.

There are two surgical approaches. In the one-stage approach, the diagnostic biopsy might be followed immediately by the removal of the tumor while you are still under anesthesia. After the operation, you can discuss whether you need additional therapy and what the most effective method or sequence would be, particularly if several therapies might be realistic alternatives.

In the two-stage approach, only the biopsy is done. You then discuss the results with your doctor. If the biopsy shows cancer, you and your doctor plan the definitive cancer treatment. If surgery is an option, the operation to remove the tumor will then be carried out.

Radiation Therapy The purpose of radiation is to make tumors shrink or disappear. Radiation does this by damaging the genetic structure (DNA) of the tumor cells so they can't grow or divide. The damage is done by a beam of X-rays, gamma rays, or electrons aimed directly at the tumor from a high-energy X-ray machine set up at a specific distance from your body or by radioactive materials placed inside or close to the tumor.

There is no pain or discomfort during radiation therapy. Undergoing treatment is much the same as having a chest X-ray, except the machine is left on for several minutes instead of a second or two. Radiation may be the only treatment needed for some localized cancers, or it might be used along with other kinds of therapy.

Chemotherapy This term is often misunderstood. What it means is treating some medical condition with chemicals (drugs). Treating cancer with 5-fluorouracil is chemotherapy. So is treating an infection with penicillin or a headache with aspirins.

Yet when chemotherapy is mentioned in connection with cancer, the term generates a lot of fear. Almost everyone has heard horror stories about serious side effects. These side effects can be unpleasant, but they are in general greatly exaggerated. It's true that a few people cannot tolerate chemical therapy at all. But most can tolerate it reasonably well. Others have moderate to significant reactions. When approaching the subject, also keep in mind that many drugs are used in chemotherapy and not all of them have serious side effects. The side effects themselves can often be reduced or controlled by anti-nausea drugs or other medications.

Surgery and radiation treat cancers that are growing in one particular place (locoregional treatment), whereas chemotherapy is generally used for cancers that have traveled through the blood and lymph systems to many parts of the body (systemic treatment). In the past, chemotherapy was used only when surgery and radiation were no longer effective. But now it is the treatment of choice for some kinds of cancer and is often used in combination with surgery and radiation, especially for localized cancers.

Biological Therapy This is a relatively new way to treat cancer. It takes advantage of recent research that shows that the immune system may play a key role in protecting the body against cancer. The immune system might even play a part in combating cancer that has already developed. Refer to chapter 9, "What Happens in Biological Therapy and Immunotherapy," which provides a more in-depth look at biological therapy.

The immune system consists of white blood cells called lymphocytes that act as a defense system against foreign organisms such as bacteria and viruses. One type of lymphocyte—the T cell—is formed in the thymus gland and is a natural killer of foreign cells, including cancer cells. Another lymphocyte—the B cell—is produced in the bone marrow and lymph nodes and makes antibodies in response to stimulation by a foreign protein. B lymphocytes can also kill cancer cells. Another white cell—the monocyte—interacts with T and B cells.

Biological therapy encompasses a number of classes of therapeutic agents, including

1. Highly purified proteins characteristic of natural proteins produced by the body, such as interleukin-2 (IL-2) and interferon, which boost the lymphocytes' cancer-killing properties. These are used in certain tumor types, such as kidney cancer and melanoma.

2. Monoclonal antibodies that target various cancer proteins. Examples include trastuzumab (Herceptin) for breast cancer; rituximab (Rituxan), yttrium Y 90 ibritumomab tiuxetan (Zevalin), and iodine I-131 tositumomab (Bexxar) for non-Hodgkin's lymphoma; gemtuzumab ozogamicin (Mylotarg) for acute myelogenous leukemia; alemtuzumab (Campath) for chronic lymphocytic leukemia; bevacizumab (Avastin), cetuximab (Erbitux), and panitumumab (Vectibix) for colorectal cancer; bortezomib (Velcade) in multiple myeloma and mantle cell lymphoma; cetuximab for head and neck cancer; dasatinib (Sprycel) for various forms of leukemia; and sorafenib (Nexavar) for renal cell cancer. In some cases, the monoclonal antibody is attached to chemotherapy drugs ("chemolabeled"), attached to radioactive particles ("radioimmunotherapy"), or attached to toxins ("immunotoxins"). Active research, including clinical trials, is in progress to discover the best way to use these new treatments, especially in combination with chemotherapy.

3. Cancer vaccines, which are specifically directed against cancer cells. These are created by various methods, some relatively nonspecific and others directed against specific proteins preferentially expressed on cancer cells. Similar in principle to vaccines used against various infectious diseases, vaccines are designed to stimulate a person's immune system to attack and destroy the foreign agent (in this case, cancer cells).

Combination and Adjuvant Therapies

Twenty or thirty years ago, it was common to think about treating cancer only by surgery *or* radiation *or* chemotherapy, depending on the stage of the disease. Two or all three therapies might be used, but usually only one at a time and in the sequence mentioned—surgery if the tumor was localized, then radiation if there was an actual or potential recurrence, then chemotherapy if the cancer involved vital organs or had spread so far that surgery or radiation had to be ruled out.

Recently there has been great interest in using what is called combination or multimodality therapy. Multimodality therapy incorporates two or three of the standard treatment methods with the goals of increasing response rates, reducing the likelihood of tumor recurrence, and, of course, improving survival. For many malignancies, there is no universal agreement on the best combination or best sequence, but several broad principles have emerged:

• When tumors are large, locally aggressive, and touch adjacent structures, radiation and/or chemotherapy might be given before surgery. The goals here are to shrink the tumor and make the surgical procedure much simpler. This is called neoadjuvant therapy. In hospitals with special radiotherapy equipment, radiation will sometimes be given during surgery (intraoperative radiation) to kill invisible or microscopic tumor cells that might cause the cancer to come back in the future.

• Radiation and/or chemotherapy may be given after surgery, referred to as adjuvant therapy. Radiation is given to reduce the chances of local recurrence of the tumor (recurrence in the area that the tumor originated), especially for tumors that are large and where surgical margins were close or positive. Chemotherapy is given to reduce the chances of systemic recurrence (metastases elsewhere in the body), by wiping out tumor cells that may be too small to be visible right now but that might cause a recurrence later on. For example, evidence is clear that adjuvant chemotherapy benefits women who have undergone surgery for breast cancer, especially those whose cancer has spread to the lymph nodes under the armpit (axilla).

• Radiation and chemotherapy have also been combined in an attempt to produce a more powerful antitumor effect than either treatment can produce alone. Certain chemotherapy agents act as *radiosensitizers*—they enhance the effects of radiation to make its cell-killing abilities even more potent. The dosages of both modalities, however, may sometimes have to be reduced to prevent major side effects that could result from their simultaneous administration.

• The new biological therapies, as listed earlier, are being blended with standard radiotherapy and chemotherapy. But research on these combinations is still in an early stage. We are still testing this form of therapy to discover what sequence, dosage, or combination is the most helpful and how adding biological therapies to the others can be made more effective than today's standard treatments.

How Your Physician Decides on the Best Treatment

Making the decision on which treatment to use is a stepwise process. It really begins with the suspicion of cancer aroused by signs or symptoms, then proceeds through the diagnostic process outlined in chapter 2, "How Cancer Is Diagnosed." Once the diagnosis is confirmed by a positive biopsy, several factors have to be considered.

The Stage How far along the tumor is in its development is the most critical factor. Sometimes the stage isn't known until a surgeon actually has a look at the tumor. But there are other ways to find out what stage the malignancy has reached.

During the staging process, many parts of the body will be searched for evidence of cancer. Tests will discover the extent of the spread and the involvement with other tissues at the primary site. This will involve blood tests to see how organs such as the kidneys and liver are functioning. Imaging techniques such as chest X-rays and CT scans will be used to see if there is any involvement of the lungs either directly or by spread.

Other specialized tests will be ordered according to the primary site and the type of tumor being investigated. Each type of cancer has a typical pattern of spread, so different specific areas of the body will be investigated in each case.

Prostate cancer, for example, can spread to bone, so bone scans, bone

X-rays, and blood tests may be important diagnostic tests for advanced stages of the disease. Lung cancer can spread to the center of the chest (mediastinum), an area that can be mapped with a CT scan and looked at directly through a scope (mediastinoscopy). Cancers of the stomach and bowel commonly spread to the liver, so CT scans of the abdomen and blood tests will be needed to investigate those areas.

It is important to understand that *when a cancer spreads, it remains the same cancer.* A breast cancer that spreads to the bone does not become bone cancer. If it spreads to the lung, it does not become lung cancer. Wherever it lands, it grows as breast cancer. It's like blowing the seeds off a dandelion—whether the seed lands in a field, a forest, or a crack in a sidewalk, what grows is still a dandelion.

This is important because the choice of cancer treatment is guided more on where the tumor starts than on where it lands.

The Biology of the Disease An analysis of the disease—its cell type, biology, and expected behavior—is an important factor to consider. The tumor's biology strongly affects the likelihood of a particular therapy slowing down or stopping the disease.

State-of-the-Art Alternatives Once the staging process is completed, your doctor has to consider all the treatments that might be appropriate considering the type of tumor, the site of origin, and the stage of spread. In some cases, only one specific therapy may be generally accepted as appropriate. But in many cases, a variety of approaches might be used.

Cancer treatment is always evolving. Every year new discoveries are made and old methods are modified or discarded. It's hard even for specialists to keep up with all the developments in the field. But there are several ways your primary physician can find out about the most current treatment methods that are considered state-of-the-art.

• Cancer specialists (medical oncologists) are often consulted at this stage. So are surgeons or specialists in radiotherapy.

• The most recent medical literature can be reviewed, perhaps along with a computer search of your disease via a database like PDQ (see chapter 47, "Cancer Information").

• Physicians and specialists attend many of the hundreds of cancer meetings that take place every year where important research findings and other cancer information are presented.

Tumor Boards Another way for your doctor to review your case, get information, and discuss the best treatment, especially with unusual types of cancers, is to attend a meeting called a tumor board. These boards are held frequently in all hospitals where cancer treatment is offered. They allow a group of doctors specializing in cancer to meet, discuss particular cases, and give their opinions about the advantages and disadvantages of treatment alternatives. It is very common at such a meeting for biopsy results to be presented and explained by the pathologist and for the radiologist and nuclear medical specialists to present all the X-rays and scans.

Your primary physician or oncologist will present your case (anonymously) so that each physician there has the same information your doctor has in making his or her decision.

In many larger hospitals there are specialty tumor boards that review cases in one particular field—breast cancer, urologic cancer, gynecologic cancers, or head and neck cancers, for example.

When it comes to recommending treatment, then, your doctor has had the benefit of input and ideas from a wide range of professionals.

Personal Factors: Benefits and Risks
Which treatment is finally recommended will also depend on such personal factors as your age, your other medical problems (which might make surgery risky), and especially the possibility of significant side effects with one or another treatment.

Age comes into the decision because the patient who is forty years old may be able to tolerate the aggressive chemotherapy drugs that bring about a substantial rate of remission. The same drugs given to an eighty-year-old could be risky. At that age, the kidneys don't function as well as they do earlier in life and the risk of therapy could outweigh the potential benefit. But each case has to be decided on its own merits.

Both you and your doctor have to consider the relative advantages and disadvantages of each therapy. You have to weigh the chances of achieving remission or cure against the risks and side effects of treatment. You and your family are partners with your physician in this decision-making process.

Your Decision In making the final decision on treatment, nothing replaces a good discussion between you and your doctor. He or she should be able to explain to you the staging process, the tests that were done, their results, and all the available methods of treatment.

He or she may present the information from any tumor board that was held. Or he or she can sometimes pass on the consensus of the informal consultations with other doctors that often take place in medical groups having several physicians involved in the cancer field. Your doctor should also have alternative forms of therapy in mind and should outline what could be done if your tumor doesn't respond to treatment or if some other problem comes up.

Informed Consent There may be legal principles regarding "informed disclosure" that come into play during these discussions. In the state of California, for example, patients with breast cancer must be given a pamphlet published by the state describing the various methods of primary treatment and the advantages and disadvantages of each. Although this document appears to be comprehensive, its coverage of many important areas may be incomplete and outdated.

A brochure certainly cannot replace the important and key discussion between physician, patient, and family. Nothing can. This initial comprehensive discussion about deciding on therapy is *the most important single meeting* that you have with your physician. It forms the basis for all of the decision making that follows.

When and How to Ask for a Second Opinion

Even after you have met with the physician who has outlined your treatment plan (for example, the medical oncologist or surgeon), you may still feel insecure about the treatment options you've been given. You might want to discuss them with another physician. This is a perfectly acceptable, rational, and appropriate thing to do.

There should be no hesitation on your part in asking your doctor if he or she would have another specialist review all the material relating to your case. Second opinions are not unusual. Some insurance companies require them.

In view of your need for a continuing relationship with your primary physician or specialist, it would be helpful to express your satisfaction with his or her decision and care. You can simply say that you wish to have someone else review the case to assure yourself that your decision to accept treatment will be made on the most thoroughly informed basis possible.

Whom to Consult You may have a certain consultant in mind or you might ask your doctor to select a senior specialist in your city or at a major medical center, depending on your diagnosis. Many times, your oncologist may recommend a second opinion and refer you to a local specialist or a specific cancer center where researchers with a special interest in your disease are working. Your doctor should have no hesitation in making your case material, including pathology slides and X-rays, available to the second-opinion consultant. This consultation is generally done fairly quickly so it does not delay treatment.

It is not a good idea to get a second opinion "in secret." Ultimately, it is not in your best interest. Second-opinion consultations are done by physicians for physicians. They are done to review and help improve your medical care. Consultants cannot evaluate your case properly unless they have at least the same information your primary doctor has, including the slides, X-rays, and results of laboratory tests and other procedures.

Don't think your doctor will take offense or feel hurt. Your doctor should welcome the opportunity to satisfy your need for a second opinion. Please read chapter 5, which is dedicated specifically to second opinions, as this is a very important topic for you to know about.

Considering a Clinical Trial

Depending on the type and stage of your cancer, your doctor might recommend a new kind of treatment. The word *investigational* might come up. Or *experimental* might be the term used. If the standard treatment options available to you aren't likely to be effective, your doctor might simply suggest that you take part in a *clinical trial.*

All these terms might make you feel more than a little anxious. They shouldn't. Investigational treatments that are being given in a clinical trial are used only under very stringent conditions. They are important in moving the medical field forward and wouldn't be used at all if there wasn't some hope they might be as effective as or more effective than currently available treatments, especially if standard treatment options are limited.

What a Clinical Trial Is Advances in cancer treatment are rarely made by one scientist or physician working with a single or even a few patients. Advances usually come about because of some innovative idea or concept for a new therapy, based on an expanding understanding of cancer biology. This idea is eventually tested in a large number of patients to find out two things: Is it effective? And is it as good as or better than conventional treatments?

It takes several hundred and sometimes several thousand patients to prove quickly and reliably whether a new treatment will work and is worthwhile. It is almost impossible to conduct a trial in any single hospital or cancer center. The concept of cooperative clinical trials was developed for just this reason. The rules and procedures for clinical trials are standardized and specific.

The Clinical Protocol A clinical trial consists of an exact written description of a treatment program that is called the clinical protocol. This is formulated and written with great care. Not only do the researchers need to be sure that the trial will answer the two main questions about effectiveness, but the rights of the patients being treated have to be safeguarded, too. The risks involved have to be minimized and disclosed.

The clinical protocol outlines the criteria for patients who might participate in the trial. It also describes what tests will be done and how the researchers will determine if a tumor is responding. Systems for monitoring the patient and checking for any adverse effects will be detailed. And there will be provisions for informed consent.

Who Approves the Trial The entire project has to be approved by a human use committee made up of physicians and nonphysicians who have no relationship with the study (commonly referred to as an IRB, or institutional review board). The members of this committee certify that the patients' rights are protected, that the trial is reasonable and logical, and that the study will answer the question it is supposed to answer. This same committee reviews the study again during and after completion of the trial as originally proposed. The Cancer Therapy Branch of the National Cancer Institute also keeps watch on these investigational studies.

The Importance of Clinical Trials Almost every advance in cancer treatment over the past several decades has come about because of clinical trials. In fact, just about every chemotherapy drug and radiation treatment now considered standard therapy was first given in a clinical Phase I trial. These treatments were given to patients who were willing to be in the forefront of advances in medical knowledge.

The willingness of thousands of women to participate in clinical trials by the National Surgical Adjuvant Breast Project (NSABP), for example, has resulted in answers being given to extremely important treatment questions. These trials have formed the basis for adjuvant chemotherapy in breast cancer patients with a high risk for recurrence even though no apparent tumor is left after surgery. This has saved many lives.

The Three Phases of Clinical Trials Whether for surgery, chemotherapy, radiotherapy, or biological therapy, clinical trials are always conducted in three phases.

A chemotherapy clinical trial, for example, proceeds this way:

• *Preliminary (Preclinical)* After a new anticancer drug has been found to be effective against one or more experimental tumor systems in the lab, it is tested in rats or other small animals to find out which dosage might be both effective and reasonably safe.

• *Phase I* About twenty human patients are treated with the same drug. There is no assurance or certainty that a significant tumor response will occur, although, again, every single anticancer drug now useful in therapy was initially a Phase I agent.

Patients selected for these trials are almost always in cancer research centers and have already received all known effective anticancer therapy. After the proposed treatment is explained to them, they may volunteer to receive the new treatment. Phase I studies are often not tumor specific; that is, patients with breast cancer, lung cancer, and colon cancer may all enroll in the same Phase I study of a new agent. Since there is "nothing to lose," it is hoped that this specific new agent may in fact prove effective.

This phase will often involve a "dose escalation" scheme, in which different patients receive increasing doses of the study medication(s). The primary objective here is to test for safety (but also to get some sense of the potential efficacy). The study is completed when no unusual problems or toxic effects have been found and the maximal tolerated dose has been determined. The study can then move to the next phase.

• *Phase II* This phase of clinical trial typically enrolls patients with one particular type of tumor. The goal here is to get a clearer picture of how effective the new agent or treatment regimen is against a certain type of cancer, by looking at the percentage of patients who respond to the therapy. The safety of the drug(s) being tested continues to be an important objective to evaluate. Phase II trials generally enroll twenty to fifty patients and can involve one or several medical centers.

• *Phase III* In this phase, the new therapy is compared with standard treatment (patients are randomly selected to receive one treatment arm or another) to see if there is an improvement in the response or if the same response rate is achieved but with less-toxic side effects.

A therapy tested in a clinical trial may involve a drug already in clinical use. A new treatment often consists of standard drugs used in a new combination or a new sequence, in new dosages, or even simply given in a new way. But if a new drug is involved and the Phase III trial is successful, the National Cancer Institute will approve the drug for general use. Eventually, the new therapy might become the standard therapy.

Clinical Trials and the "Approved" Uses of Drugs Every drug comes with an official package insert detailing what dose to use for what illness. This information is also listed in the *Physician's Desk Reference*. These summaries usually contain only the information "passed" by the government's approval agencies. This is important to know because many drugs

in standard use may not specifically be approved for a particular indication, even though experience with patients has shown they are effective. Oncologists will often use these drugs "off-label." About half of all the current uses of anticancer drugs in the United States and Canada, in fact, are not given in the official inserts.

Since the inserts do not necessarily reflect the most up-to-date cancer research, the current standard use of these drugs, or even their optimum use, your doctor should not be restricted to printed drug-listing materials. In fact, appropriate uses of anticancer drugs may not be listed in such official sources.

That being said, there are three important points to consider: (1) A responsible physician should make treatment recommendations based on compelling evidence that has been presented or published, not just by "reaching off the shelf" for what he or she thinks might possibly work. (2) Insurance companies may or may not cover the cost of drugs that are being used off-label, especially with some of the newer agents that are extremely costly. (3) Some of these newer agents do carry significant risks, so should not be given cavalierly, especially beyond their known indications. Make sure you discuss these considerations with your physician carefully, so that you understand the rationale behind the treatment plan that is being recommended.

— 5 —

Second Opinions

Ernest H. Rosenbaum, M.D., Andrew H. Ko, M.D.,
Malin Dollinger, M.D., and Richard and Annette Bloch

■ ■ ■ ■

Does Everyone Need a Second Opinion?

Ernest H. Rosenbaum, M.D.

When cancer patients come in for their initial consultation, they bring a multitude of problems. Usually they come for a diagnostic work-up after they have already been given a diagnosis of cancer. They arrive at an oncology office in a state of alarm and fear. They also have grave questions about their future life.

The first problem I find is the way in which they were given the diagnosis. Usually, it is through a follow-up call after a biopsy and/or test to tell them that they have cancer. Receiving the diagnosis produces a strong emotional reaction. Most people are shocked and devastated, and need more time to fully comprehend the meaning of cancer.

Most cases are usually straightforward. A diagnosis is made and treatments are initiated. Thus, many patients may not need a second opinion. But when a diagnosis of cancer is made, there is much fear, misunderstanding, and many questions about therapy. All these factors can determine whether a person may live or die—thus it is not unreasonable for a patient to want to have another point of view, what is called a second opinion.

After analyzing the cancer data, the most important thing a physician can do for a concerned patient or family is to explain, in simple terms, all the pertinent issues. Patients wish for state-of-the-art medical care, but they may have doubts about what is the best way to proceed. Although this is when a second opinion can be very helpful, most patients are reluctant to offend their primary physician by doing so. Many patients do not realize that getting a second opinion is standard practice.

Unless emergency treatment is needed, I feel it is very important for patients and their families/friends to allow themselves time to learn exactly what the diagnosis means. They need to gather information on how it can be treated (surgery, radiation, or chemotherapy), weigh the options (such as watchful waiting for a few months for a less aggressive approach versus immediate treatment in the next few days), and understand the prognosis and the chances for a cure.

Most patients are now better informed—often having gathered information from the Web (e.g., PDQ [Physician Data Query/ Cancer Net]), newspapers, magazines, or well-meaning friends. This information can be very mixed and confusing.

It often takes time and several explanations going over the same questions for an anxious and fearful patient to understand and be satisfied with the medical recommendations. Often there are several approaches to a problem, and sometimes there is no definitive answer, given the limitations of current medical science.

To help patients make proper decisions, I make a point of informing them and their families/friends at the initial visit that I have two rules in my practice (included on the tape recording that I do for all my consultations):

• *Rule 1* If I am uncertain or have any questions about the diagnosis or treatment, I will advise them that I would like them to get a second opinion. I state that I would be glad to recommend the person and place that I think would offer the most beneficial consultation to add additional information on how to proceed with their oncology evaluation or therapy, or they can choose a consultant of their choice.

• *Rule 2* If at any time they wish to seek a second opinion, as is their right, I would be glad to provide my records, test results, X-rays, and pathology report to whomever they wish. If they would like me to select and help arrange a second-opinion consultant, I would be available to do so.

If they are coming for a second opinion, I also clarify that they will continue their care with their primary oncologist.

I can recall a case where mine was the ninth opinion. This reflects how it may take multiple discussions with your doctor or with another independent unbiased physician to arrive at a conclusion on diagnosis and therapy that can give you peace of mind and satisfaction about which is the most appropriate therapy.

Following are several points of view about second opinions as a part of the supportive care process:

Do Not Be Afraid to Ask for a Second Opinion

Andrew H. Ko, M.D.

As an oncologist at a major academic medical center, I see patients as a second (or third, or fourth) opinion all the time. Conversely, sometimes I am the first oncologist to see a patient, and after their consultation, they ask whether they should seek a second opinion (or tell me in a straightforward manner that they are planning to do so).

You should not worry about your oncologist taking this as a personal affront in any way. In fact, I almost always support, and usually encourage, a patient to obtain a second opinion, for several reasons. Many times, a second physician will confirm and reinforce the recommendations of the first physician, and that in and of itself can provide reassurance to the patient and family that the treatment being offered is sound practice. On the other hand, in some instances, there may be honest differences in opinion from one physician and one medical center to the next. This may not necessarily mean that one person is right and the other person is wrong but could reflect different styles of practice, different personal philosophies and thresholds of when it is appropriate to treat or not (for example, one physician may be very aggressive and take a "treat at all costs" approach, while another may be less willing to offer therapy if there is a very low likelihood of a patient's responding), or the simple fact that there may be different and completely equally valid ways of approaching the same situation in a given individual. Finally, it may be the case that one medical center or office has a particular clinical trial that you may be interested in and qualify for, but that is not available through the first physician you see (so, in general, it makes little sense to seek a second opinion within the same hospital or same group practice that you are already in).

In thinking about whether you should seek additional medical opinions, here are a few practical points to note:

1. If there is any ambiguity or debatable points about your diagnosis or treatment plan, you can ask your physician

whether he or she participates in a tumor board and whether your case can be presented at the next tumor board meeting. These tumor boards are held at most academic medical centers as well as at many community medical practices and are attended by many physicians and health care providers of different specialties. This way, you are actually indirectly soliciting the opinions of many physicians at the same time, which may provide some assurance that your treatment plan has been discussed, formulated, and agreed upon by a multidisciplinary team of doctors—not just one physician who may have his or her own unique biases.

2. While it is useful to seek a second opinion for all the reasons outlined above, I have seen occasional patients who have traveled nation- and worldwide after they have been diagnosed, seeking one opinion after the next. In so doing, they delay starting treatment for a long period of time and often are paralyzed with indecision because they have difficulty processing so much information with so many varying opinions. At a certain point, this becomes counterproductive. Set your plan ahead of time: For example, you will seek one or two additional expert opinions within a given time frame and then make your best-informed decision of how to proceed based on this information.

3. Ask your original physician whether he or she can guide you in your decision making of where to seek additional opinions. As noted above, your physician will (or should) not take offense at your request and may be able to direct you to a particular center where there is particular expertise or where exciting clinical trials are going on that you may be eligible for. Additionally, he or she may be able to put into appropriate context some of the stuff you are looking up on the Internet—what you are coming across that is worthy of exploring further and what may not be.

4. In general, it is difficult to get and unwise to ask a physician to provide an opinion on your case without actually seeing you. Most physicians try to avoid such consultations, where a patient asks them to review all their records and then suggest a treatment plan without a direct meeting. There are many reasons for this, including medicolegal and practical (most physicians simply don't have the time to perform such tasks, which can be quite time-consuming, in the midst of other patient responsibilities). However, the most compelling reason is that for a physician, nothing beats meeting and talking to a patient face-to-face to best be able to put together a treatment plan that is most appropriate for that given person.

5. Make sure you know ahead of time whether your insurance provider will cover the cost of a second opinion (especially if it is out of network); if not, make sure you know how much that outside consultation will cost you out of pocket.

6. It's always a great idea to bring extra copies of your records, your treatment summary to date, and any diagnostic tests (including actual X-ray and CT scans, not just dictated reports)—even if the office of your original physician is responsible for sending this information to the consulting physician ahead of time. We've seen a number of patients in second opinion where materials were lost in transit, and without adequate background information available at the time of your visit, the quality of the consultation suffers. Also, bring the contact information of your original physician with you to give to the consultant, so that there can be direct and easy communication between the physicians involved in your care.

7. For most patients, requesting a second opinion will primarily be motivated by a desire to get a different perspective on their situation, to hear about clinical trial possibilities, or to learn about different treatment options, especially if their case is unusual. On occasion, though, there will be instances where a patient just

might not "connect" with the first physician he or she sees, there is a clash in personalities, or communication is simply lacking. You have every right at that point to seek care from another provider, as a trusting patient-doctor relationship is so critical to your well-being and health. At the same time, try to avoid too much "doctor-shopping" or "doctor-hopping," as continuity of care and a longitudinal relationship with a physician and his or her health care team are valuable assets. Often, trust builds over time.

Second Opinions: A Valuable Part of Supportive Care

Malin Dollinger, M.D.

None of us are prepared to be told we have cancer. It's like a membership in a new club . . . one we didn't know existed, didn't apply for, and don't want to belong to. Everyone seems to treat us differently. Life and all of our old priorities suddenly change. We need to know right now what is going on—how bad the cancer is, where it is, where it has spread. What are the choices for treatment? How successful is each one? What are the risks and side effects of each treatment? Is one better than another? Why? What should I do? How much time do I have to decide? For that matter, how much time do I have?

Thank God you have never had to ask and answer these questions before. Somewhere in the back of your mind, you are worried about having an auto accident or breaking a bone, or needing an operation, but you have absolutely no training or experience in having cancer. How do you make decisions about what to do? You find a physician you trust. Usually a cancer specialist (oncologist) is involved in your care. This makes sense. Oncologists know about cancer. However, there is so much information about cancer. Some of it is valid and reliable, in books and medical literature and from your doctors. Some of it may not be reliable: what your

friends or the Internet tells you. How do you tell the difference?

First, believe what your doctor tells you. He or she has spent years training, learning, and understanding this process we call cancer. Second, read all you can. However, making these vital and critical decisions about your cancer care is different from most decisions you have made in your life. Almost always, you choose between two things you like: Steak or chicken? A Ford or a Chevy? Buy this house or that one? Fact is, it wouldn't be the end of the world no matter which of these decisions you made. Both choices, then, are in a sense "positive."

When making a decision about cancer treatment, your choices are things you *don't* want, instead of things you do want. You don't want an operation (no matter which one your physician suggests). You also don't want radiation therapy. You don't want chemotherapy. You don't even want a biopsy!! Much less the blood tests and CT scans and all the doctor visits. So you are not used to making choices about things you don't want. It feels strange, and it is strange.

That's why it is so important to be able to talk to a health care professional about these choices. . . . Best is someone who knows what the choices mean—good and bad. Often your "main-M.D."—perhaps your oncologist—can explain all these choices to you. You may be quite happy and satisfied with these discussions. However, you have no prior experience with making these choices, or making this kind of choice, about things you don't want.

So a second opinion is one way of exploring the choices. It's an important one, to help you be very sure that you understand what the choices mean. Some choices in life are very clear: It does not require a second opinion to know the significance of pulling a parachute rip cord or not pulling a rip cord. However, before you go up in an airplane to go skydiving, would it be important to know which brand of parachute (and parachute "packer") is reliable? Of course!! You do this before the plane takes off.

In cancer treatment, even though there is a great emotional need to "get going"—you want the treatment yesterday—there is rarely an emergency medically. Most of the time, nothing bad will happen if a few weeks go by while you make sure you understand the difficult decisions that you need to make. If you have a need for additional discussion (and maybe you aren't even sure if you do), a second opinion is one way of being sure you understand the choices.

This should not be a threat to your regular doctor. You should be "partners" in your care, and you can simply explain, "Yes, I am really pleased with your care, and I want you to continue to take care of me . . . and I would also love to have some additional input from someone who maybe has a different perspective or angle."

After all, who is the one that is most important to please and to satisfy? You are! Don't worry about hurting the doctor's feelings. He or she is a professional, and this is not the first time another physician has "looked over" his or her care. It begins in early training, and happens every day, in some way. As a matter of fact, your physician should welcome the opportunity to have another consultant review and approve your care decisions or perhaps suggest a novel idea that might be to your benefit. Either way, you win. Yes, there may be some instances when you have some basic disagreement with your physician or there isn't the "fit" that there should be. Sometimes you do need to change physicians. But that isn't the usual reason for a second opinion. Most of the time, you simply want to be sure that there is "no stone left unturned" in your care. Few people change oncologists—he or she becomes a really important person in your life.

What does the second-opinion consultant do? He or she wants to know everything about your previous diagnosis and treatment. You usually bring copies of all your X-ray films and all your records. It's a good idea to have a copy of all your records anyway, in case you travel and are away somewhere and become ill. Often the consultant will wish to look at the pathology slides to verify the type of cancer that is present. You need to have copies of your previous consultations and opinions, hospital records and discharge summaries, and especially the pathology reports (these reports give the cancer diagnosis) and the operative reports of any surgery you may have had for the cancer. The consultant reviews all this material and examines you. Often you will bring your spouse, your significant other, family members, or a close friend with you, to share in the discussion and to help you remember the discussion and make decisions. It may be helpful to bring a pad to take notes, and a tape recorder to keep a record. The consultant will then go over all of the findings with you and discuss and emphasize the current and future decisions to be made. It will be especially helpful if you bring questions of your own, to be sure you have no unanswered questions or problems when you are done. The consultant will then prepare a written report, which will be sent to your physician, and often to you as well. He or she may call your primary doctor on the phone to have an immediate discussion of your findings; this is especially important if you are about to have surgery or begin a new treatment program and are waiting for "agreement."

Should you tell your present physician about the second opinion? Yes! It is in your best interest that all of your doctors know all the facts and opinions. Your health is at stake, and unless you have had a major disagreement with your physician and are using the second opinion as a pathway toward changing doctors, it is to your advantage to share all the information. Your physician is your partner on the pathway toward success.

Specialists usually make cancer treatment decisions, and their training is relatively uniform and sophisticated. There are seldom any major differences in the standard ways of treating various cancers, and cancer specialists generally know what the choices are and what the risks and complications are. There may be advantages and disadvantages of each treatment choice. What a consultant may help with is

1. Deciding with you which choice makes the most sense

2. Reassuring you that your own doctor has made the best choice for you at this time

3. Outlining some of the choices that will need to be made later, should there be a need for other treatment or different treatment

4. Defining a new treatment or pathway that may not generally be known or available, such as a center or physician with special research in your cancer, or with a special program, protocol, or clinical trial or promising new treatment

Many insurance and health care companies, who will pay for such opinions, have acknowledged the importance of second opinions. It is becoming the "normal" and appropriate thing to do. My experience is that second-opinion consultants are very respectful of the hard work and dedication of your principal doctor and are careful to be entirely professional and to give appropriate credit and validity to those decisions already made. After all, their patients have obtained second opinions, too!

Multidisciplinary-Second-Opinion Fundamentals

Richard and Annette Bloch

Doctors other than oncologists diagnose most cancers. They are diagnosed by family doctors, gynecologists, ear-nose-and-throat doctors, and so on. Some of these doctors do not encourage their patients to seek second opinions. These doctors may be afraid of losing revenue or threatened by having their patients believe some other doctor is more knowledgeable, or they just may not want to bother consulting with other physicians. The patients of these doctors are probably most in need of the second opinion.

The critical element in successfully treating cancer is in promptly receiving the proper treatment. We know that cancer comes in a hundred different varieties. There is no relationship between breast cancer and brain cancer other than the term *cancer* and the fact that they both involve rapidly dividing cells. It is impossible for one primary physician to be informed on the latest and best treatment for every type of cancer. Furthermore, it is impossible for one specialist, such as a surgeon, radiotherapist, or oncologist, to know the very latest and best treatment in his or her own specialty for every one of the more than one hundred different types of cancer.

At lunch with a medical oncologist, we asked how often he treated a patient for cancer without a second opinion. This man, in his sixties, replied that he had never in his career treated a cancer patient without a second opinion. Furthermore, he always insisted on a second opinion from someone other than an associate of his. This was the rationale:

1. Cancer is a very serious disease that grows exponentially. If it is not diagnosed properly the first time, there is often no second chance.

2. The doctor is human and could make a mistake.

3. Someone else could see something that one doctor doesn't see.

4. Someone else could know something that one doctor doesn't know.

We thought this was a profound statement and wished that every doctor treating a cancer patient could hear this. Our conclusion from this statement is that any doctor treating a cancer patient without a second opinion is not practicing medicine, but trying to play God. We thought it was only God who was supposed to be perfect, know everything, and never make a mistake.

These thoughts were substantiated in the May 1985 publication of the National Institutes of Health entitled *Cancer Control Objectives for the Nation, 1985–2000*. It states, "The application of the state-of-the-art treatment is complex. At all levels of the health service delivery system—from the primary care physician who has initial contact with the patient to specialists directing the cancer treatment—physician knowledge is not yet optimal. That knowledge should include an appreciation for state-of-the-art treatment information and an interest in ensuring early multidisciplinary decision making. . . . For about 70 percent of cancers, optimal therapy derives from multidisciplinary discussions. The relative rarity of some of the most responsive tumors means that proficient treatment can be maintained only at some major cancer centers. . . . Malpractice

considerations may result in physicians selecting 'safe' therapy, which neither offers significant risk nor the chance of cure. . . . A major determinant of outcome for most newly diagnosed cancer patients with curable disease hinges on early multidisciplinary treatment planning and the availability of expertise and resources to carry out such a treatment plan."

A multidisciplinary panel (tumor board) is an excellent way to obtain other opinions as well as advice for treatment planning. The purpose of the panel is to review the referring doctor's proposed treatment and approve it or recommend additions or alternatives. The recommendations of the panel are discussed in front of the patient. The panel's comments are written down for the patient and a copy is sent to the referring doctor.

This idea of holding all discussions openly and frankly in front of the patient and any relatives or friends he or she cares to bring is unique in the medical world. Not only do a majority of patients leave with a recommended course of medical treatment, but every patient also leaves with an improved state of mind. They all feel better and more confident about what lies ahead.

— 6 —

What Happens in Surgery

Erik K. Nakakura, M.D., Ph.D., Carlos A. Pellegrini, M.D.,
David R. Byrd, M.D., and Sean J. Mulvihill, M.D.

■ ■ ■ ■

If you have cancer, there is a very good chance that you will see a surgeon during the course of your treatment. Surgery plays a crucial role in treating the disease. It is the oldest form of treatment and also the most effective. More cures are achieved by surgery than by any other form of therapy.

Surgery's role in cancer treatment has expanded considerably over the past few years. Better understanding of the natural history of many tumors, safer anesthetic techniques, and improved preoperative and postoperative care have led to fewer postoperative complications and better long-term survival rates. Surgeons can now also plan operations more effectively because a tumor's size and location can be determined more precisely with modern imaging techniques.

Surgery can support other treatment methods as well. For example, the development of pumps and similar devices that allow precise, continuous, and comfortable delivery of drugs has added a new dimension to cancer treatment. So has the implanting of radioactive seeds to deliver measured doses of radiation to internal tumors. Surgery is critical to the effective use of these techniques.

Why Surgery Might Be Recommended

Since surgery is used in the diagnostic, treatment, and posttreatment phases of cancer management, your primary physician or oncologist might suggest surgery in a variety of circumstances. The many different types of surgery each have their own goals. In general, there are eight reasons why surgery might be recommended.

• *To prevent or lower the risk of developing cancer* Some benign diseases associated with a high risk of developing cancer are commonly referred to as precancerous conditions. To avoid the risk of cancer, therefore, it may be beneficial to remove an organ affected by one of these diseases.

Ulcerative colitis, for example, is a benign inflammatory condition of the large bowel. Colon cancer develops in about 40 percent of people whose large bowel has been affected by the disease for over twenty years. If a younger person has ulcerative colitis affecting the entire colon, then it *may* be appropriate to remove the colon before cancer appears.

Any operation performed to prevent cancer—commonly called prophylactic surgery—calls for a detailed discussion between you and your doctor. The risks of developing cancer have to be weighed carefully against the risk of surgery itself and the permanent changes that surgery will cause. The situation may not always be clear and other options may be possible. In such cases, you, the surgeon, and your oncologist have to study all the facts and decide on a course of action that takes your preferences into account.

As an example, consider that several risk factors significantly increase the chance that some women will develop breast cancer. A double mastectomy would significantly decrease the likelihood of breast cancer developing but would also result in the loss of both breasts. Whether to perform the surgery is up to the woman. Some women may feel more comfortable avoiding surgery at an early stage and living with the risk. Others may feel otherwise.

• *To diagnose or stage the disease* Although many nonsurgical techniques can diagnose cancer accurately, in most cases it is still necessary for an oncologist planning therapy to have a sample of tissue to analyze. A surgeon can remove a small amount of tissue by inserting a very fine needle into the area of the tumor and drawing out a few cells to be examined under a microscope. This fine needle aspiration (FNA)—or aspiration cytology—is the easiest and most comfortable technique used to obtain sample cells, but the very small amount of tissue involved may not be enough for an accurate diagnosis.

When more tissue is needed, a larger needle can obtain a "core" of tissue for microscopic examination. If that sample is still not enough, a small operation—an incisional biopsy—may be performed to remove a portion of the tumor. When the tumor is small, the surgeon might do an excisional biopsy, meaning that the entire lesion is removed rather than just a sample of it. This is very common with skin lesions, where the doctor has to know whether the lesion is a benign condition or a malignant melanoma or some other skin cancer.

To stage the disease properly, a more formal operation may be needed to obtain tissue from several areas of the body. This is in rare cases done for lymphomas,

where a staging laparotomy—opening and examining the abdomen—is done to sample tissues from the liver and lymph nodes and to remove the spleen.

It is important to remember that diagnostic surgery is just that—an operation designed to obtain tissue to confirm a diagnosis or to help plan adequate treatment. The goal is not to cure the cancer.

There has been a recent explosion in the development of minimally invasive surgery in both the diagnosis and treatment of solid malignancies. Videoendoscopic surgery is now frequently used to stage cancers in the abdomen (laparoscopy) and the chest cavity (thoracoscopy), and often eliminates the need for a major exploration of the abdomen or chest when unsuspected disease is found by these techniques. These procedures are most commonly performed under general anesthesia, and involve small incisions, which allow rapid recovery and return to normal activity. This technology is rapidly evolving and is commonly used for the resection of some solid tumors.

• *To remove the primary tumor* For many cancer patients, removal of the tumor may be the best form of treatment. In some cases, surgery leads to a cure. This form of surgery is referred to as surgery for the primary lesion. For this to be possible, the tumor has to be localized in an organ or area of the body that can be safely removed.

This type of surgery generally involves a major operation requiring admission to the hospital, general anesthesia, and several days for recovery. The surgeon tries to remove the affected organ or area along with an adjacent area—called the margin—of normal-looking tissue. This margin is important because cells and small parts of the tumor may extend beyond what the surgeon can see as obvious cancer.

The lymph glands connected to the organ with the tumor might also be removed, since most tumors spread to lymphatic glands quite early. Removing the nodes along with the tumor improves the chance of removing all the cancer and, therefore, the chance of cure.

After the operation, the surgeon passes the entire specimen—the "gross" (visible) cancer, the margin, and the lymphatic glands—to a pathologist for examination under a microscope. The pathologist will be able to find out the exact kind of tumor involved and how far it extends into normal tissues and glands. The extent of the tumor determines the prognosis and the need for additional forms of therapy. It usually takes two or three days for a specimen to be processed and examined, so the surgeon will not usually be able to discuss the final diagnosis or prognosis with you or your family for a few days after surgery.

• *To remove other tumors* Besides removing the primary tumor, surgery may also be performed for residual, metastatic, or recurrent lesions. Surgery for "residual" tumors means that the operation has been preceded by radiation therapy or chemotherapy. The idea is that certain tumors shrink or even disappear with radiation or chemotherapy and that the surgeon can then remove the rest of the affected organ.

In other cases, after the original tumor is removed, the surgeon may remove the metastases, which are small cancer cells that have broken off the tumor and spread to other organs. For example, patients with colon cancer who develop metastases to the liver and in whom there is no other evidence of disease may benefit from the removal of the metastatic tumor.

Finally, if the tumor has returned at the original site—"recurrent" disease—the surgeon may attempt a second removal of the tumor. This operation may be performed with some melanomas or breast cancer, for example.

• *To relieve symptoms* Some tumors produce symptoms such as pain and bleeding, or cause other problems, such as obstruction and bowel perforation. In some patients, surgery can help relieve these symptoms. In the stomach and intestines, for example, a tumor may become large enough to cause blockage, preventing food from moving properly through the system. Tumors can also block the biliary tract, causing jaundice. In these situations, it may be useful to operate to remove the tumor or bypass the blockage, even if cure is not possible. This kind of surgery is referred to as palliative.

Other symptoms caused by tumors can also be palliated. Some cancers can bleed or cause pain. If the tumor is extensive and the presence of metastases makes surgery for cure impossible, the tumor may still be removed solely to stop the bleeding or control the pain. In these cases the operations are also considered palliative.

• *To reconstruct or rehabilitate* Removing an organ or tumor can sometimes produce some deformity or functional problem. When that happens, surgery can often improve appearance, function, and the quality of life. Excellent techniques provide reconstruction for women who have had a radical mastectomy. There are also ways to restore appearance and function after head and neck surgery.

It is not unusual for both doctor and patient to focus so sharply on treatment that they simply accept some of the crippling results of major surgery and overlook alternatives that can improve the quality of life. So be aware of this form of surgery and discuss the alternatives for reconstruction with your oncologist, surgeon, or other doctor involved in your treatment.

• *To support chemotherapy and radiation therapy* Surgery is often used to support other forms of cancer therapy. If you need to have drugs administered intravenously, for example, you may have a port, catheter, or pump surgically implanted. Ports and catheters are implanted under local anesthetic in an operating room or in a radiologic suite, although general anesthetic can be given to people who prefer less discomfort.

A port is essentially a small chamber placed under the skin, usually near the shoulder. The chamber connects to a small tube inserted in a vein and threaded through it into larger veins. Access to the port is easy for the person injecting the drug and avoids the pain and discomfort often associated with intravenous injections.

Catheters may sometimes need to be placed into large veins through the skin. The catheter differs from the port in that its end is left outside the skin; the tube enters the body through a small puncture. Catheters usually have up to three inner lines so that different solutions—medication or nourishment, for example—can be given.

Pumps are more sophisticated devices. They have a large chamber that is filled with a drug, usually 1 to 1½ ounces (30 to 50 ml). The pump has a mechanism, driven by the body's heat, that allows the drug to be delivered constantly through a small catheter inserted into a vein or artery without the need for a stay in the hospital. It is sometimes possible to target a specific organ such as the liver and deliver large amounts of chemotherapy drugs directly to it through an artery.

To support radiation therapy, an operation can be performed to implant catheters that are subsequently loaded with a radio-emitter. Surgery is also used to expose a tumor so that a large dose of radiation can be given directly to the tumor or the tumor bed (see "Intraoperative Radiation Therapy (IORT)," in chapter 7, "What Happens in Radiation Therapy").

• *To treat complications* Tumors or their treatments often suppress the immune system. This can lead to infections, bowel perforations, or obstructions that may require surgical treatment.

Preparing for Surgery

Before you have surgery, your doctors will study the kind and extent of the tumor involved, then discuss what kind of surgery

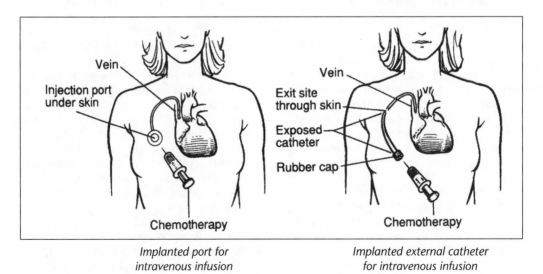

Implanted port for
intravenous infusion

Implanted external catheter
for intravenous infusion

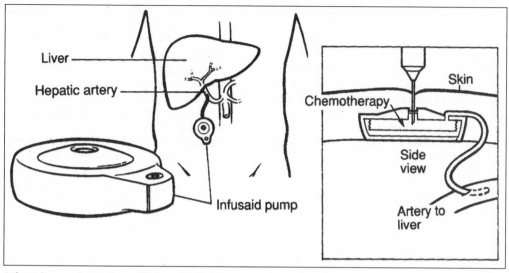

Infusaid pump for prolonged internal infusion

you need. The intensity of preparation for the surgery will depend on the kind of operation planned. If the surgery is for diagnosis and will involve a needle biopsy, there may only be a need to make sure your blood will clot so that bleeding from the needle puncture will stop quickly.

Preparation is much more elaborate for a major operation. Assuming that the tumor has already been studied thoroughly, two areas will be given special attention—the identification of any abnormalities or associated diseases and their correction before the operation. Patients are examined more or less comprehensively depending on the type of operation planned and their age. As people get older, they tend to develop diseases of the heart, lungs, and other organs that can jeopardize their recovery from an operation.

Diagnosis of Associated Diseases It is important for your surgeon to know if you have diabetes, if you are being treated for some other disease, what medications you are taking, how many white and red blood cells are in circulation, how well your blood clots, and so on. Much of this information can be obtained through blood tests. Blood-clotting abnormalities can be discovered with tests, but the best indicator of an increased risk of bleeding during surgery is a history of bleeding problems.

Similarly, a chest X-ray will give the surgeon an idea of the state of your lungs and an electrocardiogram (ECG) will help evaluate the state of your heart. If necessary, more sophisticated tests of lung and heart function will be performed. These will not only help evaluate the overall risk of surgery but also help determine the kind of anesthetic and other drugs you may need.

Correction of Associated Diseases Once problems have been identified, as many abnormalities as possible should be corrected. High blood pressure (hypertension), for example, should be treated before the operation. Infections can be treated with antibiotics, blood can be replenished if the blood counts are not high enough, and there may be ways of improving pulmonary function.

One of the most common problems people with cancer have is malnutrition. It is very important to correct this before the operation, since good nutrition gives your body the strength to get through the trauma of the operation and to heal properly. If necessary, additional feedings through a small tube in the stomach or an intravenous line can provide your body with an extra 2,500 to 3,000 calories a day.

What You Can Do to Prepare

While your doctor will look after most of the abnormalities noted above, there is a lot you as a patient can do to improve the outcome of the operation.

First, if you smoke, stop. Whether or not you intend to stop forever (which is always beneficial), you should stop as soon as the decision to operate is made. Lung and breathing problems are the most common type of complication after surgery, and they can be minimized if the pulmonary system is working well. Clearing the lungs for as many days as possible before surgery will significantly improve your chances of not developing these problems.

Second, become as physically fit as possible. This will make both the operation and your recovery a lot easier. Eating appropriately and losing weight if you are overweight will also help. And any form of exercise, including walking, will be beneficial because it improves both circulation and pulmonary function.

Third, make sure to discuss with the surgeon the details of the operation and what you can expect afterward. Knowledge of the hospital, the intensive care unit, the staff, and the procedures to be followed will help you prepare for the operation emotionally.

Fourth, discuss the use of blood. Most major surgery requires administering blood, and there is some risk involved, albeit a small one. That risk can be completely abolished if you use your own blood. If your blood count is high enough and the state of your tumor permits, it may be appropriate to store your own blood two weeks before surgery so it can be returned to you if needed (see chapter 17, "Blood Transfusions and Cancer Treatment").

Finally, arrange for family or friends to help you in your recovery after you return home from the hospital. When you return home, you will likely be eating by mouth, walking, and able to care for most of your personal needs. Even so, you will need help with preparation of meals, shopping, and housekeeping chores. If the planned surgery is extensive, or if you are weak even before surgery, additional help, such as a visiting nurse or even a temporary stay in a rehabilitation facility, may be in order. It is helpful to outline plans for these needs with your surgeon before surgery.

Anesthetics

Modern anesthetic techniques have greatly increased the safety of major cancer surgery and the ability of surgeons to combat cancer. Anesthesia is safe and comfortable. Each form of surgery requires a different form of anesthetic, the major kinds being local, regional, and general.

• *Local anesthesia* is used for procedures that are short and superficial—in other words, near the skin. A biopsy or catheter placement, for example, can be performed under local anesthetic. The surgeon injects a drug such as lidocaine that numbs the site. You will remain awake and will usually feel some pressure as well as minor pulling of tissues in the area. If you do feel any pain, tell the surgeon so you can get additional anesthetic.

• *Regional anesthesia* involves giving the anesthetic agent near the spinal cord.

The drug may be given by a single injection (called an epidural) or continuously through a small catheter tube placed directly into or near the spinal canal (peridural).

This form of anesthesia is excellent for operations in the lower part of the body, especially the lower extremities and the pelvis. The main advantage of regional anesthesia is that it gives you complete pain relief for many hours and that it wears off slowly, allowing you to take other forms of pain relief as needed after the operation. Another advantage, especially if you have lung problems, is that you stay awake throughout the operation, eliminating the interference with breathing that takes place with general anesthetic. Remaining awake, however, may be considered a disadvantage by some people.

• *General anesthesia* is used in most major operations for cancer. Anesthetic agents are given by intravenous injection, through a breathing mask, or both. They act directly on the brain to produce a temporary loss of consciousness. In most cases, the anesthesiologist will also use muscle relaxants to produce a profound relaxation of the body. This will make the surgery easier to perform and will mean less pain afterward. Because your muscles will not be functioning, you won't be able to breathe spontaneously. But a tube will be placed in your windpipe (trachea) and connected to a machine (ventilator) that will deliver air to your lungs every few seconds.

The anesthesiologist monitors breathing by periodically checking the concentration of oxygen in the blood. The anesthesiologist is also in charge of administering fluids intravenously, including blood when needed. The amount and the quality of the fluids are regulated carefully to maintain adequate blood pressure, an adequate amount of circulating blood, and adequate blood flow to the body's organs.

After the Operation

Contrary to popular belief, waking up from general anesthesia is not always unpleasant. In fact, it is not too different from waking up from any deep sleep. You will usually wake up in a recovery room, although you may not remember the experience.

Depending on the operation, you may find upon awakening that one or more intravenous lines are running into your body. You may also find drains in some body cavities. You may feel some discomfort and not be able to eat for a few days. The surgeon will have covered all these points with you before the operation.

Pain Control Most patients worry about pain after the operation, but there are several relatively easy ways to control it. If mild pain relievers (analgesics) like acetaminophen (Tylenol) and codeine won't do the job, pain can be controlled by the injection of stronger analgesics, the most potent being narcotics like morphine. These drugs provide relief from pain for three to four hours and should be re-administered by the clock or as soon as the pain reappears.

In the past, patients had to call a nurse each time they felt the need for an injection, but patients themselves can now activate devices that deliver the analgesic. The patient-controlled analgesia (PCA) device has a compartment for the morphine, a trigger button to press, and a small computer that delivers a fixed dose of the drug. There is also a lockout period set by the doctor and nurse—usually six to ten minutes—to make sure the drug isn't administered too often. The main advantage of this form of pain control is that the pain can be relieved as soon as it is felt, which usually means that smaller amounts of medication are needed.

Another way to control pain is with morphine or a local anesthetic administered into the spinal canal, just like the epidural given during the operation. This will control the pain completely but usually causes bladder malfunction. A catheter, therefore, will be needed to drain the bladder of urine.

These options should be discussed and a basic plan devised before the operation. The main point to remember is that pain can be controlled and that there is no need to suffer. It's also useful to note that taking liberal doses of morphine or other analgesics in the postoperative period does not lead to drug addiction.

What Are the Risks?

It is important for you to discuss with the surgeon before the operation the risk of anesthesia, the risk of the surgical procedure itself, and any potential complications. You should also discuss the operative mortality—usually defined as a death that occurs within thirty days of an operation—that can result either from the underlying disease or from complications that develop during the operation.

• *The risk of anesthesia* is related to your age, the magnitude of the operation, and the presence of associated diseases. The American Society of Anesthesiology has devised a formula to classify the status of patients, divided into five classes. As the age or the associated diseases increase, the number of the class increases to indicate a greater risk. Class 1 patients, for example, are young to middle-aged with no significant associated diseases who have a localized process requiring a limited operation. Class 2 patients have mild associated diseases that do not limit their activities. Class 3 patients have severe systemic disturbance from other diseases, such as low pulmonary function, vascular complications, or heart disease. Class 4 patients have severe disorders that threaten life. Class 5 patients are critically ill and are not expected to survive without surgery. The overall risk of anesthesia is very small, especially for Class 1 and 2 patients.

• *The operative risks* vary greatly with the kind of operation performed. They are usually divided into immediate risks (occurring within a few days or weeks of surgery) and late risks (occurring months or years after the operation). Just as in the case of anesthesia, the immediate risks are increased by the presence of other diseases.

Bleeding is usually quoted as a common risk of surgery, but very few patients suffer much from it. The most common immediate complications are pulmonary and usually result from earlier lung disease, a history of smoking, or the fact that postoperative pain and being in bed prevent the lungs from expanding. These complications can be prevented or minimized by vigorous coughing, as a nurse may request, and by getting up and walking around as soon as possible.

Another complication that may occur after a prolonged period in bed is the development of a clot in the legs brought on by poor circulation. The major risk is that part of the clot might break loose and lodge in the lungs. This is called a pulmonary embolism and is a potentially serious complication that can be prevented by walking or by moving your legs, particularly the calf muscles, while in bed.

Other common complications in the postoperative period have to do with the operative wound. Infection can set in around the incision, but infections can easily be treated and shouldn't cause you much physical or emotional discomfort.

Late complications of surgery have to do with the scarring that is an inevitable part of the healing process. Scarring in the abdomen can occasionally lead to a bowel obstruction or some other form of mechanical blockage.

Choosing a Surgeon and a Medical Facility

This is not usually an overwhelming problem. In most cases, your oncologist or the primary care doctor who diagnosed your cancer will recommend someone whom he or she knows and has worked with before. In other cases, you may know of a surgeon personally or by reputation and can use him or her either directly as the surgeon or as a source of information.

If you want to make the choice yourself, it is a good idea to get information from the local medical society about doctors who are board certified in surgery. While certification by the American Board of Surgery does not necessarily mean outstanding performance, it does have implications about a surgeon's level of knowledge, training, and adherence to certain standards. Most reputable surgeons are also Fellows of the American College of Surgeons, which can also help you with names of surgeons practicing in your community. Write to American College of Surgeons, 55 E. Erie Street, Chicago, IL 60611, or telephone 312-644-4050.

When the procedure you are facing is minor or has to do with one of the more common forms of cancer, chances are that the operation can be performed successfully by most surgeons. But if your oncologist says your disease is out of the ordinary or if the operation you need is a major or complex one, it is usually best to seek out the services of an experienced surgeon working in a sizable hospital or other medical institution. His or her experience is an important asset, but more important is that the specialists, sophisticated equipment, and advanced techniques that may be needed to react to problems during and after an operation are available only at large medical centers.

Once you have made a preliminary decision about a surgeon, it is a good idea to arrange a meeting. Decide for yourself whether he or she is the kind of person you want to entrust your life to. If you feel positive about it, follow through. If not, it is easy enough to find another surgeon who can perform the operation just as well.

At this point, you might also want to get a second opinion. Another opinion can be very useful, especially with a case that is difficult, complex, or uncommon. You will be able to compare the two approaches to the disease, and that may give you more confidence as you face your operation.

When all this has been done, you are ready for surgery.

— 7 —

What Happens in Radiation Therapy

Daphne A. Haas-Kogan, M.D., Lawrence W. Margolis, M.D.,
T. Stanley Meyler, M.D., and Eugene T. Morita, M.D.

■ ■ ■ ■

About half of all people with cancer need radiation therapy as part of their overall treatment plan at some point in their illness. It is often recommended as the primary treatment but can also be used along with chemotherapy or surgery. When used with surgery, it might be given before, during, or after the operation. When used with chemotherapy, it may be given before or after the program begins or at the same time as chemotherapy.

There are two main goals in radiation therapy:

• *Cure the cancer.* This usually requires a long and complex course of treatment.

• *Relieve symptoms (palliation).* Treatment to achieve this goal is usually less complex and takes less time.

How It Works

Radiation therapy—which is also called radiotherapy—uses high-energy X-rays, electron beams, or radioactive isotopes to kill cancer cells without exceeding safe doses to normal tissue.

Radiation accomplishes its purpose by killing cancer cells through a process called ionization. Some cells die immediately after radiation because of the direct effect, though most die because the radiation damages the chromosomes and DNA so much that they can no longer divide.

The key to successful treatment is getting the appropriate amount of radiation to the tumor in the most effective way. There are several technical ways of doing this. The most common way is by external radiation, in which a radiation beam is directed at the tumor from a machine. Internal or systemic radiotherapy delivers radiation by giving a radioactive source intravenously or by injection—intravenous radioactive iodine or radioactive gold into the abdominal cavity, for example. With intracavitary radiotherapy, an applicator containing radiation seeds is placed in an organ such as the uterus. In interstitial radiotherapy, the sources are placed directly in the tumor. Radiation can also be administered during surgery in a technique termed intraoperative radiation therapy (IORT). These methods are usually used in combination with external radiation.

Planning the Therapy

All radiation treatment is supervised by physicians who are generally board-certified specialists trained to evaluate and treat cancer patients using radiation. Your specialist may be called a radiation oncologist, radiotherapist, radiation therapist, or therapeutic radiologist.

Whatever the term used in your particular hospital, this specialist is an important member of your cancer team. He or she may be consulted at any time during your treatment, from immediately after the diagnosis to well along in your therapy. At whatever stage the radiation oncologist joins your team, the treatment-planning process follows several standard steps.

The Goal The first thing the radiation oncologist has to do is thoroughly evaluate your case. He or she will acquire your medical history, perform a physical examination, review all scans, diagnostic X-rays, pathology slides, and operative reports, and then will discuss your case with your primary physician, medical oncologist, or possibly a surgeon. After the evaluation has been completed, a decision will be made on what role radiation therapy will play—will the goal of treatment be curative or palliative? At this point, the radiation oncologist will also decide on the method of radiation to be used—external, the various internal methods, or a combination. Then the detailed planning starts.

The Simulation If external radiation is going to be used, the first step in the detailed planning stage is called a simulation, performed on a special X-ray machine built to resemble the machine that will ultimately be used. Certain contrast agents or probes may be used to aid in the simulation. The point of the exercise is to make all the necessary measurements to fix the precise location of the tumor. Marks will be made on your skin with a colored ink to outline the target the radiation oncologist will be aiming for—the "radiation port"—which has to be the same every day.

While the simulation is being done, the radiation oncologist may use the services of a clinical physicist and dosimetrist. The physicist is specially trained in the clinical application of radiation therapy and will give advice on technical matters that the radiation oncologist will incorporate into the plan. A dosimetrist is a person who,

with the use of computers, helps design the specialized treatment plan developed for each individual.

Following the simulation, you will be ready to start treatment either that day or possibly several days later if your case is complex. The reason for the delay is that all the data from the simulation will be fed into a computer. The treatment team will need time to study the various plans and tailor any shielding or blocking devices that may be needed to keep radiation away from your healthy tissues.

The Dosage The amount of radiation you receive is measured in units that used to be called rads. The term used now is *centigray* (cGy), but since 1 gray equals 100 rads, the two terms are interchangeable.

Deciding what dosage of radiation to give is a critical part of the treatment plan. Careful planning allows the radiation oncologist to deliver the maximum effective dose to the visible tumor and any invisible tumor cells that might be nearby while protecting the surrounding normal tissues as much as possible.

Calculating a dosage figure that balances these two goals can be complex, since the size and stage of the tumor have to be taken into account and since different tissues tolerate different levels of radiation. The liver, for example, will tolerate 3,000 cGy, the lungs 2,000, and the kidneys 1,800. Higher doses can be delivered to small parts of one of these organs, but if the entire organ is given higher doses than these, normal tissues will be harmed.

The radiation oncologist prescribes the total dose necessary to destroy the tumor, then calculates the daily dose over a specific period. This is called the fractionation schedule. Throughout, the radiation oncologist works with a figure called the therapeutic ratio, defined as a comparison of the damage to the tumor cells compared with normal cells. The therapeutic ratio can be enhanced in a number of ways—by using altered time fractionation schedules, careful treatment planning, selection of the optimum radiation energy for the specific problem, and by the use of specialized techniques such as high linear energy transfer (LET) radiation or chemical modifiers that either make the tumor cells more sensitive to radiation or better protect normal tissues.

The Number of Treatments Radiation is usually given daily five days a week. That schedule can continue for two to eight weeks depending on the tumor, the kind of treatment being used, and the dosage required. The point of using multiple treatments instead of a single treatment is to give normal cells a chance to recover and repair themselves.

The Delivery Method Radiation oncologists now have a variety of ways to deliver the most effective amount of radiation to specific tumor cells. Which method to use is based on many factors, including the biology of the tumor involved, the possibility of side effects or complications, the physical characteristics of the various sources of radiation, and how these different sources affect the body's many different cells, tissues, and organ systems. The methods can be broadly divided into external and internal radiation, with several options available within each category.

Types of External Radiation Therapy

External radiation therapy—the delivery of the dosage from a source outside the body—can vary according to the photon energy of the machines involved, the type of beams produced (electrons, X-rays, gamma rays), when the treatment is given, and the number of beams involved in the treatment procedure.

High- and Low-Energy Radiation External-beam treatment uses special equipment that uses either low energy (orthovoltage machines) or high energy (megavoltage machines). All the machines used today are quite precise about where they deliver the radiation dose.

Orthovoltage Equipment Orthovoltage X-rays are produced in a tube in which a filament is heated to a high temperature. Electrons are emitted and strike a tungsten target, producing X-rays with energies up to 300 kilovolts. This type of machine delivers its maximum dose on the surface of the skin and has a very limited range of penetration. These days, orthovoltage machines are used only for surface tumors such as skin cancers.

Megavoltage Equipment These are high-energy machines with energies greater than 1,000 kilovolts. Megavoltage machines let the radiation oncologist treat internal tumors without giving an excessive dosage to the skin. Commonly used megavoltage machines include cobalt 60 and linear accelerators that produce the maximum dose at an internal depth determined by the energy of the machine. A 25-megavolt betatron, for example, delivers its maximum dose almost 2 inches (4.5 cm) beneath the skin.

• Cobalt 60 became available in the 1950s and is still used. This machine contains a radioactive source housed in a specially designed lead container. As the cobalt isotope decays over time, it produces a beam in the megavoltage range.

• The linear accelerator, one of the most popular machines now being used, is available in energies ranging from four to thirty-five megavolts. Many of these machines can treat patients with X-rays or electrons or a combination of both. The combination is called a mixed beam and allows the radiation oncologist to tailor the treatment to a specific tumor and reduce the dose to surrounding tissues.

The machine works by producing electrons that are accelerated along a wave guide to a high velocity. These electrons can be directly used for treatment in the electron mode, or they can be directed at a target within the machine to produce the X-rays that are then used for treatment. The high-energy electrons used in the electron mode have a specific range of penetration into tissue, determined by the energy of the beam selected. The higher the megavoltage, the greater the penetration. Because an electron therapy beam produces a high skin dose, the whole course of treatment will seldom be given with only the electron beam unless you are being treated for cancer near or involving the skin.

Intraoperative Radiation Therapy (IORT)
People with localized tumors that can't be completely removed or have a high risk for a local recurrence—carcinoma of the pancreas, for example—may be candidates for IORT, a treatment carried out during surgery. The surgeon localizes the organ containing your tumor and removes as much of the tumor as possible. He or she then moves the normal tissue out of the path of the radiation beam. Radiation equipment may then be brought into the operating room, or you may be wheeled to a radiation department. A treatment cone connected to a linear accelerator is placed directly over the tumor, which is then treated with a single high dose. Normal tissues are spared, since they are outside the beam.

Stereotaxic (Stereotactic) Radiosurgery

This was introduced in the 1950s by Dr. Lars Leksell of Sweden, who found that he could treat deep-seated blood vessel malformations within the brain by using a number of cobalt sources. This is sometimes called a gamma knife.

If you are receiving this treatment, your head will be placed in a special frame that helps to maintain alignment and localize the treatment volume. With the frame in place, you will have a CT or MRI scan or an angiogram study. Technical information from the scan is then fed into a treatment-planning computer, and a dose distribution is calculated for the linear accelerator. You will then be transported to the linear accelerator, which will direct high doses of radiation from specific angles outside your head so that they converge on the target area. Surrounding tissues are for the most part spared.

The computer revolution and the availability of linear accelerators have made this form of treatment especially useful for vascular malformations, meningiomas, acoustic neuromas, and some malignant brain tumors.

Types of Internal (Systemic) Radiation Therapy

Modern radiation treatment makes extensive use of methods that deliver radiation to cancer cells not from a distance but by being inserted directly into or around the tumor. Radioactive sources can be injected, housed in special applicators, or implanted in the form of needles or seeds. With this type of treatment, radioactive isotopes are given intravenously or placed in an organ such as the bladder or abdomen.

Treatment with Radioactive Compounds

Radioactive tracers are unique in their ability to target specific tumors by being incorporated into their metabolism (e.g., thyroid cancer), finding antibody sites on tumor sites (e.g., lymphoma), localizing to tumor receptor sites (e.g., neuroendocrine tumors), or using the body's own response to the tumor to deliver a treatment dose (e.g., strontium-89). The membrane of tumors may have specific antibody sites where antibodies (monoclonal antibodies) can react or may have nonspecific receptors (neuroendocrine tumors).

For many years, nuclear medicine physicians have treated patients with radioactive iodine-131, for both overactive thyroids and cancerous thyroids. Iodine is essential to the metabolism of the overactive as well as the cancerous thyroid, since the uptake of iodine is a requirement to make thyroid hormone. The treatment for an overactive thyroid is quite benign, leaving patients usually feeling normal within several months after treatment. Some patients will become underactive in their metabolic function and may require supplemental thyroid hormone. No long-term ill effects causing such problems as cancers have been reported out of the ordinary in patients with overactive thyroids treated with radioactive iodine.

Most thyroid cancers can be induced to take up radioactive iodine sufficient to treat this type of cancer. The radioactive iodine uses the mechanisms of the tumor's metabolism to direct treatment. Treatment can be effective in destroying thyroid cancer. Long-term follow-up of these patients has shown that when the tumor is destroyed in this fashion, the outlook is substantially better than for those whose tumors were not destroyed.

More recently, tumors that have spread to bone and are causing pain can be treated with radioactive tracers such as strontium-89 and samarium-153. Frequently, tumors cause a significant local response, so bone scans show an intense bright spot. Tumors that spread to bone and cause such a response can be treated using the aforementioned radioactive tracers. Tumors such as prostate, breast, and lung cancer have been effectively treated. Although not curative, treatment can relieve pain in about 80 percent of patients with prostate cancer. In 10 percent of these patients, the pain reduction can be dramatic.

Some radioactive tracers have compounds that incorporate into the metabolism of the tumor and thus treatment can be rendered. A class of tumors called neuroendocrine tumors can be treated with a precursor that is incorporated into the metabolism of this type of tumor. Radioactive I-131 attached to this precursor is used. The predominant use of this precursor is for neuroblastomas. In neuroendocrine tumors, another mechanism is used by having radioactive tracers go to receptors on the membranes of these types of tumors. Other tumors such as lymphomas are now being treated by utilizing monoclonal antibodies on tumor sites.

Treatment with radioactive materials will grow because of the unique localization that can occur in many tumors. Utilizing mechanisms such as the metabolism, antibody sites on tumors, other types of receptor sites, and the body's own reaction are being actively used in treatment.

Interstitial Radiation Therapy This method, also called brachytherapy, places the source of radiation directly in the tumor and surrounding structures. It is most commonly used in tumors of the head and neck, the prostate, and the breast. It is also usually used in combination with external radiation.

There are two types of implants:

• A permanent implant involves small radioactive seeds such as gold or iodine placed directly in the affected organ. I-125 seeds, for example, are used for prostate cancer. Over several weeks or months, the seeds slowly deliver a specific dose of radiation to the tumor.

• A removable implant is the most common method of interstitial radiation therapy. The operation, usually carried out under general anesthesia, involves placing narrow, hollow stainless steel needles through the tumor. Once the placement seems satisfactory, Teflon tubes are inserted through the needles, and the needles are then removed, leaving the tubes in place. The operation is then terminated and you are returned to your room, where a small ribbon of radioactive seeds will be inserted into the tubes in a procedure called afterloading.

With computerized treatment planning, the specific strength of each seed can be selected, thereby providing the desired dose to the tumor volume over a specific period. Once the dose is reached, the tubes and the seeds are removed. This type of implant is commonly used for tumors of the head and neck or as a boost after external beam radiation of breast cancer after a lumpectomy.

Most interstitial radiotherapy is done with multiple tubes or seeds left in place for typically two to three days.

Another method of treatment is to use a single source. This is a tiny high-intensity source on the end of a flexible wire. The source shuttles in and out of the treatment applicators, stopping in predetermined spots for designated times under the control of a computer. In this way, the whole treatment can be given in five to ten minutes on an outpatient basis.

Today, some centers are using high-dose-rate insertions. After the patient is sedated, the applications are inserted using a remote-control machine under a physician's guidance. Radioactive sources of intense activity are placed in specific locations for a few seconds each. This method requires several insertions over several weeks. The main advantage is that there are no associated risks, such as the complication of blood clots in the lungs from prolonged bed rest.

Intracavitary Radiation The most common use of this method is in gynecologic tumors, such as carcinoma of the uterus. Specially designed hollow applicators are placed in the uterus under general or spinal anesthesia. X-rays are taken in the operating room to determine correct positioning, and once the placement is satisfactory the operation is ended. After you

are returned to your room, a small plastic tube containing the required number of sources of radioactive isotope of a specific strength is inserted into the hollow applicators. The sources and applicators are left in place for forty-eight to seventy-two hours, during which time you have to stay in bed. The seeds deliver the dose over the specified time, and once the dose is reached, the applicators and the sources are removed.

The advantage of this method is that a very high dose of radiation can be delivered to the tumor, while the rapid falloff in the dose gives maximum protection to the surrounding structures.

Intraluminal Radiation Therapy This method has limited use with some tumors in hollow organs like the esophagus and biliary tract. In esophageal carcinoma, for example, a specially designed tube is placed in the opening (lumen) of the esophagus. Then under X-ray visualization—fluoroscopy—several small radioactive sources are placed in the tube opposite the tumor. The tumor receives a high dose of radiation, while the dose to the surrounding structures is minimized. Intraluminal therapy is often used in combination with external radiation.

New Techniques to Improve Radiotherapy

Today's researchers are exploring several ways to make radiation therapy more effective, building on important advances in biology, physics, and engineering. Some have already produced significant results.

Three-Dimensional Conformal Radiation Therapy (3-D CRT) This method adds a significant degree of accuracy and allows better coverage and dosage to the tumor volume while decreasing dosage to normal surrounding tissue. It is a treatment technique based on CT scan anatomy, where beam shapes are determined by a beam's-eye view of patient anatomy.

Intensity-Modulated Radiation Therapy (IMRT) An additional degree of precision is obtained by adding intensity variation across those same fields by using computer-controlled treatment planning and dose deposition.

Hyperthermia The effect of heat on some types of cancer has been observed for more than 100 years. In 1893, W. B. Cooley reported that high temperatures had an effect on thirty-eight patients, twelve of whom had a complete regression of their cancers. Many malignant cells show a therapeutic response to high temperatures. And even moderate hyperthermia (108°F [42°C]) can destroy malignant cells.

Compared to radiotherapy alone, the combination of heat plus radiation has increased the response rate of certain tumors such as melanomas, and there are also promising preliminary results from treating brain tumors using interstitial implants plus heat.

Researchers are now studying the use of a new "multimodality" treatment—the combination of radiation therapy, chemotherapy, and heat—which may increase the response rate for some tumors (see chapter 11, "Hyperthermia").

Clinical Modifiers Research continues in the hope of finding chemical compounds that will modify radiation effects. Since radiation is more effective in cells with a good oxygen supply, one of the first approaches to modifying radiation sensitivity was through the use of hyperbaric oxygen chambers. Patients were placed in a closed chamber so they could breathe air with a higher than normal concentration of oxygen.

Recently, radiation-sensitizing agents that have an effect similar to oxygen have been developed. Other compounds now being investigated are "radioprotectors" that may decrease damage to normal tissues.

High Linear Energy Transfer (LET) Radiation Radiation with accelerators that use heavy particles or subatomic particles rather than electrons, X-rays, or gamma rays is now being studied in many centers. Several types of heavy particles are under investigation, including protons, helium ions, and neutrons. Two features seem to make this type of radiation—called high linear energy transfer (LET) heavy particle radiation—more effective: First, it can kill poorly oxygenated cells better than standard radiation can. Second, tumor cells are less able to repair sublethal damage from high LET radiation.

Several tumors have been identified that may benefit from high LET heavy particle radiation—sarcomas of bone and soft tissue, salivary gland tumors, some head and neck tumors, and melanomas of the eye—and the search is on to find others. In the past few years, high LET radiation has been used with patients with advanced malignant disease. But it is still an investigational treatment and is available only in a few facilities in the United States.

Hyperfractionation In recent years there has been considerable interest in hyperfractionation, in which patients are given radiation treatment twice daily rather than the conventional once daily. By using multiple smaller doses of radiation, a higher overall dose can be delivered. The treatments are usually given at least six hours apart to allow for tissue repair. Preliminary data suggests an improvement in the control of head and neck tumors without significant difference in acute toxicity. These altered fractionation schemes are being extensively studied in head and neck, brain, and lung tumors.

Intensity-Modulated Radiation Therapy (IMRT) Sophisticated planning techniques have significantly improved our ability to tailor the radiation field to the desired treatment region. IMRT is one such novel technique that allows the radiation oncologist to optimally manipulate the intensities of individual rays within each beam. IMRT requires highly specialized technology and software that are not available at every radiation oncology center.

IMRT offers a new approach to delivering high doses to the tumor while sparing normal tissues in the body. The precise position of the tumor may move, both during a given treatment session and between days of treatment. Such movement may result from shifting internal organs such as during breathing or digestion as well as from small alterations in the exact position of the patient on the treatment table. Tumor movement may cause portions of the tumor to receive less radiation than prescribed or may cause normal structures to receive more radiation than intended.

Therefore, the keys to effective use of IMRT are accurate demarcation of the tumor and normal structures and patient immobilization. To address patient immobilization and daily positioning, some centers are using image-guided techniques. These new approaches allow the radiation oncologist to confirm the tumor location every day. One of the most exciting techniques to minimize tumor and patient movement is the use of a computerized tomography (CT) image of the patient using the "cone beam" technique, which allows the generation of an image of the tumor and all surrounding normal structures using the same linear accelerator with which the patient is being treated. Appropriate adjustments can then be made daily to ensure that the tumor is receiving the appropriate dose of radiation and that normal tissues are receiving doses within their tolerance range.

The emerging concept of image-guided motion management is taking hold within the radiation oncology community, and many centers are learning not only to optimize patient immobilization techniques but also to utilize novel technology to ensure ever-increasing accuracy in radiation delivery.

Dealing with Side Effects

The common side effects of radiation therapy can be divided into generalized (systemic) and localized effects. What the effects are and how severe they become generally depend on the area treated, the size of the radiation port, the daily dose rate, and the total dosage delivered.

Not everyone who has radiation therapy suffers side effects. Many people go through treatment experiencing only minimal effects or none at all. But for some people, the side effects can be significant and uncomfortable.

Systemic Effects One of the most common systemic side effects is fatigue or malaise. This is especially common among patients receiving treatments to large areas, such as the whole abdomen and in total lymph node radiation.

A lot of people associate nausea and vomiting with X-ray treatments, but both these symptoms are unusual in radiotherapy patients. Again, it depends on the area being treated. Nausea and vomiting may occur in patients receiving radiation to the upper abdomen, but it is rare in patients getting radiation to the head and neck, chest, or pelvis. Even when you are receiving treatment to the abdomen, nausea and vomiting can usually be controlled by adjusting the dosage, changing the diet, or using antinausea medications.

Localized Side Effects As certain parts of your body are treated, you may experience several common localized side effects. Your radiation oncologist will go over these with you before treatment and will give them individualized attention if they occur.

• *Skin* All radiation has to pass through the skin, but with today's high-energy machines and daily treatment techniques using multiple ports, the side effects on the skin are seldom a problem unless the treated area actually involves the skin.

Most skin reactions appear as a redness called erythema. This is similar to sunburn and goes through the same stages—redness, gradual tanning, then peeling. Once the condition is treated, the reaction will usually go away within a week to ten days. If the dose has been high, late skin changes may appear in the form of increased pigmentation, which may be more noticeable in people of dark complexion.

If you develop any of these symptoms, it is important not to put any creams or lotions on your skin without the approval of your radiation oncologist.

• *Head and Neck* One of the most significant side effects is irritation of the membranes lining the body cavities, such as the lining—or mucosa—of the mouth. If you are being treated for a cancer of the head and neck, the mucosa surrounding the tumor may become red. And as treatment progresses, quite a few small superficial ulcers may develop. This can cause a lot of discomfort and will probably interfere with swallowing and nutrition. Fortunately, the effect is temporary and will disappear as soon as the treatment is finished.

Radiation to the head and neck may also interfere with taste if your tongue is in the primary radiation beam. And the amount of saliva produced can be significantly reduced if the salivary glands happen to be in the treatment beam (see "Special Problems of Radiation Patients" in chapter 23, "Maintaining Good Nutrition").

• *Chest* Most patients receiving chest radiation will not have any local symptoms. But the esophagus, which carries food from the mouth to the stomach, passes through the chest and may develop a mucosal reaction similar to that described for the mouth. If this happens, you may develop heartburn-type symptoms, which can be relieved by taking a liquid antacid such as Amphojel, Gelusil, Maalox, Mylanta, or Riopan.

• *Abdomen* The most significant side effects of radiation are associated with treatment to the abdomen. The larger the radiation port and the higher the dosage, the more likely you are to experience these effects.

Radiation to the upper abdomen can cause nausea and vomiting, usually during the first few days of treatment. As the treatment progresses, the symptoms often diminish.

• *Pelvis* Treatment to the pelvis can be associated with cramps, perhaps followed by diarrhea during the second and third weeks of treatment. A low-residue diet or an antidiarrhea medication such as Lomotil, Imodium, or Kaopectate will usually control the problem.

Most patients getting radiation treatment to the pelvis do not develop any significant bladder problems. But it is not unusual to have to urinate often, to feel an urgency to urinate, or to feel some pain when urinating. Fortunately, these symptoms are usually temporary and will go away soon after the treatment course is completed. In the meantime, a medication such as phenazopyridine (Pyridium) or flavoxate (Urispas) will usually ease the problem.

• *Hair Loss* Only hair within the radiation port will be affected by treatment. So you will lose scalp hair only if you are receiving radiation to your head, usually for tumors involving the brain. If the entire brain needs to be treated, the radiation can affect the entire scalp. But only a part of the scalp might be affected if a smaller portion of the brain is radiated.

Whether the hair loss is temporary or permanent depends on the dosage (see "Hair Loss," in chapter 20, "Coping with the Side Effects of Chemotherapy").

— 8 —

What Happens in Chemotherapy

Robert J. Ignoffo, Pharm.D., Ernest H. Rosenbaum, M.D.,
and Malin Dollinger, M.D.

■ ■ ■ ■

More than half of those diagnosed with cancer receive chemotherapy. For many people, chemotherapy helps treat their cancer effectively, enabling them to enjoy full, productive lives.

A chemotherapy *regimen* is a treatment plan that usually includes drugs to fight cancer and drugs to help support completion of the cancer treatment at the full dose on schedule. Most experts agree that staying on your chemotherapy plan gives you the best opportunity for a successful result.

The term *chemotherapy* means the treatment of cancer using specific chemical agents or drugs that are selectively destructive to cancer cells and tissues. The treatment of cancer with chemical agents or medications has been around since the days of the ancient Greeks. Yet the practice of modern cancer chemotherapy as it's known today really only began in the late 1940s, when nitrogen mustard and antifolate drugs were made available to fight tumor cells. Over the ensuing twenty years, chemotherapy was used, but essentially as an investigational treatment.

In 1965, perhaps still the most important breakthrough in cancer therapy occurred. Drs. James Holland, Emil Freireich, and Emil Frei hypothesized that cancer chemotherapy should follow the strategy of antibiotic therapy for tuberculosis, with combinations of drugs, each with a different site of action. The

cancer cells could conceivably mutate to become resistant to the single agent, but using different drugs *simultaneously* would make it extremely difficult for the tumor to develop resistance to the combination. Since then, cancer drug development has exploded into a multibillion-dollar industry. Antitumor drugs that are more effective have been developed and become mainstream, and other new drugs and supportive techniques have been developed, in particular, to reduce the side effects of the cancer-killing agents.

Furthermore, the genome has been mapped and many advances in new technologies have occurred leading to a greater understanding of the nature of cancer and how chemicals interact with cancer cells. Either alone or in combination with other treatments, chemotherapy can now cure several common forms of cancer, including breast cancer and testis cancer, leukemia, choriocarcinoma, Hodgkin's disease and non-Hodgkin's lymphomas, and some cases of ovarian cancer. Many types of drugs are used and can be classified as cytotoxic, hormonal, targeted, or biologic agents.

The Range of Drugs For many years, researchers have tried to find a single drug—a "magic bullet"—that would cure cancer. This has yet to be found, but the targeted-therapy revolution has arrived and may herald new hope for a cure. Today, about 100 anticancer drugs are available on the market and many others are under investigation in a variety of cancers. These investigational drugs are supplied to clinical trial investigators under a special government license. Furthermore, to make drugs obtainable earlier for therapy, some drugs with an established role in treatment are also made available to practicing oncologists, even though they are not yet on the retail market.

The Goals and Possible Results of Therapy

Your doctor might recommend chemotherapy for several reasons. The goal might be

- to cure a specific cancer,
- to control tumor growth when a cure isn't possible,
- to relieve symptoms such as pain,
- to shrink tumors before surgery or radiation therapy, or
- to destroy microscopic metastases after tumors are removed surgically.

While surgery and radiation therapy are used to treat localized tumors, chemotherapy treats the whole body. It destroys malignancies of the blood, the bone marrow, and the lymphatic system (leukemias and lymphomas). It destroys cancer cells that have broken off from solid tumors and spread through the blood or lymph system to various parts of the body.

Neoadjuvant Therapy This form of chemotherapy involves giving drugs before surgery or radiation therapy and is intended to shrink tumors so that surgery or radiation will be more effective. Neoadjuvant chemotherapy usually involves combinations of drugs known to be effective against particular tumors. The drugs are given in the highest dosages the patient can tolerate. If the patient's tumor responds and gets smaller, the ability to completely remove the tumor

is enhanced. For example, neoadjuvant therapy is commonly used in patients with breast cancer who have large, difficult-to-resect breast masses and who desire breast reconstruction later on in the course of their care. Note that the same drugs can often be used effectively after definitive surgery or radiation is performed.

Adjuvant Therapy When chemotherapy is used to eliminate small invisible metastases after surgery or radiation therapy, it is known as adjuvant therapy. This is given when there is a high risk of a cancer recurring because small cells that couldn't be detected during surgery or any other way may remain and later grow back.

Adjuvant chemotherapy usually involves combinations of drugs known to be effective against particular tumors. The active drugs are given after recovery from surgery (usually within four to eight weeks) in full dosages according to patient tolerance, since the longer the delay, the less chance of cure. Radiation is sometimes used as a component of adjuvant therapy as well.

What Chemotherapy Can Achieve There are four possible results of chemotherapy given for visible or known areas of cancer:

- *Complete Remission* The tumor may seem to disappear completely, meaning that there is a complete response to the drugs. This clearly indicates the treatment is working, but it will most likely be continued for several more cycles so that any "hidden" cancer cells can be destroyed. Current detection methods can miss an internal tumor smaller than half an inch (about 1 cm) and if treatment is stopped too soon, there is a high chance for a relapse.

Some remissions, especially for very responsive tumors, may be permanent, while others may be temporary, lasting for months or even years, only to reappear or begin to grow again. Complete remission, therefore, is not necessarily the same as a cure. *Cure* usually means the lack of any sign of cancer for at least five years, but how it's defined really depends on the kind of cancer being treated and on the individual patient.

• *Partial Remission* The tumor may shrink by more than half its size but not disappear. This is obviously a good result, but therapy has to be continued until the tumor either completely disappears or stops shrinking. If it simply stops shrinking, the drug regimen may be changed or surgery or radiotherapy may be used to remove or try to wipe out the remaining tumor or tumor cells.

• *Stabilization* The tumor may neither shrink nor grow. This can be looked on as a favorable result of therapy, but the oncologist will prefer that the treatment causes the tumor to shrink, especially if the goal is complete remission. If the response is stabilization, the effect may be brief and the tumor may start growing again. The period of stabilization can sometimes last for months or years.

• *Progression* The tumor may keep growing despite therapy. Sometimes the response to treatment is slow, meaning that it may take several cycles for the treatment to work. For some tumors, like breast cancer or ovarian cancer, it often requires at least three cycles of treatment before one can say that the therapy is not working. The task of the oncologist is to discover this as soon as possible after the therapy has had a fair trial. Then an alternate treatment regimen can be planned.

How Anticancer Drugs Work

Like normal, healthy cells, cancer cells go through a continuous process of change. Each cell divides into two daughter cells. These cells grow, rest, and then divide again. The drugs used in chemotherapy are powerful chemicals designed to interrupt this cycle and either stop the cells from growing or alter their growth rate.

Several different types of drugs are used in chemotherapy. Each type kills cells at a different stage of the cell's life cycle. Each does its job in a different way.

• *Antimetabolites* attack the cells during the growth process of the cell cycle, when they are more easily killed. The antimetabolites imitate normal cell nutrients (nucleotides) and get incorporated into the important cellular components, particularly DNA and RNA. The "antivitamin" methotrexate, for example, resembles the normal vitamin, folic acid. The cancer cell consumes the drug— "thinking" it's getting a good meal—but instead starves to death because of lack of essential folic acid.

• *Alkylating agents* attack all the cells in a tumor whether they are resting or dividing. These drugs bind with the cells' DNA in various ways to prevent reproduction.

• *Antitumor antibiotics* insert themselves into strands of DNA. They either break up the chromosomes or inhibit the DNA-directed synthesis of RNA that the cell needs to grow.

• *Alkaloids* prevent the formation of chromosome spindles necessary for cell duplication.

• *Hormones* such as estrogen and progesterone inhibit the growth of some cancers, although how they work is not clearly understood.

• *Targeted drugs* attack cells by targeting molecular abnormalities that are present in tumor cells but not normal cells. Some agents target the environment of the tumor cell, the stroma or extracellular matrix, while others may prevent new blood vessels from forming, all of which are vital for tumor growth. Other targets include cell receptors on the surface or within the cell that signal downstream events, such as cell growth, angiogenesis (new blood vessel growth), and changes in genes.

Drug Combinations Combination chemotherapy uses two or more drugs given according to a plan designed to inhibit or kill as many cancer cells as possible.

Drugs that attack tumor cells at every stage of their life cycle—called noncell-cycle-specific drugs—may be given first to reduce the size of the tumor. This may activate the remaining cells to divide. When they do, cell-cycle-specific drugs that attack dividing cells will be given. Other sequences of other drugs can also be devised to maximize the therapeutic effect.

This is much like fighting a war, making sure you use all your forces on several fronts with repeated attacks. Your chances of winning the battle are greatly improved.

Drug Resistance Another advantage to giving drug combinations is that it reduces the chance that resistance to any one drug will develop.

Resistance is one very common reason why these agents fail to do what they're supposed to. A course of chemotherapy is often quite successful at first. The cancer responds, leading to a remission. But then, even though the drugs are still being given, there is a relapse and the cancer starts to grow again. A resistance to therapy has developed just like the resistance to penicillin or other antibiotics that can develop when treating an infection.

When this happens, the drugs in the treatment program have to be changed. Unfortunately, if you develop resistance to one drug or group of drugs, there may be less chance that your body will respond to another drug program.

Why Resistance Develops One of the mysteries of cancer therapy is why some people respond well to a treatment while others do not. Over the past two decades, research on drug resistance led to speculation that multiple resistances developed during therapy and that this was responsible for progressive and uncontrollable metastatic disease.

More recent research has begun to explain how cancer cells become resistant to drugs. There is a protein called P-glycoprotein on the surface of a cancer cell. This protein acts like a pump, regulating the passage of drugs into and out of the cancer cell. Tumor cells with larger amounts of P-glycoprotein may not allow any drugs to enter. This, of course, makes chemotherapy ineffective.

There are now ways to measure the amount of this protein, so it can often be predicted whether a cancer will be resistant to chemotherapy. P-glycoprotein genes have also been discovered, which may explain why some cells in a tumor are resistant to drugs while others are not. This in turn may explain why some drugs are not effective when administered, even when a drug sensitivity test indicates that the tumor *should* be sensitive to a certain drug. Researchers are trying to overcome drug resistance related to P-glycoprotein.

How the Drugs Are Given

The drugs used in chemotherapy are very powerful. The line between a therapeutic and a toxic dose is so fine and the consequences of the wrong dose so severe that general physicians without special training don't prescribe them. Chemotherapeutic agents are usually given only by oncologists, usually medical or pediatric oncologists (specialists in the medical treatment of cancer) and hematologists (specialists in diseases of the blood), although some surgical and gynecological oncologists also give chemotherapy.

Delivery Routes and Methods The drugs can be delivered to your circulatory system by many different routes. They can be taken orally in capsule, pill, or liquid form; given by injection through a syringe into a vein, artery, or muscle; given intravenously through an IV infusion device; given by intrathecal or intraventricular injection, which means a shot into the fluid surrounding the spinal cord or brain; or by intraperitoneal injection, directly into the abdomen.

Single or multiple drugs can also be injected directly into an organ such as the liver, using a small pump to ensure a constant flow. An external pump might be used, although internal pumps can now be surgically implanted and remain in the body for several weeks or months or permanently (see chapter 6, "What Happens in Surgery," for illustrations of catheters, ports, and pumps).

Each delivery route has its advantages and disadvantages.

• *Intravenous* For intravenous delivery, you have to have a vein that can be entered easily without causing a lot of discomfort. This isn't always easy. Some people naturally have small veins. Sometimes the veins get "used up" after several chemotherapy sessions.

If a vein isn't easily accessible, a temporary plastic tube (catheter) can be implanted under the skin in the chest or in an arm or leg. These catheters, or central lines, as they are called, extend into larger veins. They provide an access point either for injections or for the slow drip (continuous infusions) of therapy over hours or even days. All kinds of fluids can enter the vein through the catheter—chemotherapy drugs, nutritional formulas, antibiotics, blood or platelet transfusions, antinausea drugs, or morphine or other painkilling narcotics.

The catheters avoid any discomfort from vein "sticking" and also any worry about having shots of irritating drugs that might leak out into the tissues. They can't be pulled out with an average pull or jerk, so they are quite safe. And they are simple to care for. They just need occasional cleaning and changing of the injection cap and periodic injections of heparin, a drug that prevents blood clotting in the catheter.

• *Implanted Infusion Ports* Another type of catheter is completely under the skin. It is called an infusion port, and it's filled by placing a special needle through the skin into the chamber. The chamber contains a rubber or Silastic cover that can be punctured thousands of times with a special needle to deliver therapy, antibiotics, or nutrients directly into a large vein.

The advantage of the implanted system is that since it is completely under the skin, no dressings or cleaning is needed and care is much simpler. Heparin injections won't be needed so often either. The disadvantage is that there is a slight risk of the drug leaking out. Also, a port can occasionally get out of position and become more difficult to enter.

• *Ambulatory Pumps* Small portable pumps that deliver chemotherapy while you go about your normal activities are called ambulatory pumps (*ambulatory* just means you can walk around).

These devices are often about the size of a deck of cards. They hold the drug supply, a mechanism for injecting it slowly and smoothly into an attached catheter, a battery to power the mechanism, and controls for regulating the rate of drug delivery. Many of the pumps have become very sophisticated. Some have alarms to alert you to problems. One of the systems can deliver four separate drugs in a preset time sequence.

Several types are available. The balloon pump (Travenol infuser) is the cheapest and simplest, consisting basically of a large plastic reservoir. The pump is filled, then attached to a port or catheter. The pump empties automatically when it's connected.

• *Intrathecal or Intraventricular (Central Nervous System) Delivery* Some patients, such as those with acute leukemia, need chemotherapy drugs injected into the spinal fluid. This can be done by repeated lumbar punctures (spinal taps), but the preferred method is to use an Ommaya reservoir, a rubber bulb device usually placed under the scalp. A tiny tube connects the reservoir to the spinal fluid compartment. This requires a minor operation to put the reservoir bulb and tube in place. Drugs are injected through the skin into the reservoir. Infection in the reservoir area is a possibility, so patients are usually monitored for side effects such as tenderness, inflammation, fever, stiff neck, and headaches.

• *Intraperitoneal or Abdominal* This technique, which involves delivering drugs directly into the abdominal cavity, is sometimes used for ovarian or abdominal metastatic cancer. A catheter is connected to a chamber, usually on the chest or abdominal wall. The drugs are injected into the chamber, which releases them into the abdominal cavity. This eliminates the need to put a new tube into the abdomen every time drugs have to be given. High dosages can be given this way, higher than would be possible with any other method of delivery.

• *Intra-arterial Drugs* These drugs are often given to a specific area such as the liver, head and neck, or pelvis through the artery supplying that area. This is usually done in the hospital, where the delivery system can continuously infuse chemotherapy over a specific time. The drugs are given through a pump that can overcome arterial pressure.

• *Implantable Pumps* These special pumps were developed to be surgically implanted in the abdomen, usually over a lower rib. The pump is shaped like a hockey puck and has two chambers—one for the drug, the other for a fluid that forces the drug into the catheter. It also has a side port for chemotherapy injections. The pump can deliver a drug for as long as two weeks, then the chemotherapy solution can be replaced with salt water to give your system a rest.

Which Route to Use This decision depends on several factors, mainly the type of tumor and the drug being used. There are many questions to answer. Can the drug be absorbed in the stomach? How big a dose is required? What are the side effects? Are they tolerable?

Ultimately, the decision will be made on the basis of what is the most effective way to get the highest dosage of the right drug to the right place. Whichever route is chosen, your doctor will give you and your family or friends complete information on the usual effects of the drug, its side effects, any safety precautions to take, and what reactions to report.

Where the Drugs Are Given

Most injectable drugs are given by oncology nurses in an infusion clinic or the doctor's office. However, intravenous or peritoneal administration of some drugs requires a stay in the hospital for a few days. Some injections may be given by oncology nurses as part of a home care service.

If pills, liquids, or capsules have been prescribed, prescriptions may be filled in a community or specialty pharmacy. Oral drugs can be taken at home or at work. Even if you are taking the chemotherapy orally, however, you will still have to visit your doctor's office every so often so the tumor's response can be monitored and your blood counts analyzed. Some drug programs require more frequent office visits because the schedule can be fairly complex.

How Long Treatment Lasts

Cancer therapy is a fast-changing field, with new treatment schedules always being tested in clinical trials. Although new chemotherapeutic drugs are being developed, it is often the same standard drugs in new combinations or given on different schedules that make the difference between success and failure in destroying cancer cells.

So there are few hard-and-fast rules on how often drugs are given or how long treatment lasts. Apart from the ever-changing recommended treatments, every person is different, every tumor is different, and every chemotherapy program is tailored to fit the situation.

Chemotherapy is given in cycles of treatment. A cycle of therapy may consist of one drug being given for one or several days and last one, two, three, or four weeks. A course of chemotherapy may last four to six cycles.

It may take a relatively short period of time to receive some chemotherapy drugs, while it may take hours to receive others. It all depends on the treatment regimen that your doctor prescribes.

The length of treatment varies with different treatment programs.

• For programs that may be able to cure certain forms of cancer, even if widespread, the therapy is typically given for no more than about six months or up to a year in a few cases. This is true of Hodgkin's disease, some lymphomas, cancer of the testis, and adjuvant therapy for breast cancer and colon cancer.

• Where a remission has been achieved in various forms of metastatic cancer, treatment will be given until the maximum effect has been observed and then for a little while longer in an attempt to destroy hidden tumor cells. If therapy is stopped—unmaintained remission—it may be a long time before the tumor begins to grow again and more therapy is needed. But sometimes chemotherapy is continued indefinitely—maintained remission—until a relapse occurs, at which time the drug program will be changed.

• For programs in which chemotherapy is combined with radiotherapy, specific rules and formulas apply to each treatment protocol—prescribed doses, schedules, and drug combinations—which are generally followed exactly.

• There are similar standards for adjuvant chemotherapy programs for patients who have a high risk for recurrence. The therapy to wipe out small nests of cancer cells that cannot be detected is generally given for six months to one year.

Selecting the Right Drugs

Which drugs to use, alone or in combination, is decided on the basis of many factors, including the extensive guidelines for treatment in the cancer literature. Yet each treatment program is, in a sense, an experiment, since the results in a particular patient cannot be predicted. There are no guarantees. It is not possible to state ahead of time whether a certain drug or combination of drugs will stop or slow down tumor growth in a certain individual.

Doctors are able to estimate, for example, that perhaps 30 or 55 or 73 percent of patients can be expected to respond to a particular drug program for a particular tumor. But they cannot know until they conduct the treatment trial whether any one individual will respond with the hoped-for tumor shrinkage.

What *Response Rate* Means A misconception often arises when a doctor says that a drug has, say, a 60 percent response rate. Patients sometimes think this means that the drug will be at least partly effective against tumors in all treated patients. But to say a drug has that response rate is like saying that a diaphragm or condom is a 95 percent effective way of preventing conception. That figure doesn't mean that all women will become 5 percent pregnant. It means that those contraceptives work in 95 percent of the people who use them and don't work for the other 5 percent.

Similarly, a drug with an average response rate of 60 percent means that 60 percent of the patients receiving it will respond. But 40 percent will not, although tumor growth might be delayed in some of them.

Devising the Plan As with any plan for cancer treatment, the chemotherapy program your doctor recommends will be tailored to the precise stage of your particular kind of tumor, your age, your physical condition, and any other medical problems. He or she will generally be guided by some specific information.

• *What's Worked in the Past* Oncologists rely primarily on experience from clinical trials involving many patients with similar tumors. They will usually consult reports in medical journals and the research findings presented at cancer meetings. Since more and more literature on drug treatment is being produced every month, the updated cancer information provided by the Physician Data Query (PDQ) system of the National Cancer Institute should also be consulted. Such computer databases are now essential for physicians who want to keep track of the rapid changes in the field.

Many state-of-the-art treatments are part of clinical trial protocols available at major cancer centers as well as some community hospitals.

• *Drug Sensitivity* A great deal of research over the past two decades has been devoted to finding ways of predicting which drugs would kill which tumor cells most successfully. This research has involved growing an individual patient's cancer cells in the laboratory and testing a whole battery of anticancer agents on them.

This drug sensitivity test program—called a clonigenic assay—may give a doctor some guidance on which drugs to use. But it's especially useful for indicating which drugs *not* to use. If a drug doesn't kill single cancer cells in the lab, then it probably won't be effective in the body. So any drugs that are inactive in a laboratory test of a patient's tumor cells would not usually be used with that patient.

These tests may be useful in selected patients but are not yet the final solution to the problem of drug selection. Their usefulness is limited by a number of factors:

• The tumor may not grow in the laboratory, or only certain drug-sensitive cells may grow.

• There may be differences between the way the drug works in the body and the way it works in a test tube. In the body, the drug can be bound and inactivated, be eliminated by the kidneys, or not be allowed to get through the P-glycoprotein "gate" on the cell surface.

• These test procedures apply only to one or, at most, two drugs tested one at a time. But chemotherapy cures are generally produced only by combinations of many drugs.

• *The Possibility of Using Other Therapies* There is no one absolutely right choice in cancer therapy, and the treatments recommended can change over the course of the illness. One reasonable choice at a particular time may not be appropriate at a later time.

A woman whose breast cancer recurs in a nonvital place, for example, may have several options. Her doctor may recommend surgery, radiation treatment to the region to possibly control the cancer for years, hormone treatments, simple chemotherapy, complex chemotherapy, or even doing nothing until the cancer grows and starts to bother her in six months' or a year's time.

Each treatment option has advantages and disadvantages, and there may be more than one option that is sensible.

Selecting the Right Dosage

Larger doses of chemotherapy drugs may result in more cancer cells being killed, but a balance has to be struck between improved therapeutic effects and unacceptable toxic effects. It may *not* be a kind act for your doctor to limit the dosage to avoid toxic effects. For those tumors that can potentially be cured with chemotherapy or have a good chance of going into remission, reducing the dosage to minimize toxicity will also reduce the possibility of cure or remission. The kindest act is to provide the maximum safe dose for cure, even at the cost of some toxicity. When the risks are weighed against the benefits, it doesn't make sense to take all the risks yet fail to get the benefits because the dosage was too low.

When Therapy May Be Stopped Because of Side Effects There is no reason to stop therapy when the drugs produce few problems and the control of the tumor is very satisfactory or even barely satisfactory. But major or objectionable side effects or complications can only be justified by a very significant and pronounced antitumor response.

The decision to stop therapy really depends on how you and your doctor define *objectionable* and what you are willing to put up with. Most men with metastatic testis cancer, for example, can be cured with less than six months of chemotherapy. Naturally, both doctors and patients are usually willing to put up with more discomforting side effects in that case because of the improved chance of cure. The alternative would be fatal.

What is important is for the doctor to give an adequate dosage of drugs—one that would be expected to produce results if that particular tumor in that particular patient happens to be sensitive. Then, after waiting an appropriate time—often about two or three months—tests will show if the tumor is shrinking.

High-Dosage Chemotherapy A variety of exciting programs for high-dosage chemotherapy continue to be tested in major cancer centers. The hope is that greatly increased dosages may cure some malignancies that may not be curable with standard dosages. Various supportive measures may be used with these programs to decrease the toxic effects of the higher dosages, although in some cases, it is known that increased dosages may be given without the need for additional measures.

A very aggressive supportive measure is removing early blood-forming cells—called stem cells—from the body before very high dosage chemotherapy is given. These stem cells are preserved, then reinjected to reestablish normal blood production and blood counts. This procedure used to be called bone marrow transplantation. A more appropriate term is *bone marrow protection*.

Patients with high-risk cancer (e.g., acute leukemia) may receive high-dosage chemotherapy and transplanted bone marrow to replace the diseased tissue or cancer-affected normal organ. In the case of high-dosage chemotherapy, the early blood-forming cells do not replace any diseased tissue. The anticancer treatment is the chemotherapy, not the removal and reinjection of early blood cells.

Peripheral stem cells can now be removed from veins using special equipment. Although bone marrow may also be collected as a backup, many high-dosage chemotherapy programs depend primarily on stem cell removal and subsequent administration. Research is determining the role of high-dosage chemotherapy with stem cell protection in treating several potentially curable malignancies (see chapter 15, "Bone Marrow and Blood Stem Cell Transplantation").

Measuring the Response

There are several ways to tell if a tumor is responding to treatment. They are often the same methods used to diagnose the tumor in the first place—physical examination, X-rays, blood tests, and scans. These same tests will have been done before treatment to establish a baseline for future comparisons.

• A lump or a tumor involving lymph nodes can be felt and measured directly. The size of the liver, the spleen, and other organs can also often be determined by physical examination. Your doctor will record these measurements in your chart and compare them from time to time to see if the size of the tumor is decreasing.
• Some tumors, such as those involving the lungs, show up on X-rays. If new X-rays are taken at one-, two-, or three-month intervals, the size of the tumors on the X-ray film can be measured with a ruler.
• Internal tumors, such as those involving the liver or other organs, are more difficult to measure. Special techniques need to be used—scanning using radioactive tracer isotopes, CT, or MRI. Again, the size of the tumor as shown on the image can be measured directly at various intervals.
• Some tumors produce a substance that can be detected in the bloodstream. For example, colon cancer produces carcinoembryonic antigen (CEA), and ovarian cancer produces cancer antigen 125, or CA-125. These tumor markers can be used to assess response to treatment or progression.

Monitoring Blood Counts

Cytotoxic drugs used in chemotherapy are growth inhibitors. They are especially good at turning off cells that are growing very quickly. Unfortunately, the drugs are not selective in their action. They turn off every fast-growing cell. There is no way the drugs can tell an abnormal cell from a normal one.

The most important rapidly growing normal cells affected by the drugs are the blood cells. The red cells that carry oxygen are not usually affected very much. But the levels of the white cells (which fight infection) and the platelets (which stop bleeding) usually fall during chemotherapy.

There are no symptoms of a minor decrease in blood counts. A slight decrease isn't harmful anyway. In fact, blood counts are expected to fall. This ensures that the drugs are being given in the maximum possible safe dosage. The lowered counts also show your doctor that the drugs are doing what they are supposed to do—stop fast-growing tissues from growing. If there is enough drug in your system to stop white blood cells, then there is enough to have a potential effect on other rapidly growing cells, namely the cancer cells.

Still, it is very important that your doctor keep a close watch on the blood cells. The blood counts have to be measured regularly, usually before each chemotherapy treatment. If the counts are normal, it may be safe to give the standard dose or even increase the drug dosage. If one of the counts is too low, a drug dose can be modified or even put off for a while. When a therapy session is skipped because of low counts, this does not mean that the cancer cells will get out of control. The rest period is a normal part of the therapy, done for safety reasons.

The Danger of Infection A very low white blood cell count could lead to serious infections, and a very low platelet count could lead to bleeding. If the white blood count or platelet count falls lower than is safe, a rest period will allow the blood counts to recover. If you have fever, chills, or any other sign of infection, like a cough or sore throat, during chemotherapy, call your doctor so therapy can be stopped until the infection has been treated effectively. Chemotherapy may suppress your immune system, making it harder for you to fight off infections. Any infection might spread and could become serious.

Minimizing Infection To lessen the chance of a serious infection developing, it is sometimes useful to administer a colony-stimulating factor (CSF) such as G-CSF (filgrastim [Neupogen] or pegfilgrastim [Neulasta]) or GM-CSF (sargramostim [Leukine]). This practice minimizes the time when the white blood cell count is low. These agents are also used to improve a low white blood cell count after an infection has already developed.

Certain aggressive chemotherapy programs may incorporate CSFs into the treatment plan. This may allow for the safer use of higher dosages of chemotherapy. It may also increase what is called dose intensity. This means that the chemotherapy schedule can be completed without any delays caused by low white blood cell counts. Improved dose intensity has improved the remission rate in a number of responsive cancers.

Dealing with Side Effects

The prospect of chemotherapy can be frightening. This is not surprising, seeing as how the side effects have been portrayed so horrifically in the popular press. Word of mouth hasn't helped either. Everyone seems to know of an uncle of a friend of someone at work who had just a terrible time. But the side effects are usually not nearly as bad or troublesome as your friends may have told you or as you may have read about or seen on TV.

Many people tolerate chemotherapy very well and have few negative reactions. The person who visits the doctor's office, gets a shot for colon or breast cancer, then goes home or back to work and functions fairly well rarely appears on television or gets written up in the papers (see chapter 20, "Coping with the Side Effects of Chemotherapy," and chapter 19, "Living with Cancer").

Taking the Right Approach More than 100 drugs are used in cancer chemotherapy. Some produce very few side effects and are easy to take. Others can cause major problems that have to be combated with appropriate medications. It is also important to remember that some of the most active drugs against cancer are also the ones that provoke the most side effects.

You should try hard to put any fears behind you. Fear of treatment and fear of side effects is a major problem, for anxiety can make the reaction worse. Supportive care, counseling, and antianxiety drugs may become vital to making sure therapy continues. A more relaxed attitude toward chemotherapy may well lead to fewer bad experiences.

Approach chemotherapy with the knowledge that it is impossible to attack cancer cells with drugs without also affecting normal tissues. As mentioned earlier, the drugs are most effective against rapidly growing cells. Tumor cells grow rapidly. So do hair follicles, the bone marrow, and the cells in the lining of the gastrointestinal tract—mouth, stomach, and bowel.

There are basically two kinds of side effects of chemotherapy, immediate and chronic.

Immediate Side Effects These are mainly nausea and vomiting. Both can occur soon after treatment, but both usually go away fairly quickly. Fortunately, a number of very effective antinausea medications have been developed over the years. They are often given two, three, or four at a time, sometimes intravenously, and can usually prevent major problems with both nausea and vomiting. Very often, your doctor will have to try different combinations of antinausea medications if the first combination isn't working as well as you both would like.

Sometimes these nausea medications produce their own side effects, mainly sleepiness or general fatigue. But these minor effects are well worth the trade-off if you can avoid feeling sick. Treatment schedules can also be arranged so that the medication does not disrupt your life too severely. Chemotherapy may be given on a Friday, for example, so that any tiredness will wear off enough by the following Monday and you can return to work.

Chronic Side Effects Since fast-growing cells are affected the most, there may be some hair loss, sore mouth, nausea, diarrhea, lowered blood counts, or secondary cancers.

Hair Loss This problem occurs with some chemotherapeutic drugs, but not all. The amount of hair loss can vary from a slight thinning to baldness. The loss may be gradual or sudden. Sometimes all body hair—that of the head, eyebrows, legs, armpits, and pubic areas—may be lost. Depending on the drug used (and on the individual), hair loss on the head can be reduced by using a tourniquet or an ice cap. These narrow the blood vessels in the scalp so that less drug reaches the hair follicles.

The hair loss will be less upsetting if you plan ahead. Before treatment, get a short haircut so the loss won't be so noticeable. Get fitted for a scarf, turban, or wig. And keep in mind that hair loss is always temporary. Many people find that their hair starts growing back while they are still getting chemotherapy.

Sore Mouth A sore mouth or sores in your mouth are side effects of some drugs but last only a few days. Your doctor can prescribe medication to relieve any pain. Choosing soft, bland foods, rinsing

frequently with mild mouthwashes, and using a soft toothbrush will help.

Delayed Nausea Some drugs (cisplatin [Platinol], carboplatin [Paraplatin], cyclophosphamide [Cytoxan], and doxorubicin [Adriamycin]) may cause nausea that begins two to five days after administration.

Diarrhea Some drugs, such as fluorouracil, capecitabine (Xeloda), and irinotecan (Camptosar, CPT11), frequently cause diarrhea. Severe cases have been reported and have led to dehydration and electrolyte loss. Prophylactic antidiarrheals (Imodium) may be needed to prevent or treat severe diarrhea.

Low Blood Counts Depressed blood counts can have several effects, depending on which blood component is low.

• Low red cell counts may lead to a general feeling of weakness. You can offset this effect by making sure you get enough rest and not overtaxing yourself in your daily activities.
• Low white cell counts leave you vulnerable to infection, so it will be important to avoid people with colds or the flu and to take other preventive measures (see chapter 20, "Coping with the Side Effects of Chemotherapy").
• Low platelet counts may lead to easy bruising and bleeding, so you'll have to take care to avoid cuts, burns, and injuries and to avoid aspirin and alcohol. If the platelet count is very low, you can get a transfusion. The bone marrow will usually return to normal in two or three weeks.

Some drugs have very specific side effects. Your doctor can spell these out for you, indicating your chance of having them and outlining special measures you can take to minimize or prevent them (see chapter 20, "Coping with the Side Effects of Chemotherapy"). For information on the latest drugs being used in clinical trials, see chapter 42, "The Impact of Research on the Cancer Problem: Looking Back, Moving Forward").

Late Development of Other Cancers Since most anticancer drugs can produce cell mutations, which can themselves produce cancers, a very small percentage of cancer patients receiving chemotherapy may years later develop secondary cancers from the chemotherapy. The most common type of such secondary cancer is acute leukemia, which may occur many years after usually prolonged and lengthy treatment with alkylating agents (e.g., cyclophosphamide [Cytoxan] and phenylalanine mustard [Alkeran]). Now that this problem has been recognized, oncologists limit the dosage of these drugs to the absolute minimum required to control the cancer and whenever possible may be able to substitute other types of chemotherapy agents. Although the risk of developing acute leukemia after treatment with alkylating agents is very low, using them is sometimes justified, since the advantages are great and the risks are small. For additional information, see *Everyone's Guide to Cancer Supportive Care* by Ernest H. Rosenbaum, M.D., and Isadora R. Rosenbaum, M.A., and the Web site *www.cancersupportivecare.com.*

— 9 —

What Happens in Biological Therapy and Immunotherapy

John W. Park, M.D., and Malcolm S. Mitchell, M.D.

■ ■ ■ ■

Biological therapy, also referred to as immunotherapy, is a relatively new way to treat cancer. The term *biological therapy* is sometimes used to refer to all of the therapies outside of surgery, radiation, and chemotherapy and thus can mean targeted therapies more generally. This chapter will focus primarily on immunotherapy; please refer to chapter 44, "Investigational Anticancer Drugs," and chapter 14, "Antiangiogenesis," for more details on other classes of novel agents.

Immunotherapy is based on the idea that the human immune system, which is designed to eliminate and destroy any foreign substance found inside the body, can play a role in targeting and killing cancer cells.

There are a number of obstacles to successful immunotherapy. One of the most challenging is that the immune system doesn't always treat cancer cells as "foreign." It is relatively easy for our immune system to recognize bacteria or viruses, since they are quite different from normal human cells. But the difference between a tumor cell and a normal cell is small.

Significant progress has been made, however, and immunotherapy is now an accepted treatment for some cancers. Current immunotherapy includes treatment with immune system proteins, including cytokines and antibodies. Cytokine therapy is designed to activate the immune system and help it do its job more effectively. Interferon and interleukin-2 (IL-2) are the best known of these cytokines. Monoclonal antibodies, which are artificially produced versions of the body's antibodies, are typically used to go after specific targets on cancer cells. Other types of immunotherapy, including cancer vaccines, are under active study.

How Your Immune System Works

To understand the role that biological agents play in cancer treatment, it helps to know how the normal immune system works.

When something foreign, such as a bacteria, virus, or tumor cell, gets into your body, several kinds of cells go into action (the "immune response").

• *Antigen-Presenting Cells* These cells include macrophages, dendritic cells, and other white blood cells. These are the body's front line of defense. They are the first cells to recognize and engulf foreign substances (antigens). They break down these antigens, then present the resulting smaller proteins to the T lymphocytes (which results in the production of antibodies and T cell–mediated immune responses).

• *Lymphocytes* These are members of the body's white blood cells, and include the B and T cells.

B lymphocytes produce antibodies—proteins (gamma globulins) that recognize antigens and attach themselves to them.

T lymphocytes are the cells programmed to recognize, respond to, and remember antigens. When stimulated by the antigenic materials presented by macrophages, the T cells make lymphokines that signal other cells. The T cells are also able to destroy cancer cells on direct contact.

Subsets of T cells—called helper or suppressor T cells, depending on their function—are involved in stimulation or inhibition of antibody production in collaboration with B lymphocytes.

• *Other White Blood Cells* Other cells involved in the body's defenses include *neutrophils*. If you have an infection, their number increases rapidly. They are the major constituents of pus and are found around most common inflammations. Their job, like that of macrophages, is to "eat" (ingest) and destroy foreign material, especially bacteria and fungi.

How Immune Cells Interact The immune response is a coordinated effort. All these immune cells have to work together and therefore require communication with each other. They do this by secreting special protein molecules called cytokines that act on other cells.

There are many different cytokines—interleukins, interferons, tumor necrosis factors, prostaglandins, and colony-stimulating factors, for example. Some immunotherapy strategies involve giving large doses of these proteins, either alone or in combination. This is done in the hope of stimulating the cells of the immune system to act more effectively against the tumor.

Types of Immunotherapy

Cancer immunotherapy can be classified into the following types of strategies:

• *Active versus Passive* Therapies seeking to improve the immune response against cancer can either stimulate the patient's existing immune system or provide new components to replace or add to the patient's immune system. The first strategy is called "active" immunotherapy and includes treatment with immune system modulators such as "adjuvants," as well as vaccines. The second strategy, called "passive" or "adoptive," involves transferring to the patient certain immune system components, such as antibodies or cells.

• *Specific versus Nonspecific* Immunotherapy can be directed against a particular target (the "antigen") on cancer cells, in which case it is referred to as antigen-specific therapy. Examples of antigen-specific strategies include most cancer vaccines and all monoclonal antibodies. Alternatively, immunotherapy can seek to augment or improve the immune system's effectiveness in general, which is a nonspecific approach because the therapy is not directed against a particular antigen. Nonspecific strategies include treatments with cytokines such as interferon and interleukin-2.

Biological Agents

The most notable types of biological agents are discussed below:

Interferons (IFNs) There are three main types of interferon: alpha, beta, and gamma. Interferon-alpha was among the first of the cytokines shown to have an antitumor effect, both a direct effect on cancer cells and indirect effects by activating the immune system.

Studies have shown that interferon-alpha can help to fight a number of different cancers, including malignant melanoma, kidney cancer, and chronic myelocytic (myelogenous) leukemia. For example, interferon-alpha has been approved for use in postsurgical treatment of melanoma with positive lymph nodes (Stage III). Treatment at a high dose for a year was shown to be helpful for this stage of the disease, meaning that fewer patients experienced recurrence of melanoma if they received this treatment (see the chapter "Melanoma").

Interleukins This is a rather large family of protein molecules, which are all part of the communication network used within the immune system. Thus far, the only one approved by the FDA is IL-2, which has been used for treatment of kidney cancer and melanoma. IL-2 increases the activity of T lymphocytes, especially killer T cells that can identify and destroy tumor cells. Optimal therapy involves intravenous treatment with high doses of IL-2. This treatment can occasionally provide long-lasting effects against cancer but can also cause a number of serious side effects.

Colony-Stimulating Factors (CSFs) The CSFs are not directly effective against tumors, but they do play a major role in increasing the number and the activity of neutrophils and/or macrophages.

One area in which CSFs have been particularly helpful is in boosting the bone marrow against the effects of cancer treatment. It is well known that chemotherapy dramatically reduces the number of white blood cells (mainly neutrophils) that fight infection, making chemotherapy patients vulnerable to certain bacterial and fungal infections. It is for this reason that the dosage of chemotherapy often has to be kept low, thwarting any attempts to give higher and potentially more effective doses. Today the number of neutrophils can be increased by using colony-stimulating factors (such as G-CSF [granulocyte–colony-stimulating factor] and GM-CSF [granulocyte macrophage–colony-stimulating factor]), which directly stimulate the production of new neutrophils from the bone marrow. Infections are

therefore less common and less severe. The CSFs allow greater doses of chemotherapy to be given, which in turn may lead to more effective treatment.

T Cells Some investigators are studying the use of T cells in the fight against cancer. For example, many tumor vaccines are designed to activate T cells in the body. Another approach is to remove a large number of T cells from a patient—either from the bloodstream or from within the tumor itself—in order to stimulate them in the laboratory and then reintroduce them into the patient as an "autologous" (from same patient) treatment. Although this approach is still being researched, there have been some promising results in animals and in small studies with humans. Once again, melanoma and kidney cancer seem to be the most readily affected.

Cancer Vaccines One type of immunotherapy that has been studied for years and is only now coming of age is "active specific immunotherapy," more commonly known as the use of cancer or tumor vaccines. As discussed above, cancer vaccines are "active" because they seek to stimulate the patient's own immune system, and are "specific" because they are usually designed to boost the immune response against particular antigens present in the tumor.

Cancer vaccines would in theory work the same way as vaccines for measles, smallpox, and other infectious diseases. However, a major difference is that cancer vaccines are being developed for use *after* someone has cancer rather than as a preventative. Cancer vaccines can be given to prevent recurrences or to get the body to reject existing tumors, although this is easier said than done. Nevertheless, encouraging results have now been obtained in a variety of cancer types. For example, in melanoma, certain vaccines have produced some degree of clinical response. Advances in cancer vaccines include more sophisticated techniques to stimulate key immune cells, such as antigen-presenting cells and T cells.

Antiangiogenesis (Blocking Blood Vessel Formation) This targeted therapy attempts to starve the tumor by preventing it from generating new blood vessels (see chapter 14, "Antiangiogenesis"). A tumor has to make many new vessels to support its growth, whereas normal organs do not—this gives doctors a selective strategy against the cancer. Antibodies and drugs have been designed to block the substances produced by the tumor or their target on blood vessels, making it possible to inhibit tumor growth.

Gene Therapy Gene therapy, the technique of inserting genes into tumor cells, immune cells, or other cells, is in its infancy. Gene therapy has been used in experimental systems to improve the immune response against cancer, as part of a vaccine or as a treatment directed to the patient's immune system. Also, in many cancers, an abnormal (transformed or mutated) oncogene and/or the absence (deletion) of tumor suppressor genes causes the cancer to develop. Replacing defective or absent genes with properly working ones in susceptible people could stop the disease from progressing (see chapter 45, "Advances in Cancer Biology").

Monoclonal Antibodies Antibodies are proteins that are produced by B lymphocytes. Every B lymphocyte produces one kind of antibody that recognizes a foreign structure, or antigen. If the antibody comes into contact with the antigen, it will become attached to it.

The field of biotechnology has produced man-made antibodies in the laboratory, also known as monoclonal antibodies (MAbs). This invention allows researchers to clone B lymphocytes from mice immunized against specific antigens. Each clone produces a specific antibody, which is thus called a "monoclonal" antibody. These antibodies react against tumor-associated proteins on the cancer cell surface and can be used to see where the tumor is in the body or to direct attached killer molecules—such as radioisotopes or chemotherapy drugs—to the vicinity of the tumor. Another biotechnology advance is the production of MAbs (which originally came from mice) that are more similar to human antibodies. This means it is now possible to avoid many of the allergic side effects the mouse antibodies used to cause. Longer courses and larger, repeated doses of the antibodies can also be given.

Monoclonal antibodies can be used by themselves as a treatment against cancer cells. They can target specific cancer-promoting processes such as those associated with oncogenes (see chapter 45, "Advances in Cancer Biology"). They can also work in concert with the immune system to reject tumors. This is based on the principle that a tumor cell surrounded by antibodies is more vulnerable to destruction by cells of the immune system.

MAbs can also be programmed to deliver other anticancer agents, such as chemotherapy drugs or toxins, to the tumor. This is antibody-guided treatment. The monoclonal antibody homes in on the cancer cell, latches onto it, and lets the payload of drugs or toxins do their work.

Caution and Hope

Many promoters of unproven and useless anticancer treatments claim that their product or therapy improves the immune system and so will probably cure cancer. As an educated consumer of health care services, you should beware of any such false claims about new agents that augment the immune system. Except for some rare tumors such as Kaposi's sarcoma and some lymphomas that often result from immune suppression, there is as yet no definite proof that most cancers are caused by failure of the immune system. Furthermore, rather simple solutions (certain kinds of diets, vitamins, etc.) to the complex questions of immunity and cancer are not scientifically sound.

This does not mean, however, that stimulating the immune system will not treat cancers effectively. After many years of intensive investigation, therapies involving cytokines and monoclonal antibodies have become standard and important treatments for a number of cancer types. Research on these and other approaches, including cancer vaccines, is ongoing and has the potential to yield more and better treatments in the fight against cancer.

— 10 —

Laser Therapy

V. Raman Muthusamy, M.D., Carlos A. Pellegrini, M.D., and David R. Byrd, M.D.

■ ■ ■ ■

Laser therapy involves the use of high-intensity light to destroy tumor cells. Lasers have increasingly been used as part of the anticancer arsenal, and their role in the treatment of malignancy is now better defined. Laser therapy can completely eliminate cancer in some patients who are diagnosed early in their disease. However, this technique is mainly used to relieve serious symptoms such as bleeding and obstruction, especially in advanced cancers that can't be cured by surgery, radiation, or chemotherapy. In addition, it is often used when standard treatment isn't viable because of advanced age, poor nutritional status of the patient, or heart or pulmonary disease.

Increasingly, there is data suggesting that laser therapy can destroy precancerous tissue with replacement of this tissue with normal tissue during the healing phase. Successful treatment of early cancer of the esophagus has also been reported, but whether this can be used routinely as standard therapy for such tumors is still under investigation.

How Lasers Work

The word *laser* is an acronym for "light amplification by stimulated emission of radiation." The light is produced by devices that can "excite" substances such as carbon dioxide, argon, and neodymium:yttrium-aluminum-garnet (Nd:YAG) to a higher energy state. As these substances return to their "resting" state, they release their extra energy in the form of a powerful light with a special "energy" that is capable of vaporizing human tissue, including tumor cells.

What makes this type of energy so useful in cancer treatment is that it can be aimed so precisely. Lasers focus on very small areas with extreme accuracy.

Endoscopic Laser Therapy Laser therapy is usually given by activating the special light beam through a flexible tube called an endoscope, the same instrument used to diagnose many cancers. The scope can be passed through any opening in the body—the mouth, nose, anus, or vagina.

A laser operator looking through the scope can see the tumor directly and aim the light beam precisely into the target tissue. The operator then activates the device and the energy is produced. On contact with the tissue, the laser beam produces an intense heat. At 140°F (60°C), this heat can coagulate protein. At 212°F (100°C), it can vaporize tissue. The tissue usually burns for just a few seconds, giving off a bit of smoke and leaving a hole or ulcer.

Destroying a tumor with a laser beam is not as effective as removing it with conventional surgery. A surgeon can remove all the visible tumor, including the tumor below the surface of the organ and a wide margin of tissue on each side. The laser operator removes only the visible tumor on the organ's surface. However, tumors can be like icebergs, with the top being just the tip of a much greater mass below the surface. Thus, with some tumors, residual tumor may be left behind. In addition, since the tumor is destroyed and not removed, proof that all cancerous tissue has been removed or destroyed cannot be obtained after treatment. Rather, only by observation over time can we determine the true effectiveness of tumor ablation therapy.

Photodynamic Laser Therapy In some cases, laser therapy can be used to destroy tumors by activating a drug in the target tissues by simply shining light of a certain wavelength on a region of the tumor. Thus, the laser here destroys the tumor not by direct heat energy, but by a chemical reaction that starts with the activation of the drug by the laser light. This form of therapy is known as photodynamic therapy, and has increasingly replaced thermal laser techniques in the treatment of cancers, particularly gastrointestinal tumors. The chemical is usually injected two days before the laser treatment is planned, so that the drug can be absorbed by the target tissue and can then make this tissue more sensitive to light. Malignant tissues, because they divide more rapidly than noncancerous tissues, have increased absorption of the chemical. The chemical is activated by light at a specific wavelength and thus is called a photosensitizer. After a tumor is sensitized by a chemical such as hematoporphyrin, a type of photosensitizer, the laser light is selectively applied only to the intended treatment region, leading to very precisely localized tissue destruction.

When Laser Therapy Might Be Recommended

Laser therapy is used primarily to treat cancers of the skin, trachea, lungs, esophagus, stomach, colon, rectum, anus, and bladder. Traditionally, it has been used to complement surgery, radiation, or chemotherapy as a definitive cancer treatment. However, recent select cases in patients with small tumors suggest that for cancers at a very early stage, treatment such as photodynamic therapy may be curative.

Direct laser therapy to cancer of the skin or cervix can be very successful. But the usual objective of laser therapy, particularly heat-generating lasers, is to help relieve an acute obstruction. This might be done so that surgery, radiotherapy, or chemotherapy can be used effectively. Or it may be done to keep some vital body tube open—the esophagus for swallowing, the trachea for breathing, or the colon, rectum, and anus for eliminating stool.

The benefits are usually short-term, however, and there are technical limitations. The best results are usually obtained in centers where the procedure is performed frequently by highly experienced endoscopists.

Planning the Treatment

Before laser therapy is even attempted on the trachea, bronchi, or gastrointestinal tract, the first thing to decide is whether an endoscopic biopsy needs to be done to verify the diagnosis.

The next step is a thorough clinical assessment. This may involve specific kinds of X-rays (such as a barium swallow or barium enema), CT or MRI scans, and ultrasound (either transabdominal or endoscopic). These imaging studies are needed to estimate the risk of bleeding and to map the exact shape and size of the tumor and any sharp angles (as in the colon or esophagus) that will have to be dealt with.

Endoscopic ultrasound is of great value, since it allows the tissue beneath the surface to be assessed at the time of endoscopy with the use of ultrasound. This technique has been shown to provide greater accuracy than CT, MRI, or other radiology tests in determining the depth of invasion of GI tumors. It is very important to know how much of the tumor is within the opening, or lumen, of the body tube and how much of it has extended through the wall of the lumen into surrounding tissues. The status of the lymph nodes is important, too, and this information is also obtained by both endoscopic ultrasound and radiology studies such as CT and MRI.

Treating an Obstruction in the Trachea

Tumors in the windpipe (trachea) can't be treated very successfully with standard treatments. Less than 30 percent of patients are candidates for surgical removal of the tumor, and radiotherapy has few long-term survivors. Yet if the goal of treatment is palliation of symptoms of airway obstruction or bleeding, laser therapy is a reasonable alternative.

Tracheal and endobronchial cancers can be directly seen through an endoscope and can be treated with an Nd:YAG laser (direct thermal laser) or via photodynamic therapy with the use of the light-sensitizing hematoporphyrin-type agents. The tumor usually grows back and another treatment will be needed within a few months. With intrabronchial lesions, this interval can be stretched out by "afterloading" iridium-192. This involves placing empty catheters next to the tumor through an endoscope, then inserting the radioactive materials into the catheters to deliver a specific dose of radiation. Thus, this is a form of localized radiation therapy.

Treating Colorectal Cancer and Anal Cancer

Laser treatment may also be curative in a few cases of colorectal cancer and anal cancer diagnosed at a very early stage. However, surgery, radiation, and chemotherapy remain the primary therapies for these cancers. As a result, the goal of laser therapy is usually for relief of obstructive or bleeding symptoms.

Colorectal Cancer If the purpose of laser treatment is to diminish or stop bleeding or to diminish the bulk of a tumor, one or two treatments will usually be enough.

When the obstruction is large, it may be hard to get the endoscope into the tumor. It may be necessary to pass a guide wire through the tumor mass and use a smaller scope. An alternative is to use a guide wire to insert a balloon to dilate the constricted area, which will also allow a small scope to be passed to accomplish laser treatment. In cases of severe obstruction where laser therapy is cumbersome or not successful, the placement of a metal mesh stent through the endoscope across the obstruction may be needed, and this therapy can often provide immediate relief of obstruction and its symptoms.

• The most successful treatments occur when the tumor is growing inward, extending into the bowel lumen rather than outward toward the layer of the colon or rectum beneath the inner surface (submucosa and muscularis layers).

• Short or smaller tumors and straight rather than curved or angulated areas of the colon are more successfully treated, because it is easier to point the laser and destroy the targeted area when the tumor is short and without angulation.

• The therapy is not curative and will require follow-up treatment to keep the lumen open every several weeks to a few months, depending on how fast the tumor is growing.

• In rare instances, an obstruction of the bowel from colorectal cancer may be decompressed by endoscopic laser therapy. This may allow surgery or other therapies to be planned on an elective rather than an emergency basis. Again, endoscopic stenting also plays an important role in achieving this goal when laser therapy is ineffective because of the size or location of the tumor.

Anal Cancer Anal lesions that are typically treated are a growing polyp or an obstructing cancer when surgery, radiotherapy, and chemotherapy are not appropriate treatments. Again, the best results from laser treatment are when the tumor is within the lumen rather than extending through the wall to adjacent tissues. A well-differentiated cancer that is small (less than 1 inch [2.5 cm]), nonulcerating, and growing into the lumen typically responds the best to laser therapy.

The procedure is the same as for colon cancer and can be repeated after a few days if you are in the hospital or a few weeks later if you are being treated as an outpatient. Several treatments might be needed to completely remove the obstruction. Of note, laser therapy is particularly useful in treating obstruction in this situation, as endoscopic stenting of the anus is not recommended due to the pain from the stent's metal mesh prongs pressing against the perianal area.

• Fluid might accumulate in the tissues from the laser therapy, which may temporarily intensify the obstruction or require pain-relieving medications.

• Retreatment is usually necessary several weeks to a few months after the obstruction is first relieved.

• Many studies have shown that the obstructed lumen can be kept open in approximately 90 percent of cases. Bleeding can be controlled in over 85 percent of cases.

Laser Therapy and Esophageal Cancer

Theoretically, laser therapy might be the only form of treatment needed for a very small tumor in the esophagus that could be completely vaporized via a thermal laser. More often, photodynamic therapy is used for such lesions.

While in the past, surgery was the treatment of choice, today patients with early esophageal tumors have a variety of treatment options. Many more tumors are being found at early stages, due both to the increased use of endoscopy in general and to screening programs that follow patients at elevated risk for developing certain esophageal cancers, such as those with Barrett's esophagus. In addition, these tumors can be very accurately staged with the use of endoscopic ultrasound and CT and PET scans. Thus, we can now have a good idea if a tumor is localized to the esophagus and is a good candidate for localized therapy, such as laser therapy (typically photodynamic therapy) along with localized resections of the tumor with the endoscope (called endoscopic mucosal resection). However, surgery with or without chemoradiation is recommended for patients with more advanced lesions that have spread beyond the surface layers of the esophagus or for patients with early tumors who do not want to undergo follow-up endoscopies, which are necessary to ensure complete tumor eradication in patients who receive endoscopic laser therapy.

But if the cancer can't be cured by surgery (and advanced esophageal cancer can seldom be cured), lasers can still help relieve the symptoms. When the tumor becomes so large that the opening of the esophagus—the lumen—gets blocked, swallowing food or sometimes even saliva is not possible. About 50 percent of patients can maintain their ability to swallow throughout their illness if a laser is used to restore the lumen by vaporizing the tissue blocking it. In addition, laser therapy can be useful in relieving repeat obstruction in patients who have previously been endoscopically stented and who have since had tumor regrow around or through the metal mesh of the stent.

Laser versus Endoscopic Stent Placement

As mentioned above, although laser therapy provides a safe and effective option for relief of esophageal obstruction, there are alternatives to laser therapy in treating swallowing problems. A tube, or stent, placed in the esophagus can achieve an esophageal opening for swallowing in more than 95 percent of patients. This procedure carries minimal morbidity and mortality with currently used stents. These stents are typically made of metal with flare ends to help them grip the esophageal tissue and stay in position. They may or may not have a covering on them, which is intended to prevent tumor regrowth through the mesh. Generally, these stents provide immediate relief of obstruction and may last six months or more. Repeat stenting within a stent can be performed if obstruction recurs, or laser therapy can be done with the stent to relieve obstruction.

The use of these stents does have some drawbacks. If the stent crosses the gastroesophageal junction, severe reflux (heartburn) symptoms and regurgitation may develop. In addition, the stent may dislodge or move down the esophagus or slide into the stomach, although this usually occurs only when chemoradiation is being performed. Should this happen, the stent can usually be retrieved with an endoscope during an endoscopic procedure and a new stent is reinserted. Lastly, stents are not typically used for upper esophageal tumors because of the discomfort caused by the metal prongs in the back of the throat.

Endoscopic Laser Treatment Pretreatment evaluation will again involve mapping the exact geometry of the tumor and staging the disease. The size, depth of penetration of tumor invasion, and lymph node status as determined by endoscopic ultrasound, CT, and PET will determine whether the tumor is operable and whether preoperative chemotherapy and radiation therapy is needed.

In the procedure itself (usually photodynamic therapy using a nonthermal laser and a photosensitizer), the endoscope will be passed through the mouth and down the esophagus to the tumor site. Only the top layers of the area illuminated by the laser will be affected. An opening of up to ½ inch (1 cm) can be achieved with a single treatment. However, several sessions might be needed to achieve an opening large enough to allow for eating most solid foods. These sessions are often spaced at forty-eight-hour intervals to allow tissue destruction to occur and to determine what additional therapy may be needed. For photodynamic therapy, as the photosensitizer is in the body for only a short time, treatment must be done within forty-eight to ninety-six hours of drug injection to have maximal benefit. Otherwise, reinjection of the photosensitizer is needed prior to retreatment. The laser technique chosen (thermal versus photodynamic therapy) and the specifics of the treatment (amount of energy used, length of area treated, etc.) vary based upon the specifics of the tumor and are determined by the treating physician.

Some general points that influence the choice of treatment are listed below:

• Lasers are most useful in the middle and lower esophagus, which is straight, and least valuable for tumors outside the esophageal wall.

• For direct thermal therapies, it is difficult to know how deep to go into the submucosa, since there are no good landmarks.

• There may be very narrow spaces (strictures) involved, which makes laser treatment more difficult. Dilating the esophagus first may help to allow the laser to enter the narrow space and target the most obstructive regions.

• There is a sharp corner (acute angulation) at the junction of the esophagus with the stomach that makes laser therapy in this area very difficult.

• Since only the tumor within the lumen is removed, tumors usually come back quickly. The therapy may have to be repeated every several weeks to keep the passage open.

• Laser therapy can help control bleeding as well as open a passageway to allow foods to be swallowed.

Finally, it should be noted that patients receiving photodynamic therapy have some side effects unique to this treatment modality. Because the photosensitizer is distributed at a small level in all tissues of the body (even though it is present in greater amounts in the cancerous tissue), exposure to the sun can cause a severe sunburn that is not prevented by sunscreen lotions. This is because the photosensitizer most often used requires light at 630 nm to be activated. However, sunlight (but not indoor lighting) contains this wavelength of light as well. As a result, patients receiving photodynamic therapy (but not thermal laser therapy) should not go out in the sun uncovered for a period of thirty to sixty days to avoid this sunburn. Other side effects of photodynamic therapy include short-term pain, fever, nausea or vomiting, and the possibility of stricturing of the esophagus of 20 to 40 percent when early nonobstructive cancer is treated.

Combining Lasers and Other Treatments

Different degrees of swallowing difficulty merit different approaches. Dilation of the esophagus before using chemotherapy or radiotherapy to help shrink the tumor may be the best way to get a functional esophageal opening that will improve the quality of life.

• Obstruction may occur with squamous cell esophageal cancer or with an adenocarcinoma of the stomach that grows upward to obstruct the esophagus.

Lasers might be used in combination with standard treatments for these cancers.

• There may be a longer survival for squamous cell carcinoma with laser therapy combined with radiation therapy. Squamous cell carcinoma and adenocarcinoma have the same results for laser treatment, with tumors on the surface (Stage I) being easier to treat than tumors under the surface (Stage II).

• Results are better if the lesions are less than 2 inches (5 cm) in diameter. In one study, lasers gave almost all the patients (97 percent) an open passageway, but only 70 percent could eat satisfactorily.

• After the obstruction is removed, radiotherapy with seed implants may help prolong the swallowing interval.

Laser Therapy and Bladder Cancer

The primary treatment for patients with carcinoma of the bladder is radical surgery. However, for patients unable to tolerate major surgery, lasers offer a minimally invasive palliative strategy. These tumors tend to grow and block the flow of urine in and out of the bladder and often bleed. Sequential laser treatments through a scope can shrink these tumors and eliminate their complications for extended periods of time.

The most promising use of lasers in management of tumors involving the bladder, ureter, and collecting system of the kidney (renal pelvis) is the use of photodynamic therapy by adding the photosensitizers mentioned above to laser therapy. This promises to give the maximal treatment to a "sensitized" tumor by lasers with the least injury to surrounding normal tissue, as tissues not exposed to the laser light are left undisturbed.

— 11 —

Hyperthermia

Penny K. Sneed, M.D., and I-Chow Joe Hsu, M.D.

▪ ▪ ▪ ▪

The idea of using heat to help destroy tumors has been around for a long time. In the early 1800s, there were medical reports that some people with cancer showed signs of tumor shrinkage after they developed high fevers. By the end of the 1800s, there were reports of some complete remissions because of high body temperatures. But the biology behind the use of elevated temperature—"hyperthermia"—for cancer treatment wasn't studied in depth until the 1960s and 1970s. Clinical trials of hyperthermia in cancer patients began in the 1970s, so this is a fairly new anticancer treatment modality.

Hyperthermia is usually combined with radiation therapy or chemotherapy. It is not applicable to all types of tumors and it is not widely available, but results have been very promising in certain studies.

How It Works

Mild-temperature hyperthermia in the range of 102 to 107°F (39 to 42°C) may improve the body's immune response against tumors and improve blood flow and oxygen supply to a tumor, potentially making the tumor more sensitive to radiation therapy and allowing better delivery of chemotherapy, immunotherapy, or gene therapy to a tumor. When temperatures rise above 106°F (41°C), the heat starts to damage cells. The amount of damage done depends on the temperature and the length of the exposure to

heat. Very high temperatures above 122°F (50°C) are sometimes used in a carefully controlled manner for tumor ablation. However, the temperatures that have generally been used for cancer treatment range from 106 to 113°F (41 to 45°C) for about an hour at a time.

Combining Hyperthermia with Other Therapies Heat is particularly effective when combined with radiation because heat is especially destructive to two types of cells that tend to be resistant to radiation:

• cells making DNA in preparation for division and
• cells that are acidic and starved for oxygen (poorly oxygenated). Unlike normal tissue, many tumors are likely to have poorly oxygenated cells. These cells may be three times more resistant to radiation than normally oxygenated cells, but they are particularly susceptible to hyperthermia.

Heat also makes cells more sensitive to radiation by preventing them from repairing radiation damage. Heat and radiation work best together when the two treatments are given simultaneously or within perhaps an hour of each other. Hyperthermia treatments are often given only once or twice weekly, because after cells are exposed to heat, they may become somewhat resistant to subsequent heating for up to three days.

Heat also seems to improve the effect of some of the drugs used in chemotherapy, such as bleomycin (Blenoxane), cisplatin (Platinol), cyclophosphamide (Cytoxan), doxorubicin liposomae (Doxil), melphalan (Alkeran), mitomycin-C, and the nitrosoureas.

Heating Techniques During the past thirty years, devices have become available to heat tumors directly.

Hyperthermia treatment techniques can be divided into four broad categories—superficial, interstitial, regional, and whole body heating.

• *Superficial heating* of tumors in or near the skin is often performed using an external applicator. This square or round box is placed on the outside of the body over the tumor. The applicator is connected to equipment that supplies different types of energy—microwave, radiofrequency, or ultrasound—that will heat the tumor region.

• *Interstitial (inside the tumor) hyperthermia* requires placement of needles or plastic tubes directly into the tumor, under anesthesia. Heat sources are then inserted into the plastic tubes, or radiofrequency current is passed through the needles. Interstitial techniques often raise the tumor temperatures much higher than could be done with external techniques and without doing much damage to surrounding normal tissues.

• *Regional hyperthermia* involves using radiofrequency or microwave applicators to heat large volumes of tissue deep inside the body.

• *Whole body heating* can be accomplished by using hot-water blankets, specialized ovenlike devices, or other methods. This procedure is safe for temperatures up to 107°F (42°C). This temperature may not be high enough to be effective in combination with radiation

therapy alone, but may become useful with chemotherapy or immunotherapy. Whole body and/or regional hyperthermia can also be combined with localized hyperthermia to improve tumor heating.

Although hyperthermia treatment may be given externally, the temperatures inside the tumor usually have to be carefully monitored to control the treatment properly. This often means that tiny thermometers have to be placed in the tumor region, usually inside one or more small needles or tubes that are gently inserted through the skin under a local anesthetic.

Side Effects Hyperthermia does not cause any marked increase in radiation side effects or complications. Hyperthermia by itself, however, can cause discomfort or even significant local pain in about half the patients treated. It can also cause blisters, which generally heal rapidly. Less commonly, it can cause burns, which tend to heal very slowly and occasionally need surgical repair.

How often blisters or burns occur depends on whether the tumor involves the skin and on the degree of skin cooling used during the treatment. In one study, heat blisters occurred in 10 percent of the superficial areas treated, but normal tissue ulceration occurred in less than 1 percent of cases. This indicates that burns can normally be avoided with careful monitoring and control of surface temperatures.

When Hyperthermia Is Appropriate

As a form of treatment, hyperthermia has had very limited success when used by itself. In one study, only 13 percent of superficial tumors treated with hyperthermia alone had a "complete response"—in other words, disappeared completely. But many studies in patients with superficial malignancies have shown benefits when hyperthermia is added to radiation therapy.

Randomized trials in Europe have proved the benefit of superficial hyperthermia in combination with radiation therapy for chest wall recurrences of breast cancer, as well as metastatic melanoma in the skin, lymph nodes, or tissues just under the skin.

A recent North American trial of radiation with hyperthermia for a variety of superficial cancers used a small test heat session before randomizing the "heatable" tumors to radiation without further heating versus radiation with twice-weekly hyperthermia for one or two hours. About 90 percent of tumors were found to be "heatable," and the complete response rate was 42 percent for radiation without additional hyperthermia compared with 66 percent for radiation with twice-weekly hyperthermia. The largest benefit was seen in patients who had been treated previously with radiation to the same area.

Interstitial hyperthermia has been used for some tumors in the head and neck, breast, pelvis (such as cervical and prostate cancer), skin or soft tissues, and for malignant brain tumors.

Regional hyperthermia has been used with radiotherapy for certain soft-tissue sarcomas and for pelvic tumors. In the Netherlands, a randomized trial showed the benefit for cervical cancer and bladder cancer.

New Directions Many exciting areas of investigation could make clinical hyperthermia more useful in the future. There is now a better understanding of how much hyperthermia is necessary to improve the results of radiation treatment, but many more studies are needed to explore mild-temperature hyperthermia along with chemotherapy, immunotherapy, and gene therapy. Technological advances are being made in the equipment needed to perform hyperthermia and to monitor temperatures noninvasively, to make hyperthermia safer, easier, more effective, and more widely applicable.

— 12 —

Cryosurgery

Katsuto Shinohara, M.D. (Prostate),
Terry Sarantou, M.D., and Leland J. Foshag, M.D. (Liver)

■ ■ ■ ■

Cryosurgery is a surgical treatment method using extreme cold (freezing). The term *cryotherapy* is often used interchangeably with *cryosurgery*, but *cryotherapy* has a broader meaning that includes the use of cold temperatures for many therapeutic purposes, such as relieving pain or reducing swelling or fever with cold packs. Many people are familiar with the use of cryotherapy by dermatologists for treating warts and by gynecologists for external tumors of the cervix.

Cryosurgery is a form of cryotherapy that uses special instruments to freeze tissues. The response varies from a mild inflammatory reaction, as would follow a minor freezing injury, to the destructive response that follows a severe cold injury, like frostbite.

Cryosurgery in Cancer Treatment

The effects of cold on tissue have been known since ancient times, with cold water and ice applications being used to treat such things as wounds, bleeding, infections, and external ulcers.

Cryosurgery as a treatment for cancer has a relatively short history. Iced saline (salt) solutions were first used in England in the 1850s to treat advanced cancers of the breast and cervix. The development of refrigeration agents and the mechanisms to deliver them safely led to the current practice of using hollow stainless steel vacuum-insulated probes (cryoprobes) to freeze structures either inside or on the surface of the body.

These probes are placed in a tumor. Liquid nitrogen (or argon gas) flows through the probes, freezing the surrounding tissue to a temperature of –320°F (–196°C). Current cryosurgery devices use pressurized argon gas as a refrigeration agent because it offers more effective and controllable freezing than liquid nitrogen. The rate of cooling, the lowest temperature achieved, and the number of freeze-thaw cycles performed are important factors for tissue destruction. An ultrasound device monitors the extent of the freezing. After the freezing is complete, the frozen tumor tissue thaws and is left to form scar tissue, which is not harmful to the body. Treated tumors inside the body are taken care of by the body's own reabsorbing process. Tumors on the surface are left to dissolve and form a scab.

In the United States, cryosurgery is currently used for primary and metastatic tumors of the liver and prostate, as well as kidney cancer and some bone and gynecologic malignancies. Encouraging results have been reported for tumors of the breast, lung, and brain, as well. Physicians in Europe and the Far East have used cryosurgery to treat some other types of tumors.

Cryosurgery for Liver Tumors

Cryosurgery offers a new therapeutic approach for primary and metastatic tumors of the liver that cannot be surgically removed.

Primary Tumors Primary cancer that starts in the liver (hepatocellular carcinoma, or HCC) is rare in the United States but very common among people from Asia. It is associated with exposure to the hepatitis virus, which is common in Asia and causes cirrhosis of the liver. The degree of underlying cirrhosis compromises the normal function of the liver, which limits the surgical options because of the possibility of liver failure after surgery. This cancer also frequently occurs in the form of multiple tumors that cannot be surgically removed because of the extent of disease at the time of diagnosis.

Cryosurgery is useful in these situations because it can limit the destruction of unaffected liver tissue.

Metastatic Tumors In the United States, the most common tumor to spread (metastasize) to the liver is cancer of the colon and rectum. More than 160,000 Americans develop colorectal cancer every year, with up to one-fourth of them having metastatic disease to the liver at the time of diagnosis. Liver metastases are also detected in many more patients after the diagnosis, such that by the time of death, up to 70 percent of patients with colorectal cancer have metastatic disease to the liver.

Other tumors that predominately metastasize to the liver, although less frequently, include kidney cancer, breast cancer, gastrointestinal carcinoma and sarcomas, neuroendocrine tumors, and

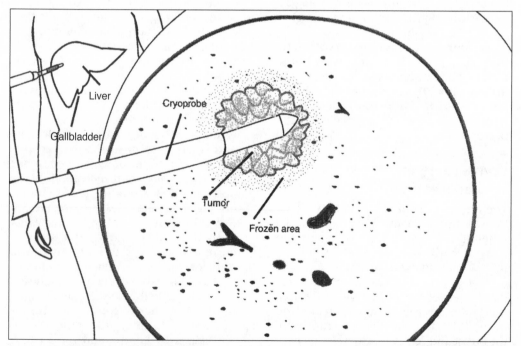

A cryoprobe inserted into the liver can kill a tumor by freezing it. The procedure is monitored by ultrasound, which can distinguish between frozen and normal tissue.

adenocarcinoma with unknown site of origin. Many people with these cancers die from the spread of cancer to the liver rather than lack of control of the original tumor.

In these cases, therapeutic options have been limited.

• Surgery offers the best chance for cure, but only about one in four patients is a candidate because there is often extensive disease, including multiple metastases involving both lobes of the liver and lesions near major blood vessels or bile ducts. Such patients cannot tolerate surgery.

• Of those who successfully undergo surgery to remove cancer deposits in the liver, about 30 percent survive five or more years without further treatment.

• When complete removal of the tumor with the potential for cure cannot be performed, palliative surgery has no significant benefit, except in patients with neuroendocrine tumors.

• Systemic chemotherapy (whole body) and/or chemotherapy targeted directly to the liver (via a hepatic artery catheter) has been the standard treatment for colon carcinoma that has metastasized to the liver and cannot be removed surgically. Although some chemotherapy trials have produced encouraging response rates, many chemotherapeutic agents carry substantial risks of serious complications. Overall survival is disappointing.

When Cryosurgery Is Appropriate

Cryotherapy and its role in treating liver tumors continue to evolve. But cryosurgery should not be considered an alternative to standard surgery, which should always be performed whenever possible. When used alone or in combination with standard liver resection, however, cryosurgery can significantly increase the number of patients who can undergo surgery.

Evaluation A high-quality dynamic CT scan and/or MRI of the abdomen should be performed to evaluate the extent of disease in the liver as well as outside of the liver.

The diagnosis of a primary or metastatic malignant liver tumor can be made by either a needle biopsy done with ultrasound, CT, or MRI guidance or a biopsy done during surgery. The diagnosis can also be made using the combination of rising levels of the tumor markers alphafetoprotein (AFP) and carcinoembryonic antigen (CEA) and the appearance of the lesion on ultrasound, CT, or MRI of the liver.

Eligibility Cryosurgery for liver tumors, either primary or metastatic, can be considered under the following conditions:

• Patients should be in reasonably good overall health, with minimal to moderate liver malfunction.

• The tumor cannot be removed with conventional surgery because of technical considerations: The tumor may be large or in a difficult area, there may be multiple lesions on both sides of the liver, or there may be underlying cirrhosis. There are limits to the extent of tissue that can be safely frozen with cryosurgery. Generally, 30 to 40 percent of the liver may be frozen if involved with tumor. The more tumor tissue that is frozen, the more likely there will be complications associated with cryosurgery.

• The malignant tumor should be confined to the liver and not involve other organs. Encouraging results have been reported by surgeons in Europe performing cryosurgery in patients with tumors that have spread to the liver with a small amount of disease outside the liver that was also completely resected surgically. In general, patients who also have disease outside the liver have a poorer prognosis and should be considered for cryosurgery on an individual basis.

• Patients who have had previous treatment with surgery and/or chemotherapy or chemoembolization can be considered for treatment, including those whose disease has progressed while on chemotherapy and those who have had a decrease in tumor size and may benefit from cryosurgery when their tumors are smaller.

• Systemic chemotherapy and/or hepatic arterial infusion chemotherapy can be given after cryosurgery to the liver.

• Patients who develop new tumors confined to the liver can safely undergo repeat cryosurgery.

In Combination One of the most common uses of cryosurgery for liver tumors is to combine the technique with conventional surgery. Cryosurgery can also be combined with radiofrequency ablation (RFA) (see chapter 13, "Radiofrequency-Generated Heat Treatment").

• Cryosurgery may help in cases where conventional surgery is successful but there is concern that a few cancer cells remain where the edge of the cancer was removed. A flat "disk" probe can be used to freeze the cut liver edge.

• A patient with multiple liver tumors may be best served by removing the portion of tumor that can surgically be removed and freezing the portion that cannot. Large unresectable liver tumors are usually treated with cryosurgery, while small tumors can be treated at the same time with RFA.

• Cryosurgery should be considered for patients who will receive postoperative chemotherapy. Investigators are combining cryosurgery and the concurrent placement of hepatic artery catheters to be connected to pumps that deliver concentrated chemotherapy directly into the liver. The rationale is to destroy all visible disease with cryosurgery while the subsequent chemotherapy will control any microscopic cancer deposits.

Future studies will assess the benefits of combined treatments on overall survival. In a number of tissues, cryosurgery causes an immune response to substances from the frozen tissue. This is not yet well understood, but may provide an added benefit in enhancing a patient's own immune response to control cancer.

Cryosurgical Technique

This type of surgery should be performed by surgeons familiar with hepatic anatomy and surgery. The surgery is performed in a similar fashion to that of conventional liver surgery. A special warming blanket is placed over the head, upper chest, pelvis, and legs to keep patients warm during the procedure.

The abdominal cavity is explored to detect any tumor deposits outside the liver. The liver is left in place but freed from some of its attachments to other structures. The surgeon feels the liver between both hands and also uses a handheld ultrasound device to locate and determine the extent of the tumors.

Ultrasound scanning can help diagnose masses deep within the liver that are normally difficult to feel and provide the surgeon with a road map of major blood vessels and bile ducts. With ultrasound guidance, the tip of the stainless steel probe is passed into each tumor and liquid nitrogen is circulated through the probe. As the tumor tissue is frozen, an "ice ball" develops. Ultrasound is used to monitor the extent of freezing, assuring the destruction of only a small rim of normal liver tissue around each tumor. For larger tumors, up to five probes can be used simultaneously.

After the freezing cycle is completed, the probes are rewarmed and, after several minutes of thawing, are removed from the frozen tumor. The frozen cryoprobe tracts are packed with a cellulose material to prevent bleeding. The frozen tumor is left in place in the liver and is absorbed by the body. Once the procedure is completed, the patient is transferred to the intensive care unit for postoperative monitoring.

After the Procedure Most patients spend only one night in the intensive care unit. Nearly all are able to breathe completely on their own within several hours of surgery.

Patients with very large tumors that require extensive freezing may occasionally need a blood transfusion.

The morning after surgery, patients are encouraged to sit up in a chair and can take some fluids by mouth later the same day. Postoperative pain can be individually controlled with the help of a special pain pump. Patients are discharged about six days after surgery.

Complications Cryosurgery of liver tumors is considered relatively safe, with very few procedure-related deaths reported. The incidence of major complications is less than 5 percent.

- A small drop in body temperature (about 4°F [2°C]) can be expected during the freezing procedure, but this should not cause any complications.
- Most patients show an increase in liver enzymes of up to about twice the normal values, but normal levels quickly return.
- Postoperative liver failure is rare.
- Common complications indirectly related to cryotherapy include an increase in the white blood cell count and low-grade fevers that resolve quickly.
- Complications directly related to hepatic cryosurgery include bleeding from the liver, which can be controlled with pressure and/or packing; short-term abnormalities in blood-clotting factors; fluid collections around the lungs; abnormal leakage of bile from the liver; liver infections; and a temporary decrease in kidney function.

Results Survival depends on many factors, including tumor type and bulk. Investigators have reported survival rates of 15 to 22 percent of patients with primary liver cancer after five years and up to 60 percent of patients with colon and rectal cancer metastases to the liver after two years.

Physicians treating these patients are looking at new combinations of treatment. In some patients, cryosurgery is now combined with placement of a hepatic artery catheter to deliver chemotherapy to the liver after surgery. This may help to control disease that is too small to be detected at the time of surgery. Most patients who are undergoing cryosurgery of the liver at this time have had previous chemotherapy that no longer can control tumor growth. Physicians are studying the benefits of applying cryosurgery to the liver when metastatic disease is first detected and proceeding with chemotherapy afterward. Further studies in larger patient populations will determine if this approach is better.

Very encouraging results have been reported in cryosurgery for neuroendocrine tumors that have spread to the liver. These tumors produce chemical substances that cause disabling symptoms of skin flushing, increased heart rate, and diarrhea (see, for example, the chapter "Carcinoids of the Gastrointestinal Tract"). The liver is often extensively involved with tumors. Cryosurgery can decrease the tumor bulk, thereby reducing these symptoms. Then these patients can be treated with chemotherapy and/or future cryosurgery.

Cryosurgery and RFA have expanded the possible treatment of either primary or metastatic cancer of the liver, with a small but real influence on outcome and survival.

Advantages and Disadvantages

Cryosurgery has many advantages over standard surgical removal of the liver tumor. One of the main advantages is the minimal damage suffered by normal liver tissue because only a relatively small area is frozen.

Conventional surgery also carries the risk of hemorrhage and damage to the bile ducts. Large blood vessels can tolerate freezing extremely well because the passage of warm blood disrupts the freezing. Careful placement of the cryoprobes with ultrasound guidance should help ensure adequate destruction of tumor tissue adjacent to blood vessels.

Disadvantages of cryosurgery for liver tumors include the need for an open surgical procedure, technical limitations, and the complications previously listed. Continued technical advances will limit these complications and allow hepatic cryosurgery to be performed in a less-invasive manner.

The continued application and evaluation of cryosurgery and RFA techniques provides the surgeon with the opportunity to affect the outcome of a much larger proportion of patients with unresectable liver tumors.

Cryosurgery for Prostate Cancer

There are many options for managing localized prostate cancer, including surgical removal of the gland (radical prostatectomy), external-beam radiation therapy, and interstitial radiation therapy (also known as brachytherapy or radioactive seed implant). The treatment decisions are based on a patient's age and health, the grade and stage of the disease, and individual patient preferences. Cryotherapy is one option.

Eligibility Patients with low-risk features—that is, low-serum prostate-specific antigen (PSA; a tumor marker for prostate cancer defined by a blood test), low aggressiveness of cancer defined by biopsy, and low clinical stage of tumor—have the best outcomes with cryosurgery. Patients with large prostate glands exceeding 3½ cubic inches (60 cc) are difficult to treat and may need hormone therapy to downsize the gland. Patients for whom preservation of erectile function is a high priority are less appropriate candidates, as explained in a later section on potency.

Salvage Treatment Few localized treatment alternatives are available for patients with recurrent cancer in the prostate after radiation therapy. Cryosurgery has been established as a viable option for this condition. Patients for salvage cryotherapy must have a life expectancy of more than ten years and local recurrence of cancer confirmed by biopsy. They should also have various X-ray studies to rule out any evidence of metastatic disease.

Procedure Freezing of the prostate is carried out using a multiprobe cryosurgical device. Current devices use small needle-shaped probes with a size of 0.06–0.09 inches (1.5–2.4 mm) in diameter. They can be placed directly into the prostate through the skin between the anus and scrotum (perineum) under ultrasound guidance, in a way that permits ice balls to overlap and destroy the entire prostate.

The freezing is monitored using transrectal ultrasound (a small probe inserted in the rectum). The edge of the freeze zone is clearly visible. Two freeze-thaw cycles are routinely performed, which enhances tissue destruction. If the ice ball does not extend to the top (apex) of the prostate, the cryoprobes are pulled back into this area and a third freeze-thaw cycle is carried out.

As the temperature at the visible edge of the ice ball is higher than needed to destroy cancer cells completely, the ice ball is allowed to extend 3–4 mm beyond the prostatic capsule into the surrounding tissue. Behind the prostate, freezing is extended as far as the muscle layer of the rectum, which allows adequate freezing of that part of the prostate but does not damage the rectum.

Precautions are taken to minimize risk or damage to the urethra, the tube that carries urine out of the body. A urethral warmer during the procedure protects the urethra near the urination muscles and bladder neck. Inadequate urethral warming may result in the separation of the lining of the tube (urethral slough-ing) and urinary retention because of sloughed tissue obstructing the tube.

After the Procedure Patients are released from the hospital on the same day of the procedure. A tube to drain urine (Foley cath-eter) is inserted into the bladder through the urethra and is kept in place for the fol-lowing seven to ten days. Minimum pain is generally involved in the area of freezing or needle insertion. A PSA test is obtained every three months in the first year and every six months thereafter. Prostate biopsy to confirm the efficacy of treatment is usu-ally performed a year later.

Complications Immediate postoperative complications of cryosurgery are very low; blood loss is negligible, and most patients are discharged within forty-eight hours of surgery. More than one month after cryotherapy, however, there are sometimes significant complications related to the procedure. These compli-cations have been greatly reduced with recent and more advanced technologies and improvement of technique.

• Incontinence (loss of urinary control) occurs in 3 to 4 percent of patients.
• Urethral/prostatic sloughing used to be a common problem when an effective urethral warmer was not available, and 23 percent of patients in one study needed additional surgery (transurethral resec-tion of the prostate, or TURP) to remove obstructing tissue. Currently, the inci-dence of tissue sloughing is reported to be 3 to 5.5 percent. Transurethral resection of the damaged prostate after cryotherapy carries a significant risk of incontinence.

• The incidence of urinary retention and incontinence falls with the use of better urethral warmers and improved smaller multiprobe systems.

The Effect on Potency Most patients are impotent following cryosurgery. To treat prostate cancer adequately, it is usually necessary to allow the ice ball to extend on both sides of the prostate into the tis-sue that contains the nerves and blood vessels that facilitate erection. Potency may recover with time, especially if freez-ing next to the prostate is less aggressive. One study reported an impotence rate of 90 percent at six months but only 41 percent after one year. Despite the recent improvement of devices, impotence rate after cryosurgery remains high. Eighty-six to 95 percent of previously potent men were impotent six months after cryother-apy. Significant injury to the nerves on one or both sides is probably inevitable if cryosurgery is performed in a manner that holds out the best chance of cure, especially in patients with extension out-side the prostate capsule.

Evaluating Cryotherapy Results in Prostate Cancer

Local Control A number of disease- and treatment-related factors have been shown to predict rates of local control. Low-risk patients were those with a PSA of less than or equal to 10 ng/ml, a Gleason score of less than or equal to 6, and clinical stage T1 or T2a disease; intermediate-risk patients had a PSA greater than 10 ng/ml, a Gleason score of less than or equal to 7, and clinical stage T2b or higher; and high-risk patients had two or three of these adverse risk fac-tors. The positive biopsy rate was 18 per-cent overall: 12 percent among low- and intermediate-risk patients and 24 percent among high-risk patients.

The use of two freeze-thaw cycles, the use of thermosensors during treatment, and increasing the number of probes all contribute to the improvement of local cancer control.

Biochemical Failure PSA levels following cryotherapy initially rise sharply and then fall, reaching a nadir (lowest point) within three months after treatment in most patients. Because this treatment modality does not ablate every gland in the prostate at the microscopic level, a persistently detectable PSA following cryosurgery may not indicate persistent disease. In a pooled analysis, with a median follow-up of twenty-four months, the actuarial five-year biochemical disease-free survival (PSA not rising) rates were 60, 45, and 36 percent for low-, intermediate-, and high-risk patients using a PSA threshold of 0.5 ng/ml to define failure, and 76, 71, and 45 percent using a threshold of 1.0 ng/ml. Another report of a single institute with the largest series of patients to date stated that using an absolute PSA threshold of 0.5 ng/ml to define failure, as is done in many surgical series, the biochemical disease-free survival (PSA not rising above 0.5 ng/ml) rates were 61, 68, and 61 percent for low-, intermediate-, and high-risk patients. Adapting the American Society for Therapeutic Radiology and Oncology (ASTRO) definition of failure—three successive rises in PSA—the biochemical disease-free survival (PSA not rising) rates were 92, 89, and 89 percent, respectively.

Despite these promising early results, some principles should be emphasized.

• Postcryosurgical biopsies of many patients show benign epithelial cells. Since some normal prostate cells remain, it is possible that parts of the prostate have not been completely treated.

• The significance of a detectable PSA after cryotherapy in a patient with negative biopsies is not fully known at this time. It seems, however, that in most patients, a PSA of less than or equal to 0.5 ng/ml one year after cryotherapy indicates absence of disease.

• The surgical mortality rate for patients undergoing cryotherapy for prostate cancer is extremely low.

New Directions Cryotherapy holds promise for cancer cure, with most patients having negative follow-up biopsies and very low levels of PSA on early follow-up. However, longer follow-up is required to define the long-term cancer cure rates.

The best results appear to be in patients with disease confined to the prostate, the same patients who would be expected to do well with radical prostatectomy or radiation therapy.

Since prostate cancer in early stage may involve a part of the gland, partial cryosurgery in order to preserve sexual function and to avoid other complications is proposed and is under investigation.

The technology is still evolving, and better results with reduced complications may be possible with further refinements in urethral warming devices and in freezing techniques.

— 13 —

Radiofrequency-Generated Heat Treatment (Radiofrequency Ablation)

Stanley J. Rogers, M.D., and Allan E. Siperstein, M.D.

■ ■ ■ ■

Radiofrequency ablation (RFA) is a promising new therapeutic modality that is now used to gain control of primary and metastatic tumors. While there is growing experience using RFA to treat tumors located throughout the body, the technique is most commonly used to treat tumors in the liver. Therefore, RFA of liver tumors will be the main focus of this chapter, although similar principles apply using this modality for tumors located in the lungs, the pelvis, and other body sites.

Treatment of primary and metastatic liver tumors poses a significant therapeutic challenge in the United States and worldwide. The gold standard remains surgical resection of the tumor with intent to cure. Overall, however, few patients undergo such surgery and even fewer are cured by this treatment modality. Eighty percent of recognized tumors are not surgically resectable at the time of diagnosis, and many patients are not good surgical candidates due to associated comorbidity. Multiple options are available in the treatment arsenal for hepatic neoplasms (see Table 1; see also the chapter on liver cancer). These include systemic therapy (chemotherapy), regional therapy (hepatic artery infusion chemotherapy, chemoembolization, hepatic artery ligation), and local therapy (tumor ablation via ethanol injection, cryotherapy, and, more recently, radiofrequency ablation).

Radiofrequency ablation uses heat generated by radiofrequency waves (electricity). Radiofrequency energy, which is commonly used in conventional operating room electrosurgical cautery units, is delivered through specially designed probes to heat tumor tissue. Heat is well known to be a very effective way to kill viable cells and tissue and is routinely used in sterilization procedures to kill cellular and subcellular microorganisms. At the cellular level, as temperature rises above 113°F (45°C), proteins are permanently denatured, producing membrane fusion, loss of cellular function, and ultimately

---

Table 1. **Treatment Options for Hepatic Neoplasms**

1. Systemic therapy
   a. Chemotherapy
   b. Immunotherapy

2. Regional therapy
   a. Hepatic artery infusion chemotherapy
   b. Chemoembolization
   c. Hepatic artery ligation

3. Local therapy
   a. Tumor ablation via ethanol injection
   b. Cryotherapy
   c. Radiofrequency ablation

cell death. The process is rapid, requiring only minutes for irreversible protein denaturation and coagulative necrosis of cells in tissue.

How It Works

The production of heat from radiofrequency energy occurs when high-frequency electric current passes from an electrode probe into tissues. The current causes the ions (charged atoms in tissues) to vibrate in an attempt to align themselves with the current. The ions move back and forth so rapidly, they create friction, which in turn generates heat. Since the heat is generated from within the tissue itself, the RFA probe tip is not significantly hotter than the surrounding tissues.

The amount of heat generated is the difference between heat production and heat dissipation (see Table 2).

• Heat production is the result of three variables: distance from the electrodes, density of the radiofrequency current, and duration of the application.

Table 2. Variables in Heat Generation

1. H_p: Heat production determinants
   a. Distance from electrodes
   b. Radiofrequency current density
   c. Duration of heat application

---

2. H_d: Heat dissipation determinants
   a. Convection (primarily)
      i. Local blood flow
      ii. Regional blood flow
   b. Conduction
      i. Source tissue density
      ii. Target tissue density

---

3. H_g: Heat generated equals heat production minus heat dissipation ($H_g = H_p - H_d$)

• Heat dissipation is determined mainly by *convection* and, to a lesser degree, by *conduction*. Convective tissue cooling is a function mainly of local or regional blood flow, while conductive tissue cooling is determined primarily by the density of source and target tissues.

Depending on the power applied and the electrical resistance, or impedance, of the tissue, electrical energy and therefore heat dissipate rapidly as the distance increases from the electrode tip. The size of the ultimate ablation lesion is determined largely by the size of the probe, with a sharp boundary occurring between dead tissue and unaffected surrounding tissue.

Current Procedures

Studies in laboratories and in animals have sought to determine the ideal electrode configuration and rate of energy delivery. With the electrode configuration currently used, radiofrequency ablation lesions of 2 to 2¾ inches (5–7 cm) in diameter may be produced in ten to fifteen minutes.

The ablation catheter is typically a needle that contains several prongs that are inserted into and then deployed in the tissue to be treated. These prongs will deliver electrical energy to the tissue and also serve to fix the ablation catheter firmly in place during treatment. Thermocouples may be incorporated into each of the tips of the prongs to allow continuous dynamic monitoring of tissue temperature. In addition, tissue resistance, or impedance, and ultimately ablation efficacy, may be determined and used to guide the ablation process.

Ultrasound is used to visually monitor the progress of ablative treatment. As tissues are heated, dissolved gases (primarily nitrogen) form microbubbles within the tissue. Ultrasonographically, a hyperechoic or echogenic focus is created by the accumulation of these microbubbles, which reflect sound waves back to the ultrasound transducer. This process typically begins at the center of the ablation lesion and expands to the periphery as the ablation cycle progresses.

Results The initial studies of radiofrequency ablation technology were produced by Italian researchers who used ultrasound-guided percutaneous placement of ablation catheters in liver tumors. They mainly evaluated patients with centrally based hepatocellular carcinoma lesions rather than peripheral tumors located near the liver surface and adjacent to diaphragm or visceral structures. These tumors were successfully ablated, as shown by follow-up angiography or cross-sectional imaging. Moreover, they reported little to no bleeding or other complications.

Laparoscopic Techniques

The radiofrequency technology has since been adapted for use with laparoscopy and other minimally invasive surgical techniques. Laparoscopic surgery specifically uses long, thin instruments passed through small incisions in the abdominal wall. Several clear advantages exist with the use of the laparoscopic radiofrequency ablation of liver tumors:

• Each laparoscopic procedure starts with a diagnostic laparoscopy, which, in comparison to radiologic imaging, allows for an improved evaluation for extrahepatic peritoneal-based metastatic disease.

• Laparoscopic ultrasound of the liver allows for the most accurate detection of additional areas of metastatic disease within the liver, frequently identifying small lesions not noted on preoperative imaging studies.

• Most important, with the laparoscopic use of radiofrequency ablation technology, tumors near the surface of the liver may be successfully treated by isolating the ablation process from surrounding structures, including diaphragm, chest wall, and visceral structures. This is not possible with percutaneous ablation, where conduction of electrical energy would put adjacent structures at risk.

Clinical Trials Multiple clinical trials have demonstrated the safety and efficacy of radiofrequency thermal ablation, and in particular using the laparoscopic approach. Current studies are ongoing to demonstrate the long-term results of this technology in comparison to other available treatments and to identify a survival benefit with the use of this treatment modality.

Laparoscopic Radiofrequency Ablation Technical Study Protocol

• In the operating room under general anesthesia, a diagnostic laparoscopy is performed, with biopsy of any suspicious tissue found outside the liver.

• Laparoscopic ultrasonography of the liver is then performed, and all suspected metastases are mapped.

• Color flow studies of the metastatic lesions assess their blood supply.

• Under ultrasound guidance, biopsies are performed of the suspected neoplasms.

• The radiofrequency thermoablation catheter is placed through the skin under ultrasound guidance into the lesion, and the prongs are inserted directly into the neoplasm.

• The ten- to fifteen-minute ablation cycle is monitored by the thermocouples at the tips of the prongs and by microbubble formation detected by ultrasound.

• A laptop computer connected to the electrical generator allows accurate records to be kept of each cycle.

• At the completion of an ablation, the temperatures are monitored for another one to two minutes to ensure adequate heating even at the periphery of the lesion.

• A postablation duplex color-flow ultrasound examination of the lesion is then performed to document the lack of blood flow within the expected volume of ablated tissue.

Results Laparoscopic radiofrequency thermoablation of liver tumors shows great promise in the treatment of both primary liver cancer and metastatic neoplasms of the liver, though longer follow-up is needed to determine whether this treatment significantly improves survival or quality of life.

— 14 —

Antiangiogenesis: Inhibition of Blood Vessel Growth as a Strategy for Treating Cancer

Emily K. Bergsland, M.D.

■ ■ ■ ■

Angiogenesis is the process by which new blood vessels sprout from an existing vascular (blood vessel) bed. Although new blood vessels grow rapidly in the developing embryo, in normal adults, blood vessel growth rarely occurs. There are "switches" in the body that normally turn blood vessel growth on and off. The process is tightly controlled by an array of stimulatory and inhibitory factors, with intense bursts of new blood vessel formation largely restricted to the menstrual cycle, pregnancy, and wound healing.

Interestingly, there is a large body of evidence suggesting that abnormal angiogenesis contributes to the development of a variety of diseases, including diabetic retinopathy (changes in the back of the eye), psoriasis, rheumatoid arthritis, and cancer. Hence, therapies designed to inhibit the growth of new blood vessels may be useful treatments in cancer and other diseases. In cancer, blood vessels probably "feed" the tumor, allowing it to grow beyond an initially small size. Now that we are beginning to understand how small tumors recruit new blood vessels, we can use this information to develop therapies to stop the formation of these new blood vessels and "starve" the tumor (antiangiogenesis). Bevacizumab (Avastin) was the first dedicated antiangiogenic agent to be approved for human use.

Dozens of other antiangiogenic agents are in development.

Antiangiogenesis and Cancer

It is now generally accepted that tumor growth and spread to distant organs (metastasis) require growth of new blood vessels. Prior to the recruitment of new vessels (termed the angiogenic switch), tumor size is limited to about the size of a pinhead. New capillaries are required for tumor growth because they provide a mechanism for waste and nutrient exchange, as well as a route for metastasis. Some studies have shown that the angiogenic switch is activated during early (precancerous) stages of tumor progression in many cancers, even before invasion has occurred. Consequently, researchers think that antiangiogenic agents may someday be used to prevent, as well as treat, invasive cancer. The available data suggest that this type of therapy may be more effective when combined with chemotherapy, radiation, or other biologic agents than when given as a single agent. In addition, antiangiogenic agents may potentially prove most effective in the treatment of early cancer, or in preventing the growth of new cancers after cancer surgery. In patients with advanced disease, these agents may be more likely to stabilize disease than to cause a major shrinkage.

Regulation of Angiogenesis

The process of angiogenesis involves multiple steps, such as breakdown of the tissue surrounding the blood vessel by proteins called proteases, production and proliferation of new blood vessel lining (endothelial cells [ECs]), and migration of ECs to generate a new capillary sprout that eventually matures into a tube that forms the new tiny blood vessel. The regulation of angiogenesis appears to be accomplished by many regulators working together in our bodies. During the past two decades, dozens of stimulatory and inhibitory counterparts (see the table below) have been discovered. The balance of regulators at any one time in a given tissue probably determines whether or not angiogenesis occurs.

Antiangiogenesis

Why Should It Work? There are several reasons why we think that inhibiting blood vessel growth may be beneficial in patients with cancer. New capillaries appear to be required for tumor growth and metastasis. Furthermore, antiangiogenic agents may preferentially target vessels in the tumor, since normal adult blood vessels are essentially dormant. Additional differences probably exist between normal endothelial cells and those associated with a tumor. These alterations can theoretically be exploited to develop cancer-specific antiangiogenic agents, thus potentially avoiding the toxicity associated with traditional cancer therapies like chemotherapy and radiation. Finally, drugs in this class might be broadly useful across a variety of tumor types, since the blood vessels are targeted rather than the cancer cells themselves (which are prone to mutations and perhaps more likely to develop resistance to anticancer drugs).

Treatment Strategies A number of approaches to antiangiogenesis are being explored, all of which stem from advances in our understanding of the process by which angiogenesis is regulated:

1. Block activity of factors that normally stimulate angiogenesis.

2. Increase activity of inhibitory factors by administration of extra factor made outside the body or by gene therapy to enhance production of the factor within the patient.

3. Interfere with the normal relationship between endothelial cells and the surrounding tissue.

4. Inhibit an integral step of angiogenesis (e.g., by specifically blocking endothelial cell migration, division, or tubule formation so new blood vessels can't form).

5. Employ endothelial-specific toxins. Agents in this class would be designed to bind endothelial cells in order to deliver a toxin such as chemotherapy or radiation.

Examples of each of these classes of inhibitors are already being tested. Many others are in various stages of development.

Examples of Regulators of Angiogenesis Inside the Body

STIMULATORY	INHIBITORY
VEGF	IL-12
aFGF	Endostatin
bFGF	Angiostatin
IGF-I	Interferon-2a
Angiogenin	Platelet factor-4
HB-EGF	Thrombospondin
IL-8	TIMP-1 and TIMP-2
Thymidine phosphorylase (PD-ECGF)	Angiostatic steroids
HGF	16 kD prolactin
Proliferin	

Clinical Experience Dozens of antiangiogenic agents have already entered the clinic for testing in patients with cancer (see the table on pages 116–117). Combinations with chemotherapy, radiation, and/or other biologically based therapies are also being explored.

Many of the antiangiogenic agents under evaluation are directed against vascular endothelial growth factor (VEGF), which has emerged as a central therapeutic target in cancer. VEGF is a potent, positive regulator of angiogenesis that signals through receptors on the surface of endothelial cells. VEGF, as well as its receptors, are often overexpressed in cancers; levels of expression often inversely correlate with patient outcome. In addition to direct effects on endothelial cells, experimental evidence suggests that VEGF inhibitors may help to "normalize" the aberrant tumor blood supply, thus potentially improving delivery of chemotherapy and other therapeutic agents.

To date, the most impressive results have been associated with the use of a humanized monoclonal antibody designed to bind and inhibit VEGF function called bevacizumab (Avastin). Bevacizumab was approved by the United States Food and Drug Administration (FDA) in 2004 for use in in patients with previously untreated metastatic colorectal cancer (in combination with chemotherapy). Recently, it also gained approval for use in the first-line treatment of advanced lung cancer. Numerous other trials with this agent are ongoing.

In addition to antibody-based strategies, significant efforts have been placed on generating small molecule inhibitors of VEGF receptor signaling. While many different inhibitors are in development (which vary in terms of specificity, potency, and oral bioavailability), two agents in this class (sorafenib [Nexavar] and sunitinib) have already been approved for use in human cancer. Many other VEGF inhibitors, as well as numerous other antiangiogenic strategies, are being explored.

Bevacizumab (Avastin) Bevacizumab is a recombinant humanized monoclonal antibody directed against VEGF. The approval in colorectal cancer stemmed from a Phase III clinical trial showing that patients with previously untreated metastatic colorectal cancer (mCRC) who were randomized to receive 5-fluorouracil + leucovorin (LV) + irinotecan (IFL) chemotherapy plus bevacizumab lived nearly five months longer than patients treated with chemotherapy alone. Use of bevacizumab was also associated with statistically significant increases in radiographic response rate and time to tumor progression (the time it takes the tumor to grow or new tumors to form). Bevacizumab was given intravenously every two weeks and was generally well tolerated, although treatment-associated high blood pressure was seen. In addition, small but clinically significant increases in gastrointestinal perforations and arterial thromboembolic events (like strokes and heart attacks) were observed.

Subsequent studies showed that bevacizumab improved the activity of oxaliplatin-based chemotherapy in the second-line setting, and of 5-FU/LV chemotherapy in the first-line treatment of patients with mCRC. Taken together, these data led to the approval of bevacizumab in combination with 5-FU–based chemotherapy in the first- and second-line treatment of patients with mCRC. Ongoing studies are aimed at exploring the incremental benefit of bevacizumab in the adjuvant setting (i.e., after potentially curative removal of the primary tumor), and in combination with other treatment regimens (including ones that incorporate oral 5-FU drugs and other biologically based agents).

The ECOG 4599 trial was designed to evaluate the use of bevacizumab in combination with chemotherapy (carboplatin/paclitaxel) in patients with previously

Selected Antiangiogenic Agents in Clinical Trials

AGENT	STAGE OF TESTING	SPONSOR
Anti-VEGF antibody (bevacizumab)	Phase IV (approved in lung and colon cancer)	Genentech
Lenalidomide (thalidomide analog)	Phase IV	NCI, Celgene (commercially available)
Thalidomide (immunomodulatory, anti-inflammatory and anti-angiogenic properties)	Phase III	Celgene (commercially available)
SU11248 (sunitinib) (receptor TKI)	Phase III (approved for GIST and RCC)	Pfizer
Sorafenib (Bay 43-9006) (receptor TKI)	Phase III (approved for RCC)	Bayer
Celecoxib (Celebrex) (Cox-2 inhibitor)	Phase III	Pfizer (commercially available)
AZD2171 (receptor TKI)	Phase II/III	Astra Zeneca
AVE0005 (VEGF Trap)	Phase II/III	Regeneron Pharmaceuticals/ Sanofi-Aventis
GW786034 (pazopanib) (receptor TKI)	Phase III	Glaxo Smithkline
ZD6474 (receptor TKI)	Phase III	AstraZeneca
PTK787/ZK222584 (receptor TKI)	Phase III	Novartis
AMG706 (receptor TKI)	Phase I/II	Amgen
ABT-510 (thrombospondin analog)	Phase I/II	NCI

untreated metastatic nonsmall cell lung cancer. The addition of bevacizumab improved progression-free and overall survival in these patients (by around two months), leading to the FDA approval of bevacizumab for this indication. The relative efficacy of this combination compared to numerous other potential first-line treatment regimens for this patient population is unknown, and is the subject of ongoing clinical trials.

The preliminary results of a large, randomized clinical trial for patients with previously untreated metastatic or locally recurrent breast cancer have also been reported. The study showed that patients who received bevacizumab in combination with standard chemotherapy with paclitaxel had a longer time period before their disease worsened compared to patients who received chemotherapy alone. The study results suggest that bevacizumab has activity in breast cancer, however, the drug has not yet been approved for use in this disease. Interestingly, a previous study in patients

AGENT	STAGE OF TESTING	SPONSOR
ATN-224 (2nd generation tetrathiomolybdate)	Phase I/II	Attenuon
Combretastatin (tumor vascular-targeting agent)	Phase II	NCI
PI-88 (heparinase inhibitor)	Phase I/II	Progen
PXD-101 (histone deacetylase inhibitor)	Phase II	CuraGen/TopoTarget
AG-013736 (receptor TKI)	Phase II	Pfizer
Tetrathio-molybdate (TM, copper chelator)	Phase II	University of Michigan
Panzem (2-ME) (estradiol metabolite with antiangiogenic activity)	Phase II	EntreMed
SU-014813 (receptor TKI)	Phase II	Pfizer
FR901228 (histone deacetylase inhibitor)	Phase II	NCI
BMS-582664 (receptor TKI)	Phase II	Bristol-Myers Squibb Company
M200 (volociximab) (anti-alpha5 beta 1 integrin antibody)	Phase II	Protein Design Labs
EMD121974 (cilengitide) (Cyclic peptide, inhibits alpha(v)beta(3) and alpha(v)-beta(5) integrins)	Phase I/II	NCI
AMG 386 (Fc-peptide fusion protein, angiopoietin inhibitor)	Phase I	Amgen
NPI-2358 (vascular disrupting agent)	Phase I	Nereus Pharmaceuticals, Incorporated

Adapted from the National Cancer Institute database, *www.cancer.gov/clinicaltrials* (updated March 2007).

assigned to a different chemotherapy (capecitabine [Xeloda]), with or without bevacizumab, failed to show that bevacizumab improved the outcome. The fact that the study was designed for women who had received prior chemotherapy for advanced disease may be significant and suggests that the benefit of bevacizumab in breast cancer may depend on the extent of prior therapy and/or the agent(s) with which bevacizumab is combined.

The approval of bevacizumab for use in humans validated VEGF as a target for therapy in cancer and fueled interest in antiangiogenesis as a therapeutic strategy. However, the potential benefits of bevacizumab must be carefully weighed against the potential risks. The cumulative data with this drug suggest that it is associated with high blood pressure, an increased risk of gastrointestinal perforations (overall incidence of about 1 percent), and spilling of protein in the urine. Treatment with bevacizumab increases the risk of stroke and heart attack (especially in patients older than sixty-five and with a prior history of similar events). Use of bevacizumab has also been associated with two types of bleeding: (1) minor bleeding, usually in the form of nosebleeds and (2) massive, sometimes fatal, bleeding. While gastrointestinal bleeding has been observed, the association with potentially fatal bleeding from the lungs is perhaps most concerning. Patients with squamous cell lung cancers and central, cavitary lung cancers seem to be particularly at risk; the safety of bevacizumab in this population has not been established. Furthermore, bevacizumab impairs wound healing in animal models and should be discontinued several weeks before elective surgery (it takes weeks to months to clear from the body). It should not be resumed until the surgical incision is fully healed (at least twenty-eight days after major surgery). Its use in patients with brain metastases or significant underlying heart disease has not been studied. Finally, bevacizumab may impair fertility and, if possible, should not be used in pregnant women.

Sunitinib Sunitinib is an oral, small molecule receptor tyrosine kinase inhibitor (TKI) of VEGF receptor signaling (VEGFR-1, -2, -3). In contrast to bevacizumab, sunitinib is a pill and is not specific for VEGF. It also inhibits the activity of the platelet-derived growth factor (PDGF)–alpha and PDGF-beta receptors—both of which are also known to be involved in the regulation of angiogenesis. In addition, it inhibits signaling through the c-Kit, RET, and FLT3 genes, which might also be valid therapeutic targets in cancer.

In 2006, sunitinib received FDA approval for the treatment of renal cell carcinoma (RCC), as well as gastrointestinal stromal tumor (GIST). GIST is a rare form of stomach and intestinal cancer that is exceedingly resistant to chemotherapy. Advances in our understanding of the molecular mechanisms underlying tumor progression led to the discovery that tumor growth is dependent on abnormal c-Kit receptor function. Treatment with the small molecule inhibitor imatinib mesylate (Gleevec) revolutionized the treatment of patients with advanced disease. However, until sunitinib, no treatment was available for patients with imatinib-resistant disease or intolerance to imatinib. Sunitinib was approved based on the results of a study suggesting that it delays time to tumor progression in these patients.

RCC (a form of kidney cancer) is unusually dependent on VEGF. A quarter of patients with RCC have locally advanced disease at diagnosis; one-third of patients have metastatic disease at presentation. The disease is inherently resistant to chemotherapy, and until recently, the mainstay of therapy was cytokine therapy with interleukin-2 (IL-2) and interferon. The results of two small studies exploring second-line treatment with single-agent sunitinib showed a 30 to 40 percent response rate and a median time to disease progression of eight to nine months. A planned interim analysis of a Phase III study of interferon versus sunitinib (as first-line therapy for patients with metastatic RCC) subsequently showed that patients assigned to sunitinib experienced a higher response rate (34 percent versus 6 percent) and improved time to tumor progression (eleven months versus five months) compared to interferon.

Of note, bevacizumab has also shown activity in RCC but is not approved for this indication. Like bevacizumab, treatment with sunitinib is associated with hypertension. Other common side effects include diarrhea, hand-foot reaction (redness and tenderness of the palms and soles), skin rash, and fatigue.

Sorafenib (Nexavar) Sorafenib, like sunitinib, is a receptor TKI that interferes with VEGF receptor signaling. It is also oral, and not entirely specific. While originally developed as an inhibitor of c-Raf kinase, it also inhibits VEGF receptors (VEGFR-1 and -2), PDGFR-beta, FLT3, and c-Kit. In addition to direct effects on tumor cells, sorafenib inhibits angiogenesis in experimental models. The drug was approved for the treatment of RCC in 2005 based on the results of two studies suggesting that treatment with sorafenib delays disease progression. It has a side-effect profile that is fairly similar to that of sunitinib.

Future Considerations

Over the past several years, we have witnessed an explosion in the number of antiangiogenic agents in development. A myriad of approaches are under investigation—the majority involving the inhibition of VEGF, a potent regulator of angiogenesis. Several large Phase III trials have validated VEGF as a target for therapy in cancer. Bevacizumab (Avastin) has received FDA approval for the treatment of patients with advanced lung cancer or metastatic colorectal cancer in combination with chemotherapy. The small molecule receptor tyrosine kinase inhibitors, sorafenib (Nexavar) and sunitinib, have antiangiogenic activity and were also recently approved for use in humans.

Future efforts will be aimed at identifying safer and more specific inhibitors of angiogenesis; improving patient selection (i.e., predicting response to therapy and/or toxicity); and optimizing the best approaches to treatment (stage of disease, duration of therapy, type of disease, dose, schedule, and combinations with other agents/treatment modalities). *Hundreds* of clinical trials are ongoing, in which the use of antiangiogenic agents in a variety of diseases, and in combination with a range of other agents, are being studied.

— 15 —

Bone Marrow and Blood Stem Cell Transplantation

Marcel P. Devetten Jr., M.D., James O. Armitage, M.D., and Elizabeth C. Reed, M.D.

■ ■ ■ ■

Bone marrow contains immature (or stem) cells that are capable of continuously producing new blood and bone marrow cells. This is what helps make bone marrow the "factory" for normal mature blood cells—the red cells that carry oxygen, the white cells that fight infections, and the platelets that help blood clotting.

Doctors long ago realized that the availability of bone marrow stem cells opened the possibility of replacing diseased or defective bone marrow with normal marrow from another person. Over the past thirty years, medical knowledge has advanced to the point where effective bone marrow transplantation techniques have been developed. In many cases, stem cells are not obtained from the bone marrow, but are derived from the bloodstream. In this chapter, we will consistently refer to the procedure as bone marrow transplantation; however, the term *stem cell transplantation* can be used interchangeably. Bone marrow transplantation is now considered the treatment of choice for many patients with malignant (cancerous) conditions, and even for some patients with nonmalignant bone marrow disorders.

Why a Bone Marrow Transplant Might Be Recommended

Although most bone marrow transplant procedures are no longer considered experimental, there are still serious risks associated with undergoing bone marrow transplantation. Bone marrow transplantation is not a procedure that can be recommended lightly. If a patient can be cured with treatment that does not involve a bone marrow transplant, that would almost always be the preferred approach. However, bone marrow transplantation offers a unique possibility of cure for some patients and the potential to significantly increase the time lived without cancer for many others.

We now believe that bone marrow transplantation works through a combination of two mechanisms: The effect of the administration of high doses of chemotherapy and/or radiation therapy (doctors refer to this treatment as the "conditioning" regimen) and the direct effect of transplanted bone marrow cells against cancer cells. This second effect occurs only in patients who receive a bone marrow graft from another individual (brother, sister, or unrelated donor). The second effect is commonly referred to as the "graft-versus-malignancy" effect.

Some patients are considered too old or too sick to withstand the serious side effects from the high-dose conditioning regimen. Those patients are commonly treated with a "reduced intensity" conditioning regimen (also known as a mini transplant). As the name implies, the reduced-intensity conditioning regimen is less intense, and the effect from the transplant procedure relies almost completely on the direct graft-versus-malignancy effect. Alternatively, some patients are treated with a high-dose conditioning regimen followed by transplantation of their own bone marrow cells (see the section on autologous transplantation in "Types of Bone Marrow Transplants," in this chapter). Those patients rely completely on the action of the conditioning regimen for the outcome of their transplant procedure, and they do not get the additional benefit of the graft-versus-malignancy effect.

The highest likelihood of curing cancer is achieved when the action of the high-dose conditioning regimen is combined with the action of the graft-versus-malignancy effect. Unfortunately, this also results in the highest risk of serious side effects. Matching the risk of a particular transplant procedure with the risk of serious side effects and the risk of the cancer is a complex procedure that is best done by doctors with a special expertise in bone marrow transplantation.

Types of Bone Marrow Transplants

Transplanting any organ—a heart, kidney, lung, or bone marrow—from one person to another is a complicated procedure. The immune system is designed to destroy foreign tissues, and "graft rejection" is always a possibility. The risk of rejection can be reduced by matching as much as possible the tissues of the donor and the tissues of the person receiving the transplant. An additional problem is one that is unique to bone marrow transplant procedures (i.e., it is not seen in patients who receive a kidney, lung, or heart transplant): The donor bone marrow cells can start an immunologic reaction against the body of the recipient. This complication is known as graft-versus-host disease or as "reverse rejection" (the recipient

body does not reject the graft, but the graft rejects the recipient body). There are only two situations where the problems of rejection and graft-versus-host disease don't play a role: when the recipient's own bone marrow cells are used for transplantation (autologous transplantation) and when the recipient receives bone marrow from an identical twin brother or sister (syngeneic transplantation).

Depending on the availability of appropriate donors, there are three types of bone marrow transplantation that can be attempted:

1. Autologous Transplantation If someone receives his or her own bone marrow after high-dose chemotherapy or radiotherapy, or both, we call the procedure an autologous transplantation. This can be done by removing marrow before therapy and keeping it in cold storage (cryopreservation) until treatment is complete. This procedure is particularly useful to treat a number of cancers that are very sensitive to chemotherapy or radiation therapy, but that cannot be cured with conventional doses of chemotherapy or radiation. Increasing the dose of chemotherapy or radiation increases the likelihood of curing the cancer. The increased doses of chemotherapy or radiation would normally destroy a patient's bone marrow, and recipients of such high-dose therapy would likely die from the lack of functional bone marrow. However, by first harvesting and storing the bone marrow stem cells and then returning these bone marrow stem cells to recipients after they have received their high-dose chemotherapy or radiation, it is possible to "bypass" this problem.

Autologous stem cell transplantation can therefore be thought of as a trick that doctors use to safely give patients very high doses of chemotherapy or radiation therapy. Because the donor and the recipient are the same individual, there is no risk of rejection or graft-versus-host disease. But it adds the risk of possibly reinfusing cancer cells that were inadvertently stored along with the marrow. And, of course, the procedure is helpful only for patients with cancer that is very sensitive to chemotherapy or radiation therapy.

2. Syngeneic Transplantation In rare instances, someone who needs a bone marrow transplant has an identical twin brother or sister. Because identical twins have the exact same immune composition, there is no risk of rejection or graft-versus-host disease when bone marrow is transplanted from one twin to the other. And, of course, there is no risk that the bone marrow from the donor twin contains contaminating cancer cells. A syngeneic transplantation is therefore more effective than an autologous transplant. Obviously, very few patients have an identical twin brother or sister.

3. Allogeneic Transplantation This type of bone marrow transplant involves the transfer of marrow from one individual to a completely different individual. The marrow donor is selected through a process known as HLA (human leukocyte antigen) typing. Each individual has unique proteins that appear on cell surfaces and are involved in cell self-recognition: the HLA antigens. These antigens can be identified in the laboratory through a blood test. This makes it possible to tell whether cells from two individuals have the same ("matched") HLA antigens or differ (are "unmatched") in their HLA antigen composition.

Because HLA antigens are inherited through parents (with half of the HLA type coming from the mother and the other half coming from the father), individuals with the same father and mother (e.g., brothers and sisters) have a chance of inheriting the same HLA type. This explains why doctors usually recommend HLA typing of brothers and sisters when they are searching for a possible bone marrow donor. The chance of any two siblings matching is one in four. Thus, if a person has one sibling, the chance for a match is 25 percent, with two siblings it is 44 percent, with three siblings it is 58 percent, and with four siblings it is 69 percent.

Unfortunately, many patients who could benefit from bone marrow transplantation do not have an HLA-matched brother or sister. Those patients rely on the identification of an unrelated volunteer bone marrow donor. Given the extraordinary complexity and diversity of HLA antigens—there are more than a billion possible combinations—finding matched but unrelated individuals is very difficult.

The National Marrow Donor Program (NMDP) operates in the United States and cooperates with similar registries in other countries to find unrelated donors. This registry has made it possible to identify donors for many patients with common HLA antigens. Yet it is still hard to find donors for patients with uncommon antigens. Adding to the problem is the uneven distribution of HLA antigens among people with different genetic backgrounds. Because most of the volunteer donors so far are of European ancestry, it is especially hard to find donors for patients with African, Asian, or other ancestry. (If you are interested in participating in the National Marrow Donor Program, contact your local Red Cross Blood Center for information about how to volunteer.)

The Source of Cells

There are small numbers of cells circulating in the blood that are as capable of replenishing the bone marrow as cells from the bone marrow itself. It has been shown that if sufficient numbers of these cells can be collected, they can be used for successful "bone marrow" transplantation. This procedure is often called a peripheral blood stem cell (PBSC) transplant. Both approaches are effective in restoring normal marrow function. Today most autologous transplants and an increasing number of allogeneic transplants are being done with cells derived from the blood.

A relatively new source of stem cells is blood from the umbilical cord. Cord blood is rich in stem cells, but the volume is small and the cell dose obtained is usually only adequate for engrafting children or very small adults. The availability of cord blood from cord blood banks has made it possible to perform stem cell transplants for patients who do not have an adequately matched related or unrelated donor.

How Stem Cells Are Obtained

In newborn children, essentially all bones have active marrow. In adults, active marrow is found mainly in the center of the pelvic bones, ribs, spine, and collarbone. When an appropriate donor is identified, active marrow can be removed from these bones with needles and a syringe. Alternatively, it is possible to remove stem cells from blood.

Getting Cells from the Bone Marrow Most bone marrow transplants involve extracting bone marrow from the bones of the pelvis by repeated needle punctures. The donor is usually under general or spinal anesthesia during this process, because it takes 150 to 200 needle punctures to remove enough marrow for a transplant— 500 to 1,000 ml (1 to 2 pints). Most donors who undergo a bone marrow harvest from the pelvic bones experience a sore back for a few days after the harvest procedure. Other complications are rare.

Getting Cells from the Blood Immature blood stem cells can be obtained from blood by a procedure called apheresis. This involves drawing blood into a machine that works like a cream separator. The machine skims off the peripheral blood stem cells, and the remaining blood cells are returned to the donor. The procedure has to be repeated several times to get enough cells for transplantation. Each procedure usually lasts two to four hours. Prior to the apheresis procedure, the number of immature cells in the blood usually has to be increased by the administration of various drugs (usually hematopoietic growth factors), allowing more rapid collection. Both allogeneic and autologous transplants can be done in this way. Peripheral blood stem cell collection does not require any type of anesthesia, and there is usually no soreness at the completion of the procedure. There may be side effects from the administration of hematopoietic growth factors or other drugs. And it usually takes longer to collect cells from the bloodstream than to harvest them from the bone marrow.

Obtaining Cord Blood Cord blood is obtained from the umbilical cord immediately after delivery of a baby. The cells are then processed and frozen for future use. Because the cells are removed after the delivery, there is no risk to the mother or the newborn baby.

Complications and Risks

Any transplant procedure is fraught with risk. Anyone undertaking this risky venture usually does so because the alternatives are less attractive. The specific risks are related to the phase of the procedure and can be divided into effects that are delayed or immediate.

Delayed Effects Long-term toxic effects of high-dose therapy can include cataracts in people receiving total body radiotherapy. Exposure to irradiation also increases the chance of developing other cancers, such as skin cancers and certain types of leukemia. Girls who receive radiation during puberty are at an increased risk of developing breast cancer later in life. Radiation exposure can inactivate the function of the thyroid gland (hypothyroidism) several years later. And both radiation and chemotherapy can result in sterility of men and women who are still fertile prior to their bone marrow transplantation.

Immediate Risks Much more threatening are the risks during and soon after the transplant procedure. The high-dose therapy itself, the damage to the immune system, and the reaction of the immune system to the transplanted marrow can all cause dangerous complications.

• *Toxic Reactions from Drugs and Irradiation* High-dose therapy occasionally has an acute toxic effect on the heart, lungs, liver, or kidneys that can be life-threatening, although this is quite rare.

• *Infections* After the transplant, there will be a period of one and a half to four weeks during which the new bone marrow cannot manufacture red cells, white cells, or platelets. Though it is fairly easy to transfuse red cells and platelets, it is nearly impossible to transfuse white cells. Going without them for any time is dangerous, because the risk of infection is high when blood counts are very low. So anyone getting a transplant will usually be given liberal amounts of antibiotics. Sometimes these are given before any signs of infection appear and are usually not discontinued until the blood counts have returned to a more normal level. They are always given at the first sign of a fever. Most of the time, infections can be controlled until normal white cells return. But certain infections—such as fungal infections—can still prove fatal.

• *Pneumonia* The lung seems to be the organ most sensitive to the adverse effects of transplantation. It has been suggested that the lung is to bone marrow transplantation what the quarterback's knee is to the football game. A lot can go wrong. The lung can be injured because of infection, because of the toxic effect of high-dose chemotherapy or radiation, or because of some unknown cause.

When severe pneumonia develops after a bone marrow transplant, death often—but not always—results. The most common pneumonia after transplant is caused by aspergillus, a particularly severe pneumonia that can develop during or several months after the transplant. Previously, reactivation of cytomegalovirus frequently caused life-threatening pneumonia after an allogeneic transplant. That complication has been decreased by the prophylactic use of an antiviral drug, ganciclovir.

• *Bleeding* Platelets can usually be transfused easily, but for a few patients it is difficult to transfuse enough of them. For these patients, serious bleeding is a possibility.

• *Graft Rejection* This is a serious risk for people having an allogeneic bone marrow transplant for aplastic anemia. The risk seems greater for those who have unrelated or less well-matched allogeneic transplants. What usually happens is that the marrow function starts to come back, but then it disappears. This is a serious complication, but it can sometimes be overcome by a second transplant.

• *Graft-Versus-Host Disease* After an allogeneic bone marrow transplant, the immunologically active cells in the new marrow can recognize the "host"—the patient receiving the transplant—as foreign and start an attack. The most commonly damaged organs are the skin, liver, and intestines.

Medicines have to be given after a transplant to reduce the possibility of graft-versus-host disease but are not always 100 percent effective. If the condition nevertheless develops, it can occur soon after the return of white cells (acute graft-versus-host disease) or much later (chronic graft-versus-host disease).

The two types are similar in some ways, though each has distinctive features. The acute form often doesn't last long but can be quite severe. If it is severe, the prognosis for survival is very poor. Chronic graft-versus-host disease is usually not immediately life-threatening but can be severe enough to affect quality of life. Patients with chronic graft-versus-host disease often suffer from dry eyes, mouth sores and swallowing difficulty, skin rashes, and lack of flexibility of the skin and joints. Less commonly the liver or lungs can be affected. Chronic graft-versus-host disease is difficult to treat, and the treatment often has to be continued for many years.

Choosing a Transplant Center

If there were a simpler way to cure cancer, there would certainly be no call for bone marrow transplantation. Having the procedure will sometimes involve traveling a considerable distance to a marrow transplant center. Which center to choose is often a difficult decision, with such factors as convenience, the center's experience with the disease, and insurance issues all affecting the decision.

Experience When facing a treatment as dangerous as bone marrow transplantation, most people want to be sure they are treated at a highly experienced center so the risk can be minimized. With certain cancers, it might be appropriate to choose a transplant center that has a special interest and extensive experience with your particular type of tumor.

The American Society of Clinical Oncology, the American Society of Hematology, and the American Society of Blood and Bone Marrow Transplantation have made joint recommendations for the *minimal* criteria for a center to perform the procedure. You and your doctor may want to consult one of these organizations.

Costs Bone marrow transplantation is expensive and, in the United States, all transplant centers, before they will allow admission, will want some guarantee that the cost of the treatment will be reimbursed. Most health insurance companies in the United States now have contracts with selected transplant centers, and full reimbursement is usually available only for patients who undergo their transplant procedure in one of those selected institutions. Unfortunately, some patients will be denied this treatment altogether because their insurance company will refuse to pay for it.

Getting Started If you are referred to a particular transplant center, you will usually have to go to the facility for a "transplant interview." The center has to decide whether you are a good candidate for the treatment. You have to decide whether you feel comfortable undergoing treatment at that center.

Once this decision has been jointly made, there will be other decisions such as whether more "traditional" therapy might be done to improve the chance for success. An allogeneic donor may have to be found or stem cells will have to be taken and stored for an autologous transplantation.

A Summary of the Steps to a Successful Transplant

For a successful bone marrow transplant to be performed, your medical team will have to complete a number of steps in sequence. Each step involves critical decisions and potential risks.

1. Determine that the cancer is sensitive to high-dose therapy and cannot be cured with simpler treatment.

For both doctor and patient, this is the hardest part of the procedure. The candidate for a transplant has to have a disease serious enough that a treatment as risky as bone marrow transplantation is a reasonable option.

What makes the decision particularly difficult is that transplants are much more successful when patients are referred for treatment early in the course of their disease. Early on, they are more likely to be healthy, there is less cancer, and it hasn't become highly resistant to therapy after repeated treatments. But transplant-related deaths are least acceptable in these early stages. The easiest course would be to refer a patient for transplantation only when all other therapies have failed. Unfortunately, at that point bone marrow transplantation is not likely to be beneficial.

The best approach, then, is to identify those who might benefit from the procedure and refer them for the treatment as soon as it seems clear that they cannot be cured with a simpler therapy.

2. Identify a donor to obtain stem cells.

Once the decision to have a transplant is made, the next difficult decision is what type of donor to use. As previously explained, autologous transplantations are generally less risky. But if the bone marrow is extensively involved by tumor, an allogeneic or syngeneic transplant or a peripheral blood stem cell transplant will be the only choice. There may be other problems that preclude the use of autologous transplantation. In that case, a bone marrow donor will have to be found: an HLA-matched brother or sister, a partially matched relative, or a matched but unrelated donor for an allogeneic transplant or an identical twin for a syngeneic transplant. The identification of a suitable donor can take as long as several months.

3. Decide on the type of conditioning regimen.

The purpose of the conditioning regimen is to destroy the cancer and to suppress the recipient immune system enough for the new bone marrow cells to grow. The choice between a traditional high-dose conditioning regimen and a reduced-intensity ("mini") conditioning regimen usually depends on factors like the age and underlying disease of the recipient.

4. Infuse the marrow stem cells intravenously.

In a typical bone marrow transplant unit, the day on which the marrow is given is referred to as day 0 (zero). The other days spent in the hospital are numbered as either a plus or a minus, counting from the day the marrow is infused.

5. Manage the complications until the marrow produces enough normal blood cells and, in an allogeneic transplant, until graft-versus-host disease is controlled.

The period after the marrow infusion is the most dangerous. This is when the bone marrow cells begin to proliferate, ideally to the point where the marrow will produce enough red cells, white cells, and platelets. This is also when there is a high risk of infections, bleeding problems, and graft-versus-host disease. Most patients who don't survive long after a bone marrow transplant die from infections or the effects of graft-versus-host disease after the new marrow starts to grow. Most patients have to stay in close proximity to their transplant center until the risk of such complications has decreased enough to safely return home.

Effectiveness of Bone Marrow Transplantation for Selected Cancers

The information below summarizes the results of allogeneic and autologous bone marrow transplantation as a treatment for a variety of cancers. These results are only summaries and certainly vary with specific clinical situations. In general, younger age, well-matched donors, healthy recipients, and absence of disease at the time of transplant are associated with better outcomes.

It is also important to recognize that bone marrow transplantation as a treatment for cancer is a fast-changing field. New high-dose therapies or improved transplant techniques might change the results with a particular disease in a very short time.

Acute Leukemia Both adults and children with acute leukemia are often treated with bone marrow transplantation. Some patients with acute leukemia might benefit from autologous bone marrow transplantation, but the majority of transplant procedures for acute leukemia in the United States are allogeneic transplantations.

Adults with acute myelogenous leukemia (AML; the most common acute leukemia in adults) or with acute lymphoblastic leukemia (ALL) are usually offered an allogeneic bone marrow transplantation if they have AML or ALL that is characterized by a high risk of disease recurrence after standard chemotherapy treatment. The risk of recurrence can be assessed by special tests that are usually done at the time the leukemia is diagnosed. These tests are known as cytogenetic studies, and the results determine who is most likely to benefit from an allogeneic transplantation. Adults with high-risk AML or ALL who undergo an allogeneic transplantation as part of their initial treatment have a cure rate of 40 to 50 percent. Transplants that are performed later in the course of the disease (when the leukemia has recurred) are less successful, with a cure rate of 20 to 30 percent.

Many children with ALL can be cured without any transplantation. However, for some children with high-risk ALL or recurrent ALL, an allogeneic transplantation is the treatment of choice. Most children with AML are offered an allogeneic transplantation as part of the initial treatment. Outcomes in children are generally slightly (5 to 10 percent) better than in adults.

Chronic Leukemia Allogeneic transplantation used to be the treatment of choice for patients with chronic myelogenous leukemia (CML). The cure rate for patients treated early after diagnosis is approximately 80 percent. However, new treatments that do not involve transplantation have recently become available. Early results of treatment with the drug imatinib mesylate (Gleevec) look very promising, and allogeneic transplantation is now often reserved for patients with advanced disease at the time of diagnosis or patients who do not respond well to treatment with imatinib. There is only limited experience with the use of allogeneic transplantation for patients with chronic lymphocytic leukemia (CLL). Patients with CML or CLL are usually not treated with autologous transplantation.

Non-Hodgkin's Lymphomas and Hodgkin's Disease Lymphomas are among the tumors most responsive to chemotherapy and radiation, so it is not surprising that these tumors are among those most likely to respond to high-dose therapy accompanied by a bone marrow transplant. Because these diseases often respond well to high-dose chemotherapy and radiation, they are most commonly treated with autologous transplantation procedures. For a small percentage of patients with non-Hodgkin's lymphoma or Hodgkin's disease (for instance, patients with recurrent disease after previous autologous stem cell transplantation), allogeneic transplantation can still offer a possibility for cure. There are many different types of non-Hodgkin's lymphoma, and the success rates depend on the exact type of lymphoma that is treated. Following are some of the more commonly treated lymphomas:

Aggressive Non-Hodgkin's Lymphomas (mostly diffuse large B cell lymphomas) These can be cured between one-third and one-half of the time with primary therapy. But if there is a relapse after initial therapy, autologous stem cell transplantation will cure 30 to 50 percent of patients. In addition, certain patients with advanced disease at the time of diagnosis might benefit from autologous transplantation early in the course of their disease (immediately following standard chemotherapy treatment).

Follicular Non-Hodgkin's Lymphomas These malignancies are rarely cured with standard therapies, although they are associated with a long average survival. But an average survival of even ten years is not good enough for people who are thirty or forty years old at the time of diagnosis. For this reason, several centers have recently begun to treat follicular lymphoma patients with high-dose therapy and bone marrow transplantation early in the course of their disease. Allogeneic transplantation has also been increasingly used for this disease. The results so far show that these patients tolerate the transplant process well and a large proportion of them stay in remission for extended periods.

Mantle Cell Non-Hodgkin's Lymphoma This lymphoma is very difficult to cure with standard doses of chemotherapy and/or radiation therapy. Some recent studies have shown very promising results with the use of autologous transplantation and reduced-intensity allogeneic transplantation for patients who are transplanted as part of their initial treatment.

Hodgkin's Disease Patients with this cancer do so well with standard treatment approaches that physicians in the past have been reluctant to refer them for transplantation early enough in their disease for a transplant to be beneficial.

But patients who relapse after high-quality combination chemotherapy have a poor outlook with more standard therapy. And when these patients are referred for high-dose therapy and bone marrow transplantation soon after their relapse, 50 percent or more seem to be long-term, disease-free survivors—in other words, probably cured. The cure rate is much less (10 to 20 percent) when they have the transplant after failing many chemotherapy regimens.

Multiple Myeloma Autologous stem cell transplantation does not cure patients with this blood cancer, but it can significantly increase survival. Most patients are therefore offered an autologous stem cell transplant as part of their initial therapy. Allogeneic transplantation with high-dose conditioning is generally not well tolerated by patients with multiple myeloma, but reduced-intensity allogeneic transplantation appears better tolerated. The optimal transplant strategy for patients with myeloma (autologous, allogeneic, or both) is still being investigated. In addition, new drugs have been developed for the treatment of myeloma that might result in outcomes that are just as good as or better than the outcomes achieved with stem cell transplantation.

Solid Tumors in Adults Bone marrow transplantation has been used in a wide variety of so-called solid tumors—carcinomas and sarcomas—in adults. It can cure some men with advanced testicular cancer, for example, a predictable result given the extraordinary responsiveness of testicular cancer to chemotherapy. A small number of patients with soft-tissue sarcomas have also had long remissions after high-dose therapy and a bone marrow transplant.

Unfortunately, many common solid tumors such as lung cancers and gastrointestinal cancers aren't sensitive enough to high-dose chemotherapy and radiation to make the bone marrow procedure beneficial.

One of the most common carcinomas in the United States—breast cancer—is reasonably sensitive to chemotherapy and radiotherapy. Clinical trials with high-dose therapy and autologous bone marrow transplantation suggest that increased doses of drugs active against breast cancer can increase the response rate. However, a large randomized trial in metastatic disease showed no difference in disease control or survival between conventional chemotherapy and autologous transplant. Studies determining the benefit of adjuvant transplant for breast cancer are too early to be conclusive. Recently regression of renal cell cancer after nonmyeloablative allogeneic stem cell transplant was reported in patients with tumor unresponsive to conventional therapy.

Solid Tumors in Children Most pediatric solid tumors are sensitive to chemotherapy and can sometimes be cured by chemotherapy without bone marrow transplantation. But, as might be expected, high-dose therapy and autologous or allogeneic transplantation can cure some children who can't be cured with standard therapy. Neuroblastoma is the pediatric cancer in which the procedure has been most carefully studied. It appears that some children can have long-lasting remissions—in other words, can probably be cured—with high-dose therapy and bone marrow transplantation. But, as with many other diseases, the optimal timing and treatment procedures have not yet been identified.

Aplastic Anemia Aplastic anemia is a disease that results in complete absence of normal bone marrow activity. Allogeneic bone marrow transplantation is the procedure of choice for younger patients (generally up to forty years) with a matched sibling donor. The outcomes are excellent, with cure rates well over 80 percent. Unfortunately, the cure rates for older patients and for patients undergoing unrelated donor transplants are not as good.

The Future of Transplantation

Bone marrow transplantation is a rapidly evolving field that is likely to become more important in cancer treatment. The advances over the past several decades have been remarkable. As a result of improved recognition and treatment of infections, the risk of dying from an autologous stem cell transplantation is now well below 5 percent in most experienced transplant centers. Allogeneic transplantation remains more risky, but the introduction of reduced-intensity transplant procedures has made this procedure available to many patients for whom the procedure was previously considered too risky. Basic research has vastly improved our understanding of the complex immunologic interactions that occur after allogeneic stem cell transplantation. The expectation is that this will result in more "targeted" transplant strategies that selectively eliminate cancer cells without harming healthy normal cells. The use of well-designed clinical research trials will have to show the efficacy of these new approaches.

— 16 —

Integrative Oncology:
Complementary Therapies in Cancer Care

Barrie R. Cassileth, Ph.D., and K. Simon Yeung, Pharm.D., M.B.A.

■ ■ ■ ■

The terminology in this area of patient care has been unfortunate, as there are both good and bad therapies called by the same words: *alternative; complementary; questionable; complementary and alternative medicine (CAM);* and so on. This has created a great deal of confusion. This chapter aims to provide some clarity and to review therapies that can safely and effectively help you through cancer treatment and beyond. Dangerous products and those that are not effective are also discussed.

"Alternative" Medicine

"Alternative therapies" are typically promoted as independent, viable treatments for cancer, literal alternatives to mainstream care such as surgery, chemotherapy, and radiotherapy. Such "alternatives" are not viable options at all. They are often invasive and biologically active, unproven or disproven, expensive, and potentially harmful.

They may harm directly through biologic activity, or indirectly when patients postpone receipt of mainstream care. Examples include the metabolic therapies available in Tijuana, Mexico; high-dose vitamins and other products sold over the counter or delivered intravenously in alternative clinics; electromagnetic cures; and many other products and regimens.

Therapies promoted for use instead of mainstream care do not work and should not be used.

Unfortunately, information available to the public varies widely in accuracy, and misinformation about health issues is widespread. Many Web sites and publications that seem to be objective are actually sponsored by commercial groups that promote and sell the products they report on. In 1999, the U.S. Federal Trade Commission (FTC) identified hundreds of Web sites promoting and selling phony cures for cancer and other serious illnesses and has worked to remove them. Today, however, there are still literally millions of Web sites about alternative or complementary cancer therapies, some accurate and many not.

It is difficult, if not impossible, for most people to distinguish between reputable sources of information and those backed by vested interests. However, one quick clue is to look at the source of the information. If it is a major cancer center, the American Cancer Society, the National Cancer Institute, or another part of the National Institutes of Health, you know it will provide accurate and useful information. On the other hand, if the book or Web site is selling a cancer treatment that is not offered in your hospital's cancer program, or if it is claiming to cure cancer, view it with great caution (reputable

Web sites are listed at the end of this chapter).

The physicist Dr. Robert L. Park, in his *Voodoo Science: The Road from Foolishness to Fraud,* notes seven signs of voodoo science, on which the following list on voodoo medicine is based:

1. The proponent pitches his or her claim directly to media.
2. The proponent claims that a powerful establishment is suppressing his or her work.
3. The evidence is anecdotal rather than based on solid published data.
4. The proponent works in isolation.
5. The proponent says his or her belief is true because it has endured for decades or centuries.
6. Any benefit is at the very limit of detection.
7. New laws of nature are offered to explain how it works.

Look out for these claims and avoid therapies associated with these kinds of statements.

Integrative Oncology

Integrative oncology is a synthesis of the best of mainstream cancer care and complementary therapies. There is an important difference between complementary therapies and false "alternatives." Complementary therapies are used along with mainstream treatment, primarily to manage physical and emotional symptoms, as detailed further below.

Complementary Therapies According to a large survey, all but a tiny fraction, perhaps about 2 percent, of people who use complementary or alternative remedies do so to complement, not to replace, mainstream care. That is, they correctly use complementary therapies, not alternatives. Virtually all studies conducted of cancer patients and of the general public

internationally show that those who use complementary therapies tend to be better educated, of higher socioeconomic status, female, and younger than those who do not. They also tend to be more health conscious and to use more mainstream medical services than people who do not.

National Activity The Office of Alternative Medicine (OAM) was established at the National Institutes of Health by congressional mandate in 1992, its stated purpose to investigate unconventional medical practices. In 1998, Congress elevated the OAM to the National Center for Complementary and Alternative Medicine (NCCAM), allocating more money for its research. In 1998, the Office of Cancer Complementary and Alternative Medicine (OCCAM) was established at the National Cancer Institute (NCI) to coordinate and help support good research related to cancer.

In addition, numerous hospitals, medical centers, and major cancer centers have developed research and clinical service programs in complementary therapies. These helpful, evidence-based therapies include meditation and other mind–body relaxation therapies, massage therapies, acupuncture, exercise, fitness and nutritional guidance, counseling on the use of herbs and food supplements, yoga classes, and more. Research often addresses these topics as well. Helpful complementary therapies are listed in Table 1 and discussed in the following sections.

Mind–Body Techniques The potential to influence our health with our minds is an appealing concept in the United States. It affirms the power of the individual, a belief common in American culture. Some mind–body interventions, such as hypnosis, meditation, and relaxation techniques, have moved into mainstream medicine as their merits have been studied and

Table 1. Complementary Therapies to Smooth the Way During Cancer Treatment and Recovery

ANXIETY AND STRESS

Acupressure: Use the fingers of one hand to press inside the wrist of the other hand. Press for a minute or two approximately 2 inches above the hand crease. Pressing this acupoint relieves nausea as well as anxiety and stress.

Aromatherapy: Put a few drops of essential oil of rosemary, lavender, or chamomile (available at health food stores and pharmacies) in the bath, or light a scented candle while relaxing. The fragrance is luxurious and calming.

Meditation and other relaxation techniques: These are opportunities for minivacations in the mind. Close your eyes and see yourself in a pleasant, peaceful place. Breathe deeply and slowly. Or lie down, eyes closed. Start at the tips of your toes and gradually move up your body as you consciously relax each body part. Your body and mind will relax accordingly.

Music therapy: Music has important physiologic as well as emotional benefits. It calms, distracts, and soothes at a very fundamental level of being.

Therapeutic massage: Visit a licensed, certified massage therapist experienced with people undergoing cancer therapy, or arrange for that person to visit you. Or have a friend or family member gently massage your neck and shoulders, hands, and feet. Weekly therapeutic massages will keep you feeling good.

Valerian: Make a tea from 1 to 2 teaspoons of the dried root from this herb. You may prefer capsules, because the tea does not have a pleasant odor (health food stores and pharmacies have both). It is nonaddictive and effectively reduces anxiety and brings about sleep.

Yoga: Take a class, rent a videotape, or borrow a book, and practice postures along with deep-breathing techniques. Anyone can do it—even while bedridden. It is said to bring mind, body, and spirit together in a peaceful union. However it works, yoga relaxes.

BACKACHE OR MUSCLE ACHE

Capsicum cream: Hot red peppers contain a powerful pain-relieving chemical called capsaicin. It is the active ingredient in many rub-on pharmaceutic pain relievers. Blend or mash a red pepper. Add some of the mashed red pepper to white body lotion or cold cream until the mixture turns pink. Rub it on the sore areas.

Hydrotherapy: A warm bath or Jacuzzi should help.

Massage: Try a professional massage by a licensed, certified massage therapist or a careful muscle massage by a friend or relative. Patients with lymphatic cancers should avoid touch massage.

Willow bark tea: The bark of the willow tree contains salicin, the active ingredient in aspirin. (Avoid this herb if aspirin causes upset stomach, if you take an anticoagulant such as warfarin (Coumadin), or if your doctor told you to use an aspirin substitute.)

COLDS AND FLU

Garlic: Eat raw or cooked garlic, or try deodorized garlic capsules.

Eucalyptus or camphor: Place in a steam vaporizer and inhale. This may help to reduce symptoms of congestion.

Zinc lozenges: Studies show they may reduce the duration of a cold or flu.

CONSTIPATION

Fluid extracts or capsules of senna: These work well. Plantago seed, also called psyllium seed, is an effective herbal bulk laxative. Take it with plenty of water.

Prune juice: Alone or flavored with apple juice, lemon, and honey, this is a delicious way to solve the problem.

Water (6 to 8 glasses a day) and fiber (fruit, bran cereal, prunes): Consumed regularly, these should keep the problem away, and regular exercise is also helpful.

DEPRESSION

Light therapy: This consists of bright-light boxes placed at eye level on a desk or table. Light boxes are made specifically to reduce depression, and they are especially effective in northern parts of the world where sunlight is rare or during winter months in the Northern Hemisphere. Light boxes are used in mainstream medicine and recommended by psychiatrists to treat seasonal affective disorder (SAD).

Meditation and yoga: Both of these are very helpful for depression as well as anxiety (see "Anxiety and Stress," above).

Tai chi: This is a gentle exercise program practiced daily by millions of older Chinese and popular in the United States as well. Follow the slow motions, which typically mimic animal movements, as displayed in books, videos, or classes. Research shows that tai chi not only lifts depressed mood, but also improves bodily balance, reduces falls, and increases physical strength.

DIARRHEA

Peppermint tea, and yogurt.

HEADACHE

Acupressure: Press the acupoint(s) between the eyebrows or in the hollows at the base of the skull on both sides of the spine.

HEARTBURN

Herb teas, especially ginger and peppermint.

NAUSEA

Acupressure: Press inside the wrist with the fingers of the other hand (see "Anxiety and Stress," above).

Peppermint tea.

Ginger tea, capsules, or candy: Shave peeled fresh ginger and add it to boiled water to make tea, or add sugar and gelatin to the boiled ginger water and let it cool. Cut it into cubes and eat it as candy. Ginger ale or cookies, if made with real ginger and not flavoring, works, too. Ginger capsules are available at health food stores and pharmacies.

PAIN, CHRONIC

Acupuncture: See your yellow pages for a licensed, accredited acupuncture doctor. Properly trained acupuncturists use disposable stainless steel needles and do a virtually painless job.

(continues)

Table 1. **Complementary Therapies to Smooth the Way During Cancer Treatment and Recovery** *(continued)*

PAIN, CHRONIC

Biofeedback: This requires equipment and a trained biofeedback therapist. Check the phone book. Many pain clinics and pain management experts in hospitals use biofeedback or can make referrals.

Useful herbs: These include external capsicum (see "Backache or Muscle Ache," above), and willow bark tea (avoid if you should not take aspirin or are on anticoagulants).

Hypnotherapy: Some people can get rid of chronic pain, or reduce it substantially, with hypnosis. Pain clinics, the phone book, and your nurse or doctor are good referral sources for certified hypnotherapists.

Therapeutic massage (see "Anxiety and Stress," above).

SLEEP PROBLEMS

Hydrotherapy: Relax in a warm bath scented with lavender oil.

Therapeutic massage (see "Anxiety and Stress," above).

Meditation (see "Anxiety and Stress," above).

Tea of fresh or dried lemon balm or valerian root (see "Anxiety and Stress," above).

published. Randomized trials have demonstrated the positive effects of relaxation therapy on anxiety, depression, or mood in cancer patients. Relaxation training and hypnosis decrease anxiety during treatment procedures, such as chemotherapy and bone marrow aspiration, in most randomized trials. In addition, hypnosis can effectively treat anticipatory nausea in children. Research has also generally found hypnosis and relaxation training to help relieve chemotherapy-related nausea in adults.

Some proponents argue that patients can use mental attributes and mind–body work to prevent or cure cancer. This belief is attractive because it ascribes to patients almost complete control over the course of their illness. But, unfortunately, it is not true. Psychological health is an important part of good cancer care. Support groups, good doctor–patient communication, and the emotional and instrumental help of family and friends are vital. However, the idea that patients can influence the course of their disease through mental or emotional work is wishful thinking, and it has been proven wrong in many studies. That idea is also counterproductive, because it can evoke feelings of guilt and inadequacy if disease continues to advance despite one's best spiritual or mental efforts.

Traditional Medical Systems Ancient healing systems, such as Ayurveda from India and traditional Chinese medicine, have given us complementary therapies that can enrich our lives today. The term *ayurveda* comes from the Sanskrit words *ayur* ("life") and *veda* ("knowledge"). Ayurveda's ancient healing techniques are based on the classification of people into one of three main body types. For each, there are specific remedies for disease and prescriptions to promote health. This system has a strong mind–body component and uses techniques such as yoga and meditation to keep the body in balance, techniques that are as helpful today as when they were first developed some 3,000 to 4,000 years ago.

Traditional Chinese medicine explains the body in terms of its relationship to the environment and the cosmos. Qi (pronounced "chee"), the life force said to run through all of nature, flows in the human body through vertical energy channels known as meridians. It is believed that qi must flow in the correct strength and quality through each of the meridians and organs for health to be maintained. Illness is thought to result from blockages to the free flow of qi. Acupuncture, the insertion of needles at special points on the meridians, is used to eliminate the blockages and restore the free flow of the life force. Given modern understanding, acupuncture points appear to correspond to physiologic and anatomic features such as nerve junctions or trigger points.

Although the very existence of qi or a "vital energy force" has never been proven, there is a great deal of scientific research that supports the value of acupuncture for the relief of pain and other symptoms. Evidence from randomized trials indicates that acupuncture is effective for both acute and chronic pain. Studies report that approximately half of patients in significant pain despite receiving good pharmaceutical management gain persisting pain relief from acupuncture. One explanation for the pain-control effects of acupuncture is that it stimulates release of the body's own narcotics and other chemicals sent out by the brain. Functional MRI technology is now used to examine the specific nervous pathways involved in acupuncture. Acupuncture can produce activity in certain areas of the brain that are involved in pain perception.

Another carefully studied problem is nausea and vomiting, where randomized, placebo-controlled trials consistently support the effectiveness of acupuncture as an antinausea treatment in pregnancy, after anesthesia, and during chemotherapy, and to prevent postoperative vomiting in pediatric patients.

In addition to acupuncture, acupressure, qigong, and tai chi also come from traditional Chinese medicine. Tai chi is a well-documented, effective, gentle exercise technique, particularly useful in preventing falls among the frail or elderly. The wisdom of the ages still proves helpful today.

Touch Therapies Hands-on therapeutic massage has important benefits, documented in randomized trials. These studies suggest that massage therapy reduces anxiety in many groups, including cancer patients. Data also indicate that massage relieves depression and fatigue, as well as pain and anxiety. Touch is a valuable therapy.

"Therapeutic touch" is another popular manual healing method that, despite its name, involves no direct contact. Instead, healers move their hands a few inches above a patient's body and sweep away "blockages" to the patient's energy field. A study published in the *Journal of the American Medical Association (JAMA)* showed that experienced therapeutic touch practitioners were unable to detect the investigator's "energy field." Mainstream science does not accept the ideas on which no-touch "therapeutic touch" is based.

Herbal Remedies for Cancer Herbal remedies are an essential part of traditional and folk healing methods with long histories of use. Herbal treatments for illnesses have been found in virtually all areas of the world and across cultures throughout time. Although many prescription medications, including several chemotherapeutic agents, come originally from natural products, few unrefined herbs in their natural state have been found useful when they have been submitted to actual study. Although many herbal and other natural products are promoted and sold over the counter as anticancer agents, very few are found to work.

Essiac is one example. It has remained popular for decades, especially in North America. Developed initially by a native healer from southwestern Canada, it was popularized by a Canadian nurse, Rene Caisse (*essiac* is Caisse spelled backward). Essiac is made of four herbs: burdock root, Turkey rhubarb, sheep sorrel, and slippery elm bark. Researchers at the National Institutes of Health and elsewhere found that it has no anticancer effect, but it is still widely promoted.

Another example is Iscador, a derivative of mistletoe. This is a popular cancer remedy in Europe, where it is said to have been in continuous use as a folk treatment since the druids danced around Stonehenge. Survival benefit has not been shown in good studies.

Selected vegetable (SV) soup is an opposite example. This is a formula of nineteen vegetables from traditional Chinese medicine developed by a New York laboratory scientist who wanted it to be studied properly. The antitumor activity of SV soup was studied by adding it to the diets of twelve patients with Stages III and IV nonsmall cell lung cancer. Thirteen clinically similar patients who did not receive SV soup served as controls. All patients received conventional therapies. The median survival of control patients was 4 months (mean 4.8 months). The median survival of patients who received the vegetable remedy was 15.5 months (mean 15 months). Because this nontoxic vegetable brew seemed to improve survival and quality of life in nonsmall cell lung cancer, the National Institutes of Health support a study that is currently under way at Mount Sinai Hospital in New York City.

This study is an example of how herbal cancer remedies, pretested to ensure purity and consistency of product and studied carefully, may produce potentially useful, nontoxic cancer treatments. The difficulty with most time-honored herbal remedies is that they are rarely tested for purity, examined for consistency, or studied carefully.

Nonetheless, unwarranted promotional claims are often made for these products and they remain readily available.

Cancer patients are often tempted to try over-the-counter herbal products, including those promoted as viable cancer treatments. It is therefore important to recognize herbal remedies that may help (see Table 1) and those that are toxic or interact with other medications (see Table 2). Because neither the FDA nor any other governmental agency examines herbal remedies for safety and effectiveness prior to their marketing, few products have been formally tested for benefits, side effects, or quality control, but information is beginning to emerge from public experience with over-the-counter supplements.

Recent reports in literature describe severe liver and kidney damage from some herbal remedies. These reports underscore the fact that "natural" products are not necessarily safe or harmless. Many people are not aware that herbs are dilute pharmaceuticals, natural drugs that contain scores of different chemicals, most of which have not been documented. Effects are not always predictable. Herbs and other natural products can keep blood from clotting or increase the intensity of prescription medications or produce other unwanted results.

Furthermore, possible herb–drug interactions are of serious concern. Patients on chemotherapy should stop using herbal remedies before and during treatment. Similar cautions are necessary before radiation, as some herbs photosensitize the skin and cause severe reactions. Patients scheduled for surgery should be aware that some herbs produce dangerous blood pressure swings and other unwanted interactions with anesthetics. Herbal supplements such as feverfew, garlic, ginger, and ginkgo interfere with clotting of the blood and should be avoided by anyone on warfarin (Coumadin), heparin, aspirin, or related agents. The risk of herb–drug interactions appears to be greatest for patients with kidney or liver problems.

Dietary Supplements Nonprescription dietary supplements, which include vitamins and minerals, homeopathic remedies, herbal treatments, antioxidants, and other over-the-counter products, are commonly used today by cancer patients as well as by the public in general.

No legal standards exist for the processing or packaging of herbs. Quality-control standards and reviews are needed. Because they are not mandatory, however, few food supplement companies voluntarily self-impose quality evaluation and control. Consumer protection and enforcement agencies cannot provide protection against contaminated or falsely advertised products. Current federal regulations do not permit such oversight, and full policing and analysis of the estimated 20,000 food supplement items now sold over the counter is logistically and financially prohibitive.

In Summary

Fraudulent products and regimens abound; there are no viable "alternatives" to mainstream cancer care. Complementary therapies, conversely, are rational, evidence-based therapies used along with mainstream cancer care to relieve symptoms and enhance quality of life. Massage therapy, acupuncture, music therapy, meditation, self-hypnosis, and other mind–body therapies are examples of complementary interventions that effectively reduce physical and emotional symptoms associated with cancer and its current treatments. These helpful complementary therapies should be sought from certified practitioners trained to treat patients with cancer. Herbal remedies, many of which hold great promise and are currently under study, should be avoided by patients under active treatment or on prescription medication.

Sources of Reliable Information

National Cancer Institute Office of Cancer Complementary and Alternative Medicine: *www.nci.gov/occam*

National Institutes of Health National Center for Complementary and Alternative Medicine: *www.nih.gov/nccam*

Memorial Sloan-Kettering Cancer Center (information about herbs, vitamins, and other over-the-counter products): *www.mskcc.org/Aboutherbs*

Table 2. **Dangerous Herbs**

HERB	WHAT PEOPLE USE IT FOR	ADVERSE EFFECTS
Chaparral tea	Pain	Liver failure
Comfrey	Bruises, ulcers	Toxic to the liver and can lead to death
Kava kava	Anxiety, insomnia	Liver failure
Ma huang (ephedra) (banned by FDA)	Asthma, weight loss	Heart failure and stroke
Saint-John's-wort	Depression	Interferes with chemotherapy and other prescription medications
Yohimbe	Sexual dysfunction	Seizures, kidney failure, and death

National Council Against Health Fraud:
www.quackwatch.org

American Society of Clinical Oncology:
www.asco.org

— 17 —

Blood Transfusions and Cancer Treatment

Nora V. Hirschler, M.D., Herbert A. Perkins, M.D., and Kim-Anh Nguyen, M.D.

■ ■ ■ ■

Blood is a complex living tissue. It is made up of three kinds of cells that are manufactured in the blood cell "factory"—the marrow cavity of our bones. All these cells are suspended in a liquid called plasma, and each cell plays a critical role in keeping us alive.

• Red blood cells carry oxygen to our tissues.
• White blood cells—leukocytes—help us fight off infections.
• Platelets are necessary to form the blood clots that stop bleeding.

Blood transfusions play a crucial role in cancer treatment. The disease can reduce the marrow's ability to produce blood cells, sometimes so severely that the cells have to be replaced by transfusion. Some forms of cancer—leukemia and multiple myeloma—grow in the marrow cavity, leaving no space for the development of normal blood cells. These normal cells will then have to be provided by transfusion.

But most of the people with cancer who need blood transfusions need them because of the aggressive approaches used to treat the disease. If blood transfusions weren't available, most of the remarkably effective cancer treatments available today could never have been introduced—the chemotherapy used to kill cancer cells, for example, which may also kill developing blood cells in the marrow. Also, many cancers can

be cured or at least helped by surgery, and that surgery may result in loss of blood by hemorrhage to the point where it has to be replaced. No other form of medical treatment can make such a difference between life and death as blood transfusions can.

Weighing the Risks

In the vast majority of instances, blood transfusions are very safe, and the benefits far outweigh the risks. However, as with other forms of treatment, transfusions can bring about complications. Most of these are not serious and are easily controlled. However, serious and potentially fatal complications may occur in rare instances.

Infection There is always a very slight risk that you could be infected by some organism.

AIDS The risk foremost in everyone's mind is the possibility of being infected with the human immunodeficiency virus (HIV) that can lead to acquired immunodeficiency syndrome (AIDS). But the risk of getting AIDS from a single-unit transfusion is now so low—1 in 2 million, and possibly lower—that it should have almost no effect on the decision to have a transfusion.

Hepatitis The number one infectious risk associated with transfusion is, and has always been, hepatitis. Despite the medical histories taken from blood donors and the tests performed, hepatitis B virus may be present in approximately 1 in 200,000 donations. The vast majority of patients infected with hepatitis B virus (95 percent of adults) recover without any harmful effects. Hepatitis C virus may be present in approximately 1 in 2 million donations. Eighty-five percent of infected recipients have a persistent asymptomatic infection, and 20 percent of those develop clinically significant disease—usually after a period of twenty to thirty years.

Cytomegalovirus (CMV) Cytomegalovirus is a virus present in about half of the general population. Persons with a normal immune system have no symptoms. However, patients whose immune systems have been severely suppressed because of disease or treatment for it and who have not previously been exposed to CMV can develop a serious illness if infected with CMV by a blood transfusion. CMV-negative or leukocyte-reduced blood components may be recommended for some cancer patients by their physicians.

West Nile Virus (WNV) West Nile virus is a disease transmitted by mosquitoes. The transmission risk varies from one season to the other and from one geographical region to another, and it is difficult to predict. The majority of infected people are asymptomatic; however, immunosuppressed patients can experience more severe cases of encephalitis or meningitis. A blood donor screening test for WNV is performed on every unit, reducing the transfusion risk to a minimum.

Bacterial Infection from Platelet Transfusions Rarely, sepsis can be caused by bacterially contaminated transfused platelets. Platelets are stored at room temperature, thus favoring the growth of common bacteria such as skin organisms. Currently, all platelets are tested for the presence of bacteria, greatly decreasing the risk of transfusion sepsis.

Other Infections Blood banks test for syphilis and HTLV-1 and -2 (human T cell lymphotropic virus, type 1, is a virus that may occasionally cause leukemia). Other infections are rarely transmitted.

Reactions to Differences in Donor Blood
Unless you are transfused with your own blood or have an identical twin who donated blood for you to use, the blood you receive will contain many things that are foreign to you. This is true even when the blood is correctly cross-matched. (A cross-match is a test to see if the serum of the patient recognizes anything in the donor blood cells as foreign.)

The donor's blood—the red and white blood cells, platelets, and even plasma proteins—will have antigens (proteins) your body will never have come in contact with before. What usually happens when you are exposed to foreign antigens is that your immune system reacts. After all, the system is designed to recognize and try to destroy anything foreign that gets into our bodies, especially invading germs such as bacteria and viruses. Fortunately, the immune system rarely recognizes most of the differences between a donor's blood and your own.

Differences in Red Blood Cells These are the most critical. While there are more than 400 recognized differences, only 3 are commonly of practical importance: the A, B, and D antigens that determine your ABO and Rh blood types.

Antibodies are part of the immune response to foreign antigens. If you have type B blood, you have anti-A antibodies, so if you are transfused with type A red cells, those cells will be destroyed. Not only will the transfusion not accomplish its purpose, but you may experience chills, fever, aches and pains, and in rare cases shock, bleeding, and even death. Blood banks and hospital transfusion services do repeated tests and checks to be sure patients don't receive blood with the wrong ABO type.

Red blood cells are also either Rh positive or Rh negative, depending on whether you have one of the Rh antigens called D. The D antigen is easily recognized as foreign by an Rh-negative patient, whose system then makes an antibody against it.

Blood banks always test red blood cells from donors and transfusion patients to see if they contain A, B, and D antigens. They also test the serum (a form of plasma) to see if it contains antibodies to these antigens. The hospital transfusion service also checks the serum of each patient who will be transfused to see if it contains antibodies to other red cell antigens. If it does, the blood bank must provide donor blood lacking these antigens. As a final check, the transfusion service does a cross-match.

Differences in White Blood Cells The white cells have an entirely different set of foreign antigens than the red cells do. The most important are called HLA antigens. These are the same antigens that a laboratory looks for when tissue typing to select an organ donor for a transplant.

Antibodies to white blood cells develop fairly easily through transfusion or pregnancy. They rarely cause serious harm, but they do explain the chills and fever experienced by about 3 percent of patients receiving transfusions. If you have such reactions to an uncomfortable degree, your doctor can prevent or minimize them in future transfusions by ordering red blood cells from which most of the white cells have been removed (leukocyte-reduced red blood cells) or by transfusing blood through a filter that removes white cells. Many hospitals now transfuse only leukocyte-reduced blood components. Occasionally, antibodies from the blood donor can react with the white cells of the patient, causing a transfusion reaction called TRALI (transfusion-related acute lung injury). Symptoms of this reaction are severe shortness of breath and difficulty breathing. Prompt recognition of the symptoms and supportive treatment fortunately results in recovery in the majority of cases.

Differences in Platelets Donor platelets have the same HLA antigens as the white blood cells, plus they have antigens unique to platelets. If you have to have repeated platelet transfusions, your immune system may form antibodies that will attack and destroy the donor platelets, making the platelet transfusions useless. These antibodies can also cause chills and fever when they react with donor platelets.

Differences in the Plasma Reactions to donor plasma in the form of hives happen in up to 5 percent of patients. Hives can sometimes be severe to the point of generalized swelling, and in rare cases, the reaction can result in a life-threatening obstruction to breathing. Allergic reactions to plasma can usually be simply treated or prevented with antihistamines. And if you do have a severe reaction, future transfusions can be given without causing a reaction by washing the blood cells with a saline (salt) solution to remove the plasma.

What Gets Transfused and When

When someone donates blood, one pint of blood is usually drawn into a plastic bag. The bag contains a solution that keeps the blood from clotting and helps preserve the red cells. Each bag, with its attached tubing and the needle that goes into the donor's arm, comes as a sterile unit in a sealed pouch and is used only once.

The blood is stored in a refrigerator under carefully controlled conditions until it's used. If it isn't used within five or six weeks, the blood has to be discarded because changes in the red blood cells during storage make it less effective and possibly dangerous, although in special circumstances, red blood cells can be frozen and stored for years. What part of this stored blood is transfused depends on your condition and your needs.

Whole Blood This is used only when a patient is hemorrhaging large amounts of blood in a short time. Almost always, the blood bank separates each unit of blood into red cells, platelets, and plasma.

Red Cells Because of your cancer or your treatment, you may become anemic to the point where breathing becomes difficult, your heart pounds, or you become very weak. If that happens, red blood cells will be transfused. If your marrow is not doing its job, it may be necessary to transfuse red blood cells every three to four weeks. Red blood cells will also be transfused when there is a lot of bleeding, as there may be during surgery.

Platelets When your marrow can't produce enough platelets on its own, a platelet transfusion might be necessary to prevent bleeding. Moderate drops in the platelet count do not need treatment. But very low counts—less than 10,000 without bleeding, a little higher with—will require platelet transfusions, often every two to three days.

At least 70 percent of patients who get repeated platelet transfusions will make antibodies to foreign platelet antigens, making the transfusions less and less effective. Blood banks can solve this problem by providing platelets that have the correct HLA type or by doing many cross-matches with donor platelets.

The Apheresis Technique Modern cancer treatment has led to such a voracious need for platelets that the need cannot be met just by making a platelet component

from each whole blood donation. So blood banks have turned to a procedure known as apheresis. In this process, a donor's blood is taken from a vein, passed through an apheresis (or separating) device, and returned to the donor. The device skims off and saves the blood platelets, while the red blood cells and plasma are returned. When patients no longer respond to the platelets of random donors, family members are often asked to donate platelets by apheresis, since they are much more likely than random donors to have the same platelet antigens as the patient.

Plasma The plasma component of whole blood is used in a variety of ways:

• It may immediately be frozen (fresh frozen plasma) and then used to transfuse missing plasma proteins into patients with unusual deficiencies of clotting factors.
• It can be processed into cryoprecipitate, a special product used to treat certain bleeding problems.
• It can be made into albumin to treat shock, gamma globulin to prevent hepatitis, and clotting factors to treat patients with deficiencies in specific clotting factors.

Donating Blood to Yourself

Since any blood bank component can transmit infections or cause reactions, the safest blood donor is yourself. Getting your own blood is called an autologous transfusion. It is not always possible for people with cancer to donate blood, since it is certainly not appropriate if you are likely to have cancer cells in your blood. But it is worth asking your surgeon whether any of the following approaches are possible or advisable:

Predeposit Donation Many cancer patients can provide their own blood before surgery if time permits and a few basic conditions are met. In this "predeposit autologous donation," your blood is taken exactly as it is from a standard blood donor. The usual age limits for donors don't apply, but you can't be too anemic or have certain types of serious heart disease. It is usually possible to collect two, three, or four units of blood in the five- to six-week period that blood can be stored. Since you will be giving blood much more often than is permitted for the usual blood donor, your doctor will usually prescribe iron so that red cell production is not slowed down by iron deficiency.

Hemodilution This is another approach to autologous transfusion. Instead of blood being gradually donated before the operation, several pints are taken in the operating room just as surgery is about to begin. A saline solution is transfused at the same time so that your total blood volume doesn't change. Your blood is then transfused during the surgical procedure or after the operation as the salt solution escapes from your circulation.

Cell Salvage This approach is possible when fairly large amounts of blood escape into a body cavity during surgery. The blood can be removed, washed with a saline solution, and later returned to you. Cell salvage may not be possible, however, if there is a risk that cancer cells will be returned to your system.

Blood from Other Donors

If you can't donate blood for your own use, you will have to rely on blood supplied by volunteer blood banks or on blood donated from a relative or friend.

Directed or Designated Donations Directed donors may be selected by a patient or a patient's family in the belief that their blood will be safer than that from the usual blood bank volunteer. Usually, this belief is not correct.

Why Directed Donors Are Riskier There are logical reasons why directed donors are less safe on the average.

• People asked to donate for a relative or friend may, because of embarrassment or for reasons they wish to keep confidential, not want to confess that they are ineligible.
• Directed donors are usually first-time donors, while more than two-thirds of routine donors have given in the past, most on many occasions. With each donation, there was a chance that the medical history or laboratory tests would uncover some reason for ineligibility or that an investigation of an infection in a transfused patient would identify the donor as a possible source.

Despite the arguments against the use of directed donors, most patients and families are convinced that *their* relatives and friends are safer than routine donors. For the peace of mind of the patients and families, most blood banks accept requests for directed donations. In some states, they are required by law to do so.

Blood donated by a first- or second-degree relative must be irradiated to prevent the potentially lethal complication known as graft-versus-host disease. This occurs when living cells in the donor blood remain alive after transfusion to the patient (much more likely with related donors), recognize the patient's tissues as foreign, and attack them. This complication is prevented by irradiating the donor blood component before transfusion.

Community Blood Bank Donors These donors are volunteers who have no reason to donate their blood other than the pleasure it gives them to help their fellow humans.

Each blood donor (and this applies to directed donors as well) must read an information sheet that details reasons why a person should *not* donate blood. If the donor concludes that he or she is eligible, a medical history is then obtained using a series of very detailed questions, a number of which are specific about sexual practices.

The donor is also given the opportunity to indicate confidentially that the blood he or she donates should not be transfused. This procedure takes care of situations in which the donor knows he or she is not eligible but does not wish this to become apparent to relatives, friends, or coworkers.

Finally, the blood donated is tested for a whole series of infectious agents—HIV, hepatitis B, hepatitis C, HTLV, West Nile virus (WNV), and syphilis, as well as cytomegalovirus (CMV) in special circumstances. The result is the safest blood supply by far that this country has ever known.

The Need for More Donors Greater than 90 percent of transfusions use blood from volunteer donors in the community. The rest are autologous or directed. If blood isn't available when a patient needs it, that patient could die. Yet serious blood shortages, which require rationing of the available supply, are frequent in many communities.

There are many reasons for the shortage of blood donors. Most people who do not give blood fail to do so because they just ignore the need or assume someone else will do it. A quarter of the population has the completely mistaken notion that it is dangerous to donate blood, that one might become infected with AIDS. And a very large number of people are not eligible to be blood donors anymore, based on the strict criteria used and tests performed.

People with active cancer cannot donate blood for others. Yet cancer patients should have a heightened awareness of the need for an adequate blood supply. Carry the message to your relatives and friends to become regular blood donors. Then, if you need a transfusion in an emergency, the blood will be there waiting for you.

— 18 —

Oncology Nursing

Deborah Hamolsky, R.N., M.S., O.C.N., A.O.C.N.S., Josefa Azcueta, R.N., O.C.N., and Margaret Hawn, R.N.

■ ■ ■ ■

Cancer nurses have many diverse roles across all of the settings where cancer care is delivered. Across the continuum of care from preventive care through active treatment and supportive care, through survivorship or hospice care, people's lives will be touched by their encounters with specially educated oncology nurses.

The professional commitment from these specially trained nurses is to share their knowledge and expertise in order to decrease suffering and to improve health outcomes and quality of life. Oncology nursing is committed to deliver this expertise with compassion, empathy, and cultural sensitivity. We have learned from our greatest teachers, those people with cancer who have entrusted us with their care, that cancer medicine and nursing is most meaningful when given with intelligence and from the heart.

Professional Training

Nursing studies have shown that people with cancer have expectations of the nurses caring for them. Competency is the most important expectation. People care that the nurse can start the IV and give chemotherapy, change a dressing, insert a urinary catheter, provide education about medications and treatments, communicate effectively with their physician colleagues, and know how to respond to an emergency.

Nurses have diverse educational backgrounds and you may meet many people who are "nurses":

• Nurse's aides or hospital attendants complete a training program and may have many years of experience. They can give you direct hands-on care but do not give medications.
• Licensed vocational nurses (L.V.N.s) and licensed practical nurses (P.N.s) complete an educational program and can give medications and direct care. They work collaboratively with registered nurses (R.N.s).
• R.N.s receive their education from an associate degree program, a hospital training program, or a bachelor's degree program at a college or university. R.N.s are licensed by the state within which they practice. Many hospitals have different clinical levels of expertise and authority where R.N.s progress over time, based on merit and continuing education.
• Advanced practice nurses have master's or doctorate degrees and may work as nurse practitioners, clinical nurse specialists, administrators, consultants, researchers, or academic faculty. They may choose to continue to work as staff nurses at the bedside. In advanced clinical practice, these nurses teach and act as role models for other nurses, take part in advanced problem-solving, participate in clinical research trials, and provide leadership.

When you are getting treatment for your cancer, you obviously want reassurance that you are in the hands of an expert who is aware of the most up-to-date treatment methods.

Professional Organization

In the United States, the national organization of oncology nurses is the Oncology Nursing Society (ONS). It was founded in 1975 and had grown to more than 33,000 members in 2006. There are 224 chapters and 30 special interest groups. ONS is dedicated to professional development; promotion of excellence in clinical practice; research; education; and public health and policy advocacy. The award-winning Web site (*www.ons.org*) has an excellent component of patient education, particularly on symptom relief (*CancerSymptoms.org*).

Certification Oncology nurses may be certified through the Oncology Nursing Certification Corporation (ONCC). Certification is designed to inform people with cancer that the nurse, based on testing and ongoing education, has a standard knowledge base. There are both the basic (oncology certified nurse [O.C.N.] and certified pediatric oncology nurse [C.P.O.N.]) and the advanced levels of certification (advanced oncology certified nurse [A.O.C.N.]). In 2005, the advanced certification exam became more specialized with the A.O.C.N.P. for nurse practitioners and the A.O.C.N.S. for clinical nurse specialists.

Oncology nurses build on their basic medical and nursing knowledge with additional education in

- giving chemotherapy and newer targeted therapies and providing symptom relief for side effects such as fatigue, nausea, vomiting, and hair loss;
- controlling cancer pain;
- managing cancer emergencies;
- providing emotional and practical support to patients and their loved ones;
- patient education and care before and after surgery;
- care and teaching of long-term intravenous (IV) devices such as Hickman catheters, Groshong catheters, and ports;
- participation in clinical research teams or independent nursing research;
- managing new technology and treatments—such as bone marrow transplants, targeted therapies, and genetic counseling and testing—as they evolve; and
- prevention and screening.

Nurses can also develop their knowledge in several subspecialties such as radiation oncology, surgical oncology, medical oncology, palliative (comfort) care, cancer prevention and early detection, and genetic counseling. In addition, there is specialized experience within the spectrum of cancer care settings: inpatient nursing, hospice, home care, research, ambulatory and office nursing, and managed care. Some nurses, particularly in large regional cancer centers, may develop an even more specific area of interest such as breast, colon, or prostate cancer or pain control. Some skills—for example, patient education or systems coordination or navigation—can cross many areas of care. Cancer nurses are skilled at coordinating care with and providing referrals to physicians, social workers, psychologists, physical and occupational therapists, nutritionists, and other health care professionals and services.

Radiation Therapy As one example of further education, nurses who specialize in radiation oncology work primarily in radiation therapy departments, either in hospitals or with independent practices. Their specialized knowledge of radiation treatment for cancer includes

- how the machines and treatments work;

- radiation safety;
- what can be expected from the treatment planning, treatment, and follow-up care;
- which treatment courses are expected to cause side effects, and managing those side effects—fatigue, skin changes, diarrhea, sore mouth—when they do occur;
  - emotional support and education;
  - referrals as needed; and
  - nutritional counseling and support.

The nurses work in collaboration with radiation oncologists, radiation physicists, radiology technicians, social workers, psychologists, psychiatrists, physical and occupational therapists, and clinical dietitians to carry out the treatment plan prescribed by the radiation oncologist for each individual patient.

External-beam radiation, delivered by a machine in the outpatient department, is given in divided doses over a set number of weeks. If you need a radiation implant (radiation delivered into a specified place in the body), you will be hospitalized, usually in an oncology unit, for as long as the implant is in place. In either case, oncology nurses, collaborating with the treating team, can help you and your family with symptom management, information, and coping strategies during the course of your treatment.

The Nurse-Doctor Team

Effective cancer treatment requires a team effort. Your oncologists (surgical, medical, and radiation) are responsible for the diagnosis and planning of effective treatment. A professional collaboration between oncology physicians and nurses continues to grow. Oncology nurses will make decisions about your care within their scope of practice, depending on the level of education, experience, and professional certification.

In the hospital, the staff nurses are with you twenty-four hours a day, seven days a week. Your doctor will often ask the nursing team for updates on your condition. Nurses may make "walking rounds" with the doctor to find out how you are doing and to make plans for the upcoming day. It is the oncology nurse at the hospital who monitors your vital signs, gives medication, assesses lab work and physical findings, evaluates your needs, and calls the physician when necessary. Clinical nurse specialists are clinical leaders who work to improve nursing care. Nurse managers are the nurse leaders who work to make the unit function.

On an outpatient basis, in the office or in an ambulatory care setting, the nurse will work with you over the course of treatment. The doctor maps out the treatment plan; the doctor and oncology nurse carry it out. Nurses may help the doctor plan and decide the most effective way to deliver chemotherapy drugs. Nurse practitioners have an independent role, which varies with the scope of practice in different states.

Nurses and doctors, often with other disciplines, often hold patient care conferences to discuss your treatment. Nurses can point out changes in your condition that your doctors might not be aware of, some of which could possibly change the treatment plan.

In the research field, oncology nurses may work independently or collaborate with physicians. There is a growing body of nursing research in symptom management and quality of life. The research nurse conducts clinical trials involving new therapies, collecting data, and assessing responses and side effects. There is a greater acknowledgment of collaboration as more studies are coauthored in journals.

Over the course of your treatment, you may spend a lot of time with your oncology nurse. A special relationship may develop, forged in the terrifying moments of new diagnosis, the ongoing familiarity created from weekly or monthly visits, the follow-up phone calls to check on symptoms, and the everyday quality of sharing stories.

Your care and treatment is truly a team effort by your oncologist, the oncology nurse, and others. It is you who benefits most from this collaboration.

Nursing in the Hospital, Clinic, and Office

While there are many nursing roles in the office, the hospital, the home, and hospice, the majority of cancer nurses work in hospitals. Most cancer centers and many community hospitals have units devoted to cancer treatment—oncology units—staffed by oncology nurses.

Hospital staff nurses provide direct care to patients over eight-, ten-, or twelve-hour shifts. During your hospital stay, you will probably come in contact with a great variety of nurses with different levels of training and responsibility.

The Ambulatory Care/Office Nurse You will likely receive much of your cancer treatment outside a hospital. Therefore, you might find yourself in a comprehensive cancer center, an outpatient clinic, an ambulatory care center, or a private office.

One major reason for this shift out of the hospital is health care cost. There is a great push to shorten hospital stays because outpatient care is more cost-effective for patients, insurance companies, and health care plans. But more important, you benefit by going to an office or clinic, getting your treatment, and then going home to recover in your own home and sleep in your own bed.

Antinausea treatments have become so sophisticated that many of the negative side effects that used to mean a long stay in the hospital for treatment have been eliminated. Of course, specialized or research cancer treatments still usually have to be given in the hospital so your condition can be closely monitored. But even then, you

can spend more time outside the hospital than used to be the case.

Outpatient nursing includes giving all types of chemotherapy treatments ranging from a rapid injection to a five- to seven-hour infusion. Outpatient nurses learn the latest treatment protocols and investigational studies and can give you and your family important information about your disease, treatment, possible side effects, and how to manage your medications. These nurses are experts at starting IVs and peripherally inserted central catheter (PICC) lines or caring for any of the surgically implanted catheters such as the Hickman, the Port-a-Cath, and the Infusaid pump, to name a few. Their job may include mixing and preparing the chemotherapy drugs, syringes, IV bags, or bottles.

Administering and Monitoring Chemotherapy

If your doctor prescribes chemotherapy that needs to be given intravenously, your oncology nurse will be the person to administer the medication. There are many things you can do as a partner in your care to make the infusion experience easier. Communicating clearly your fears, anxieties, and expectations with your nurse is very important. In order to make this experience tolerable, your oncology nurse needs to know the following: Have you had any previous experience with receiving IVs? Do you have any needle phobias? Have you ever fainted or felt lightheaded when receiving an injection? Have you been told your veins "roll" or "collapse"? Do you have any particular sites you prefer? Answers to all these questions will help the oncology nurse tailor his or her activities to your needs.

If you are very anxious or are very fearful about receiving IVs, oftentimes anxiety-reducing activities can help.

• Exploring complementary therapies such as massage and acupuncture

- Listening to soothing music
- Closing your eyes
- Holding a loved one's hand
- Smelling a pleasant fragrance such as lavender or lemon oil
- Reading an engrossing book (ideally not about cancer)
- Listening to books-on-tape
- Bringing a "comfort object" from home such as a blanket or pillow
- If needed, speaking to your nurse or doctor about whether or not medication might be helpful

Some offices even provide televisions with VCRs or DVD players. Ask your medical office if these are available to you.

What Does It Feel Like to Receive Chemotherapy? Receiving intravenous chemotherapy should not be a painful experience. Having a needle placed may provide initial discomfort, but this should subside after the needle is taped down. There are some chemotherapy agents that can be irritating as they are infused. Be sure to let your oncology nurse know if you have any discomfort. There are many ways to alleviate the discomfort some chemotherapy agents can cause. Warm wet towels wrapped around the IV site can provide immediate relief. If it is not contraindicated, diluting the solution or slowing the infusion rate can help decrease discomfort.

Most often patients report a cold feeling radiating from the needle insertion site. This is simply the solution infusing into your veins. Solutions tend to be room temperature and subsequently feel cold as they infuse into a warm body. This cold feeling usually subsides after a few minutes. If you find this bothersome, a warm towel wrapped around the site can bring relief.

Many chemotherapy agents are infused over a long period of time, possibly an hour or more. Other chemotherapy agents are manually pushed into the vein using a syringe. There is a class of chemotherapy medications called vesicants. Your oncology nurse or doctor pushes these medications directly into the vein. These drugs can cause burning of the surrounding tissues if they leak outside of the vein. Be sure to ask your nurse if you are receiving a vesicant chemotherapy. Always immediately report any burning, stinging, redness, or swelling you may notice at the needle insertion site.

During the time it takes for you to receive your chemotherapy, you may have your vital signs (blood pressure, pulse, temperature) checked. This is just an assessment made by the nurse to be sure everything is stable. After your chemotherapy infusion is finished, the nurse removes the needle and places a bandage on the site. You will need to monitor the site for the next few days for any signs of inflammation or infection.

Vascular Access Devices There are ways to access the venous system other than putting a needle directly into a vein. Some patients have very small veins or have had chemotherapy in the past, making it very difficult to place a needle. Your oncology nurse or doctor may recommend a venous access device (VAD). These devices come in many different forms. Some are external catheters that are placed in a major vein and then exit the body, usually in the upper chest area. This looks like a clear or white tube exiting the body. Blood can be drawn out of and infusions given directly into this tube.

External catheters require daily maintenance, which is usually performed by the patient or caregiver. This includes daily dressing changes, cleaning of the skin around the catheter exit site, and flushing heparin and sterile saline through the catheter. It is also a good idea to keep the site dry at all times. The site needs to be assessed daily for redness, drainage, or swelling. Any of these findings must be reported immediately to your doctor.

Another type of VAD is placed under the skin. This is referred to as a mediport or Port-a-Cath. It is usually placed under the skin in the chest area and looks like a 1½- to 2-inch bump under the skin. A needle is required to access the device; however, it is usually one quick stick! Implanted devices must be flushed with sterile saline and heparin every four weeks when not in use. This will be done by your oncology nurse.

VADs allow the patient with small or scarred veins an opportunity to receive chemotherapy and other supportive infusions as well as give blood samples with a minimum of discomfort. Like any foreign device placed in the body, VADs carry the risk of infection and increased blood clot formation. Your doctor and oncology nurse will discuss with you in detail the advantages and disadvantages should this become a choice for you.

Nursing in the Home and Hospice

For the same reasons that outpatient treatment has become more widespread, home care is becoming an important part of oncology care. There are now a variety of home care agencies that are staffed by oncology nurses. Many people choose this type of treatment simply because they prefer to get their chemotherapy in the privacy of their own homes with family and friends close by.

Home Care Generally, nursing care within the home varies with the treatment intensity and duration. Chemotherapy is not the only treatment you can get at home. Under the direction of the oncologist, the oncology nurse can provide you with wound care, central venous (CV) line care and teaching, intravenous (IV) hydration, IV antibiotics, and total IV nutrition.

Hospice Care Hospice can be an important alternative if your cancer becomes very advanced. In the end stages of cancer, hospice care gives you the choice of spending the weeks or months not at a hospital, but at home with loved ones by your side.

As with other oncology specialties, hospice nurses are closely involved with both you and your family. Under your doctor's guidance, the hospice nurse provides support and education regarding symptom control, including pain medication by many different routes.

They teach family and friends how to care for their loved ones and decrease their distress. The hospice nurse, with a team of medical social workers, chaplains, volunteers, and bereavement specialists, also helps the family deal with the impending death and handle the bereavement period that follows. During that time, the hospice nurse spends many hours with the family and is available at all hours of the day or night.

Support for You and Your Family

The role of the oncology nurse varies depending on where and what kind of care is needed at any particular moment. But improving the quality of life for people with cancer is a primary goal of cancer nursing practice. To reach that goal, the oncology nurse is devoted to reducing your physical discomfort and providing emotional support to you and your family.

Managing Symptoms Cancer and the side effects of treatment may have symptoms that are distressing or affect your day-to-day life. Your health care team has to work together to identify and relieve these symptoms. There is now a great deal of nursing knowledge that lets the oncology nurse evaluate, advise on, and effectively take the edge off symptoms like nausea and vomiting, pain, constipation, diarrhea, mouth sores, shortness of breath, loss of appetite, and emotional distress.

Support Groups and Other Resources It is important that whatever needs you have for emotional support be matched with the resources available in your community. These needs often change over the course of an illness and may depend on individual cultural and religious differences and the availability of family, friends, and community support.

There are nurses, social workers, psychologists, and psychiatrists in private practice who have a special interest in and experience with people who have cancer. Most oncology nurses and social workers will be able to give you information about support resources. Nurses are especially active in referrals for support services, particularly the cancer support groups that are widely available. These groups can be led or facilitated by social workers, psychologists, or psychiatrists. Many are co-facilitated by nurses. There are many groups led by professionals who have themselves been diagnosed with cancer.

Not everyone with cancer wants or needs to take part in a structured support group. Many patients successfully use friends and family members as a source of strength. Some people choose individual psychotherapy, either along with or instead of a support group. Yet you should be aware that many people with cancer have credited their support groups with fostering hope and supporting their recovery.

A Special Relationship Many cancer nurses choose to specialize in oncology because they want to make a difference. They want to establish ongoing and meaningful relationships with people who have cancer and their loved ones. The oncology nurse truly touches many lives in many different ways. The nurses who specialize in oncology develop the technical skills needed for cancer care. They will support and inform you and your family throughout your illness. They will be your advocates.

Simply stated, oncology nurses strive to treat you with kindness and caring, expertise and competence, warmth and good humor, and, above all, dignity.

As a wise woman completing therapy said to the nurses caring for her: "Being diagnosed with cancer felt like jumping off the edge of a cliff. Thank you for teaching me to fly."

PART TWO

Supportive Care

— 19 —

Living with Cancer

Ernest H. Rosenbaum, M.D., Malin Dollinger, M.D.,
Isadora R. Rosenbaum, M.A., and Lenore Dollinger, R.N., Ph.D.

Cancer used to be thought of as a virtual death sentence. Yet more and more people have learned to view this disease in a very different light. Many now recognize that living with cancer means learning to live with a chronic disease. It means learning how to manage symptoms and treatments while returning to as many of the normal activities of daily living as possible.

It's important to have life go on as usual or at least as close to usual as you can make it. Maybe you won't be able to take a planned vacation. Maybe you won't be exercising or playing sports or making love as vigorously or as often as you used to. Then again, maybe you will. The point is that a cancer diagnosis doesn't have to be absolutely devastating—although it can be if you let it.

The key is not to feel as though you are a helpless victim of blind fate. Do that and you may easily lose the will to live. If you're going to be cured, go into remission, or even just improve the quality of your life, *you have to take an aggressive stance.*

Fighting cancer is a joint effort, a shared responsibility between you and your medical team. This partnership is based on honesty, communication, education, and a willingness to do your part. The medical team assumes responsibility for planning the most effective treatment and giving therapy and support. You have to assume responsibility for working on proper nutrition, proper physical exercise, and the proper mental attitude.

Do your part and the result will be a much greater ability to cope, a strengthened will to live, and a much more enjoyable life. Sometimes it may seem like a struggle, but you—just like many people before you—can learn to live with cancer.

Talking to Family and Friends

Not too many decades ago, some illnesses were never discussed openly, even among family and friends. Tuberculosis was rarely mentioned in front of other people, for example. And any mention of cancer was made in hushed tones more suitable to talking about bubonic plague. *Cancer* gradually became the most feared word in the English language. It still is. Today, many people remain reluctant to talk about it, even though it is now a rather common disease and often a curable one.

How open you should be about the fact that you have cancer or about how your treatment is going is entirely up to you. There is no single "right" way to talk about it. There are no "right" words to use. Like everyone else, you will have to find your own comfort zone and the words you're most comfortable using. If you would rather talk about your "malignancy" or "tumor" or "growth" or "lump" or "problem" than keep using the word *cancer* all the time, so be it.

Deciding Whom to Tell Some people prefer to keep their cancer a very private matter, not telling anyone outside the family. One person in our experience had breast cancer metastatic to her liver and bones for twenty-six years, and no one knew but her husband and her daughter. She continued to work, run track, and remain active in the community. One of the reasons she survived is that she was *living* with her cancer. For her, this approach was a very positive one. She wanted to forget about it and get on with her life.

Others who need outside help pick one or two close friends who have indicated that they would be available emotionally to provide comfort and support when they are needed.

Deciding What to Say Although it can be hard, it makes sense to be open and direct with your family and close friends if you feel comfortable doing that.

Without candor and openness, concerned relatives and friends are left with their own darkest imaginings. They have their own fears and frustrations that will only grow into terrifying phantoms if they are left behind a veil of secrecy and ignorance of what you are really experiencing. A mutual confrontation of fears is a good way of keeping your own fears and the fears of others under control.

Being open doesn't mean that you have to start every conversation with the story of your latest aches and pains. Nor, if someone asks how you feel, do you necessarily have to answer with a long detailed description. The litany of the person who wants sympathy or empathy—"I've got it bad. It hurts here and here. I've got to get this treatment"—makes a lot of people want to avoid you. People with cancer are often avoided because, by their own conversation, only bad things seem to happen to them.

Another person in our experience—a military man and pharmacist who had lymphocytic leukemia and, concurrently,

colon cancer—was a very open, extroverted person. But if someone said to him, "How do you feel?" he always said, "I never had it better in my life." For him, this was a great opener, ending any conversation about his cancer that he could have found depressing, demoralizing, or inappropriate. It also made the association with others far less uncomfortable and much warmer because no one was made uneasy.

Short-circuiting painful conversations like this is one way of coping and getting on with your life. But, again, it is not the only way. What is right for you is your own decision. For you, it might not be helpful to just say "fine" if someone asks how you are doing. Such an automatic social response might be appropriate for friends, relatives, or coworkers you are not particularly close with, but not for someone close who is trying to be supportive.

The same caution applies the other way. When you are feeling low physically or mentally, many people will try to buck you up by telling you, "Don't worry, everything will be fine." This is a common, socially acceptable statement we are all taught to say to show support. But the true message seems to be, "Don't tell me that you don't feel good; tell me you're okay."

When you really aren't feeling so good, this kind of support obviously contradicts what you know to be true. At such times, it is especially nice to have a close friend or relative who can say, "I'm sorry you're feeling down, and I'm glad I'm here for you." For that special someone to be there for you, you have to be able to communicate truthfully how you really feel.

Coping with Special Family Problems

Cancer is a personal disease, but everyone close to you suffers in some way. Cancer is especially hard on family members, particularly when you are in the hospital for an extended time. The period of separation can be traumatic.

Family caregivers are often very stressed. Everyone in the family wonders where you will be in a month or two months down the road—in the hospital, a nursing home, at home and needing nursing care? They are afraid you will have great discomfort or pain.

Very often, the family struggles with questions about how needs can be met and care arranged in such a way that insurance companies will pay for it. They wonder how other caregivers can become involved so they can get back to work. Relatives who live some distance away may have to make plans for the care of their children so they can come and provide help for a few weeks or a month. Schedules may have to be rearranged, but people are often uncertain about when they should come.

And all members of the family have fears of losing someone who is an important part of the family's life.

The Needs of Children When you are away in the hospital or when you are back home but feeling tired from treatment, it is not unusual for children to feel lost or neglected. You and other family members have to reassure them often that they are still loved. With younger children, you may also have to quickly eliminate any notion that they somehow caused this illness.

Teenagers are especially vulnerable to stress. They have all the same worries that other members of the family have. They have the same needs for reassurance as younger children. And at the same time, they may be burdened by having to take on adult responsibilities around the house. If all this becomes too much to bear, they can rebel by cutting the number of visits to the hospital, not doing their new chores at home, or even drinking alcohol or taking drugs.

Strained Relationships Not all families are supportive all the time. Realistically, not everyone is able to be open, loving, and intelligently supportive in a crisis. Families sometimes feel death before it even happens. Oncologists have seen patients take a turn for the worse, then have seen family members decide emotionally and psychologically that all is over and stop coming to the hospital for visits. The family goes into mourning while the patient is still trying to get better and have hope. It's sad to say, but oncologists sometimes see family members fighting at the bedside over wills and codicils.

But even close families and stable relationships can be threatened by the pressures of a long-term illness. Emotional and physical exhaustion, frustration, and constant worry and care can all take their toll. Anger and guilt can surface in sudden attacks, recriminations, or indifferent or oversolicitous behavior. Other problems that may have been latent in a relationship for years can suddenly emerge.

All these possible strains just emphasize the need for everyone to look after his or her own needs. You have to do all that you can to look after yourself. Your family members have to be reminded that they need time for themselves. They need moments of rest and relief to keep themselves on an even keel emotionally and psychologically.

Both you and your family may be suffering from the same feelings of inadequacy, the same burdens of guilt, the same quiet anguish, the same sheer tedium of prolonged illness. Any or all of these can break the spirits of the most loving and courageous people.

No one can or should be blamed or criticized for the ways he or she responds to the crisis of cancer or the threat of change or loss. Some people and some relationships grow stronger. Some waver but hold fast. Some collapse. Some experience new heights of love, respect, and understanding.

Dealing with Negative Emotions

Nothing can undermine your will to live and your "battle-ready" posture so much as the negative emotions that are so often the response to a cancer diagnosis—anger, fear, loss of self-esteem, and feelings of isolation. These emotions have to be resolved. If they aren't, helplessness, futility, and resignation can easily take over.

Resolving Your Anger How you react to the cancer diagnosis depends on your personality and how you usually adapt to life's problems. If you are the sort of person who looks on adversity as one more problem to be attacked with determination or as simply something you have to make the best of, then your normal positive attitude will probably carry you through the initial shock of the diagnosis and the tough times ahead. But if you usually react to adversity by asking, "Why me?" you may spend most or all of your emotional energy being angry at the disease, the "gods," or other people for bringing this catastrophe down on your head.

Anger is a normal reaction. In some ways, it can help you through the period of grieving that comes after the diagnosis. In fact, if you don't feel some anger and find some way of expressing it, you may be setting yourself up for a period of depression. But there is a time for anger and a time to put anger aside.

If anger stays unresolved, it takes away the energy that could be channeled into coping with the disease and living life as fruitfully as possible. The first step in resolving it is to recognize why you are angry. If you don't, you may find yourself taking out your anger on others, finding fault with friends or family, making a big deal about trivial matters, or flying off the handle at the slightest provocation. The result may well be that you drive needed people away just when you need them most. But if you recognize your anger for what it is, you will be getting your mental attitude set to cope with it.

It's important to let your anger out. Talk about it. Scream. Punch a pillow or throw things around—anything to help release anger's hold on you. Then work to apply that energy in a positive and useful direction. Tell the world you just ain't ready to go, and put your anger to work to make sure you don't have to.

Coming to Terms with Fear Most people hear the word *cancer* and immediately think of suffering, prolonged disability, or the phrase "Nothing can be done." These responses may be okay for the movies, but except in unusual circumstances, they don't have a lot to do with the reality of cancer treatment today. Something can almost always be done. Pain and other side effects of treatment can be controlled. Disability is not inevitable. Most people are surprised to learn that their ideas about cancer are much more pessimistic than the facts warrant.

But no one with cancer has any experience or training in how to deal with the sometimes scary events that happen day to day, week to week, or month to month. Even if the surgeon "got it all out" or the radiation or chemotherapy seems to be working, there is always a fear that the cancer will come back.

Fear is a terrible master if you let it get a grip on your life. You can literally be "frightened to death." It is a documented phenomenon in modern medical practice that people who accept a cancer diagnosis as a death sentence can die quite quickly, long before the disease has progressed far enough to cause death by itself.

A diagnosis of cancer is not a death sentence. The first question people usually ask when they get the diagnosis is, "How long have I got?" Unfortunately, some doctors still answer with an unqualified "six months" or "a year" or "two years." Specific predictions like these are simply not valid. Such figures may be published averages for people with a specific type of cancer, but they are only averages. Obviously, some people did not live as long as the estimate and some lived longer. By definition, half of the people live longer than the "average." No estimate of *individual* survival can be made until therapy has begun and the response to it has been established. Until then, predictions are, at best, guesswork and uncertainty that can only stifle hope and the will to live.

Knowledge and understanding are the keys to freeing yourself from unreasonable fear. If you want to know the truth about cancer, talk to oncologists and other members of your health care team. Don't listen to what friends, relatives, or acquaintances tell you or take reports in the press as gospel. Fears can be resolved if you understand clearly the problems you face, if you understand the treatments and supportive measures that might be taken, and if you have a reasonable and realistic estimate of the discomfort or inconvenience you can expect.

Dealing with the Fears of Others Even if your own fear is under control, well-meaning friends or family members can communicate their fears to you. Unless you are prepared for this, you might find your reserves of emotional energy drained and a depression coming on.

The only way out of this situation is to either hide the fact of your cancer or make sure your family and friends understand your disease and treatment. You may even want to include some of them in your consultations with your doctor so they can become part of your "informed" support team. This may also help your doctor, for, from the doctor's point of view, many of the problems in communication come from the family— the husband or wife, the sister or brother, the cousin or friend, who has heard about a cure somewhere or about someone who's had better treatment. By making sure that all interested parties are kept informed, everyone can focus their energies and efforts on the most constructive channels.

Overcoming a Loss of Self-Esteem Your self-esteem can be threatened by the very idea of having cancer. Unfortunately, it's not unusual to feel that if you were somehow a better or more complete person, you wouldn't have been stricken in the first place, or that the cancer is some sort of divine punishment. These are all superstitious beliefs that, sad to say, still cling to the word *cancer*. But having cancer doesn't mean that you are unworthy in any way or that you are guilty of some terrible wrongdoing. Cancer can happen to anyone. It will happen to one out of every four Americans. Even if you don't fall victim to these superstitions, however, cancer can take away or change some of the things that have always given you a sense of self-esteem.

Your Body Image Changes to your body as a result of surgery, radiotherapy, or chemotherapy can have a devastating effect on your self-esteem, especially if the changes are visible to other people. If you lose some part of your body, if you have scars or skin changes, or if you lose your hair or a lot of weight, everyone can't help but notice. And you're bound to feel uncomfortable when they do, at least at first. If you have to have an ostomy, you may feel humiliated by having to collect your body wastes in a bag. If you have surgery to your genitals, you may feel that you are no longer a "real man" or a "real woman."

But your body is not your self. Your true self is your spirit and your soul. It may be hard for you to accept this truth, but you can come to accept it with help and encouragement. Become involved with a support group and get to know other people who have had similar body changes. Just as you will be able to relate to them, so other people will be able to relate to you just as you are. The volunteers who work with groups or other social agencies can help you adjust emotionally. You, in turn, may eventually be of value to others going through the same changes.

Loss of Independence and Control To some extent, this is inevitable for anyone with cancer. In the beginning, you will have to depend on the medical system for your very life. When you are in the hospital, other people may well determine when you eat, sleep, bathe, walk, or even go to the bathroom. You may feel uncomfortable or humiliated by having to use a bedpan or having your body exposed to doctors, nurses, and medical staff.

When you get home, you may have to depend on family, friends, or social service agencies for help around the house, personal body care, or meeting your financial obligations. You may start to feel "useless" or feel guilty about being a burden to people you care about.

You may simply have to accept your loss of independence for a while, but your sense of self-esteem can be improved if you take as much responsibility as you possibly can in the areas you *can* handle.

• Look after as many self-care tasks as you can.
• Be methodical and dedicated about eating the right foods and doing regular exercises to increase your strength and mobility.
• Keep charts of your progress to help you feel a sense of accomplishment.
• Carefully choose some little job you can do around the house, whether it's

tending plants or caring for a pet or finding some other outlet for your ability to nurture.

Your self-esteem can also be improved if you get involved in a range of supportive programs such as special group counseling and patient support organizations. If there are no support groups in your area, talk to your local medical staff, social workers, clergy, and other people with cancer and start one yourself.

Avoiding Isolation Our society likes to think that it is compassionate and willing to rehabilitate people who are disabled or suffering from chronic diseases. The reality is that disabled people are often shunted aside or even shunned. Employers and coworkers can keep their distance. Family and friends, attentive and sympathetic at first, can drift away over time as they deal with their own problems and live their own lives. Everyone can feel uncomfortable talking to someone who is seriously ill, not knowing quite how to relate or what to say. At times like these, it is easy to feel abandoned and lonely.

Even when you are surrounded by caring friends and family, you may feel cut off. Any life-threatening disease can put you in touch with the essential aloneness humans feel when contemplating their own mortality. Some people turn their attention and energies inward to such a degree that they lose contact with life and the rest of humanity.

Isolation and loneliness can often be self-inflicted. If you focus on grieving or feeling sorry for yourself or if you accept the diagnosis as a death sentence, you may snip your ties to the world and live as though you already belong to the dead. When that happens—just as when isolation comes from the outside and old connections are broken by others—you have to make new connections, building new bridges to people and activities that can renew your energy and zest for living.

You may be frightened or pessimistic about taking the first steps toward making a new life. But you *can* change direction. The benefits of doing so make the effort more than worthwhile.

Support Groups

Some people need special help to cope with their cancer, and their doctors can't always provide it. Doctors are as interested in their patients' emotional well-being as they are in their physical well-being, yet medical appointments are usually taken up with talks about treatment problems, side effects, precautions, and complications.

Doctors do recognize the importance of dealing with emotional concerns and can often refer you to the many external support groups and systems available to you. These groups give all cancer patients the kind of help that only interested and dedicated people, often sufferers of the same disease, can provide.

At the Hospital Many local hospitals, especially those with cancer treatment centers, have support groups that are run by health professionals and often meet every week. These are groups designed just for individuals with cancer and for family members. Some of these groups are specialized, dealing only with the common physical and emotional problems of people who have been treated for specific tumors. For example:

• People who have had ostomies—artificial openings created in the colon, intestine, or bladder—have to learn what they can do to live as normal a life as possible.
• People who have had their larynges, or voice boxes, removed have to learn how to speak all over again.
• Women who have had a mastectomy have specific emotional problems. So do men with testicular cancer.

Outside the Hospital The American Cancer Society and other professional organizations have programs that help deal with physical, emotional, and mental problems associated with having cancer. The Reach to Recovery program for women with breast cancer and the I Can Cope program of weekly seminars are two examples. Both include a comprehensive educational process for cancer patients and their families.

The Wellness Community is another example of an organization devoted to improving the quality of life of people with cancer. It features educational programs, seminars, and discussion groups and provides the opportunity for everyone with cancer to relate to others with the same fears and worries. Many people find the approach of this rapidly expanding organization—which encourages you to become an active participant in your fight for recovery—extremely helpful (see chapter 32, "The Will to Live").

Depending on where you live, there may also be organizations designed to meet the needs of young adults, who do not always feel comfortable in other support organizations.

How the Groups Work There are great advantages to taking part in a group when you feel well enough to participate. A group of people in circumstances similar to yours can offer companionship and the chance to discuss many concerns and feelings.

How the support groups are designed and structured and what they cover vary. But they all have in common the gathering together of people with similar experiences. In these groups, you can tell your story, sharing your experience of cancer and its effect on your life. You can hear the stories of others, support their similar experiences, and decrease their sense of isolation, fear, and loneliness. You can also share information and resources that will help you and others cope with specific problems.

Each group functions for better or worse, depending on the members and the leadership. *Not everyone is suited for a group.* Some people prefer and would do better not participating in a group. But many people with cancer have given credit to their support groups for helping them maintain hope and setting them on the road to recovery.

Where to Find the Right Group Local chapters of the American Cancer Society usually have a current listing of which groups are offered. Many cancer newsletters contain this information, and most oncology nurses and social workers can help you find support resources.

Getting Back to Work

Many people don't realize how much their feelings of self-worth depend on their being active, productive, and capable of taking care of themselves and others. Then an illness strikes and it soon sinks in just how important all that is. Of course, a job is pretty much essential for financial well-being. But it can also be essential for psychological well-being.

This is especially true when you have cancer. The loss of self-esteem that often follows a cancer diagnosis or treatment can be magnified by sitting around doing nothing while you depend on family and friends for personal care, financial assistance, and help around the house. So it is vital to your peace of mind to find ways of returning to productive work in some capacity. It might mean getting back to your old job. It might mean learning a new skill, studying or even simply doing work around the house (see chapter 30, "Home Care").

Keeping a Positive Attitude Admittedly, getting back to work can sometimes be a problem. You may be disabled in such a way that you can no longer do the same job you had before treatment. And you may have to confront some discrimination in the job market or prejudice in the workplace.

It's unfortunate, but there is still some stigma attached to having cancer. Employers and coworkers may react out of a vague fear of or uneasiness about cancer in the abstract. Coworkers can stay at arm's length either because they just don't know what to say or because they have the irrational and completely mistaken notion that they'll catch something terrible if they go near you. Employers might be afraid of decreased production or financial losses because of the time you might need to take off for treatment (see chapter 33, "Living with Mortality: Life Goes On").

A study by the American Cancer Society in the 1970s showed that cancer patients did face some discrimination in hiring, firing, job assignments, benefits, and attitudes. Almost a quarter of the people who took part in the study reported either being rejected for jobs because of cancer treatment or being the target of negative attitudes. Slightly more than half described at least one illness-related problem.

But the good news was that 46 percent said they had *never* had problems at work because of their cancer. And over three-quarters said that after treatment, they had earned salary increases because of promotions or increased responsibilities. Since that study was done, many states have passed legislation to outlaw discrimination because of medical conditions, including cancer.

What is absolutely essential is that you keep a positive attitude despite some rejection. Medical social workers, physical and occupational therapists, and vocational counselors can all help ease the transition back into the workforce. They can help you match your skills with available jobs or help you get retraining if that is necessary. But learning to live with cancer is the key. Your positive attitude will strengthen your resolve and also just might rub off on employers and coworkers.

Your Need for Recreation

Recreation is an important part of living. We all need a break from the routine and stress of daily life to keep us steady even in the best of circumstances. Although it is sometimes hard to summon up the energy or the will, recreation is even more important when we are sick. Engaging in some kind of recreational activity helps relieve tensions and bring on a feeling of relaxation. It also contributes to feelings of self-worth and well-being.

When you are being treated for cancer, you may forget about recreation. Or you may think it's not important, inappropriate, or just too hard to pursue. It is none of these. No matter what your limitations, you can start many activities while you are in the hospital and continue when you go home.

Being with a Group Working with a group or simply working on your own among other people engaged in the same activity has a lot of advantages. The companionship can give you the opportunity to talk about any problems or concerns you have. Better yet, it gives you the chance to talk about all kinds of things that have absolutely nothing to do with cancer. Either way, being with others can lift your spirits and calm your anxieties.

If you are up to it, you can arrange outings with one or more companions. You might want to do something as simple as take a walk in the park with an old friend or take in something entertaining like a movie or a play. If you are involved with craft work, go on an outing to a museum or library to pick up new information or broaden your appreciation of craft activities.

There are many outside resources you can contact, both for learning opportunities and companionship—the YMCA/ YWCA, local clubs, schools, colleges and universities, community centers, religious organizations. And keep looking in local newspapers and magazines for recreational activities that change from week to week.

Things to Do on Your Own If you feel more comfortable with solitary pursuits, check out the library in your neighborhood or at the hospital for suggestions. There are many games, crafts, and other activities that you can become involved in no matter what your limitations in strength and energy. The list of possibilities is almost limitless.

- Start a scrapbook. Put all your loose photos and mementos into some pleasing arrangement. Divide them by subject or theme and write captions or amusing comments. Maybe you could devote part of the layout to tracing your family tree.
- Take up sketching, painting, or some other artistic activity. If you have no experience with art, start with line drawings of still life. Once you've got the basic contours of the object on paper, fill in details and shadings and add color. Experiment with various materials. You might find you have talents you never dreamed you had.
- Listen to music. It not only soothes the "savage breast," it can raise your spirits, help you sleep, relieve pain, and make mealtimes more pleasant and satisfying. Listening to music is not only enjoyable, it's downright therapeutic.
- Rent funny movies. If you have a VCR or DVD player, watch as many comedies as you can. Whether your taste for humor is satisfied by Charlie Chaplin, the Marx Brothers, the Three Stooges, or Monty Python, many comedies are available at your local movie rental outlets.
- Watch comedians. Let Jay Leno, David Letterman, Robin Williams, Jerry Seinfeld, Bill Cosby, or anyone else you

like, tickle your funny bone. Laughter can change your whole outlook on life.

• Crochet or knit. Both activities can be very entertaining. And you can see the results of your labors quickly. Even if you've never done either before, you can easily learn to make simple afghans, scarves, shawls, or hats for yourself or as gifts for others.

• Collect stamps, coins, figurines, recipes, sports cards, or anything else that catches your interest. Collecting gets your mind working on organizing, classifying, and physically arranging your collection, as well as on what you need to make the collection more complete.

• Set up a golf putting course in your home or yard. A very simple arrangement is all that's needed. It will give you an opportunity to stay active and give you a challenge every day.

What kind of recreational activity you pursue is entirely up to you. But whatever you choose as a diversion should be just that—something enjoyable and fun that diverts your mind away from your illness. The relief from stress and the positive attitude fostered by enjoyment can be critically important to your recovery.

The Goal of Total Rehabilitation

Overcoming your anger and fears, developing the right attitude, getting your support system in place, and arranging for productive work and recreation are just the start of your rehabilitation and recovery. All these "set the table" for all you have to do during the tough times ahead.

Once you have made the critical decision that you want to get well, you have to be willing to make sacrifices and believe that achieving the goal is worth the effort. You will have to pay attention to all kinds of things that are detailed in the next few chapters—coping with side effects, maintaining good nutrition, getting enough exercise, learning how to relax, becoming secure enough to express yourself sexually, and many more.

You will have to know your strengths and limitations and be able to set realistic goals. And you will have to be willing to compromise, to accept what cannot be changed and move on from there. Having cancer means that your life has to be restructured if you are going to get as full a rehabilitation as possible. This doesn't mean that you have to change the habits of a lifetime, even if you could. But it does mean you will have to make adjustments in your daily living patterns so that your time can be used in the most efficient and constructive ways.

If you pay attention to your mind and body and spirit, you will be well on your way not only to living with cancer, but to achieving the highest level of success possible in the given circumstances.

— 20 —

Coping with the Side Effects of Chemotherapy

Robert J. Ignoffo, Pharm.D., Ernest H. Rosenbaum, M.D., Malin Dollinger, M.D., John P. Cooke, M.D., Ph.D., and Andrzej Szuba, M.D., Ph.D.

■ ■ ■ ■

When you are ill, your overriding goal is to get well and return to an active life. If you are going to reach that goal, every part of your rehabilitation program is important—from the psychological and social dimensions to the nutritional aspects to the pain control. However, unless the side effects of treatment are looked after, you might not have the energy or even the desire to get back to normal activities. Side effects can be debilitating. They can sap your strength, weaken your resolve, and generally just make life unpleasant.

With support from the medical team and your family and friends, you can manage these side effects and eventually overcome them. It may take some effort on your part, but the benefits will be well worth that effort.

Nausea and Vomiting

Nausea is a subjective feeling of stomach distress or wooziness accompanied by a strong urge to throw up. Vomiting is the process of eliminating stomach or duodenal contents.

Uncontrolled nausea and vomiting can interfere with the patient's ability to receive cancer treatment and to care for him- or herself by causing chemical changes in the body, loss of appetite,

physical and mental difficulties, a torn esophagus, broken bones, and the re-opening of surgical wounds. Constant vomiting naturally makes it impossible to eat or take fluids and can lead to dehydration and electrolyte/mineral loss, so whatever can be done to reduce nausea should be done *before* vomiting starts. Paying attention to nausea's psychological causes and using antinausea drugs will help control what can be disturbing events.

Fortunately, nausea and vomiting are temporary side effects of both chemotherapy and radiotherapy. They can also be brought on by an obstruction in the intestine, irritation of the gastrointestinal tract (gastritis), or brain tumors. It is very important to prevent and control nausea and vomiting in patients with cancer.

Types of Nausea and Vomiting Nausea and vomiting caused by cancer treatment can be classified into four types:

- Anticipatory
- Acute
- Delayed
- Chronic

Not all chemotherapy causes nausea and vomiting. Each patient is different in his or her reaction to chemotherapy.

Table 1 lists chemotherapy drugs according to their potential to cause nausea or vomiting. Getting three or four drugs at a time, which is often the case, can make the reaction even more severe. The dosage and the number of cycles to be given can also be contributing factors.

You and your caregivers will receive instructions from your doctor, nurse, or pharmacist about the type of chemotherapy you'll be getting. For each drug, a program will be established that will allow you to have some control over the situation. With psychological factors playing such a big part, it is very important that you be a participant in preventing nausea and vomiting.

Anticipatory Nausea and Vomiting If a patient has had nausea and vomiting after several previous chemotherapy treatments, he or she may experience anticipatory nausea and vomiting with subsequent treatments. The smells, sights, and sounds of the treatment room may remind the patient of previous episodes and may trigger nausea and vomiting before a new cycle of chemotherapy (or radiation therapy) has even begun. This is referred to as anticipatory nausea and vomiting (ANV), with nausea occurring in about 30 percent of patients and vomiting in about 11 percent of patients. This can set up such a psychological pattern that it affects the amount of chemotherapy that can be given and makes it much harder to control nausea and vomiting before and after treatment.

Anticipatory nausea and vomiting is the result of a conditioned reflex. This means that if chemotherapy made you throw up before, then you will feel nauseated whenever you take the treatment or even when something triggers the very idea of treatment. This conditioned aversion often takes hold after three to four chemotherapy sessions and can last a long time. A common story among doctors is one about a patient who meets her oncologist on the street years after therapy and throws up on the spot.

Your anxiety state, how you feel about yourself and your cancer, and how you respond to stress and disease may all be important factors in setting up this psychological pattern. Furthermore, once the pattern is established, all kinds of stimuli can trigger feelings of nausea— the colors or odors in the room where the chemotherapy is given, the smell of alcohol used to prepare you for the IV needle, the sight of the nurse entering the room.

The following characteristics seem to be associated with the development of ANV. If you have three or more of these characteristics, you may be at risk for ANV.

1. Age under fifty years.
2. Nausea and/or vomiting after last chemotherapy session.
3. Posttreatment nausea described as moderate, severe, or intolerable.
4. Posttreatment vomiting described as moderate, severe, or intolerable.
5. Feeling warm or hot all over after the last chemotherapy session.
6. Susceptibility to motion sickness.
7. Sweating after the last chemotherapy session.
8. Generalized weakness after the last chemotherapy session.
9. Female gender.
10. High state of anxiety (anxiety reactive to specific situations).
11. Greater reactivity of the autonomic nervous system or slower reaction time.
12. Patient expectations of chemotherapy-related nausea before beginning treatment.
13. Percentage of infusions of chemotherapy followed by nausea.
14. Postchemotherapy dizziness.
15. Lightheadedness.
16. Longer latency of onset of posttreatment nausea and vomiting.
17. Emetogenic (vomiting) potential of various chemotherapeutic agents. Patients

Table 1. **Chemotherapy Drugs and Their Potential to Cause Nausea or Vomiting**

HIGHEST POTENTIAL	INTERMEDIATE POTENTIAL	LOW OR MINIMAL POTENTIAL
Carmustine (BiCNU)	Carboplatin (Paraplatin)	Bevacizumab (Avastin)
Cisplatin (Platinol)	Cyclophosphamide (Cytoxan) < 1,500 mg/m^2	Bleomycin (Blenoxane)
Cyclophosphamide (Cytoxan) > 1,500 mg/m^2	Doxorubicin (Adriamycin)	Bortezomib (Velcade)
Dacarbazine (DTIC-Dome)	Cytarabine (Cytosar) > 1 g/m^2	Capecitabine (Xeloda)
Dactinomycin (Cosmegen)	Daunorubicin (Cerubidine)	Cetuximab (Erbitux)
Mechlorethamine (nitrogen mustard) (Mustargen)	Doxorubicin (Adriamycin)	Chlorambucil (Leukeran)
Streptozocin (Zanosar)	Epirubicin (Ellence)	Cytarabine (Cytosar) < 1 g/m^2
	Idarubicin (Idamycin)	Etoposide (Etopophos)
	Ifosfamide (Ifex)	Fluorouracil (5-FU)
	Irinotecan (Camptosar)	Gemcitabine (Gemzar)
	Procarbazine (Matulane)	Hexamethylmelamine (Hexalen)
		Hydroxyurea (Droxia)
		Melphalan (Alkeran)
		Mercaptopurine (Purinethol)
		Methotrexate (Mexate)
		Mitomycin-C (Mutamycin)
		Mitoxantrone (Novantrone)
		Paclitaxel (Taxol)
		Rituximab (Rituxan)
		Thioguanine (Thioguanine Tabloid)
		Trastuzumab (Herceptin)
		Vinblastine (Velban)
		Vincristine (Oncovin)
		Vinorelbine (Navelbine)

Adapted from Kris. *J. Clin. Oncol.* 24 (2006):2932–2947.

receiving drugs with a moderate-to-severe potential for post-treatment nausea and vomiting are more likely to develop ANV.

18. Morning sickness during pregnancy.

To deal with this problem, you will have to take steps both to relax before your chemotherapy and not to inadvertently set up situations that become associated with nausea.

• Try to relax in a quiet, darkened room before your treatment sessions.

• Use behavioral techniques to help you relax and control any triggering stimuli—hypnosis, relaxation therapy, imagery, or listening to your favorite music or a relaxation tape.

• Perhaps try acupuncture or acupressure, which have been effective in controlling nausea or vomiting in some cases.

• The time of day when you get treatment can sometimes make a difference. If you have a problem with either the morning or the afternoon, try to change your appointment schedule.

• Avoid eating hot, spicy foods or other dishes that might upset your stomach or gastrointestinal tract.

• Eat slowly, so you don't develop gas or heartburn.

• Try to avoid cooking odors that may bring on nausea by having friends or family prepare meals at their own homes and bring them over to you.

• Always avoid your favorite foods when you are getting chemotherapy. You might start to associate these foods with treatment, nausea, and vomiting and develop a strong aversion to them.

• Controlling acute nausea and vomiting are important factors in the preventing subsequent episodes of ANV.

Acute Nausea and Vomiting After Treatment
Nausea and vomiting (emesis) that occur one to six hours after treatment with chemotherapy or radiation therapy are referred to as acute nausea and vomiting.

Like anticipatory nausea, posttherapy nausea and vomiting can have significant therapeutic implications. You may start to fear therapy, a fear that can gnaw at you and make you want to avoid treatment. It may also make problems such as pain control and maintaining an overall good quality of life much harder to deal with.

Fortunately, there are several newer antinausea medications (antiemetics) that if used properly are very effective, completely preventing vomiting in about 70 percent of patients. Commonly used antiemetics are discussed below.

Delayed Nausea and Vomiting (DNV)
Nausea or vomiting that occurs two to five days after chemotherapy is referred to as delayed nausea and vomiting. DNV is more difficult to control than acute nausea and vomiting. A few of the antiemetics discussed below are effective against DNV.

Antinausea Medications (Antiemetics) A wide variety of antinausea drugs have been developed over the past fifteen years that have improved the control of nausea and vomiting. Your doctor can work out a program to combat your nausea, although if one drug or drug combination doesn't work as well as you would both like, you may have to experiment with different programs.

Generally, antiemetics should be taken thirty to sixty minutes before chemotherapy so that they have time to take effect.

• If vomiting has already started and you can't keep a pill down, antinausea suppositories such as prochlorperazine (Compazine) or trimethobenzamide (Tigan) may help. Long-acting prochlorperazine extended-release capsules (Compazine Spansules) can be very helpful, since they work for six hours. Thiethylperazine (Torecan) is sometimes used rather than prochlorperazine. If these agents are not useful, haloperidol (Haldol) may be helpful.

Table 2. **Common Antiemetics**

	ORAL	IM (INTRAMUSCULAR)	IV	SUPPOSITORY
Aloxi (palonosetron)			x	
Anzemet (dolasetron)	x	x		
Ativan (lorazepam)	x	x	x	
Benadryl (diphenhydramine)	x	x	x	
Compazine (prochlorperazine)	x	x	x	x
Decadron (dexamethasone)	x	x	x	
Emend (aprepitant)	x			
Haldol (haloperidol)	x	x		
Kytril (granisetron)	x	x		
Reglan (metoclopramide)	x		x	
THC (marijuana tablets, Marinol)		x		
Tigan (trimethobenzamide)	x	x		x
Torecan (thiethylperazine)	x	x	x	x
Zofran (ondansetron)	x	x		

• Lorazepam (Ativan) may help with anticipatory nausea and vomiting. Lorazepam can be taken under the tongue for rapid absorption during severe nausea. Lorazepam is also an antianxiety drug and sedative that can cause short-term amnesia, which might take the edge off any memory of vomiting once the episode is over.

• Marijuana and dronabinol (Marinol) —the natural delta-9-tetrahydrocannabinol (THC) and the synthetic form of THC—may successfully control nausea and vomiting by working on the higher brain centers. But they can also cause drowsiness, dry mouth, dizziness, a rapid heartbeat, and sweating.

• Dexamethasone (Decadron) may be helpful for controlling both acute and delayed nausea and vomiting. For patients receiving intermediate- or high-potential chemotherapy, dexamethasone will usually be combined with other drugs, especially the 5-HT-3 antagonists.

• The 5-HT-3 antagonists—Ondansetron (Zofran), granisetron (Kytril), dolasetron (Anzemet), and palonosetron (Aloxi)—are the most significant drugs used for controlling nausea and vomiting caused by intensive chemotherapy and radiotherapy. They work by linking to the 5-hydroxytryptamine-3 receptor and preventing the release of serotonin, which stimulates the vomiting center. They may be needed when you are receiving highest-potential chemotherapy drugs or when you cannot get relief with other antinausea agents. They are often given with dexamethasone (Decadron) IV. They suppress vomiting in 60 to 80 percent of patients and are even more effective in combination with other antinausea drugs.

• Aprepitant (Emend) is an NK-1 antagonist. The NK-1 receptor is also important in the mechanism for delayed nausea and vomiting. It is used for preventing both acute and delayed nausea and vomiting from high-emetogenic chemotherapy drugs, especially cisplatin (Platinol), cyclophosphamide (Cytoxan), carboplatin (Paraplatin), and doxorubicin (Adriamycin). Aprepitant is usually combined with dexamethasone and a 5-HT-3 antagonist. It should be given orally for the first three days of chemotherapy. If you are on the blood thinner warfarin (Coumadin), your INR should be monitored more frequently, as there is a drug interaction with aprepitant.

Sore Mouth

The lining, or mucosa, of the gastrointestinal tract—which includes the inside of the mouth and throat—is one of the most sensitive areas of the body. Many chemotherapy drugs can inflame the lining, a condition called mucositis. Many drugs can also cause small ulcerations or sores to develop. Radiation delivered to the head and neck can irritate the lining and cause sores, too, and so can mouth or throat infections, especially fungus infections like monilia (thrush). All these can be very painful or at least uncomfortable.

If you are going to get over your mucositis, mouth care is very important. You will have to make sure your mouth stays clean and moist and that you eat the proper foods and get medication for any infections that develop.

Oral Hygiene A good oral hygienic program includes dental cleaning and scaling, followed by daily brushing and flossing to reduce plaque.

Any scaling, cleaning, tooth extractions, or repair of cavities should be done before your cancer therapy begins. Extractions especially should be completed at least two weeks before therapy to give your mouth a chance to heal. Ill-fitting dentures should be fixed or replaced.

Before any dental work is to be performed, your blood counts should be checked to be sure that counts are adequate to take care of any possibility of infection or bleeding (low white cell counts can lead to infections, and a low platelet count may lead to bleeding). So any periodontal or dental work has to be coordinated with your oncologist. If you have any mouth injury because of a dental procedure, antibiotics are certainly recommended.

The following daily steps will help your mouth stay in good shape:

• Use a soft-bristle toothbrush and soften it more by soaking it in warm water. Brushing with a paste of baking soda and water may be less irritating than commercial toothpaste.
• If brushing your teeth is painful, use either a cotton swab or commercial Toothettes, a sponge-tip stick impregnated with a dentifrice.
• Avoid commercial mouthwashes. Some of these have ingredients (especially alcohol) that can irritate your mouth even more. Lemon glycerin swabs may make your mouth feel clean, but they are not recommended, because glycerin will make your mouth drier.
• A Water Pik to cleanse your mouth is helpful.
• Peridex (oral rinse) will help gum inflammation and bleeding.

Dry Mouth Chemotherapy and radiation to the salivary glands can make your mouth very dry. This can make your mucositis or mouth sores more painful, so you should do everything you can to keep your mouth moist.

• Commercial preparations such as Moi-Stir or MouthKot—an oral natural saliva substitute—may help.
• You can make your own mouthwash with liquid Xylocaine, baking soda, and salt dissolved in 1 quart (1 l) of water.
• Sucking sour-lemon hard candies, a Tic Tac, an ice pop, or flavored or plain ice cubes can help.
• Use lip balms or lipstick for lips.

Mouth Sores If the soreness in your mouth becomes severe, there are quite a few anesthetic agents you can use on a short-term basis. If your symptoms persist, you should have a complete dental hygienic evaluation.

• Benadryl elixir, lozenges, and analgesics may help reduce mouth pain.
• Swishing and swallowing the anesthetic jelly viscous Xylocaine or spraying Hurricane spray can also help you eat if you have pain in your mouth, pharynx, or esophagus.
• It may help to swish diluted milk of magnesia, sucralfate (Carafate) slurry, or Mylanta around your mouth.
• Orabase—with or without Kenalog—is a dental salve that covers mouth sores while they are healing. You may have to apply it several times a day.

Infections Mouth infections can be dangerous and have to be cared for. You should examine your mouth every day for any irritation or early fungus growth (white spots inside your mouth that don't wash off). Look under your tongue and at the sides of your mouth and report any changes to your doctor. If you do get an infection, it should be treated promptly.

• If you have a herpes virus—acute or recurrent—your doctor may prescribe oral acyclovir (Zovirax).
• Monilia requires antifungal agents, including Mycostatin oral suspension, Nizoral tablets, Mycelex Troches, or Mycostatin Pastilles.
• You can freeze Mycostatin liquid in medicine cups in the refrigerator and let it melt in your mouth.

Nutrition A normal high-protein, high-calorie diet—with supplements as needed—will help your sore mouth or tongue heal faster. Drinking lots of fluids will also help the healing process as well

as help make your mouth sores more comfortable.

A high-protein, high-calorie diet would include scrambled eggs, custards, milkshakes, malts, gelatins, creamy hot cereals, macaroni and cheese, and blenderized or pureed foods. Commercial supplements such as Ensure, Sustacal, and Carnation breakfast drink can also be helpful.

Until your mouth sores heal you should avoid

• very hot or very cold foods;
• tomatoes and citrus fruits such as grapefruit, lemons, and oranges, which can burn your mouth;
• salty foods, which can cause a burning sensation;
• hot, spicy, coarse, or rough foods, including toast, dry crackers, and chips;
• alcoholic beverages and tobacco, both of which irritate the lining of the mouth; and
• any medications such as mouthwashes or cough syrups that contain alcohol.

Loss of Appetite

Loss of appetite, called anorexia, is one of the most common side effects of chemotherapy. It can also result from radiation therapy, stress and anxiety, depression, and the cancer itself.

For the sake of your health, your strength, and your ability to fight cancer, you have to get enough nutrition. But it's hard to keep your appetite when your mouth and tongue are sore or you have trouble swallowing. Fortunately, these side effects are usually short-term, lasting only three to eight days. But even after they go away, you still might have trouble getting your normal appetite back.

You can talk to a dietitian, a nurse, or your doctor about ways to improve your appetite. If you don't seem to be making

---

Tips to Increase Appetite

- Plan your meals in advance and arrange for help in preparing them. You might also better tolerate meals prepared by friends or relatives, since cooking at home might produce offensive odors that will put you off food.

- Make your mealtimes a pleasant experience.

- Stimulate your appetite by exercising for five or ten minutes about a half hour before meals.

- Have an aperitif such as a small glass of wine before meals. It will help you relax and stimulate your taste buds.

- Relax for a few minutes before meals, using relaxation exercises.

- Eat frequent, small meals and have snacks between meals that appeal to your senses.

- Add extra protein to your diet. Fortify milk by adding 1 cup (250 ml) of nonfat dry milk to each quart (liter) of whole milk or milk recipe. Be creative with desserts. And use nutritional supplements.

---

too much progress, you might also ask your doctor about medications that can stimulate your appetite, such as

- prednisone, a corticosteroid hormone, when given in small doses of 10 to 20 mg a day (there are side effects to consider);
- megestrol acetate (Megace), 400 mg two to three times a day (it may take two to three weeks to observe an increase in weight); and
- dronabinol (Marinol), a legally available synthetic form of marijuana in capsule form. It is usually used as an antinausea drug, but stimulation of appetite is a positive side effect.

Taste Alterations

Many chemotherapy drugs can change your sense of taste and smell. What these changes are depends on the individual, but they are most common with foods that are either very sweet or very bitter. Oddly enough, sweet foods might taste sour and sour foods taste sweet. Chewed meat may have a bitter taste because of the release of proteins in your mouth. Sometimes there is a continuous metallic taste in your mouth after chemotherapy,

which naturally enough can affect what you eat and how you eat.

Taste changes may not last long. But while you are experiencing them, you can do several things to lessen their effect:

- Brush your teeth several times a day and use mouth rinses such as diluted bicarbonate of soda.
- If foods and beverages taste bitter, add sweet fruits, honey, or NutraSweet.
- If meat tastes bitter, substitute bland chicken or fish, eggs and mild cheeses, or tofu. All of these might taste better if you use them in casseroles or stews.
- It will also help if you marinate meats, chicken, or fish in pineapple juice, wine, Italian dressing, lemon juice, soy sauce, or sweet-and-sour sauce.
- Add whatever flavorings you enjoy, but avoid spicy, highly seasoned foods.
- You might find that starchy foods such as bread, potatoes, and rice have a more acceptable taste if you eat them without butter or margarine.

Constipation and Impaction

Constipation means infrequent bowel movements. It also means a collection of dry, hard stools that get "stuck" in your rectum or colon. When you are constipated, you will often feel bloated and not have much of an appetite. If constipation persists, it may cause a stool "impaction"— a very large hard stool that you will have great difficulty passing.

It is important to try to prevent constipation and stool impaction, for both can cause great distress and pain. Patients with heart, respiratory, or gastrointestinal diseases can be especially aggravated by the discomfort and pressure of an impaction.

Causes All kinds of things can make you constipated—lack of exercise, emotional stress, various drugs, or simply a lack of high-fiber or bulk-forming foods in your diet.

Chemotherapy drugs such as vincristine (Oncovin), vinorelbine (Navelbine), and vinblastine (Velban) are often constipating as well as narcotic analgesics (morphine, oxycodone [Percocet, Percodan, Oxycontin], and codeine), gastrointestinal antispasmodics, antidepressants, diuretics, tranquilizers, sleeping pills, and calcium- and aluminum-based antacids.

When prescribing these drugs, your doctor should anticipate the need for a stool softener and/or a mild laxative. Enemas or suppositories might also be needed.

Laxatives and Stool Softeners If you become constipated, talk to your doctor about a laxative program. It is essential that you take laxatives, suppositories, and enemas only under your doctor's supervision. Don't try to diagnose and treat yourself, since there may be more to the situation than you may realize. For example, diarrhea can occasionally develop at the same time as a stool impaction, with the liquid stools moving around the impaction. If you decide to take antidiarrheal drugs, you can make the situation much worse.

There are many different ways to treat a wide variety of conditions, and your doctor may recommend several kinds of medications depending on your condition and other personal factors.

• *Stool softeners* help the stool retain water and so keep it soft. Stool softeners—docusate sodium (Colace), 100 to 240 mg per day with a full glass of water—should be used early, before the stools become hard, especially as it can be days before any effect is noticeable.

• *Mild laxatives* help promote bowel activity. Examples are milk of magnesia, Doxidan, cascara sagrada, and mineral oil (a lubricant).

• *Stronger laxatives* such as Fleet Phospho-soda, magnesium citrate, senna (Senokot), or bisacodyl (Dulcolax) suppositories or tablets cause increased bowel activity.

• *Contact laxatives* such as castor oil cause increased bowel activity.

• *Bulk laxatives* include dietary fiber, bran, methyl cellulose (Cellothyl), and psyllium (Metamucil).

• Laxatives with magnesium should be avoided if you have kidney disease. Laxatives with sodium should be avoided if you have a heart problem. Laxatives that contain magnesium can also cause diarrhea.

• If you are taking narcotics you should use stool softeners and mild laxatives rather than bulk-forming laxatives, because the combination can cause high colon constipation.

• A nonstimulating bulk softener such as Colace helps to soften the stool, and mineral oil or olive oil can be used to loosen the stool.

• Glycerin suppositories or Dulcolax suppositories may be used to stimulate bowel action as a contact laxative. (Dulcolax may cause cramping.)

• A bowel stimulant such as metoclopramide (Reglan) may be useful.

• Lactulose is an acidifier that softens the stool and increases the number of bowel movements.

Hints to Prevent and Relieve Constipation

- Eat foods that are high in fiber and bulk. These include fresh fruits and vegetables (raw or cooked with skins and peels on), dried fruit, whole-grain breads and cereals, and bran. Avoid raw fruits and vegetables, including lettuce, when your white blood cell count is lower than 1,800. *Note:* You should start a high-fiber diet before taking a chemotherapy drug that causes constipation.

- Drink plenty of fluids—eight to ten glasses a day. Avoid dehydration. Try to drink highly nutritional fluids (milkshakes, eggnogs, and juices) rather than water, since liquids can be filling and may decrease your appetite.

- Add bran to your diet gradually. Start with 2 teaspoons (10 ml) per day and gradually work up to 4 to 6 teaspoons (20 to 30 ml) per day. Sprinkle bran on cereal or add it to meat loaf, stews, pancakes, baked goods, and other dishes. Dietary bran is helpful.

- Avoid refined foods such as white bread, starchy desserts, and candy. Also avoid chocolate, cheese, and eggs, since these can be constipating.

- To make your bowel movements more regular, take prunes or a glass of prune juice in the morning or at night before bed. Prunes contain a natural laxative as well as fiber. Warmed prune juice and stewed prunes will be the most effective.

- Eat a large breakfast with some type of hot beverage, such as tea, hot lemon water, or decaffeinated coffee.

- Get enough rest and eat at regular times in a relaxed atmosphere.

- Get some exercise to stimulate your intestinal reflexes and help restore normal elimination.

All laxatives should be used with care. If you use them continually, you might develop a gastrointestinal irritation that can make it difficult to regain your normal bowel habits once you stop taking them. Increasing doses can also make your colon and rectum insensitive to the normal reflexes that stimulate a bowel movement.

Treating Stool Impaction A stool impaction develops when all of a stool doesn't pass through the colon or rectum. The stool gradually gets harder and harder as water is absorbed by the bowel. Then the stool gets larger and larger. If you can't pass it, it may partially obstruct the bowel or cause irritation of the rectum or anus. If you do pass it, it may cause small tears or fissures in the anus.

The primary treatment is to get fluids into the bowel to soften the stool so it can be passed or removed. Using enemas—either oil-retention, tap water, or phosphate (Fleet)—may help accomplish this goal. Sometimes it might be necessary for a health professional to use a gloved finger in the rectum to break up a large bulky mass or to extract the stool.

Diarrhea

Diarrhea is a condition marked by abnormally frequent bowel movements that are more fluid than usual. It is sometimes accompanied by cramps.

You may get diarrhea because of chemotherapy, radiation therapy to the lower abdomen, malabsorption due to surgery to the bowel, or a bowel inflammation or infection. Some antibiotics, especially "broad spectrum" antibiotics, can cause diarrhea, and it might develop because of an intolerance to milk.

Chemotherapy drugs that frequently cause diarrhea include irinotecan (Camptosar) and capecitabine (Xeloda). Aggressive antidiarrheal therapy is recommended for treating the first sign of increased stool frequency caused by these drugs, in order to prevent severe dehydration.

Treating Diarrhea Effective treatment depends on finding the cause. A good general approach is to limit your diet solely to fluids to allow the bowel to rest. Drink plenty of mild liquids, such as fruit drinks (Kool-Aid and Gatorade), ginger ale, peach or apricot nectar, water, and weak tea. Hot and cold liquids and foods tend to increase intestinal muscle contractions and make the diarrhea worse, so they should be warm or at room temperature. Allow carbonated beverages to lose their fizz—stir with a spoon—before you drink them.

When you are feeling better, gradually add foods low in roughage and bulk—steamed rice, cream of rice, bananas, applesauce, mashed potatoes, dry toast, and crackers—eaten warm or at room temperature.

As your diarrhea decreases, you may move on to a low-residue diet. Frequent small meals will be easier on your digestive tract. Low-residue nutritional supplements are also available from most pharmacies.

Replacing What Is Lost Diarrhea can cause dehydration, so you will have to drink plenty of fluids. To replace the fluid, sugar, and salt you will lose, a good general formula is 1 quart (1 l) boiled water, 1 teaspoon (5 ml) salt, 1 teaspoon (5 ml) baking soda, 4 teaspoons (20 ml) sugar, and flavor to your taste. As with any specially prepared concoction, however, you should check with your dietitian or doctor to make sure you can tolerate the particular ingredients.

Potassium is also lost in diarrhea. It is a necessary mineral, and it must be replaced.

Foods high in potassium include bananas, apricot and peach nectars, tomatoes, potatoes, broccoli, halibut, asparagus, citrus juices, cola drinks, and milk. Supplementary potassium tablets sometimes have to be taken.

Foods to Avoid Many types of foods are likely to aggravate your diarrhea and should be avoided. These include

• fatty, greasy, and spicy foods;
• coffee, regular (nonherbal) teas, and carbonated beverages containing caffeine;
• citrus fruits such as oranges and grapefruit;
• foods high in bulk and fiber, such as bran, whole-grain cereals and breads, popcorn, nuts, and raw vegetables and fruits (except apples); and
• beverages and foods that are generally served very hot or very cold.

Milk Intolerance Some people are born with lactose intolerance and some develop it as they grow older. The intolerance results from a deficiency of lactase, an enzyme that digests milk sugar (lactose) in the intestine, and is marked by cramping and diarrhea.

A lactase deficiency can sometimes develop after intestinal surgery, radiation therapy to the lower abdomen, or chemotherapy. Because you can no longer digest milk sugar properly, you feel bloated and experience cramping and diarrhea.

• If your diarrhea is caused by milk intolerance, you should avoid milk and milk products such as ice cream, cottage cheese, and cheese. Depending on how sensitive you are to milk, you may also have to avoid butter, cream, and sour cream.
• If you are very sensitive, look for lactose-free, nonfat milk solids. You can even make your own lactose-free milk by adding Lactaid—a tablet containing

Diarrhea Medications

- **Kaolin-pectin emulsion (Kaopectate).** Take 2 to 4 tablespoons (25 to 50 ml) after each loose bowel movement.

- **Diphenoxylate (Lomotil).** One to two tablets every four hours as needed. You can take Lomotil with Kaopectate or Imodium. Maximum eight Lomotil tablets per day.

- **Loperamide (Imodium).** Two capsules initially, then one to two capsules every two to four hours. Maximum sixteen capsules per day.

- **Paregoric.** Take 1 teaspoon (5 ml) four times a day. It may be used with Lomotil.

- **Cholestryamine (Questran).** A bile-salt sequestering agent. One packet after each meal and at bedtime.

- **Belladonna alkaloid (Donnatal) or glycopyrrolate (Robinul).** Anticholinergic, antispasmodic agents for bowel cramping. One to two tablets every four hours as needed.

- When all else fails, try psyllium (Metamucil) plus Kaopectate.

---

lactase—to your milk and keeping it in the refrigerator for twenty-four hours before using it.

- You can use buttermilk or yogurt because the lactose in them has already been processed and is digested. You might also tolerate some processed cheeses.

- You might try Mocha-mix, Dairy Rich, and other soy products, or some lactose substitutes like Imo (an imitation sour cream), Cool Whip, and Party Whip.

Swollen Limbs (Lymphedema)

Lymphedema—the medical term for swelling caused by the buildup of fluid (lymph) in the soft tissues—develops because of some blockage of the lymphatic system. Most lymphedema in cancer patients results from scarring after the surgical removal of lymph nodes or after radiation therapy. It usually involves areas next to large collections of lymph nodes in the armpit (axilla), pelvic region, and inguinal (groin) areas. The lymphatics (lymph vessels) are obstructed and swelling in the arms or legs is the result.

In its early phase, the swelling of the limb will "pit" with finger pressure. Elevating the arm or leg or using an elastic support arm glove or stocking will help reduce the swelling and improve the lymphatic flow.

Acute and Chronic Lymphedema Acute lymphedema may be a temporary condition. It can happen after a radical surgical procedure with lymph node dissection or after an acute inflammation such as an infection in the limb. More often seen in cancer patients is chronic lymphedema. Sometimes it results in only minor swelling and discomfort. But occasionally it can lead to grave disability and disfigurement.

Chronic lymphedema is more difficult to reverse than the acute variety because the more the limb swells, the harder it is to drain the fluid adequately. People with chronic lymphedema are also more susceptible to infections or local injuries, which results in more scarring and additional lymphedema. Infections of the limb—known as cellulitis—often develop after even minor cuts or abrasions and they can often only be controlled with long-term antibiotics.

Occasionally lymphedema becomes prolonged and severe. It can be aggravated by poor protein intake that may result from loss of appetite or nausea and vomiting from chemotherapy. It can also be aggravated by a decrease of the protein in the blood called albumin. The decrease results in leakage of water into the tissues, which leads to additional arm or leg swelling.

Who Gets It A small number of people with cancer develop lymphedema. It is not unusual after treatment for several common cancers:

• Breast cancer. Primary radiotherapy to the breast is rarely associated with lymphedema. It is more common if you are treated with radiotherapy after surgery to the regional lymph node areas.

• Malignant melanomas with lymph node dissection and/or radiation involving an extremity.

Hints for Preventing and Controlling Lymphedema

1. Whenever possible, keep the swollen arm or leg elevated, preferably above the level of the heart. When you are sitting, put your leg on a chair or stool.

2. Clean and lubricate your skin every day with oil or skin cream.

3. Do everything you can to avoid injuries and infection in the affected limb.
   • Use an electric razor to shave the underarm or leg to avoid skin cuts.
   • Wear gloves when gardening or doing housework and wear a thimble when sewing.
   • Suntan gradually, if at all, and use a sunscreen.
   • Avoid walking barefoot, particularly on the beach, or wading in water.
   • Use insect repellents and wear protective clothing to avoid insect bites.
   • Clean any breaks in your skin with mild soap and water, then apply an antibacterial ointment.
   • Use gauze wrapping instead of adhesive bandages on any skin wounds.
   • If you develop a rash, consult your doctor.
   • Try to minimize all the "invasive" procedures for drawing blood and giving medications— injections, finger pricks, and IVs—on the affected arm or leg.
   • Take good care of your nails and don't cut the cuticles.
   • Cut your toenails straight across.
   • See a podiatrist for any foot care problems.
   • Keep your feet clean and dry and wear cotton socks.
   • Avoid extreme hot or cold—ice packs or heating pads, for example—on the swollen limb.

4. Avoid constrictive pressure on your arm or leg.
   • Don't cross your legs while sitting.
   • Wear loose jewelry and clothes with no constricting bands.
   • Carry handbags on the nonswollen arm.
   • Don't use blood pressure cuffs on the swollen limb.
   • Wear only elastic bandages or stockings without constrictive bands.
   • Don't sit longer than thirty minutes without changing position.

5. Check the limb daily for signs of change. Especially watch for signs of infection—redness, pain, heat, swelling, or fever—and call your doctor immediately if any signs appear. Be sure to report any sensation of swelling or sudden increase in fluid.

6. Practice your drainage-promoting exercises faithfully.

7. After the limb has healed, *gradually* return to your normal activity. But always practice protective procedures—edema can come back if you get an injury.

• Prostate cancer or gynecologic cancers after surgery, with or without radiation.

• Testicular cancer with lymph node dissection, with or without radiation.

• Patients who have had several courses of radiotherapy to the axilla, shoulder, or groin, especially if surgery has also been performed there to treat recurrent cancer.

Preventing Lymphedema If you have had any of the above procedures, you will have to take extra-special care of the limb that might be affected. You should treat your arm or leg with the same care and attention you give to your face.

You can do a lot to prevent lymphedema—good nutrition with a high-protein diet, active physical exercise to help your muscles pump the lymphatic fluid, control of obesity. You should also try hard to avoid infections from small cuts you might get from working around the house or by doing physical work that might damage or injure the skin on the affected arm or leg.

Even if you follow a prevention program faithfully, lymphedema can occasionally develop years after surgery. This often happens after a local infection, although sometimes it happens for no apparent reason at all. If you develop any evidence of inflammation or infection (cellulitis) with redness or increased swelling, report it to your doctor. He or she can evaluate your condition and prescribe any necessary antibiotics. You may have to stay on antibiotics for several weeks or even months.

Milking Your Muscles Exercising your muscles is vital if you want to prevent lymphedema. It is just as vital if you want to control it. The compression of your muscles helps to milk the fluid in the lymphatics back toward your heart.

Physical therapists can recommend the most appropriate exercises for you. Many people are often encouraged to walk or ride a bicycle to help improve the lymphatic flow. Breast cancer patients are usually instructed to go through a series of hand and arm exercises after surgery. A similar program is used by patients with melanomas involving the limbs. Therapists can instruct you in the use of lymphedema milking pumps that can reduce your swelling; this can be an effective approach for chronic lymphedema.

Hair Loss

Losing your hair (alopecia) can be quite an emotional experience. As the most visible side effect of cancer treatment, it is often the most upsetting. In fact, you may find it helpful to have your mate or a close friend or relative with you when you talk to your doctor about the potential for hair loss.

Why You Might Lose Your Hair Chemotherapy drugs circulate throughout your body, and they aren't selective about which cells they affect. They change normal as well as malignant cells and have an especially destructive effect on rapidly growing cells like your hair and the cells lining your mouth and gastrointestinal tract. So hair loss is a common side effect of chemotherapy, especially with drugs such as cyclophosphamide (Cytoxan), doxorubicin (Adriamycin) and vincristine (Oncovin). Your chances of losing your hair are increased if you are getting combination therapy.

When You Lose Your Hair You may not lose all your hair. It may just become thin or patchy. The loss might also be sudden or gradual. It usually happens within the first cycle (usually around week 3), but it may not happen until the second cycle. And, whether the loss is partial or complete, you may develop some scalp irritation, dermatitis, or scaling that will need medical attention.

The hair almost always comes back. It may take three to six months, or it might come back while you are still on chemotherapy. When it does come back, it might have a slightly different texture or color or curl.

Hair Loss and Radiation You might lose some hair after radiation therapy to the skull or brain. This may be total and permanent, but if lower doses are used, the hair sometimes comes back within two or three months.

Preparing for Hair Loss This is one side effect you can plan for well in advance. There are several things you can do before you begin treatment that will make losing your hair not quite as upsetting:

• Get a short haircut so that the hair loss won't be as noticeable either to others or to you when you look in the mirror.
• Treat your hair and your scalp gently by avoiding hairsprays, perms, and dyes.
• Select hair covers that you'll need during the period of hair loss—turbans, scarves, hats, wigs, and scarves with hair fringes that look like your own hair. Many insurance companies will pay for a hairpiece or wig, since they are a "part" of treatment, so ask your doctor for a prescription. To get the best possible match, buy a wig before you lose your hair.

Tourniquets and Ice Caps Scalp tourniquets and ice caps can be used to prevent or reduce hair loss. But they are not very useful when the chemotherapy drugs tend to stay in the bloodstream for several hours or if the drugs are taken orally, which leads to the same time effect. Even so, using caps and tourniquets during therapy might make you feel better by reducing anxiety.

Tourniquets and ice caps are not recommended if you are being treated for cancers that are likely to have hidden scalp metastases—melanoma, kidney cancer, leukemia, lymphomas, and tumors that spread in the bloodstream.

Allergic and Dermatologic Reactions from Chemotherapy

Chemotherapy can cause several skin reactions. Vesicant drugs (nitrogen mustard [Mustargen], vincristine [Oncovin], etoposide [Etopophos], doxorubicin [Adriamycin], mitomycin [Mutamycin], and others) can blister and also produce local skin reactions when accidentally injected outside a vein or port. But precautions and antidotes can minimize these reactions. Vinorelbine (Navelbine) may cause burning along the vein during injection. In some cases, blisters along the vein have been reported. Your nurse will administer vinorelbine in a more dilute solution if it causes localized burning or blistering. Specific drugs (bleomycin [Blenoxane], paclitaxel [Taxol]) have the potential of causing allergic reactions. These reactions can be minimized with adequate antiallergic medications taken before chemotherapy. Patients receiving tretinoin (Retin-A) can experience redness, dryness, itching, and increased sensitivity to sunlight, and thus should take adequate precautions. Finally, the hand-foot syndrome is a painful redness, irritation, and fissuration of the hands and soles seen with fluorouracil, capecitabine (Xeloda), and liposomal doxorubicin (Doxil). Treatment of this syndrome is mainly support and moisturizing of the affected regions with creams and emollients.

Fertility Effects of Chemotherapy

Today, many young patients are cured of cancer after receiving chemotherapy. However, alterations in gonadal (reproductive) function are now recognized as a common complication of cancer chemotherapy. Women may experience premature gonadal failure, menopause, sterility, and even osteoporosis (from estrogen deprivation). Men may have low sperm count and infertility. Other issues concerning cancer survivors are risks of complications of pregnancy, birth defects, and malignancy in their offspring.

Although many questions remain to be answered, your doctor will provide counseling and use newer strategies to prevent gonadal complications from chemotherapy. One approach is to use alternative hormonal therapies or preservation of sperm or eggs for future use.

Chemotherapy (especially cyclophosphamide [Cytoxan]) given to boys before or during puberty has resulted in 1 percent and 67 percent gonadal dysfunction, respectively. MOPP (nitrogen mustard [Mustargen] + vincristine [Oncovin] + procarbazine + prednisone) chemotherapy used in Hodgkin's disease inhibits virtually 100 percent of sperm function in men. Gonadal damage after puberty is usually assessed by analyzing the seminal fluid. The effects of various chemotherapy regimens on male spermatogenesis are shown in Table 3. It appears that the major drugs that cause gonadal dysfunction are the alkylating agents such as cyclophosphamide, thiotepa, nitrogen mustard, and chlorambucil (Leukeran). For patients in whom fertility is spared, the outcome of pregnancies has not shown a higher incidence of congenital anomalies, spontaneous abortion,

Table 3. Chemotherapy and Male Fertility

DISEASE	REGIMEN	PERCENT LOW SPERM COUNT
Hodgkin's	MOPP (nitrogen mustard [Mustargen] + vincristine [Oncovin] + procarbazine + prednisone)	85 percent
Hodgkin's	ABVD (Adriamycin + bleomycin + vinblastine + dacarbazine)	0 percent
Testes cancer	Cisplatin, vinblastine, bleomycin	14–28 percent
Sarcoma	Doxorubicin + cyclophosphamide	65 percent

Table 4. Chemotherapy and Amenorrhea (Loss of Menstrual Periods)

DISEASE	REGIMEN	PERCENT LOSS OF MENSTRUAL PERIODS
Ovarian cancer	Cisplatin, vincristine, methotrexate, etoposide, actinomycin D	6 percent
Breast cancer	CMF (cyclophosphamide + methotrexate + 5-fluorouracil)	85 percent
Breast cancer	Cyclophosphamide	83 percent
Breast cancer	Fluorouracil	9 percent
Hodgkin's	MOPP	24 percent
Hodgkin's	COPP (cyclophosphamide + vincristine [Oncovin] + procarbazine + prednisone)	57 percent
Hodgkin's	ABVD	0 percent

The two tables above are modified from M. Perry, *Chemotherapy Source Book*, 2nd ed., Williams and Wilkins, 1997, pp. 813–832.

or neonatal mortality. There are fewer studies of fathers surviving cancer. In men with germ cell tumors, there has not been an excess of congenital anomalies and chromosomal abnormalities in their offspring. In addition, there was no difference in growth maturation. In pregnancy, fetal exposure to multidrug chemotherapy has been associated with minimal risk when chemotherapy was after the first trimester.

Effects of Chemotherapy during Pregnancy

Surprisingly, chemotherapy is fairly safe to both the child and mother when given during the second and third trimesters of pregnancy. Although there have been reported cases of fetal malformations, these are not any more frequent than the general population. However, chemotherapy should be within near term and given after birth, if possible. Chemotherapy should generally be avoided during the first trimester, especially with methotrexate therapy. Both cyclophosphamide (Cytoxan) and doxorubicin (Adriamycin) have been given safely during any trimester of pregnancy.

Cardiac (Heart) Toxicity from Chemotherapy

Some chemotherapy drugs, such as doxorubicin (Adriamycin), daunorubicin (Cerubidine), epirubicin (Ellence), and idarubicin (Idamycin), or radiation therapy to the chest can have an adverse effect on the heart. Such reactions as cardiac congestion and decreased exercise tolerance are generally seen with prolonged treatment, but can also occur early on. Your doctor may obtain special cardiac studies (ejection fraction) and may record an echocardiogram of your heart before and throughout the treatment. In case of damage to the heart, the drug may be stopped or modified. Dexrazoxane (Zinecard) can be given to minimize the effects of chemotherapy on the heart muscle. An alternate method to minimize the cardiotoxic effect is to administer the liposomal form of doxorubicin (Doxil), substantially lowering the effect on the heart.

— 21 —

Fatigue

Ernest H. Rosenbaum, M.D., Barbara F. Piper, D.N.Sc., R.N., A.O.C.N., F.A.A.N.,
and Pat Kramer, M.S.N., R.N., A.O.C.N.

■ ■ ■ ■

Fatigue is the feeling of being tired after resting or a good sleep. Affecting up to 90 percent of cancer patients, especially those undergoing therapy, it is one of the most common side effects of the disease and its treatment. It can occur on the same day, or for several days, or for long periods of time during and after therapy. Fatigue affects quality of life, the ability to function, and the capacity to live a productive, satisfactory existence.

Fatigue can be a major problem during and after therapy, and an active program for fatigue reduction may be required. Both rest and exercise help in controlling debility and fatigue. In addition to treatment effects, fatigue can also be caused by emotional stress, anxiety, depression, pain, and insomnia, as well as a hormonal problem such as hypothyroidism (low thyroid function) or anemia due to cancer or its treatment.

Anemia occurs when there is a shortage of red blood cells produced by the body or a decrease in the hemoglobin level, resulting in a decrease in the oxygen-carrying capacity of the blood. Symptoms of anemia are tiredness, weakness, shortness of breath, dizziness, and possibly a decrease in heart function. It is commonly diagnosed with a very simple blood test with instruments that measure the level of hemoglobin and/or count the number of red cells.

The bone marrow is a "factory" that produces white cells, red cells, and plate-lets. When red blood cell production is reduced because of cancer, chemotherapy, immunotherapy, or radiation therapy, the level of functioning red cells in the body is deficient. Thus, there are fewer red cells to carry oxygen, which can be one of the causes of fatigue.

In addition to reduced bone marrow function from cancer therapy, lack of iron, vitamin B_{12}, and folic acid can also be causes of anemia and can easily be tested. Fortunately, there are drugs that can help correct the anemia.

It is believed that proinflammatory mediators (immunological chemical cytokines, including tumor necrosis factor [TNF]) are triggered by malignant diseases, chemotherapy, immunotherapy, or radiotherapy, thereby contributing to fatigue. In a new approach, agents that block cytokine (chemical) production are used in clinical research trials to diminish fatigue and its symptoms. In progress are pilot research studies that use cytokine blockers of tumor necrosis factor–alpha (TNF-α) to reduce fatigue from chemotherapy.[1] A TNF-α antagonist, infliximab, is being tested in clinical research to help alter fatigue in breast cancer survivors.[2]

Modafinil (Provigil), a drug for treating sleeping disorders, has been shown to improve cognitive function (memory and attention) and mood and to reduce fatigue in patients with brain cancer. Memory and attention span improved by 21 percent, mood improved by 35 percent, and fatigue levels were reduced by 47 percent, thus improving quality of life.[3]

Modafinil has recently been reported (by the Multinational Association of Supportive Care in Cancer [MASCC] meeting in 2006) to have positive effects by significantly reducing cancer-related fatigue in a one-month trial. It was effective in women with breast cancer who had had fatigue for up to two years after treatment.[4]

The Management of Fatigue

Fatigue is one of the most common problems seen in cancer patients. The two basic rules for combating fatigue are rest and exercise. When you find that you are not able to function well because of fatigue, getting extra rest is important. At the same time, an exercise program can be very beneficial in helping to maintain and build up muscles that will help you in your everyday activities. You may need an aid to daily living (ADL) such as a cane or walker, and if you're unable to do your housework, for example, you may need assistance for cleaning and cooking. You may also need help getting your family to their daily activities and functions.

The M. D. Anderson Cancer Center has developed the Brief Fatigue Inventory (BFI), using a scale of 0 to 10 (with 0 being no fatigue and 10 being severe fatigue), to rate and give a general assessment of the level of fatigue. The BFI can be found at *www.mdanderson.org/topics/fatigue/*.

Tips on managing fatigue include

• eating frequent small meals and snacking on high-protein foods;
• incorporating nutritional supplements, such as Ensure, Boost, and Scandishake, into your diet;
• maintaining good fluid replacement with liquids and electrolyte-positive drinks; and
• planning your day so that strenuous activities are done at times of optimal strength.

Do not be shy; being able to accept help during this period is important. Fortunately, for most people, there is recovery, and as you regain strength, fatigue will hopefully subside, making the normal demands of daily life easier to meet.

Try to schedule yourself throughout the day to do necessary tasks when you have more energy. Try to be more organized—for example, plan your shopping trips with a list that is coordinated with the aisles in the store you use. Or, if necessary, use a shopping service that delivers to your home. Accept help in carrying shopping bags to your car and from your family and friends when you get home. Shopping on-line is another option. Cooking is often a chore when you have fatigue. Thus, cooking in larger quantities and freezing portions can make meals available that are easy to prepare so you can save your strength for other activities. Accept help in cooking and housekeeping as needed.

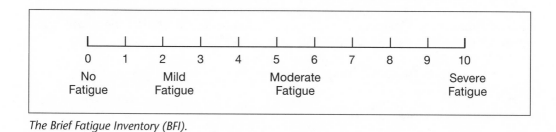

The Brief Fatigue Inventory (BFI).

Because you may be unable to do a full day's workload, planning and scheduling shorter but more productive hours in the office may help you in maintaining a satisfactory and productive effort at work.

Try to enjoy hobbies and activities, both inside and outside the home, such as movies, concerts, and art exhibits, as well as fun projects with family and friends. Use relaxation techniques such as biofeedback and meditation, not only to save energy, but also to help promote a sense of well-being.

Cancer-Related Fatigue and Sleep

There appears to be an association between cancer-related fatigue and disturbance in sleep patterns. A survey by Sarvaes and colleagues[5] noted that 40 percent of breast cancer survivors had fatigue problems posttherapy, most of which returned to a normal state with time. Psychological factors such as depression and anxiety were also noted as contributing to fatigue, in addition to physical symptoms and sleep disturbances. Those who received chemotherapy had more significant symptoms with greater sleep difficulties. There is also a relationship between fatigue and social, cognitive, and behavioral factors.

Research is under way to further elucidate the relationship between cancer-related fatigue and sleep disturbances, assessing a symptom cluster including pain, anxiety, and depression. The consequences of this combination of cancer-related fatigue, cardio-respiratory disturbances, and sleep disturbances include lack of concentration, difficulty making decisions,

and irritability, all of which can impact family, school, work, and social life.

Ongoing research (currently under assessment) to define the causes of cancer-related fatigue, such as cytokine (cell chemical products) and hormonal imbalances, will hopefully lead to less debilitating cancer treatments. Also under assessment are efforts to establish a balance of exercise, work, and other activities that may benefit fatigue and sleep patterns. Ways of better controlling pain, anxiety, and depression are being developed with improved treatment plans, as well as symptom management.

Notes

1. Monk JP, Phillips G, Waite R, Kuhn J, Schaaf LJ, Otterson GA. Assessment of tumor necrosis factor alpha blockade as an intervention to improve tolerability of dose-intensive chemotherapy in cancer patients. *J Clin Oncol* 2006;24(12): 1852–9.

2. Bradbury J. Taking fatigue out of cancer. *The Lancet Oncol* 2006 Jun 7(6):457.

Collado-Hidalgo A, Bower JE, Ganz PA, Cole SW, Irwin MR. Inflammatory biomarkers for persistent fatigue in breast cancer survivors. *Clin Cancer Res* 2006;12(9):2759–66.

3. Thomas Kaleita, PhD, UCLA.

4. Morrow GR, Ryan J, Kohli S, et al. Modafinil (Provigil) for persistent post-treatment fatigue, Poster presentation at MASCC meeting, Toronto, Canada, June 24, 2006.

5. Servaes P, Verhagen S, Bleijenberg G. Determinants of chronic fatigue in disease-free breast cancer patients: a cross-sectional study. *Ann Oncol* 2002; 13(4):589–98.

— 22 —

The Role of Sleep in Health, Disease, and Therapy

David Claman, M.D.

■ ■ ■ ■

Our knowledge about sleep and sleep disorders has increased dramatically since the 1950s, which is when REM (rapid eye movement) sleep was first described in the medical literature. Sleep is now viewed as an active state, with highly regulated physiologic processes. Compared to a century ago, the average person today probably sleeps about one hour less per night, which makes sleep deprivation a common issue. Many people in society have disrupted sleep schedules, shift-work schedules, or sleep a shortened number of hours. Many medical conditions may cause pain or discomfort that can disturb sleep.

Cancer patients have many potential physical and psychological issues. The sleep of cancer patients may be disturbed not only by physical pain or discomfort, but also by psychological issues such as anxiety and depression regarding their condition or prognosis.

Stages of Sleep

A normal sleep pattern goes through the various REM and non-REM stages of sleep. People go through wakefulness; Stages 1, 2, 3, and 4 of non-REM sleep; and then REM sleep. When you go to sleep, you will be awake for a few minutes and then go through non-REM sleep. The deepest sleep is in Stages 3 and 4 of non-REM, and the longest period of Stages 3 and 4 occurs during the first one to two hours of sleep. This is the time period that young children are likely to have night terrors and sleepwalking. Following this period of deep sleep, the first period of dreaming, or REM sleep, occurs. At one- to two-hour intervals more, REM periods occur through the night of sleep, such that by the early morning, most people have had between four and six separate dreaming periods. People usually remember the dreaming episodes only if they wake up immediately afterward, but the average person will have four to six dream periods a night.

A review article in the *New England Journal of Medicine* about sleep in the elderly showed the normal patterns of sleep as the population ages. In the first few years of life, there is a much larger number of hours slept per day, but this slowly decreases through the age of twenty, by which time most people have settled into a stable pattern of sleep hours and sleep stages. The amount of REM sleep as a percentage of sleep time remains fairly constant for many decades and may have only a slight decrease in the elderly. The total time in bed increases around the time of sixty to seventy years of age, which is when many people retire from work. People have the luxury of going to bed earlier and tend to be in bed awake for longer periods of time. It's not that the number of minutes that people sleep is decreasing, but that they're awake in bed for longer periods. Sleep stages stay pretty constant over time, and sleep duration does not change significantly during later years.

The More Common Sleep Disorders

Purposeful Sleep Deprivation Many of us undervalue sleep and take shortcuts when it comes to going to bed and getting up, so that we're not getting a full 7 ½ to 8 hours of sleep per night. The most common cause of sleepiness during the daytime is purposeful sleep deprivation.

Insomnia Insomnia is far and away the most common sleep disorder reported in the population. From a survey done for the National Sleep Foundation back in the early 1990s on how frequently insomnia was reported in the U.S. population, we know that approximately 36 percent of the population has experienced either occasional insomnia or chronic insomnia. Nine percent of people currently report chronic insomnia.

Insomnia is a very subjective complaint. The first step in evaluating insomnia is asking whether the trouble is getting to sleep at bedtime, waking up frequently as the night goes on, or waking up at three A.M. and unable to get back to sleep at that hour. The insomnia complaint can be a combination of these different issues. If you can't get to sleep at bedtime, it may be that caffeine is keeping you awake. Or perhaps you're worried or tense about different issues related to work, family, or your health that usually come up at bedtime. If you're waking up frequently at night, there may be physical or emotional issues behind this. Waking up early in the morning could be related to stress or depression. Emotional causes are less common than physical problems, but those really depend on the individual person, the issues involved, and the medications being prescribed.

There are four main categories of causes of insomnia: medical, psychiatric, situational, and pharmacologic. The more medical problems people have, the more frequently they complain of insomnia. This is an important area to focus on for patients who may be waking up with shortness of breath from lung problems, with ulcer pain, or with chronic arthritis pain in the hips or knees or hands. Hopefully, treating these medical problems will improve the sleep-related problems. Psychiatric issues are common causes of insomnia, especially in patients with depression, anxiety, or schizophrenia. It is estimated that about one-third of the patients with chronic insomnia may have anxiety disorders or some problem with depression. The next category is situational issues, such as tests, public-speaking engagements, and job changes, which can also cause insomnia. Most people with stressful situations that cause insomnia don't seek medical attention for it and hope that when the situation resolves, their sleeping will improve. Pharmacologic causes of insomnia may occur because many medications, both prescription and nonprescription, have sleep-related side effects. The two most common substances to disturb sleep are caffeine and alcohol. If you drink caffeine in the evening, it may keep you awake at bedtime and be a cause of insomnia. If you drink alcohol at bedtime to get to sleep, and the alcohol wears off two or three hours later, you may find yourself waking up in the middle of the night and not being able to get back to sleep.

Sleep Issues Specific to Cancer Cancer patients may develop insomnia, as they may suffer from issues relating to their cancer, to psychiatric disorders, to adapting to their new situation or condition, or to drugs used to treat their cancer or their symptoms. Patients may not receive adequate sleep due to anxiety in anticipation of a doctor visit or treatment. Patients awaiting surgery, chemotherapy, or radiation treatment tend to suffer from insomnia. Chemotherapy has also been shown to disrupt brain chemistry and some cognitive functioning, which in turn will interfere with sleep. Pain may be due to the underlying cancer, surgery, radiation therapy, or other treatment. Pain can make it more difficult to get to sleep or to stay asleep, or it may interfere with sleep quality. Effective relief of pain may improve all of these issues. Breathing issues are frequently important to cancer patients. Breathing may be more difficult due to either the underlying cancer or other conditions such as asthma, emphysema, or congestive heart failure. Treatment focused on improving breathing should improve sleep quality and help a cancer patient feel more rested. Anxiety and depression can seriously disturb sleep, especially for cancer patients. Fear of dying during sleep also prevents many cancer patients from getting adequate rest. These issues that cause depression can be treated by medications, but improved sleeping habits (see "Sleep Hygiene," in this chapter) may improve sleep without a need for medications. Lastly, medication side effects can disturb sleep, particularly when cancer patients are frequently treated with multiple medications. Examples of this would include pain medicines causing daytime drowsiness and antidepressants causing insomnia. Caffeine and alcohol may also disturb patients' sleep quality. Medications like Decadron (dexamethasone) (acts as a stimulant) and tamoxifen (Novadex) (acts as an antidepressant) make changes to brain chemistry and will often interfere with sleep patterns. A detailed review of medications and potential side effects is often of value. Talk to your pharmacist, doctor, or nurse.

Important Factors in Insomnia The factors that affect the development of insomnia can be broken down into several different groups: predisposing factors, precipitating factors, and perpetuating factors. Predisposing factors include personality type, sleep-wake cycle, and age, because as the population ages, insomnia is very frequently a subjective complaint. All of us struggle with occasional precipitating factors, such as changes in situation or environment, medical or psychiatric illnesses, or new prescription or nonprescription medication. Most people will struggle with some amount of predisposing and precipitating factors, will have a brief episode of insomnia, but will slowly improve over time, and won't necessarily become a person with chronic insomnia or need to see a doctor about the problem. Most people who have chronic insomnia also have some contribution from perpetuating factors that reinforce the insomnia problem. Negative conditioning about sleep is particularly common. For example, people who say, "I'm so tense about my sleeping problem that as soon as I go into my bedroom, I'm worried sick that I'm not going to be able to sleep, and I lie awake for hours," can very often lie in bed and sleep poorly. How can you relax and get to sleep when you are filled with tension and worry? Substance abuse, whether it's with sleeping pills, caffeine, alcohol, or illegal drugs, can precipitate sleeping problems. Performance anxiety—for example, "If I'm not asleep in the next ten minutes, I won't be able to do my job tomorrow"—is a common issue. Last on the list of perpetuating factors is poor sleep hygiene.

Sleep Hygiene The best intervention for insomnia is a behavioral approach called sleep hygiene, a term that refers to good and bad sleeping habits. The goal is to practice good sleeping habits so you sleep better and to avoid bad sleeping habits, which will make you sleep more poorly.

For good sleep hygiene:

• Maintain a regular schedule for going to bed and waking up, regardless of your "weekend" versus "weekday" schedules.

• Avoid excessive time in bed. Spending too much time in bed can lead to frustration at not sleeping, and that will add to the insomnia problem.

• Avoid taking naps during the day. Taking a nap to catch up on sleep during the day means less sleep that night, reinforcing the bad sleeping pattern at night. Depending on your reasons for being sleep-deprived, naps can be either beneficial or detrimental to the insomnia situation.

• Use the bed and bedroom for sleeping and sex only. Make the bed a pleasant place to be, not one filled with anxiety. Sleeping and sex are pleasant activities that will be associated with positive conditioning.

• Do not watch the clock while in bed, because this reinforces how much time has gone by and exacerbates worry about not sleeping.

• Do something relaxing before going to bed.

• Make the bedroom quiet and comfortable.

• Avoid taking the troubles of the day to bed with you.

• Avoid alcohol and caffeinated beverages.

• Try to get regular exercise, but not within two hours of bedtime.

• Avoid using sleeping medications, if at all possible, unless it's truly necessary.

Most people can make significant improvement by focusing on their sleep hygiene.

Obstructive Sleep Apnea Obstructive sleep apnea is estimated to affect 2 to 4 percent of the general population. *Apnea* means not breathing; thus, sleep apnea is not breathing while you're sleeping. In adults, sleep apnea is almost always obstructive, meaning that the airway closes off and blocks breathing. The chest tries to breathe and makes greater and greater efforts to do so. Finally, the mind

interrupts the sleeping pattern to get the breathing going again. The airway opens and the breathing resumes, but this causes a disturbance in the brain-wave sleeping pattern so that the person is not rested in the morning. Generally, there is a reduction in the blood oxygen level as a physiologic outcome of the absence of breathing, because the body continues to do all its normal metabolic activities and uses up oxygen during the time that you're not breathing. Obstructive sleep apnea is a fairly common disorder, and one that is diagnosable and treatable. The expert witness in cases of sleep apnea is often the sleeping partner, and it's very important in the sleep clinic to talk to the sleeping partner. The patient is usually unaware of the sleep apnea issues, and the sleeping partner can often provide reliable information about the presence of snoring and episodes of interrupted breathing.

Treatment for Obstructive Sleep Apnea
There are a number of different treatments that can be given for obstructive sleep apnea:

1. Weight loss is commonly recommended in sleep apnea, because most patients with sleep apnea are overweight. Weight gain causes deposits of tissue in the neck. This accumulation makes the airways smaller and predisposes patients to sleep apnea. Those patients who do lose weight will generally reduce the severity of their sleep apnea.

2. It is also recommended to avoid alcohol and sedatives near bedtime. Alcohol relaxes the muscles in the windpipe, making it more likely that the airways will close off and block breathing.

3. Postural training involves sleeping only on your side, instead of sleeping on your back. Many people with sleep apnea have more breathing problems when they sleep on their backs, and patients are encouraged to sleep on their sides. If

sleeping on your side does help, sew one or two tennis balls in back of an old T-shirt, so that if you roll over onto your back, you'll feel the tennis balls and roll back over on your side.

4. Continuous positive airway pressure, or CPAP, is a mask treatment using an air compressor to blow a balloonful of air into the airway. CPAP is the most common form of therapy for sleep apnea.

5. Oral appliances are plastic bridges that fit the upper and lower teeth to hold the jaw in a more forward position. They are worn during sleep on an ongoing basis to provide some improvement.

6. Lastly, surgery can be done for sleep apnea. Surgery offered a lot of promise originally, but we have learned that surgery is not always successful, so CPAP is often used as the first treatment option. Surgery for sleep apnea raises a complex set of issues, which depends on the severity of the sleep apnea and the anatomy. Despite the risks and potential failure of surgery to cure apnea, surgery is clearly appropriate for some patients.

CPAP remains our most effective treatment. It involves wearing a mask that covers the nose and is held in place by straps. The attached air hose is connected to a small air compressor that sits at the side of the bed. During sleep, the muscles relax and the airway locks shut. Putting a mask over the nose and blowing a balloonful of positive airway pressure into the windpipe helps keep the airway open to maintain normal breathing. CPAP treatment, although cumbersome, can actually eliminate 90 to 100 percent of the sleep apnea in affected individuals. There are a number of treatments available for obstructive sleep apnea, but CPAP treatment is probably the most commonly recommended and most effective therapy.

Disrupted Circadian Rhythms Circadian rhythms are rhythms of behavioral and physiological processing, which occur approximately every twenty-four hours. The strongest stimulus for circadian rhythms is sunlight, which makes sense from an evolutionary point of view, although social cues and exercise can also have an effect. This is how your mind and body know when to lie down and go to sleep and after you sleep 7 ½ or 8 hours, when it's time to wake up. Circadian rhythms do get confused in two situations: jet lag and shift work. In jet lag, both the physical stimulus of bright sunlight and the social interactions encourage realignment, and most people can adjust their circadian rhythms one to two hours per day according to sunlight and social activity.

In shift work, the physical stimulus—the light—and the social stimuli of family and friends are oriented to keeping you awake during the daytime. Most people with shift work try to sleep during the daylight hours several days per week but sleep at night on the weekends. The most effective way to perform shift work from a sleep point of view is to sleep during the daytime seven days a week. If you go back and forth, you will essentially be getting jet lag from weekend to weekend, and your circadian rhythms will usually stay oriented toward being awake during the sunlight hours and being asleep at nighttime. Most people in their twenties and thirties can handle shift work, but when they reach their fifties or sixties, it becomes too difficult. Jet lag and shift work are an interesting contrast to each other in terms of the different issues with realigning circadian rhythms and sleeping at a time that your body is going to be able to rest the most effectively.

Your need for sleep will vary, depending in part on your activities and habits (not all people require eight hours of sleep nightly). Prolonged lack of sleep reduces efficiency and the ability to function. How you sleep is important, too. If sleeping pills or pain medications are helpful in obtaining an adequate night's rest, they should be used. Resolving any perplexing and annoying emotional problems helps immeasurably. The use of relaxation techniques, meditation, and biofeedback is often invaluable.

Sleeping Medications

If behavioral therapies (e.g., sleep hygiene) and symptom-specific treatments (e.g., controlling pain with appropriate medications) are ineffective for treating insomnia, then a range of medication options are available. These include hypnotics, sedatives, and antidepressants. Hypnotics are typically shorter-acting medications with less chance of causing morning drowsiness. Sedatives typically have a longer duration of action and are more helpful if anxiety is also present. Antidepressants can be given either to help relieve depression and anxiety

(in order to help reduce insomnia) or to act as a sedative at bedtime. It would be important to discuss with your physician which of these medications might be most helpful for your situation.

In Summary

Understanding the multitude of physical and psychological issues that can disturb the sleep of cancer patients is the first step in finding appropriate assistance from the medical team or from family and friends. The first step in improving insomnia is the framework of good sleeping habits outlined in the list of sleep hygiene recommendations. Sleep disorders are diagnosable and treatable and may be worthy of discussion with the medical team. Improved sleep can be quite helpful in coping with physical and psychological issues that occur in the setting of cancer.

— 23 —

Maintaining Good Nutrition

Natalie L. Ledesma, M.S., R.D., Ernest H. Rosenbaum, M.D.,
and Malin Dollinger, M.D.

■ ■ ■ ■

Good nutrition is vital to each and every one of us all the time. It is impossible to stay in good health without consuming the right foods in the right amounts. Good nutrition provides us the energy and the building blocks our bodies need in order to function properly and stay in good repair.

Good nutrition is even more necessary when you have cancer. Your body is fighting disease, and food is a critical weapon in this fight. You will need even more nutrients than usual—a metabolic necessity about 20 percent higher than that of a healthy person who engages in moderate activity. The extra nutrients will provide your body more energy, repair damaged tissues, help boost your immune system, and create a feeling of general well-being.*

The Best Approach to Eating

What you will need may be an entirely different approach to eating. Forget the signals that have always told you when to start eating and when to stop. They may no longer be a reliable guide. You will have to approach eating as a necessary part of your therapy and may need to eat even when you're not hungry.

Food has many meanings for us in our world. It is associated with good times and friends, comfort, culture, pleasure,

and hence nourishment—not just in the physical sense, but as "food for the soul." Oftentimes we may not be able to eat or enjoy food in the same way due to taste changes, loss of appetite, and other symptoms and surgical conditions. This is the time to try new foods or prepare foods in different ways—your eating may possibly be dictated by a need for a specific diet. The following are basic guidelines; your personal guidelines will depend on the treatment you are on or what your individual goal is. Research is ongoing to determine the "optimal" diet to treat cancer or its recurrence and to prevent cancer. Many studies are currently under way.

Common Problems

Many people with cancer have a difficult time maintaining good nutrition, since the cancer therapies or the cancer itself can make it challenging to eat enough food. There are several major common problems:

• *Loss of Appetite* This is the most serious problem. Pain, nausea, vomiting, diarrhea, constipation, or a sore or dry mouth can easily make you lose interest in food. You may also tend to eat less because of fear, anxiety, or depression about having cancer.

*For more expanded information, see *Everyone's Guide to Cancer Supportive Care*, Ernest H. Rosenbaum, M.D., and Isadora R. Rosenbaum, M.A., 2005.

• *Malabsorption* For a number of reasons, nutrients may not be absorbed normally into the bloodstream from the gastrointestinal tract. Cancer of the pancreas can cause a decrease in the digestive juices that regulate absorption. Abnormal connections between surgically created loops in the intestine may divert food from parts of the intestine where nutrients are usually absorbed. The intestine may become less able to absorb nutrients if your normal food intake is reduced for a lengthy time.

• *Physical Problems* Tumors in the mouth and neck areas, as well as radiation therapy directed to those areas, can make it difficult to swallow or can cause pain in the mouth or throat. Radiation directed to the abdomen or the removal of part of the stomach or intestinal tract can cause diarrhea, cramps, or decreased nutrient absorption. Gastrointestinal or gynecological cancers sometimes lead to intestinal blockages or obstructions.

• *Changes in Smell and Taste* Chemotherapy or radiation to the neck and mouth can distort the perception of smell and taste, and the loss of taste tends to be greater if the tumor is more advanced. Some foods can start to taste bitter or rancid, especially meat, which might taste bitter and metallic. Individuals with a deficiency in zinc also experience a metallic taste. It is common to develop strong aversions to foods such as meat, eggs, fried foods, and tomatoes. These changes lessen your appetite, making it even more difficult for you to avoid weight loss.

• *Early Filling* The feeling of being full after taking only a few bites of food is a common problem and will lead to weight loss if you try to stick to the usual three meals a day.

• *Nausea and Vomiting* Various chemotherapy and radiation therapy regimens cause nausea and/or vomiting. Some patients benefit from meditation, acupuncture, or seasickness wristbands. Be sure to eat and drink slowly and consume smaller, more frequent meals. Nausea can be heightened with an empty stomach. Overly sweet foods and beverages and fatty foods oftentimes lead to or increase feelings of nausea. Ginger may help alleviate nausea. Your doctor can also prescribe certain types of drugs and medications that help with nausea and vomiting. These include ondansetron (Zofran), granisetron (Kytril), palonosetron (Aloxi), aprepitant (Emend), lorazepam (Ativan), and dexamethasone (Decadron).

Because of all these problems, many people with cancer become malnourished almost to the point of starvation. And malnutrition can have very serious effects.

The Dangers of Weight Loss and Malnutrition

Malnutrition affects your whole body, making you steadily weaker. It can also decrease your immunity and make you more susceptible to infections. It can promote tissue breakdown that can lead to "fistulas"—leakage from the natural gastrointestinal tract—and poor healing of any surgical wounds. Malnutrition can also worsen any problem of malabsorption of food you may have as a side effect of treatment, resulting in cramping, bloating, and diarrhea.

Excessive weight loss is a concern so often seen in cancer patients. Losing a great deal of weight unfortunately sets up a vicious cycle. You can reverse that cycle! A decreased appetite and weight loss lead to fatigue and depression. Depression and progressive weakness lead to reduced activity and an even smaller appetite. Further weight loss and weakness lead to a lower resistance to disease and a decrease in immunity. Lower resistance may limit

How Many Calories and How Much Protein Do You Need?

Your normal weight _____ pounds

Your desirable weight _____ pounds

- Your minimum daily protein requirement: desirable weight (pounds) x 0.5. _____ grams

- Your minimum daily calorie requirement: desirable weight (pounds) x 15.5 (men)_____ calories

    (x 18 if you have already lost weight)

    desirable weight (pounds) x 13.5 (women)

    (x 16 if you have already lost weight).

- Keep a daily record of your weight (and your protein and calorie intake).

If you are losing weight, increase your protein and calorie intake to

protein grams: desirable weight x 0.7 _____ grams

calories: desirable weight x 20 (men) = _____ calories

calories: desirable weight x 18 (women) = _____ calories

---

the amount of chemotherapy, radiation therapy, or surgery that can be delivered, leading to a poorer prognosis.

Good nutrition can increase immunity, promote feelings of well-being and a better mood, lessen toxicities of treatment, and increase the quality of your life. Good nutrition enables you to have more energy to do the things you enjoy and love.

Planning for Improved Nutrition

The key to keeping this cycle at bay is to do everything in your power to prevent malnutrition from occurring in the first place. Once weight loss begins, it is hard to reverse. The time to start thinking and planning for proper nutrition is not when you have already lost a lot of weight, but when the diagnosis is made or your treatment gets under way.

If you lose more than 5 percent of your usual weight, you and your doctor should consider the loss significant. Losing 10 percent of your normal weight is a danger signal. A 15 percent weight loss may result in a further decrease in your appetite, depression, fatigue, and progressive weakness that will limit your chance of recovery.

Good nutritional management and careful food selection may also be necessary to avoid gaining a substantial amount of weight. Some patients, especially those receiving chemotherapy, tend to use eating as a way of managing nausea. Some of the hormones used to manage breast cancer can also stimulate the appetite.

Nutritional Components

- If you are losing a lot of weight, you can increase your caloric intake. Choose nutrient-dense foods to provide a significant amount of calories and nutrition yet avoid the need to consume a large volume of food. Nutrient-dense foods include fruit smoothies made with protein powder, dried fruits, unprocessed nuts, nut butters, eggs, avocados, coconut milk, olive and canola oils, and energy bars. You may also consider increasing your fat intake, as fat is the most calorically dense food substance. However, choose healthy fats, such as those foods listed above. Avoid trans-fatty acids, or hydrogenated oils, that are found in certain margarines and processed foods.

• Include a comfort food in your diet to help you accept your need for a certain diet during this time. Ask your dietitian how your favorite comfort food or a food that evokes good feelings can be incorporated into your diet. Also remember that if you are trying new foods, you can learn to enjoy a food once a habit is formed.

• Lower your dietary intake of fat to approximately 20 percent of your diet, unless you are losing weight, are on a treatment that your health care team deems a risk for weight loss, or are awaiting surgery. Choose lean cuts of meat, chicken, and fish, if you eat these, and reduce portion sizes to about three ounces per meal. Consider using meat and poultry raised without hormones or pesticides.

• Eat more plant-based protein and less animal-based protein—choose more beans or legumes if you are able to tolerate these. Products on the market (e.g., Beano) may improve tolerance to gassy foods.

• If you use dairy products, consider using non-BST (growth hormone) treated cows. We don't know the effects that growth hormone from animals has on cancer, as more research is necessary. However, it may be wise to choose dairy products without this hormone. Fortunately, hormone-free dairy is becoming much more readily available.

• Generally have the following:
– Six grain portions daily (one serving, for example, equals one slice whole-grain bread or ½ cup barley, pasta, or cooked cereal). Opt for whole grains!

– Three to five vegetable portions daily (this is standard, but five or more servings are suggested); one serving equals ½ cup cooked or 1 cup raw (if allowed). You can also use vegetable juices such as carrot juice and low-sodium V8 to increase your vegetable intake or if you can't tolerate the vegetables.

– Two to four fruit portions daily (one serving equals one small banana or medium fruit, or ½ cup juice).

• Increase fluid consumption. Aim for eight to ten 8-ounce glasses of water per day. Remember that foods such as low-salt broth, weak teas and herbal teas, juices, soups, and ice pops, are also considered fluids.

Nutritional Support Such support is usually best directed by your physician and dietitian, preferably at the start of therapy. The hospital nutritionist, however, can plan an individualized program for you after two or three days of observation and analysis of any deficits in your intake of calories, protein, or fat. You and your family can be instructed in basic nutritional requirements (the concept of four food groups is outdated).

The nutritionist can also discuss how to handle special dietary problems associated with cancer and cancer therapy, such as anorexia, bloating, heartburn, constipation, diarrhea, nausea, vomiting, sore or dry mouth, indigestion, and loss of taste or taste changes.

Special Diets Your nutritional needs may change during therapy. After surgery, for example, you may need to go on a liquid diet and work your way up through a soft diet before getting back to your regular foods. You may need a lactose-restricted diet, a high-fiber diet, and/or a high-protein diet. You might also need nutritional supplements, either with or between meals, to increase your daily intake of nutrients.

These might include lactose-free, high-calorie, high-protein drinks such as Resurgex, ProSure, Support, Ensure, Resource, Boost, and Nutren. For some patients, the sweetness of these beverages increases nausea or causes diarrhea. Alternatively, you may consider making your own smoothie with fruit, protein powder, tofu, and milk, soy milk, or yogurt.

Some chemotherapy drugs can prevent absorption or cause the depletion of certain vitamins and minerals. Your doctor or dietitian may advise you to take oral supplements to counter the depletion of magnesium caused by cisplatin (Platinol). 5-fluorouracil may cause a loss of potassium, which can be replaced with medication and/or a diet rich in fresh produce, such as apricots, bananas, oranges, and potatoes.

There are diets to prevent kidney stones from forming and diets to prevent diarrhea, constipation, nausea, and vomiting. There are diets to help improve taste and appetite. All of these preventive and palliative techniques, including occupational therapy to improve your ability to swallow, can be used along with other supportive programs to control depression, relieve pain, and promote physical activity.

Fad diets may be very tempting and appear to follow sound medical principles, but oftentimes they can be dangerous. They may not supply the macro- and micronutrients you need during this special time.

A Team Effort With guidance from your doctor, the nutritionist, and a few good pamphlets and brochures, you and your

---

Guidelines for Overcoming Weight Loss

- Help ease the problem of early filling by eating smaller portions of food more frequently throughout the day and by drinking fluids between meals instead of with food.

- Eat by the clock at regularly scheduled times. Your appetite signal may not be reliable at this time.

- Snack between meals with high-protein diet supplements, fruit smoothies, avocados, energy bars, and nuts.

- Add extra calories to your diet by adding coconut milk or olive or canola oil to soups, cooked cereals, and vegetables.

- Add extra protein to your diet by using protein powder in various foods, fortified milk, soy milk, peanut butter, chopped hard-boiled eggs, and tofu.

- Taste blindness makes it important that you do everything you can to enhance the smell, appearance, and texture of food. Cook dishes that appeal to your sense of smell. You may try something very tart, such as a squeeze of lemon, to increase salivary secretion and taste.

- Choose comfort foods that are within the dietary restrictions your doctor or nutritionist provides as guidelines.

- Exercise about half an hour before meals to stimulate your appetite.

- Make mealtimes pleasant by doing relaxation exercises beforehand to reduce stress, by setting an attractive and colorful table, and by eating with family or friends.

- Plan daily menus in advance. If possible, prepare many portions of food and have them frozen and ready to heat and serve.

family should be able to handle most nutritional problems at home.

And remember that good nutrition is a team effort. It requires not only the expertise of nutritionists and the medical team, but the tact and concerned attention of family and friends. Your support team should know that you will be more likely to respond to enjoyable company and gentle encouragement than to harassment and manipulation. The preparation, serving, and sharing of food expresses the concern of caregivers, family, and friends. And that concern can have a direct effect on your sense of well-being.

Also remember that planning for good nutrition early in your disease not only may result in your being able to take more intensive therapy, but can also make the difference between survival and death.

So eat often and well. You will feel better mentally and physically. You will heal faster after surgery and have fewer unpleasant side effects from radiation or chemotherapy. You may be able to tolerate more chemotherapy. Your radiotherapy will not have to be interrupted as often. Your immune system will be better able to resist infection. And, last, but not least, you will be able to lead a more active and enjoyable quality of life.

Tube and Intravenous Feedings—Oral Supplements

The *ideal* way to get enough food is by eating normally—put the food in your mouth, chew it well, and swallow. The food is absorbed naturally, using a functional gastrointestinal tract to meet nutritional needs. This is also the least expensive method of nutritional support.

However, there are times when normal eating just isn't practical. You may experience problems with swallowing, nausea, vomiting, or diarrhea, or you just might not be able to consume enough calories. Your mouth, throat, esopha-

gus, or stomach might be so inflamed that you can neither chew nor swallow. You might also have some obstruction or irritation in the gastrointestinal tract. These kinds of problems are not unusual after certain surgeries, chemotherapy, or radiotherapy. And it is when you have these kinds of problems that the possibility of malnutrition becomes a critical concern.

Enteral Nutrition As long as your stomach and bowel are still working properly, enteral—or tube—feedings can be a practical and low-cost way of providing good nutrition.

Feeding tubes can be placed

- through your mouth (orogastric),
- through your nose (nasogastric), or
- directly into your stomach through the abdominal wall (gastrostomy) or the small bowel (jejunostomy). This can be done during or after surgery, when the need for high-calorie and high-protein nutrition is most critical. There is also a technique called percutaneous endoscopic gastrostomy (PEG) that allows a stomach tube to be placed through the skin into the stomach without the need for major surgery.

Oral and Enteral Formulas Obviously, solid food can't be delivered to your stomach or jejunum (small bowel) through a tube. So you will need enteral feeding of liquid formulas, which can be prepared by pureeing food, or you can buy any of the nutritionally complete formulas your physician or nutritionist might prescribe. The specific formula to use depends on your individual situation. There are special formulas for lactose intolerance (lactose-free) and for high-calorie, high-protein intake. Alternatively, you may need a low-residue and/or chemically defined liquid diet. There are also formulas for diabetics and patients with liver or kidney failure.

- Resurgex, ProSure, Support, Ensure, Resource, Sustacal, and Meritene are soy-based, lactose-free, low-residue, high-calorie, high-protein supplements in beverage form.
- Lactose-free (unflavored) supplements used mainly for tube-feeding diets include Nutren, Isocal, Osmolite, and Jevity. All except Jevity are also low residue.
- Vital HN, Vivonex TEN, and Peptamen are low-residue, lactose-free chemically defined diets with hydrolyzed protein and crystalline amino acids and/or dipeptides. These are useful when you have malabsorption problems or an inflammatory disease like gastroenteritis.
- Glucerna and Vitaneed are special supplements used for tube feedings for diabetics.
- Nepro (high protein) and Suplena (low protein) are specific electrolyte-controlled supplements used in cases of renal deficiency. Glucerna, Nepro, and Suplena can also be taken by mouth.

Possible Side Effects of Enteral Feeding
Though effective in delivering enough nutrition, feedings through nasogastric tubes can produce some side effects:

- You may suffer some throat irritation, nausea, or vomiting.
- Some formulas, including cold or concentrated formulas, may cause diarrhea. The formula may have to be changed to lactose-free isotonic solutions at room temperature.
- Impaction and constipation can occasionally develop, possibly leading to an obstruction in the intestine.

Parenteral Nutrition When neither oral nor enteral nutrition methods are appropriate, you can still get all the nutrients you need through a process called total parenteral nutrition (TPN), formerly called hyperalimentation. What it means is that you get all the proteins, carbohydrates, fats, vitamins, and minerals you need intravenously.

The goal of TPN is to support the patient who is, or will become, nutritionally deficient after surgery or radiotherapy, or secondary to chemotherapy. It has not been shown to improve the quality of life for terminal patients. While you are receiving TPN, if approved by your physician, you may also eat solids and drink fluids. However, TPN sometimes decreases the appetite.

Special Problems of Radiation Patients

Radiation oncologists try to select the most effective dose of radiation to destroy a tumor while still protecting normal tissues. Nonetheless, there are often acute effects during treatment, mainly on rapidly growing tissues that are in the radiation field such as the skin, the mucous membranes (mucosa) in the esophagus, the bladder, the small intestine, and the rectum. These tissues usually heal within a few weeks after radiation. There may also be late chronic effects that can result in the formation of scar tissue, ulcerations, or damage to an organ.

Depending on which part of the body is irradiated, you may develop special problems that will affect your ability to get enough nutrition. But many of these problems can be prevented or eased by careful planning and treatment. Your close cooperation with your radiation oncologist and dietitian will let you complete your treatment with as few side effects as possible.

Mouth Problems Radiation to the mouth and throat may result in painful sores on membranes (mucositis), dry mouth, dental problems, and taste changes or the loss of taste.

Dental Problems If you are getting radiation to the oral cavity or pharynx, a complete dental evaluation is essential before treatment. Your teeth should be X-rayed and any decayed teeth either repaired or removed. If you have to have a tooth extracted, the site must be completely healed before treatment to avoid late and irreversible bone damage. Radiation treatment should generally not start until about fourteen days after any extraction. Your other teeth should be treated daily with a topical fluoride to help prevent cavities.

Mucositis Radiation mucositis frequently occurs with radiation to the head and neck. If the membranes lining your mouth and throat are inflamed, you will need a nourishing soft diet. Sharp-edged or salty foods, such as pretzels and potato chips, should be avoided. Additionally, extremely hot or cold, acidic or spicy, foods may irritate the membranes further. You should also stop drinking alcoholic beverages and smoking or chewing all forms of tobacco immediately, since they can irritate the mouth and throat.

When you have mucositis, good oral hygiene is crucial. Frequent use of a gentle mouthwash can help reduce discomfort or pain, especially if you use a solution of baking soda and salt dissolved in warm water instead of commercial mouthwashes that might irritate the mucosa.

Natural enzymes in papaya or 100 percent papaya juice have been shown to help with mucositis. Pineapple also works well but burns due to the acid. Some patients find relief with mixing about 1 tablespoon (15 ml) honey in a cup of warm water. Research has found that glutamine powder is also helpful in reducing mouth sores. Patients can swish and swallow 5 to 10 gm glutamine powder mixed with water three times daily.

If the mucositis is severe and interferes with eating or drinking, you can use a topical anesthetic such as viscous lidocaine (Xylocaine) solution, gargling 1 teaspoon (5 ml) before meals. A slurry of sucralfate (Carafate)—prepared by dissolving sucralfate in water and sorbitol, which is available at most drugstores—can also coat the oral membranes and soothe any discomfort.

Your radiation oncologist will have to check your mucositis carefully and often to rule out monilia (fungus) infection. These infections can be treated locally or systemically with nystatin (Mycostatin) oral suspension or tablets, ketoconazole (Nizoral), or fluconazol (Diflucan).

Dry Mouth Xerostomia, or dry mouth, isn't unusual after radiation to the mouth or pharynx, since you can't produce as much saliva after irradiation of the salivary glands. This may be a temporary condition, though if the total dose exceeds 4,000 cGy, you may have some degree of permanent mouth dryness. You can minimize symptoms by using an artificial saliva such as Salivart, moisturizing gels such as Oral Balance, and a special dry-mouth toothpaste such as Biotene. It will also help if you increase your intake of fluids, particularly with meals, and if you use creams, gravies, and sauces to moisten dry, hard food.

Loss of Taste Irradiation of the taste buds can make you lose your sense of taste. The decrease in, or the thickening of, saliva from irradiation of the salivary glands can contribute to the problem, too. Taste will usually come back within two months after radiation treatment is completed.

Problems in the Esophagus Radiation is frequently delivered to the upper chest (thorax) to treat lung cancer, esophageal cancer, and lymphoma. And the esophagus usually has to be within the radiation port. If you get doses over 3,000 cGy in three weeks, the lining of your esophagus may react, causing some pain when you swallow. The reaction will go away gradually, but it is possible that the daily

Enteritis: Hints on Food Tolerance

Foods to Avoid

- Whole-grain or high-bran breads and cereals.
- Nuts, seeds, coconut, beans, and legumes.
- Fried, greasy, or fatty foods, which may be hard to digest.
- Fresh and dried fruit and some fruit juices (such as prune juice).
- Raw vegetables.
- Rich pastries.
- Popcorn, potato chips, and pretzels.
- Strong spices and herbs.
- Chocolate, coffee, tea, and soft drinks containing caffeine.
- Alcohol and tobacco.
- Milk and milk products. Exceptions are buttermilk and yogurt, which are often tolerated because lactose is altered in the presence of lactobacillus. You may use milkshake supplements such as Resurgex, ProSure, and Ensure, which are lactose-free.
- Sugar-free foods that contain "sugar alcohols," such as maltitol and sorbitol.

Foods to Enjoy

- Fish, poultry, and meat (preferably broiled or roasted).
- Bananas, peeled apples, and apple and grape juices.
- White bread and toast.
- Macaroni and noodles.
- Baked, boiled, or mashed potatoes.
- Foods high in soluble fiber—including bananas, white rice, oatmeal, and barley—which act as binding agents and should help to produce a more solid bowel movement.
- Cooked vegetables that are mild, such as asparagus tips, green and wax beans, carrots, spinach, and squash.
- Mild processed cheese, eggs, smooth peanut butter, buttermilk, and yogurt.

Helpful Hints

- Eat foods at room temperature.
- Drink twelve glasses of fluids per day. Allow carbonated beverages to go flat before you drink them. You can help the process along by stirring the drink until the bubbles disappear.
- Add nutmeg to food. This will help to increase motility of the gastrointestinal tract.
- Start a low-residue diet on day 1 of radiation therapy.

---

dose can be reduced or your treatment interrupted for a short period to allow rapid healing.

In the meantime, a soft, bland diet, antacids, and a topical anesthetic such as a viscous lidocaine (Xylocaine) solution will often minimize the symptoms. A slurry of sucralfate (Carafate) will coat the esophagus and soothe the discomfort, as it does in the mouth. Probiotic supplement powders may also help to heal the esophagus, hence reducing the discomfort. If symptoms persist, you may have a candida infection, which can be effectively treated with ketoconazole (Nizoral) or nystatin (Mycostatin).

Problems in the Bowel (Radiation Enteritis) With their rapidly dividing cells, the membranes lining the large and small bowel and the rectum are quite sensitive to even low doses of radiation. Thus, any radiation delivered to the upper abdomen or pelvis can cause an irritation of the bowel known as radiation enteritis.

Only 5 to 15 percent of people treated with radiation to the abdomen will develop chronic problems, and the severity of the symptoms will depend on several factors—how much of the abdomen or pelvis is irradiated, the daily dose, the total dosage required, and the possible use of chemotherapy at the same time. People with a history of abdominal surgery, pelvic inflammatory disease, atherosclerosis, diabetes, or hypertension are also more likely to suffer radiation injury.

Symptoms If you are getting radiation to the upper abdomen, you may experience bouts of nausea and vomiting. Pelvic irradiation is more likely to cause irritation in the rectum, frequent bowel movements, or watery diarrhea. These disturbances to the intestinal mucosa may change the way your gastrointestinal tract absorbs nutrients from the food you eat. It may become much more difficult to absorb fat, bile salts, and vitamin B_{12}, for example.

Your doctor will evaluate the extent of the enteritis by assessing how often you have diarrhea, the character of the stools, whether you have any rectal bleeding, and whether your abdomen is enlarged (distended). He or she will also watch for possible dehydration or an electrolyte mineral imbalance in your blood resulting from diarrhea and/or malabsorption.

Managing Enteritis The medical management of radiation enteritis includes dietary changes, medication, and, in severe cases, an interruption of radiation treatment. If you are getting abdominal or pelvic radiation, you may need to start on a low-fat, low-fiber, low-residue diet right from the beginning of treatment.

Some patients, however, do not experience significant gastrointestinal distress. Be sure to make dietary changes gradually to avoid gastrointestinal distress. For example, if you currently consume a high-fiber diet, decrease the fiber content a few grams daily.

Medications If radiation enteritis persists despite changes in your diet, it may be necessary to reduce the daily dose of radiation to the abdomen and pelvis. You may also have to use medications such as the following:

• Kaolin-pectin emulsion (Kaopectate; 2 to 4 tablespoons [25 to 50 ml] after each loose bowel movement).
• Diphenoxylate (Lomotil; one to two tablets every four to six hours as needed, to a maximum of eight tablets a day). Most patients find they need only two or three tablets per day after the diarrhea has been controlled.
• Loperamide (Imodium; two capsules initially, followed by one capsule after each loose stool, the total dosage not to exceed sixteen capsules per day). Loperamide is also available in a liquid form (half-dose strength) that does not require a prescription.
• Belladonna alkaloid or glycopyrrolate (Donnatal or Robinul; one or two tablets every four hours for abdominal cramping).
• Paregoric (1 teaspoon [5 ml] orally every four hours for diarrhea).
• Prochlorperazine (Compazine; 10 mg every four hours), lorazepam (Ativan; 1 mg every two to four hours), or metoelopramide (Reglan) tablets or liquid (10 mg four times daily, thirty minutes before each meal and at bedtime) can usually control nausea.

Things to Remember

The times when you are weak and feel bad, and do not feel like eating, are the times when you most need the energy, protein, and protective factors from foods.

Do

- plan your meals,

- have a positive attitude,

- prepare a shopping list, and

- prepare foods and meals when you are feeling better.

Remember that during this time, you may be eating differently. It is okay that while being treated, your energy needs temporarily override other needs. After treatment, you will have time to adjust your diet.

Realize that the food problem will most likely be temporary and a few weeks or months from now, you will be focusing on the joy you are receiving from feeling better and from being able to advance your diet.

— 24 —

Controlling Pain

Wendye R. Robbins, M.D., and Ernest H. Rosenbaum, M.D.

■ ■ ■ ■

Pain remains a major problem where 30 to 50 percent of cancer patients undergoing active cancer treatment suffer with pain and 70 to 90 percent of patients with advanced cancer suffer with moderate to severe pain.

Pain intensity is generally correlated to the site and size of the tumor mass. Typically, tumors that compromise bone or neural structures are the most painful. Particularly in cases of bony metastases, pain and functional loss are frequent complaints. While the incidence of primary bony tumors is relatively low, the rate of metastasis to bony structures is high (especially in primary tumors of the breast, lung, prostate, and kidney). Pain may be caused by direct bony destruction or deformation. Furthermore, irritation or entrapment of sensory nerves or networks of nerves (plexuses) may cause unpleasant electrical or shooting sensations.

Pain can have a terrible effect on a cancer patient's life. It can lead to depression, loss of appetite, irritability, withdrawal from social interaction, anger, loss of sleep, and an inability to cope. In addition to producing painful sensations and feelings, pain can also cause limited mobility, decreased appetite and energy, and generalized deconditioning. Patients with pain are also at risk for other morbidity, including pneumonias, hypoventilation, hypercalcemia, and disorders of blood clotting. If uncontrolled, pain can strain relationships with loved ones and erode the will to live.

Ask any group of cancer patients to describe their greatest fear. Chances are that they will say, "Pain and suffering—not death." This is not an unreasonable response. Pain can be terrifying and debilitating.

Pain can occur at any time in the course of dealing with some forms of cancer—during treatment that leads to remission or cure, as well as in the terminal phase. However, 90 to 95 percent of most pain problems can be controlled, according to the Committee on Pain of the World Health Organization (WHO), with existing medicines. Yet many cancer patients are still not receiving adequate pain relief. Why?

Among the obstacles to giving and receiving appropriate pain medication is widespread misunderstanding about the effects of medications, including opioids; poor communication between patients and caregivers; and a need for increased awareness, among patients and caregivers alike, of the causes and ramifications of different types of pain. In developing individually tailored pain-relief programs, patients and caregivers also need to ensure that they are well informed about the various pain-relief options through frequent consultation with pain specialists.

Barriers to Effective Pain Control

Patients, families, and friends are often terrified of what will happen in the future if pain becomes worse, yet there are several barriers to pain control:

1. Patients may be reluctant to report their pain. They often underreport the level of pain so as not to appear weak, vulnerable, or out of control.

2. They may wish to give the impression of beating their disease—the wish to be "a good patient."

3. Fear that increased pain may reflect disease progression induces some patients to take smaller amounts of pain medications.

4. There may be a fear of side effects and of being called an addict.

5. Pain control sometimes has a lower priority, or care providers may not ask the right questions.

6. Pharmacies often do not stock potent opioids for fear of being burglarized.

7. Cost of pain medications could be prohibitive for many patients.

Common Misunderstandings About the Use of Opioids for Pain Control Opioids are drugs originally derived from the poppy plant. Although morphine (MS-Contin, Kadian) is the best-known member of this class, many similar molecules (including oxycodone [Percocet, Percodan, Oxycontin], hydromorphone [Dilaudid], fentanyl [Duragesic], hydrocodone [Vicodin, Lortab], and methadone) have been synthesized to produce effects similar to those of morphine. Unfortunately, many people adhere to certain myths about the use of opioids for pain control, with the result that they take insufficient doses or refuse to take them at all. Following are five of the most prevalent myths:

• *Myth 1: Opioids should be administered only as a last resort to the gravely ill or those near death.* Not true! Opioids are often highly effective in the disease process when severe pain calls for strong medication. They may be used as single agents or as part of a drug "cocktail" to relieve suffering. Many patients will use opioids successfully for months or years without ill effects. Some patients are able to return to work while on opioids.

• *Myth 2: The use of opioids for pain leads to addiction.* Definitely not! Addiction is a compulsive need to take a substance despite a known risk of harm. Opioids used for pain control do not cause self-destructive behavior. Patients do not become drug-crazed or switch to street-drug abuse, and they do not misuse them. However, they can become *physically* dependent on opioids if they take them over a long period of time. When such people achieve a cure through therapy, they can reduce their opioid intake slowly to avoid withdrawal symptoms.

• *Myth 3: People who take opioid medications develop a tolerance for them, leading to a need for increasingly larger doses.* This is sometimes true. Tolerance, if it occurs at all, does not develop suddenly. If it does occur, it is true that physicians will respond by increasing the dose; however, when administered correctly, opioid medications are safe even at very high doses.

• *Myth 4: Opioids are dangerous because they make it harder for terminally ill patients to breathe.* Morphine and other opioid drugs are *not* dangerous respiratory depressants in patients with advanced cancer and pain. In fact, because of tolerance, depression of respiration almost never occurs. Instead, patients will relax and often sleep because they are finally comfortable. Opioids can be more dangerous if coadministered with other drugs (sleep medications or antianxiety medications) that depress the central nervous system.

• *Myth 5: Patients should take opioids by injection because they are poorly absorbed when taken orally.* Most opioids are absorbed very well when taken orally. However, since a fair amount of an oral dose is lost to nontarget body tissues, oral doses are usually larger than those given intravenously or intramuscularly. Newer formulations of oral opioids allow for continuous release from the gastro-intestinal tract, release across the skin, release under the tongue, or release after inhalation. These drugs may be taken on a less frequent basis.

Poor Communication Between Patients and Caregivers Good communication between patients and caregivers is essential to achieving optimal pain relief, and the failure to achieve it can lie with either or both parties. Patients' attitudes are a mélange of their past and current experiences with pain, cultural and religious teachings, the attitudes of family and friends, and their own personal values and coping mechanisms. As a result of one or more of these influences, many people feel they should be able to tolerate pain and are therefore ashamed to discuss the extent of suffering or discomfort with their physicians.

Another reason for poor communication is that pain has its own vocabulary, making it difficult for many people to accurately articulate the quality, texture, and intensity of their pain. Is it sharp? Dull? Electric? Sporadic? Insistent? Moreover, the memory of pain is inexact. Between attacks of pain, people tend to forget about the level of intensity and other specifics. To compound the problem, some caregivers may not be sufficiently experienced at eliciting this crucial information from their patients.

For example, pain can be either somatic (originating in the tissue, bones, or organs) or neuropathic (resulting from damage to, or pressure on, nerves)—or a combination of the two. Somatic pain is often described as "achy, dull, and localized" when it results from a broken bone associated with tumor involvement, or as "crampy and diffuse" when it results from an obstruction in the intestine or urinary tract.

Neuropathic pain, on the other hand, is usually described as "sharp, burning, electrical, shooting, or buzzing." These sensations typically occur in areas served by the injured nerves, which can be either in the peripheral nerves or in the central nervous system. Such an injury can be caused by the direct spread of a tumor, such as that of colon cancer in the pelvis where the nerves to the legs or pelvic structures reside. It can also be caused by pressure on nerves, as when spinal tumors pinch or press on nerves to the arms or legs. Other types of neuropathic dysfunction include hypersensitivity of the skin or an exaggerated, painful response to nerve stimuli (even a simple touch) and an occasional motor change such as weakness or atrophy of an affected muscle group. Surgery, various chemotherapeutic drugs, and radiation treatment can also produce temporary side effects of somatic and/or neuropathic pain or discomfort.

Progressive Pain-Relief Measures

In recommending palliative measures for pain, physicians use guidelines set forth by the World Health Organization (WHO), which include standard treatments for mild, moderate, and severe pain—sometimes given with adjuvant medications. For those who fail to benefit from these standard procedures, physicians can try one of several means of direct intervention. And, to augment all of these options, patients can also experiment with any of several methodologies that enlist the mind and emotions in reducing the stress that exacerbates pain.

World Health Organization Guidelines An expert committee convened by WHO's

Progressive Pain-Relief Measures

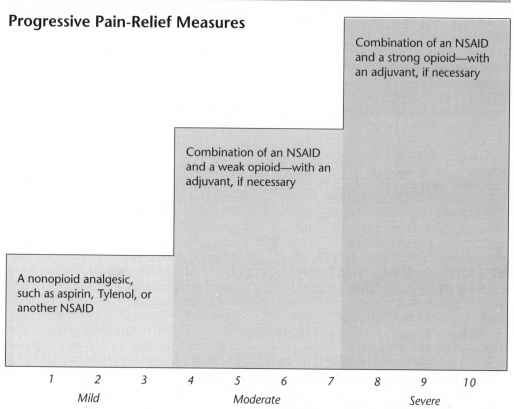

Combination of an NSAID and a strong opioid—with an adjuvant, if necessary

Combination of an NSAID and a weak opioid—with an adjuvant, if necessary

A nonopioid analgesic, such as aspirin, Tylenol, or another NSAID

| 1 | 2 | 3 | 4 | 5 | 6 | 7 | 8 | 9 | 10 |
| Mild | | | | Moderate | | | | Severe | |

Adapted from the World Health Organization's analgesic ladder for the management of cancer pain.

Cancer Unit developed a "pain ladder" on a scale of 1 to 10 to aid physicians in assessing the source, quality, and intensity of pain and in determining the most appropriate relief measures. The goal is to keep pain down to a level of less than 4 through continual reassessment of the cause of the problem and the effectiveness of the means of control. "Effectiveness" requires that a balance be maintained between the administration of any necessary increases in the strength of a medication and the production of toxic side effects, such as delirium, confusion, constipation, nausea or vomiting, allergies, and skin rashes.

Primary Pain-Relief Measures The following medications are recommended for different levels of pain, as determined by the pain ladder scale:

• *Mild Pain* Nonnarcotic medications such as aspirin, acetaminophen (Tylenol), and other aspirin-like drugs—known as nonsteroidal anti-inflammatory drugs (NSAIDs)—rofecoxib (Viox) and celecoxib (Celebrex).

• *Moderate Pain* A combination of NSAIDs and weak narcotics, such as codeine, hydrocodone (Vicodin, Lortab), oxycodone (Percocet, Percodan, Oxy-Contin), and propoxyphene (Darvon).

• *Severe Pain* Strong opioids such as morphine (MS-Contin, Kadian), meperidine (Demerol), hydromorphone (Dilaudid), fentanyl (Duragesic patches), and methadone in combination with an NSAID. When administered correctly, increasing opioid medications is safe even at very high doses.

The guidelines also suggest adding an adjuvant medication to these narcotic and nonnarcotic medications when appropriate. These medications—which include steroids; bone-forming, antidepressant, and anticonvulsant medications; antihistamines; and sedatives—are often useful in treating opioid-resistant pain. For whatever reason, they do relieve pain, although they are not usually labeled as pain relievers.

A simple measure such as aspirin or acetaminophen, with or without codeine, or ibuprofen (Motrin, Advil) may do the job well enough. But when pain is severe, the dosage has to be increased or the drug has to be taken more frequently. If these simple measures don't help, then it is important to increase the strength or potency of the medication. Sometimes, just the addition of an adjuvant medication is all that is needed.

Other Pain-Relief Options For the 5 to 10 percent of people who do not receive adequate pain control under WHO's guidelines, there are other options. Pain specialists can prevent pain stimuli from reaching the central nervous system by the delivery of local anesthetic procaine (Novocain) or lidocaine (Xylocaine), steroids, toxins, or nerve-destroying agents. They can also use an alternative delivery system, such as the administration of opioids and other drugs subcutaneously or into the spine, or use a local spinal anesthetic. Transcutaneous electrical nerve stimulation (TENS) and ultrasonic stimulation may also be viable options.

Many people find that the ancient arts of acupuncture and acupressure or the application of hot and cold compresses can relieve pain, as does exercise—which not only helps maintain strength and flexibility, but actually changes muscle cells, making them less sensitive to pain. Finally, to decrease the loneliness and stress that exacerbate the experience of pain, others harness the power of their minds and emotions with biofeedback, psychotherapy, family counseling, and listening to music—a proven, highly effective therapy.

Anticonvulsants such as carbamazepine (Tegretol), phenytoin (Dilantin), and gabapentin (Neurontin) may help in pain relief, especially neuropathic pain. Other techniques include epidural spinal injections, peripheral nerve blocks, radiofrequency neurolysis to destroy nerves with radio waves, or alcohol nerve injections. Control of anxiety with lorazepam (Ativan) or alprazolam (Xanax) may assist in pain control. Radiation treatments to bone or soft-tissue cancer areas can offer palliative pain relief.

Supportive Techniques for Pain Control Emotions and psychological issues are also components of pain. Psychological support through counseling can help reduce a sense of loneliness and isolation. Counseling can help you come to terms with your situation and help in planning for the future. Talking with clergy or other trusted spiritual advisers may also reduce anxieties and fears that can be factors that contribute to pain.

Exercise, massage, transcutaneous nerve stimulation, biofeedback, acupuncture, and acupressure may all be of help in controlling pain. When you are relaxed and less tense, you may find that the pain is more easily controlled.

One very effective pain control device may be as close as your stereo. Music has been rated to have an analgesic effect twice that of a plain background sound.

So listen to your favorite musical works and artists. Music can help you relax, raise your spirits, give you great joy, and help you control your pain.

Good Pain Control and Pain Palliation A 90 to 95 percent success rate in pain control can be achieved when people learn to articulate the quality and intensity of their pain (physicians are not mind readers). Likewise, caregivers must sharpen their assessment skills. And, both cancer survivors and caregivers must continually reevaluate the effectiveness of their chosen pain-relief program, creatively incorporating adjuvant and other therapies as well as stress-reduction techniques.

— 25 —

Guarding Against Infections

Lawrence Mintz, M.D., and W. Lawrence Drew, M.D., Ph.D.

Everyone with cancer runs a risk of developing some sort of infection. This is because many cancers, and the methods used to treat them, affect the immune system defenses that normally keep infections at bay.

Our first line of defense against infection is the outer and inner linings of the body—the skin and the mucous membranes. Both these barriers are punctured by the invasive procedures necessary to diagnose or treat cancer problems. Chemotherapy and radiation are particularly damaging to mucous membranes. Needles used to draw blood for testing, urinary catheters, intravenous (IV) lines, and infusion pumps used for delivering IV medications all create potential ports of entry for infectious organisms.

Once infecting organisms enter our bodies, one of the most important defenses—white blood cells (WBCs) called neutrophils—usually goes into action. Neutrophils can attack, ingest, and destroy organisms, usually bacteria and some yeasts, that live extracellularly—that is, outside of the cells of our body tissues. They can recognize organisms as "foreign" on their first encounter with them, and they thus serve as the first line of defense against invading microorganisms. However, the number of neutrophils is dramatically reduced by chemotherapy, radiation therapy, leukemia, and bone marrow transplants. As the WBC count decreases, the risk of infection increases.

Another defense mechanism is known as cell-mediated immunity, in which specialized WBCs called T lymphocytes attack invading organisms. These cells require a certain amount of time (usually a few days to a week or so) to recognize organisms as foreign and to begin attacking them. Once sensitized to an invading organism, however, the T lymphocytes retain "immunologic memory," so the next time they encounter the same type of organism, they mobilize and begin their attack much more quickly. Although T lymphocytes do not initially react as quickly as do neutrophils, they do have the ability to recognize and destroy organisms such as viruses and some bacteria and fungi that live intracellularly—that is, inside the cells of our body tissues. Some cancers, such as Hodgkin's disease and other types of lymphoma, can cause defects in cellular immunity, as can chemotherapy, radiation, and drugs that suppress the immune system.

Another part of the immune defense system is known as humoral immunity. Here other specialized WBCs called B lymphocytes produce and secrete proteins called antibodies to fight organisms they have previously encountered. When these specific organisms enter the body again, the antibodies circulating in the bloodstream recognize and attach to them, helping to destroy them. This part of the immune system can be damaged in cases of multiple myeloma and chronic lymphocytic leukemia, or when the spleen is damaged by disease or surgically removed.

We all carry (are colonized by) "resident" bacteria, called normal flora, that live on our skin and mucous membranes and in our intestines. These organisms are usually harmless, but they can cause serious infection when our defenses are down. We can try to prevent infections, but nevertheless they do occur.

The Different Types of Infections

Infections are defined by the location in the body where they occur and by the type of organism involved. For example, many different types of organisms can infect the lungs, but the disease they all produce is called pneumonia.

The clinical course of an infection, the treatment regimen needed to cure it, and the ultimate outcome all depend not only on the location of the infection in the body, but also on the specific type of organism causing the infection. Most common organisms fall into three broad categories:

Bacterial Infections The major sources of these infections are bacteria normally found on our skin and mucous membrane surfaces and in our gastrointestinal tract. Bacteria on the skin can gain access to the body if, for example, an IV line is in place, resulting in a local soft-tissue infection called cellulitis or, if the bacteria enter the bloodstream, in a serious system-wide infection called sepsis. Similarly, normal oral or intestinal bacteria can reach the bloodstream if the mucous membranes or lining of the gut are damaged by radiation or by certain types of chemotherapy. This therapy-induced tissue injury is called mucositis (inflammation of the mucous membranes).

Other types of bacteria do not generally colonize the body, and many of these are inherently "pathogenic." That is, they will cause infections when encountered, even in otherwise healthy individuals. One example of a pathogenic organism is the bacterium that causes tuberculosis.

We usually acquire these organisms by direct face-to-face contact with people who are already infected with them, and the illnesses they cause are thus considered contagious. Patients with depressed immune systems are generally more susceptible to and suffer more serious infections from these pathogenic organisms than do exposed but otherwise healthy people.

Fungal Infections Yeasts and fungi do not, in general, normally invade the body when host defenses are normal. In fact, most fungal infections develop only after *several* abnormal circumstances exist. For example, the use of broad-spectrum antibiotics may kill off much of the normal intestinal flora, creating an ecological "vacuum" that is filled when the gut becomes heavily overgrown by antibiotic-resistant yeast. This alone does not generally cause invasive yeast infection. However, the added "insults" to the body caused by chemotherapy-induced mucositis; by the use of steroids and other immunosuppressive drugs; and by the presence of invasive devices such as urinary catheters, intravenous lines, and nasogastric "stomach" tubes may then allow the yeast colonization to progress to localized and then disseminated yeast infection. Because infections like this only occur if they are given the opportunity to do so by multiple bodily "insults," they are collectively referred to as *opportunistic infections*.

Viral Infections Unlike bacteria and fungi, viruses are not technically "living" organisms. They consist of small packets of genetic material (DNA or RNA) surrounded by a protein coat or shell. In order to multiply, they *must* enter and reside within living host cells. There, the protein coat is stripped away, and the "naked" DNA or RNA takes over control of the cell, giving it genetic instructions to manufacture and assemble more viral particles. A cell whose functions have been taken over by a virus no longer performs its normal activities. Furthermore, after the cell has produced hundreds or thousands of new virus particles, it ruptures and dies, releasing the new viruses to infect still other cells.

As previously noted, T lymphocytes and related cells of the cell-mediated immune system are able to detect the presence of viral infection within host cells. The lymphocytes then attack and destroy the infected host cells before they can produce more viruses and spread the infection.

When immunity is depressed by either cancer or chemotherapy, new viruses can readily establish infections in your body, and old, dormant viral infections can be reactivated. Cold sores, for example, are caused by the herpes simplex virus. This virus can persist within your body indefinitely, although it can have long quiescent periods. When cellular immunity is depressed, the virus can flare up and produce a severe bout of cold sores. Another type of persistent herpes virus—called varicella-zoster virus (the same one that causes chicken pox)—can reactivate and cause shingles, or herpes zoster, which can become widespread and even life-threatening.

Signs and Symptoms

There are several common signs and symptoms of infection. Some might be caused by something other than an infection, but you should consult your doctor as soon as any of them appear.

• Fever (greater than 101.3°F [38.5°C]). This is a very reliable sign of infection and has to be attended to immediately, especially if your neutrophil count is low.
• Shaking chills.
• Severe night sweats.
• Nausea and vomiting, especially if accompanied by fever.
• Diarrhea, especially with a fever or with blood in the stool.

• Burning or pain when urinating, which could indicate a bladder infection.
• Shortness of breath, chest pain on breathing, or persistent coughing (with or without sputum production), either of which may be the first sign of pneumonia or bronchitis.
• Sore throat.
• Tenderness, redness, swelling, pain, or discharge at the site of a temporary or permanent intravenous catheter used for chemotherapy (such as a Port-a-Cath or Hickman catheter).
• Headache or neck stiffness with fever. This could indicate meningitis, a very serious infection of the nervous system that should be treated immediately.

Diagnosis

Once you notice any of these signs and symptoms, your doctor will start searching for the origin of the infection. He or she will take a medical history, including detailed questions about your symptoms, which helps point the way toward determining where the infection may reside. A physical examination can confirm the clues provided by your symptoms and may lead to the discovery of abnormalities you may not be aware of.

Once the history and physical examination are completed, your blood, sputum, and urine will be analyzed. Stools, spinal fluid, and skin lesions might be tested, too, depending on your history and physical-examination findings. Depending on the results of the laboratory tests, you may undergo other diagnostic studies such as chest X-rays, CT, MRI, or PET scans, or nuclear medicine studies such as gallium or indium scans.

Treatment

There is a huge array of antibiotic, antifungal, antiviral, and immune-modulating therapies available to fight infections.

Which to use depends on the organism involved and the site of infection.

In an ideal world, the infecting organism would be identified quickly and the most effective drug against it would immediately be given. But cultures and laboratory test results may take twenty-four to forty-eight hours or longer. While the offending organism still isn't known, what is called empirical therapy will begin, meaning that broad spectrum drugs will be directed against the most likely culprits. The choice of drugs will be guided by the specific symptoms and physical findings, the underlying cancer or immunosuppressive condition present, and the type of anticancer therapy being used.

Once the organism is identified, treatment can be modified, if necessary. The broad spectrum drugs may be replaced by a specific antibiotic most effective against the causative organism. A combination of antimicrobial agents may be used if they are likely to be most effective.

Length of Treatment When to stop antibiotic treatment depends on the situation. If you've had fever and a low white blood cell count, but neither the organism nor the site of infection can be identified, then antibiotics will usually be continued until the fever is gone and your WBC count is returning to normal.

If the site of infection is known—as in pneumonia, for example—and your temperature and WBC count is normal, antibiotics will be continued for one to two weeks.

If cultures have isolated the organism, your fever is gone, and your white count is back to normal, antibiotics will usually be stopped five to seven days after the fever disappears.

The Issue of Antibiotic Resistance

The development of new and improved antibiotics during the 1970s led some to speculate that all infectious diseases would soon be eradicated. However, microorganisms were not about to give up that easily. The lessons learned from Darwin about "survival of the fittest" apply not just to plants, animals, and man, but to microbes as well.

When exposed to an antibiotic, vast numbers of microorganisms die, but a few may develop a random genetic mutation that confers resistance to the antibiotic. This genetic trait will be passed on to subsequent generations. Since bacteria can reproduce as quickly as every fifteen minutes, or approximately 75 to 100 generations a day, it is not difficult to appreciate how quickly resistance to antibiotics can spread within the population of microorganisms. The more heavily antibiotics are used, the greater the likelihood that antibiotic resistance will emerge and spread throughout the bacterial world.

In recent years, we have witnessed the rise of many new mutations and combinations of mutations that allow certain bacteria to resist the effects of nearly all available antibiotics. Infections with these multiply-resistant organisms pose a huge challenge to treatment, especially for immune-suppressed individuals in whom infections may progress with alarming speed.

What You and Your Doctor Can Do to Avoid Infections

There will be certain times during the course of your illness when you will be more susceptible to infections, particularly when your WBC count is at its lowest. This point is called the nadir. Infections are most likely to develop when the nadir falls below 1,000 cells per cubic millimeter. When the nadir falls below 500, infections can progress much more rapidly, and when it is below 200, they can reach critical stages in just a few hours. You should do everything you can to avoid possible sources of infection at all times, but especially when your susceptibility is greatest.

To help prevent the development and spread of antibiotic resistance, it is vital that antibiotics be used sparingly and with great care. Antibiotics should be used only when necessary. The use of antibiotics to treat common colds is an example of the misuse of antibiotics, since colds are caused by viruses that are not susceptible to antibiotics.

To keep their normal flora as antibiotic-sensitive as possible, it is particularly important that immune-suppressed individuals avoid any unnecessary exposure to antibiotics. This applies not only to the patient him- or herself, but also to household contacts of the patient. If a patient's child or spouse is receiving antibiotics, he or she might develop resistant intestinal bacteria that can contaminate the home environment and spread to the immune-suppressed patient. If the patient later develops an infection with one of these resistant bacteria, the choices of antibiotics available to treat the infection become much more limited.

It has become standard practice in many chemotherapy programs to raise WBC counts by giving a colony-stimulating factor (CSF) such as G[granulocyte]–CSF filgrastim (Neupogen) or GM [granulocyte macrophage]–CSF sargramostim (Leukine). These are synthetic forms of substances the body naturally secretes to stimulate bone marrow to produce WBCs. CSFs are very effective and are used with chemotherapy to shorten the length of time that the WBC count remains extremely low. Raising the count decreases significantly the risk of serious infections.

Much has been learned from the AIDS epidemic about giving antibiotics to people at risk before any infection has developed. Prophylactic antibiotics have many benefits. Ciprofloxacin (Cipro), for example, can decrease bacterial infections when the WBC count is low. During periods of profound immune suppression in bone marrow transplant recipients, the prophylactic use of the antiviral drug ganciclovir (Cytovene) can prevent cytomegalovirus infections, and the oral antifungal drug fluconazole (Diflucan) can prevent fungal infections. However, as noted above in the section on antibiotic resistance, prophylactic antibiotics have many drawbacks as well. They should be used only if specifically ordered by your physician, and even then it is reasonable to ask your physician if he or she believes the benefits of their use outweigh the risk of emerging resistance.

The external environment contains innumerable bacteria that can cause infectious problems in people whose immune systems are suppressed or whose WBC counts are low due to cancer or chemotherapy. Plants and soil contain many bacteria, fungi, and spores. Gardening or otherwise working in soil can expose individuals to skin nicks, cuts, and thorn pricks that can introduce dangerous organisms into their systems. For this reason, during periods of immune suppression, it is best to avoid all gardening activities. Simply put, don't play in the dirt.

Cut flowers in vases are colonized with many potentially dangerous organisms, particularly a bacterium called pseudomonas. The growth of this organism in vase water is the principal reason the water becomes turbid, and its presence is the reason that hospitals discourage or prohibit flowers and plants in immune-suppressed patients' rooms.

Hand Washing

The single best preventive measure you can take against infection is to wash your hands often and thoroughly. Hand washing should be performed after using the toilet, before preparing food, after handling raw meat or poultry, and at any other time when the hands might be contaminated or are visibly soiled. It must be practiced by those caring for patients (medical staff, other caregivers, household members, and visiting friends), as well as by patients themselves. Although hand washing was proved effective 160 years ago, it is grossly under-utilized. Even today, numerous hospital studies have confirmed that only a quarter to a half of all caregivers regularly and appropriately wash their hands. Hand washing is such a critical issue in preventing infection that it will be discussed here in considerable detail.

History In 1846, Ignaz Semmelweis, a twenty-eight-year-old Viennese-trained Hungarian physician, was serving as the senior house officer at the obstetrical clinic in Vienna. At that time, a disease called puerperal fever, or childbed fever, was rampant among women giving birth in hospitals. Semmelweis observed that nearly 20 percent of the women on his ward, in the first division of the clinic, died of childbed fever. On the other hand, the maternal death rate in the second division of the clinic was only 2 percent. Both divisions had the same equipment and used the same delivery techniques, but, Semmelweis noted, the first division was used to train medical students, while the second division was used to train midwives.

In 1847, a friend and colleague of Semmelweis's died from an infection after cutting his finger with a knife while performing an autopsy on a childbed fever victim. His colleague's autopsy revealed features similar to those of women dying from puerperal fever. Semmelweis put these observations together and realized that the medical students performed autopsies on their expired patients while the student midwives did not. He further noted that following autopsies, medical students often went directly from the dissecting room to the maternity ward without washing their bloody, contaminated hands.

Although the germ theory of infection would not be developed for several more decades, Semmelweis concluded that the physicians and medical students must be carrying some unknown infecting particles on their hands from the cadavers to the patients they examined during labor, thereby causing childbed fever.

To test his hypothesis, Semmelweis mandated that on his ward, hands must be scrubbed with a brush in a solution of chlorinated lime between autopsy work and the examination of patients. Maintaining meticulous records, he showed that the death rate from puerperal fever dropped precipitously from nearly 20 percent to under 2 percent. The following year, he extended his washing protocol to include all instruments used on patients in labor, and childbed fever was virtually eliminated from his hospital ward.

Despite the seemingly "incontrovertible proof" that his theory was correct, doctors rejected Semmelweis's findings and did not adopt his practices. Many were offended by the implication that doctors were killing their patients. Semmelweis was ridiculed and fired from his job.

In the 1870s and 1880s, the germ theory of infection was conclusively proven by Louis Pasteur in France, Joseph Lister in England, and Robert Koch in Germany. Even so, their findings were only slowly accepted by the general medical community. The pioneering theories of Ignaz Semmelweis were ultimately vindicated several decades after his death. Today, hand washing is considered the cornerstone of infection prevention, yet, as noted above, it is grossly underutilized by many health care professionals in both inpatient and outpatient settings.

The Mechanism of Skin Contamination
Human skin is not sterile. A number of relatively benign, or nonpathogenic, bacteria normally colonize the skin surface, where they reside in minute skin creases

and crevices. The hands, as well as the armpits and groin areas, generally harbor 10 to 20 percent more bacteria than other skin areas. The highest accumulation is typically under the fingernails. These "normal" skin bacteria adhere quite tightly to the surface of skin cells and are not easily removed. More problematic, however, are the pathogenic, or disease-causing, bacteria that may contaminate the hands after contact with infected wounds, fecal material, and other contaminated substances. Fortunately, these bacteria (such as *Staphylococcus aureus*, salmonella, and pseudomonas) do not adhere as avidly to skin cells and are more easily removed. Bacteria do not penetrate intact skin. However, once on the hands, pathogenic bacteria can enter the body by touching open wounds or even normal but sensitive areas such as the mucous membranes of the eyes, lips, mouth, and nose. Even the "benign" skin bacteria can cause infections if they gain access to normally sterile areas of the body. This occurs most frequently upon insertion or manipulation of medical devices that enter sterile sites, such as intravenous lines and urinary catheters.

Viruses, particularly those that cause respiratory diseases like the flu and the common cold, can also be carried on the hands. They are acquired by touching animate or inanimate surfaces that have been contaminated by infected individuals. Examples include shaking hands with an infected person or touching door-knobs or other objects recently handled by such people. Like bacteria, respiratory viruses do not penetrate intact skin, but are introduced into the body when contaminated hands or fingers touch mucous membranes. Unlike some bacteria, viruses do not adhere firmly to skin cells. Thus, even the simplest hand washing will readily remove these viruses.

Hand-Washing Techniques Proper hand washing consists of lathering the hands with warm water and plain soap, rubbing them vigorously (using friction) for fifteen to thirty seconds, then drying them thoroughly. The detergents in soap remove loose dirt, grime, viruses, poorly adherent pathogenic bacteria, and dead skin cells with their adherent normal skin bacteria. For the general population, including most cancer survivors, hands should be washed as above after using the toilet, touching potentially contaminated surfaces, contact with plants or soil, handling uncooked meats and poultry, and at any other time the hands might be contaminated or are visibly soiled.

For caregivers and patients who will be manipulating open wounds, catheters, or other bodily invasive medical devices, more thorough hand washing is necessary. In these situations, high-level disinfection or "sterile technique" is called for. On your doctor's recommendation, you may need to use soap containing an antibacterial product such as chlorhexidine or an iodine-containing substance such as povidone iodine. These products are usually available only by prescription. Before using these products, rings, watches, and other jewelry should be removed. After wetting the hands, the medicated soap should be lathered with friction on all surfaces, including the wrists and lower third of the forearms, for a full thirty seconds, followed by a thirty-second rinse with warm running water. Hands should be dried with a clean, disposable towel, which is then used to turn off the faucets. Blotting rather than wiping the hands is preferable in order to avoid irritation and chapping. Again, on your doctor's advice, clean or sterile vinyl or latex gloves should be put on after hand washing and before certain procedures are carried out (e.g., changing a dressing or flushing an intravenous catheter). After the procedure, gloves are removed by peeling them off inside-out and discarding them in a suitable receptacle where they will not be touched again by you or others. Aside from performing sterile procedures as noted above, antibacterial hand washing is generally only necessary for patients whose immune systems are depressed by persistent or recurrent cancer or due to chemotherapy. Once again, the type of hand washing needed should be guided by the advice of your health care provider.

Another type of hand-washing product comes in the form of alcohol-based rinses, foams, or gels. These are most commonly used in hospitals, where they are found in wall-mounted dispensers in patient rooms or just outside their doors. Because they can be applied in about fifteen seconds and dry automatically by evaporation, they offer speed and convenience. They do have drawbacks, however. They do not kill spores (thick-walled, dormant forms of certain bacteria), and they do not remove debris and dead skin cells as well as does washing with soap and running water and friction. Because the alcohol evaporates quickly, it does not leave any residual antibacterial activity on the hands, as do most of the medicated antibacterial soaps. Thus, they are a temporary measure for convenience only. Hospital personnel who use these alcohol rubs must also frequently wash their hands in the typical manner, especially before and after performing any procedure requiring high-level skin disinfection or sterile technique. Patients may also carry small alcohol gel dispensers for use in situations when there is no access to soap and running water, but these products are not a substitute for frequent, routine hand washing.

Many over-the-counter soaps for home use are labeled "antibacterial." They usually contain a chemical called triclosan, which is listed on the bottle label. Earlier studies suggested that exposure of bacteria to triclosan might lead to the emergence of triclosan-resistant organisms that could then colonize household areas such as sinks, faucet handles, drains, and countertops. More disturbing still, there was evidence that exposure to triclosan could also induce bacteria to become resistant to many important antibiotics. The results of more recent studies are less clear-cut on this issue, although it is still possible that resistant bacteria may emerge with frequent and longer-term exposure to triclosan. Therefore, it would seem advisable for patients and their household members to avoid routine use of triclosan-containing hand-washing soaps (unless directed to do so by their physicians) until more definitive evidence of these products' efficacy is available.

Immunization

Immunization or vaccination is a procedure by which components of an infectious organism are given to a person (usually by injection but sometimes orally or by nasal spray) in order to stimulate the production of protective antibodies against that infection. Most immunizations are made from killed organisms or from proteins or other molecules from these organisms. Since these types of vaccines do not contain live organisms, they do not multiply within the body and are therefore incapable of causing infection in and of themselves.

Certain vaccines consist of live, attenuated (weakened) organisms that do multiply within the body. Because they are attenuated, they do not cause symptomatic infections in otherwise healthy people. However, they should generally not be given to immune-suppressed patients because they may multiply unchecked in the body and cause potentially serious side effects or even death. Examples of live, attenuated vaccines include measles, mumps, rubella (German measles), smallpox, chicken pox, and the related shingles vaccines, as well as the new live, attenuated influenza vaccine given by nasal spray. The standard injectable influenza vaccine contains no live virus. Except for the nasal influenza and shingles vaccines, all the immunizations discussed below are safe to administer to immune-compromised individuals.

More information on the diseases and vaccines described in the following sections can be obtained on-line by searching for the disease or vaccine at the CDC's Web site, *www.cdc.gov.*

Influenza Influenza ("the flu") is a viral respiratory illness that recurs annually in the winter months. Outbreaks vary in severity from year to year. In a mild flu season, 15,000 to 20,000 Americans may die from flu or its complications, while in severe epidemic years, 50,000 to 70,000 deaths may occur. Those most at risk of dying from influenza or its complications are the very young, those over sixty-five years of age, and those with chronic medical conditions, including depressed immune systems.

Influenza viruses genetically mutate each year. The greater the degree of genetic mutation, the more likely it is that immunity from prior infections or vaccinations will be ineffective in providing protection against the current mutated strain. Therefore, vaccine manufacturers change the vaccine composition each year, based on the genetic changes noted in the virus during the previous year. For optimal protection, people should receive the latest vaccine preparation each year.

Since it takes about two weeks to develop protective antibodies after vaccination, influenza vaccine should be taken between mid-October and early November, several weeks before flu is expected to arrive in the community.

In general, flu vaccine is up to 85 percent effective in preventing or decreasing the severity of influenza. Because of a weakening of the body's immune response with increasing age, the vaccine tends to be less effective with advancing age, although one is never too old to obtain some benefit from vaccination.

Since the vaccine is produced in chicken eggs, people with severe egg allergy, or those who have had a well-documented allergic reaction to a previous flu shot, should not be vaccinated. Aside from some mild discomfort at the injection site and a possible low-grade fever during the twenty-four hours following the immunization, the vaccine is extremely safe. The mild side effects noted above should not be interpreted as an allergic reaction and should definitely not discourage people from receiving future annual influenza vaccinations.

A common misconception holds that the flu vaccine can actually cause influenza. This is not true. Shortly after vaccination, some people might coincidentally come down with a different viral illness, or even the flu itself, if it was already incubating at the time the vaccine was received. Similarly, since the vaccine is not 100 percent effective (especially in years when the virus undergoes a major mutation, rendering the current vaccine less effective), an individual may still come down with the flu after being vaccinated. In neither case, however, is the vaccine the cause of the subsequent illness, and this should never be a reason for refusing an annual influenza vaccination.

The above discussion applies for the traditional, nonlive, injectable forms of influenza vaccine. Recently a new live, attenuated, nasal-spray influenza vaccine has become available (FluMist). It is indicated only for use in otherwise healthy individuals between the ages of five to forty-nine years. It should *not* be given to people with impaired immune systems.

Pneumococcal Pneumonia Pneumonia, an infection of the lungs, can be caused by several different types of organisms. About 10 to 25 percent of all pneumonia in the United States is caused by the bacterium *Streptococcus pneumoniae* (pneumococcus), and it is estimated to cause about 40,000 deaths annually. There are some ninety different strains of pneumococcus. These organisms are often carried transiently (for a few days or weeks), and without symptoms, in people's throats—a situation referred to as colonization. Pneumonia occurs when the bacteria colonizing the throat enter the upper airway, or trachea, and travel down into the lungs, where they produce infection.

In general, mechanical defense mechanisms such as coughing and the constant upward flow of tracheal mucus toward the throat and mouth sweep these bacteria out of the trachea and help prevent them from entering the lungs. In certain instances, however, these defense mechanisms can be bypassed in a process called aspiration, which can occur during vomiting, during choking on foods or liquids that "go down the wrong tube," or even during sleep, when the cough reflex is somewhat suppressed and small amounts of oral secretions may trickle past the defense barriers and enter the lungs. Aspiration most commonly occurs in elderly or debilitated people with diminished cough and gag reflexes.

People are also protected against developing pneumococcal pneumonia by other host defenses such as antibodies, bacteria-destroying white blood cells, and the action of the spleen, which filters pneumococci out of the blood. Patients with certain conditions may lack some of these defenses. For example, cancers such as multiple myeloma, chronic lymphocytic leukemia, and Hodgkin's disease and other lymphomas impair antibody production. Other conditions, such as diabetes, cirrhosis of the liver, and chronic kidney disease may lead to low WBC numbers or function, as may cancer chemotherapy and chronic steroid therapy. Patients whose spleens are damaged or surgically removed (splenectomy) and patients with bone marrow transplants, chronic debilitating diseases, malnutrition, asthma, chronic pulmo-

nary disease, and HIV infection are also at increased risk of pneumococcal pneumonia. Acute influenza infections and smoking also increase the risk of pneumococcal pneumonia.

A pneumococcal vaccine (Pneumovax) induces antibody production against twenty-three different strains of pneumococcus, which, together, account for the vast majority of cases of pneumococcal pneumonia. The vaccine is 60 to 70 percent effective in preventing or decreasing the severity of pneumococcal pneumonia. It may be less effective in the very elderly, in those with defective antibody production, and in those with other high-risk factors for infection. Even so, it should be given to people in all these risk groups.

The vaccine contains no live organisms and can thus be given safely to all immune-compromised individuals. About half of those receiving pneumococcal vaccine develop very mild side effects, such as brief pain or redness at the injection site. Less than 1 percent of those vaccinated may experience muscle aches or low-grade fever lasting a few days.

Pneumococcal vaccine should be given to all adults sixty-five years of age or older, as well as to all people of any age with high-risk factors such as those mentioned above. People who need to have their spleens surgically removed or those about to start chemotherapy or long-term steroid therapy should, if possible, receive the vaccine two weeks or more before surgery or drug therapy is begun.

Vaccine-induced antibody levels persist for five years or more in healthy young adults, but they decline with time, especially in the elderly. The U.S. Centers for Disease Control and Prevention (CDC) currently recommends that a second dose of pneumococcal vaccine be given five years after the first dose to those at high-risk for pneumococcal pneumonia. They also recommend a second dose to those over sixty-five years of age if they received their first dose five or more years previously and were under the age of sixty-five when they received that dose.

Tetanus and Diphtheria Everyone should receive a tetanus and diphtheria booster immunization every ten years. Tetanus toxoid (T) is combined with low-dose diphtheria vaccine (d) in a preparation known as Td vaccine. Like the influenza vaccine, Td contains no live organisms and can safely be given to immune-compromised patients.

Recently, a highly contagious and serious childhood infection called pertussis (whooping cough) has been found to infect adults to a much greater degree than previously suspected. Accordingly, the CDC now recommends that all adults under sixty-five years of age receive a single dose of a special combined tetanus-diphtheria-pertussis vaccine (Tdap), marketed as Adacel, at the time of their next routine tetanus booster dose. Thereafter, adults can return to their regular schedule of routine Td booster vaccinations every ten years.

Shingles Shingles, or herpes zoster, is a viral disease that manifests itself as a painful, blistering rash in a bandlike distribution on one side of the body, usually on the trunk. The rash generally extends from the back, near the spine, and around the body, stopping at the midline in front. It lasts several days and then slowly heals as the blisters scab and fall off over the course of ten to fourteen days or longer. The pain can be intense and, in a significant proportion of patients, can last weeks, months, or even years—a condition called postherpetic neuralgia.

Shingles is caused by varicella-zoster, the virus that causes chicken pox. Eighty-five percent of people develop chicken pox during childhood. Although virtually all children easily recover from the infection, the virus never completely leaves the body. Some virus survives in the nerve roots that emerge from the spinal cord, but the body's immune system keeps the virus suppressed and dormant. As immunity wanes with age, particularly after age sixty or so, the virus in a single nerve root may reactivate and travel down the nerve, where it emerges on the skin supplied by that nerve in the form of the rash described above. By age eighty-five, approximately half of all adults will have experienced an attack of shingles. About a million new cases of shingles occur each year in the United States.

Shingles is particularly common in cancer survivors whose disease or chemotherapy suppresses their immunity. Treatment with antiviral drugs, if given within seventy-two hours of the onset of rash, may reduce the severity and duration of the pain by half or more.

In May 2006, the Food and Drug Administration (FDA) approved a new shingles vaccine (Zostavax) for people sixty years of age and older. When given to those in their sixties, the vaccine was 50 percent effective in preventing attacks of shingles and over 67 percent effective in preventing postherpetic neuralgia. When administered to those eighty years of age and older, the vaccine was 18 percent and 39 percent effective, respectively, in preventing shingles and postherpetic neuralgia. A single vaccination is effective for at least four years, but longer-term studies are needed to determine the full duration of its protective effects.

Although the vaccine is now licensed and available, it is quite expensive (about $150 per dose); it remains to be seen whether insurance companies will cover its cost. In addition, it is a live-virus vaccine and should therefore not be given to those with impaired immunity, such as people with AIDS or immunosuppressive cancers like lymphoma and certain leukemias, and those receiving immunosuppressive chemotherapy. It can, however, be given to currently immune-competent individuals who are expected to become immunosuppressed, such as patients with early, asymptomatic HIV infection and those with cancers and other conditions who plan to receive chemotherapy and other immune-suppressive therapies in the future.

Hepatitis B Hepatitis B is a viral infection transmitted by exposure to blood from, or sexual contact with, infected individuals. Those at greatest risk of acquiring hepatitis B in the United States are people with multiple sexual partners (including gay men), monogamous sexual partners of hepatitis B carriers, injection-drug users, and household contacts of hepatitis B carriers. The infection can also be transmitted from an infected woman to her newborn at the time of delivery. A single drop of blood from an infected individual can contain tens of millions of infectious viral particles. Thus, since even minute amounts of infected blood are capable of transmitting the infection, sharing toothbrushes or razors with an infected household member poses a risk of infection. Blood transfusions were once a great risk for infection, but with the current screening and blood testing practices used by blood banks, this risk has been reduced to less than 1 in 5,000 transfusions.

The symptoms of infection (jaundice, fatigue, loss of appetite, and upper right abdominal discomfort, pain, or tenderness) occur in 30 to 80 percent of acutely infected adults, whereas infected infants and young children rarely develop any symptoms at all. Most symptomatic people recover clinically in about one to three months and completely clear the virus from their liver and blood within six months, thus developing lifelong immunity to reinfection. However, about 5 percent of infected older children and adults fail to clear the virus and become chronic carriers of the virus in their blood. The rate of chronic infection rises to about 30 percent for children infected between one and five years of age. For infants infected at birth, an astounding 90 percent or more become lifelong chronic viral carriers.

Patients with chronic hepatitis B may initially be asymptomatic or may exhibit only a mild, nonspecific symptom such as fatigue. However, the virus causes ongoing and slowly progressive liver damage. After five years, up to 20 percent of adult patients will have developed cirrhosis of the liver, and this percentage increases further with time. Cirrhosis usually results in progressive loss of liver function (i.e., liver failure), at a rate of 20 to 25 percent of patients per year. Once liver decompensation occurs, only about a third of patients will survive for five years.

Up to 15 percent of chronic hepatitis B patients with cirrhosis will develop hepatocellular carcinoma, a liver cancer that is highly fatal. Chronic hepatitis B patients who drink alcohol have a four times greater risk of liver cancer than those who do not drink. Overall, 15 to 25 percent of patients with chronic hepatitis B will die from chronic liver disease (cirrhosis, liver failure, and/or liver cancer).

Fortunately, vaccination against hepatitis B prevents acute infection as well as the chronic complications of cirrhosis, liver failure, and liver cancer. Thus, hepatitis B vaccine, introduced over a quarter century ago, was the first vaccine shown to prevent cancer (specifically hepatocellular carcinoma). In the United States, routine hepatitis B vaccination is now recommended for all individuals. Ideally, the first dose should be given at birth; the second, one to two months later; and the third, six months after the first dose.

For those in whom vaccination was not begun at birth, and who do not belong to high-risk groups for acquiring hepatitis B, a three-dose vaccination series can be begun at any age, using a similar vaccination schedule of 0, 1 to 2, and 6 months. Of course, the later the vaccine series is begun, the greater the chance the individual might already have become infected. Once a person has acquired hepatitis B infection, vaccination will provide no benefit.

For people at high risk of acquiring hepatitis B (those with multiple sexual partners, sexual contacts of hepatitis B carriers, injection-drug users, and household contacts of hepatitis B carriers), it is more cost-effective to screen them first with a blood test for the presence of hepatitis B infection. If the screening test is negative, the vaccination series should be begun without delay.

One other group deserving special mention is those who have just been exposed to infectious hepatitis B. This group includes people with very recent exposure to an infected or high-risk individual, such as through sexual contact, needle-stick exposure, blood splash to a mucous membrane (eye or mouth), or birth to an infected mother. In these individuals, the hepatitis B virus has already entered their bodies but has not yet become established. Treatment of these people is called postexposure prophylaxis. In addition to beginning the vaccine series, these individuals must also receive an intramuscular dose of hepatitis B immune globulin (HBIG), a serum with extremely high levels of antibody against hepatitis B. These antibodies will begin to neutralize the hepatitis B virus already introduced into their bodies during the time it takes for the vaccine to stimulate their immune systems to produce their own antihepatitis B antibodies. To be effective, HBIG should be given within twenty-four hours (and preferably within twelve hours or less) of the time of exposure. The first dose of hepatitis B vaccine should be given at the same time but at a separate site on the body from the HBIG injection. The second and third doses of hepatitis B vaccine should be given at the time intervals described above.

Cervical Cancer Cervical cancer is the second most common cancer in women worldwide. Each year, nearly 10,000 women in the United States are newly diagnosed with cervical cancer and nearly 4,000 women die from it. Infection with the human papillomavirus (HPV) is now known to be the primary cause of cervical cancer (see the chapter "Cervix").

Of the more than 100 types of HPV, about 40 are known to be spread by sexual contact. Approximately 6 million genital HPV infections occur annually, making it the most common viral sexually transmitted disease in the United States. Over half of all sexually active men and women become infected with one or more types of HPV at some point during their lifetime. The most common condition caused by sexually transmitted HPV is genital warts, which are acquired by up to half a million Americans annually. Ninety percent of these warts are caused by HPV types 6 and 11.

Of greater concern is the association of genital HPV infection with cervical cancer. Although several HPV types can cause cervical cancer, types 16 and 18 account for 70 percent of all cases.

In about 90 percent of people infected with genital HPV, the virus is eliminated from the body within two years, leaving them immune to reinfection with that specific HPV type. The 10 percent of women who develop persistent HPV infection constitute the risk group for subsequent cervical cancer. Persistent infection with high-risk types of HPV in women and men is also associated with the development of at least some cases of cancer of the vagina, vulva, penis, and anus. Fortunately, these cancers are far less common than cervical cancer.

In June 2006, the FDA licensed Gardasil, a vaccine that protects against the four major types of HPV discussed above (types 6, 11, 16, and 18). The vaccine was tested in over 11,000 girls and women nine to twenty-six years of age.

During five years of follow-up, the vaccine proved to be virtually 100 percent effective in preventing cervical, vaginal, and vulvar precancerous lesions caused by HPV types 16 and 18, as well as 100 percent effective in preventing genital warts caused by HPV types 6 and 11. It is not known, at present, how long vaccine immunity will ultimately last. Longer-term follow-up studies will determine whether and when vaccine booster doses might need to be given.

The vaccine is remarkably safe. The predominant side effect is mild pain at the injection site. Because the vaccine contains no live virus, it can safely be given to immune-suppressed individuals; however, immune compromise might decrease the vaccine's efficacy. The vaccine contains no thimerosal or mercury.

Like the shingles vaccine, Gardasil is quite expensive ($120 per dose; $360 for the full three-dose series). The details of insurance coverage for this vaccine remain to be determined.

Ideally, the vaccine should be given before sexual activity begins. The CDC's Advisory Committee on Immunization Practices (ACIP) recommends the vaccine be given to girls and women nine to twenty-six years of age, preferably at ages eleven to twelve years. It can also be given to older adolescents and adults. It will provide no benefit against any of the four HPV types with which a woman might already have become infected, but it will protect against the remaining types. It offers no protection against any of the other HPV types not included in the vaccine.

Limited studies reveal no ill effects when the vaccine is given to pregnant women. Until more extensive studies are conducted, however, it is currently recommended that pregnant women delay vaccination until after delivery.

A second HPV vaccine, Cervarix, has been developed to prevent cervical cancer in women over twenty-five years of age. It provides protection only against HPV types 16 and 18, the strains responsible for 70 percent of cervical cancer. It is expected to be approved by the FDA in 2007. There is no reason to believe that Gardasil would not be effective in this age group as well. The only reason Gardasil is not licensed for women older than twenty-six years is that it was studied only in girls and women up to that age.

Despite the availability of the HPV vaccine, women should still receive routine cervical cancer screening with a standard Pap smear or the newer liquid-based Pap test. A new test that detects the presence of HPV DNA in cervical cells is also available. The reason for continuing routine screening is that 30 percent of cervical cancers are caused by HPV types not included in the current vaccines. By the same token, women whose Pap smears show precancerous changes or whose DNA tests are positive for the presence of HPV virus are still eligible to receive the HPV vaccine, since their current infection might be due to an HPV strain other than the ones present in the vaccine.

Other Infection-Prevention Measures

Other practices to avoid infection in general, and particularly during periods of immune suppression, include the following:

• Stay away from people with colds or the flu. Many respiratory viruses can also be spread by hand-to-hand contact, so also avoid shaking hands with people with respiratory infections, or wash your hands immediately after doing so. Similarly, to prevent respiratory infections, avoid public areas where there is little ventilation, such as airplanes, theaters, and other crowded enclosed spaces.

• Avoid intimate contact with people who have open sores such as cold sores or other infections.

• Protect your skin from cuts and abrasions. Cut your nails carefully to avoid small nicks. Shave with an electric razor rather than a blade. Use gloves for protection when doing physical work that might damage the skin.

• Avoid dental work or cleaning that can cause gum bleeding if you are receiving chemotherapy or if your white blood cell or platelet count is low (less than 3,000 WBC or less than 100,000 platelets).

• Avoid raw vegetables and any fruit that can't be peeled. Vegetables can harbor enormous numbers of potentially dangerous bacteria on their surfaces. Fruits with intact skins that can be peeled are safe. However, you should either have someone else peel the fruit for you or wash your hands thoroughly after you peel the fruit yourself. Avoid lettuce and raw spinach completely when your WBC count is very low. There is no way to clean bacteria from the surfaces of these leafy vegetables.

• Don't eat undercooked meat or poultry or raw eggs. Raw meat products can contain dangerous microorganisms such as *Listeria, Toxoplasma,* and *E. coli* O157: H7. Nearly all uncooked poultry contains salmonella. Chicken eggs can also harbor salmonella internally, even though their shells are intact.

• Cutting boards and other kitchen surfaces that come in contact with raw meat or poultry should be thoroughly washed with hot, soapy water and dried before other foods are placed on them.

• Don't clean cat litter boxes or birdcages. Avoid all contact with animal stool and urine. Cat feces can contain *Toxoplasma,* and the droppings of certain birds can contain yeasts, molds, and the organism responsible for psittacosis, a rare but severe bacterial pneumonia.

• Avoid constipation, using a stool softener if necessary. The act of straining can cause small tears in the anus and the lining of the lower bowel. This is dangerous when the WBC count is low. Also avoid rectal thermometers and any other manipulation of the anus or rectum.

• If your WBC count is less than 2,000 or you are otherwise immune suppressed, ask your physician if there are any other restrictions or precautions that apply.

Conclusion

Infections pose a serious threat to cancer survivors during periods of immune suppression. Signs and symptoms of infection must carefully be watched so that work-up and treatment can begin as quickly as possible. In the current climate of growing antibiotic resistance among microorganisms, treatment options must carefully be chosen. Indiscriminate use of antibiotics should be avoided, as should the use of over-the-counter antibacterial soaps, in order to reduce the risk of becoming colonized with resistant organisms.

There are a number of other commonsense procedures that, if followed conscientiously, can help reduce the risk of infections. Among these, frequent hand washing is the most important and effective. Immunization can help protect against a variety of infections and, in the case of hepatitis B and HPV vaccines, can actually prevent liver and cervical cancers, respectively. In the face of immune suppression, it is not always possible to avoid all risks of infection, but with good hygiene and diligence in watching for signs of infection when they arise, most life-threatening infections can be either avoided or successfully treated.

— 26 —

Living with an Ostomy

Kerry Anne McGinn, R.N., N.P., M.S.N.

■ ■ ■ ■

Some of my good friends just happen to have ostomies.

Like Virginia. She's the one stretching her four-foot-ten-inch self so that her head shows above the lectern for the speech she's giving. After ten years with a colostomy—ten years of energetic work as an organizer, a publicity person, and a grandmother—she says, "My colostomy's just part of me."

Like Joe. "My urostomy is a positive asset. When we go camping and everyone has a little beer, I'm the only one who doesn't have to get up in the middle of the night to trudge to the Porta-John."

Like Carol. She may be hard to find, between her trips to Australia and Finland, her teaching, and her writing contracts. She says, "My ostomy is a minor nuisance. I barely remember it most of the time. Actually, I did have to be a little extracautious when I ran the marathon in Helsinki."

These three are a few of the hundreds of thousands of people who have had a passageway constructed through the abdominal wall as an exit for feces or urine. This change becomes necessary if the normal outlet cannot be used because of disease, trauma, or birth defect. Without their ostomy surgeries, none of these people would be alive. With their ostomies, each is happily, comfortably, normally alive.

A Few Definitions

An ostomy is the surgical creation of an "opening into" some organ to connect it with the skin. There are various kinds of ostomies—a tracheostomy, for example, can be performed to improve breathing. Most ostomies, however, are performed to allow the elimination of body wastes through the abdominal wall.

Ostomy is the word for the total change the surgeon makes. *Ostomate* is one common term for a person who undergoes this change in personal plumbing. The new opening that can be seen on the abdomen is called a stoma.

There are three general categories of these abdominal exit ostomies:

- *Colostomy* is the rerouting of the colon, or large intestine. This change may be permanent or temporary.
- *Ileostomy* is such a detour in the ileum, the last section of the small intestine.
- *Urostomy*, or urinary diversion, covers a number of surgical procedures that redirect urine to the outside of the body when the bladder or another part of the urinary tract has to be bypassed or removed.

Colostomies

A colostomy is the most common ostomy. Surgeons perform colostomies for colorectal cancer, for other cancers of the abdomen or pelvis that press on or invade the large intestine, and for conditions that have nothing to do with cancer.

In this surgical procedure, part of the colon is removed or disconnected and all or part of the rectum may be removed as well. The end of the remaining colon is brought to the surface through the skin of the abdomen, folded back like a turtle-neck, and stitched in place to form the stoma.

Adjusting to the Ostomy How does your body change when you have a colostomy? What stays the same?

Everything we eat, from apple pie to zucchini, must be broken down into tiny particles and changed to simpler chemical substances that can be absorbed into the bloodstream. The resulting nutrients make their way to cells throughout the body, providing constant fuel and materials for energy, growth, and rebuilding. This complex process of digestion takes place in the long—28 feet (8 m) or longer in an adult—twisting channel that starts at the mouth and ends at the anus.

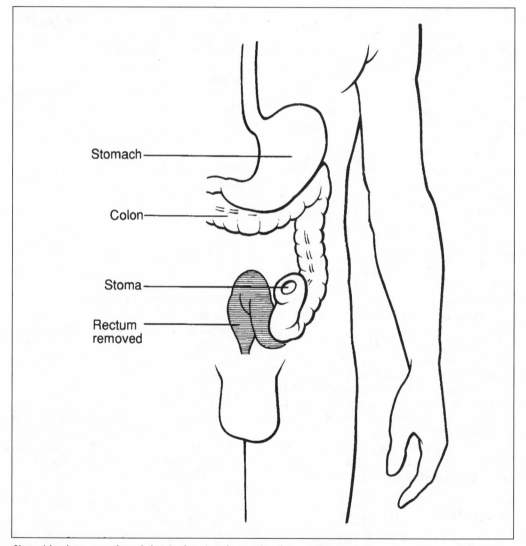

Sigmoid colostomy, after abdominal-perineal resection for rectal cancer.

By the time food reaches the colon—the last 6 feet (2 m) of the channel—most of the nourishment has been absorbed. Here the major tasks are absorbing water and some mineral salts in the first portion of the colon, then transporting and storing the indigestible remains of the food in the rest of the colon and the rectum. At the far end is the anus, a ringlike sphincter muscle that opens to release feces.

The body adjusts quite nicely to a shortened digestive tract. If your ostomy occurs near the end of the colon, as it does in many colostomies, you've lost only a storage area and a sphincter to release feces. If your ostomy is higher up in the digestive tract, you may lose part of the ability to absorb water, so the discharge will tend to be less formed, more liquid. (This is much more of a problem for the person with an ileostomy, who has no colon and may have a problem absorbing mineral salts also, but ileostomy surgery is rare for cancer.) The remaining intestine eventually takes over some of the water-absorbing function. The kidneys, the major regulators of water and mineral salts, handle the rest of the adjustment.

Temporary and Permanent Colostomies

With new surgical techniques available, surgeons are performing fewer "permanent" colostomies—in which the rectum and anus are removed—than they did in the past.

But if a cancer occurs near the very end of the digestive tract, this may be the best way to remove all the cancer and save a life. An abdominal-perineal (A-P) resection is the usual surgery, with the surgeon making incisions in both the abdomen and the perineal area around the anus to remove the cancer and construct the colostomy.

Often, a surgeon constructs a "temporary" colostomy, which can sometimes last for years. This operation involves bypassing, but not removing, the rectum and anus. For instance, a surgeon might cut out a colon cancer but want the area to heal without feces passing over it. Or a large tumor that can't be removed causes pain because it's blocking the passage of stool. Using one of several techniques, the surgeon can form a colostomy using the colon ahead of the affected section, leaving the problem area alone. Stool can then pass out of the body but through a new exit. Later, the colostomy may be reversed so that stool moves through the anus again.

How the Stoma Functions The stoma that results from a colostomy could be described as a soft valve. Since it is made from the digestive tract that winds from the mouth to the anus, it is the same red-pink color as the mouth and is lined with essentially the same kind of soft, velvety mucous membrane. It stretches to permit waste to be expelled. During inactive periods, the tissue pulls together rather like puckered lips (*stoma*, in fact, means mouth). Although it expands and contracts, the stoma does not have the firm muscle control of the anal sphincter. So voluntary control of a bowel movement must be replaced by something else.

For many people with colostomies, that "something else" is a pouch (also called an appliance or a bag). This is made of thin flexible plastic or rubber, which adheres to the skin over the stoma to hold feces until a convenient time for disposal. These are comfortable, odorproof, and secure.

An alternative for many colostomates with fairly solid stool is "irrigation," a kind of enema through the stoma done every day or two. This permits them to empty the bowel at a convenient regular time. They wear only a tiny pouch or a soft pad over the stoma the rest of the time.

Urinary Diversions

Urinary diversions, or urostomies, are often performed for cancer in the urinary tract.

Normally, once the kidneys have filtered wastes out of the blood, they flush excess fluid and wastes as urine through narrow tubes to an expandable storage area—the bladder—and then out of the body. At least some kidney function is essential for life, but any other part of the urinary tract can be removed or bypassed. Because reasons for urostomies vary from birth defects to bladder cancer, the age range of urostomates is wide, as is the range of different surgical techniques.

Making the Conduit To treat bladder cancer, surgeons may create an ileal conduit (also called an ileal loop or Bricker loop). The surgeon removes the bladder or sometimes just bypasses it. A section a few inches long is cut away from the last part of the small intestine (the ileum), keeping the blood and nerve supply intact. This section is closed at one end, the narrow tubes from the kidney are attached to it, and the open end is brought through the abdominal wall to form a stoma.

The remaining ends of the intestine are reconnected and resume their function of moving feces out of the body. If the surgeon prefers to use a section of colon rather than ileum, the ostomy is called a colonic conduit.

The conduit is not an artificial bladder. It doesn't store urine. It is simply a passageway, and urine continues to drip out of the stoma all the time. This means that if you have this kind of urinary ostomy, you wear a pouch at all times and drain it into the toilet as needed.

Taking Care of Your Stoma

Although the stoma usually shrinks somewhat in diameter as postoperative swelling subsides and you resume your normal diet and exercise, the red-pink color remains.

Unlike an incision, a stoma requires little healing. A urostomy stoma starts to expel urine immediately, even before the new urostomate has left the operating room. Colostomies start discharging feces in a few days, usually with a lot of gas and watery stool until the bowel settles down after surgery.

Stomas come in many shapes and sizes, depending on the kind of ostomy and the person who owns it. Since it is made from the large intestine, a colostomy stoma will be wider than an ileal conduit urostomy stoma made from the small intestine. Some "temporary" stomas may be quite large and have two openings in one stoma or two stomas near each other. Most stomas should protrude from the skin enough so that feces or urine discharge away from the skin rather than pooling around the stoma.

At first, it's a temptation to feel overprotective about a stoma. You might feel that it is so fragile, it might be damaged by a breeze or a bump. While reasonable protection is essential, the stoma is surprisingly tough. It is not harmed by water, by contact during sex, or even by gentle bumps against furniture. But it does bleed easily, even from as little cause as an overzealous wipe with a washcloth, because many tiny blood vessels are very close to the surface of the stoma. A pouch or a soft pad will protect it from the friction of clothes.

Getting Support

When you have an ostomy, you can eat, work, and play normally. But there are new skills to learn. Fortunately, there are many resources to help and give you moral support.

An enterostomal therapist (ET nurse or stoma nurse) is a registered nurse with special training in the care of ostomies and ostomates. ET nurses work in hospitals or have private practices. With their knowledge and caring, they are a godsend for both new and long-time ostomates. Ask your doctor for the name of the ET nurse in your hospital or community. (Some of these nurses are called WOC nurses because their role has grown to include wound care, ostomies, and continence problems.)

The United Ostomy Association (UOA) is an organization of many thousands of people with ostomies. The association holds local meetings and provides ostomy visitors—volunteers matched for sex, age, and type of ostomy—for the new ostomate. Some people come to the meetings for information, some for moral support, and some for the social contact. Some people come because they are having problems, others because they have solved problems and are happy to pass on their experience.

Some are desperate, discouraged, depressed. Many of them find answers, and all of them find support and a place where they can talk freely about what concerns them. Local chapters of UOA may be listed in the phone book or can be located through the American Cancer Society. The national organization publishes a quarterly journal and holds regional and national conferences.

Keeping a Positive Attitude

Hearing that you have cancer and need an ostomy is a double jolt for anyone. It takes time, information, and support to adjust. But it is definitely not the end.

I'll never forget Roger. A year before I met him, the doctor in his small town had diagnosed rectal cancer and had recommended colostomy surgery. "No way," stormed Roger. "You're not going to see me with one of those awful bags."

Despite his doctor's urging, Roger refused surgery. He underwent radiation and chemotherapy, but the tumor spread. When Roger came to our big-city hospital and, by some administrative quirk, to my orthopedics floor, he was deathly ill. But he was still adamantly opposed to "those damned bags."

I was scarcely an ostomy expert at the time, but I knew someone with a colostomy—my mother. I knew people could be happy with a colostomy, bleak as Roger's chances seemed to be. So Roger and I talked. Just quiet talk. I passed on what information I had and my own confidence that ostomy surgery might make him feel much better. Meanwhile, his bowel became totally blocked, his pain became agonizing, and his temperature soared. The bowel had burst and infection had set in. Too ill to protest much, Roger agreed to surgery. The doctors did minimal surgery, creating a "temporary" colostomy so that stool would no longer spill into his abdomen.

To our astonishment, Roger survived both the surgery and a very rocky postoperative course. As he grew stronger, we started teaching him about caring for his ostomy, created in haste and none too neat. Remembering my mother's experiences with the United Ostomy Association, I asked the doctor's permission to call UOA for an ostomy visitor to see Roger, a real boost indeed. Eventually, still with his "temporary" colostomy, Roger was well enough to go home to his hometown hundreds of miles away, where we alerted the UOA chapter to expect him.

After he left, I wondered how he was, what had happened to him, whether he was still alive. His chief pleasure at home, besides his family, had been riding his horse, but I rather doubted that he'd ever be able to do that again.

Nine months later, he returned to our hospital and was again admitted to our floor.

"Roger! What's the matter?"

"You'll never believe it, Kerry," he said, with a fine combination of sheepishness and pride. "I was at the rodeo."

"Hey, that's great! You've been getting out of the house some. Have you been able to ride at all?"

"Sure, that's what I was doing, roping cattle at the rodeo."

I took a deep breath. "But, Roger, what about your colostomy?"

"No problem. The pouches you gave me stick on fine. You know, I just wish I'd known back then how easy a colostomy is. If only I'd known."

"Why are you here?"

"Well . . . I took a tumble from the horse and broke my ankle."

— 27 —

The Look Good . . . Feel Better
Cosmetic Program

The Washington, D.C. Cosmetic, Toiletry, and Fragrance Association Foundation

■ ■ ■ ■

Just about anyone's quality of life is seriously diminished during cancer treatment. Fatigue and changes in daily routine and in physical appearance; personal emotions; and reactions from family, friends, and colleagues can all weigh heavily on cancer patients.

If you are a woman getting cancer treatment, you may find that physical changes are especially hard to bear. Your personal appearance directly affects your self-image and your psychological well-being. And if you are experiencing some of the common side effects of radiation or chemotherapy, you may start to believe that you're in worse medical shape than you really are. The face you see in the mirror each morning is a harsh reminder of your disease. Every day, you can't escape your loss of hair, eyelashes, and eyebrows or the changes in the tone and texture of your skin.

Looking in that mirror, you may start thinking that you couldn't possibly lead a "normal" life. But in today's world, leading a normal life—with all the household, work, and social demands normal life involves—is essential while you are getting cancer treatments. What you need to get back to a good quality of life is help in overcoming the changes in appearance that cancer treatments bring.

Fortunately, to help you do just that, Look Good . . . Feel Better (LGFB) is a free

national public service program designed to teach women with cancer—through practical and hands-on experience—the beauty techniques that help restore their appearance during chemotherapy and radiation treatments.

So while your medical treatment helps heal the inside of your body, the Look Good . . . Feel Better program helps you renew your self-esteem by enhancing your "outside" appearance. It encourages you to pay attention to yourself during a time of dramatic physical changes.

How the Look Good . . . Feel Better Program Works

Look Good . . . Feel Better started in 1989, when three national organizations pooled their resources to develop the service and make it available to women across the country. The program was founded and developed by the Cosmetic, Toiletry, and Fragrance Association (CTFA) Foundation—a charitable organization supported by the members of the cosmetic industry's trade association—in collaboration with the American Cancer Society (ACS) and the National Cosmetology Association (NCA). NCA is a national organization that represents hairstylists, wig experts, aestheticians, makeup artists, and nail technicians, among others.

Look Good . . . Feel Better provides

• free beauty tips and techniques to cancer patients—through group workshops or individual sessions—by volunteer cosmetologists and beauty advisers,
   • complimentary makeup kits for everyone participating in a group program, and
   • free self-help program materials.

The Look Good . . . Feel Better program is administered nationwide by ACS and is designed to meet the needs of local communities. NCA organizes volunteer cosmetologists who can evaluate your skin and hair needs and who will teach you the appropriate beauty techniques to deal with the appearance-related side effects of cancer treatments. The CTFA Foundation provides the makeup, materials, and financial support for the program. Look Good . . . Feel Better is "product neutral" and does not promote any specific cosmetic product line or manufacturer. All volunteers for Look Good . . . Feel Better are trained and certified for participation by ACS at local, state, or regional workshops. The purpose of this training is not only to discuss important hygienic guidelines and helpful cosmetic tips, but also to promote sensitivity and understanding about what a cancer patient goes through during treatment. This is a necessary step for each volunteer.

Group Sessions Each group session usually consists of six to ten women led through a two-hour program by beauty professionals. Through practical hands-on experience, the women learn a twelve-step makeup program and are shown beauty tips about hair, wigs, turbans, and scarves. To ensure that every participant gets the same working tools, each woman in a group program receives a complimentary bag of makeup containing twelve items, which match the

twelve-step program: cleanser, moisturizer, concealer, foundation, powder, blush, eyeshadow, eyeliner, eyebrow pencil, mascara, lip liner, and lipstick.
   Look Good . . . Feel Better group programs are located in comprehensive cancer centers, hospitals, ACS offices, and community centers.

Personal Consultation A free one-time consultation in a salon by a participating volunteer may also be available, depending on where you live. The makeup kit is not provided at one-on-one consultations. A list of volunteers willing to provide this service is compiled and distributed to all ACS divisions as well as to the Look Good . . . Feel Better toll-free number, which provides program information (1-800-395-LOOK).

Look Good . . . Feel Better for Teens

Look Good . . . Feel Better for Teens was launched in 1996. This program is designed to address the needs and concerns that teenage cancer patients, both girls and boys, have about the appearance side effects of treatment and the frequently resulting low self-esteem. Like LGFB for adult women, the teen program includes instruction on skin care and makeup, as well as alternatives for coping with hair loss—all geared to teens. In addition, the teen program addresses some of the important social, fitness, and nutritional issues unique to teenagers battling cancer.
   Look Good . . . Feel Better for Teens is offered as a group program in eighteen designated children's hospitals. Information about the teen program can be obtained through the national LGFB toll-free number, 1-800-395-LOOK. Look Good . . . Feel Bettter for Teens information is also available on-line through *www.2bMe.org,* or through *www.lookgoodfeelbetter.org* by clicking on "Teens."

How and Where to Find Programs in Your Community

Many doctors, nurses, social workers, and other medical professionals recognize how important outward appearance is to their patients. And with their help, Look Good . . . Feel Better is now reaching out to tens of thousands of women across the United States.

The growth of the program has been remarkably rapid and widespread. Two pilot programs were successfully operated at the Memorial Sloan-Kettering Cancer Center in New York City and the Vincent T. Lombardi Cancer Research Center at Georgetown University Hospital in Washington, D.C., in the fall of 1988.

By March 1989, the program was off and running. Since then, Look Good . . . Feel Better has been implemented in all fifty states and the District of Columbia and most of the National Cancer Institute–designated comprehensive cancer centers. Group programs served 50,000 women with cancer in 2005. LGFB materials are also available in Spanish, and bilingual programs are available in some cities.

For more information, or to find out about programs in your area, call your local office of the American Cancer Society or the Look Good . . . Feel Better toll-free number at 1-800-395-LOOK, or visit the Look Good . . . Feel Better Web site at *www.lookgoodfeelbetter.org*.

— 28 —

Becoming Sexually Active Again

Christine M. Derzko, M.D., David G. Bullard, Ph.D.,
Ernest H. Rosenbaum, M.D., and Malin Dollinger, M.D.

■ ■ ■ ■

Cancer affects all aspects of your life. So it's not surprising that it can affect your sexual feelings and the ways you express those feelings. You and your spouse or partner remain sexual beings and may have much the same needs and desires as you had before the illness struck.

Sexuality can be expressed in many ways—in how we dress and how we move and speak, as well as through kissing, touching, masturbation, and intercourse. Changes in body image and tolerance for activity as well as anxieties about survival, family, or finances can strain the expression of sexuality and can create concerns about sexual desirability. But if you were comfortable with and enjoyed your sexuality before your illness, the chances are excellent that you will be able to keep or regain a good sexual self-image despite any changes brought about by cancer.

Many people, and in particular those dealing with an illness, find that being sexually active is not important to them to maintain a loving, intimate relationship. This can be a healthy, normal choice for any individual or couple. However, the loss of interest may be transient for others, and they may be quite distressed either by their loss of libido (sexual interest) or by their inability to respond or perform sexually as they had in the past. If sexual intimacy has been a joy and comfort to you, you may want to resume or continue being sexually active even

though your cancer has been diagnosed, is being treated, or has been treated.

This may require some adaptation of your normal sexual patterns, and it might be a challenge to change them. Support groups can give understanding and encouragement, and open, comfortable communication with your partner is essential. Make a point of sharing your concerns with your partner: He or she wants and needs to help sort out the problems. You may also need specific information and guidance from your doctor. But the subject of sexual health for people with chronic illnesses, especially cancer, has been neglected for far too long. Members of your medical team may find it hard to initiate discussions about sexual problems. Nevertheless, don't make the mistake of trying to be a "good" patient by not complaining and simply suffering in silence. Sexuality is a legitimate area of concern. Don't be shy: Take the initiative and ask your doctor any questions you have about your sexuality. Seek referral to a sex counselor if needed. You can overcome many problems, reduce tensions, and get much more sexual satisfaction.

The Phases of Sexuality

Understanding the phases of sexuality and how cancer can affect one or more of them can help you increase your satisfaction with sex.

• **Desire** This varies from person to person, ranging from an uninterested, indifferent attitude that may or may not change with time to a very active desire for sex. Desire can often be increased by physical, visual, or fantasy stimulation. The initial emotional impact of a cancer diagnosis and its treatment may leave little or no energy left for sexual desire. Depression or certain classes of medications can directly lower desire, as can treatment that alters hormone levels. Discussing your lack of interest with your doctor is important. It may be that alternative medications can be prescribed that do not have such a negative effect. Indeed with some conditions, hormonal replacement therapy, which may correct or at least improve the symptoms, may be appropriate. The important thing to remember is that you do have options. Explore them!

• **Excitement** The body reacts to stimulation with increased blood flow in the sex organs and increased heart rate and blood pressure. Sexual interest and stimulation are popularly thought to be characterized by an erection in men and increased vaginal lubrication in women. On the other hand, particularly after cancer therapy, a person may feel desire yet those physiological responses may not follow.

Sexual problems often occur during the excitement phase. This can lead to considerable anxiety and distress. Men may lose the ability to get or keep an erection. Women may not have enough vaginal lubrication for comfortable penetration, making intercourse difficult or painful.

• **Orgasm** This is a peak of pleasurable expression followed by a gratifying relaxation. It is both a physical release and an emotional high.

Some men might ejaculate only after prolonged stimulation. Sometimes nothing happens despite prolonged effort. Or the ejaculate might be reversed into the bladder (retrograde) rather than going forward and out through the penis. In this case, orgasm still occurs, but there is no semen or liquid.

For women, the painful intercourse (dyspareunia) that sometimes follows cancer treatment can inhibit both enjoyment and orgasm. There are a number of treatments available, so don't give up before you have explored the possibilities available to you.

• **Resolution** Many people feel relaxed and satisfied after sex regardless of whether or not they reach orgasm. For others, who experience problems during the desire, excitement, or orgasm phase, the satisfying resolution may be replaced by sexual tension, discomfort in the pelvis, or emotional frustration.

Sexuality and Cancer

Treatment for some cancers may have little effect on sexuality beyond the effects of fatigue, pain, weakness, or other temporary side effects. However, there are two distinct questions and concerns that may arise. First, in the younger patient, will the treatment of your cancer affect or impair your ability to have a family in the future, and if so, what can you do about it? Second, will the treatment directly affect your ability to function sexually? It is important to recognize that lengthy treatments and impaired fertility may cause marital stress unless both partners are encouraged and willing to communicate their feelings.

Cancer and Fertility The improved long-term survival rates and cures following treatment for many cancers have made future fertility a question to be considered in young, reproductive-age patients, preferably even before the actual cancer treatment is begun. The importance of this question has been recognized, and while the existing options are currently limited, particularly in women, this is an area of active research and it is likely that in the near future other options will become available.

What Can Be Done to Preserve Fertility?

Clearly, cancer treatment that requires surgical removal of the testes or the ovary will render the patient sterile. When preservation of fertility is an important consideration, particularly in minimally invasive disease, sometimes the surgeon may suggest alternative surgical treatment that is less radical and still may be a reasonable possibility. Alternatively, the question may arise about the possibility of collecting sperm or ova (eggs) prior to cancer treatment (surgical, radiation, or chemotherapy).

In men, radiation and chemotherapy may cause long-lasting or permanent damage to sperm-producing cells. So, younger men who will require radiation and/or extensive chemotherapy might consider sperm-banking before treatment in case the sperm count and quality do not return to normal. While this option deserves to be considered, it is important to realize that there is no guarantee that a sperm sample collected once any illness, particularly cancer, has struck will be of good quality. Furthermore, in addition to the illness itself, some of the early less radical therapies may themselves adversely affect both the sperm count and the quality.

In women, the damage done to ovaries by cancer treatment is dependent on a number of factors, including the patient's age at the time of treatment, the dose and particular chemotherapeutic drug used, and the dose and fractionation schedule of radiation given. Sometimes, to protect them from radiation, the ovaries may be surgically moved out of the area to be radiated or they may be shielded from radiation.

A question that frequently arises is "Can I 'bank my eggs' just like men can bank their sperm?" Unfortunately, at the present time, this is not routinely possible. However, in a few select centers, it is being tried on an experimental basis under the strict supervision of the institutional research committee. While hopeful for the future, currently the relatively poor survival of frozen eggs after the rethawing process, and the low pregnancy yield, make freezing of ova obtained prior to cancer treatment not available as a clinical option. However, advances are being made in this area that are of considerable research interest, so it is likely that "egg banking" may be a therapeutic possibility in the near future.

A second approach currently being looked at is that of freezing ovarian (or testicular) tissue in the hope that later, after successful treatment of the cancer, it can be transplanted back into the patient and still function. A concern remains, however, that when replaced, this frozen ovarian (or testicular) tissue may carry with it some of the cancer that was present in the individual, prior to the tissue removal.

Currently, what is available and what has been shown to be successful is the freezing of embryos. Thus, in patients whose cancer treatment can be delayed for at least several weeks and in whom exposure of the cancer to the high levels of estrogen that may necessarily occur with treatment can be tolerated, the ovaries can be stimulated and the ova obtained following the usual IVF (in vitro fertilization) protocols. Following fertilization with the partner's sperm (or when acceptable, by donor sperm), the embryos can successfully be frozen and at a later date thawed for transfer into the patient (or even a surrogate).

The Sexual Problems Associated with Specific Cancers and Their Therapies

The treatment of several kinds of cancer may directly affect sexual function.

Bladder Cancer Surgical therapy for bladder cancer can lead to decreased desire, a reduced ability for men to get an erection, retrograde ejaculation, and orgasm problems, including a lower intensity. About half of women who have this therapy end up with a shorter and narrower vagina, making penetration more difficult. Communication with your partner will become especially important in such cases, as will the use of lubricants such as K-Y jelly, Astroglide, or Crème de la Femme.

Breast Cancer Psychological counseling and support groups are helpful for many women treated for breast cancer, given the symbolic sexual significance of the female breast. Thirty to 40 percent of women who have a modified radical mastectomy report sexual concerns; fewer sexual problems are reported if a lumpectomy is required, which results in less change to body image; but even 10 percent of women who have a *benign* biopsy may want to discuss sexual concerns.

Premature menopause following chemotherapy, hormone replacement therapy, or radiation can contribute to a woman feeling a loss of desire or even an aversion to sex. When it can be done safely, treatment with low doses of testosterone cream (not commercially available, but it can be prepared by a compounding pharmacy) applied vaginally may help women regain desire and sexual enjoyment. It is hoped that women may soon have another option: the testosterone patch, which has been widely tested and shown to be effective in both naturally and surgically menopausal women distressed about their low sexual desire.

Taking more time with sexual activities other than intercourse, using vaginal lubricants, reading erotic literature or watching erotic videotapes or DVDs, and using sensory enhancements such as music, scented candles, and massage lotion are additional things to try. Of course, having a warm, caring, and communicative relationship with your partner is one of the best enhancers of sexual pleasure. The same applies to people without a partner, who can and should treat themselves with love and nurturing.

Colon Cancer There is twice the amount of sexual dysfunction after surgery for colon cancer as there is after surgery for a benign cause such as an ileostomy for ulcerative colitis. Some preliminary data suggest that following endoscopic colectomy, there may be less sexual dysfunction because there is less surgical disruption of pelvic innervation. People with ostomies may have embarrassment or worry about their partner's reaction that might interfere with their sexual responsiveness. Direct communication with and reassurance from a partner can be very helpful.

Gynecological Tumors A woman having gynecological cancer surgery with removal of the ovaries will have a sudden loss of estrogen resulting in premature menopause. Sudden loss of ovarian function is associated with very intense symptoms of menopause: severe hot flashes, joint and muscle aches and pains, mood swings, sleeping problems, anxiety, and depression. Sexual partners often have a hard time coping with these changes. All this can reduce a couple's ability to have sex or their inclination to even think about it. With the feelings of abandonment and rejection that often follow, the relationship can definitely suffer. But the right kind of help and counseling can assist the couple in talking about and coping with these problems. Seeking this help may be an important first step. Hormonal replacement therapy may also resolve some of these issues.

Hysterectomy and radiation treatment to the female genitals may lead to problems in the excitement phase. The surgery might also affect orgasm, and painful intercourse can be the result of lack of hormone (estrogen), caused by the premature failure of the ovaries that we discussed earlier, or from the radiation effects on the tissues. Consequently, the frequency of intercourse might be reduced. Some women who have had hysterectomies for benign disease report similar problems—a decrease in sexual desire especially in the first six months after the operation, with desire often returning to normal within a year.

Radical surgery to the vagina and vulva can so change the physical aspects of the genitalia that sexual activity can become very difficult both physically and psychologically because of the fear of pain or bleeding during intercourse. Plastic surgery to reconstruct the organs, along with sex counseling, can be very helpful to some, while others may learn to enjoy lovemaking without intercourse.

Hodgkin's Disease About 20 percent of men and women with this type of cancer lose energy and interest in sex. Hodgkin's disease doesn't usually affect the ability of men to get an erection, but in women, premature failure of the ovaries with the resulting lack of circulating estrogen may cause vaginal dryness, leading to painful intercourse. While the ovarian failure may be permanent, return of ovarian function particularly in young women may occur, even several years later. In general, the shorter the treatment, the lower the dose, and the younger the patient, the better the chance is that (some) recovery of ovarian function will occur.

Cancer of the Penis and Testicles As challenging as it sounds, men who lose part of their penis may still be capable of getting erections, having orgasms, and ejaculating. Removal of the whole penis can naturally cause very severe sexual difficulties. But orgasm may still be possible with stimulation of the bones, pubis, perineum, and scrotum, and ejaculation through a urethrostomy.

With testis cancer, the sexual problems depend on the type of tumor. With non-seminoma, removal of a testicle and the lymph nodes in the area usually results in a decrease in fertility and sexual activity. Some men with seminoma who have had a testicle removed plus radiation therapy report low or no sexual activity, decreased desire, problems with erections and orgasms, and decreased volume of semen. Others continue to function and enjoy their sexuality—individual responses vary considerably, as in any aspect of sexuality.

Prostate Cancer The diagnostic biopsy might result in less seminal fluid in the ejaculation. Surgical removal of the prostate can cause similar problems and, with hormonal therapy, the ability to get an erection and ejaculate may be lost or diminished.

Radiation produces problems, too, but only half as many as the surgical approach. When the pelvic lymph nodes are removed and a radiation implant is used for localized tumors, 15 to 25 percent of men have difficulties with erections and about 30 percent have a retrograde ejaculation. New "nerve-sparing" surgical approaches and new chemotherapy treatments help reduce erection and ejaculation problems. The PDE-5 inhibitors, such as tadalafil (Cialis), vardenafil (Levitra), and sildenafil (Viagra), may help men regain erectile functioning after prostate cancer treatment.

For some men following treatment such as surgery, urinary incontinence might be a problem, but this usually resolves over the course of six months, while a few men may take up to eighteen months to heal. It is important to consult with a urologist about "aggressive therapy" for erectile functioning following prostate surgery. This might entail injections or oral medication to help the erectile tissue heal.

Drugs That Affect Sexual Desire and Activity Most cancers occur in people over fifty, many of whom may already have experienced some decrease in sexual activity. The diagnosis of cancer itself may result in a significant reduction in sexual desire, as can such diseases as diabetes and alcoholism and/or psychological problems. Furthermore, it is important to know that a great many drugs can lower sexual desire and activity and can therefore lead to sexual dysfunction.

If You've Had Treatment to the Genitals or Reproductive Organs Even the prospect of surgery or radiation treatments for these cancers can make you intensely concerned about your body image. But it is usually impossible to predict the effects of treatment for any one person. Treatment can affect some people's ability to get erections, to ejaculate, or to have intercourse. The same treatment for someone else might result in little or no change in sexual functioning.

Anxiety Sexual problems that seem to be the physical results of treatment may actually be due to anxiety. You can reduce your worry by discussing potential problems and possible solutions prior to or following treatment with your doctor, other members of the health care team, or support group members who have gone through similar experiences. This discussion will also reassure you that if problems do come up, there are ways of handling them. Since in most situations physical and emotional causes of sexual problems interact, your exploration and experimentation about what you can do is very important. Your diagnosis does not dictate what is possible for you sexually.

Use of Some Medications in the Following Categories May Be Associated with Sexual Difficulties

It is always important to take the medication your medical provider prescribes for you. But if you are experiencing some sexual difficulties and you are taking any drugs from the following categories, you should be aware that the problem may be related to your medication. So, it is worthwhile to ask whether your problem is drug related and if an alternative preparation or drug is appropriate and available and could be tried.

Alcohol	H_2-receptor antagonists
Anticancer drugs and hormones	Hallucinogenic drugs
Anticonvulsants	Hormone blockers
Antidepressants	Nonsteroidal anti-inflammatory agents
Antihypertensives including beta-blockers (at high dosage)	Opiates
Carbonic anhydrase inhibitors	Pain medications
Codeine or other narcotics	Psychedelic drugs
Cytotoxic drugs	Recreational drugs
Digitalis family	Sleep medications
Diuretics	Tobacco
	Tranquilizers

Painful Intercourse Women may find that intercourse is painful not only after treatment for a genital cancer, but also if pelvic or total body radiation has been part of your therapy. There are four common reasons why this problem may arise:

• Infection of the bladder or vagina (this may be a recurring problem)
• Lack of lubrication
• Vaginal shortening
• Anxiety with resulting spasm of the vaginal muscles

Have a gynecological examination to find the cause.

• *Infection* Vaginal or bladder infections are common and may cause painful intercourse in any woman, including a woman recovering from cancer therapy. These conditions are readily treatable: Vaginal infections may be treated either *locally* (vaginal cream or suppositories) or *systemically;* bladder infections are treated with systemic antibiotics. A yeast infection (with or without a discharge) may occur as a result of treatment with some systemic antibiotics, and this possibility should be considered when intercourse becomes uncomfortable or painful during or after a course of antibiotics.

• *Lack of Lubrication* The vagina may feel "dry" in the presence of a yeast infection. But if this cause is excluded, commonly there are two reasons: (1) inadequate estrogen effect and (2) lack of adequate sexual arousal.

Estrogen is produced normally during reproductive life by the ovaries. Surgical removal of the ovaries permanently deprives the body of this natural source of female hormones. Chemotherapy and radiation therapy may temporarily or permanently stop the production of estrogen. This removal of estrogen may be an important and necessary part of the treatment of the primary cancer (e.g., breast cancer and uterine [endometrial] cancer, but not cervical cancer). Your doctor will be able to tell you for sure about this, and you should therefore feel free to discuss the question with him or her.

Unless estrogen deprivation* is essential to your management, and particularly if you are in your forties or younger, hormonal therapy with an estrogen (ET) or an estrogen plus a progestin or progesterone (EPT) is almost certainly appropriate for you and can be prescribed by your doctor. This may even be true following breast cancer therapy, particularly if the disease is receptor negative. However, any decision to initiate hormone treatment must be made in conjunction with your oncologist.

Hormone Replacement Therapy (HRT) may be in the form of either systemic medications such as pills, patches, gels, injections, or implants; or local vaginal applications such as estrogen-containing creams, vaginal rings, or vaginal tablets or suppositories. Often, despite use of adequate systemic doses of hormones, additional vaginal estrogen therapy is required to relieve symptoms of vaginal dryness (see "Hormonal Replacement Therapy in Women," in this chapter).

It may take many months for hormone treatment, local and/or systemic, to return the vagina to normal and improve lubrication. A change of dose (systemic)

---

* Even if your cancer treatment involves estrogen deprivation and thus treatment with systemic estrogens is considered inappropriate, your doctor may permit use of an estradiol vaginal ring (Estring), which releases a tiny amount of estrogen to the vagina daily; or a small amount of estrogen cream (less than the amount of toothpaste you would use on your toothbrush) applied with your finger to the vaginal and urethral openings, perhaps once every one to two weeks. This may be quite adequate to relieve itching and irritation and may make the tissues softer and more pliable and therefore allow penetration to occur.

or frequency of use (local vaginal application) is sometimes required to achieve a more rapid relief from symptoms. More commonly, though, healing brought about by time is what is needed. Keep in mind that many couples—even those without any health challenges—find that they need to use a vaginal lubricant for intercourse. Estrogen cream is not meant to be used for this purpose. Treatments and products that may be appropriate are noted below.

If the cause of dryness is not enough lubrication, use of saliva, a natural lubricant, or products such as water-soluble lubricants or baby oil can reduce friction. Artificial lubricants such as K-Y jelly, Astroglide, and Jergens lotion and other creams may make coitus possible where the lack of circulating estrogens has caused dryness. Replens (a non-hormonal vaginal gel that is available without prescription in both the United States and Canada) is a vaginal moisturizer that is applied three times a week and may improve lubrication for sexual arousal and intercourse. In some cases, small amounts (one-third to one-half an applicator) of a poorly absorbed estrogen like Premarin or Ortho-Dienestrol (dienestrol; no longer available in Canada) may help restore lubrication and atrophy of the vagina. However, if breast cancer has been diagnosed, use of even small amounts of estrogen may be discouraged. Do discuss this with your doctor.

• *Vaginal Shortening* Surgery or radiation therapy can cause shortening of the vagina or make the vagina less elastic. Either situation may make intercourse difficult. Your doctor may recommend dilators to exercise and stretch the vagina. Getting back to intercourse soon after treatment can also help prevent these problems. Different positions during intercourse, especially sitting or lying on top of your partner, may let you move in pleasurable ways. Although significant improvement can be expected after the first month of treatment with local estrogen-containing products (e.g. Premarin cream, estradiol vaginal tablets [Vagifem], or an estradiol vaginal ring [Estring]), often six to twelve months, or more, are required to fully restore the genitourinary tract to its normal state. This time lag also occurs when systemic therapy is used.

Vaginal dilators require prolonged regular use before they achieve maximal lengthening and stretching of the vagina. If treatment is begun early, a more rapid response can be expected. The penis is an excellent dilator; therefore repeated attempts at intercourse with adequate lubrication (natural or artificial), gentleness, and persistence are likely to succeed.

Do not be discouraged if initial attempts at penetration or complete penetration are unsuccessful or painful. Several months of treatment with hormone creams may be needed before the tissues soften adequately to allow penetration to occur.

• *Anxiety* Fear and anxiety may prevent the normal flow of vaginal fluids in response to sexual stimulation. Correction of this situation requires a number of combined treatments: application of a lubricating cream or gel plus relaxation plus and (most important) communication with your partner. Taking a little more time to enjoy foreplay may promote relaxation, enhance sexual response, and increase vaginal lubrication.

Sometimes anxiety can lead to a spasm of the pelvic muscles, which blocks the vaginal passage and prevents penetration. Forceful attempts at penetration may be both painful and frustrating. Consultation with a sex counselor may help you overcome the problem. This condition is readily treatable, so do not be discouraged if your initial attempts are unsuccessful.

Time, patience, sharing your feelings with your partner and support group members, and seeking help from your doctor and possibly also a sex counselor are your best guarantees of improving the quality of your sexual and intimate experiences.

Expressing Yourself Sexually After Treatment

With all the possible effects of cancer treatment, the prospect of having a normal sex life may seem out of reach. But whatever your cancer, there are steps you can take that will help you increase your sexual enjoyment.

If You've Had an Ostomy People with ostomies and their partners have to learn about ostomy appearance, care, and control. Women may be comfortable wearing special undergarments that cover a pouch while still permitting sexual stimulation. Specially designed and aesthetically attractive pouches are available.

If You've Had a Laryngectomy Laryngectomy patients should be acquainted with how to deal with sounds and odors escaping from their stomas. Wearing a stoma shield or a T-shirt will muffle the sound of breathing and will minimize your partner's feeling the air that is pushed through the stoma.

If You've Had a Mastectomy After a mastectomy, you may be worried about how you look. Undressing in front of your partner or sleeping in the nude may feel awkward and uncomfortable. That's natural, especially in light of the overemphasis our culture places on the sexual significance of breasts. Grieving over what you have lost is important. But with time and patience, most women overcome their self-consciousness and feel secure and comfortable with their bodies again.

Some women have found it helpful to explore and touch their bodies, including the area of the scar, while nude in front of a mirror. You may want to try this alone at first and then with a spouse, lover, or close friend. Share your feelings about your new body.

Be aware that your partner may not know what to say. Your spouse or lover may not know how or when to bring up the topic of sexuality and so may wait for you to do it. Your partner may be afraid of hurting or embarrassing you and want to protect your feelings. Sometimes this "protection" may feel like rejection. Although you might feel that it's risky to break the ice and approach the topic yourself, most patients as well as their partners feel relieved once they've done it.

You both may also worry about pain. If your incision or muscles are tender, minimize the pressure on your chest area. If you lie on your unaffected side, you can have more control over your movements and reduce any irritation to the incision. If your partner is on top, you may protect the affected area by putting your hand under your chin and your arm against your chest.

If you feel any pain, stop. And let your partner know why you are stopping. If he or she knows that you'll speak up when you notice any pain, you will both feel more relaxed and less inhibited in exploring and experimenting. Taking a rest or changing position may help you relax, and relaxing will usually decrease any pain. With communication and cooperation, you can work together to find positions and activities that give you the most pleasure.

Experimentation and time seem to be the keys to finding satisfactory ways of adapting to the loss of such a symbolically important part of the body as the breast. Talking with other women who have had mastectomies—women from the American or Canadian Cancer Society's Reach to Recovery program, or support groups, for example—can provide support and encouragement as well as suggestions about clothes and prostheses.

Some women find breast reconstruction important for their emotional well-being, while others find that they learn to love and appreciate their altered bodies over time.

If You're Having Trouble Reaching Orgasm
The natural interruption in the ability to experience sexual pleasure after an illness may make having orgasms more difficult for some women. If this is a problem for you, learning to re-explore pleasurable body sensations may be helpful.

It is important to do this when you can be alone and not distracted by having to please or perform for your partner. So find a comfortable place where you can be alone—your bedroom or bathroom—and a time when you won't be interrupted. Undress slowly and gently stroke your whole body. Then focus on the most sensitive areas—your neck, breasts, thighs, genitals, or any other area that feels good to you.

Use different kinds of touch, soft and light, firm and strong. Try moistening your hands with oil, lotion, or soap. Pay attention to the sensations you feel, and discover which ones are most pleasurable. Learning which kinds of touch feel best will help you heighten your sensation and will give you information to share with your partner. There are many excellent books on women's sexuality that can help to make you comfortable with this kind of exploration.

If You're Having Trouble with Erections
Since some drugs can temporarily interfere with the ability to have erections, you may want to ask your physician about possible side effects of your treatment.

Physical and Emotional Causes If you can get an erection by masturbating or you wake up with an erection in the night or morning, it is most likely that anxiety or "trying too hard" is the cause, and it's not a physical problem. If you are not sure of the cause, ask your doctor to refer you to a urologist or sex therapist or both for evaluation and treatment.

Taking the Pressure Off The more options you have for sexual expression, the less pressure there is on having erections. This in turn makes it more likely that they will happen. Many couples report that they have learned to have very pleasurable sexual experiences without erections or intercourse. Many kinds of sexual expression and stimulation do not require an erect penis. It may be reassuring to know that to have an orgasm, many women need or prefer direct stimulation by hand or mouth on or around the clitoris. This is stimulation that even an erect penis in a vagina can't provide.

If you explore other kinds of sexual touching and expression for a while, you may discover that erections will return with time or that the increased variety of sexual options satisfies both you and your partner. Patience, communication, and time are critical factors in developing pleasurable sexual experiences.

Counseling If erections don't come back and intercourse is important to you and your partner, ask your doctor to refer you to a sex therapist for counseling. Counseling will help you with relaxation techniques, with planning time for proper stimulation, and with methods for using visual stimulation and fantasy. Other cancer survivors who have had the same problem report that group counseling can also help.

A number of new medications for erection problems have come on the market in the last few years. Taken before a sexual encounter, these medications increase blood flow to the penis, resulting in an erection. The first of these, sildenafil (Viagra), became available in late 1997, followed by vardenafil (Levitra) and tadalafil (Cialis). They differ in onset of action, duration of action, and interaction with food. Sildenafil and vardenafil should be taken on an empty stomach for optimal effect, have an onset of action of thirty to sixty minutes and a duration of action of about four hours. On the other hand, tadalafil can be taken without regard to meals, has an onset of action of about forty-five minutes and a duration of action of twenty-four to thirty-six hours. Side effects include headaches, visual disturbances, and flushing. While considered generally safe for most men (including those using most blood pressure medications), sildenafil, vardenafil, and tadalafil should not be used by men taking nitrates. Medical clearance is essential prior to use of these drugs. Other medications are becoming available, so discuss the appropriateness of their use in your case.

If even with the help of these medications you are still not getting erections, the counselor may refer you to a urologist. Together with you and your counselor, the urologist can explore another option, such as use of a vacuum pump, injection therapy, or a penile implant.

Hormonal Replacement Therapy in Women

Estrogens from Reproductive Life to Menopause From puberty to menopause, the ovaries produce estrogen (estradiol), and when ovulation occurs, progesterone is added. The ovaries also produce the male hormones testosterone and androstenedione. Estrogen and progesterone act on their target organs, so called because they contain specific receptors or receiving areas where these hormones can enter the cells and produce the required effect. The target organs for estrogen and progesterone are the breasts, vulva, vagina, uterus, urethra, bladder, skin, and parts of the brain that control mood, sleep (insomnia), and temperature (hot flashes).

After menopause, the ovaries secrete very little estradiol, so the total amount of estrogen in the body drops to only a fraction of that produced during reproductive life. As a result, an alternative though small source of estrogen becomes significant. Male hormones continue to be produced by the adrenal gland—and, important, also by the ovaries—for about five years after menopause (the increased facial hair that women report in the early postmenopausal years is the result of the male hormones that continue to be secreted). These male hormones are carried to the skin, liver, body fat, and brain, where they are converted to a weak but effective estrogen, estrone. Body fat is a particularly important site of estrone production; it has long been recognized that women with more body fat have higher circulating estrone levels.

Why Is Estrogen Important? The degree to which estrogen affects the tissues becomes evident after menopause, when levels of estrogen drop. Following menopause, the deficiency in estrogen causes obvious symptoms such as hot flashes, insomnia, vaginal dryness, increased urinary frequency, increased incidence of bladder and vaginal infections, and in the long-term osteoporosis and a predisposition to arteriosclerosis. Hormonal replacement therapy (HRT) provides symptomatic relief whenever it is begun and is particularly important when the production of estrogen stops prematurely (before the age of forty)* because the long-term consequences (bone loss

---

* The Women's Health Initiative (WHI) studied the effects of menopausal hormone use in women fifty to eighty years of age and provided no guidance as to hormone use in women with premature ovarian failure.

and cardiovascular problems) are often even more significant.

What Are Menopause and Premature Ovarian Failure? Menopause means that the periods ("menses") have stopped ("paused"). Menopause occurs naturally around age fifty. However, radiation, chemotherapy, or surgical removal of the ovaries before menopause will result in ovarian hormone deficiency even earlier. In younger women who have experienced premature ovarian failure as a result of chemotherapy or radiation therapy, the ovaries may later begin to function again. Although we are unable to predict whether this will occur, factors that appear to play a role are age and type and amount of chemotherapy or radiation. Until ovarian function resumes, these women should be on hormonal replacement therapy and, if pregnancy is not desired, also on some form of contraception.

Hormonal therapy prescribed after menopause is often called estrogen therapy (ET) or hormone replacement therapy (HRT), which usually means estrogen with progestin therapy.

HRT Medications There are many possibilities for hormonal replacement therapy. Nonsmoking reproductive-aged women with premature ovarian failure (POF) are often best treated with birth control pills (oral contraceptives), which contain adequate amounts of both estrogen and progestin. The advantages of this approach are that the higher dose of hormones in birth control pills is what is often needed to control estrogen-deficiency symptoms in younger women, and that at the same time, it provides contraceptive protection should the ovaries begin to function again.

When vaginal or urinary symptoms persist despite systemic hormonal therapy, local hormonal therapy may be added. This may be in the form of an estrogen vaginal cream like Premarin or Ortho-Dienestrol (dienestrol; no longer available in Canada), estradiol vaginal tablets (Vagifem), or an estradiol vaginal ring (Estring).

Standard hormonal therapy consists of estrogen preparations, which include oral estrogens such as conjugated estrogen tablets (Premarin), estrone (Ogen), and estradiol (Estrace); an estradiol gel (EstroGel); and a transdermal estradiol patch (Estradot, Estraderm, or Climara). Women who have not had a hysterectomy need to add a progestin—either medroxyprogesterone acetate (Provera), norethindrone (Norlutate), or progesterone (Prometrium). Estrogen-progestin combinations may be used together, continuously (nonstop) or cyclically (i.e., estrogen alone for about two weeks, then estrogen with the addition of a progestin for an additional ten to fifteen days). Two products that contain a combination of both estrogen and progestin are available: CombiPatch, a transdermal estradiol-norethindrone patch, and FemHRT, an oral pill that contains ethinyl estradiol and norethindrone.

Another possibility is an implant under the skin (subdermal implant) of nomestrol acetate (Uniplant), which needs to be replaced every six months. This preparation currently is not available for use in Canada. For many years, a popular form of postmenopausal replacement therapy has been an injection of Duratestin, which is a combination of estradiol and testosterone that is given intramuscularly every six weeks. This preparation not only treats estrogen-deficiency symptoms, but also may improve libido as a result of the testosterone in the mixture. Occasionally, a small dose of testosterone is prescribed alone, specifically to treat problems of decreased libido. Oral tablets of Andriol (testosterone undecanoate) may be used two to three times per week and are available on prescription in Canada. Testosterone creams and gels in doses appropriate for women are not commercially available but can be compounded by some pharmacies for topical transdermal applications. A testosterone patch (Intrinsa) has been widely tested in North America and found to be effective in the treatment of women distressed about their problem of low libido. The testosterone patch is currently under review by Health Canada, and it is hoped that they will approve the use of this product in the near future.

Treatment Routines Estrogen with or without a progestin may be given cyclically (resulting in "menstrual periods") or in a continuous combined nonstop regimen (no "menstrual periods"). A common routine using both estrogen and progestin is to give estrogen alone for fourteen to fifteen days, then add progestin (such as medroxyprogesterone acetate [Provera]) for seven to fourteen days. Both hormones are then stopped, and a period follows in one or two days. The cycle is repeated monthly.

Similarly, if continuous estrogen is given and progestin is added only for twelve to fourteen days, a period is expected one or two days after the progestin is stopped. This routine is commonly used with transdermal preparations.

For women who do not wish to have a period but want and need HRT, a combined routine of estrogen and progestin is given continuously. After a short adjustment period (approximately six months) during which some vaginal bleeding may occur, most women enjoy all the benefits of HRT, including relief of hot flashes, insomnia, and vaginal and urinary symptoms.

Effects of HRT HRT has numerous normal effects, not all of which are welcomed by women. These effects, addressed below, are the result of estrogen's effects on the target organs and tissues. Obvious early benefits include a reduction in hot

flashes and night sweats and more restful sleep. Some women also report a greater sense of well-being.

After a few months' treatment, women may notice other beneficial effects. The vagina and cervix can be expected to become healthier and more moist with increased vaginal secretion and better lubrication during intercourse. Many women also report increased sexual awareness and enhanced sexual response after starting hormone replacement therapy. In addition, fewer bladder and vaginal infections occur.

However, there may be some normal but undesirable effects as well, including increased sensitivity and sometimes tenderness of the breasts, increased vaginal discharge, and the return of vaginal bleeding, or "menstruation."

Is Hormonal Replacement Therapy (HRT) for You? Whether or not systemic HRT is appropriate or likely to prove beneficial for you can best be decided by your doctor. Talk to him or her about the possibility of this treatment. You may be an ideal candidate. This is particularly likely if your periods have stopped and menopause has occurred in your early forties or before. On the other hand, you may want or need to manage your symptoms without hormones.

Management of Menopausal Symptoms Without Hormonal Replacement Standard estrogen therapy may not be safe or appropriate for some; thus, it is heartening that considerable research has been directed to finding other, nonhormonal and nonmedical approaches that can improve sexual functioning and menopausal symptoms after breast cancer. These include giving patients access to educational pamphlets discussing menopause, estrogen replacement therapy, urinary incontinence, tamoxifen (Nolvadex), and sexuality and teaching them the use of slow abdominal breathing (for hot flashes), the use of Kegel pelvic-floor-muscle exercises (for urinary incontinence and sexual response), and the use of moisturizers such as Replens and lubricants such as Astroglide (for vaginal dryness). Also, patients with particular psychosocial stressors benefit from referral to counseling or to support groups.

General Guidelines for Resuming Sexual Activity

Whenever you are sick, your usual sense of control over your body may be shaken. You may feel inadequate and helpless. An illness can change the way you experience your body or it might actually change the way you look because of surgery, amputation, scarring, or weight loss or gain.

These changes can create painful anxiety. You wonder whether you'll be able to function in your usual social, sexual, and career roles. You wonder what people will think of you. This anxiety—and the depression and fatigue that often go along with it—understandably make sexuality seem less important. But once the immediate crisis has passed, sexual feelings and how to express them may become important again.

Feeling anxious about resuming sexual activity is normal and natural. It is easy to "get out of practice." You may have questions about whether sexual activity will hurt you in some way. You may wonder how you will be able to experience sexual pleasure, and your partner may share the same worries. He or she may be especially concerned about tiring you out or hurting you somehow.

But once you resume sexual relations, your comfort and confidence should gradually increase. If not, sex counseling may help you discover ways to deal with whatever problems you are having. For many people, a "new start"—by themselves or through counseling—is refreshing. It might even create opportunities

for greater intimacy and sharing than ever before.

What to Do When You Are in the Hospital
Your cancer treatment might involve long stays in the hospital and long separations from those you love. Hospitals or rehabilitation facilities don't usually provide much privacy, so there may be little opportunity for sexual expression unless you speak up.

Although health care facilities are rarely designed to ensure patients' privacy, there is no reason why you and your partner can't have time for intimate physical contact in the hospital. With a little friendly intervention, your doctor might be able to arrange for a special room where you and your loved one can spend some time alone. Or you can always make a sign reading "Do Not Disturb Until ___ o'clock" or "Please Knock" and hang it on the door to your room. The nurses will respect your wishes.

If this sounds important to you, ask your doctor to speak to the hospital staff and help foster a caring and respectful attitude toward your need to express your sexuality with guaranteed privacy. It takes some education and maybe a change in the "way things are always done around here," but may be well worth the effort.

Developing Helpful Attitudes and Practices Whenever you are ready to become sexually active again, there are a few things you should keep in mind.

• *You are loved for who you are, not just for your appearance.* If you were considered lovable or sexually desirable before you got cancer, chances are that you will be afterward, too. Your partner, your family, and your friends will still love you and value you, as long as you let them.

• *We are all sexual beings.* Whether we are sexually active or not, sexuality is part of who we are. It is not defined just by what we do or how often we do it.

• *Survival overshadows sexuality.* If you've lost your good health, it is normal and natural for stress, depression, worry, and fatigue to lower your interest in sex. Just coping with basic everyday decisions can seem like a burden. But take one day at a time and be patient. Sexual interest and feelings will probably come back when the immediate crisis has passed.

• *Share your feelings.* Making relationships work is a task we all face, but it can be made more difficult by worries about our worth and attractiveness. Whether you are looking for a new relationship or already have a regular partner, you may find yourself in the position of having to share your sexual feelings with someone, perhaps for the first time.

This sharing may feel awkward at first. Learning how and when to talk about sexual issues may not come easily. You may feel shy or nervous about exploring new and different ways of finding sexual pleasure. You may be waiting for your partner to make the first move, while your partner is waiting for you to make the advances. This familiar waiting game is often misunderstood as rejection by both people. It may be frightening to think of breaking the silence yourself. Yet a good move is to make the first move. Try sharing some of the myths or expectations you grew up with about sexuality. Often this is humorous and may break the ice in starting a frank discussion about your sexual needs and concerns. Try not to make broad, generalized statements. Talk about what is important to *you* and about how *you* feel. The payoff is greater understanding of each other's needs and concerns, and that is worth the effort.

• *Expect the unexpected.* The first time you have sex after treatment, physical limitations, worry about your performance or appearance, or fear of rejection may keep you from focusing on the sheer pleasure of physical contact. On the other hand, you may be surprised by unfamiliar pleasurable sensations. If you expect some changes as part of the natural recovery process, they will be less likely to distract you from sexual pleasure if they do happen.

• *Give yourself time.* You and your partner may be frightened of, or even repulsed by, scars, unfamiliar appliances, or other physical changes. That's natural, too. But such feelings are usually temporary. Talking about them is often the first step to mutual support and acceptance. Don't pressure yourself about having to "work on sex." A satisfactory and enjoyable sex life will happen one step at a time. You may want to spend some time by yourself exploring your body, becoming familiar with changes, and rediscovering your unique body texture and sensations. Once you feel relaxed doing this, move on to mutual body exploration with your partner.

• *Take the pressure off intercourse.* Almost all of us were brought up to believe that intercourse is the only real or appropriate way of expressing ourselves sexually. Yet sexual expression can encompass many forms of touching and pleasuring that are satisfying psychologically and physically.

When you resume sexual activity, try spending some time in pleasurable activities—touching, fondling, kissing, and being close—without having intercourse. Reexperience the pleasure of playing, of holding, and of being held without having to worry about erections and orgasms. When you feel comfortable, proceed at your own pace to other ways of being sexual, including intercourse if you like.

Experiment and explore to discover what feels best and what is acceptable. If radiation therapy, for example, has made intercourse painful, try oral or manual stimulation to orgasm, or intercourse between thighs or breasts. If you are exhausted by the disease or movement is painful, just cuddling or lying quietly next to your partner can be a wonderfully satisfying form of intimacy.

• ***Don't let your diagnosis dictate what you can do sexually.*** Your sexuality cannot be "diagnosed." You will never know what pleasures you are capable of experiencing if you don't explore. Try new positions, new touches, and above all new attitudes.

• ***Your brain is your best and most important sex organ!*** And its ability to experience sensation is virtually limitless.

• ***Plan sex around your changing energy levels.*** Life with cancer can be exhausting. Fatigue, depression, and just feeling sick are almost normal for cancer patients at certain times. The amount of energy you have for all kinds of activities, including sex, can vary from day to day or week to week. So plan sexual activities to coincide with the times when you think you will feel best.

• ***Ask for help if you need it.*** Don't hesitate to seek counseling or information if you have problems. Help is available from a wide range of sources. If you want to discuss any problems, bring them up with your health care providers. Ask them to recommend competent sex counselors or therapists in your area. There may also be other resources available nearby, such as people who have had both cancer and experience in talking about sexual concerns.

• ***Be patient.*** The important thing is to be patient, with both yourself and your partner. You won't adjust overnight. Give yourself time to explore and share

your feelings about your body changes and time to again see yourself as a desirable sexual being. When you can accept the way your body looks and recognize your potential for sexual pleasure, it will be easier to imagine someone else doing the same.

The satisfaction and good feelings—emotional and physical—that can come from a sexual relationship require patience, communication, respect, cooperation, and a willingness to remember that in some respects the relationship must be learned all over again, physically if not emotionally.

Everything may not work properly at first. Everything may not be enjoyable at first. But for those for whom sexuality is still an important component of their intimacy, continuing to have the courage and confidence to keep trying should bring healing results.

BIBLIOGRAPHY

Books

Alterwitz R. *Intimacy and Impotence: The Couple's Guide to Better Sex After Prostate Disease.* Cambridge, Mass.: Da Capo Press, 2004.

Written in an honest, compassionate style by a patient with prostate cancer and his wife. Discusses impotence in nonmedical terms, with information on commercial treatments. Gives practical advice about making love. Includes everything from getting into the mood to commonsense suggestions for having sexual satisfaction and intimacy when erections are not possible.

Barbach L. *For Yourself*, revised. New York: Signet, 2001.

———. *For Each Other*, revised. New York: Signet, 2001.

Classics that empower women to enjoy their own sexuality, with suggestions for women who want to learn to become orgasmic alone and with a partner.

———. *Loving Together: Sexual Enrichment Program*. New York: Signet, 1997.
Self-help workbooks for men and women.

Barbach L, Geisinger D. *Going the Distance: Finding and Keeping Lifelong Love*. New York: Plume, 1993.
Wonderful and realistic book on maintaining intimacy.

Bostwick D, MacLennan G, Larsen T. *Prostate Cancer: What Every Man—and His Family—Needs to Know*, revised. New York: Villard, 1999.

Brownworth V (ed.). *Coming Out of Cancer: Writings from the Lesbian Cancer Epidemic*. Seattle: Seal Press, 2000.

Dackman L. *Up Front: Sex and the Post-Mastectomy Woman*. New York: Viking, 1990.
Moving and insightful account of one woman's experiences.

Fincannon J, Bruss K. *Couples Confronting Cancer: Keeping Your Relationship Strong*. American Cancer Society, Atlanta Chapter, 2003.

Gottman J. *The Seven Principles for Making Marriage Work*. New York: Simon & Schuster, 1999.
———. *Why Marriages Succeed or Fail . . . and How You Can Make Yours Last*. New York: Simon & Schuster, 1994.
Results of over twenty-five years of research pointing out the danger signals for troubled marriages, with suggestions to help marital communication.

Hefferman M, Quinn M. *The Gynaecological Cancer Guide: Sex, Sanity, and Survival*. Melbourne: Michele Anderson Publishing, 2003.

Written by an Australian patient and her physician to show that a good life after cancer is possible. Includes anatomy and function of female reproductive organs, gynecological cancers and their treatment, and thoughtful and comprehensive strategies about sexual survival during and after cancer therapy.

Keen S. *To Love and Be Loved*. New York: Bantam Books, 1997.
Beautifully and simply written book on the various aspects of loving relationships; how to establish and maintain intimacy in communication.

Kydd S, Rowett D. *Intimacy After Cancer: A Woman's Guide*. Redmond, Wash.: Big Think Media, 2006.
Based on the personal stories shared by cancer survivors and nurses, oncologists, and psychiatrists treating cancer patients; for more information, see *www.intimacyaftercancer.com*.

Ogden G. *The Heart and Soul of Sex*. Boston: Trumpeter Books, 2006.
Discussion of national survey of ethnically diverse women ages twenty-one to eighty-five years in expanding the view of sexuality, intimacy, spirituality, and religion. Suggests various strategies to enhance and explore women's sexuality.

Schover L. *Prime Time: Sexual Health for Men over Fifty*. New York: Holt, 1984.
Provides validation and useful suggestions for men and their partners.

———. *Sexuality and Fertility After Cancer*. New York: John Wiley & Sons, 1997.
A useful book covering various issues about sex and fertility. Helpful in learning how to enjoy sex again and to make informed choices about pregnancy after cancer treatment.

——. *Sexuality and Cancer: For the Man Who Has Cancer, and His Partner.* American Cancer Society, 1988.

——. *Sexuality and Cancer: For the Woman Who Has Cancer, and Her Partner.* American Cancer Society, 1988.

Excellent, comprehensive booklets.

Smith W. *A Portrait of Breast Cancer: Expressions in Words and Art.* Oklahoma City: Project Woman Coalition, 1996.

Wainrib B, Haber S. *Men, Women, and Prostate Cancer: A Medical and Psychological Guide for Women and the Men They Love.* Oakland, Calif.: New Harbinger Publications, 2000.

Welwood J. *Perfect Love, Imperfect Relationships: Healing the Wound of the Heart.* Boston: Trumpeter, 2006.

Eloquently describes how our deepest longing for love is in fact the key to healing our personal wounds and the wounded nature of the world at large . . . echoing Buddha, with the message that we have direct access to the love and happiness we most long for, as our very essence.

Zilbergeld B. *The New Male Sexuality,* revised. New York: Bantam, 1999.

A commonsense, practical discussion of the fantasy model of sex and myths of male sexuality and the importance of an individual's conditions for good sex; with specific self-help chapters dealing with common male and couples' sexual problems.

— 29 —

Staying Physically Fit

Francine Manuel, R.P.T., Ernest H. Rosenbaum, M.D.,
Jack LaLanne, and Isadora R. Rosenbaum, M.A.

If you were involved in an exercise program before you became ill, you will probably be open to the idea of getting involved in an active program all through your recovery. But if you have never been involved in an organized exercise routine, you may need some encouragement. Welcome this encouragement if you get it. If you don't get it, seek it out, because getting and staying physically fit should be one of your most important goals.

Why You Should Exercise

Physical fitness is healthy for everyone, of course. But it is essential for all cancer patients. Even though it's hard to find the energy to exercise when you are sick, the benefits of keeping your body in an active state are too great to ignore. When you participate in a daily exercise program you will reap the following rewards:

1. You will improve your prognosis.

If you are in good physical condition, you may tolerate therapy better. This, in turn, may allow you to have more aggressive treatments and so stand a better chance of remission or cure. It is well known that successful treatment and an improved prognosis depend directly on physical status. The simple truth is that if you are physically fit, you may live longer and enjoy a more active life.

2. You will stop your muscles from wasting away.

When we are healthy, we all usually exercise our muscles one way or another—by walking up and down stairs, doing housework, going shopping, taking part in athletic activities like golf and tennis, or simply by walking as we go about our business. Even a low level of activity helps to maintain muscle tone and strength. But during an acute or chronic illness, prolonged bed rest is often necessary. Muscles shrink in size and strength when they're not used for a long time. An exercise program will make sure that that doesn't happen to you.

3. You will recover faster.

If you do not exercise after surgery or while you're undergoing radiotherapy or chemotherapy, your muscles will get weaker and weaker. The tissues that may be broken down by therapy will not be repaired as quickly as they should be. By exercising, you can help your tissues rebound and you can minimize any deterioration in your joints. You might also help prevent complications such as bone softening, blood clots, and bedsores. And, not least, you'll get some relief from the boredom and depression that often come with being confined to bed.

When to Start

Become physically active as soon as possible after treatment. It is now the general practice within one day of surgery to get out of bed and at least sit in a chair. Even this minimal activity helps reduce the loss of muscle mass and increase strength.

True, pain can limit physical exercise after a mastectomy, bowel surgery, or some other major operation. And you may be depressed by a change in your body image and not feel like doing anything. You may need help to get going. But with appropriate timing, you should turn your attention to rehabilitation.

In the Hospital At least a gentle exercise program should begin while you are still in the hospital. This may involve simple muscle tightening while you lie in bed or passive muscle exercises administered by a physical therapist or taught to your family. As your strength returns, different forms of physical activity—isometric and isotonic exercises and rhythmic repeated movements for various muscles—will help get you on the path to improved fitness. Massage therapy can complement these activities, helping you relax your mind and body and improving your circulation.

You might think all this will involve too much of an effort while you're still in the hospital. But you will feel much more confident when you do go home if you have already started to regain your strength. You will also be less prone to falls or other accidents that might result from a weakened condition.

Planning a Program

Before you leave the hospital, physical therapists can assess your physical condition and come up with an appropriate set of exercises. Everyone has different wants and needs, so programs are usually customized. They will also be flexible,

taking your energy level into account. The staff of the physical therapy department can also instruct you, your family, and other caregivers on how to proceed with your program at home. Their recommendations on an appropriate program may be essential to your recovery.

Safety Rules When you begin exercising, keep in mind a few simple rules for safety:

• Ask your doctor if you're ready to exercise. Let him or her set limits to your activity.
• Have someone join you. This will make the exercise more enjoyable and safer, especially when you are just getting out of bed and may feel dizzy.
• Stop and rest if you feel tired or if your muscles are sore.
• Leave out any exercises that seem too difficult and try them another day when you feel stronger.
• Try to repeat each exercise three to five times at first, then gradually increase the repetitions to ten or twenty.
• Try to exercise at least twice a day, more often if you feel up to it.

The most important rule is to start out gradually. Don't overdo it. Muscles that haven't been used for days or weeks will strain very easily. Light warm-up exercises several times a day will be useful, both as a starting point for your program and as a daily prelude to more vigorous exercises later on.

When you start your exercise program, you might experience some fatigue, dizziness, or even nausea. Discuss any problems with your doctor or physical therapist. But these side effects usually pass fairly quickly.

Working Through the Stages A graduated program may take you through three stages, or you can use all three stages depending on how you feel:

• *Stage 1—Beginning-to-Move Exercises* These are simple exercises that help you maintain and increase your range of motion. They don't require much exertion and can be done while you are lying in bed.

• *Stage 2—Increased-Activity Exercises* A small weight (up to 2 pounds [1 kg]) is used to increase resistance. These exercises can be done when you are spending part of the day out of bed sitting in a chair.

• *Stage 3—Up-and-About Exercises* These exercises will build up your strength when you are able to stand, walk, and spend the whole day out of bed. (For more detailed information, consult *Rehabilitation Exercises for the Cancer Patient*, by Ernest H. Rosenbaum, Francine Manuel, Judith Bray, Isadora R. Rosenbaum, and Arthur Cerf, available from Bull Publishing, PO Box 208, Palo Alto, CA 94302.)

Setting a Regular Routine Once you are back on your feet and approaching your normal level of activity, you can establish a set routine, naturally within any limitations or restrictions identified by your doctor. A very enjoyable workout program can be created.

Aerobic programs are a helpful addition to the three-stage program. You take your pulse before beginning, then take it again halfway through and at the end of the routine. The aim is to roughly double your heart rate, although your physician may set a specific rate that you should not exceed.

There are a great number of aerobic programs to choose from. You may even alternate programs to avoid boredom. A variety of TV shows can take you through an aerobic workout every day, although aerobic programs need only be done for twenty minutes, three times a week, to achieve maximum benefits. If you have

a VCR or DVD player, Jane Fonda or other celebrities can take you step by step through a program with their videos. These videos are widely available and offer an ideal way to work up to a full routine. Some of the videos show a slower group on one side and a faster-paced group on the other. You can also stop the video or limit the number of repetitions. Most sport stores and movie rental stores carry these tapes and DVDs. Some carry used tapes and DVDs at a discounted price.

If aerobics are not for you, there are all kinds of machines—stationary bikes, stair climbers, treadmills, rowing or skiing machines, and so on—that use weights or hydraulics to build all your muscles. Home equipment is worthwhile if you have a busy schedule and want to work out at your own pace at your own convenience. Some of these units are expensive, but some can be purchased at a more reasonable price, during special sales.

You can go to a health club if you want a variety of equipment to choose from and to be with people who are also working out. Or, if you don't feel comfortable with a formal program, there are always the options of stair climbing and brisk walking. You can go up and down your stairs at home for fifteen to twenty minutes every other day or take a long walk, perhaps during your lunch hour if you have returned to work, every other day. Whatever your routine, staying active will build up your body's reserves so that if you do need a temporary period of bed rest, your energy stores won't be depleted.

While you should think of your program as being as much a part of your recovery as visits to the doctor, try to enjoy yourself. Exercising can be a lot of fun. And it can be very stimulating. If you have days when depression and boredom get you down and exercising seems like too much of a burden, just remind yourself of all the benefits of exercising regularly. Your program will improve your energy level and stamina, improve your appetite, help you relax, and help you sleep at night. The more you exercise, the better you will feel.

— 30 —

Home Care

Barbara J. Buckley, M.S.W., L.C.S.W., Susan Sweeney, R.N., Ph.N.,
Ernest H. Rosenbaum, M.D., Malin Dollinger, M.D., and Isadora R. Rosenbaum, M.A.

■ ■ ■ ■

The trend in providing more care at home has continued to accelerate over the past decade. There are many reasons for this. Hospital stays are getting shorter, in part due to changes in medical practice. Some surgical techniques have changed, resulting in less time needed for recuperation. Most chemotherapy is done outside the hospital, with fewer side effects than in years past. Medical staff recognize that the hospital is not always the best place for healing. And the rapid changes in health insurance, with attendant regulations and insurance oversight, have also contributed to the changes in medical practice.

Most people feel much more comfortable in the warm, familiar surroundings of home than they do in a hospital or rehabilitation center. Medical facilities can seem strange, antiseptic, regulated, and sometimes forbidding. Yet some cancer patients may wish to prolong their hospital stay. Why? Because they or their caregivers are afraid they won't get proper treatment at home or be able to cope with home care problems.

These fears are understandable, but they can be overcome. Medical and nonmedical crises can be anticipated. And questions can be answered and crises sometimes avoided by education and hands-on training in the elements of home care. This education will begin before discharge from the hospital and may be continued and reinforced by the home care nurse. Both patients and their caregivers should be involved, to the extent of their ability, in learning about the patient's care at home.

Is Home Care for You? Home care can play a vital part in your healing and recovery. But it isn't for everyone. There are times when going home is just not practical. Your physical needs may be complex and require more care than is practical to provide at home. Also, you and your caregivers need to assess your ability to cope with the psychological stress of a home care situation. Support can be provided to you and your caregivers to help with the stress, but still it may be too difficult.

It may be hard for someone with cancer to endure the feelings that daily dependence on family and other loved ones can bring. And the stress of having a chronically ill person at home may be difficult for a family already overwhelmed by other responsibilities. These concerns are best addressed by good communication between all concerned, sometimes with the assistance of a neutral third party such as a counselor, clergyperson, or oncology social worker. You as a family may decide that it is not feasible to provide care at home, and another option such as assisted living, residential hospice, or a skilled nursing facility needs to be considered.

Home care is a cooperative effort. You, your caregivers, and your medical team are all involved. The decision to go home has to be made by all concerned—the attending physician, discharge planners, your caregivers, and you.

Planning to Go Home

The key to successful home care is planning. This should begin from the day of hospital admission . . . if not before! Changes may be needed in the way your home is organized. You might have to buy or rent special equipment and work out the routines necessary for proper care. All this may seem like a lot of work, maybe even too much of a burden. Yet a comfortable and workable home care environment can be devised. And it can be a helpful step in your recovery.

Discharge Planning Once you and your medical team have made the decision for you to go home, you should be able to call on the services of a discharge planner. This person may be a medical social worker, public health nurse, nurse or social work case manager, or hospital discharge coordinator. He or she will help you and your caregivers define your needs and match them with the resources available in your community.

Training Prior to your discharge from the hospital, one of your nurses will provide you and your caregivers with some education about your needs at home. This usually includes information about your medications and your physical care. If your physician orders it, this education will be reinforced and expanded by the home care nurse who sees you in your home.

For more intensive education, you and your family and other caregivers may want to look for workshops and education programs focusing on caregiver training. These may be organized by an outpatient department or cancer center, a home care company, or a national organization such as the National Brain Tumor Foundation or the Family Caregiver Alliance. The programs vary in length, but most will address both the "hands-on" technical information you may need and coping issues. Many caregivers find it especially helpful to meet with others who are going through a similar situation.

Assessing Your Resources Since the objective of home care is to keep your home life as normal as possible while still providing you with quality medical care, the first step to effective home care is taking a good look both at the support available to you and at the physical layout of your home.

Home care requires a willingness of family and friends to accept the responsibility of helping you on a sustained basis. Some key questions have to be answered:

• How much time can your family and friends commit to you?
• How will they balance providing support to you with their work and other responsibilities?
• If more than one person will be providing care, can a rotation schedule be worked out?
• Are there others (such as children or elders) in the home with demands that need to be met?
• Can each caregiver have enough free time to maintain his or her own physical and emotional well-being?
• Do you have the financial resources to hire a private nurse or home health aide to provide some of the day-to-day assistance?

In the home, you and your caregivers, with assistance from the home health care staff, should look carefully at the physical setup. Pay special attention to the bathroom and bedroom, the location of stairs, and the space available for extra equipment. You may want to remove scatter rugs or small objects on the floors. Railings or grab bars might be installed, and rubber strips attached to the tub and shower to prevent slipping.

Equipment The discharge planner, with follow-up by the home health care nurse, will also help you decide what equipment you will need.

Following are some commonly needed aids:

• Hospital beds: manual, semielectric, or electric; safety side rails; overhead trapeze bars; overbed tables
• Wheelchairs: standard folding or powered chairs—with or without footrests
• Bathroom safety equipment: bath benches, grab bars, shower attachments, elevated toilet seats, and toilet assist frames
• Patient aids: commode chairs, flotation pads, sheepskin pads, transfer lifts, and respiratory equipment
• Patient care items: foam cushion rings, bedpans, urinals, heel and elbow protectors, sitz baths, and incontinence pads and pants

Some, but not all, will usually be covered by health insurance policies. Policies vary widely, and you will need to check your own policy. Your discharge planner may also be able to help you with this. And the home health care agency or the companies who supply this equipment will also check with your insurance and obtain the necessary authorizations if the equipment is covered by your policy. (For additional information, see "Aids to Daily Living," in *Everyone's Guide to Cancer Supportive Care* by Ernest H. Rosenbaum, M.D., and Isadora R. Rosenbaum, M.A., and the Web site *www.cancersupportivecare.com*.)

Other Resources The discharge planner can also give you information about community resources, including home health agencies and private attendant care agencies. The local chapter of the American Cancer Society can also provide information about resources, support groups, and organizations devoted to specific illnesses and their problems.

Getting Treatment at Home

Why are we talking so much about getting treatment at home? In a way, things have come full circle. In the early 1900s, medicine had much less to offer in the way of specific therapies than it does now. Before the age of antibiotics, modern diagnostic tools, and effective treatment for many now curable diseases, doctors sent their patients to the hospital only when they were extremely ill. Medical care was given primarily in the home or in the doctor's office. But during the last century, as more and more technological advances and medical treatments became available, the hospital became the primary place for medical care. People were admitted for complex diagnostic studies and the initiation of therapy, especially for serious diseases like cancer.

But the pendulum has been swinging away from the hospital as the focus of medical care and back to the home and the outpatient arena. Both can be just as effective places for treatment as the hospital clinic. And both are a lot more convenient and comfortable. There are other advantages—lower cost and the ability of family and loved ones to offer direct supportive care.

Now hospitals are again used mainly for serious, life-threatening medical problems or complications, major surgery, or the start of complex therapies that require sophisticated equipment or observation that isn't available elsewhere.

Home Care Services

Home care services have expanded in many areas. A variety of important treatment procedures—including IV antibiotics, total parenteral nutrition, pain management, and some chemotherapy—can be provided in the home under the supervision of a trained nurse who is working closely with your physician. The ability to give these treatments safely at home has been greatly improved by the use of specialized venous access devices (see chapter 6, "What Happens in Surgery," and chapter 18, "Oncology Nursing").

If you are receiving these treatments at home, the home care nurse will train you and your caregivers in the techniques and procedures specific to your needs. This can include training in administering other medications through infusion or injection.

Health insurance companies are often quite willing to pay for home care, especially when the cost of providing the treatment at home is shown to be significantly less than it would cost in the hospital. Many insurance benefits, including Medicare and Medicaid, will pay for the home care services of an R.N., rehab therapists (physical, occupational, speech), a medical social worker, a nutritionist, and a home health aide. To be paid for by your insurance plan, the services need to be recommended and ordered by your physician, and they must also meet criteria established by your insurance.

Caring for Your Body

Like most people with cancer, you are probably going to have a number of problems in caring for your body. But these too can be anticipated and you can begin to deal with them before discharge from the hospital. You and your caregivers should begin receiving instructions in specific care techniques from your nurses in the hospital.

Bowel and Bladder Care You should be given a practical approach to bowel and bladder care. Special attention will be given to the problems of constipation, diarrhea, and incontinence. You and your caregivers should have a basic knowledge of laxatives, enemas, catheters, and dietary management (for more detailed information, see chapter 20, "Coping with the Side Effects of Chemotherapy," and chapter 23, "Maintaining Good Nutrition").

There are three main problems with the bowels and bladder, all uncomfortable, but all preventable in many cases:

• **Constipation** Irregular or infrequent bowel movements can be caused by many things: chemotherapy drugs, pain-controlling narcotics, changes in diet or environment, or lack of activity.

Adding foods high in fiber and bulk to your diet, such as fruits, vegetables, whole-grain breads and cereals, and bran may prevent constipation. You should also drink plenty of fluids and be as active as possible. Stool softeners, stimulating laxatives, and suppositories can help. More severe constipation can be relieved by enemas, either commercially prepared or a home mixture of 1 teaspoon (5 ml) of table salt and 1 pint (500 ml) of water. If your white blood cell count or platelet count is severely depressed, talk to your doctor about a remedy for constipation to help prevent infections and bleeding.

• **Diarrhea** Unusually frequent and liquid bowel movements can result from chemotherapy, radiation treatment, emotional stress, or sensitivity to certain foods. Your doctor can help find the cause and advise you if you need medication.

To relieve the discomfort, restrict yourself to warm fluids so your bowel can rest. Then gradually add foods low in roughage (such as dry toast, crackers, mashed potatoes, applesauce, and rice). As you slowly return to your normal diet, drink plenty of liquids to replace the fluids lost in the diarrhea.

• *Incontinence* If you have a problem controlling urination, two kinds of catheters can be used. Men can use a condom type, which fits snugly on the shaft of the penis and is attached to a gravity drainage bag. The other type is a Foley catheter, which is inserted directly into the bladder and attached to a bag that is changed regularly.

With either type, it is important to keep the skin clean and dry. With the Foley catheter, special care has to be taken to keep the connections and drainage port free of contamination. A nurse in the hospital and/or at home can show you and your caregivers the procedures to follow in handling each type of catheter. The removal or replacing of the catheter will be done by a health care professional.

Skin Care If you have to remain in bed for long periods of time, you will want to pay special attention to the condition of your skin. When some part of the body lies against a surface like a mattress for a long period, nutrients and oxygen cannot reach the skin cells. The area breaks down and the skin cells die. This creates pressure sores or bedsores. Your tailbone, hips, spine, elbows, ankles, and shoulder blades are particularly susceptible to these sores. It is especially important to prevent your skin from being damaged by this kind of chafing because the sores can become infected. Weight loss and the side effects of radiation or chemotherapy can lower resistance to infection.

Proper skin care, along with adequate nutrition, helps prevent pressure sores and will also keep you feeling refreshed. A nurse or physical therapist can instruct you and your family in the basic techniques of skin care, such as.

• frequent position changes (most important),
• dry, wrinkle-free linens,
• heat,
• gentle massage,

• good hygiene,
• the use of talcum and skin lotions, and
• the use of a foam rubber ("egg crate") mattress or a foam or sheepskin pad to cushion your body and provide better air circulation.

If bedsores occur, special nursing treatments will need to be instituted.

Mouth Care Daily care of your mouth and teeth is always necessary, but cancer treatment can create special problems. Radiation treatment affects the mouth when it is given directly to the area, and mouth sores may be a side effect of chemotherapy given for tumors in any part of the body.

You should brush your teeth daily with a soft-bristled brush. You might also floss daily to clean between the teeth, unless it becomes too irritating to your gums. Your mouth should also be kept moist, both for oral health and for comfort. If a dry mouth is a problem, your doctor can prescribe an artificial saliva or a saliva stimulant. Rinsing your mouth frequently with water and sucking on ice chips or sugarless candies can also help keep the mouth moist (see chapter 20, "Coping with the Side Effects of Chemotherapy," and chapter 23, "Maintaining Good Nutrition").

Fatigue Many people with cancer find that fatigue is a major problem and the one that most keeps them from enjoying their everyday life. There are many reasons for this. Anemia is a side effect that is experienced by some people receiving chemotherapy. If that is the case, there may be helpful medications that your physician can prescribe.

In addition, there are some other things you can do that may reduce your sense of fatigue:

• Get enough rest, including short naps during the day if needed.

• Prioritize your activities, doing only those that are most important to you.

• Be sure to ask for help with activities and chores.

• Eat a well-balanced diet.

Pain Control

Patients about to go home from the hospital are often worried about how they will deal with pain. If they have been relying on the doctors and nurses to give them their pain medication, they often wonder, "Who will give me the medicine at home?" "What if I run out of medicine?" "Suppose I need an injection?" "What if I'm alone and the pain gets worse?"

The most important thing to remember is that most pain can be relieved. There are many medications available and one or more of them will certainly help (see chapter 24, "Controlling Pain"). Also remember that pain is a complex experience that is not totally physical. Psychological and emotional factors play a major role in anyone's response to pain. Chronic pain that is relieved for a while and then returns can be very tiring. That fatigue in turn can make the pain worse. Acute or sudden pain can set off anxieties and fears.

The key to overcoming pain is to feel that you are the "expert" and that you can do something about it. Having control over pain helps you relax. Relaxation means less anxiety, and less anxiety means less pain.

Keeping Track of Your Pain When your physician recommends a program of pain medication, it will be important for you and your caregivers to keep a record of how the medication affects you. This will be the first step in gaining control over your pain.

Monitor where the pain is, what it feels like—sharp, dull, intermittent, or stabbing—how long it takes the medication to start working, how long the relief lasts, and whether there are any side effects. Grade your pain on a scale of 0 to 10, with 0 being no pain at all and 10 being the most severe pain you have felt. All this information will help your doctor make changes in the dosage or prescribe other, possibly more effective, medication. As you become more aware of how the medication is working, you will feel more confident about managing your pain control program at home.

Injections Your pain medication may be in the form of pills, liquids, patches, rectal suppositories, or injections. Pills, liquids, patches, or suppositories are usually easy to use. But many people are afraid to give themselves injections.

These fears can be overcome with help and a little training in the proper techniques from nurses at the hospital, at the infusion center, or in your home. After all, many diabetics give themselves injections every day. A nurse can show you and your caregivers how to measure the medication and draw it into the syringe, how to prepare the skin, and how to inject the needle. With a little practice, you will feel able to give a shot safely and comfortably. Once you know you can do it, you will have more confidence that you can control your pain.

Where to Give the Injection The doctor or nurse will also advise you about where to give the injection. Generally, medications that are either irritating to the skin or designed to act quickly are injected deep into the muscle tissue (intramuscular). Nonirritating medications are often injected just below the skin (subcutaneous).

The three common places of intramuscular injections are the upper outer portion of the buttocks, the thigh midway between the hip and the knee, and the upper arm about a third of the way down from the shoulder to the elbow. The most common places to give subcutaneous injections are the fleshy part of the upper arm and the abdomen.

Infusions Continuous infusions of pain medicine, either through an IV catheter such as a Hickman or subcutaneously through a small plastic needle, may be used for severe pain or pain not relieved by a variety of oral or injected medicines. Small pumps are used so you can remain mobile and as active as your condition allows. A home health nurse will instruct you and your caregivers about the operation of the pump. (For more information about ports and pumps, see chapter 6, "What Happens in Surgery," chapter 8, "What Happens in Chemotherapy," and chapter 18, "Oncology Nursing.")

Side Effects Pain medications can produce side effects such as nausea and constipation, but both can be treated. It's very important, however, that you tell your doctor about the side effects and let him or her recommend what to do about them. Treating them yourself can cause complications. If you take certain types of bulk laxatives at the same time as narcotic pain medications, for example, the laxative can actually cause rather than relieve severe constipation.

If There's an Emergency

One of the biggest fears you and your caregivers may have when planning a home care program is what will happen if there's an emergency. Your doctor, home care nurse, or social worker can help you and your caregivers prepare for emergencies. They can answer your questions about things that might come up and discuss procedures for getting help quickly. You may also want instruction in appropriate first-aid procedures. You may want to consider wearing a Medic Alert bracelet or getting an emergency response system that will call for help for you if you are alone and have an emergency.

For your own peace of mind, there are two things you can prepare that may be helpful to have at home:

• A card listing the telephone numbers of your doctor, home health agency, pharmacy, ambulance service, fire department, and police department, and a close relative or friend. Keep the card by the telephone.

• A self-care card recording important facts about your condition and medications. You may not always be able to reach your own doctor and if you or your family have to explain things to another doctor on call, you may get confused or lose valuable time if vital information isn't at your fingertips. The self-care card should include your name and diagnosis, treatments you've been getting, chemotherapy drugs and any other medications you are taking, any allergies, your blood type, and the names and numbers of other doctors involved in your care.

What to Do If an emergency does arise, you and your caregivers should follow three basic principles:

1. *Stay calm.* Remember that help is always available and will usually arrive within minutes of an emergency call.

2. *Determine the problem and call for help.* Check the pulse rate to see if it is fast, slow, or irregular. Check for breathing problems, changes in mental state, new pain or sudden increases in pain, nausea or vomiting, or injuries from a fall or other accident. If the symptoms seem to require immediate attention, call the doctor or an emergency service. 911 is the universal emergency call number.

3. *Take appropriate action while waiting for help to arrive.* The most common emergencies are heart-related problems, breathing problems, bleeding, broken bones, and falls.

Though hospital and home health agency staff can give family members some training in dealing with these emergencies, the best preparation is a first-aid course taught by the Red Cross or other community organization. These courses teach the technique of cardiopulmonary resuscitation (CPR), the Heimlich maneuver to deal with choking, how to stop serious bleeding, and what to do to keep someone comfortable when bones are broken. The most important thing for caregivers to keep in mind is, *when in doubt, call for help.*

Emotional Support for Your Family and Caregivers

If you have been in the hospital, you may feel a little frightened when you first get home. But you'll probably be eager to be sleeping in your own bed and returning to your own routines. Your loved ones will also be glad to have you home, but they may be worried, too. They will wonder about providing you with the proper care. They will have to deal with new routines, changing roles, new expectations. Also, they will have to deal with the many changes of mood and behavior you'll go through as you cope with your illness.

Home care is a major commitment for your caregivers. They give not only their physical services, but also their empathy and compassion. Many people with cancer, because of the intensity of their illness, are often able to give little emotional support in return.

So loved ones may need special emotional support. They may feel left out of critical decisions, burdened with responsibilities, afraid of what the future will bring. They may feel sad because of changes in their relationship with you and the losses they are experiencing. They may feel angry about the disruption of their own lives and guilty for any number of reasons. Children also have special needs that will vary according to their age and their relationship with you.

The Importance of Communication The emotional needs of everyone can best be met by planning and by open communication. If more than one person is involved in your care, a schedule to rotate responsibilities should be arranged. Everyone needs to have some free time for his or her own physical and emotional well-being. It is important that caregivers be helped not to feel guilty for considering their own needs as well as yours and for taking time for their own activities.

Feelings, especially fears and resentments, should be discussed as openly as possible. Bottled-up feelings can be difficult to manage and exhausting for everyone. However, every individual and family and culture has their own style of handling feelings, and these differences must be respected. But there are always some ways to have healthy communication. Usually it is easier if feelings are shared, rather than being left alone with them.

People of all ages may have particular needs, but minor children who have a parent with cancer may face some particular challenges. Often they feel confused or guilty; and in their effort to protect youngsters, adults sometimes keep children from knowing important information. There are many resources to help you deal with the special needs of your children.

Supportive individual or family counseling or support groups may also be helpful. Groups of families, spouses, or caregivers can be very useful in having a safe place to express difficult feelings and also for learning that you are not alone. Today there are many resources on the Internet that provide support to caregivers. They include facilitated support groups, information resources, and "chats" on particular subjects. Two good resources to begin with are *www.cancersupportivecare. com* and *www.cancercare.org.* And for in-person support, your doctor, nurse, oncology social worker, or the American Cancer Society can put you and your loved ones in touch with appropriate resources.

— 31 —

Palliative Care

Margaret I. Fitch, R.N., Ph.D.

■ ■ ■ ■

For some people with cancer, a cure may not be possible. The most appropriate approach in such cases is to offer treatment and care that are directed toward palliation.

Palliative care is a form of comfort-giving care, irrespective of diagnosis, that fully recognizes that cure or long-term control is not possible. The primary concern or goal of palliative care is to support quality of life as defined by the person who is dying. Palliative care is provided so that people who are dying can be helped to maintain the best possible level of physical, emotional, mental, spiritual, vocational, and social life during their remaining time, no matter how much limitation may be imposed by their advancing disease.

It is so important to understand that the phrase "There is nothing more we can do" usually means to the doctor that the disease cannot be cured. It does not mean that we have run out of ways to help and to support people. There are still many things that can be done to promote comfort and ease the distress patients and family members feel.

The Range of Services Providing palliative care requires the special skills and expertise of a variety of health care professionals. It includes close attention to controlling or managing symptoms and providing psychosocial and spiritual support. Both patient and family are involved in palliative care to ensure that the patient can live as fully as possible in the face of impending death and the most satisfactory quality of time together can be achieved. Family members benefit from such support during the illness and, later, during their time of grief and bereavement.

Another term that is sometimes used is *hospice* care. First used in England, *hospice* refers to a place where palliative care is given and also to the concept that palliative care, after curative treatment is no longer appropriate, is especially important and worthy. It now also applies to *any* palliative care, whether in an institution (hospice) or in the home (hospice care).

Palliative care/hospice care is, then, a set of ideas or beliefs about what is important when people are dying and how they can be helped. The ideas have been used to develop special programs or ways of offering help to patients and families. In some hospitals, palliative care teams of nurses, doctors, social workers, and others will visit a patient in the hospital. In some communities, palliative care experts and health professional teams will visit a person at home. There are also volunteer hospice organizations across the country that can provide support and assistance for people at home and in the hospital. The exact type of service available from place to place is apt to vary. Not all communities will offer the same services, and what is available may not be widely publicized. Patients and families may have to ask about which services are available in their communities.

The health care professionals and volunteer visitors involved in this work are trained in helping the person who is dying feel supported and cared for. However, not everyone has the same comfort level in talking about death and dying. Patients and families who want palliative care may have to request it or turn to other health care professionals than those they have known to find the support they need.

Palliative care units may be found in hospitals, long-term care settings, or nursing home settings. Sometimes there is a feeling that a palliative care unit is a "place to go to die." What is important to know is that the focus in such a unit is on *living* until death. The emphasis is on achieving comfort (freedom from pain) and maintaining as much activity as possible. Often the regulations and atmosphere in a palliative care unit are more relaxed than in a typical hospital setting. In many instances, arrangements can be made for family gatherings or visits with family pets. A palliative care unit can become "a home away from home."

The Role of Palliative Care

Hospice or palliative care focuses on life. Hospice recognizes that death is a part of life and dying is a normal process. We are human beings and death will come to each of us.

For most of us, the idea of our own death or the death of someone we love is inconceivable. In North America, thoughts of death are pushed aside. We are a death-denying society. So, when faced with the inevitability of death— our own or that of one whom we love— most of us feel ill prepared. Many of us feel overwhelmed by the situation and are not certain where to turn for help. Sometimes we are not sure what kind of help we need.

Hospice or palliative care services exist in the hope and belief that through receiving appropriate care, people who are dying and their family members might be free to discover a satisfactory degree of mental and spiritual preparation for death. The route to appropriate care is through working in partnership— patient, family, and health care team members working together—with a clear focus on issues of patient autonomy and patient and family preferences and expectations for care.

Main Goals of Palliative Care

The main goals of palliative care are

• to provide relief from pain and other distressing symptoms,
• to provide psychological and spiritual care, and
• to provide support for the family during the illness and the period of grief and bereavement that follows.

Pain and Symptom Relief Individuals with advancing disease can experience a variety of symptoms, depending on the specific type of disease. The most common symptoms include pain, loss of appetite, fatigue, weakness, weight loss, constipation, difficulty breathing, confusion, nausea, vomiting, cough, and dry or sore mouth.

The nurses and doctors may try several approaches to find the most appropriate way to achieve comfort. It is important that both patient and family members keep a close eye on the symptoms the patient is experiencing, and note whether a particular approach is helpful. If the approach is not effective, another should be tried quickly and the search continued until comfort is achieved. Keeping in touch with the family doctor is important, as the family doctor can also work with the hospital health care team to manage the pain and other symptoms effectively.

One of the most commonly experienced symptoms, pain, no matter how chronic or severe, can almost always be controlled and managed without harmful side effects. By using a variety of medications, nurses and doctors work to discover the "tailor-made" plan to relieve pain. It is important not to be discouraged if a particular approach is not helpful. Several different approaches may need to be tried before finding the most helpful one for the patient. Each patient may have pain for different reasons and respond to pain differently.

The most important medications used to relieve pain and prevent side effects are called analgesics. When milder analgesics such as aspirin and codeine are no longer effective, there should be no hesitation in using a stronger analgesic (called an opioid) such as morphine for moderate to severe pain. The dose of the opioid is exactly matched to the level of pain the person is experiencing and adjusted whenever the pain changes. In some situations, patients remain alert despite large doses of medication. The patient does not become "accustomed" to the drug or require increasingly higher doses to control the pain; nor does he or she become addicted. It is important to remember that pain is a personal experience and that the health care team will create an individual care plan based on the person's report of pain.

Medications may be given by mouth (liquid or pill), by suppository, by injection into a vein, or by continuous infusion with a "pain pump" or a patch on the skin. The first approach is to try the medication by mouth.

For chronic pain, medication must be given regularly. It is inappropriate to wait until the patient is in pain again before the next dose is given. Sometimes, taking regular doses means the patient will need to be awakened from sleep, especially at night. But it is important to maintain the schedule to prevent the pain from reappearing or "breaking through" (see chapter 24, "Controlling Pain").

Each of the other symptoms of advancing disease (constipation, cough, difficulty breathing, diarrhea, confusion, etc.) requires the same close attention that pain requires if patients are to be comfortable. It is important that patients and families discuss any symptoms with the nurse or doctor and state any preferences they may have for managing them. If patients are involved in the planning of how to treat or relieve symptoms, they are more likely to feel in control of them. This sharing process will also help patients understand the physical changes occurring to their body.

One of the changes that can occur for cancer patients as their disease advances is loss of weight and wasting of body tissues. This can be accompanied by changes in skin color and loss of appetite. Watching these changes can be difficult both for the patient and for family members. The changes are part of the normal course of the advancing disease. As the end of life draws closer, all bodily functions slow down. Weakness and fatigue can be profound, and there may be periods of confusion. Finding the energy to talk is often difficult.

As the time for death draws nearer, many people have questions about what their death might be like. Some have heard about others' experiences with dying and wonder if their experiences will be the same. In most instances, nurses and doctors can anticipate how an individual will die based on the type of disease and the symptoms. Patients and family members feel better prepared if they talk with the nurse or doctor about what bodily changes to expect and how things might feel.

Psychosocial and Spiritual Care To be faced with one's own death releases a range of emotions. Each person will react in his or her own way. There can be shock and disbelief that this could be happening, anger that it is happening at this time in one's life, or acceptance that one's appointed time has come. A range of worries will usually emerge as a person begins to imagine the ending of life and what will happen to the people he or she loves. There may be financial concerns, legal issues, and worries about how one's family will manage. As bodily changes occur and the need to depend on others for help increases, many people have concerns about not contributing to the family in their usual way and worry about being a burden.

This can also be a time when people question what their lives have truly meant and experience a range of spiritual questions. Regrets about things one did as well as things left undone can create a sense of guilt and remorse. Sometimes people feel that they are very alone, that no one could possibly understand what they are going through. This can also be a time for inner growth and reaching a sense of profound peace. As individuals review their lives, they may gain insight about themselves and an understanding about some of the events and relationships they experienced. The spiritual questions may be of a religious nature or related to another strongly held belief and practice that brings solace to the person.

Not everyone will experience all of these feelings, but they are all natural and it is helpful to talk about them. Various professionals—nurses, social workers, chaplains, and psychologists—can be of assistance in listening, as well as help with choices and assist in organizing any additional support that might be desired. Some people find it helpful to talk with their close friends or family members. Some will turn to their rabbi, minister, or priest.

As difficult as these feelings are to face and to talk about, they do not go away if they are ignored. Finding a comfortable way to acknowledge and express them will be helpful. While some people will talk to another person, others will write in a diary, paint a picture, write a poem, or compose a song. Others may find solace in listening to music, reading, or meditating. Feelings can be expressed in many ways. What is useful to one person may not be helpful to another. Each of us needs to find the way that works best for us.

Support for the Family Family and friends also experience a range of emotions. They, too, share the shock and disbelief, the feelings of unfairness and anger, and the overwhelming sense of helplessness about changing the course of events. In some instances, there may also be a sense of relief that the suffering and struggle is nearly over or relief that death brings an end to a troubled relationship. In turn, some feel guilt for holding those feelings of wanting things to be over quickly.

It is important to recognize that family may not be the biological family. It may be people who are very close to the person who is dying and are seen as family. They are able to come together and form a close, loving, and protective circle of caring for their friend.

Loved ones will experience their own concerns about the future. There is a sense of their world being suddenly changed so that it will never be the same again, and a fear about how they will face the challenge of managing alone. The world without one's spouse, partner, parent, or child is impossible to imagine. There is an overwhelming sense of dread and despair, an emerging sense of profound loss. It is difficult to concentrate or focus. Suddenly all one's priorities have shifted and the world seems turned upside down.

For some people, the time they have together can strengthen their relationship and create lasting memories. There is time to share, in a deep and profound way, what their lives together have meant. There is time to talk about the past and to make plans together. Such discussion could cover plans and dreams for children's futures, what to do about the house, what to do with finances, what the funeral should be like, or what should happen to the body. Not all people will be able to discuss these topics easily and may need assistance in doing so. Nurses, social workers, chaplains, psychologists, and palliative care volunteers may be called upon for help.

It is helpful to remember to focus on life and living until death comes. People need to live until they die. Celebrations and life pleasures are still there to be enjoyed, to be shared. Birthdays, anniversaries, graduations, and achievements offer time for families to gather and to affirm life.

On the other hand, it is important to discuss with the person who is dying what would be helpful for him or her. The presence of too many people all at the same time could be overwhelming and tiring. Perhaps the more appropriate plan would be for visitors to come in small numbers and be able to sit and talk quietly. Sometimes, too, it is the little things that can make such a difference—a trip to the countryside, listening to favorite music, sitting in the garden feeling the sun on one's face, hearing children's laughter, or seeing a sunset. Family and friends can play an important role in making these things happen.

Reactions to a family member's impending death will differ from family member to family member. Not everyone will feel exactly the same way at the same time. There is no "right way" to cope and no "appropriate" time schedule for feelings. One person may feel strong at a time when another feels most vulnerable. One may cry easily while another does not feel able to cry. One may bury himself or herself in work while another is unable to concentrate. Some will talk openly about the situation and others will remain very closed or silent. What is important is that a family can understand these differences and find ways to draw on one another's strengths. Talking with one another, or with someone else, about one's feelings can be helpful.

Young children are part of the family, and it is important that, when appropriate, they be included and involved in conversations about what is happening. It is very easy for a child to think he or she has caused the death if no other explanation is provided. There are many helpful books about talking with children about death.

Making funeral arrangements and preparing a will are two activities that, if completed before death, can make the time of death and period of mourning less stressful. Most funeral homes provide a "prearrangement" service for families; many of the details for visitation and the memorial service can be made ahead of time. This approach can also enable the individual to be involved in planning for the funeral and the disposition of his or her body. Writing a will provides a vehicle for a person to plan with certainty how his or her possessions will be dispersed. At the same time, it is important to acknowledge that sometimes a person's ethnic beliefs and values see the preplanning as a bad omen and they will not be open to these discussions.

The choice between dying in a palliative care unit or in a hospital and dying at home can be difficult for both patients and families. Both settings have benefits and drawbacks. In a unit, there is twenty-four-hour nurse and doctor support, while in the community, the nurse may visit only once or twice a day; in a unit, the patient is more separated from family and a familiar environment, whereas at home, he or she could be the center of the household; in a unit, the family can visit and provide help in some ways, while at home, the family carries the major burden of caregiving. If care is to be provided at home, it is important to ensure that medical care can easily be accessed (e.g., having a doctor available for home visits).

Before making a choice about which approach to take, the patient and family should talk over the details and explore the benefits and drawbacks with the nurse or doctor. In some instances, arrangements can be made to take advantage of both settings at different phases of the illness.

PART THREE

Quality of Life

— 32 —

The Will to Live

Ernest H. Rosenbaum, M.D., and Isadora R. Rosenbaum, M.A.

■ ■ ■ ■

As medical professionals, we have always been fascinated by the power of the will to live. Like all creatures in the animal world, human beings have a fierce instinct for survival. The will to live is a force within all of us to fight for survival when our lives are threatened by a disease such as cancer. Yet this force is stronger in some people than in others.

Sometimes the biology of a cancer will dictate the course of events regardless of the patient's attitude and fighting spirit. These events are often beyond our control. But patients with positive attitudes are better able to cope with disease-related problems and may respond better to therapy. Many physicians have seen how two patients of similar ages and with the same diagnosis, degree of illness, and treatment program experience vastly different results. One of the few apparent differences is that one patient is pessimistic and the other optimistic.

We have known for over 2,000 years—from the writings of Plato and Galen—that there is a direct correlation between the mind, the body, and one's health. "The cure of many diseases is unknown to physicians," Plato concluded, "because they are ignorant of the whole. For the part can never be well unless the whole is well."

Recently there has been a shift in health care toward recognizing this wisdom, namely that the psychological and the physical elements of a body are not separate, isolated, and unrelated, but are vitally linked elements of a total system. Health is increasingly being recognized as a balance of many inputs, including physical and environmental factors, emotional and psychological states, and nutritional habits and exercise patterns.

Researchers are now experimenting with methods of actively enlisting the mind in the body's combat with cancer, using techniques such as meditation, biofeedback, and visualization (creating in the mind positive images about what is occurring in the body). Some doctors and psychologists now believe that the proper attitude may even have a direct effect on cell function and consequently may be used to arrest, if not cure, cancer. This new field of scientific study, called psychoneuroimmunology, focuses on the effect that mental and emotional activity have on physical well-being, indicating that patients can play a much larger role in their recovery.

It will be many years before we know whether it is possible for the mind to control the immune defense system. Experiments with biofeedback and visualization are helpful in that they encourage positive thinking and provide relaxation, thereby increasing the will to live. But they can also be damaging if a patient puts all of his or her faith in them and ignores conventional therapy.

The Power of the Mind

The mind's role in causing and curing disease has been debated endlessly.

Speculation abounds, particularly in the case of cancer. But no studies have proven in a scientifically valid way that a person can control the course of his or her cancer with the mind, although patients often believe otherwise.

There are many individual cases that attest to the power of positive attitudes and emotions. One patient with high-risk cancer had a mastectomy at age twenty-nine. At thirty-one, she had advanced Stage IV cancer with widespread massive liver and bone involvement and, subsequently, extensive lung metastases. She also had an amazingly strong will to live.

"I would get out of bed every morning as if nothing was wrong," she once said. "I may have known I was going to have to face things and could feel sick during the day, but I never got out of bed that way. There was a lot I was fighting for. I had a three-year-old child, a wonderful life, and a magical love affair with my husband." Thirty years later, she is still alive, still on chemotherapy, and still living an active life.

We often ask our patients to explain how they are able to transcend their problems. We have found that however diverse they are in ethnic or cultural background, age, educational level, or type of illness, they have all gone through a similar process of psychological recovery. They all consciously made a "decision to live." After an initial period of feeling devastated, they simply decided to assess their new reality and make the most of each day.

Their "will to live" means that they really *want* to live, whether or not they're afraid to die. They want to enjoy life, they want to get more out of life, they believe that their life is not over, and they're willing to do whatever they can to squeeze more out of it.

The threat of death often renews our appreciation of the importance of life, love, friendship, and all there is to enjoy. We open up to new possibilities and begin taking risks we didn't have the courage to take before. Many patients say that facing the uncertainties of living with an illness makes life more meaningful. The smallest pleasures are intensified and much of the hypocrisy in life is eliminated. When bitterness and anger begin to dissipate, there is still a capacity for joy.

One patient wrote, "I love living, I love nature. Being outdoors, feeling the sun on my skin or the wind blowing against my body, hearing birds sing, breathing in the spray of the ocean. I never lose hope that I may somehow stumble upon or be graced with a victory against this disease."

Strengthening Your Will to Live

Unfortunately, and quite understandably, many patients react to the diagnosis of cancer in the same way that people in primitive cultures react to the imposition of a curse or spell: as a sentence to a ghastly death. This phenomenon, known as "bone pointing," results in a paralytic fear that causes the victim to simply withdraw from the world and await the inevitable end. In modern medical practice, a similar phenomenon may occur when, out of ignorance or superstition, a patient believes the diagnosis of cancer to be a death sentence. However, the phenomenon of self-willed death is only effective if the person believes in the power of the curse.

In the treatment of cancer, we've seen patients fail on their first course of chemotherapy, fail again on the second and third treatments, then—with more advanced disease—a fourth treatment is highly successful.

In all things, you have to take a risk if you want to win, to get a remission or recover with the best quality of life. Just the willingness to take a risk seems to generate hope and a positive atmosphere in which the components of the will to live are enhanced. There are many other ways of strengthening the will to live.

Getting Involved The best thing a patient can do to strengthen the will to live is to get involved as an active participant in combating his or her disease. When patients approach their disease in an aggressive fighting posture, they are no longer helpless victims. Instead, they become active partners with their medical support team in the fight for improvement, remission, or cure. This partnership must be based on honesty, open communication, shared responsibility, and education about the nature of the disease, therapy options, and rehabilitation. The result of this partnership is an increased ability to cope that, in turn, nurtures the will to live.

Helping and Sharing with Others A way to strengthen this partnership is to extend the relationship to others. The emotional experience of sharing and enjoying your family and partnerships supports your love for life and your will to survive.

As you make the transition from helpless victim to activist, one of the most important realizations is that *you* have everything to do with how others perceive you and treat you. If you can accept your condition and hold self-pity at bay, others won't feel sorry for you. If you can discuss your disease and medical therapy in a matter-of-fact manner, they'll respond in kind without fear or awkwardness. You are in charge. You can subtly and gently put your family, friends, and coworkers at ease by being frank about what you want to talk about or not talk about and by being explicit about whether and when you want their help.

Sharing your life with others and receiving aid or support from friends and family will improve your ability to cope and help you fight for your life. A person who is lonely or alone often feels like a helpless victim. There is a need to share your own problems, but helping others find solutions to or cope better with the problems of daily living gives strength to both the giver and the receiver. There are few more satisfying experiences in life than helping a person in need.

Patients can also take part in psychological support programs, either through private counseling or through group therapy. Sharing frustrations with others in similar circumstances often relieves the sense of isolation, terror, and despair cancer patients often feel.

Those who must live with cancer can live to the maximum of their capacity by

- living in the present, not the past,
- setting realistic goals and being willing to compromise,
- regaining control of their lives and maintaining a sense of independence and self-esteem,
- trying to resolve negative emotions and depression by actively doing things to help themselves and others, and
- following an improved diet and exercising regularly.

Nurturing Hope

Of all the ingredients in the will to live, hope is the most vital. Hope is the emotional and mental state that motivates you to keep on living, to accomplish things, and to succeed. A person who lacks hope can give up on life and lose the will to live. Without hope, there is little to live for. But with hope, a positive attitude can be maintained, determination strengthened, coping skills sharpened, and love and support more freely given and received.

Even if a diagnosis is such that the future seems limited, hope must be maintained. Hope is what people have to live on. Take away hope, and you take away a chance for the future, which leads to depression. When people fall to that low emotional state, their bodies simply turn off.

Hope can be maintained as long as there is even a remote chance for survival.

It can be kindled and nurtured by minor improvements or a remission and maintained when crises or reversals occur. There may be times when you will feel exhausted and drained by never-ending problems and feel ready to give up the struggle to survive. All too often it seems easier to give up than to keep on fighting. Frustrations and despair can sometimes feel overwhelming. Determination or dogged persistence is needed to accomplish the difficult task of fighting for your health.

The experience of cancer not only is destructive in a physical way, but can be a major deterrent to your fighting attitude and will to live. But even during the roughest times, there are often untapped reserves of physical and emotional strength to call upon to help you survive one more day. These reserves can add meaning to your life as well as serve as a lighthouse that leads you to a safe haven during a turbulent storm.

Hope has different meanings for each person. It is a component of a positive attitude and acceptance of our fate in life. We use our strengths to gain success to live life to the fullest. Circumstances often limit our hopes of happiness, cure, remission, or increased longevity. We also live with fears of poverty, pain, a bad death, or other unhappy experiences.

You may worry so much that you lose sight of the possibility of recovery and lose your sense of optimism. On the other hand, you may become so hopeful and confident that you lose sight of reality. Your main challenge is balancing your worry and your hope.

Hope is nourished by the way we live our lives. Achieving the best quality of life requires settling old problems, quarrels, and family strife as well as completing current tasks. Problems that have not been resolved need to have completion. New tasks should be undertaken. If the future seems limited, you can achieve the satisfaction of knowing that you have taken care of your affairs and not left the burden to your family or others. By doing so, you can achieve peace of mind, which will also help strengthen your will to live. With each passing day, try to complete what you can and have that satisfaction that you have done your best.

Be bold, be venturesome, and be willing to experience each day to the fullest to enhance your enjoyment of life. As long as fear, suffering, and pain can be controlled, life can be lived fully until the last breath. Each of us has the capacity to live each day a little better, but we need to focus on both purpose and goals and set into action a realistic daily plan—often altered many times—to help us achieve them. These resources are the foundation of the will to live. Only by using the power of the will to live—nourished by hope—can we achieve the sublime feelings of knowing and experiencing the wonders of life and appreciate its meanings through vital living.

— 33 —

Living with Mortality: Life Goes On

Malin Dollinger, M.D., and Bernard Dubrow, M.S. *

■ ■ ■ ■

We revel in life's beginning, wrestle with its challenges, and take pride in our achievements. We know deep down that we are mortal and that our lives will end some time in the future—the distant future, we hope—but we are not consciously aware of our mortality from day to day.

The media bombard us with flashes of death in stories and graphic pictures of car accidents, plane crashes, murders, and wars, but we block them out in our minds. We feel protected and safe. We can accept the death of war heroes and old people, but reject the idea of its happening to us. We focus on guarding and enjoying our lives and intuitively distance ourselves from thoughts of our mortality.

But what happens when we are jolted by the diagnosis of a possibly fatal illness such as cancer? After recoiling from the shocking news and accepting its reality, how can we cope with this new state of uncertainty? How can we adjust our life-long attitudes and renew our trust in the future? For the first time, we find ourselves in the strange and disruptive situation of having to cope with living and dying at the same time. How can we do it?

The threat of serious illness unleashes a wide range of moods and emotions. We swing back and forth between fear and hope, nostalgia and yearning, sadness and joy, self-affirmation and self-doubt,

confidence that modern medicine offers the prospect of fighting the disease and concern that treatments can fail. Religious people sense God's closeness at times and at other times feel abandoned.

Searching for Answers To avoid confusion and despair, these and other contradictory feelings have to be sorted out, faced squarely, and dealt with.

New social and economic questions also arise. Should you keep trying to fulfill your ambitions, to build and compete? Will telling your friends and coworkers that you have cancer adversely affect your prospects for success? How should you protect your family from financial disaster? How do you emerge from the loneliness that seems to accompany illness and find meaning within your silent universe?

Denial of your illness lessens your capacity to find answers to these and other vital questions. But if you retain control of the illness as much as possible, you will be able to look directly at your own mortality and deal with it.

The Five Stages of Living with Mortality

The process of living with mortality begins when you are first told the diagnosis. A new cancer "victim" develops fear,

*The editors were inspired by the insights and creativity of Bernard Dubrow, M.S. We were very saddened by his passing, in 1997, and wish to acknowledge his lasting contribution.

despair, hope, depression, anxiety, and determination to find answers. It doesn't matter if there is a 50 percent chance of a cure or an 80 percent or a 95 percent. As long as there is even a 5 percent chance that the cancer is *incurable*, the emotional turmoil persists and the need to learn how to go on living in a purposeful way, despite the fear and worry, remains.

Many people diagnosed as having a chronic potentially fatal disease react, think, and behave in similar ways, following a similar pattern. Not everyone will go through all the stages described below. Some will skip one or two or even come back to an earlier stage if a new symptom or other significant event occurs. But it is useful to become aware of these common reactions, whether or not you experience all of them yourself. Understanding these experiences will help you face your own uncertainties and fears and help you put in perspective some of the decisions you will have to make.

When faced with the threat of death or dying, many patients and their families turn for understanding and guidance to the highly regarded work of Dr. Elisabeth Kübler-Ross. She illustrates five stages—denial and isolation, anger, bargaining, depression, and acceptance—that occur during a terminal illness. But the Kübler-Ross model applies to death in the near future of weeks or months. These circumstances may not apply to cancer patients who have been told they have a *potentially* fatal illness and that they *might* die of it, but cannot know when, and, then again, may *not* die of it, but may not know that for years to come. Living with a chronic *potentially* fatal illness associated with a life span measured in years involves responses that differ in many important ways from those described by Dr. Kübler-Ross. A more apt staging might involve disbelief, discovery, redirection, resolution, and emerging victorious.

Understanding the patterns of reaction to a prolonged illness with perhaps years of remission and a significant chance of being cured will help you put your emotional survival in focus while your doctor concentrates on your physical survival. You will also realize that whatever stage you may be in, you are not alone. Your loved ones will be able to help you go on living. You will renew your confidence and zest in life, deal with fear and worry, discover new value and meaning in your life, achieve gratification, and even attain peace of mind.

Disbelief When the diagnosis of cancer is made, many people first go through a stage of disbelief. You will likely be unprepared for this sudden insult to your normal physical and emotional existence. There may be some denial involved. You may think, "The diagnosis is wrong. . . . It will go away. . . . It can't happen to me." You wish you could make a poor prognosis go away by picking up the phone and saying, "Hello, Heaven, please hold."

But you can hope—and with good justification—that you have significant time left, whether you are cured or not. The opportunity remains for you to enjoy life's pleasures. Eventually, you are able to accept the idea, "The cancer victim is really me." At that point, you can proceed to the next stage.

Discovery Now you need to know all about the kind of cancer you have. You need some details about its stage and prognosis. You have to find out, to whatever extent is personally meaningful, all that is important to know about the illness. What tests do you need? What treatments are available? Are there alternative treatments? What are the advantages, disadvantages, and risks of each? Where should you go for treatment? Is a second opinion important? What questions should you ask your doctor? You need to do whatever you have to do to be satisfied you're getting the best possible treatment.

One of the main purposes of this book is to help you with this discovery stage. Another pathway to discovery is through a connection with a key physician, sometimes your own physician and sometimes a specialist, with whom you can develop a relationship of confidence and trust. This physician will advise and guide you through the journey ahead.

Besides discovering technical information, you also have to discover your own strengths and weaknesses, your spiritual beliefs, how others can be of help, and who your friends really are. Do your relationships with others need clarification? When you have gathered this essential information and gained understanding of your situation, you are able to redefine and take charge of your life. A new phase of dealing with life begins.

Redirection You need to continue, adapt, or invent a lifestyle and an attitude that let you function physically and emotionally. This is an opportunity to redirect your life in fresh, productive ways.

The method of redirection is an individual choice and depends to a significant extent on how you have dealt with major life problems in the past. Some people need logical, sensible, step-by-step discussions and explanations, with lists of ideas and choices. Others need only minimal consultations with their physicians. Some feel protected and supported by their religious beliefs and make trust in God a major part of their redirection. Some are helped by their relationships with their family, friends, and support groups. There is no single right answer to how we should approach life; there are a number of right answers:

Balancing Worry and Hope The powerful emotions of fear, hope, despair, anger, and guilt released by a serious illness fade with recovery, but anxieties accumulate with a chronic potentially fatal disease. Tensions rise and fall and moods swing in cycles of highs and lows.

You may worry so much that you lose sight of the possibility of optimism. You may also become so hopeful and confident that you lose sight of reality. Your main challenge is how to balance your worry and your hope, integrating both into your day-to-day life without losing sight of either. As you ride this roller coaster of emotion, you should persist in finding the reality of each situation. The struggle is difficult, but great is the reward of finding peace of mind.

Controlling Negative Emotions It's just human nature to believe that if things are going well for us, we must be doing something right. We also tend to believe the opposite: If things aren't going well and some misfortune occurs, we have *not* been doing the right things.

If a construction site collapses or a power plant erupts, we feel the need to mount a thorough investigation to find out why it happened and especially to find and punish whoever was responsible for the disaster. It is not surprising that we sometimes assume personal responsibility for our own illness and single ourselves out as deserving punishment. Explaining illness as a kind of punishment for a tragedy stemming from doing something wrong is, of course, a psychological reaction, a distortion of reality arising from the destructive emotion of guilt.

There is also a reaction called survivor's guilt. By remaining alive when others have died, some survivors dare not feel too confident or reassured for fear of somehow being punished for enjoying good fortune. They may feel that they have survived at the expense of others, although obviously they have not!

The redirection stage can be a time to learn how to lessen the destructive impact of emotional issues. Some people gain support and insight from spouses, family members, or close friends. Sometimes professional help is useful, including clergy, psychologists, psychiatrists, social workers, and counselors. For some, attending group meetings where feelings can be shared in a comfortable setting can relieve many psychological stresses. This will not abolish all anxiety, but will give expression to the deep emotions—fear, anger, and guilt—that arise during a prolonged life-threatening illness. The first step toward control of negative emotions is recognizing them during this stage of living with mortality.

Affirmation During this stage, some people approach life with renewed enthusiasm, especially if a battle plan has been formulated to conquer the cancer.

You need to find ways to reaffirm your interest in life, in pleasurable activities, in your profession or your hobbies. The role of loved ones and friends is especially important. They have to give you "permission" to share your worries and fears. They can do this by encouraging you to tell them about your problems rather than turning off communication by trying to simply cheer you up. Giving blanket reassurance by saying "Everything will be okay" sends the message that they want to hear only good things. They have to affirm that they are truly interested in you as an individual going through perhaps the most critical time of your life.

This stage—which, one hopes, can last a long time—also includes key medical judgments such as the affirmation that the correct physician is in charge of your care and is making the correct decisions about treatment. Sometimes a relapse, a setback, or even an uncertain lab test or X-ray report may disrupt the redirection process. You may suddenly find yourself back in a stage of disbelief or discovery, but you will be better prepared to settle on and handle the course of action required to resolve new questions or problems.

During this stage, you will also usually be forced by circumstances to deal with physical, emotional, financial, and social effects, whether your illness is considered to be "cured," is in remission, or requires continued treatment. You must master the techniques of how to get on with your life and enjoy yourself despite problems such as denial of health insurance claims, prejudice in the workplace, and trying to find people with whom you can share your concerns.

You have to learn to retain your independence and to keep the anxieties of illness from suffocating you. Redirection helps shape your life and makes it more productive.

Resolution Finally, the stage of resolution is reached. This may occur if your cancer is cured and you are able to accept this fact and put the experience behind you. It may also occur when you realize that cure is not possible.

If your cancer cannot be cured, this stage is not necessarily associated with a sudden dismal change in attitude or depression, although certainly your spirits and emotions may be at a low ebb. Having known for months or years that someday this time might come, someone who has been dealing productively with his or her illness will have spent time getting renewed enjoyment from life in whatever way possible, perfecting relationships with significant people, and sorting through the issues that he or she finds important. You may have discovered the meaning of life in general and of your life in particular. In some cases, there may even be relief that the long-awaited catastrophe need no longer be feared in the abstract but can be dealt with directly.

You have worked through the complex and progressive emotions that the illness has created in you as well as in those you love. You know that everything possible has been done and are comforted by the fact that you have gained additional time and meaning. You know that if there is to be a brief period of ending, it will be made as comfortable and as free of suffering as possible. This may mean aggressive medical treatment to relieve symptoms, hospice care when appropriate, or the cessation of active anticancer treatment if that is appropriate.

If the previous three stages have successfully dealt with problems and needs, the fourth stage of living with mortality represents the attainment of peace of mind. It can become a validation that your struggle has been worthwhile and of value to you, your loved ones, and your close friends.

If your cancer is gone, many months or, more often, several years after apparently successful treatment—which can often be complex, difficult, and lengthy—your mind finally allows you to believe that you are cured. You can then reach the stage of resolution by regaining your belief once more that you are a normal person. You finally accept that the hoped-for goal has been achieved. You have a new awareness of the value of life and what in life holds special meaning for you.

Emerging Victorious The miracles of modern medicine have created a new dilemma for millions of people with chronic illnesses such as cancer, heart disease, and stroke. Prolonged illness, especially if potentially fatal, generates anxiety, tension, and worry that may be more troublesome than the illness itself.

Those who have cancer are labeled "cancer patient" and often agree somehow to accept this new identity that has been forced upon them. Loved ones and friends treat you differently—not to mention employers, insurance companies, and everyone else who hears the news that you have cancer.

You want to get on with your life. You want to feel and look normal. Your doctor has told you that you are okay now. But that's hard to believe when every trip to the doctor's office, even for a checkup, reawakens old fears. Anxiety will not disappear completely, but thinking about and understanding the emotional stages cancer patients face will help you cope with the awareness of mortality that cancer evokes.

For some of us, the threat of death increases our creative energies. Friends and family can draw closer and long-standing conflicts can be resolved. In spite of, or perhaps because of, the prospect of suffering, life intensifies and takes on added importance. Time is telescoped, and greater sensitivity to the wonders of the world is often gained.

In our society, the prospect of dying makes most people shrink and hide from a significant part of life. But you have to think positively. You have to recognize the potential within each of us even during prolonged illness.

It is unfortunate that our society shuns the thought of dying and turns away from the large segment of the population marked with the stigma of a chronic potentially fatal illness like cancer. We deny the self-worth of millions of capable and active people. We have to learn to recognize that medical technology has greatly extended life by offering effective treatments to people who are seriously ill. Such people are living full lives and deserve full acceptance by society. When a chronic and potentially fatal illness is not dealt with effectively by patients, family, or friends, emotional problems will inevitably mount and social fears will continue to fester. But if the threat to life by disease is accepted, understood, and dealt with, life, not death, will be the winner.

— 34 —

New Hope in Managing Distress with Cancer*

Mitch Golant, Ph.D.

■ ■ ■ ■

Distress and Cancer

We know that distress is common for people with cancer. In fact, virtually everyone becomes distressed coping with the diagnosis and treatment of cancer—it is the most underreported and common side effect of cancer. Distress is a normal reaction that in recent years has been validated through research. Fortunately, oncology professionals now have a better understanding of the emotional challenges faced by cancer patients and their families.

Distress may interfere with your ability to cope effectively with cancer, its physical symptoms, and its treatment. Forty-seven percent of cancer patients have distress severe enough to be diagnosed with a mood or anxiety disorder.

There are many symptoms of distress, including a spectrum of feelings that runs from sadness, vulnerability, fearfulness, anger, and unhappiness to severe depression, panic, and debilitating anxiety. It is important to monitor the severity of these symptoms. But this can sometimes be tricky. There are *reliable* symptoms such as persistent depressed or angry mood and lack of pleasure in activities. However, there are also *unreliable* symptoms such as fatigue, insomnia,

eating disturbances, and decreased sexual desire. These symptoms are considered unreliable because they can mimic side effects of the cancer treatment itself. But no matter what their source, the bottom line is that these distress symptoms decrease your quality of life.

In general, people tend to cope with cancer much like they coped with problems before cancer. If you were a nervous, anxious person before cancer, you are likely to develop anxiety symptoms during the illness. If you were generally a person with good coping skills and a strong support system before cancer, you will most likely cope reasonably well with cancer and its treatment.

Sometimes, the type and severity of the cancer and/or its treatment can impact your level of emotional distress. For example, in a study published in 2001 by Jim Zabora, then at Johns Hopkins University, lung cancer patients (as a group) experienced the highest levels of emotional distress after diagnosis, followed by patients with brain tumors and those with pancreatic cancer. In fact, a 2005 Institute of Medicine report entitled *From Cancer Patient to Cancer Survivor: Lost in Transition* underscores the need for patients to be given not only a road map for medical treatment, but also

* Adapted from the *Frankly Speaking About New Discoveries in Cancer* program, produced by The Wellness Community. *http://www.thewellnesscommunity.org/programs/frankly/newdiscoveries/ newdiscoveries_home.htm.*

a plan for managing the psychological and emotional effects of the illness. Just as scientists are working to discover how to detect cancer earlier, psychosocial oncology professionals (psychologists, psychiatrists, social workers, oncology clinical nurse specialists, and other mental health professionals) would like to help you identify emotional distress shortly after diagnosis so that you can get the support you need to actively participate in treatment and maintain a good quality of life during and after treatment.

The Distress Management Thermometer

A simple way to assess your distress is by using the NCCN's Distress Management Guidelines, including a Distress Management Thermometer. The NCCN Guidelines are created by professional consensus on currently accepted approaches to treatment and are updated as often as new significant data become available. The most recent and complete version of the guideline is posted on-line at *www.nccn.org.*

Psychoneuroimmunology: The Mind-Body Connection

Psychoneuroimmunology (PNI) is a recent scientific discipline that studies the link between the mind and the

NCCN Distress Management Thermometer

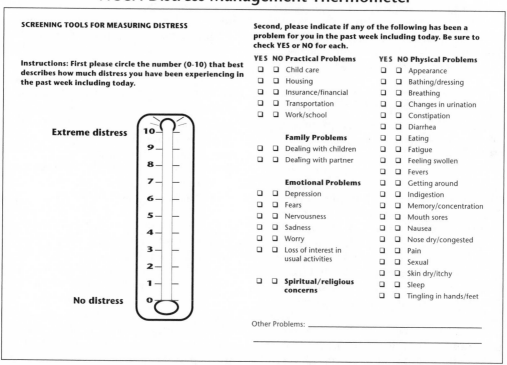

SCREENING TOOLS FOR MEASURING DISTRESS

Instructions: First please circle the number (0-10) that best describes how much distress you have been experiencing in the past week including today.

Extreme distress — 10

9

8

7

6

5

4

3

2

1

No distress — 0

Second, please indicate if any of the following has been a problem for you in the past week including today. Be sure to check YES or NO for each.

YES NO **Practical Problems**
☐ ☐ Child care
☐ ☐ Housing
☐ ☐ Insurance/financial
☐ ☐ Transportation
☐ ☐ Work/school

Family Problems
☐ ☐ Dealing with children
☐ ☐ Dealing with partner

Emotional Problems
☐ ☐ Depression
☐ ☐ Fears
☐ ☐ Nervousness
☐ ☐ Sadness
☐ ☐ Worry
☐ ☐ Loss of interest in usual activities

☐ ☐ **Spiritual/religious concerns**

YES NO **Physical Problems**
☐ ☐ Appearance
☐ ☐ Bathing/dressing
☐ ☐ Breathing
☐ ☐ Changes in urination
☐ ☐ Constipation
☐ ☐ Diarrhea
☐ ☐ Eating
☐ ☐ Fatigue
☐ ☐ Feeling swollen
☐ ☐ Fevers
☐ ☐ Getting around
☐ ☐ Indigestion
☐ ☐ Memory/concentration
☐ ☐ Mouth sores
☐ ☐ Nausea
☐ ☐ Nose dry/congested
☐ ☐ Pain
☐ ☐ Sexual
☐ ☐ Skin dry/itchy
☐ ☐ Sleep
☐ ☐ Tingling in hands/feet

Other Problems: _____

body—how thoughts, feelings, and attitudes positively or negatively affect illness or health. Scientists explain that long-term unremitting stress diminishes the positive impact of the immune system, while positive emotions enhance the immune system.

Since the first line of defense against disease progression is the immune system, enhancing its power by reducing stress and increasing positive emotions—at the very least—improves quality of life and *may* enhance the possibility of recovery. In thinking about this possibility and especially the notion of *enhancing the power of the immune system by reducing stress,* several questions immediately come to mind: What are the most significant stressors for people with cancer? Which emotions are positive and should be boosted? Which are negative and should be diminished? Which stressors should be reduced? And how do we reduce the negative and enhance the positive?

The Value of Support Groups

Imagine yourself sitting in a room with ten other people who have cancer. Just last week, your doctor as well as other patients in his or her waiting room suggested you attend such a gathering because you were so upset and worried. The group begins with the professional facilitator asking you to share your cancer experience. Perhaps you might explain what type of cancer you have, when you were diagnosed, what treatments you are going through. You may also choose to share what you are feeling and how cancer has impacted your life. In the moment before you answer, you pause and reflect: Why am I here? Will participating in a support group help me—and if so, how?

Over the last twenty-five years, there has been extensive research on the positive effects of support groups. Research has shown that they help reduce the three most significant stressors associated with cancer: unwanted aloneness, loss of control, and loss of hope. For example, in controlled studies at Stanford University and the University of California, Los Angeles, psychological distress and pain were significantly reduced, while quality of life significantly improved, in women who participated in breast cancer support groups.[1] Some studies have even shown increased survival as a result of support group participation.[2] More recently in a replication of previous research, Pamela J. Goodwin, M.D., and her colleagues found that although women in professionally facilitated support groups did not survive longer, they experienced significant quality-of-life improvements—they were less distressed and suffered less pain.[3]

Community-based (rather than hospital- or university-based) cancer support programs also lend further evidence that support groups can be beneficial.[4] Less tightly controlled studies of community-based cancer support programs have found that participants generally rate their experiences as positive and beneficial.[5] In a study done at The Wellness Community (TWC) with Stanford University, findings suggest that community support groups that encourage preparing for the worst while hoping for the best may reduce cancer patients' overall distress.[6]

Although TWC is awaiting final outcomes from this study, the women in the community-based support groups benefited at about the same rate as those who participated in the more formal Stanford University study in terms of reduced depression and trauma symptoms, and improved social support, emotional coping, and post-traumatic growth. Moreover, those women in the study who participated in the community group were empowered to make changes in their lives that they thought important, to develop a new attitude toward the illness, to create a better partnership with their physicians, and to more readily access cancer-related information and resources. This is encouraging news for people participating in professionally facilitated community-based cancer support groups—especially at TWC with its wide geographic reach.

The Wellness Community (TWC) Model
Founded in 1982, TWC currently provides services to more than 5,000 people with cancer each week. Thirty-thousand cancer patients make about 200,000 visits to its twenty-one national facilities each year, attending support groups and educational and wellness programs—including physician lectures, and meditation, exercise, and nutrition workshops—all free of charge. The support groups are led by licensed psychotherapists specially trained in TWC's unique program methodology.

The program is based upon founder Dr. Harold Benjamin's seminal idea, the Patient Active Concept: *People with cancer who participate in their fight for recovery from cancer will improve the quality of their life, and may enhance the possibility of their recovery.* It combines the will of the patient with the skill of the physician.

TWC's Patient Active program focuses on an empowerment model; patients are supported in making active choices in their recovery—making changes in their lives that *they* think are important, partnering with their physicians, accessing resources, and developing a new attitude toward the illness. Moreover, the program emphasizes reducing the three most significant psychosocial stressors faced by people with cancer: feelings of isolation, loss of control, and loss of hope. It is these aspects of The Wellness Community model that are important new discoveries in improving quality of life for people with cancer and their loved ones.

The Wellness Community paradigm links the findings from psychoneuroimmunology (PNI) with its application to psychosocial support. Support groups, educational programs, physician lectures,

stress-reduction workshops, and camaraderie during social events—holiday parties, joke-fests, and informal get-togethers—all help to reduce stress and improve quality of life by providing cancer patients with the kind of support that they need.

Help with Expressing Emotions Psychosocial oncologists have learned that the expression of emotions is an important component for managing the diagnosis and treatment of cancer. In particular, primary negative emotions—fear, anger, and sadness—are normal and adaptive. Research has shown that the process of accessing, expressing, integrating, and reframing your emotions within a support group or in individual psychotherapy improves quality of life. However, if these same emotions are repressed, it can lead to aggressiveness, hostility, and irresponsible and inconsiderate impulses.

On the other hand, restraining hostile, impulsive, irresponsible, and thoughtless behavior is associated with improved quality of life, lower levels of distress, and better social functioning.[7] (Restraint should not be confused with suppressing your emotions. Suppressing emotions means blocking them entirely and is associated with negative mental health.) So, learning to express a whole range of emotions within a support group or other therapy can lead to decreases in hostility, greater self-confidence and -assertion, greater expressions of support, empathy, interest, and humor, and better physical health and physiological functioning.[8] And honing these skills may enable you to balance the expression of strong emotions without alienating others— especially family and friends.[9]

The Challenge of the "Positive Attitude"

People with cancer have long been told that having a positive attitude increases their chances of survival. How true is this? Is it important to have a "positive attitude" in order to battle cancer and improve outcomes? And, conversely, will a "negative attitude" mean a worse outcome or earlier death?

In a 2004 study by Penelope Schofield and her colleagues at Peter MacCallum Cancer Centre in Melbourne, Australia, that involved 204 lung cancer patients, there was no evidence that a high level of optimism prior to treatment enhanced survival. However, the study underscored the importance of optimism in relation to quality of life: Those patients who were more optimistic were less depressed and more likely to adhere to treatment.

Other researchers are examining the biological underpinnings of optimism by studying immune function and stress hormones. So far, findings similar to those in the Schofield study indicate that successful coping isn't necessarily about having a positive outlook or striving for a cheery disposition. Rather, coping in a way familiar to you (which could involve anything from stress relief to exercise) can prove beneficial. Indeed, if someone is a natural curmudgeon, then continuing to be a curmudgeon may be the very thing to help lower stress, bolster the immune system, and, possibly, influence the success of the cancer treatment.[10]

This new research does not focus so much on patients' tendencies to look at the glass as half full or half empty and how that may influence survival outcomes. Instead, researchers are examining how different coping styles may affect biological indicators of disease-fighting ability such as cortisol rhythms (a measure of stress levels) and natural killer cell counts (a measure of immune response). With better understanding of these biological variables, there may be ways (such as muscle relaxation, stress reduction exercises, and problem solving) to help patients manage stress and maintain natural killer cells at levels that improve their chances of extending survival.

For instance, scientists are measuring cortisol concentrations in women's saliva and counting the circulating natural killer cells. In an ongoing study, preliminarily published in 2000 in the *Journal of the National Cancer Institute,* researchers found that women with breast cancer whose cortisol levels were flat and didn't follow the typical pattern of decline throughout the day died sooner than women with normal, fluctuating cortisol patterns. Researchers believe that this finding indicates psychological intervention may boost one's disease-fighting ability––a notion that in the past has driven the focus on "staying positive."

Researchers are now realizing that people cope with stress in vastly different ways. Individuals need to identify solutions that match their natural temperament and personality. The next step is finding the mechanisms that enable patients to keep their cortisol patterns and natural killer cells at optimum levels and hopefully extend their survival. For some patients, this may happen by being uncooperative and unpleasant rather than positive.

For example, at Ohio State University, an ongoing study is measuring not only survival rates, but also endocrine responses and biological markers of immunity in women with breast cancer. Participants are learning muscle-relaxation, problem-solving, and time-management techniques. They are making dietary changes, such as reducing fat intake and increasing fiber intake, and exercising, all in the hope that some of these methods will strengthen their ability to fight and ultimately beat the disease.[11]

In alignment with these findings, research at The Wellness Community indicates that participants in TWC's support groups are encouraged to make changes in their lives that they think are important, develop a new attitude toward the illness (but not just a positive attitude), access resources and information about cancer, and partner with their physicians.

In essence, people with cancer should be encouraged to develop realistic expectations about their illness so they can make good decisions about their care, not be pressured to be blindly positive. The important distinction is that optimism should not exclude sadness, anger, sorrow, grief, and hurt. You can decide to go on in the face of all that, knowing the outcome is not under your control.

The Difference Between Optimism (Positive Attitude) and Hope

Jerome Groopman, M.D., author of *The Anatomy of Hope*, explains that a positive attitude, or optimism, is the thought that "everything is going to turn out for the best." But life isn't like that. Sometimes bad things happen to wonderful people. Hope, in contrast, does not make that assumption, but rather in a clear-eyed manner assesses all the problems, challenges, or obstacles, and through information and education, seeks and finds a possible realistic path to a better future. This future is often unknown and unknowable but is constantly re-assessed based upon new information. A person with true hope will experience a wide range of emotions, including fear, anger, and sadness, and through it all will try to move forward through all the difficulties.[12]

At TWC, hope is understood to be something participants gain from each other. After all, there is no person a cancer patient would rather see than a cancer survivor. The ability to make pragmatic decisions in the face of cancer based upon being with others who know what you are going through is an essential ingredient at TWC. Participants learning from each other can increase hope as well as reduce some of the stress associated with cancer.[13] If longer survival is not possible, then it is reasonable to hope for other meaningful outcomes—like hoping for a peaceful death or the resolution of family conflicts. And gaining information and support from others with cancer may lead to positive immunological and stress hormone responses.

The Internet and Cancer Support

Today, it is hard to imagine what life would be like without e-mail and access to the Internet. We take it for granted. But the idea that you could receive support and information via the Web that is as helpful as the support or information you receive via a face-to-face support group or workshop is revolutionary. And this revolution is taking place today, backed up by research to support its value.

To capture the immensity of this health-information revolution, consider these facts about the Internet:

• A February 2004 Harris Poll found 74 percent of Internet users—76 million Americans—had visited a Web site that provided health-related information or support.
• 25.2 million had contacted a support group for help.
• 4.9 million had participated in some form of support group.
• 70 percent of those who had sought health information reported that the information they received influenced their treatment decisions.

Have you ever considered joining an on-line support group or chat room? Have you wondered whether these Internet-based support groups actually help? An important 2003 research study found that women with breast cancer who participated in professionally facilitated on-line support groups scheduled in "real time" (modeled after TWK's face-to-face support groups) experienced significant decreases in depression and negative reactions to pain, as well as significant increases in spirituality and zest for life.[14] Another study offering professionally moderated support groups that were not in real time and included semistructured topics also showed significant decreases in depression, perceived stress, and cancer-related trauma.[15]

In a comparison of face-to-face to on-line support groups, both offered through TWC for women with breast cancer, participants in both groups derived similar support and access to information. Similarly, the facilitators in both settings played near identical roles helping participants express emotions, reframe experiences, and learn from each other.[16] So, while there is need for continuing research, it appears that those participating in TWC on-line support groups are receiving similar benefits to those participating in face-to-face groups. These results are promising in that many more people with cancer—especially those who are too sick or too distant from support services—can now be helped.

In fact, as a result of these findings, in February 2002, TWC launched The Virtual Wellness Community (TVWC) at *www.thewellnesscommunity.org*. The Web site mirrors a brick-and-mortar wellness community with free, professionally moderated support groups. It hosts physician lectures, mind-body programs, and other services for cancer patients and their loved ones. The Wellness Community creates homelike settings for their participants, and we wanted The Virtual Wellness Community to do the same. There is a mind-body room, a library, and a kitchen filled with nutrition information.

Currently, there are on-line support groups at The Virtual Wellness Community and other Web sites, for people with a variety of diagnoses, including breast, prostate, lung, ovarian, pancreatic,

and colorectal cancers and lymphoma, and for caregiver groups as well. TWC also offers similar program services in Spanish (*http://espanol.thewellnesscommunity. org*). As of May 2004, TVWC had received more than 4.5 million hits since its introduction and over 71,000 unique visitors, while serving 129 people in on-line support groups.

Following are other valuable Web sites that provide ongoing education and support:

• People Living With Cancer by the American Society for Clinical Oncology (*www.plwc.org*)
• Cancer*Care* (*www.cancercare.org*)
• The American Cancer Society (*www. cancer.org*)
• The National Cancer Institute (*www. cancer.gov*)
• GroupLoop, for teens with cancer, by The Wellness Community (*www. grouploop.org*)

While there are a multitude of places on the Internet to find information and engage in discussion with other survivors, it is important to be careful about what information you may be receiving. For on-line support groups or chat rooms, ask if the sessions are professionally facilitated or moderated, if they are password secure, and if there is a way to screen participants for cancer. This can help to create a safe environment that is a good place to share information and feelings.

Other Helpful Activities for Managing Distress

Along with participation in support groups, managing difficult emotions, and reducing feelings of isolation and loss of hope, there are several other ways to increase control and actively cope with cancer. Research shows that the following skills not only improve quality of life, but may actually enhance immune function, too:

• Managing stress through muscle relaxation, self-hypnosis, mindfulness meditation, directed visualization, and other stress-reduction methods
• Problem solving (especially for difficult decisions) by breaking down the issue into its component parts: definition, brainstorming solutions, prioritizing, choosing a course of action, and evaluating the results
• Managing pain by treating it promptly and sufficiently
• Reducing fatigue by managing your expectations during and after treatment
• Treating lingering depression, since it impedes your ability to cope with the illness and follow treatment recommendations

Hope for the Future

There are nearly 10.5 million cancer survivors today! It is true that there are many actions people with cancer can take that may have a beneficial effect on the fight for recovery. We are in an exciting era where new discoveries in cancer treatment—targeted therapies and findings from the Human Genome Project—are not only prolonging life, but improving quality of life. We have learned that access to high-quality cancer-related information and support are the building blocks for coping with the illness. We have outlined evidence-based skills that you can use that can and will make a difference. You are not alone, and we hope this information will provide you with the tools to help you help yourself!

Notes

1. Spiegel et al., 1981; Spiegel and Bloom, 1983; Cain et al., 1986; Trijsburg et al., 1992; Fawzy et al., 1993; Berglund et al., 1994; Classen et al., 2001.

2. Spiegel et al., 1989; Fawzy et al., 1993.

3. Goodwin PJ, et al. The effect of group psychosocial support on survival in metastatic breast cancer. *N Eng J Med* 2001, Dec;345:1719–26.

4. Taylor et al., 1986; McLean, 1995; Glajchen and Moul, 1996; Gray et al., 1998; Helgeson et al., 2000.

5. Taylor et al., 1986; McLean, 1995; Glajchen and Moul, 1996; Gray et al., 1998; Helgeson et al., 2000.

6. Cordova, Giese-Davis, Golant, et al., 2003.

7. Giese-Davis, 2002.

8. Greenberg et al., 1993 and 1996; Salavoy et al., 2000.

9. Giese-Davis, 2002.

10. Marcus AD. "Fighting Cancer with a Frown." *Wall Street Journal,* 6 April 2004: D1.

11. Marcus AD. "Fighting Cancer with a Frown." *Wall Street Journal,* 6 April 2004: D1.

12. Groopman J. *Anatomy of Hope.* New York: Random House, 2003.

13. Benjamin H. *The Wellness Community Guide to Fighting for Recovery from Cancer.* New York: Tucher, 1995.

14. Lieberman M, Golant M, Giese-Davis J, Winzelberg A, Benjamin H, Humphreys K, Kronenwetter C, Russo S, Spiegel D. Electronic support groups for breast carcinoma: A clinical trial of effectiveness. *Cancer* 2003;97(4):920–925.

15. Winzelberg A, et al. Evaluation of an internet support group for women with breast cancer. *Cancer* 2003;98(5);1164–1173.

16. Golant M, Lieberman M, Giese-Davis J, et al., *Facilitating online vs. face-to-face support groups.* 6th World Congress of Psycho-Oncology, Alberta, Canada, April 2003.

— 35 —

Survivorship Guidelines
for Cancer Patients and Their Families

*Ernest H. Rosenbaum, M.D., Patricia Fobair, L.M.S.W., M.Ph.,
and David Spiegel, M.D.*

■ ■ ■ ■

Cancer Is a
Life-Changing Event!

A cancer survivor is defined as one living from the time of diagnosis, throughout the remainder of his or her life, with and beyond cancer. Understanding the long-term physical and psychosocial effects of cancer and cancer therapy can help patients and their families better deal with potential complications associated with being a cancer survivor.

Currently, there are over 1.4 million new cases of cancer diagnosed each year in the United States; by the year 2030, this number is expected to double. The National Cancer Institute (NCI) and American Cancer Society (ACS) project that about one-third of women and one-half of men will have cancer in their lifetime. One in four people are expected to die from the disease.

At the same time, the survival rate is increasing, rising from 3 million survivors fifteen years ago to over 10 million survivors in the year 2006. This rate will continue to increase with advances in diagnosis, treatment, and care. It is estimated that by 2030, there will be over 20 million survivors. Cancer has become a *chronic* disease.

Unfortunately, many survivors experience lasting adverse side effects of treatment. Although the current five-year survival rate is 64 percent (compared to 50 percent twenty-five years ago), the estimated follow-up needed is at least ten to twenty-plus years, the remainder of the survivor's life. Susan Sontag's cancer experience provides a good example of the potential for productivity, wellness, and longevity in survivorship—diagnosed and treated for metastatic breast cancer at age forty-five, she subsequently died at age seventy-one of a new cancer.

Despite advances and innovations in cancer diagnosis and treatment, the consequences for survivors remain serious. Over 50 percent of cancer survivors have residual side effects; over 25 percent experience recurrence or develop new cancers. It is estimated that 75 percent of survivors can have health deficits related to their treatment.[1]

There is also overwhelming evidence that "cancer patients die of noncancer causes at a higher rate than persons in the general population."[2] Added to known cancer-specific vulnerabilities, the increased risk of additional illnesses (referred to as comorbid conditions) makes the need for follow-up programs for cancer survivors even more urgent. Common comorbid conditions that threaten the lives of cancer survivors include well-known entities such as coronary artery disease, congestive heart failure, and diabetes.

Age is a major risk factor that has recently been shown to correlate to functional decline. Sixty-one percent of cancer survivors are over the age of sixty-five. In the United States, 12.4 percent of the population (35 million people) is currently over sixty-five, and this demographic is expected to double by 2030 to 70 million (20 percent). As people's life expectancies continue to increase, a natural result is that they often must deal with more comorbidities.

Survivors are also at risk for psychological and physiologic changes, which include potential organ dysfunction, an impaired immune system, sexual dysfunction, cognitive changes, fatigue, depression, anxiety, and family distress, as well as economic challenges related to insurance, job security, and monetary survival.

The Challenge

The greatest of the many barriers to effective long-term survivorship care is the lack of awareness. While many cancer patients seek better ways to reduce their risk and improve their survival through better health and lifestyle practices, some patients, after completing their therapy, wish to distance themselves from their cancer and do not wish to continue in a follow-up program.

The challenge for health professionals is to provide and implement ways to improve lifestyle changes and health outcomes. Cancer survivors need to be made aware of the new conditions and risks that follow cancer and its treatment, as well as strategies they can implement to reduce their vulnerabilities. Oncologists and the medical team (primary physicians, general practitioners, nurse specialists, etc.) can play a key role in cancer detection, treatment, surveillance, and prevention for patient care. Unfortunately, only about 20 percent of oncologists actively guide survivors on better health practices and lifestyle changes. In addition, physicians often do not have access to current standards of care and clinical guidelines.

A multidisciplinary team approach and a variety of delivery systems are needed to address the medical, psychosocial, and lifestyle components of survivorship care. The American Society of Clinical Oncology (ASCO), Institute of Medicine (IOM), National Coalition for Cancer Survivorship (NCCS), and ACS are currently working together on a task force to provide specific guidelines for therapy, screening, and prevention. The following is a list of actions identified to improve health and longevity:

1. Collect statistics on comorbid health and follow-up screening of survivors, assess treatment results and quality of life, and promulgate "best practices"[3]

2. Collect and analyze data on disability and dysfunction due to age to identify ways to improve function and quality of life[4]

3. Promote better lifestyles (e.g., diet, exercise, smoking cessation, limited alcohol, and reduced sun exposure) and screening for comorbid diseases, cancer recurrence, new cancers, and comorbidities

4. Reduce and improve side effects of therapy and cancer (e.g., lymphedema, sexual dysfunction, fatigue, cognitive/memory problems, and mucositis) and late aftereffects, or sequelae (e.g., cardiac dysfunction, osteoporosis, pulmonary fibrosis, and kidney failure)

5. Improve survival by reducing comorbidities and treatment side effects (using improved treatments such as sentinel node biopsies and adjuvant therapies and new drug treatments to promote longevity, quality of life, and survival)

Recommended "Road Map" for Survivors

Healthy survivorship requires implementation of a healthy lifestyle, measures to reduce comorbid risks, and a *cancer care plan* with recommendations for follow-up for each patient. An ideal care plan includes a review of the patient's medical history, diagnosis, and treatments and a set of follow-up recommendations to help guide both patient and caregivers over the next twenty-plus years with appropriate surveillance and interventions to minimize, and hopefully prevent, further problems. The patient should be provided with the following:

1. Information about potential late- and long-term side effects of cancer and cancer therapy and the possibility of recurrence or a new cancer
2. A standardized program highlighting potential future problems and prevention measures such as follow-up observational and screening programs
3. Information about lifestyle changes that can reduce the risk and severity of side effects and comorbidities
4. Psychosocial and group therapy support for anxiety, fear, isolation, and depression problems
5. A list of community resources to aid in obtaining benefits, insurance, employment protection, and life-support needs
6. Ongoing communication of new advances in medicine and current research that could help reduce the sequelae of both cancer and cancer therapy

By providing patients with a *cancer care plan*, oncologists make it possible for survivors to truly understand the lifelong scope of their condition and become "partners" in their medical care. Although many survivors wish to forget their cancer experience at the end of their therapy, many others need the reassurance of having a plan and knowing how to recognize what may later be side effects of their disease or its treatment.

There is no specific follow-up schedule, as each patient is different and will require different follow-up program guidelines depending on the type of cancer he or she has. However, there are generalized elements that should be included, outlined on page 291.

Side Effects of Cancer and Its Therapy

With the current five-year survival rate of 64 percent, the majority of cancer patients will live years and decades longer. At the same time, they face various challenges following curative or remission therapy, which in turn can affect personality, emotions, and social relations. There are also possible physical changes due to surgery, radiation therapy, chemotherapy, and immunotherapy, causing physical limitations and challenges to quality of life. While there are a number of side effects associated with cancer and its therapy that should be discussed with the physician, late effects, long-term effects, recurrence, second tumors, infertility, and fatigue are addressed below.

Late Effects Late effects of therapy involve unrecognized toxicities that occur many years posttherapy. Information about potential latent side effects of cancer therapy can arm survivors with knowledge and a plan. By providing and promoting lifestyle interventions, it is possible to reduce the rate of current and late comorbidities and adverse therapy related to toxic side effects.

Often, there may be changes that occur months or years after treatment. An example of this is heart problems following therapy with drugs such as doxorubicin (Adriamycin) and trastuzumab (Herceptin). Research is ongoing to evaluate better and safer treatments and also ways of coping with and reducing these delayed side effects.

Many times, late complications from toxic side effects of therapy not only bring back fears and physical problems, but also may require specialized treatments and care to help improve and ameliorate

An Example of a Cancer Survivor Follow-Up Plan

1. Patient name: _____ Address: _____ Telephone: _____

2. Medical record number: _____

3. Hospital(s) where treated: _____

4. Diagnosis

   Type of cancer: _____

   Pathology and grade: _____

5. Doctors involved in care: _____

   Addresses: _____

   Telephone numbers: _____

6. Brief History

   Clinical evaluation: _____

   X-rays: _____

   Lab tests: _____

7. Treatment: _____

   Surgery report: _____

   Radiation Therapy Report

      Type: _____

      Dose: _____

      X-ray field: _____

      Where performed: _____

   Chemotherapy and/or Immunotherapy Report

      Protocol: _____

      Drugs: _____

      Dose: _____

      Frequency: _____

(continues)

An Example of a Cancer Survivor Follow-Up Plan (*cont.*)

8. Potential short- and long-term consequences of therapy (such as delayed cardiac toxicity and delayed physical impairment) and side effects: _____

   _____

   _____

9. Suggested posttreatment plan for potential second malignancies or recurrence: _____

   _____

   _____

10. Follow-Up Recommendations for the Next Ten to Twenty-Plus Years

    Intervals for follow-up doctor visits: _____

    Tests needed: _____

11. Provide resources for supportive care for:

    • group or family support,

    • occupational therapy and/or physical therapy,

    • home care,

    • psychosocial support for survivors, and

    • physical care (pain, nutrition, fatigue, or sexual dysfunction).

12. Provide information on insurance, employment protection, and community resources.

these symptoms. For example, thyroid failure (hypothyroidism) can occur years following neck radiation involving the thyroid gland. Knowing that this could happen can help reduce anxiety by assuring the patient that this is not a recurrence of the cancer, but a delayed side effect from treatment.

Long-Term Effects Long-term effects are side effects or complications of therapy that persist when therapy is completed, requiring patients to develop compensatory treatment programs to relieve or

control these symptoms. This is in contrast to late effects, which occur months or years posttreatment.

For example, peripheral neuropathy (pain, numbness, tingling, loss of sensation, or heat or cold sensitivity in the extremities or the body) is often a long-term side effect in patients receiving particular chemotherapy agents such as platinum compounds (carboplatin [Paraplatin], cisplatin [Platinol], oxaliplatin [Eloxatin]), vincristine (Oncovin), and taxanes (paclitaxel [Taxol], docetaxel [Taxotere]). Surgery, radiation, or chemotherapy can cause damage to vital organs, such as the heart, lungs, kidneys, and gastrointestinal tract. Older persons over the age of sixty-five may have preexisting heart, lung, kidney, gastrointestinal, or liver problems that are exacerbated by anticancer therapy, as these organs may be more susceptible to side effects from treatment.

Cardiac dysfunction problems can occur early or late with anthracycline drugs, including doxorubicin (Adriamycin), daunorubicin (Cerubidine), epirubicin (Ellence), and mitoxantrone (Novantrone). Long-term follow-up is recommended for possible congestive heart failure up to twenty-plus years after treatment. For those who already have cardiac problems, radiation to the heart and treatment with these drugs can also cause progressive cardiac problems. Protective drugs are being developed to delay or prevent damage. In addition, lifestyle changes of diet and exercise are important for promoting better health and disease prevention.

Platinum compounds can cause decrease in kidney function, and this can also be accentuated when there is abdominal radiation involving the kidneys. Platinum compounds can also cause high-frequency hearing loss. For those receiving radiation therapy to the head, common problems may include cataracts, dry eyes, and dry mouth. Abdominal radiation can cause chronic diarrhea, malabsorption, milk/lactose intolerance, bowel dysfunction, and weight loss.

Recurrent and Second Tumors Survivors also need to be followed for many years for the possibility of developing either a recurrence of their original cancer or a completely separate, second primary cancer relating to their prior therapy. It's been estimated that up to 25 percent of patients may face a problem such as bone marrow failure, myelodysplasia (bone marrow dysfunction), or a new cancer. Lifestyle practices can be helpful in reducing the risk of comorbid conditions and possibly second cancers or delayed recurrences.

Fertility Problems Infertility is a serious concern for patients wishing to have children. Infertility can occur with patients receiving radiation to the testes. However, it has been noted that hormone levels in irradiated children usually remain normal as they go through puberty. Radiation to the abdomen and chemotherapy may also affect the reproductive organs (ovaries or testes), resulting in infertility. While chemotherapy can cause infertility, not all drugs have this effect. The alkalating agents, such as nitrogen mustard (Mustargen), cyclophosphamide (Cytoxan), chlorambucil (Leukeran), and ifosfamide (Ifex), have been implicated, but the effects depend on the dose and administration of the drugs. Methods to preserve fertility are therefore an important consideration for those wishing to have children (see chapter 20, "Coping with the Side Effects of Chemotherapy").

Fatigue Fatigue is one of the major problems during therapy and posttherapy, requiring an active program for fatigue reduction. Both rest and exercise help in controlling debility and fatigue problems. In addition to treatment effects, fatigue can be caused by emotional stress, anxiety, depression, pain, and problems sleeping, as well as a hormonal problem such as hypothyroidism (low thyroid function) or anemia due directly to cancer or as a result of treatment.

Preventive Measures

It is as important to make and implement positive recommendations for cancer prevention as it is to diagnosis and treat cancer. Given the increase in risk of developing side effects and comorbidities, as well as the potential recurrence of other cancers, prevention measures are critical for the cancer survivor.

Consensus guideline templates are being developed to promote wellness and quality of life, from the time of diagnosis through the current standard of five years' surveillance posttreatment and into long-term follow-up for ten to twenty-plus years beyond that.

Follow-up care is essential and in reality will most likely be delivered by primary care physicians or a nursing team. There is a need for experience in long-term follow-up for chronic conditions, even for individuals who seem to have recovered completely from their cancer and associated treatment.

The three levels of prevention are described below with examples pertinent to cancer survivors. The patient's *cancer care plan* should provide a detailed list of recommended screening tests and frequency, as well as suggestions for staying healthy.

Primary Prevention Primary prevention refers to lifestyle changes aimed at preventing cancer from occurring. Examples include a prudent-type diet, smoking cessation, reduction of alcohol use, reduction of sun exposure, and exercise.

Secondary Prevention Secondary prevention involves implementing screening programs to detect cancer at its earliest stages, usually before a person notices anything wrong (e.g., screening tools for cervix, breast, colon, prostate, and skin cancers). This includes vigilance in detecting secondary malignancies after original cancer therapy (e.g., increased risk for breast cancer many years following chest mantle radiotherapy for Hodgkin's disease therapy merits long-term follow-up for detection of breast cancer at its earliest stages). Additionally, secondary prevention involves early detection of nonmalignant conditions

that may result from cancer treatment, such as osteoporosis.

Tertiary Prevention Tertiary prevention is directed toward individuals who already have a disease (e.g., cancer), to prevent further damage, pain, and debility and to improve their overall functional status. This includes management of late and long-term toxicities related to cancer therapy. Examples include using drugs such as dexrazoxane (Zinecard) to reduce the risk of cardiac toxicity from anthracyclines; administration of bisphosphonates for patients with bony metastases to reduce the risk of fractures and other skeletal complications; and optimizing pain management in patients with pain due directly to their cancer or as a result of cancer treatment.

Lifestyle Changes

A cure does not mark the end of the healing process. Sometimes, it is a difficult transition from the state of illness to the state of well-being. While the goal is to resume as normal a life as possible, there are major changes following the crisis of a cancer diagnosis and treatment. Physical, psychological, and social problems may come to light or persist following the completion of cancer treatment.

To promote better health and reduce the risk of premature morbidity and mortality, survivors need to improve both the physical and emotional quality of life. Thus, it is necessary that survivors acquire and adopt lifestyle changes to help reduce the risk of future morbidity. As patients grow older, new risk factors are constantly evolving that require new solutions, constant vigilance, and care.

Functional status deteriorates during cancer therapy but usually recovers posttherapy with time. Older cancer patients who have one comorbidity have twice the risk of experiencing functional debility; with two comorbidities, the risk increases fivefold. Some of the problems survivors face after surgery, chemotherapy, and/or radiation therapy include a decrease in immune functioning, cardiopulmonary toxicity, and, in many cases, weight gain.

The diagnosis of cancer not only poses a challenge for survivors, but also necessitates many changes in lifestyle for both the patient and the family. Improving lifestyles reduces comorbid health risks and can help reduce therapy side effects. Preventive and healthy activities should be implemented, including psychosocial support, a healthy diet, exercise, sun protection, osteoporosis prevention, smoking cessation, and alcohol abstinence. Physicians and nurse specialists are best situated to recommend the screening and preventive medicine programs that will promote a better quality of life for posttherapy cancer patients.

Adopting a Prudent Diet Diet modifications made post–cancer diagnosis are common in 30 to 60 percent of survivors. These changes generally include decreased consumption of red meat,

saturated fat, and trans fats and increased consumption of fruits, vegetables, and whole grains. Decreased calorie intake combined with increased exercise is important for weight control, longevity, and survival.

In particular, survivors need to acknowledge lifestyle dangers and changes due to obesity. Obesity increases the risk for diabetes, cardiovascular disease, and certain cancers, including breast (postmenopausal), prostate, colon, kidney, esophagus, and endometrial cancers. In fact, 20 to 30 percent of cancers in the United States can be attributed to obesity and lack of exercise. In addition, the diseases associated with obesity, diabetes, and cardiovascular disease are responsible for an increased number of non-cancer-related deaths among survivors. In survivors, fully one-half of non-cancer-related deaths are related to noncancer comorbidities.

The proportion of newly diagnosed obese cancer patients is increasing, as is the number of patients who gain weight during therapy and post–cancer therapy. Thus, weight control through diet and

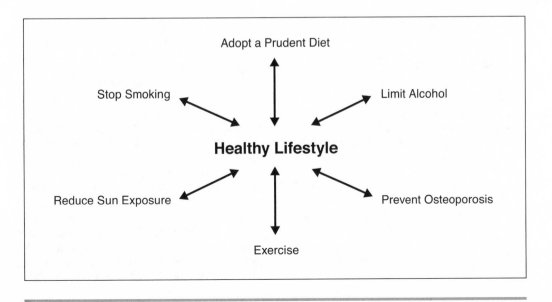

exercise is crucial for healthy survivorship. Survivors need to work toward the goal of a body mass index (BMI—weight [kg] divided by height [meters] squared and multiplied by 703) of less than 25 to avoid obesity. Unfortunately, older males and people who are less educated are less likely to adopt changes necessary to avoid obesity. It has been estimated that only 25 percent to 42 percent of survivors consume adequate amounts of fruits and vegetables, and that 70 percent of breast and prostate cancer survivors are overweight or obese.

Diabetes is also a common, chronic disease in cancer survivors. It can lead to eye disease, kidney disease, and nerve damage and is a risk factor for cardiovascular disease. Most people with diabetes are overweight and have type 2 diabetes, or non-insulin-dependent diabetes mellitus. Although excellent control of blood sugar levels can decrease the risk of the above complications, prevention of this type of diabetes through lifelong diet modification with exercise remains the best option for a healthy life.

A prudent diet that will help prevent obesity and diabetes, as well as potentially increase longevity, is all of the following:

- A well-balanced diet.
- A low-fat diet (less than 25 percent fat calories).
- Limit saturated fats to 8 percent of calories.
- Decrease animal fats and processed meats.
- Increase fish intake.
- Use low-fat dairy foods.
- A high-fiber diet (30 to 35 g per day).
- Increase whole-grain foods (breads and cereals).
- A variety of eight to ten portions of fruits and vegetables daily.
- Increase cruciferous vegetables (e.g., broccoli, cauliflower, turnips, and kale).

In addition, limit salt-cured, smoked, and nitrate-cured foods, as well as fried and barbecued foods. Alcohol should also be limited to one or two drinks a day.

Exercise Exercise plays a key role in reducing cancer risk and can be very beneficial in promoting survival and longevity. Exercise is correlated with improved quality of life, improved physical functioning (oxygen capacity, strength, flexibility, and general health), and improved blood pressure, heart rate, and circulating-hormone-level control. It is now well established that for breast and prostate cancers, exercise helps promote longevity and potentially disease control. The risk reduction has been confirmed in many studies, which also provide an understanding of the physiological mechanisms by which exercise effectively reduces breast and prostate cancer risk, as well as fatigue, and improves quality of life.

Exercise helps reduce obesity and not only improves long-term health, but also reduces the risk of several comorbid conditions, including disease progression, possible second primary cancers, osteoporosis, cardiovascular disease, diabetes, and functional physical decline.

Exercise is a vital component to losing weight. Aerobic exercise is the most effective and involves rhythmical use of the large muscles of the legs and arms to elevate the heart rate within a certain range. Examples are brisk walking, jogging, swimming, bicycling, gardening, dancing, playing actively with children, and sexual activity.

Preexisting comorbidities (arthritis, cardiovascular disease, chronic obstructive pulmonary disease) may limit physical and social functioning. For survivors with these conditions, alternate exercise programs such as tai chi, qi gong, and yoga can help promote muscle strength, flexibility, coordination, balance, and body function. Also, tai chi has been shown not only to improve health-related quality of life, balance, and self-esteem, but also to contribute to prolonged longevity. Tai chi also promotes psychosocial support for improving health-related quality of life.

Physical-activity programs help improve cardiorespiratory fitness during and after treatment and at the same time help lessen fatigue and promote improved vigor with better quality of life and less depression and mental distress.

Tobacco in Survivors The use of tobacco is diminishing. Fewer cigarettes were sold in 2005 than in 1951, and more places are now designated as nonsmoking areas. There are now more nonsmokers than smokers.

Unfortunately, however, more children in the eighth grade are now smoking. Quitting rates for lung and head and neck cancer survivors are about 40 percent versus about 4 percent for breast cancer patients. Sadly, younger survivors often continue to smoke. Smoking has been causally related to lung, bladder, head and neck, cervix, kidney, and esophagus cancers, as well as cardiovascular disease and chronic obstructive pulmonary disease.

Cessation efforts are necessary for survivors. Even five minutes of a physician's advice on how to stop smoking can be very critical in a patient's success.

Alcohol in Survivors In over 100 studies, alcohol has been shown to be a small to modest cancer risk factor, where one drink a day increases the risk 8 to 10 percent and two drinks a day may increase the risk up to 25 percent.

Research suggests that the effect of alcohol on breast cancer risk is greater in postmenopausal women with estrogen-positive tumors. How and why this is remains unknown at this time but may be related to increased estrogen levels. Alcohol increases the need for folic acid; thus 400 mcg per day is suggested for those who consume alcohol.

The majority of habitual alcohol drinkers do not eat a nutritious diet, resulting in an additional health deficit. The alcohol abstinence rate for head and neck cancer survivors is about 50 percent; for breast and lung cancer survivors, the abstinence rate is 8 to 16 percent.

Reducing Sun Exposure Excess sun exposure can damage the skin, causing premature aging and sometimes leading to various forms of skin cancer. A skin protection program is vital.

Preventing Osteoporosis Loss of ovarian or testicular function may also contribute to osteoporosis by decreasing hormone levels (estrogen or testosterone) with subsequent bone weakness and/or fractures. This problem necessitates the use of calcium, vitamin D, hormonal replacement therapy (estrogen or testosterone), and possibly biphosphonate therapy.

Short- and Long-Term Psychological Effects

All patients and survivors not only have medical problems from cancer and its therapy, but also have emotional and social well-being challenges. The stress of coping with a cancer diagnosis ranges from mild to severe, often depending on the severity of the diagnosis and treatment and the prior mood of survivors. A third or more of patients report psychological distress during the early months of treatment.[5,6,7] The prevalence of psychological distress in one study of 4,496 cancer patients at the Johns Hopkins Kimmel Cancer Center was 35 percent.[8]

Mood usually improves over time for many survivors.[9] Although some patients adjust their lives and actually feel better, others have anxiety, depression, and feelings of isolation, as well as problems interacting with friends and family. Subgroups of survivors remain vulnerable to distress or depression for a long period of time. Clinical depression affects 18 to 21 percent of survivors at various points of time.[10,11] Cancer survivors who were depressed prior to their diagnosis are at a heightened risk for shortened survival time.[12]

Cancer survivors are vulnerable to both acute and post-traumatic stress, a result of the life threat and loss of control experienced following diagnosis and treatment. These responses are similar to those of the acute and post-traumatic stress syndromes seen in soldiers on the battlefront or returning from war, or among those who have experienced extreme psychological or physical problems.

Clinical evaluation, counseling, and educational programs offered immediately postdiagnosis and following treatment can reduce stress and lead to a better adjustment to the consequences of having cancer and receiving therapy. The cancer center at Stanford University (where the authors work), for example, has been a leader in offering group support, individual counseling, massage, medical qi gong, tai chi, restorative yoga, healing and guided imagery, expressive art and imagery, creative writing, healing touch, and exercise. Educational programs are provided, such as Managing and Understanding Your Chemotherapy and Look Good . . . Feel Better, as well as nutritional consultations. Group therapies are provided for patients with breast, brain, ovarian, and colorectal cancers, leukemia and lymphoma, and multiple diagnoses, and for husbands of women with cancer.

Psychological Support

Patients facing a diagnosis and treatment for cancer often have anxiety, depression, psychological distress, loss of control, and fear. These emotions are better controlled with psychological support such as individual counseling and group therapy.

Psychosocial Spiritual and Religious Support

It is of interest that an association between spirituality and improved survival has been observed in some studies. Cardiovascular research has shown that patients who gain comfort and strength from religion and/or spirituality and who participate in social and community groups have a lower mortality rate during the six months following cardiac surgery than those who are lacking in these categories.

In a recent article in the *Mayo Clinic Proceedings,* Edward Creagan, M.D., wrote that "cancer survivors may be spared for reasons that are not clearly understood," and that "among the coping methods of long-term cancer survivors, the predominant strategy is spiritual. It is still recognized that the biology of a cancer is the most important determinant in the life history of a cancer course, but it is now becoming recognized that religion or spirituality may also influence the course of the cancer."[13]

Community Resources Many people do not understand that cancer is not contagious, and their fears may be transmitted and cause problems for cancer survivors in the work area. Misconceptions and prejudices can influence how employers and coworkers treat survivors. The fear that a worker will be less productive has been refuted. In a study by MetLife Insurance and Bell Telephone, a survivor's job performance showed no difference when compared to nonsurvivors. In fact, survivors often work harder to prove their worth.

As a cancer survivor, you need to look at changes directed by superiors at the job, often because of fears that responsibilities cannot be effectively met. There is a social readjustment with coworkers and superiors, who may treat you differently or not promote you as merited. Keeping notes on these problems is important: If you are discriminated against and legal action is necessary, you will need documentation.

The Americans with Disabilities Act of 1990 makes it illegal to discriminate against any qualified applicant who is disabled, has a history of disability, or is perceived to have a disability. Thus, survivors have recourse if they have legitimate complaints (Equal Employment Opportunity Connection, 1801 L Street, NW, Washington, D.C., 20507).

A good resource is the National Coalition for Cancer Survivorship, Silver Springs, Maryland (*canceradvocacy.org*).

More information is also available in

- the Institute of Medicine/National Research Council report *From Cancer Patient to Cancer Survivor, Lost in Transition*, published in November 2005, and
- *A Cancer Survivor's Almanac: Charting Your Journey* by Barbara Hoffman, J.D., National Coalition for Cancer Survivorship, published in 2004.

These two references also have extensive information about health insurance and employment issues for survivors.

Additional information can be found at *www.cancersupportivecare.com* and *www. canceradvocacy.org*.

Notes

1. Haylock PJ. The shifting paradigm of cancer care. *Nurs* 2006;106(3) supplement:16–19.

2. Brown BV, Brauner MC. Noncancer deaths in white adult cancer patients. *J Natl Cancer Inst* 1993;85:979–97.

3. Hewitt M, Greenfield S, and Stovall E, eds. *From Cancer Patient to Cancer Survivor, Lost in Transition*. Washington, D.C: The National Academies Press, 2005.

4. Sweeney C, Schmitz KH, Lazovich D, et al. Functional limitations in elderly female cancer survivors. *J Natl Cancer Inst* 2006;98(8):521–9.

5. Bodurka-Bevers D, Basen-Engquist K, Carmack CL, et al. Depression, anxiety, and quality of life in patients with epithelial ovarian cancer. *Gynecol Oncol* 2000;78(3 Pt 1):302–8.

6. Trask PC, Paterson A, Riba M, et al. Assessment of psychological distress in prospective bone marrow transplant patients. *Bone Marrow Transplant* 2002; 29(11):917–25.

7. Carlson LE, Angen M, Cullum J, et al. High levels of untreated distress and fatigue in cancer patients. *Br J Cancer* 2004;90(12):2297–304.

8. Zabora J, Brintzenhofeszoc K, Curbow B, Hooker C, Piantadosi S. The prevalence of psychological distress by cancer site. *Psychooncology* 2001;10(1):19–28.

9. Ganz, PA, Desmond KA, Leedham B, Rowland JH, Meyerowitz BE, Belin TR. Quality of life in long-term, disease-free survivors of breast cancer: A follow-up study. *J Natl Cancer Inst* 2002;94(1):39–49.

10. Bodurka-Bevers D, Basen-Engquist K, Carmack CL, et al. Depression, anxiety, and quality of life in patients with epithelial ovarian cancer. *Gynecol Oncol* 2000;78(3 Pt 1):302–8.

11. Fobair P, Hoppe RT, Bloom J, Cox R, Varghese A, Spiegel D. Psychosocial problems among survivors of Hodgkin's disease. *J Clin Oncol* 1986;4(5):805–14.

12. Brown KW, Levy AR, Rosberger Z, Edgar L. Psychological distress and cancer survival: A follow-up 10 years after diagnosis. *Psychosom Med* 2003;65 (4):636–43.

13. Creagen ET. Attitude and disposition: Do they make a difference in cancer survival? *Mayo Clin Proc* 1997;72(2):160–4.

— 36 —

Late Effects of Cancer Treatment

Anna T. Meadows, M.D.

■ ■ ■ ■

More than a decade ago, the recognition that there were millions of individuals in the United States (now almost 10 million) who had survived cancer prompted the director of the National Cancer Institute to establish the Office of Cancer Survivorship. The mission of the office was to support research and education that specifically addressed the needs of survivors. It enabled specific resources to be set aside to answer critical questions dealing with the effects of cancer and its treatment on this ever-increasing population. Since then, the importance of dealing with the problems of cancer survivors has been recognized. The Institute of Medicine has convened expert panels and published their findings and recommendations in two separate volumes: (1) Hewitt M, Weiner SL, Simone JV (eds), *Childhood Cancer Survivorship: Improving Care and Quality of Life* (Washington, D.C.: The National Academies Press, 2003), and (2) Hewitt M, Greenfield S, Stovall E (eds), *From Cancer Patient to Cancer Survivor: Lost in Transition* (Washington, D.C.: The National Academies Press, 2005).

The majority of survivors will be cured, and many more will live for years and decades. Some of the obstacles to achieving optimal quality of life were discussed in the previous chapter; they are in the realm of personality, emotions, relationships, and society. But the disease and its treatment can also impose specific medical, physical, or physiologic limitations that affect the quality of life for cancer

survivors. What are they and how are they related to the previous disease or treatment? Can there be effects of therapy that are not recognized immediately after treatment is complete? Can lifestyle practices exacerbate or ameliorate these effects? Are they inevitable consequences of cure—a Pyrrhic victory? Some of the answers to these questions are already available, but many require more time and dedicated patients and researchers before the answers will be known.

More than three decades ago, pediatric oncologists recognized that the treatment for childhood cancer was becoming very successful. Many children and adolescents were expected to be long-term survivors. In fact, that prediction has been borne out. At least two-thirds to three-quarters of children diagnosed with cancer are now able to be cured with modern therapy. The term *cure* began to be used in the early 1980s, when there were enough survivors who had remained free of any recurrence for some period of time from diagnosis. For some childhood cancers, it was as early as three years and for others, perhaps six or seven years from diagnosis.

Tumors of children are quite different from those that occur in adults; for example, the majority of children with leukemia have acute lymphocytic leukemia, a kind of leukemia that is rare in adults. Their other cancers are primarily derived from tissues that are still immature and undifferentiated. These cancer cells are more readily destroyed by chemicals and radiation than are the common adult-onset cancers. Since most survivors had been treated with radiation and chemotherapy, and since the drugs and radiation were also known to have effects on normal tissues, investigators began to be concerned that adverse outcomes might limit the quality of life for these children years later. This led researchers to begin the study of children and adolescents who were long-term survivors. It has taken many years to recognize that the very same treatment that worked so well to destroy cancer cells and produced such remarkable cure rates could also affect normal cells and tissues and lead to chronic problems many years later. Research in this area has led to a large body of literature concerning the effects of cancer treatment on children and adolescents.

What about adults? Until recently, the most common adult cancers were usually treated with surgery alone, and surgery may be responsible for medical effects years from treatment. Lymphedema is one such late complication that limits the quality of life for breast and prostate cancer survivors. Colostomies, amputations, and disfiguring surgery can sometimes interfere with activities of daily life or self-confidence.

During the past decade, oncologists have discovered that, for many cancers of adults, there is indeed great benefit from chemotherapy and radiation. Many cancers of adults have now been shown to respond well to the same treatment that has been so successful in children and adolescents during the past thirty years. These include leukemia, lymphomas (including Hodgkin's disease), testes cancer, breast cancer, and ovarian cancer.

Concern is now being expressed that survivors of adult cancers could be left with effects similar to those that were found to be troubling to children. Recently it has been possible to conduct long-term studies of the many adult survivors of those cancers for which chemotherapy

and radiation are widely used. Some of the long-term complications in children do not occur in adults, since they are fully grown and their organs are more resistant. However, recent studies have shown that other complications are a problem for some survivors.

Some of these are described in this chapter, but for a more comprehensive personal summary, survivors should discuss their specific risks with their oncologists. A referral may be made to a specialized clinic that deals with issues of concern to survivors. Information is also available through the National Coalition for Cancer Survivorship and the National Cancer Institute's Office of Cancer Survivorship.

Late Effects of Therapy on Growth and Development

For children, some of the most serious long-term effects concern growth and development. When immature bones are exposed to radiation, they fail to grow to their full potential. So children treated with radiation, depending on the dose and the age at which they are treated, may experience problems with linear growth if they have radiation to the chest, abdomen, spine, or legs. They also develop learning problems if their brains are in the field of radiation, especially if they are less than ten years of age at the time of treatment.

Chemotherapy has not been shown to affect the growth of children, but some drugs can act in a way that effectively increases the dose of radiation given to a particular part of the body. So a dose that would be considered unlikely to limit bone growth can do so if treatment also included so-called radiomimetic drugs, such as dactinomycin and doxirubicin (Adriamycin).

For adults whose growth is complete, radiation to long bones and to the spine will not affect linear growth. However, radiation to the brain, even in adults, may cause some short- or long-term memory problems. Knowing that this could happen before it does may help reduce the anxiety that often accompanies problems in people who have had cancer. It is quite natural to think the worst and to believe that every problem means that cancer has come back. Experience with children who are treated with brain radiation suggests that learning new ways of "learning" and remembering during the treatment period often reduces the severity of the memory problems.

Growth can also be affected by hypothyroidism (failure of the thyroid gland to produce adequate amounts of thyroid hormone). Hypothyroidism occurs when the neck has been treated with relatively large doses of radiation, such as the doses necessary to treat carcinomas, sarcomas, and lymphomas of the chest or head and neck.

Late Effects of Therapy on Fertility and Offspring

Radiation to the testes can cause boys to become infertile. However, except in cases where the dose has been very high, they are able to go through puberty normally and retain normal hormone levels. Harvesting sperm may be very important to some young men who wish to become fathers.

There is yet no well-established way to preserve eggs from females who may become infertile. Girls whose abdomens have been treated with radiation are almost always able to continue to have normal periods, and can become pregnant, unless they have received high doses to both ovaries. Women who have had abdominal radiation and become pregnant are considered to be "high risk." Their babies are sometimes small for dates, and their obstetricians should be informed of their past history. Radiation to the pelvis can affect the functioning of the ovaries and does lead to menopause earlier than the age at which it

normally occurs. Knowledge concerning these effects of radiation has been crucial in counseling young female survivors concerning family planning. The risk of osteoporosis and subsequent fractures is also increased following menopause and usually prompts a discussion concerning the benefits of hormonal replacement therapy (see chapter 28, "Becoming Sexually Active Again," and the chapter on breast cancer).

Chemotherapy can also lead to infertility. Not all drugs have that effect. Drugs known as alkylating agents, such as nitrogen mustard, cyclophosphamide, ifosfamide, and others in that class that are less widely used, can prevent both men and women from having children. The dose of drug is also critical; women are much more resistant to these effects than are men. While six months of treatment may affect most men, women can receive up to five times more drug and still have normal periods and will be able to have normal children. Again, however, menopause may occur earlier than usual, depending on the drugs and the doses.

Unlike children and adolescents who have not yet had children of their own, most adult cancer survivors would not be troubled by the infertility that accompanies abdominal, pelvic, or testes radiation or chemotherapy. Young men with testes cancer (the most common cancer in twenty- to forty-year-old males) are now being cured in large numbers, even when the cancer cells have spread (metastasized). If radiation or any of the chemotherapeutic drugs that are known to affect sperm production are to be part of the planned therapy, men in their early twenties and thirties may wish to inquire about saving sperm before treatment begins.

Many young cancer patients worry that their treatment will affect unborn children. While radiation and many drugs can affect an embryo or fetus in utero, this is quite different from any effect that these same treatments have on sperm or egg cells. There are some survivors whose cancer developed because of a genetic predisposition. This includes children with retinoblastoma and adults diagnosed with colon cancer who have the gene for polyposis coli. In those cases, it is not surprising that offspring have also developed the same tumor after inheriting the same gene. However, studies of thousands of childhood and adolescent cancer survivors have been done. It is reassuring to know that none of the studies has shown an excess of adverse pregnancy outcomes after therapy was complete that could be ascribed to the therapy.

Late Effects of Therapy on Vital Organs

Until recently, the idea that radiation and chemotherapy would damage vital organs such as the heart, the lungs, the kidneys, and the gastrointestinal tract was considered applicable only to children and adolescents. In fact, young people are likely to be at risk for more late toxicity than adults for several reasons. Their tumors usually require treatment with many drugs at relatively high doses, and some of the effects take decades before becoming apparent. Older persons may have underlying damage to their hearts, kidneys, lungs, or livers from other causes. They would then be more susceptible to additional problems caused by chemotherapeutic agents or radiation. One of the long-term effects for adults compared to children is that of peripheral neuropathy following treatment with the platinum compounds. Treatment with drugs such as amitryptyline (Elavil) and gabapentin (Neurontin) is often helpful in reducing symptoms of this complication.

Cardiac dysfunction is a particular consequence of therapy with a class of drugs known as the anthracyclines. This class includes daunorubicin, doxorubicin (Adriamycin), idarubicin, and mito-

xantrone (Novantrone), as well as others. Children who were treated with doses that exceeded those we now consider relatively safe can develop congestive heart failure five to twenty years after treatment. Adults with underlying cardiac problems who have received these drugs or radiation to the heart need to be followed regularly. Early signs of problems will enable the initiation of preventive therapy. Administering these drugs by prolonged infusions may reduce the late toxicity, and newer drugs, called radioprotectants, such as dexrazoxane (Zinecard) and amifostine (Ethyol), that have been developed for administration with the anthracyclines also may prevent or delay damage. Following healthy lifestyle practices involving diet and exercise is especially important for individuals who have had anthracyclines.

Patients treated with radiation therapy that included the kidneys or who received chemotherapy with any of the platinum compounds are at risk for kidney problems. Platinum compounds can also result in some hearing loss, especially for high-frequency sounds, rather than those in the speech range.

Radiation has long-term effects on other organs and tissues. The lungs may be affected by radiation to the chest, and also by bleomycin, a drug that affects the lungs. The pulmonary toxicity following therapy with either bleomycin or radiation will be increased in cigarette smokers. Cataracts, dry eyes, and dry mouth can be a consequence of radiation to the head. Decreased thyroid hormone, with a need for lifelong replacement, can result from radiation to the neck. Abdominal radiation can cause malabsorption, chronic diarrhea, lactose intolerance, and subsequent discomfort and weight loss.

Long-Term Psychosocial Effects

Much has been written about the psychosocial effects of having had cancer.

This summary can only touch on some of the most pervasive conclusions from numerous studies. Although few survivors are seriously affected by late medical complications, the experience of having had cancer is likely to leave its mark on the emotional and social well-being of all survivors.

Some individuals have reported major changes for the better. They have learned to appreciate every aspect of life more fully and with more positive feelings. Others are constantly troubled by anxiety and depression; many feel isolated from friends and family. Difficulties with employment and financial stress may add to feelings of insecurity and worthlessness.

Studies of childhood and adolescent survivors and their families have described a syndrome similar to post-traumatic stress that affects many patients and parents. The syndrome is characterized by intrusive flashbacks of unpleasant experiences, withdrawal or avoidance behavior, and physiologic changes similar to those experienced during threatening situations.

Programs of education and counseling after diagnosis have been shown not only to reduce stress during active treatment, but also to improve long-term psychological adjustment. Counseling services for survivors are now available at cancer centers and at most large treating institutions.

Second Tumors

Survivors of cancer live with the threat of recurrence. Sometimes that "recurrence" is not the reemergence of the original cancer, but rather the development of another type of cancer. It should be stressed that the most powerful factor predisposing to cancer is age. Therefore, as people live longer and their tissues and cells are exposed to a host of environmental influences, more cells are likely to become transformed and more cancers can develop. Cancer requires more than a single exposure, event, or "hit" to develop and often takes many years to become evident after exposure to cancer-causing agents. The vast majority of cancers, therefore, occur in individuals who are over the age of sixty years.

Once an individual has developed a malignant tumor, the possibility that another, second cancer can occur is increased. This is probably less true for children, since most childhood cancers result from chance events. The probability that a second cancer will occur depends on some well-known lifestyle practices and environmental exposures, on the therapy received for the first cancer, and, rarely, on certain genes that impart susceptibility for more than one tumor type. Many kinds of malignant tumors are related to cigarette smoking. The development of one cancer caused by smoking (e.g., lung) does not protect against cancer of the mouth, pancreas, or bladder, since all are increased in smokers. Workers exposed to asbestos, especially smokers, have an increased risk for lung cancer and mesothelioma, a cancer of the covering of the lungs and the abdominal organs.

Our knowledge of treatment-related second cancers comes primarily from studies of children who began to be cured in large numbers beginning in the early 1970s. After it was found that childhood cancers responded especially well to chemotherapy and radiation, many more children were cured. Hence, they were able to live for long enough periods following treatment for other cancers to develop. It has been known for some time that radiation is a potent carcinogen, or cancer-causing agent. It is a powerful destroyer of malignant cells and is therefore an essential tool in the oncology therapeutic armamentarium. But the same rays that destroy cancer are also capable of making changes in surrounding cells and tissues that increase the potential for malignant transformation.

Certain chemotherapeutic agents have also become associated with new cancers, but unlike radiation, which may lead to solid tumors in the field, drugs are implicated in the development of secondary leukemias. Alkylating agents are the most commonly used class of drugs that can lead to leukemia. Different members of this class have different leukemogenic potential. Dose is often an important factor in determining risk. Leukemias associated with alkylating agents occur principally between three and seven years, and almost never occur later than ten years after treatment. Another group of drugs, the topoisomerase inhibitors such as etoposide and teniposide, have also been associated with secondary leukemias. These latter occur earlier than those following alkylating agents, typically within three to five years of treatment, sometimes even earlier.

A small fraction of individuals who develop cancer do so because of genes, and those genes sometimes predispose to more than one type of cancer. Breast cancer is rarely genetic, but carriers of mutations in BRCA1 and BRCA2 may develop cancer of the ovary as well as the breast. Some of the genes associated with an increased risk for colon cancer may also increase the probability that cancers of other tissues will develop. Children who have the genetic form of retinoblastoma are at increased risk for tumors of bone and other tissues, especially during adolescence, and of other cancers as well throughout their lives. If they were treated with radiation therapy, the risk is increased for tumors in the area encompassed by the radiation field. Neurofibromatosis type 1 is another genetic condition that predisposes individuals to more than one tumor, and one in which radiation may also increase that risk.

Individuals with family histories suggestive of an inherited predisposition should seek genetic counseling to determine whether there is a responsible gene involved. This knowledge can be important in counseling survivors regarding their risk for second cancers, and in counseling family members, such as offspring, parents, and siblings.

Conclusion

All cancer survivors should receive a summary of their treatment and information regarding what is known about the potential consequences of that treatment. Many of the long-term complications of treatment described above occur in only a small fraction of people, but some are inevitable consequences of successful therapy. Most can be anticipated and treated. When physicians who care for survivors are aware of the potential long-term effects, appropriate surveillance and interventions to reduce or prevent further problems can be initiated. Patients who are aware of the therapy they received, and who remain actively involved in their own follow-up care, are their own best advocates.

— 37 —

Infertility Problems in Cancer Survivors

Mitchell P. Rosen, M.D.

■ ■ ■ ■

Infertility is a common problem for those who have had cancer and cancer therapy. In recent years, improvements in cancer treatments have been developed to both prolong life and reduce the risk of infertility. New treatment options are making fertility a possibility for many cancer survivors.[1]

The human reproductive system is complex and unique for both sexes. The reproductive system is affected by many cancer-related therapies, with the end result of difficulty conceiving. Cancer therapy effects on fertility depend on the patient's age, type of cancer, and method of treatment. In order to understand the causes of infertility related to cancer and cancer therapies, we will review the reproductive system and processes of ovulation, sperm production, and fertilization.

Reproductive System

The reproductive axis is made up of the pituitary gland, the gonads (ovaries or testes), and the reproductive tract (the vagina, uterus, and fallopian tubes in women and the epididymis, vas deferens, penile urethra, and glands in men). In men, the seminal vesicles and prostate are the major glands responsible for semen production.

Women A woman's oocytes (eggs) are completely formed during fetal development and stored in a resting pool in her two ovaries. After birth, the oocytes do not regenerate but rather decline with age; their depletion results in ovarian failure (menopause). The oocytes continually leave the resting pool, enter the growth phase, and die. When a woman reaches puberty, a complex cyclic process begins—the menstrual cycle—which rescues one of the oocytes from death and causes ovulation, which culminates in either pregnancy or a period (menses). The ovulatory cycle continues until menopause, which occurs on average at fifty-one years of age. Ovulation is controlled by follicle-stimulating hormone (FSH) and luteinizing hormone (LH), which are produced by the pituitary gland. Once expelled from the ovary, the oocyte is captured by the fallopian tube and is ready to be fertilized. If it is fertilized, the resulting embryo moves into the uterus and attaches to the uterine lining to continue development. During the ovulatory cycle the ovaries also produce estrogen and progesterone, which prepare the lining of the uterus for the embryo, thereby facilitating implantation and maintenance of a pregnancy. If the oocyte is not fertilized, the lining of the uterus is shed, resulting in a period.

Men In contrast to the female reproductive system, in the male reproductive system sperm production is initiated at puberty and continues throughout life. The testes contain stem cells that continually replenish the sperm pool. The ability to produce sperm depends on adequate amounts of FSH, LH, and testosterone. The sperm are stored in the epididymis until ejaculation. During intercourse, the sperm are transported through ducts along with secretions from the glands and are ejaculated through the penile urethra. The process of ejaculation requires intact nerves in the pelvis. The testes also produce testosterone, which controls sex drive and the ability to achieve an erection.

Cancer Therapy and Reproduction

Cancer therapies can cause a spectrum of damage to the reproductive axis. The damage may be severe and result in sterility (ovarian or testicular failure) or partial injury resulting in early menopause and infertility (inability to conceive within twelve months). Symptoms of ovarian failure include absence of menses, hot flashes, and vaginal dryness. Testicular failure can lead to loss of sex drive and ejaculation or erection difficulties.

The treatments for cancer that can affect the reproductive system include the following:

- Surgery on the reproductive organs
- Chemotherapy
- Radiotherapy to abdomen and pelvis

Surgery Operations for cancer that do not involve the reproductive axis do not affect a woman's ability to achieve pregnancy. However, if the operation involves removing parts of the reproductive system, it may cause sterility or infertility. For example, treatment for gynecological cancer may involve the removal of the uterus (a hysterectomy), ovaries (a bilateral oophorectomy), or some portion of the reproductive tract such as the cervix, vulva, or vagina. Some operations may involve these organs but spare reproductive function. However, the scar tissue that develops after surgery may hinder conception. The surgery that is performed will depend on the type of cancer and whether it has spread to other organs.

For a man, surgery may involve removing both testicles (a bilateral orchidectomy), which results in sterility. Operations that spare one or both testicles preserve the capacity to conceive; however, other surgeries that involve removing the prostate, bladder, or bowel or that cause damage to the nerves in the pelvic area can result in infertility or erectile dysfunction. Surgery in the pelvic area involving the lymph nodes may result in ejaculation difficulties.

Chemotherapy Chemotherapy targets tissues with actively dividing cells, such as skin, hair, the digestive tract, and the reproductive organs. The sperm and supporting cells of the oocyte divide during development. Therefore, all chemotherapies are potentially damaging to the ovaries and testes and may reduce the number of oocytes and sperm. Whether chemotherapy results in infertility depends on the patient's age, the type of chemotherapeutic drugs used, and the dosage of drugs given.

Results of a recent study showed that chemotherapy-induced amenorrhea (lack of menses) is a probable risk in the first year after treatment.[2] The incidence of no menses after chemotherapy in women under forty years of age ranges from 5 to 54 percent, and for those over forty years of age, it ranges from 76 to 92 percent. However, menses may return several years after treatment. The chance of return after two years of follow-up is 28 percent for those younger than forty years old and 8 percent for those over forty years of age. At age forty-five, women who undergo chemotherapy have about an 85 percent chance of going into permanent menopause. The younger the patient at the time of the treatment, the more likely she is to experience temporary amenorrhea and then resume normal menstrual function, although this can take several years. For prepubertal patients, the likelihood of early menopause and infertility is lower.

Alkylating agents, such as cyclophospamide (Cytoxan), are most harmful to oocytes. In one study, 42 percent of women treated with this type of chemotherapy were in premature menopause by the age of thirty-one, although some returned to normal menses.[3] Doxorubicin (Adriamycin) and docetaxel (Taxotere) are other agents also toxic to the gonads.

Of women exposed to chemotherapy, only 5–35 percent achieve spontaneous pregnancy. Resuming normal menstrual periods does not necessarily mean that a woman is fertile. Chemotherapy can result in partial ovarian injury (decreasing the number of oocytes) such that cancer survivors have normal menstrual cycles but don't realize they are infertile until they try to conceive. Cancer treatment may push patients out of the reproductive window and into the early stages of menopause with no particular signs or symptoms.

In men, alkylating agents are similarly most harmful to sperm production. However, the testosterone-producing cells (Leydig cells) are more resistant to chemotherapy than oocytes. Therefore, sterility may not be readily apparent. Damage to sperm production may result in low sperm count (oligozoospermia), however, with the end result of infertility. The damage caused by chemotherapy can be temporary or permanent. If the injury is directly to the sperm and does not destroy the stem cells, then recovery is possible, often with minimal residual effect. High dosages of chemotherapy can damage the Leydig cells, resulting in loss of sex drive and ejaculation and erection difficulties.

Radiation The gonads (testes or ovaries) can be temporarily or permanently damaged by radiation therapy. The severity of damaging effects is related to the radiation dosage, the number of treatments, the location of the treatment field, and the patient's age. Radioactive iodine does not cause infertility. In contrast to chemotherapy, prepubertal age provides no protection against radiation effects to the reproductive system.

Radiation therapy affects the number of oocytes remaining in the resting pool and stem cells in the testes. The dosage that causes ovarian failure depends on age. In younger women, more oocytes are present. Therefore, at a given dosage of radiation young women have less chance of menopause than older women. In one study, radiation dosages less than 2,000 cGy resulted in ovarian failure more often in women thirteen to twenty years of age than in girls less than thirteen years old. At dosages greater than 2,000 cGy, the incidence of ovarian failure was more than 70 percent regardless of age. In women older than twenty years, dosages as low as 800 cGy can result in menopause. However, even low dosages can be harmful for both sperm and oocytes, rendering one infertile, and this result is highly unpredictable. If pelvic radiation is given at higher dosages, the uterus is also vulnerable to muscular or vascular injury.[4] Symptoms include intrauterine growth retardation, spontaneous miscarriages, and preterm labor. Radiation at lower dosages to the testes may affect the sperm only, sparing the Leydig cells, yet still result in infertility. With normal supporting cells, children would experience normal pubertal development, and adults may have a normal sex drive and be capable of erections and ejaculation.

The Psychological Impact of Infertility

Infertility can be an emotionally devastating experience for anyone. In the case of cancer survivors, the possibility of infertility adds an additional burden to the many challenges created by the short- and long-term side effects of therapy and the potential for recurrence or a new cancer.

One of the domains of *symbolic immortality,* as described by Robert Jay Lifton, M.D., of Harvard University in his 1979 book *The Broken Connection: On Death and the Continuity of Life,* is the hope of leaving something behind through a biological family. Infertility often leads to grieving and loss, and although the goal of cancer therapy is survival, the possibility of being unable to continue one's family line threatens one of the most basic dreams of life.

Patients suffering grief, loss, or anxiety may need professional counseling and psychosocial therapy to aid in psychological adjustment. The hope is that fertility may return, reinforcing the survivor's commitment to life.

Some survivors fear having children when they are at risk for experiencing a cancer recurrence, developing a new cancer, or dying prematurely. This can cause both negative feelings and a negative approach to becoming fertile. There is also the fear that offspring conceived after cancer therapy might be born with a congenital abnormality. Thus far, a higher risk of congenital malformation is not supported by current research, which has found abnormalities in about 3.4 percent of cancer survivors' offspring, compared with 3.1 percent of cancer-free siblings' offspring. The genetic propensity for abnormalities in the general population is about 5 percent.[5]

Those fortunate enough to conceive after cancer treatment experience a greater sense of a normal life. Fertility is a high priority despite the risks, making it possible to be a parent and watch one's progeny grow and develop, one of the most valued and coveted of life's experiences.

Even for those who have not had cancer, infertility can be a major challenge, necessitating many physician visits, treatments, and often high costs that are not always covered by insurance. The distress from failures is an additional cost that is not always balanced by the gratification of success. Recently, there have been many advances in the treatment of infertility. If success cannot be achieved, adoption often is considered, although this approach also presents costs, both financial and emotional, in the struggle to find a suitable baby. Patients often go overseas, where more children are available for adoption, accepting the additional costs and risks of dealing with unfamiliar legal and medical systems. For many, however, adoption does not satisfy their desire to sustain the family and genetic life history.

Although a majority of infertile cancer survivors have considered adoption, another option is the third-party approach, in which a surrogate carries the baby. Alternatively, a cancer survivor may consider using a donated embryo, egg, or sperm. Some religions, such as Roman Catholicism and Islam, are against third-party reproduction. Having one's own biological child through use of current advanced technology is becoming a potentially more accessible approach.

Preserving Fertility

The improved long-term survival and cure rates for many cancers have made future fertility a question to be considered in reproductive-age patients, preferably before the cancer treatment begins. The importance of this question has been recognized, and although the existing options are limited, particularly in women, this is an area of active research, and it is likely that in the near future other options will become available.

Clearly, cancer treatment that entails surgical removal of the testes or the ovary renders the patient sterile. To preserve fertility, the most important step for those diagnosed with cancer is to discuss their concerns with their doctor. If possible, alternative treatments, such as different chemotherapeutic agents or radiation exposure, may help decrease the incidence of infertility. Before beginning treatment, discuss alternative options for fertility preservation with your doctor so that he or she can refer you to a fertility clinic. Some of the available options can be performed after treatment, but the most effective methods are used before cancer treatment.

Men Men have the option of freezing (cryopreserving) sperm for later use. This process is available in most major medical centers and is a simple and affordable method. Semen cryopreservation has been used successfully for more than fifty years. Sperm banking should be completed before the initiation of radiation therapy or chemotherapy in case the sperm count and quality do not return to normal after treatment. The sperm can be stored indefinitely without significant damage. When ready for use, the sperm are thawed and available for intrauterine insemination (IUI) or assisted reproductive techniques (ARTs). Unfortunately, men often are not advised of this option before therapy. It has been estimated that only 10–30 percent of patients use the option of stored semen.[6]

Men with cancer often have abnormal sperm counts before treatment. In the past, low sperm counts were a reason not to bank sperm because poor samples yield a low pregnancy rate with IUI. However, with ARTs, such as in vitro fertilization and intracytoplasmic (into egg) sperm injection, there is a high success rate for successful fertilizations and pregnancy.[7]

Boys and young adolescents who have not experienced puberty do not make sperm and therefore are unable to use sperm banking. For these patients, encouraging approaches in the experimental phase include the following:

• *Gonadotropin-releasing hormone (GnRH) agonists:* This hormonal therapy is administered by injection every month or every three months. It temporarily shuts down the reproductive system, thereby decreasing the number of dividing cells in the testes. Thus far, there are no proven studies of a GnRH agonist successfully protecting males from high-dose chemotherapy damage. Although older studies have shown no protection against chemotherapy, recent studies have suggested a possible benefit.

• *Cryopreserved testicular tissue for future transplantation:* Testicular tissue is obtained surgically and cryopreserved. When ready for use, the tissue is transplanted back into the testes, making spontaneous conception possible. This is an option for prepubertal patients. Research on this option is in progress, and to date there have been no live births from this method.

• *Testicular sperm extraction (TESE):* In men with no sperm in their ejaculate, TESE is an option. It is a well-established procedure to overcome severe male infertility and has a high pregnancy success rate. The chance of obtaining sperm is 30–70 percent. TESE may also be an option for prepubertal patients but is still in the experimental phase, with no pregnancies to date.

Options after cancer treatment depend on the severity of damage to the testes. If sperm are present, IUI and ART are available options. If there are no sperm in the ejaculate, TESE may be attempted. Hormonal therapies such as FSH and LH to increase sperm production are being investigated.

Women In women, the damage done to ovaries by cancer treatment depends on a number of factors, including the patient's age at the time of treatment, the dosage and particular chemotherapeutic drug used, and the dosage and fractionation schedule of radiation.

For women, there are a number of strategies for preserving fertility:

• *Embryo cryopreservation:* The most well-established option is embryo cryopreservation. It is a common technique used with couples to overcome infertility. It is available only for women who have experienced puberty and have a partner or are willing to use donor sperm. The success rate depends on the woman's age and the number of oocytes recovered from the ovary. The process entails a two- to six-week time commitment and should be performed before the initiation of cancer treatment. It begins with ovarian stimulation, which allows multiple oocytes to be produced. The ovarian stimulation requires FSH and LH and results in increases in estrogen production. In cases of hormone-sensitive cancer (i.e., breast cancer), techniques to reduce estrogen production are available. The oocytes are collected by a surgical procedure, using an ultrasound-guided needle that is passed through the vagina into the ovaries to collect oocytes. Once the oocytes are recovered, they are fertilized and stored for later use. When the patient is ready for pregnancy, the embryos are thawed and transferred into the uterus. In some cases, it may not be possible to delay cancer treatments long enough to do ovarian stimulation. If this procedure is desired, the patient should discuss it with her doctor as soon as possible so that the possible delay in cancer treatment is minimized.

The other options available to women are in the experimental phase and include the following:

• *Egg (oocyte) cryopreservation:* A question that often arises is, "Can I bank my eggs just like men can bank their sperm?" The process is similar to embryo cryopreservation. However, the oocyte is not fertilized. Therefore, the earlier need for a partner or donor sperm is avoided. Unfortunately, at present this is not rou-

tinely possible. However, in a few centers it is being performed on an experimental basis under the strict supervision of institutional research committees. The success depends on the woman's age and the number of oocytes recovered. The reported success is 2–4 percent live births per oocyte recovered. The lower survival rate of frozen eggs after thawing and the less than optimal pregnancy yield makes freezing of ova obtained before cancer treatment not yet widely available as a clinical option. This area is of great research interest, and advancements are continually developing, with corresponding improvements in pregnancy rates, so it is likely that egg banking will be feasible in the near future.

• *Ovarian transposition (oophoropexy):* Oophoropexy can protect the ovaries from radiation. The operation places the ovaries out of the radiation field. This technique has been used for years to shield the ovaries from radiation during pelvic irradiation, but the results are variable for fertility protection, ranging between 0 and 90 percent.[8] The variability in success is attributed to the difficulty of keeping the ovary out of the radiation field and the concurrent use of chemotherapy in addition to radiation. In the past this procedure entailed a long recovery time, thereby delaying radiation treatment. Newer oophoropexy techniques under investigation show promising results.

• *Ovarian cryopreservation (tissue freezing):* Another approach being studied is that of freezing ovarian tissue in the hope that later, after successful treatment of the cancer, it can be transplanted back into the patient and still function. This procedure is not widely available at this time. This process has no time requirement and therefore avoids any delay in cancer treatment. It does not require ovarian stimulation or a partner and is an option for prepubertal patients. The tissue is obtained surgically and cryopreserved. When the patient is ready, the tissue is transplanted (autotransplantation) by either of two methods:

• *Orthotopic transplant:* The ovarian tissue is transplanted back into the native ovaries. This process would potentially produce sex steroids, resume menstrual cycles, and allow spontaneous conception. To date, two reported live births have occurred after orthotopic transplant.

• *Heterotropic transplant:* The ovarian tissue is transplanted under the skin (e.g., in the arm). This process would potentially produce sex steroids and resume menstrual cycles but would not allow spontaneous conception. In order to conceive, ART would be needed. No live births to date have been recorded after heterotropic transplantation.

A major concern for ovarian transplantation is the possibility of reintroducing malignant cells from the ovarian tissue to a cancer survivor. The ovarian tissue removed before treatment could contain latent malignant cells, and cryopreservation does not kill cancer cells. Investigations are being performed to reliably screen for cancer cells in the ovarian tissue.

• *GnRH analogs:* This hormonal therapy is administered by injection every month or every three months. It temporarily shuts down the reproductive system, decreasing the number of dividing cells in the ovaries. Evidence suggests that GnRH agonists may be a beneficial option for postpubertal females receiving chemotherapy. The treatment should be administered before chemotherapy begins but may be beneficial even during treatment. Studies have shown that use of GnRH analogs does not protect against radiation.

• *Gynecological cancer treatments that spare reproductive function:* The options available depend on the type of cancer and whether it has spread to other places.

• *Cervical cancer:* Trachelectomy, removal of the cervix from early stage cervical cancer, takes special surgical expertise and appears to be a safe way to preserve the uterus for pregnancy.

• *Uterine cancer:* Hormonal treatments may treat early stages of uterine cancer.

• *Ovarian cancer:* Early stages may necessitate removal of only one ovary and tube.

Options after treatment include use of ARTs and surrogacy if a hysterectomy has been performed.

Pregnancy After Cancer Treatment

Follow-up studies indicate that the toxic effects of chemotherapy given to women before pregnancy do not appear to be a risk to children conceived naturally. However, animal studies suggest that natural conception within six months after treatment in females increases the chance of fetal abnormalities. In males, the only risks of fetal abnormality were found in those conceived during or immediately after chemotherapy.

Although cancer survival has continued to increase in recent years, infertility remains a major challenge for cancer survivors. Cancer patients interested in future fertility should receive appropriate psychological support and early referral to specialized fertility clinics and perinatal care services. It is important to note that there are no guarantees of preserving fertility with any of the aforementioned options. Cancer survivors unable to use their own eggs or sperm may still achieve pregnancy using donated eggs or sperm. The process of donating eggs or sperm is well established and has high pregnancy rates. The recipient has many options for donors, including various individual characteristics and genetic backgrounds.

A nonprofit organization, Fertile Hope, provides fertility resources for cancer patients and can be contacted at www.fertilehope.org, 888-994-HOPE, or by mail at 65 Broadway, Suite 603, New York, NY 10006.

Notes

1. Nieman CL, Kazer R, Brannigan RE, Zoloth LS, Chase-Lansdale PL. Cancer survivors and infertility: a review of a new problem and novel answers. *J Support Oncol* 2006;4(4):171–8.

2. Dr. Charles Shapiro, ASCO presentation, June 2006, Atlanta, GA.

3. Byrne J, Fears TR, Gail MH, Pee D, Connelly RR, Austin DF. Early menopause in long-term survivors of cancer during adolescence. *Am J Obstet Gynecol* 1992;166(3):788–93.

4. Critchley HO, Wallace WH, Shalet SM, Mamtora H, Higginson J. Abdominal irradiation in childhood: the potential for pregnancy. *Br J Obstet Gynaecol* 1992;99(5):392–4.

5. Holmes GE. Long-term survival in childhood and adolescent cancer. Five-center study: U.S.A. *Ann N Y Acad Sci* 1997;824:180–9.

6. Audrins P, Holden CA, McLachlan RI, Kovacs GT. Semen storage for special purposes at Monash IVF from 1977 to 1997. *Fertil Steril* 1999;72(1):179–81.

7. Tournaye H, Goossens E, Verheyen G, Frederickx V, De Block G. Preserving the reproductive potential of men and boys with cancer: current concepts and future prospects. *Hum Reprod Update* 2004;10(6):525–32.

8. Bisharah M, Tulandi T. Laparoscopic preservation of ovarian function: an underused procedure. *Am J Obstet Gynecol* 2003;188(2):367–70.

— 38 —

Cancer and the Family's Needs

Patricia T. Kelly, Ph.D.

■ ■ ■ ■

Individuals who are diagnosed with cancer need, in addition to good medical care, useful information about what to expect and help in coping with and making sense of the turbulent emotions that can accompany a cancer diagnosis. Often the major focus is, understandably, on the person diagnosed with cancer. The result may be that the family's information needs and help with emotional reactions are overlooked. In general, it is rare to find skilled health professionals who are responsible for the care and well-being of the family once a member has been diagnosed with cancer.

I first became aware of the needs of the children of cancer patients some years ago when I began to provide cancer risk information to adult women whose mothers had been diagnosed with breast cancer some many years before. I was surprised at the depth and often raw quality of the emotions these daughters expressed about their mothers' breast cancer diagnosis and the effect it had had on their own lives. Even many years later, these daughters were living what might be called blighted lives. That is, they were living the shadows of lives they might have had, and made statements such as "I feel like a walking time bomb," "I'm living as if there is a sword over my head," "I still feel separate and different from other people," and "I have trouble feeling close to others."

As a group, I found that adults of either sex whose parent was diagnosed with cancer when they were children often felt that they were doomed to follow the same course as their parent, were anxious about their own cancer risks, and even blamed themselves for worrying. Many felt unsure about how to proceed to set up a health care program that would keep them as safe as possible and help them to feel safe. I often heard words such as "I just feel in my bones that it will happen to me, too." As a consequence of their strong emotions about cancer, which often included hopelessness and despair, many had no medical follow-up or had inadequate medical care. In fact, some felt so sure that they were "hypochondriacs" that they had less care than women without a family history of cancer.

The parents and the spouses of those diagnosed with cancer told me of their confusion, of their feelings of loneliness, and of feeling excluded from the person with the cancer diagnosis. Some spoke of feeling betrayed by modern medicine or of being overwhelmed by the need to assume new responsibilities for such major tasks as finances and child raising.

These families benefited greatly from the following:

• *Information About and Help in "Navigating" the Medical Care System* Many do not know where to turn to get their questions answered. They do not realize that these days it is highly unlikely for any one physician to provide all of a person's treatment. Until the families knew which specialists provided what services, they were very confused. Some felt abandoned by doctors who did not provide what they had expected, though they had not verbalized their expectations or ever known what to ask. Once individuals understood the system, they could proceed with more confidence and could request what they wanted. And once they had a better understanding, a great deal of their anxiety was reduced.

• *An Accurate Assessment of the Risk of Cancer to Family Members* Most cancers are not due to strong hereditary factors. In fact, only about 10 percent of each of the common cancers is thought to be due to strong hereditary factors. Nevertheless, when close relatives are diagnosed with cancer, many quite naturally feel that they are now at "high risk." A family-history assessment by a geneticist to determine individual risk can be most useful, even for very young children, whose risk may not be imminent or is far less than they had imagined.

• *Information About Individual Risk Given in Concise Terms* A great deal of the information we read and hear is in a format designed for scientists, not for concerned individuals. This format is far less useful or may even be confusing when individuals attempt to apply it to themselves. Generally, risk information is more likely to be useful to an individual when it (a) involves a time frame (for example, a 10 percent risk in the span of one year is very different from a 10 percent risk that is spread evenly over the next ten years) and (b) is expressed in actual or absolute terms instead of as a comparison of one group's risk with that of another. (For example, learning there is a 10 percent risk that is spread over ten years is more useful than hearing that the risk is twice as high as or is 35 percent less than another risk.) When risk is presented in comparison terms, individuals don't learn what they

most want to know—the actual risk—so it is hard to make intelligent decisions based on what they have heard.

• *Information About How a Cell Becomes a Cancer Cell* An understanding of the origin of cancer can greatly reduce the mystique about cancer and help individuals think about cancer more clearly.

• *Information About the Importance of Communication with Others and How to Communicate Needs and Concerns Effectively* The more family members are able to communicate with each other and share information and their feelings about what is happening, the happier, healthier, and stronger they are and will be in the future.

Children Who Have a Parent with Cancer

The parents I see frequently underestimate the fears and questions their children have. Many worry that by talking to their children about cancer, they will frighten them. Parents may not realize how easily children pick up on the emotions of the adults around them. In most instances, there is no way to hide the fact that *something* is different once a parent has been diagnosed with cancer. Many of those I see who were children when their parents were diagnosed with cancer were either not told about their parents' cancer diagnosis or were told very little. These adults are far more likely to feel anxious and less trusting than those whose parents kept them informed about what was happening and were honest about their feelings.

When a parent is diagnosed with cancer, both parents may feel that their children are "just fine" or not that interested in what is going on. Some say, "Whenever I bring up the cancer, they say they don't want to hear about it, that everything will be just fine, or they leave the room."

In such cases, it may be helpful to put an arm around the child while explaining what is happening. There is no need for a long discussion, but there are some essential points to get across

• Mom/Dad was diagnosed with cancer.
• Not all cancers are alike.
• New and better treatments are being discovered every day.
• Mom/Dad is having good care and treatment.
• Sometimes the treatments and the diagnosis are stressful and scary, so there may be tension in the house and even sorrow or crying. This is normal for such a time. The doctors say that in a few months, life will be a lot easier, and that we will all feel much better. You can help by remembering that this is a stressful time, that it will change, and that we love you very much.
• The type of cancer Mom/Dad has is not found in children (most cancers are not). Most cancers do not run in families. By the time you are grown, doctors will be able to stop many cancers or treat them in easier ways than is possible right now.
• Mom/Dad is fine at present. The treatments are proceeding the way they should. If there is a problem in the future, we will tell you right away. I hope that if ever you don't feel well, you will tell us also. Meanwhile, it is important for you to keep doing all of the things you do every day and to tell me if you are worried. We want you to go on about your life as much as you can.

Obviously, these comments need to be modified for the age of the child and the family situation.

The Spouse or Partner of a Cancer Patient

Few appreciate the pain, fear, and confusion endured by the spouse or partner. And while attention and treatments are being given to the person with cancer, the spouse is sometimes shunted aside. Little or no time is spent giving the spouse of the cancer patient tips about how to proceed, leaving many to tell me they felt they had to "reinvent the wheel." For example, many of those who were diagnosed with cancer say that when they try to tell their partners about some of their fears, the response is, "Oh, don't worry about it. I'm sure everything will be okay." When this reply is repeated several times, the person with cancer may refrain from communicating his or her fears about the cancer diagnosis and the couple may draw apart.

Instead of remaining quiet and suffering, the person with cancer might find it useful to tell the spouse what is actually needed in direct terms, such as, "I've noticed that when I tell you I'm scared, you tell me not to worry. I'm thinking you say that because you care for me and you don't want me to worry. But when I tell you how worried I am, what would help me most is a hug and to hear you say how much you love me and that you worry sometimes, too."

In general, the more the couple can talk about the areas in which they feel they are not communicating and the more they can be direct about their wishes and needs, the more the relationship will be strengthened. Also, the more the spouse can participate in the ongoing decision making and discussions and the more experiences the couple can share, the less likely it is that they will drift apart. When it is not possible to share the experience, talking about it together later can help spouses to stay in touch. Unless this ongoing communication occurs between the person with cancer and his or her partner and children, family will be unable to know what the person with cancer is experiencing and feeling. In time, the person with cancer can begin to feel like Marco Polo—coming from afar with fantastic stories and having feelings that are hard for others to understand.

Many spouses of cancer patients are greatly helped by having an opportunity to get away from their home responsibilities on a regular basis and having someone other than the person with cancer with whom they can speak.

Friends and Relatives

After a cancer diagnosis, many people tell me that friends and even relatives don't call as often as they used to. Some even appear to be avoiding them. In time, the person with cancer may conclude that those who haven't stayed in touch just don't care. In such cases, it is not uncommon for a breach to occur in a family or for old friendships to end. It is important at such times to be aware that friends and relatives may sometimes need to be educated. Some may not call because they are afraid of saying the wrong thing or of calling at the wrong time, or because they just don't know what to say. Many of those with cancer have great success when they call a friend or relative and say straight out, "I haven't heard from you in a while and thought it might be because you don't know what to say or you thought that I might be resting. Well, you don't need to watch what you say now any more than

you did before. I'm the same person in many ways and I'm getting good care. Sometimes it's hard, but I am not too busy or too tired for old friends. I hope you won't let this come between us. Would you like to go to a movie [take a walk, etc.]?"

An Approach That Meets Families' Needs

Some of the families I've seen were fortunate enough to obtain some or all of the types of help discussed here. Others, who had less or none of this help available, endured more pain. A comprehensive service is needed for *all* families in which a parent has been diagnosed with cancer. Ideally this service would utilize the expertise of an oncologist, a geneticist, and a psychotherapist to supply information and support. In this way, questions and concerns could be addressed as they arose, before any became troublesome to the workings of the family or to the normal growth and development of the children. Spouses would have their needs met in a timely manner as well, which would enable them to provide more comfort to the person with cancer and to the children. Even when a diagnosis of cancer has occurred some years before, families would benefit by having access to this service.

— 39 —

Paying for Cancer Care

Malin Dollinger, M.D., Barbara Quinn, and Joseph S. Bailes, M.D.

■ ■ ■ ■

Paying for cancer care is in many respects different from paying for a single illness or a health event, such as an operation. Care extends over months, usually years, and involves many different doctors at many different times. Many different types of treatment are needed: diagnostic tests and biopsies, surgery, radiation therapy, chemotherapy, nutritional and physical therapy consultations, and management of other medical problems. Newly diagnosed cancer patients are suddenly confronted with critical questions about their insurance coverage. Paying for this type of medical care is especially complicated. Managed care has introduced new rules and methods of operation. There is a new vocabulary of words and initials that are confusing even to health care workers. And the vocabulary changes every year!

The insurance industry—both public and private—has its own policies, guidelines, and methods of payment specific to cancer care. Each company's rules may be different. It is important for you to understand how your insurance company's payment system works so that you will get the care you need at a cost you should be able to pay. It is especially important to know your policy restrictions. For example, you should know how your insurance plan deals with investigational therapy, or with consultations or second opinions that are "outside the system."

Group health care plans are often available through employers, labor unions, and other associations. As a rule, group plans do not discriminate against preexisting conditions, including cancer. Individual (nongroup) health insurance plans are also available. In contrast with most group plans, individually purchased plans almost always preclude or at least limit in some way coverage for preexisting conditions. Some individual plans reject people with serious preexisting conditions.

As a cancer patient, you are probably uncertain and unclear about the scope of your coverage, as well as about how you can obtain the benefits you are entitled to under your insurance contract. Not being fully informed can put you at great financial risk. You may end up paying for services that should have been covered by your insurance. In your plan booklet, there will be a telephone contact, for questions about coverage. If you have any uncertainties or questions, be sure to use this service. It helps to keep a written record of persons/dates/facilities where aspects of care have been approved or authorized, or when discussions were held about insurance matters and coverage.

Types of Health Care Coverage

There are many types of payment plans, insurance plans, and medical groups:

Medicare This government-sponsored health insurance program is for people aged sixty-five and older. It also covers people who are permanently disabled, provided they have received Social Security disability benefits for at least two years.

Medicare is divided into the following parts:

• *Part A—Hospital Insurance* This part of the program covers your inpatient hospital stay, limited skilled-nursing care, part-time home health care, and hospice care for those who are eligible. It is available without payment of a premium, although some services require a deductible or co-payment. Medicare Part A is administered by the Health Care Financing Administration (HCFA) through insurers called intermediaries.

• *Part B—Medical Insurance* This part of the program covers physician services and hospital outpatient care, such as blood transfusions, X-rays, and lab tests. There is limited coverage for medical equipment such as wheelchairs and walkers. Enrollment is optional, and the payment of a premium is required. Medicare Part B covers 80 percent of allowed charges. You are responsible for the other 20 percent of allowed charges, called coinsurance. You must also meet a yearly deductible before Medicare Part B coverage applies.

Medicare Part B is directed by the federal government through the HCFA and is funded through a monthly premium, which comes out of your Social Security check. It is administered through contracts with insurers (called carriers) throughout the United States.

• (Part C, or Medicare Advantage, is an alternative to parts A and B and will not be discussed here.)

• *Part D—Prescription Drug Coverage* Beginning in 2006, Medicare Part D was implemented. This is a method of delivery and payment for prescription drugs, designed to replace previous prescription payment plans in which the plan (e.g., Medicare Part B) included prescription medications. Medicare Part D separates the drug delivery and costs, and consumers are given the option of selecting one of a large number of prescription drug plans, each with its own features, coverage, inclusions, and exclusions. This is an extremely complex decision process, and Medicare recipients have public and private sources of information and guidance available to them, to assist them in the process of Part D–plan selection. In this regard, some of the important decisions involve, for example, the specific prescription drug formulary that is part of each plan—i.e., which drugs are covered at minimal rates and which require a significantly greater copayment. Another focus of plan selection involves a gap in coverage, between $2,251 and $5,100, called the doughnut hole, in which payment for drug costs is absent, limited, or paid-in-full, depending on the specific plan chosen. Since Medicare Part D is brand new, we expect that major revisions and hopefully simplification will allow Medicare participants to logically and reasonably select a plan that is optimal for them, without the need for extensive "research time" and consultation regarding the process of plan selection.

If you need additional information, as well as a free handbook describing the Medicare program, contact your local Social Security office.

Medigap This insurance is sold by private carriers and traditionally covers the 20 percent coinsurance you are responsible for under Medicare Part B. Federal law stipulates that there be only ten standard types of Medigap policies available (A through J). These policies vary widely in their scope of coverage. You should thoroughly familiarize yourself with the particular Medigap policy you are considering purchasing, so that you will have the coverage appropriate for your situation. Some of the plans cover prescription drugs, with varying deductibles and co-payments, but prescription coverage is now available only if you are already enrolled in a Medigap policy and are *not* enrolled in Medicare Part D.

Medicaid This is a joint federal- and state-funded program for low-income individuals. It provides coverage for inpatient care, outpatient services, diagnostic testing, drugs, skilled nursing facility care, and home health care. Each state has its own rules about eligibility for the Medicaid program. Your local social service or welfare department is the best place to obtain information about Medicaid.

QMBE This is the Qualified Medicare Beneficiary program, in which the state pays coinsurance and premiums for certain low-income Medicare Part B beneficiaries even if they don't qualify for Medicaid.

Traditional Indemnity Insurance Sometimes called major-medical coverage, this type of insurance is sold by numerous private insurance companies. It is the most common type of insurance coverage for people not eligible for Medicare or Medicaid. Such insurance plans typically pay the usual fee for service each time you see your doctor. There is usually a deductible and/or co-payment associated with traditional indemnity insurance. This means, for example, that you might pay the first $250 or $500 in covered charges each year and/or pay 10 or 20 percent of all fees. There may be limits in the policy (a maximum dollar amount that will be paid); these often apply to hospital room and nursing costs and to treatment for psychological problems. Commonly, reimbursement to a physician is based on the "usual and customary" amount, not on the physician's actual fees.

An employer will often have a plan for general insurance coverage for each employee.

Managed Care Plans Managed care usually requires individuals either to pay a fixed fee for a certain set of services or to see only certain physicians, who have agreed to discount their fees for particular services.

There are many variations of managed care plans (see also chapter 40, "Managed Care and Oncology"):

• *Health Maintenance Organization (HMO)* An HMO is a prepaid health plan that requires you to use a specific network or group of provider physicians, hospitals, and labs. For a fixed fee each month, HMOs provide care specified by your contract. This care may or may not be all-inclusive, so it is important to read and understand the contract of your particular HMO. For instance, although most do, some HMOs have no outpatient prescription drug benefit. In an HMO, you are usually required to select one physician as your primary or family doctor. This individual coordinates all of your care.

Examples of HMOs include Kaiser Permanente, Cigna Health Plans, and Blue Cross HMO plans. HMO members aged sixty-five and older should remember that the HMO plan replaces Medicare coverage, and you must stay within your HMO plan in order for your claims to be paid by Medicare.

• *Preferred Provider Organization (PPO), Exclusive Provider Organization (EPO), or Independent Practice Association (IPA)* Traditionally, PPOs, EPOs, and IPAs are groups of physicians and other participating providers who have agreed to offer a discount from their usual fees in order to participate in a particular group. Such groups function as "old-fashioned private practices" in that the physician or other provider receives a fee each time a service is performed or each time you see the physician. There are usually deductibles and/or co-payments for which you are responsible. You do have a choice of using providers or physicians who are not in the plan, but if you do, you will have to pay a larger portion of the cost.

What Does Your Plan Cover?

Your health benefits manual, your insurance representative, or the health plan manager at your place of employment should be able to answer the following questions. Because cancer treatment can be quite expensive, it is absolutely essential for a cancer patient to be totally familiar with both the benefits and the restrictions of his or her coverage. Here are some key questions to consider:

• *What is the effective date of the policy?* In other words, when does your coverage begin?

• *What is your deductible?* This is the amount you need to pay before your insurance plan starts paying the rest. Only medical care received as a benefit under your policy is calculated against your deductible. Noncovered services that you pay for do not count toward the deductible.

• *Do you have a stop loss?* This is the annual amount you must pay out of your own pocket before your insurance pays at 100 percent. Stop losses can be very beneficial where diagnosis and treatment are expensive.

• *What percentage of billed charges is paid by your insurance?* Some policies pay 80 percent or 90 percent of some costs but pay only 50 percent of other costs.

• *Do you have coverage for home care, nursing visits at home, private duty nursing (twenty-four-hour care), and care at a skilled nursing facility or convalescent hospital?*

• *Do you have coverage for custodial care?* Most insurance companies cover only skilled care. Custodial care—such as housekeeping, bathing, doing laundry, and providing assistance in getting to the bathroom or in preparing meals—is not usually covered.

• *Does your plan cover hospice care?*

• *Does your insurance provide coverage only if you go to specific providers?*

• *Is a referral or a plan authorization required for doctor's visits, hospital admissions, or outpatient testing?*

• *Are there any waivers that would preclude payment for treatment for your condition?* This might include prior treatment (within one year, for example) for the same or a similar condition.

• *What is your lifetime maximum?* This is the maximum benefit your insurance will pay in your lifetime. It can be $25,000 or $1 million or more.

• *How do you get care after hours or in an emergency?*

• *If you have group coverage through your employer, does coverage end if you are fired or laid off? If so, is there a way to continue coverage?* Ask your employer about COBRA [Consolidated Omnibus Budget Reconciliation Act of 1986], the federal law that requires certain plans to extend your group health coverage up to eighteen months after you are terminated from a job—though you must usually pay the entire premium yourself.

Why Claims May Be Denied

Even though your policy may appear comprehensive, denials for medical care claims are common. Sometimes a denial reflects only a practical problem—say, missing information or incorrect documentation. Sometimes the policy does not cover certain types of care. This is often a matter of interpretation. If this is the case, you will need to advocate with your doctor or other health care provider to establish that your care should be covered even though the insurance company's agent interprets the policy as appearing to exclude it. A rundown of common reasons for denial follows, along with recommendations for responding to the denial.

Preexisting Condition Your claim may be denied if your medical condition existed before you became eligible for or bought your policy. Be absolutely sure about how your particular plan interprets the term *preexisting condition.*

Noncovered Benefit Most policies have a section that lists illnesses or services that are excluded from coverage. Because of the possibility of noncovered benefits, it is a good idea to check your insurance plan *before* any treatment or tests are ordered. Some treatments are covered only when given or administered in the hospital, for example. In such cases, you or your physician's office may be able to make arrangements for outpatient coverage in lieu of hospitalization. Services may actually be cheaper that way.

Not an Authorized Provider Many insurance plans require that you use providers who are part of their network. Seeing a specialist usually requires that you be referred by an authorized provider for a consultation and for all subsequent treatment. Failure to go to contracted providers with a written referral can result in a complete denial of payment for all treatment provided.

Investigational Treatment Virtually all health insurance plans cover standard cancer diagnosis and treatments (e.g.,

chemotherapy, radiotherapy, surgery), but many insurers will deny claims deemed to be investigational (experimental), unnecessary, or inappropriate. While there is no guaranteed way to prevent denial of such a claim, make sure that you attempt to receive preapproval in writing for the treatment from your insurance carrier. To do this, you should have a "letter of medical necessity" from your physician documenting that the proposed treatment is medically appropriate, along with supporting clinical literature and a full description of the procedure or services to be provided. The anticipated cost and duration of the treatment should also be included.

Off-Label Treatment Your insurer may deny a claim if the drug your doctor has prescribed is used for any reason other than its labeled indication or the use listed on the drug company's package insert. The claim may also be denied if the drug is used in a new dosage or according to a new schedule, given by a different route, or combined with other drugs.

You should be aware that fully half of all uses of cancer drugs are not those listed on the official package insert or label. Such uses reflect advances in cancer treatment that occurred after the drug was released onto the market and are in fact the ordinary, proper, and accepted uses of such drugs. Not to use certain drugs for established "off-label" uses may be inappropriate.

When your health insurance plan uses "Drug use is off-label" to deny a claim, it is very important to appeal this denial to the insurance carrier. Such denials are usually reversed, especially if the use of the drug is standard in the community and is a necessary and effective treatment for your illness. Most pharmaceutical companies will provide reimbursement "hot lines" to provide assistance. Your oncologist's insurance or billing staff is usually familiar with ways to help you with this problem should denial occur. In many states, cancer physicians have formed organizations to advise insurance companies about effective new treatments for cancer, especially established drugs in off-label use.

Nonpayment of Premiums It is very difficult to obtain another insurance policy once you have a preexisting condition. Make sure that premiums on your current policy are kept up-to-date to ensure that your insurance policy is not canceled.

Submitting Claims

You must bring proper insurance plan identification on your first visit to your oncologist's office. Your insurance provider—whether it is Medicare, Medicaid, a PPO, an HMO, or a private indemnity plan—should give you an identification card. This card will have your subscriber identification number (often your Social Security number), group number, office co-pay amount, and the address to which any claims should be submitted. If your insurance does require submission of a claim form, also bring a fully completed and signed claim form to the office.

Always inform your physician's office of any changes in your address, phone number, or employment or insurance information. Notifying the office immediately will prevent unnecessary delays in claim submission, avoid the need for resubmission, and reduce possible denials of payment. It will also result in quicker payment of claims.

Your physician's office will submit the claim for some plans. This may also be true for hospitals, laboratories, and other kinds of service providers. Most oncology offices have an insurance or finance department. Their patient representatives will explain the billing procedures to you before you begin treatment. Find out whether they will submit your claim or whether you are expected to submit the claim yourself.

Always request a copy of your charges, which should include an itemization of all services and the diagnosis (including its code), for your visit.

Common Terms and Abbreviations

To better understand the procedure for submitting and processing claims, you should understand the terms and abbreviations used by most insurance carriers. Here are the most common ones:

• *ICD-9 (International Classification of Diseases, 9th Edition) Code* This code identifies your illness. All claims submitted to your insurance carrier will require the correct code. Carriers will not pay your claim if this code is not provided.

• *CPT (Current Procedural Terminology) Code* This code identifies the medical, surgical, and diagnostic services rendered by your physician. It is used by most insurance carriers to identify what services were performed. Claims are paid using these codes.

• *Deductible* This is the amount you have to pay before your insurance starts paying the rest. Only received medical care that is a covered benefit under your policy is counted against your deductible. Noncovered benefits, which you must pay yourself, do not count against your deductible.

• *Co-payment* This refers to the amount of your bill that you are responsible for. The co-payment is usually a specific dollar amount rather than a percentage of the bill. Prescription drug programs, for example, often have a co-payment, usually a fixed dollar amount per prescription. Co-payments are generally associated with HMOs.

• *Coinsurance* This is the percentage of the bill you are responsible for after you have met your deductible. If your policy has a $100 deductible and a 20 percent co-insurance, for example, you would pay your $100 deductible and 20 percent of all covered expenses. You are also responsible for paying for all services not covered by your policy. Coinsurance provisions are most commonly associated with PPO-type plans.

• *EOB (Explanation of Benefits)* This is the statement you will receive from your insurance carrier when your claim has been paid. It will show the provider of services, the place of service, and how the benefits were paid. If you have a deductible or coinsurance, this will also be stated on your EOB. If you have a secondary insurance carrier, that company will need a copy of your EOB in order to pay its portion.

• *EOMB (Explanation of Medicare Benefits)* This statement, similar to an insurance carrier's EOB, is sent to you as soon as your claim has been paid. It will state the provider of any service, the amount allowed under Medicare's fee schedule, the amount paid, and what charges were applied toward your deductible. If your physician is a Medicare provider, the check will be sent directly to his or her office. Similar to above, you will need this explanation of Medicare benefits in order for any secondary insurance carrier you have to pay its portion.

• *Assignment of Benefits* This is required by most physicians' offices. It means that you give written permission for your insurance company to send payments directly to the service provider. An assignment-of-benefits form is usually provided by the physician's office for you to sign. There is also a place for your assignment-of-benefits signature on your claim form.

• *Medicare Assignment* Any physician may accept the fee schedule set by Medicare in an individual case. A participating provider in the Medicare program has agreed to always take the set fee schedule ("assignment"). If your physician takes Medicare assignment (fees), you are then responsible only for noncovered services, for your deductible, and for your coinsurance. However, if the physician is *not* a participating provider in the Medicare program, it is possible for you to end up being responsible for *more* than the 20 percent coinsurance. If the physician's charge is more than the Medicare allowable charge, for instance, the physician will receive only 80 percent of the Medicare allowable fee, while you will be responsible for the entire rest of the bill. So if you are eligible for Medicare, make sure you *ask ahead of time* whether your physician participates in the Medicare program and will accept assignment of Medicare benefits for your care.

• *UCR (Usual, Customary, and Reasonable)* This is the fee determined by your insurance carrier to be the usual fee charged for the same service by the average provider with similar training in your geographic area. This may be different from the fee your physician charges.

• *Pre-authorization* This is a requirement by your insurance carrier that certain services be authorized before the services are rendered. If your insurance contains this requirement, make sure your physician's office is aware of it.

• *Superbill* This is a standard itemized "checklist of services" in widespread use. It will contain all the required codes (CPT and ICD-9) that will enable you to submit your claim.

• *COB (Coordination of Benefits)* When you are enrolled in two separate group insurance plans, those plans will coordinate their benefits so that your claim is paid at no more than 100 percent of the covered benefits. If you have more than one insurance plan, make sure you notify your physician's office so that the office can submit both claims for you.

New Ways of Paying for Medical Care

Our society is engaged in a great effort to reform the health care payment system. For example, despite all the numerous types of health insurance and managed care, many Americans have no health coverage.

There used to be only two players in the system: the doctor and the patient. Now there are several others: the health insurance industry, various federal and state regulatory agencies, employers (who often provide employee health care plans), and the federal government. New rules and regulations are being proposed and implemented that will change the basic concepts and practices of health care.

The patient's need for skillful, dedicated, and considerate care by the physician has never changed. From the viewpoint of the physician—now called a health care provider—what has changed is that

1. other parties and agencies have taken over some of the decision making that used to belong to the physician alone, and
2. consequently, physicians and hospitals and their staff must now interact continually with these other decision makers.

Many decisions now require outside approval. These can include the decision to hospitalize, where to hospitalize, which consultants may be called, what types of treatment may be used, and,

especially, how health care resources are to be allocated and provided. Requiring authorization before ordering tests and X-rays is just one example. Many doctors' offices now have more people handling insurance than they have nurses. Physicians will need to be increasingly accountable to outside agencies.

Managed care is one common term used to describe a coordinated effort by physicians, hospitals, and insurers—also called insurance payers—to create an optimum balance between incredibly sophisticated medical technology on the one hand and our inability as a society to afford paying for every possible treatment and diagnostic test for every person in every situation on the other hand. The clinical practice guidelines now being developed by various cancer centers and scientific organizations—e.g., the American Society of Clinical Oncology (ASCO) and the National Cancer Comprehensive Network (NCCN)—and by various insurance carriers will probably become increasingly important in how services are provided and covered.

Because the patterns of delivering and monitoring health care are complex and changing and because new payment systems are being created, it is absolutely essential that you completely understand the provisions of your health insurance plan. With increasingly expensive tests and treatments and more and more controls over payment for medical care, your best insurance is to completely understand the provisions of your own insurance.

In this rapidly changing medical world, there will have to be a greater effort and understanding by all the participants in medical care—the patient, the physician, the health care team, and the governmental/insurance payers—to provide cost-effective, state-of-the-art health care.

— 40 —

Managed Care and Oncology: New Ways to Deliver Health Care

Malin Dollinger, M.D., and Joel M. Pollack, C.P.A.

■ ■ ■ ■

Since the 1950s there has been a profound shift in patterns of payment for health care. Before World War II, we simply paid for medical expenses out of pocket. Since "high-tech" and sophisticated tests and treatment did not yet exist, the cost of medical care was relatively predictable and thrifty. There were no intensive care units, CT or MRI scans, ultrasounds, fancy blood tests, or, for that matter, specialists. General practitioners were paid directly, sometimes in goods rather than money.

In 1933, surgeon Dr. Sidney Garfield set up a makeshift hospital in the Mojave Desert to treat workers building the Los Angeles Aqueduct, providing comprehensive care at a fixed price deducted from the workers' paychecks—a nickel a day! That caught the eye of shipbuilder Henry Kaiser, one of the largest employers in the country. He set up a similar program for the workers building the Grand Coulee Dam in Washington state and for workers at shipyards in California, Oregon, and Washington. After World War II, Kaiser opened enrollment to the public, setting off a revolution in health care. Within a year, AFL and CIO members were joining at the rate of 2,000 per month.

Henry Kaiser set up an all-inclusive health care system for his employees, in which, for the first time, one plan owned and controlled the hospitals, employed the physicians and other health care personnel and providers, and managed the whole enterprise, including preventive medicine, under one roof. One monthly payment by the consumer took care of whatever medical problems occurred, at least as defined by the contract.

Kaiser's system became the first and the largest health maintenance organization (HMO). This was the first example of "managed care," which, broadly defined, is the application of business principles to the delivery of health care. More specifically, it is a system of health care delivery that provides effective utilization of services at a fair and reasonable price, and measures performance outcomes and quality of care. Today everyone involved with delivery of health care—physicians, hospitals, laboratories—needs to worry about efficiency, timeliness, satisfaction, accountability, and costs, as well as quality. Lately, the "gatekeeper," usually a generalist physician, has primary responsibility to direct health care for each participant. There has been much recent public discussion and controversy, and legal action, regarding the role and responsibilities of health maintenance organizations. Some have not succeeded in matching the medical needs of their customers with their ability to maintain continuing financial solvency.

In the so-called staff model, there is a large multispecialty group of salaried physicians, and in the case of Kaiser Permanente, the plan owns the hospitals and outpatient facilities as well. Once the

Kaiser model was successful, other HMOs began to appear. From 1960 to 1980, several health care systems existed side by side, with various combinations and variations, and consumers were able to choose between systems according to their preferences, tastes, and pocketbooks.

Traditional Health Care Payment Systems

• *Direct payment* In this system, the consumer pays for health care out of pocket. Even those with various insurance plans may need to pay some expenses themselves, such as deductibles, co-payments, or extra costs of special treatments, noncovered services, and investigational treatments. Even Medicare has a Part B deductible.

• *Fee for Service/Indemnity Insurance* This became the most common type of insurance plan during the 1960s, 1970s, and 1980s. Various health insurance companies issued policies (often in association with employers, but not always). These policies allowed the consumer to select his or her choice of physician (and indirectly the choice of hospital), and the physician/hospital would then bill the insurance company for services rendered. Through this process, a primitive form of "quality control" developed, chiefly related to the concept of "usual and customary fees," which inhibited practitioners from charging (or at least being paid) excessive amounts. Competitive market forces began to standardize the costs of hospitalization, laboratory tests, and X-ray exams, as well as every other aspect of health care (for example, physical therapy, nursing homes, prescriptions), since consumers quickly learned to walk away from providers and services that were equivalent in quality but excessive in cost.

• *Discounted Fee for Service* Competitive market forces began to create discounts for physician services as well. Doctors agreed to accept, for example, a 10 or 20 percent discount in their usual fees. It was preferable, of course, for the doctor to be given an "exclusive" for patients of a particular health plan in return for such a discount. The physician's overhead and costs continued regardless of how many or how few patients were seen, and his margin, the difference between gross income and cost of doing business, became lower unless he could obtain an adequate number of patients.

• *Medicare and Medicaid* In 1965, a major event in American history occurred with federal legislation creating the Medicare and Medicaid programs. Up until that time, health care expenditures were kept under control by prudent spending by both the physician and the consumer. But the federal spending on these new programs unleashed a new level of health care expenditures that had never been seen previously, and turned health care into a growth industry. Now the consumer had carte blanche for medical care, with the bills being paid through Uncle Sam. The impact of this increased spending led to a desire on the part of the providers to search for new ways to control costs, and they turned to managed care to find the answers.

Managed Care

In the late 1980s and early 1990s, the entire gradual and peaceful evolution of health care payment systems entered a steamroller era. Until then, the various systems existed side by side, and especially in smaller cities and rural areas, the older system of indemnity insurance persisted, in which submitted bills by health care providers were simply paid by the insurance companies. Then several things happened to radically change our health care payment systems:

• *More and more, health care came to be delivered by legal contract, between the physician, or more commonly a group of physicians, and the insurance company (which came to be called the payer).* A new doctor in town not only would announce his or her name, address, specialty, and training but would also, for the first time, need to indicate which insurance plans he or she accepted (which ones he or she had contracts with).

• *For the first time, employers began to be the primary contractors as well as decision makers for health care.* Later on, this created the problem of persons having chronic and/or preexisting conditions being unable to change jobs, for fear of losing their health insurance and being unable to replace it. On the other hand, a large employer might be able, nevertheless, to incorporate a person with a preexisting illness (e.g., a history of cancer), because of the "clout" of a large number of employees enrolled in a plan.

• *The type of health care provider relationships changed dramatically.* Physicians under certain contracts were more restricted in their referral abilities—for example, they could send patients only to physicians and consultants under contract with the same company or plan (unless consumers were willing to pay significantly increased costs for treatment with their own choice of physician). Each health plan contracted with a certain hospital or hospitals for guaranteed and often lower rates. This tended to promote increased efficiency in hospitals and tended to drive inefficient or poorly organized hospitals out of business.

• *The contractual needs in relating physicians to health plans made solo or small practices undesirable.* Such limited groups of physicians could not deliver services to large populations of potential patients (now called "covered lives"), nor could they offer the breadth of skills and specialties, and geographic availability, that came to be the standard requirements of contracting health care providers (the new term for physicians). Thus, just as hospitals merged, so did physicians. Small groups became large ones, and solo practitioners became rarities.

• *Cost and control became dominant in the 1990s.* Each segment of the health care system realized that their "piece of the pie" was in jeopardy and attempted strategies to increase their control. Hospitals either acquired the practices of generalist physicians and internists or joint-ventured with primary care physicians, and thereby "captured" the patients cared for and the income derived from their care (lately it has been recognized by both parties that this may not always be a good idea). Hospitals and physicians joined forces, so practicing medicine became a business as well as a profession. Of course, there were always bills and taxes to pay and records of expenses to keep, but the doctor mostly took care of patients and kept whatever was left over after expenses were paid. Now, his or her livelihood became directly determined by nonphysicians, who controlled which patient he or she would see, how many patients there would be, which consultants and hospitals could be used, and where laboratory tests and X-rays could be done, not to mention nursing homes, home care, and prescriptions.

In the old days, *value* was defined as "quality work done by the physician." Now value has an additional, and different, definition, borrowed from business:

$$\text{Value} = \frac{\text{Quality}}{\text{Cost}}$$

That means that as quality increases, so does the value (we always knew this), but also, and especially nowadays, for equal quality, the one who provides services at lower cost provides the greater value.

Patterns of Health Care Delivery

At the present time, there are a number of different patterns of health care delivery under managed care. These are

- HMOs—health maintenance organizations,
- PPOs—preferred provider organizations,
- POS—point of service plans, and
- IPAs—independent practice associations.

Whereas the traditional *fee for service*, or *indemnity insurance plan*, reimburses health care providers (a new name for physicians and other health care professionals) based on billing for services provided, a *health maintenance organization (HMO)* integrates the entire health care program, including physicians, hospitals, outpatient services, and other health services such as prevention and rehabilitation, under one management system. Physicians are under contract, often on a full-time salaried basis, although the HMO may also contract with PPOs and IPAs to provide contracted physicians' services at standard rates. *Preferred provider organizations (PPOs)* have a list of "approved" providers who agree to provide services at contracted rates. Hospitals usually are also contracted. A *point of service (POS)* plan, sometimes described as an "open-ended" HMO or PPO, allows enrollees to receive services from a non-contracted (out-of-network) provider, although the cost of those services is generally not covered to the same degree as in-network. An *independent practice association (IPA)* is a group of physicians that contracts with various payer organizations and insurance companies.

The Gatekeeper Concept One of the major concepts of HMOs is the dominance of the primary care physician (PCP), or generalist. Under this system, he or she has almost complete control of patient care. All members of an HMO managed care plan select, or are assigned to, a primary care physician. The PCP determines which doctors the patient will see. If a patient has a lump in her breast, the PCP will determine if she should see an oncologist and will usually direct the patient to an oncologist within the system. The primary care physician is usually referred to as the "gatekeeper" and the concept is known as the gatekeeper system.

From the patient's point of view, there are lots of new pathways and patterns of care. The idea of the gatekeeper may seem strange. You may not be used to having to go to the same physician first, before you go to anyone else. In fact, some plans specify, for example, that you may see an eye doctor or a skin specialist, or another type of specialist defined by the plan, without asking your PCP, because we all know and agree that such care is appropriate, efficient, and cheaper. The expertise is well understood and accepted by all. The cancer specialist is likewise acknowledged as an expert in an area of medicine that not only requires special training but is an area that many physicians prefer to delegate.

Managing Risk

While there are currently a number of different patterns of health care delivery, managed care is becoming the dominant force in the health care industry and is increasing its participation at a rapid rate, especially when it comes to Medicare. We are not sure what the eventual result will be. Today at least two-thirds of the U.S. population participate in some form of managed care—that is, some type of system in which the health care providers furnish care based on an integrated economic, contractual, business, and professional program, with mutual contracts between all participants, including management. Although the states of California, Florida, and Minnesota led the trend toward managed care, these new systems of health care delivery are now common throughout the country. Many smaller health organizations are merging, while some are no longer in business, having been unable to correctly estimate, project, and plan the necessary balance between premiums/revenues/expenses and control/allocation of medical care.

Not only is the trend of health care delivery moving toward managed care, but the financial risk for providing health care is being shifted from insurance companies and managed care organizations to the physician who delivers the care. Following are the major types of risk sharing:

Risk Pools Common in HMOs, there are several different versions. For example, the physician may be paid a salary or a modified salary based on his or her work time and patient allocation. Some of the earnings, however, are placed in a separate fund, to be divided at the end of each year according to a formula based on predefined factors such as productivity and/or saving money by avoiding inappropriate or unnecessary use of services like laboratory tests, X-ray examinations, or hospitalization.

Since allocation of medical care in HMOs is generally controlled by primary care physicians, quite often the set-aside fund is also used to pay specialists if a member needs to receive specialty care. There is thus an incentive to be thrifty of effort and expense.

The big question now being hotly debated nationally is whether care suffers by such methods of physician reimbursement. New federal legislation now requires physicians to disclose valid treatment options not covered by their health plan.

Capitation In this method, the health care provider is paid a fixed amount each month to take care of anyone in a plan that becomes ill and needs the specified services. There is no charge for any specific illness or event.

The provider contracts to take care of all of the "covered lives" for a certain price per member per month, to provide all required (contracted) care that might be needed in the provider's specialty.

For example, an oncology group might contract on a capitated basis to take care of 100,000 covered lives, for a certain payment per member per month for professional fees. This means that a check for the entire amount would arrive each month for any and all care that is required for all those covered persons.

We can estimate and calculate about how many people out of 100,000 would get cancer each month, how much it would cost to see them, what services would be required, and how many years of care would be needed, and thus what the total expense of providing care would be (these calculations are not simple!). Thus, if the estimate is close to being correct, the physician group might come out okay. If, for some reason, fewer people get cancer that month, there is money left over. If lots of people get cancer, particularly types of cancer that are expensive to treat, the physicians operate at a loss.

Thus, in a capitated plan, the health care provider takes all the risk. If 1 person, 10 people, 100, or 1,000, (or 10,000!) people show up for cancer care, the price is the same. There needs to be a minimum number of such persons covered to be sure that an unusual number of persons who happen to need expensive care will not overwhelm the technical and financial ability of the health care provider to provide the contracted care.

Physicians with capitated contracts usually protect themselves by obtaining "reinsurance" ("stop-loss" insurance) to cover the unusual patient or number of patients who may require very expensive care. Of course, the reinsurance company needs proof ahead of time that the care given is "standard, reasonable, efficient, and cost-effective," to minimize the need to use the reinsurance.

A good analogy would be homeowners insurance or automobile insurance. The insurance company, for a monthly fee, agrees to take care of whatever losses the homeowner or car owner suffers. The insurance company *knows* that each month there will be home thefts, fires, and other losses and there will be car thefts and accidents. It knows that on the average there will be a certain number of such events, and it is willing to take the risk that the average number will continue. To make the risk safer, the insurance company needs to insure a lot of people.

Capitated medical plans are becoming more and more prevalent. Doctors are finding that they need to understand business principles as much as medical ones, and some physicians choose to concentrate on the business aspects. Some even go to business school to secure an MBA, as well as medical school.

Package-Price Plans ("Carve Outs") In this system, there is a fixed price for a defined "episode" of care. There are already medical plans with a fixed price for certain events that are easy to define from start to finish, such as cataract surgery and coronary artery bypass grafts (and heart transplants, too, for that matter).

In a "carve out," the physician and/or organization agrees to provide all the care required—whatever that is—for a certain illness, ailment, or procedure for a defined fixed price determined before care is begun. Thus, again the physician takes all the risk. If it costs less to deliver the care, he or she comes out ahead; if it costs more, he or she loses money.

In the cancer field, there has been difficulty in creating such plans. This is due to the complexity and expense of such care, rapid changes in technology and treatments, the length of time (years) when care and follow-up are required, and the fact that many different facilities and professionals are involved, not just the primary doctor (who is usually an oncologist). It requires a complex and coordinated effort to discover and predict accurate and reliable costs of all the components of care for many different kinds of cancer, as well as to place under contract (and under risk!) the many providers and health care facilities. The M. D. Anderson Cancer Center in Houston and the Memorial Sloan-Kettering Cancer Center in New York have in fact created and initiated such plans.

One area of uncertainty in the development of such plans is how to continue to pay for the vital clinical research trials that test promising new methods of treatment. These economics may not yet "make sense," and insurance companies may not wish to pay for trials of new treatments, whose roles are not yet defined or proven. One current area of great discussion and controversy, and the subject of federal legislation, is the need to find a way to integrate into various insurance plans (for example, Medicare) a method to pay for "clinical trials" that represent the cutting edge of effective cancer treatment, though they are not yet "standard" treatment.

"Personal Care" or "Boutique" Practice Plans In the past few years, a few generalist physicians have changed their style of practice so that for a specified yearly fee, they have agreed to limit the total number of patients they serve, to thus be personally available "24/7" to care for this relatively small number of patients. Appointments can generally occur the same day as requested, and the face-to-face time available, between physician and patient, is not rushed or limited by the need to schedule a large number of patients, as may occur in a conventional medical practice. House calls are often provided as part of this service. This is an appealing practice pattern, from the point of view of the responsible physician as well as the patient, and it remains to be seen to what extent this new practice pattern will supplement or replace other practice plans. Certainly some adjustments and modifications will need to be made; for example, the physician will still have to provide coverage at times of illness or vacation. A partnership of two physicians thus seems appropriate. It does appear that this practice pattern resembles the epitome of the "good old days," when a GP (general practitioner) physician assumed total responsibility for his or her patients, wherever and whenever they became ill and needed medical care.

Managed Care Issues

Until the development of managed care, each of the various places where health care was delivered and provided—different doctors' offices, hospitals, pharmacies, outpatient care facilities—existed separately and there was no wish or need for anyone to coordinate the patterns of care or costs of these different locations.

There were, in fact, examples of repeated and excessive utilization of services, not by direct intention but inherent in the way the system developed. For example, different physicians might order the same blood tests or X-rays—which were in fact indicated and necessary, but perhaps the results were not available or shared among the different practices.

There was no standard care plan that defined which type of physician took care of certain types of problems. For example, a cancer patient could easily have been followed by four different physicians: a primary generalist or internist, the surgeon who performed the cancer surgery, a radiation oncologist who may have

been called upon to administer radiation therapy, and the medical oncologist who became a "quarterback" for cancer care and also administered chemotherapy and called other consultants.

While there was certainly great patient satisfaction in having all these professionals watching over them, it did produce a major increase in cost of care, in repetition of tests, and in duplication of some services (not necessarily at the lowest cost). In addition, it was often unclear which professional was in charge of medical care decisions.

Now, under managed care guidelines, the gatekeeper concept has emerged, in which a single practitioner determines the location and types of care. While this is often a generalist for most areas of medicine, with referral to specialists as needed, in the cancer field, the medical oncologist usually becomes the case manager. The need for specialized knowledge is too great. But with managed care concerns regarding costs and efficiency, and avoidance of duplication of effort, the medical oncologist now has the same need for standardization of care, with concerns for cost factors as well as quality and efficiency.

Feedback Effective managed care requires several other factors besides care quality and cost. There must be feedback to all parties—physician provider, insurance carrier, and payer—regarding the quality of care, the efficiency of delivery, the results obtained, and the satisfaction of patients with the care they receive. Such information must be integrated into the daily care plan and package, often nowadays by computer/electronic models.

There is also a need for feedback among all the participants, so that inefficiencies and inappropriate or unnecessary care pathways can be discovered and improved. That is why the package-price plan, or "carve out," would have such potential for improving our cancer care system. It would put all the treatment, care management, cost management, and communication into one package, to achieve the maximum value in quality and cost.

Total Health Care For the first time, we will need to look at the entire health care picture as a single activity. If a service is done better or more efficiently or is less costly out of a hospital (or, for that matter, *in* a hospital), compared with a physician's office, that needs to be determined and mandated.

For the first time, physician preferences may *not* determine how things are done. Only certain hospitals will be permitted to perform certain procedures—for example, bone marrow transplants from allogeneic donors. A track record of success and safety would be a requirement. Laboratory tests will be done at a designated contracted laboratory, or will not be paid for or reimbursed. The same will apply for X-rays and other tests and procedures. Already in many managed care markets, the physician has limited choice in these matters and even now has a limited choice of consultants—those on the same plan or contract as the patient.

For the first time in the history of our health care system, the need for total cooperation exceeds the need for total autonomy or total control. Doctors, hospitals, and other health care suppliers and facilities will need to consider the roles of all the other "players" in the system.

Managed care will develop and reward those systems and plans that are able to look at the entire spectrum of providers and facilities and distill from the entire system an efficient health care package that provides a high-quality and cost-effective care plan. This goal requires total management of every aspect of care.

We are not there yet, but development of such care packages is taking place at breakneck speed—by the action of, and in response to, the providers, payers, and consumers of health care rather than by the government. We are not sure how it will look when the complete cancer care meal is finally served, but a hint can be taken from this chapter, and from the not-so-accidental fact that one author is a physician and the other is an accountant.

— 41 —

Planning for the Future

Ernest H. Rosenbaum, M.D., Malin Dollinger, M.D.,
and Isadora R. Rosenbaum, M.A.

■ ■ ■ ■

"The best way to get something done is to begin."
—Elmo A. Petterle

The chances for living a long and healthy life are now greater than ever before. Age is just a number that measures time. As George Burns said, "You're not old until the candles on your birthday cake cost more than the cake."

Today, we have better nutrition, better physical fitness, improved living conditions, new drugs, and new advances in medical science such as transplants, bypasses, and other life-prolonging discoveries. More and more cancers are becoming curable when they are diagnosed at an early stage. Cancer treatment techniques are constantly being developed, and new therapies like immunology and genetic engineering are holding out the prospect of curing more cancers in the future.

Yet living with cancer remains a fearful, anxious time despite all the promise of medical advances. No matter how well informed you are about your cancer or all the therapies that might be used to treat it, you still feel some loss of control over your fate. You put your life in the hands of specialists and live in uncertainty, hopeful one day, gloomy the next.

Although living with uncertainty may seem uncomfortable, it does allow room for hope and positive thoughts. You may discover that life can be more meaningful. Little pleasures can become very important. You may even begin to "stop and smell the roses." Once any anger or bitterness about having cancer is put aside, you will find there is still tremendous room for enjoyment.

And, if you are like many other people faced with uncertainty, you may get your life in focus with more clarity than you have known before. Thinking about their own mortality, perhaps for the first time, many people decide to make plans for the future if the best happens or if the worst happens. In either case, the act of making plans wonderfully concentrates the mind. If you make that decision yourself, the act of planning will let you face the uncertain future with clarity, simplicity, and the comforting knowledge that your affairs are in order and that as few things as possible are left undone.

Your Legacy of Love

We all know that at some time death will take us. And each of us makes—or should make—some plans for when the time comes. Most of us buy life insurance to provide financially for the people we love. We make wills so that when death occurs, there is a clear plan for the distribution of our earthly possessions.

But beyond these basics, few of us take the time to prepare in detail for the time when we are no longer around. Making such preparations isn't pleasant. In some ways, it may be very difficult. It is something that we often put off, partly because we all consider ourselves immortal or too young to worry about death and all its implications.

But to avoid discussing or thinking about it only puts off the kind of planning that really should be done. The burden just passes on to our survivors. More than 90 percent of survivors in America are unprepared to handle the responsibilities and immediate needs when a loved one dies.

Making Your Medical Choices You should discuss with your physician any concerns you have about how your medical care should be delivered, especially during a medical crisis. In the event of a sudden drastic complication, such as a heart stoppage or cessation of breathing, hospitals are often legally required to "call a code," to resuscitate you with cardiopulmonary resuscitation (CPR). This is sometimes called a Code Blue. Many health care givers also believe they are morally and professionally obligated to call such a code.

Code status varies, however, and it is important to consider how far *you* want your physician to go to attempt resuscitation should a crisis occur.

• Full Code means that treatment and support will be very aggressive, with the use of cardiac resuscitation, breathing tubes (intubation), and machines.
• A Chemical Code calls for a less aggressive plan. Drugs and intravenous treatments will be used to save or prolong life, but if breathing or the heartbeat stop, no attempt will be made to restart it.
• If you agree to a No Code status, no extreme measures will be used for life support and resuscitation.

The decisions about what life support measures should be taken should be made by you in advance of a hospitalization or major illness. Then make your wishes known. This can take the form of an advance directive, a paper you fill out in advance with your instructions in case you have a serious illness and are not able to speak for yourself. There are also documents called living wills and durable powers of attorney. (These decisions can be reversed at any time.) These will protect you as a patient even if you are unable to convey the information at the appropriate time. They will also protect your family from the stress of making sudden medical decisions for you.

The best way to define the code status you wish and ensure that your wishes are followed is through written documents.

• A living will should include your decision on the extent of treatment in the event you become so seriously ill, you might die. You may amplify the living will with a codicil or statement of your wishes for additional pain and comfort care if the end is near and the primary goal is keeping you comfortable under all circumstances. You can include a written request for adequate doses of morphine or sedatives, for example.
• Durable powers of attorney should include a summary of your wishes on limits to preserving or extending life. Those responsible for monitoring and delivering your health care can then act in accordance with your wishes should you become physically or mentally unable to make your own medical decisions.

This information should be in the medical file kept by your doctor and in your hospital record. Always carry in your wallet a medical emergency information card containing all vital information about codes, diagnoses, and any medications you take. In some states, the code status request can be included on the driver's license organ donor card.

Planning Tools A book by Elmo A. Petterle called *Getting Your Affairs in Order (Legacy of Love)* (Petterle Publications, 3 Greenside Way, San Rafael, CA 94901) is a practical guide on how you can make life easier for the people you leave behind. Its objective is to approach the problem of potential death with compassion and sensitivity. The book was designed for everyone—young, old, rich, poor, married, single, healthy, and ill.

It was not written to scare you into thinking that your time is running out because of age or any other reason. It is simply a strategic planning tool, a workbook you fill in yourself. It deals with realities in a very practical and organized way so that your survivors know what they need to know and are properly instructed and prepared for what has to be done.

• The book introduces you to the material you will be working on, including how to start planning for your beneficiaries. It gives advice on will preparation—on what you have to do, what the priorities are, and what is not important.

• It covers the details on how you wish to be cared for if you become very seriously ill, including a living will and durable powers of attorney.

• It gives advice and a place to fill out your instructions about your choice of a cemetery or other resting place, mortuary and funeral arrangements, memorial or other types of services, and newspaper information and advice on death benefits that are available in the United States.

• It provides survivors with a list of immediate after-death contacts and phone numbers in order of importance. This is convenient at a most awkward time. In their grief, people often don't think clearly and may make errors such as being sold costly funeral services that might directly contradict your wishes, which should be honored.

• It also lists the proper contacts to be made within the first ten days, such as

instructions for the post office or motor vehicles departments, and what contacts should be made within the first month—telephone, gas and electric, water, and waste disposal companies, newspapers, credit cards, clubs and organizations, cable TV, and other organizations that deserve to be listed.

• It provides guidance and planning space to be filled out on financial plans, any investments you've made, and property and casualty insurance, as well as information about home and personal property insurance. It is amazing how ill informed many people are about life insurance policies, Social Security benefits, medical insurance, pensions, profit-sharing plans, IRAs, and Keogh provisions that have often been made years before. Working through this section may give you a few surprises.

• It lets you catalog vital information on banks, savings accounts, loans, safety deposit boxes, and so on, so that this information is available when it should be.

• It gives advice on how to deal with bureaucracies that are often insensitive to the needs of people at such personal times.

• It provides necessary information about medical history that may be important to the family, as well as about family history and where personal letters can be found.

There are other tools that can assist you in your planning. One especially helpful book is *The Diagnosis Is Cancer,* by Edward J. Larschan, J.D., Ph.D., and Richard Larschan, Ph.D. (Bull Publishing, PO Box 208, Palo Alto, CA 94302). This book covers some of the same ground as *Legacy of Love* but from a different perspective, dealing primarily with the legal arrangements necessary for survivors.

Many people unfortunately procrastinate, but books like *Legacy of Love* and *The Diagnosis Is Cancer* give all thoughtful people an opportunity to lessen the pain and suffering of their survivors, simply because they love them.

Hope and the Will to Live

Like every creature in the animal world, human beings have a fierce instinct for survival. The will to live—that instinct to fight when our lives are threatened by illness or some other crisis—is a natural impulse in all of us. Yet some people are easily destroyed by the mental and physical effects of disease, while others call on inner resources to sustain them through the experience. Why do some people respond positively to suffering, while others cannot endure? Maybe the survivors have learned to be resilient by coming through earlier crises, becoming strong, tough, and confident in the process. Maybe the small flame of gritty determination that makes us keep struggling at even the lowest ebb just burns brighter in some than in others. But the most important reason may be hope.

Many doctors have seen how two patients of similar ages with the same diagnosis and degree of illness and the same treatment program experience vastly different results. And the only noticeable difference between the two is that one person is pessimistic and the other is optimistic. Hope, courage, effort, determination, endurance, love, and faith all nurture the will to live. And the greatest of these is hope. There may be times when you feel exhausted and overwhelmed by never-ending problems, when you feel ready to give up the struggle to survive. Yet if you have hope, you can carry on.

As long as there is even a remote chance for survival, as long as there are even minor improvements, hope can be kindled and nurtured. As long as your family, friends, and support team keep a positive attitude, hope can see you through any crises or times of reversal. But hope has to come mainly from within. You can have hope if you are willing to fight for your life and if you are ready to do everything you can to improve your health. Just as soldiers have a revival of mood and spirit as they march home singing from an exhausting day, so you can find new energies and new strength.

Even at the roughest times, you probably have untapped reserves of physical and emotional strength at your command. Call on them and use them to survive another day. These resources are the foundation and the source of your recovery.

Advance Health Care Directive

The following advance health care directive is a sample from the state of California. You can download your home state's forms for free from the National Hospice and Palliative Care Organization, at *www.caringinfo.org,* or you can order them for free by calling 1-800-658-8898.

SAMPLE ADVANCE HEALTH CARE DIRECTIVE FOR THE STATE OF CALIFORNIA

WARNING TO PERSON EXECUTING THIS DOCUMENT

This is an important legal document. Before executing this document, you should know these important facts:

You have the right to give instructions about your own health care. You also have the right to name someone else (your agent) to make health care decisions for you. This form lets you do either or both of these things. It also lets you express your specific wishes, if any, regarding life-support treatments and organ donation. If you use this form, you may complete or modify all or any part of it. If there is anything on this form you do not understand, you should contact your primary care physician or an attorney.

INSTRUCTIONS

Part I—Designation of Agent

Part I allows you to name another individual as your agent to make health care decisions for you if you become incapable of making your own decisions or if you want someone else to make those decisions for you even though you are still capable. You may also name an alternate agent to act for you if your first choice is not willing, able, or reasonably available to make decisions for you. Your agent must act consistently with your desires as stated in this document or otherwise made known by you.

Your agent may not be any of the following: (a) your primary treating health care provider, (b) an operator of a community care or residential care facility where you receive care, or (c) an employee of the health care institution or community or residential care facility where you receive care, unless your agent is related to you or is one of your coworkers.

Unless the form you sign limits the authority of your agent, your agent may make all health care decisions for you. Should you become incapacitated, your agent will also have the authority to make decisions relating to your personal care, including, but not limited to, determining where you will live, providing meals, hiring household employees, providing transportation, handling mail, and arranging recreation and entertainment. This form has a place for you to limit the authority of your agent if you wish. You need not limit the authority of your agent if you wish to rely on your agent for all health care decisions that may have to be made.

If you choose not to limit the authority of your agent, your agent will have the right to:

1. **Consent or refuse consent to any care, treatment, service, or procedure to maintain, diagnose, or otherwise affect a physical or mental condition.**

2. **Select or discharge health care providers and institutions.**

3. **Approve or disapprove diagnostic tests, surgical procedures, and programs of medication.**

4. **Direct the provision, withholding, or withdrawal of artificial nutrition and hydration and all other forms of health care, including cardiopulmonary resuscitation (CPR).**

5. Authorize an autopsy, donate your body or parts thereof for transplant, therapeutic, educational, or scientific purposes, and direct the disposition of your remains.

6. Examine your medical records and consent to their disclosure.

Notwithstanding this document, you have the right to make medical and other health care decisions for yourself so long as you can give informed consent with respect to the particular decision. In addition, no treatment may be given to you over your objection and health care necessary to keep you alive may not be stopped or withheld if you object at the time.

By operation of law, your agent may not consent to committing or placing you in a mental health treatment facility, or to convulsive treatment, psychosurgery, sterilization, or abortion.

You may state in this document any types of treatment that you do not desire. A court can take away the power of your agent to make health care decisions for you if your agent (1) authorizes anything that is illegal, (2) acts contrary to your known desires, or (3) where your desires are not known, does anything that is clearly contrary to your best interests.

Your agent's authority becomes effective when your primary physician determines that you are unable to make your own health care decisions unless you indicate otherwise. You may choose to have your agent's authority become effective immediately.

This power will exist for an indefinite period of time unless you limit its duration in this document.

You have the right to revoke the authority of your agent at any time by notifying your agent, treating physician, hospital, or other health care provider orally or in writing of the revocation. Completing a new Advance Health Care Directive will revoke all previous directives. If you revoke a prior directive, notify every person and hospital, clinic, or care facility that has a copy of your prior directive and give them a copy of your new directive.

Photocopies of this document can be relied upon by the appointed health care agent and others as though they were the original. Place the original in an accessible, safe place so that it can be located if needed. Tell your agent and a family member where you keep the original. Give photocopies of the original to (1) your agent and any alternative agents, (2) your primary care physician or other health care providers, and (3) members of your family and/or any other person who might be called in the event of a medical emergency.

Part II—Instructions for Health Care

You may, but are not required to, state your desires about the goals and types of medical care you do or do not want, including your desires concerning life support if you become seriously ill. If your wishes are not known, your agent must make health care decisions for you that your agent believes to be in your best interest, considering your personal values. **If you do not wish to provide specific, written health care instructions, draw a line through Section II.**

Part III—Donation/Disposition of Organs

You may express an intention to donate some or all of your bodily organs and tissues following your death and identify the purpose of the donation.

Part IV—Signature

After completing this form, provide your signature and the date of execution where indicated.

Part V—Witness Requirements

This Advance Health Care Directive will not be valid unless it is either signed by two qualified witnesses or acknowledged before a notary public in California.* If you use witnesses rather than a notary public, **the law prohibits using the following as witnesses:** (1) the person you have appointed as your agent or alternative agent(s), (2) your health care provider or an employee of your health care provider, or (3) an operator or employee of an operator of a community care facility or residential care facility for the elderly. Additionally, at least one of the witnesses **cannot** be related to you by blood, marriage, or adoption, or be named in your will, or by operation of law be entitled to any portion of your estate upon your death.

Special Rules for Skilled Nursing Facility Residents: If you are a patient in a skilled nursing facility, you must have a patient advocate or ombudsman sign as a witness and sign the Statement of Patient Advocate or Ombudsman. You must also have a second qualified witness execute this form or have this document acknowledged before a notary public.

PART I—DESIGNATION OF AGENT

I, _____, designate the following individual as my agent
(PRINT NAME)
to make health care decisions for me:

Name: _____

Address: _____
(STREET ADDRESS, CITY, STATE, ZIP CODE)

Telephone: _____
(HOME PHONE)   (WORK PHONE)

Optional—First Alternate Agent: If I revoke my agent's authority or if my agent is not willing, able, or reasonably available to make a health care decision for me, I designate as my first alternate agent:

Name: _____

Address: _____
(STREET ADDRESS, CITY, STATE, ZIP CODE)

Telephone: _____
(HOME PHONE)   (WORK PHONE)

* This document is used in the State of California and is reproduced here for illustration. Your state will have a specific document that resembles this one.

Optional—Second Alternate Agent: If I revoke the authority of my agent and first alternate agent, or if neither is willing, able, or reasonably available to make a health care decision for me, I designate as my second alternative agent:

Name: _____

Address: _____
(STREET ADDRESS, CITY, STATE, ZIP CODE)

Telephone: _____
(HOME PHONE)   (WORK PHONE)

When Agent's Authority Becomes Effective

Choose one:

☐ My agent's authority becomes effective when my primary physician determines that I am unable to make my own health care decisions.

☐ My agent's authority becomes effective immediately.

Duration of Agent's Authority

I understand that this Advance Health Care Directive will be effective from the date I execute this document and will exist indefinitely, unless I specify a shorter time. I can revoke this document at any time by telling my health care provider and my designated agent that I no longer want it to be effective.

Optional: This Advance Health Care Directive will be effective only until the following date:

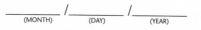

(MONTH)   (DAY)   (YEAR)

PART II—INSTRUCTIONS FOR HEALTH CARE

If you do not wish to provide specific, written health care instructions, you may draw a line through this section.

The following are statements about the use of life-support treatments. Life-support or life-sustaining treatments are any medical procedures, devices, or medications used to keep you alive. Life-support treatments may include the following: medical devices put in you to help you breathe, food and fluid supplied artificially by a medical device (tube feeding), cardiopulmonary resuscitation (CPR), major surgery, blood transfusions, kidney dialysis, and antibiotics.

Sign either of the following general statements about life-support treatment if one accurately reflects your desires. If you wish to modify or add to either statement or to write your own statement instead, you may do so in the space provided or on a separate sheet(s) of paper, which you must date and sign and attach to this form.

Optional: The statement I have signed below is to apply if I am suffering from a terminal condition from which death is expected in a matter of months, or if I am suffering from an irreversible condition that renders me unable to make decisions for myself, and life-support treatments are needed to keep me alive.

☐ I request that all treatments other than those needed to keep me comfortable be discontinued or withheld and my physician(s) allows me to die as gently as possible. I understand and authorize this statement as proven by my signature:

_____   _____
(SIGNATURE)   (DATE)

OR

☐ I request that attempts be made to keep me alive in this terminal or irreversible condition by using all available, effective life-support treatments. I understand and authorize this statement as proven by my signature:

_____   _____
(SIGNATURE)   (DATE)

Optional: My agent is authorized to make all health care decisions for me except as I state here (use more sheets if necessary):

_____

_____

_____

_____

_____

_____

_____

_____

_____

_____

_____

_____

PART III—DONATION/DISPOSITION OF ORGANS

Choose one:

☐ I wish to donate ANY needed organs, tissues, or parts.

☐ I wish to donate ONLY the following organs, tissues, or parts: _____

_____

☐ I do NOT wish to donate any organs, tissues, or parts.

Optional: My agent is authorized to make anatomical gifts, authorize an autopsy, and direct disposition of my remains, except as I state here (use more sheets if necessary):

_____

_____

_____

_____

_____

_____

_____

_____

_____

_____

PART IV—SIGNATURE

I hereby sign my name to and acknowledge this Advance Health Care Directive. By my signature, I revoke any prior Power of Attorney for Health Care or Natural Death Act Declaration. I understand that a copy of this form has the same effect as the original:

_____ at _____ , _____
(DATE)   (CITY)   (STATE)

Signature: _____

Print Name: _____ Date of Birth: _____

PART V—STATEMENT OF WITNESSES

I declare under penalty of perjury under the laws of the state of California* (1) that the individual who signed or acknowledged this Advance Health Care Directive is personally known to me, or that the individual's identity was proven to me by convincing evidence, † (2) that the individual signed or acknowledged this Advance Health Care Directive in my presence, (3) that the individual appears to be of sound mind and under no duress, fraud, or undue influence, (4) that I am not a person appointed as agent by this Advance Health Care Directive, and (5) that I am not the individual's health care provider or an employee of that health care provider, or an operator or employee of an operator of a community care facility or a residential care facility for the elderly.

Witness #1: _____   **Date:** _____
(SIGNATURE)

Print Name: _____

Address: _____

Witness #2: _____   **Date:** _____
(SIGNATURE)

Print Name: _____

Address: _____

At least one of the above witnesses must also sign the following declaration:

I further declare under penalty of perjury under the laws of the state of California that I am not related to the individual executing this Advance Health Care Directive by blood, marriage, or adoption, and, to the best of my knowledge, I am not entitled to any part of the individual's estate upon his or her death under a will now existing or by operation of law.

Signature: _____   Date: _____

*This document is used in the State of California and is reproduced here for illustration. Your state will have a specific document that resembles this one.

† **Evidence of Identity:** The following forms of identification are satisfactory evidence of identity: a California driver's license or identification card or U.S. passport that is current or has been issued within five years, or any of the following if the document is current or has been issued within five years, contains a photograph and description of the person named on it, is signed by the person, and bears a serial or other identifying number: a foreign passport that has been stamped by the U.S. Immigration and Naturalization Service, a driver's license issued by another state or by an authorized Canadian or Mexican agency, an identification card issued by another state or by any branch of the U.S. armed forces, or for an inmate in custody, an inmate identification card issued by the Department of Corrections. If the principal is a patient in a skilled nursing facility, a patient advocate or ombudsman may rely on the representations of family members or the administrator or staff of the facility as convincing evidence of identity if the patient advocate or ombudsman believes that the representations provide a reasonable basis for determining the identity of the principal.

For Skilled Nursing Facilities: Statement of Patient Advocate or Ombudsman

I further declare under penalty of perjury under the laws of the state of California that I am a patient advocate or ombudsman as designated by the State Department of Aging and am serving as a witness as required by Probate Code Section 4675.

Name/Title Printed: _____   Date: _____

Signature: _____

Address: _____

Certificate of Acknowledgment of Notary Public

Acknowledgment before a notary public is not required if two qualified witnesses have signed above. If you are a patient in a skilled nursing facility, you must have a patient advocate or ombudsman sign the Statement of Witnesses and the Statement of Patient Advocate or Ombudsman above, even if you also have this form notarized.

State of California   )
) ss.
)
County of _____)

On this _____, before me, _____,
            (DATE)   (NAME AND TITLE OF OFFICER)

personally appeared _____,
                                        (NAME OF SIGNER)

personally known to me (or proved on the basis of satisfactory evidence) to be the person(s) whose name(s) is/are subscribed to the within instrument and acknowledged to me that he/she/their executed the same in his/her/their authorized capacity(ies), and that by his/her/their signature(s) on the instrument the person(s), or the entity upon behalf of which the person(s) acted, executed the instrument.

WITNESS my hand and official seal.

_____
(SIGNATURE OF NOTARY PUBLIC)   Notary Seal

Checklist of Forms and Worksheets

The time to act is now: 93 percent of families are unprepared when a death occurs. Collecting key pieces of information and putting them in one place will help ensure that your loved ones are cared for after your death. Once you have gathered this information, be sure to tell several key people where it will be kept. Do not keep this information in a safe-deposit box (it will be sealed upon your death): Give it to your doctor, family, lawyer, agent (as designated by your medical power of attorney), and hospital medical records department.

In addition to the Advance Directive, consider putting together the following pieces of information (representative copies of these forms/checklists can be found in *Everyone's Guide to Cancer Supportive Care*):

• Additional considerations for the advance directives (gives your preferences for specific types of life-sustaining measures, such as CPR, being placed on a mechanical ventilator, or receiving a feeding tube; depending on the particular health condition—persistent vegetative state, Alzheimer's disease, etc.)

• A medical emergency wallet card (containing your contact information, diagnosis, and medications, as well as the location of your advanced directives and your do-not-resuscitate wishes)

• Medic Alert Service Form (access online at *www.medicalert.org*)

• Family information

• Location of records (your wills, financial statements, insurance policies, and personal records [passports, birth certificates, etc.])

• Review of assets and liabilities (bank accounts, stocks, bonds, and mutual funds, assets, loans, and mortgages)

• Persons to notify after death (clergy, funeral director, executor of will, life insurance agent, organ donation coordinator, attorney, etc.)

• Obituary

• Arrangements for funeral/memorial service

PART FOUR

New Advances in Research, Risk Assessment, Diagnosis, and Treatment

— 42 —

The Impact of Research on the Cancer Problem: Looking Back, Moving Forward

Amanda Psyrri, M.D., and Vincent T. DeVita Jr., M.D. *

■ ■ ■ ■

Historical Perspective: The Cancer Act and Its Implications

In 1971, the National Cancer Act was passed by the United States Congress and signed by President Nixon. The mandate of the Cancer Act, more popularly known as "The War on Cancer," was to "support basic research, and the application of results of basic research, to reduce the incidence, morbidity and mortality from cancer." In 1972, funds to support research began to flow; by the early 1980s, the annual National Cancer Institute (NCI) budget had increased from under $180 million to a little over $1 billion. Today the budget is $6.2 billion, and over $50 billion have been invested in cancer research since 1971.

Also written into the mandate of the act were instructions to apply the results of research through new programs that were not possible in 1971, "insofar as feasible," but anticipated by the authors of the act as technology was developed. With the advent of small, high-speed computers by the 1980s, the application components were eventually developed. As a consequence, in 1984 the NCI formulated goals for the reduction of cancer incidence and mortality in the United States for the year 2000.[1] These goals offered a range of targets, from realistically achievable programs to more utopian ideals—such as the application of all known scientific discoveries equally to all people. They were also *goals*, not *estimates*, as they are often mislabeled. Estimates are a best guess of what will happen if nothing changes. Goals require new programs and a maximum effort to attain them. This was the essence of the Cancer Act.

Now as the year 2007 has arrived, it is appropriate to ask about how far we have come and to address the impact of the act and the likelihood of the conquest of cancer. The answer is, we're pleased to say, that we have come further than most ever dreamed possible before the passage of the Cancer Act and that it is possible to think of a world without cancer as a major killer.

The Revolution of Molecular Biology

In 1971, cancer was a black box. We could examine it, turn it over in our hands, even weigh it, but we could not look inside. Today, thanks to the support of the Cancer Act, the lid of the box

---

*Member of the board of the ImClone Corporation, the maker of Erbitux, which is mentioned in this chapter.

has been pried open. We are gazing at an incredibly complex piece of machinery, and, what's more, we even have the blueprint for how it works.

In the seventies, the influx of research support made possible several technical advances. High on this list was the ability to examine the DNA of normal and cancerous cells at the molecular level. DNA is the genetic blueprint that provides living beings with all the information necessary for growth and development. The information in DNA is transferred from the DNA alphabet to a coded message in RNA, which in turn directs the synthesis of proteins, including enzymes that determine who each of us is as a human being. Before 1971, DNA had proven too unwieldy to study effectively. However, restriction enzymes, or "nature's scissors," were discovered as a tool for breaking DNA into manageable pieces for study, and marked the beginning of the biologic revolution as we know it.

The discovery of the value of restriction enzymes was followed by the discovery of reverse transcriptase, the enzyme that gave us new insights into biology and new ways to synthesize DNA fragments from RNA extracted from cells. All this led to "recombinant technology," the ability to sequence genes or pieces of genes and place them in bacteria to be studied and saved, and in turn to use bacteria as factories in order to produce cancer-specific biologic agents in large quantities. These and other technical advances paved the way for the major discoveries in the 1980s and gave birth to the biotechnology industry, and ultimately to the sequencing of the entire human genome that has recently been accomplished.

Angiogenesis Besides advances in molecular biology, cell biology studies performed in the 1970s shed light on mechanisms of tumor growth and metastasis. The concept of the *angiogenic switch,* a term used to describe the process by which a tumor acquires its own blood supply, was introduced in the early seventies. Tumor cells produce molecules (mainly proteins) that promote the formation of small blood vessels to and within tumors. Sustained microvessel formation is a process fundamental to continued tumor growth and metastasis. This "switch to an angiogenic phenotype" was first used to describe the development of pancreatic islet cell tumors in mice. This major discovery gave rise to antiangiogenic therapies that are currently available in the clinic.

Cell Signaling The discoveries of the eighties were grouped around the identification of specific genes associated with the course of cancer called oncogenes and tumor suppressor genes. Oncogenes promote growth and in some cases the angiogenic switch of tumor cells. Many of these genes were also found to be major components of the cell-signaling system in normal cells, the method all cells use to talk to each other. These signaling systems control normal growth and development. Thus, cancer research has turned out to be the engine of the study of developmental biology as well over the past quarter of a century. In addition, in 1980 a system of chemical modulations called protein tyrosine phosphorylation was discovered. This involves the addition of phosphate groups to proteins, a process that activates proteins from their inactive precursors. Protein tyrosine phosphorylation has proven to be fundamental in cell communication and signaling.

Cells sense signals from a variety of sources. Signals emanating from outside the cell (such as from other cells or the extracellular environment) must somehow cross the plasma membrane of the cell. This signaling process occurs via circulating elements in the blood called ligands. These ligands can be membrane permeable or can activate transmembrane receptors (proteins that span the cell membrane). The portion of the receptor on the inside of the cell, called the intracellular domain, functions as an enzyme and is turned on when the ligand binds to the receptor. These enzymes, called receptor tyrosine kinases (RTKs), add chemical phosphate groups to tyrosine subunits on proteins inside the cell. Thus, cells, in response to signals, regulate the expression and function of their proteins. RTKs control the most fundamental cellular processes, including cell growth, cell migration, and cell survival, as well as the differentiation or maturation of cells. In the past two decades, there has been dramatic progress in the characterization of these RTKs, the signaling pathways they activate, and the mechanisms underlying their regulation. The complete determination of the sequences of the worm (*C. elegans*), the fruit fly (*Drosophila*), and man (*Homo sapiens*) has made a large number of enzymes and signaling proteins accessible to biochemists and geneticists who are interested in determining the roles of RTKs in normal processes and in pathological situations. The elucidation of the signal transduction systems, or the mechanisms of "cell talk," has led to the discovery of several molecular targets in oncology that are now part of cancer treatment.

Microarrays as a Research Tool In the 1990s, there was a remarkable enhancement of the tools of molecular biology. These improvements led to many new discoveries as well as the promise of many more to come, as we were given the ability to identify and sequence the genetic codes of disease-associated genes and to identify variations in normal genes that make people more or less responsive to treatment.[2] Development of these tools made the project to sequence the entire human genome possible. Techniques including the DNA microarray (a method of analyzing genes on a small glass slide, enabling the expression of thousands of genes to be assessed at once) allow us to address and answer questions in hours that often took months or years in the past. For example, the DNA from two groups of patients with the same cancer, one curable by chemotherapy and the other not, can be flooded over the thousands of genes on a DNA microarray to determine what genes are responsible for the difference in response to treatment. Similarly, taking a step forward, proteomics (analysis of the thousands of proteins in the body at once) became available over the past few years. This protein profile is more closely associated with tumor behavior, since proteins represent the final product encoded by genes. Microarray technology enables detailed analysis of gene or protein expression patterns in response to growth factor stimulation of cells derived from normal or pathological tissues, which reveals links between signaling pathways.

Indeed our problem, to use a phrase from the old cartoon character Pogo, is that "we are faced with insurmountable opportunities" and need to solve the logistical problems associated with the flood of new information. This will be increasingly possible using high-speed computing techniques to analyze huge amounts of complex data.

How have the funds provided for cancer research been used to help patients with cancer? Since 1971, 85 percent of the NCI budget has gone into what would be defined as basic research or research done in laboratories. The remaining 15 percent has gone into the refinement and wide distribution of technology that already existed in 1971 when the Cancer Act was passed. Nobel prizes have recognized many of the technical advances and discoveries referred to here and made possible by the Cancer Act.

Advances in Cancer Treatment Have Made a Significant Impact on Patient Survival

At the turn of the last century, all cancer was incurable. With the advent of anesthesia, antibiotics, and refinements in surgical techniques, about one-third of all cancers became curable by 1950. Although radioactivity and radium were also discovered at the turn of that century, it was not until the introduction of radiotherapy equipment such as cobalt generators, which came into use in 1957 and were followed by the development of linear accelerators in 1961, that radiotherapy began to have a measurable impact. It is estimated that in 1971, when the Cancer Act was passed, no more than 36 percent of all cancers were curable by treatments such as surgery and radiotherapy directed at the site of origin of the cancer.

Therefore, two-thirds of all cancers were incurable largely because of spread beyond the local site of origin to secondary sites called metastases. Deaths of cancer patients are really caused by the growth of metastases in vital organs. The need for treatment of the entire body was apparent, and this could be accomplished by administering chemicals or drugs directly into the bloodstream to provide exposure to cancer cells wherever they were lodged. The utility of chemotherapy, or drug treatment, as an effective tool for cancer treatment was discovered in the late 1940s at the Yale Cancer Center but was not applied widely until it was proven curative for some advanced cancers, most notably childhood leukemia and Hodgkin's disease, in the late 1960s.[3] With these cures as a stimulus, chemotherapy was widely applied in common cancers after 1971, when resources were made available for widespread testing in clinical trials, the main tool for delivering new treatments to humans, as part of the U.S. national cancer program. As a consequence of the availability of surgery, radiotherapy, chemotherapy, and subsequent biologic therapies that are also given intravenously and can reach cancer cells anywhere, the survival of patients with common serious cancers in the United States increased from 36 percent in 1971 to 52 percent in 1993. The five-year relative survival by cancer site increased from 50 percent (period 1974–1976) to 65 percent (period 1995–2002) for all sites combined.[4] More important, based on the "Annual Report to the Nation on the Status of Cancer, 1975–2002," death rates in men and women combined decreased by 1.1 percent annually from 1990 through 2002 for all cancer sites combined and also for most of the fifteen most common cancers.[5] And in 2005, the overall death rates from cancers declined for the first time despite the increasing size and age of our population. We will return to some of these statistics at the end of this chapter.

The U.S. Surveillance, Epidemiology, and End Results (SEER) program, a tracking system for cancer statistics, and an offspring of the Cancer Act, is the most sophisticated national tracking system for cancer incidence, survival, and mortality in the world. It is used to trace most of the results of the national effort. There is, however, a lag in time in the published results of cancer statistics due to the delay necessitated by the collecting and analyzing of data. The most recent figures are from 2001 and measure events that occurred at least five years earlier, in 1996. This is an important point to remember when assessing the national and worldwide results of cancer treatment. Today's information is at least five years old, and so using SEER data alone, we will not accurately know how well we are doing now, in 2007, until about 2012.

Clinical Applications of Basic Science Research

It is important to know that despite improvements, the astonishing results of basic research referred to above and made possible by the Cancer Act are only now being applied to patient care. Many of these treatments are still in testing stages, so the best is yet to come in terms of making progress against cancer.

Overcoming the Problem of Drug Resistance The new biological discoveries that have come out of the basic research program have also begun to allow us to explain some perplexing problems associated with cancer. For example, we have been aware of two plateaus in cancer treatment. The first is that of patients curable by local means alone—that is, by surgery and radiotherapy—who constitute only about 36 percent of all patients. This plateau cure rate very likely reflects patients with cancers that have not yet metastasized but are susceptible to the surgeon's scalpel or radiation's beam. The second plateau is the percentage of patients curable by chemotherapy. This percentage improved steadily in the seventies and eighties but had not changed dramatically until recent work with breast and colon cancer impact on survivorship. Cure rates remain highest in tumors of lymphoid and marrow origin and in tumors of children. It is a curious observation that 90 percent of all drug cures occur in just over 10 percent of cancer types. This suggests that some types of cancer are uniquely susceptible to drugs, while others, including the more common cancers that derive from epithelial tissues, such as breast, lung, prostate, and ovary, are more resistant. One approach to overcoming drug resistance is increasing the chemotherapy dose. With the advent of techniques to stimulate the growth of bone marrow cells, such as white blood cells and the stem cells from which all other cells develop, it has become possible to attack this plateau with very intensive high-dose chemotherapy. But again, these therapies have shown limited success in a small number of chemosensitive tumor types. "Drug resistance," or the inability to effec-

tively treat a cancer with drugs, remains a major roadblock to the more effective use of systemic chemotherapy.[5]

Cancer drugs appear to exert their killing effect by stimulating cell suicide programs. This mechanism, called programmed cell death (apoptosis), is used by normal organisms for the orderly destruction of cells deemed unnecessary by the body. More curable cancers such as aggressive lymphomas are derived from cells that frequently use apoptosis to select the appropriate cells for development of the adult immune system. Epithelial-derived tumors, although they all have the same genes as lymphoid tumors, apparently cannot easily turn these genes on to respond to DNA damage caused by anticancer drugs. Some lymphoma cell types, including chronic lymphocytic leukemia (CLL), are also characterized by defects in the apoptotic machinery. Hence, these tumors frequently are not curable with chemotherapy.

Understanding the Cell Cycle The puzzle represented by drug resistance has become explainable by new information that has originated from molecular studies. The elucidation of the cancer cell cycle and systems of cell communication has both shed light on the molecular mechanisms of drug resistance.

Cancer cells kill by the failure to listen to signals that say, "Stop dividing," and by reproducing too often. To reproduce they need to go through what is called the cell cycle.[5] Information on the progression of genetic changes associated with a malignancy like colon cancer shows that a common series of changes confer malignant characteristics. These genetic abnormalities often affect genes that stand guard over the control of the cell cycle. When this guard is dropped, the abnormal growth characteristic of cancer occurs. More aggressive behavior of a tumor, for instance, is associated with mutations in genes like the well-known tumor suppressor gene p53, while cancers without changes in the p53 gene may be more amenable to cure. The p53 gene is known as the Guardian of the Genome, the genome representing our total assemblage of genetic material.

Mutations in the p53 gene, for example, allow cells to proceed in an unconstrained way through the cell cycle, and hinder the cells' ability to activate apoptosis. Such mutations are known to increase resistance to both chemotherapy and radiotherapy. For example, small cell lung cancer is initially responsive to chemotherapy due to induction of expression of the apoptotic gene BAX by chemotherapy in conjunction with p53. However, subsequent mutations render p53 dysfunctional, and cancer cells no longer respond to chemotherapy. Another gene that becomes inactive during this process is the retinoblastoma (Rb) gene. As you have read in other chapters, Rb is a tumor suppressor gene that normally controls the transcription of oncogenes. When Rb is rendered inactive (again, by the process of phosphorylation), the resulting unconstrained expression of molecules normally under its control leads to uncontrolled cell proliferation and tumor formation. These are only two examples of the kinds of information we now have that explain why more rapidly growing cancers exhibit increased resistance to chemotherapy, and thus we are provided with new opportunities for treatment by repairing, replacing, or blocking critical cell cycle genes.

Growth factor receptors that are components of cell-signaling systems have also been implicated in drug resistance. For example, the epidermal growth factor receptor (EGFR) has been linked to chemo- and radio-resistance. EGFR is a receptor that, after binding of the epidermal growth factor, activates protein targets and initiates a signaling network leading to increased proliferation, blood vessel formation, and inhibition of programmed cell death.

How can we use the information derived from molecular studies to improve the efficacy of chemotherapy? The number of targets for drug treatments has increased enormously in the past few years. One major challenge is to develop drugs that can regulate key targets in the cell-signaling systems and induce apoptosis artificially. This challenge has been taken up by academic investigators and pharmaceutical companies worldwide. If apoptosis, or the cell suicide mechanism, can easily be manipulated, the ability to affect the molecules that control the cell cycle has the potential to convert current therapy into much more effective and easier-to-use treatments for cancer very rapidly.

Targeting oncogenes or the signaling networks associated with drug resistance has been a major therapeutic strategy over the past decade. Inhibition of EGFR activation by using antibodies to EGFR or kinase inhibitors has been shown to reverse chemo- and radio-resistance; the combination of the drug cisplatin with the anti-EGFR antibody cetuximab (Erbitux) is active in a proportion of cisplatin-resistant head and neck tumors. Preventive and therapeutic strategies targeting dysfunctional p53 have also been developed. ONYX-015 is an attenuated (weakened) virus selectively toxic to cells carrying defects in the p53-dependent signaling pathways (i.e., cancer cells) and is being tested in clinical trials.

Antiangiogenesis Strategies For more than five decades, the cancer cell has been the main target for cancer therapy. However, the development of mutations hinders successful therapeutic outcomes. On the contrary, human endothelial cells, which form the lining of blood vessels, in the tumor bed are genetically stable (they do not undergo mutations) and are less susceptible to acquired drug resistance. Therefore, combined treatment of the endothelial cell (antiangiogenesis) in the tumor and the cancer cell may be more effective that chemotherapy alone. Angiogenesis inhibition is being validated as an anticancer therapy in a large number of clinical trials. The most compelling results have been reported for patients with metastatic colon cancer treated with the angiogenesis inhibitor bevacizumab (Avastin), and also for patients with multiple myeloma where the use of thalidomide (Thalomid) results in long-term (up to five years) complete remission. For more details on antiangiogenesis strategies, please refer to chapter 14.

The Paradigm of Imatinib (Gleevec) in Chronic Myelogenous Leukemia (CML)
In addition to restoring chemosensitivity in tumor cells by targeting pathways involved in drug resistance, the major challenge has been to develop drugs that can block the pivotal pathway that drives tumor growth in each cancer type.

One stunning example of this occurred in the year 2000 in a disease known as chronic myelogenous leukemia (CML).[6] In CML, there is a specific molecular abnormality referred to as the Philadelphia chromosome, resulting from a chromosomal translocation that swaps genetic material from one chromosome to another. In the 1980s, the protein produced by this translocated gene, called BCR/ABL, was characterized and its central role in the cause of CML was established. The BCR/ABL fusion protein functions as one of our old friends—a tyrosine kinase. It binds and adds phosphate groups to several intracellular proteins, leading to the activation of various signaling pathways. Chemotherapy for CML had not been very beneficial and the disease was curable in some patients only by bone marrow transplantation. Using new techniques in what is known as combinatorial chemistry, very specific drugs have been developed that block the Philadelphia chromosome abnormality. These drugs target and inactivate the

BCR/ABL fusion protein that drives tumor growth in CML. The early results are quite astonishing in that the disease treated with one of these new drugs, called imatinib (Gleevec), appears totally controllable with very modest side effects. This kind of treatment may be regarded as proof of the principle that these approaches will work against cancers with these kinds of defects, which include most cancers. However, it is essential to identify the pivotal molecular pathway that initiates and maintains tumor growth in each tumor type. There are several molecular changes that develop subsequent to this primary pivotal event; targeting these secondary changes and not "the origin" of the problem will not achieve cures.

Conclusions: Looking Ahead

As a result of the new knowledge, we have come closer to the goals the NCI originally set back in 1984 than most of us ever expected. In 1984, hundreds of consultants were involved in setting these goals. For survival targets, they used survival rate reports from two programs, the End Results Group and SEER, as baseline benchmarks. These are shown in Figure 1. The consultants concluded that when the results from clinical trials were compared with national figures, there was a difference favoring results in clinical trials, referred to as state of the art. In Figure 1, state-of-the-art estimates are shown as triangles. End results and SEER data are shown in the lower curve in Figure 1. A number of scenarios were developed by the consultants, as shown by points A through E. These scenarios involved just moving the end results closer to the state of the art by doing a better job of disseminating new information to the public (A through C) or by adding new treatments and improving dissemination (D and E) of currently available data from SEER and other sources, indicating that we have come as far as point D.[4,7]

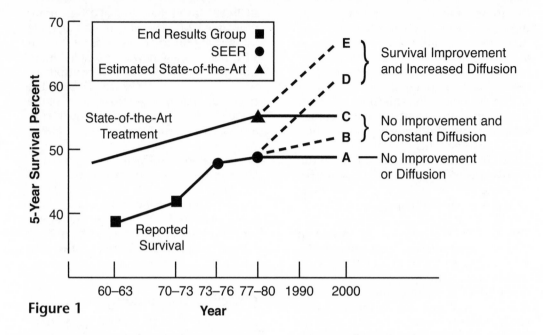

Figure 1

Improved survival is coupled with a positive change in mortality statistics as well. Figure 2 shows recent changes in mortality statistics for selected cancers.[4] It is notable that decreases have occurred in very common cancers such as prostate and colorectal cancers in men and breast and colorectal cancers in women. Declines have also been noted in lung cancers due to smoking cessation programs, although among women, death rates have increased for lung cancer. The overall reduction in mortality is due to a combination of advances in prevention, diagnosis, and treatment. For the first time in U.S. history, the number of deaths for every 100,000 people has declined over the past decade, and now overall deaths have diminished as well. However, the relative risk of death from all cancers combined in each racial and ethnic population compared with non-Hispanic white men and women ranged from 1.16-fold in Hispanic white men to 1.69-fold in American Indian/Alaska Native men. Geographic variations in stage distributions were also noted. Therefore, not all segments of the U.S. population have benefited equally from advances in prevention, diagnosis, and management.

New Initiatives In the past eight years, two new initiatives have been started to maximize the advantages that have come about because of the War on Cancer and to complete the task mandated by the Cancer Act of 1971. First, an organization called the National Dialogue on Cancer (NDC), now called C-Change, has been established under the sponsorship of former president George Bush and Mrs. Barbara Bush. The NDC, cochaired by Dr. LaSalle D. Leffall, a cancer surgeon, and Senator Diane Feinstein, has as its goal to bring together the stakeholders in the War on Cancer—the advocacy groups, federal agencies, and other private and public organizations—with a specific mission to speak with a common voice to support cancer research and to develop better ways to translate these results to patients. The 125 NDC representatives meet on a regular basis to discuss common

Annual Percent Change in Death Rates for Selected Cancers, 1992–2002

According to this year's Annual Report to the Nation, overall cancer death rates in the United States declined 1.1% per year from 1993 through 2002. The decline was more pronounced among men (1.5% per year from 1993 through 2002) than among women (0.8% per year from 1992 through 2002). Death rates for 12 of the 15 most common cancers in men decreased in that time period, as did rates for 9 of the 15 most common cancers in women.

Annual percent change in U.S. death rates for selected cancers*:

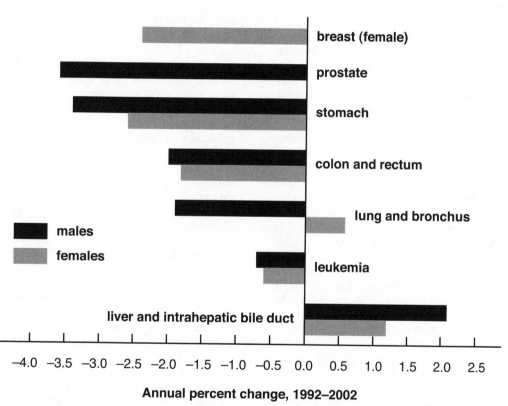

*All increases or decreases shown are statistically significant.

Source: Edwards BK, Brown ML, Wingo PA, Howe HL, Ward E, Ries LAG, et al. Annual Report to the Nation on the Status of Cancer, 1975–2002. Featuring Population-Based Trends in Cancer Treatment. *J Natl Cancer Inst* 2005;97:1407–27.

Figure 2

goals and issues. Impressed with the fruits of the Cancer Act of 1971 and the initial efforts of the NDC, Senator Feinstein asked one of the authors (V. T. DeVita) and Dr. John Seffrin, CEO of the American Cancer Society, to form a committee to develop a proposal that will serve as the basis of revised legislation for a new cancer act for the new millennium. This committee, the National Cancer Legislative Advisory Committee (NCLAC), released its report, "Conquering Cancer: A National Battle Plan to Eradicate Cancer in Our Lifetime," in September 2001.[8] The report concluded that the cancer burden can be conquered through a comprehensive strategy that not only provides greater funding for basic translational and clinical research, but also removes barriers to access to quality medical care, so that all people will benefit equally from preventive measures, medications, and technologies, providing a new overarching organizational structure to coordinate the cancer program, similar to that used for the Department of Homeland Security.

The Economic Impact of Advances in Cancer Research A valid question raised by this review of cancer research is whether the investment in cancer research has gone beyond improving the health of our nation over the past thirty years. The economic impact of cancer treatment in the United States is enormous. The "cost of cancer" each year is over $100 billion. The effect of the successful control of this disease on the country therefore could be equally enormous. This issue has been addressed by a group called Funding First, composed of eminent scientists and economists from major U.S. universities. In 2000, this group issued a startling report outlining the results of investing in health-related research.[9] Their conclusion was that while half of the economic expansion in the nineties was due to increased economic productivity, the remaining 50 percent was derived from the research

related to improvements in the health of the nation, particularly in heart disease and cancer. They also concluded that a reduction in cancer mortality of 20 percent would lead to a $10 trillion return to the economy. In fact, they estimated that total eradication of cancer would lead to a return to the economy of $46 trillion. This is a staggering figure. We have already realized a 15 percent reduction in cancer mortality in the United States. Such a reduction may already have resulted in a $7.5 trillion infusion to the economy in the past two decades, or over 1,000 times the amount of money invested in the War on Cancer.

The application of the knowledge of the molecular and cellular mechanisms of cancer progression will lead to a dramatic decrease in mortality rates. Survival improvements in CML resulting from imatinib (Gleevec) are too recent to be reflected in 1995 to 2000 statistics. However, for research advances to impact cancer incidence and deaths, the translation of the research discoveries to the widespread delivery of preventive and clinical services must be expedited.

It is interesting to note that some economists have been critical of the United States for spending a larger percent of its gross domestic product on health care (11 percent), compared with European countries, which average 7 to 8 percent in expenditure. Given the findings of Funding First, we should consider that the United States may perhaps have inadvertently stumbled on the important fact that a greater expenditure on health research and on health care can serve as a substantial economic stimulus.

Improved Access to Cancer Information by Patients Finally, a transforming and yet not often recognized impetus for cancer research and treatment over the past two decades has been the increasing knowledge of cancer as a disease by cancer patients and their families, due to the explosion of information available on the Internet. When the Physician Data Query (PDQ) was developed by the NCI in 1986, it was intended to be a tool for the use of physicians. No one could have predicted the rapid introduction to and use of the Internet by the general public in the past two decades. The computer revolution has created thousands of educated cancer patients who search out sophisticated cancer information in order to find state-of-the-art treatments for their respective diagnoses.

These educated cancer patients with their families and the increasing legions of long-term cancer survivors can be the secret weapon of support to renew the War on Cancer for the final campaign that may truly transform cancer into the most curable of chronic diseases in the first quarter of this century.

Notes

1. National Cancer Institute. Cancer control objectives for the nation, 1985–2000. *J Natl Cancer Inst Monogr* 1986; 2:3–93.

2. DeVita VT, Abou-Alpha G. Therapeutic implications of the new biology. *The Cancer Journal* 2005;6(supplement 2): S113–20.

3. Devita VT, Serpick AA, Carbone PP. Combination chemotherapy in the treatment of Hodgkin's disease. *Ann Intern Med* 1970;73(6):881–95.

4. Edwards B, Brown M, Wingo P, et al. Annual report to the nation on the status of cancer, 1975–2002, featuring population-based trends in cancer treatment. *J Natl Cancer Inst* 2005;97(19):1407–27.

5. Deisseroth AB, DeVita VT. The cell cycle: Probing new molecular determinants of resistance and sensitivity to cytoxic agents. *Cancer J Sci Am* 1995;1 (May–June):15–21.

6. Druker B, et al. *N Engl J Med* 2001; 344(14):1031–7.

7. Wingo, PA, Ries LA, Rosenberg HM, et al. *Cancer J* 1998;82:1197–207.

8. NCLAC Report Booklet 2001 (*www. cancersource/nclac*).

9. Mary Woodward Lasker Charitable Trust. Exceptional returns: The economic value of america's investment in medical research. *Funding First Monograph* 2000.

— 43 —

Cancer Risk Assessment, Screening, and Prevention

Joanne M. Jeter, M.D., and David S. Alberts, M.D.

■ ■ ■ ■

Nearly everyone will encounter cancer at some time in their lives, either through a personal diagnosis or the diagnosis of a relative or friend. Cancer is a common disease, with about 1.4 million new cases diagnosed each year in the United States alone. In fact, cancer has recently overtaken cardiovascular disease as the leading cause of death for Americans under the age of eighty-five, and it accounts for twice as many deaths as cardiovascular disease in those under sixty-five. Over a half million Americans die of cancer each year. This figure corresponds to more than 1,500 cancer deaths each day, or approximately 1 death per minute. Figure 1 shows the five leading sites of cancer incidence and their corresponding death rates in men and women.

Despite these numbers, there is reason for optimism. Even with increases in the American population, the rate of new cancer cases and deaths for all cancers combined dropped for the first time since record keeping began in the 1930s. Death rates from cancer have decreased each year from 1993 to 2002, the most recent year for which full data is available. Advances in prevention, early detection, and treatment have helped reduce death from cancer. More than 10 million people alive today with a history of cancer can attest to recent successes.

Thousands of scientists, doctors, nurses, patients, volunteers, and others have devoted themselves to conquering cancer. Their efforts have increased survival rates for all cancers combined to over 60 percent. New approaches are vital in reducing cancer incidence and deaths. New procedures are being developed to detect cancers in early and treatable stages. Genetic research and studies of the immune system continue to seek answers to why cancer cells have uncontrolled growth. New drugs attack cancer cells at specific points in their developmental pathway, before the cells become cancerous. These and future advances will one day cure cancer.

More immediate progress against cancer can be made in the areas of prevention and early detection. To achieve these goals, we must recognize that risks can be identified and reduced; tests can detect cancer in its earliest, most treatable stages; and many cancers can be prevented altogether by modifying our lifestyles.

Risk Factors

Risk factors are personal characteristics or events that may affect that person's chance of developing a disease. Lifestyle, environment, and genetic makeup, alone or in combination, help determine cancer risk.

When thinking about cancer, it is sometimes useful to think of a risk factor

Figure 1. **Five Leading Cancer Sites**

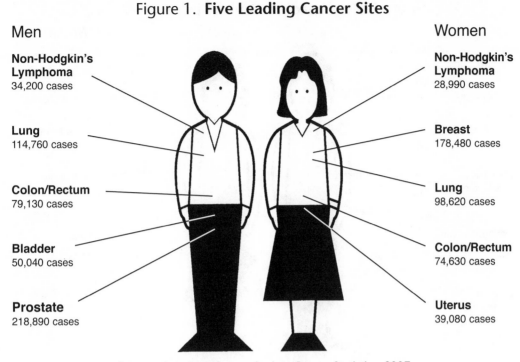

Men

Women

Non-Hodgkin's Lymphoma
34,200 cases

Lung
114,760 cases

Colon/Rectum
79,130 cases

Bladder
50,040 cases

Prostate
218,890 cases

Non-Hodgkin's Lymphoma
28,990 cases

Breast
178,480 cases

Lung
98,620 cases

Colon/Rectum
74,630 cases

Uterus
39,080 cases

Source: American Cancer Society Cancer Statistics, 2007

as something that can cause insults, or "hits," to the genetic structure of a normal cell. These hits cause normal cells to change to cancer cells by interacting with and altering a gene's normal DNA and protein products. Cancer is an accumulation of these alterations, or mutations, that result from multiple events acting together over many years or decades. It is not a one-step, one-hit process.

Certain risk factors have been identified as causing hits that start a normal cell's journey toward becoming a cancer cell. These risk factors hits include tobacco, X-rays, sunlight, industrial chemicals, some types of hormones and drugs, and certain viruses. Other hits promote the cell's continued progression to cancer; alcohol and high-fat diets are associated with these hits. It may take several promoting hits to damage a cell

beyond repair and mutate its DNA. As hits and mutations accumulate, the cell starts to grow uncontrollably, eventually becoming a cancer cell.

On the positive side, the human body does a remarkable job of protecting itself from cancer. Our cells are exposed to potential cancer-causing compounds (carcinogens) every minute of every day. Many of these compounds are by-products of normal body metabolism. The body has several lines of defense against these carcinogens, including mechanisms to protect DNA and to repair any DNA damage that occurs. Additionally, the body can alter the cell's environment to make it more difficult for an already cancerous cell to grow in an uncontrolled fashion.

Risk factors can be classified as modifiable or nonmodifiable. We can do nothing

Figure 2. **Five Leading Cancers by Death Rate**

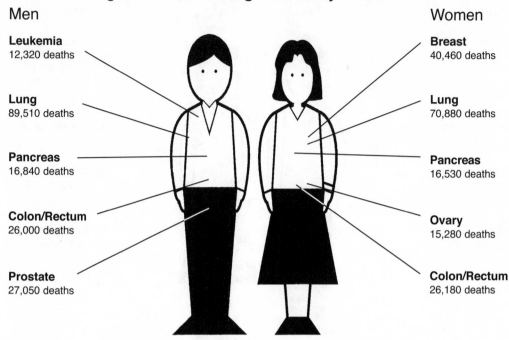

Men

Leukemia
12,320 deaths

Lung
89,510 deaths

Pancreas
16,840 deaths

Colon/Rectum
26,000 deaths

Prostate
27,050 deaths

Women

Breast
40,460 deaths

Lung
70,880 deaths

Pancreas
16,530 deaths

Ovary
15,280 deaths

Colon/Rectum
26,180 deaths

Source: American Cancer Society Cancer Statistics; 2007

about nonmodifiable risk factors, such as our gender, our race, our genes, and the hormones that are naturally produced by our bodies. But modifiable risk factors are risk factors that we can choose to change.

Nonmodifiable Risk Factors

Gender, Ethnicity, and Race Some of the gender differences for cancer are obvious. For example, the risk of breast cancer is approximately 100 times higher in women than in men. However, men are not entirely immune from this disease: Estimates suggest that more than 2,000 men in the United States will develop breast cancer in 2007. Similarly, race and ethnicity can have a significant impact on cancer risk. African-American men, for instance, are more likely to develop prostate cancer and often develop this

cancer at an earlier age than men of other races. Individuals of Ashkenazic-Jewish descent have higher rates of mutations in breast cancer susceptibility genes such as BRCA1 and BRCA2. Many researchers are trying to improve our understanding of cancer risks in different populations so that prevention efforts can be tailored to meet these needs.

Heredity When the same types of cancer appear in a family for generation after generation, a genetic alteration (inherited from the father or the mother) may be the first damaging hit to the DNA that begins the cell's change to cancer. Usually, other hits are required to sustain the cell's progression to a tumor. Approximately 10 percent of all cancers result from hereditary predisposition. Most cancers are not hereditary in nature and result from a complex interaction of genes, environment, and lifestyle.

Hormones Produced by the Body One of the most important risk factors for developing breast cancer is a woman's lifelong exposure to naturally occurring hormones. The longer a woman produces hormones, the more likely she is to develop breast cancer. Factors such as early menstruation (before age twelve) and late menopause (after age fifty-five) contribute to prolonged hormone exposure. The number of ovulatory cycles in a woman's lifetime can also affect her risk of cancer. Women who have an increased number of uninterrupted ovulations have been shown to be more likely to develop ovarian cancer. This phenomenon may explain why events that interrupt ovulatory cycles, such as pregnancy, breast-feeding, and oral contraceptive use, are associated with a decreased risk of ovarian cancer.

Modifiable Risk Factors

Tobacco It is estimated that there are approximately 45 million current smokers and more than 46 million former smokers in the United States. All of these people are at increased risk for developing cancer. Tobacco use is the single most preventable cause of death in the United States. Cigarette smoking is directly responsible for at least 30 percent of all cancer deaths each year. Smoking also causes chronic lung disease, heart disease, stroke, and vascular disease.

More than 3,000 chemicals are present in tobacco smoke, including at least 60 known carcinogens. Some of these chemicals become carcinogenic only after they are activated by specific enzymes (proteins that control chemical reactions) found in many tissues in the body. These activated compounds can then mutate DNA and interfere with the normal growth of cells. Tobacco also contains nicotine, a chemical that causes physical addiction to smoking. During smoking, nicotine is absorbed quickly into the bloodstream and travels to the brain, causing the addictive effect.

Since the release in 1964 of the first surgeon general's report on smoking and health, the scientific knowledge about the health consequences of tobacco use has greatly increased. It is now well documented that cancers of the lung, larynx, esophagus, mouth, and bladder are caused by smoking. Cigarette smoking is the most important risk factor for lung cancer, accounting for 68 to 78 percent of lung cancer deaths among females and 88 to 91 percent of lung cancer deaths among males. Additionally, smoking is known to contribute to cancer of the colon, stomach, cervix, pancreas, and kidneys.

Many people are under the impression that cigars and smokeless tobacco are safer alternatives to cigarettes. Considerable evidence shows that smokeless tobacco and cigars also have deadly consequences, including lung, larynx, esophageal, and oral cancers. Smokeless tobacco—chewing tobacco and dipping snuff—contains at least twenty-eight carcinogens. Habitual use of these products threatens the lives of several million Americans.

Children, too, are not spared addiction to tobacco. About 3 million adolescents report smoking at least once in the last month; 1.1 million report daily smoking. Nearly 4,000 young people begin smoking each day, and over 6 million people who decided to begin smoking as children will die early, preventable deaths. Clove cigarettes and flavored cigarettes are ideal "training cigarettes" for people in this age group; however, rather than being safer alternatives to regular cigarettes, these products are often unfiltered and have the same or greater health risks.

The risk of developing lung cancer, as well as other smoking-associated diseases, depends on an individual's total lifetime exposure to cigarette smoke. Such exposure is measured by the number of cigarettes a person smokes each day, the age at which smoking began, and the number of years a person has smoked. For example, in those who smoke forty or more cigarettes a day (two or more packs), the risk of death from lung cancer is more than twenty times the risk in nonsmokers.

The harmful effects of smoking do not end with the smoker. Each year, exposure to secondhand smoke, also known as environmental tobacco smoke (ETS), causes an estimated 3,400 nonsmoking Americans to die of lung cancer. ETS has also been significantly linked with nasal sinus cancer in nonsmoking adults. The surgeon general has recently issued a report that states that there is no safe level of secondhand smoke.

Quitting smoking is a critical step toward improving health. Methods and resources that can aid in quitting can be found in "How Can You Reduce Cancer Risk?" in this chapter.

Diet and Nutrition Scientific studies suggest that about 30 percent of all cancer deaths are associated with poor dietary and nutrition practices. Specific risk factors include certain types of foods; methods of cooking, processing, and storage; and excessive caloric intake of food.

Substantial evidence shows that fats and alcohol are two dietary components that, when used imprudently, can increase cancer risk. Excessive dietary fats appear to play a role in the development of cancers at multiple different sites, including the breast, pancreas, endometrium (uterus), esophagus, and colon. Although saturated fats (derived mainly from animal sources) were considered the primary culprit in the past, both saturated fats and unsaturated fats have been associated with increased cancer incidence. Similarly, overuse of alcohol has been shown to contribute to breast,

colorectal, head and neck, esophagus, and liver cancers. Risk increases with the amount of alcohol consumed and may start to rise with as few as two drinks per day. Many of the by-products of alcohol are recognized carcinogens.

Just as foods are a source for potentially dangerous carcinogens, so diet plays a role in protecting us from cancer. Populations that consume large amounts of plant-derived foods have decreased incidence of certain types of cancers, including those of the esophagus, mouth, stomach, colon, rectum, lung, and prostate. Fiber, fruit, and vegetable intake have been studied to determine their effects on colon cancer risk. Clinical trials that emphasized intake of these foods did not show a decreased rate of recurrence for colon polyps, which are considered precursor lesions for colon cancer. However, these results may be due to following the special diets for too short a time to have an effect. Intake of fiber, fruits, and vegetables is still strongly encouraged due to the other health benefits from these foods. Some of the main results from these studies are summarized in Table 1.

Levels of micronutrients may also play a role in determining cancer risk. People with higher levels of the micronutrient selenium have been found to have fewer deaths from lung, colorectal, and prostate cancers. Large studies are currently taking place to determine if selenium supplements can prevent these cancers from occurring.

Studies have shown that daily consumption of red meat may double the risk of colon cancer. One explanation for this finding may be the methods used to cook or prepare the meat. Processed meats that are salt-cured, salt-pickled, or smoked have been associated with increased risk of gastric cancer, whereas meats that have been broiled or grilled at high temperatures have been shown to have increased levels of carcinogens that can increase colon cancer risk.

Table 1. Selected Large Dietary Intervention Trials for Cancer Prevention

STUDY NAME	PREVENTION TARGET	TARGETED CHANGE	RESULT ACHIEVED	MAJOR RESULT	COMMENT
Women's Health Initiative	Breast cancer	20% dietary fat	29% dietary fat	9% reduction in breast cancer risk (nonsignificant)	Participants did not achieve the low-fat goal; may not have had long enough follow-up period to detect a difference.
Women's Health Initiative	Colon cancer	20% dietary fat	29% dietary fat	8% reduction in colon cancer risk (nonsignificant); mild reduction in colon polyps	Participants did not achieve the low-fat goal; may not have had long enough follow-up period to detect a difference.
Women's Intervention Nutrition Study	Recurrence of breast cancer	15% dietary fat	20% dietary fat	24% reduction in risk of breast cancer recurrence	May be useful for women with tumors that are negative for estrogen receptors.
Wheat Bran Fiber Study	Recurrence of colon adenoma	13.5 g fiber per day	10 g fiber per day	No difference in risk of recurrence; trend toward reduction of risk in men	May not have had a long enough follow-up period to detect a difference.
Polyp-Prevention Trial	Recurrence of colon adenoma	20% dietary fat, 18 g fiber	24% dietary fat, 17.4 g fiber	4% reduction with dietary changes (nonsignificant); trend toward reduction in men	May not have had a long enough follow-up period to detect a difference.

Other nutrition-related factors such as obesity and physical activity are part of the complex interaction of lifestyle choices that affect cancer risk. Regular physical activity seems to protect against cancer in the breast and colon, reducing risk by as much as 50 percent. Obesity has the opposite effect, increasing levels of hormones and other substances that encourage continued growth of cancer cells. For example, large fat deposits may be responsible for converting estrogen precursors to high levels of circulating estrogens. Unfortunately, current trends show that Americans are increasing their caloric intake, eating more high-fat convenience foods, and being less physically active. These trends may be related to more frequent meals away from home, sedentary lifestyle patterns, and increased media promotion of high-calorie foods.

Exposure to Sunlight Nonmelanoma skin cancer is the most common malignancy in the United States, representing 40 percent of all cancers. During the past thirty years, all types of skin cancers—melanoma, basal cell carcinoma, and squamous cell carcinoma—have increased dramatically. These skin cancers are caused primarily by overexposure to the sun's ultraviolet rays.

Solar rays can damage skin even on cloudy days. With the continued thinning of the protective ozone layer, damaging rays are becoming more intense and dangerous. Over the short term, excessive sun exposure causes freckling, sunburn, and tanning, all of which are forms of skin damage. Rather than being a sign of good health, a tan signals the skin's attempt to defend itself against solar radiation. Over longer periods of time, high levels of sun exposure can cause premature skin aging, wrinkles, and rough leathery skin, in addition to skin cancers.

Research findings suggest that intermittent intense sun exposure may increase the risk of malignant melanoma, the deadliest form of skin cancer. A history of five or more blistering sunburns can double the risk of melanoma. Because we accumulate much of our lifetime exposure to the sun prior to age eighteen, it is especially important to protect infants and children from sun overexposure.

Artificial sources of sunlight, including sunlamps and tanning booths, also increase the risk of developing skin cancer. Unfortunately, skin damage from any form of ultraviolet light is permanent and accumulates over a lifetime; however, it can be minimized by limiting sun exposure.

Geographic Patterns and Environmental Exposure The geographic patterns of cancer may provide important clues to the causes of cancer. Possible geographic risk factors include occupational exposures, regional dietary habits, ethnic background, and environmental exposures from the air or water. Additionally, geographic differences in mortality rates may reflect differences in access to medical care, such as screening, diagnosis, and treatment facilities.

Workplace exposure to chemicals such as coal-tar-based products, benzene, cadmium, uranium, asbestos, and nickel can greatly increase the risk of developing cancer. Up to 20 percent of bladder cancers may be due to chemical exposures in the aluminum, dye, paint, petroleum, rubber, and textile industries. Occupational exposures to radon and asbestos have been linked to lung cancer, and 1 to 2 percent of lung cancer deaths are attributable to air pollution.

Fertility Drugs and Oral Contraceptives Use of fertility drugs has been associated with an increased risk of ovarian cancer in some studies. However, infertility itself also increases ovarian cancer risk, thereby making it difficult to assess the independent risk associated with fertility drugs. The duration of use for some fertility drugs is restricted in order to prevent additional increases in ovarian cancer risk. Endometrial cancer is also increased in women who take fertility drugs, although separating the effect of the drugs from that of the infertility can be difficult in this case as well. Fertility drugs are not thought to increase the risk of breast cancer, cervical cancer, or colon cancer, although information in this area is somewhat limited.

The relationship between oral contraceptives and cancer risk has been controversial. Studies investigating the role of oral contraceptives on breast cancer risk have had conflicting results, but the majority of the evidence suggests that there is no increased risk of breast cancer in users of oral contraceptives. Ovarian cancer risk is decreased in oral contraceptive users in the general population, but the results are unclear for those who have an increased risk of ovarian cancer due to genetic susceptibility. Use of these medications has been shown to decrease the risk of endometrial cancer as well.

Hormone Replacement Therapy (HRT)
For years, hormone replacement therapy, consisting of estrogen alone or in combination with progesterone, has been an option for women when they reach menopause. Potential benefits of hormone replacement therapy in postmenopausal women include protection of the bones from osteoporosis (bone thinning) and relief from menopausal symptoms such as hot flashes, vaginal dryness, insomnia, and mood changes. HRT was thought to have beneficial effects against heart disease as well; however, more recent evidence now indicates that heart disease is not decreased with the use of these medications.

Initially, hormone replacement therapy was the only tool that was available to treat these conditions. In recent years,

newer drugs such as raloxifene (Evista) and alendronate (Fosamax) have become available to reduce the risk of fracture in those suffering from osteoporosis. These drugs are from a different class of medication than hormone replacement therapy and protect the bones in a different way. Nonhormonal therapies are also available to improve symptoms of hot flashes, insomnia, and mood changes.

Hormone replacement with estrogen alone has been shown to increase the risk of endometrial (uterus) cancer in women who have not had a hysterectomy. In the 1970s, women who received estrogen without progesterone were six to eight times more likely to develop endometrial cancer than women who were not on this medication. Since that time, doctors have prescribed HRT that includes low-dose estrogen and progesterone for women who have not had a hysterectomy. Progesterone counteracts estrogen's negative effect on the uterus by preventing the overgrowth of the endometrial lining, thereby reducing the risk of endometrial cancer associated with taking estrogen alone. However, the addition of progesterone to estrogen replacement therapy dramatically increases the risk of breast cancer, as discussed below. A woman who has had a hysterectomy does not need progesterone and can receive HRT with estrogen alone.

Over the past thirty years, considerable research has examined the question of whether HRT affects breast cancer risk. The research falls into two categories: observational studies, which investigate differences in cancer rates in women who are already taking HRT as compared to those who are not; and clinical trials, which randomly assign women to use HRT or to use a placebo. Because observational studies may not account for all of the differences between women who use HRT and women who do not, clinical trials are considered to provide the strongest evidence.

Some of the early studies indicated that women who used high doses of estrogen alone had an increased incidence of breast cancer. More recently, analysis of data from the Nurses' Health Study, an important large observational study comparing women who take hormone replacement therapy with those who do not, showed that prolonged use of estrogen increased the risk of breast cancer. After fifteen years of estrogen replacement, women had a 48 percent increased risk of hormone-sensitive breast cancer. After twenty years of replacement, there was a 42 percent increased risk in all types of breast cancer.

Other studies have shown that progesterone replacement may significantly increase the risk of breast cancer. One of the most important clinical trials in this area, the Women's Health Initiative, was designed to test the effects of hormone replacement therapy on heart disease, breast cancer, and colorectal cancer risks. Over 26,000 postmenopausal women were enrolled in 1991 and randomly assigned to hormone replacement or placebo. Women who had previously undergone hysterectomy were given estrogen alone or a placebo, and women who still had a uterus were given an estrogen-progesterone combination or a placebo. Results from this study showed that the combination of estrogen and progesterone was associated with an increased risk of breast cancer and a decreased risk of colorectal cancer. The women who took estrogen only did not have a decreased risk of colorectal cancer, and the effect on breast cancer risk was uncertain.

Combination HRT with estrogen and progestin has been shown to increase breast density, as seen on mammograms. Studies have shown that women ages forty-five and older whose mammograms show at least 75 percent dense tissue are at increased risk for breast cancer. Increased breast density makes it more difficult to interpret mammograms; and follow-up procedures must sometimes be done, including mammograms, ultrasounds, and biopsies. The Women's Health Initiative found that women who took estrogen alone also required increased numbers of mammograms.

Use of hormone replacement therapy in women who have a history of breast cancer or endometrial cancer remains controversial. At present, the standard of care is to use medications other than hormone replacement to treat menopausal symptoms and prevent osteoporosis in these women. Only in the most extreme situation of uncontrolled, severe hot flashes should estrogen replacement therapy be considered in this setting.

Sexual Activity Cervical cancer is caused by infection with a sexually transmitted virus called the human papillomavirus (HPV). Although most women are exposed to this virus in their lifetime, infection is usually transient. When this virus cannot be cleared by the body, cervical cancer may develop. Individuals who have multiple sexual partners or have a compromised immune system are more susceptible to the virus for this reason. HPV is also thought to play a role in cancers of the penis, vagina, and anus.

Risk Assessment

Just by virtue of becoming older, we all develop some risk for cancer. However, some people may be at even greater risk because of their combinations of modifiable and nonmodifiable risk factors. Individuals with a cancer risk that is three to five times that of the general population are considered at high risk. To identify people at high risk for cancer, risk assessment programs have been developed at many cancer centers. To enter a program, the participant completes a questionnaire that asks detailed questions about life history, personal and family medical history, work history, and lifestyle habits. A physical examination, blood work, and imaging studies may be part of the assessment as well. The questionnaire responses are analyzed to produce cancer risk scores, which are then interpreted. Participants receive results of the assessment, along with risk-reduction recommendations. These results are often forwarded to the participant's primary care provider as well.

Some risk assessment questionnaires focus on specific types of cancer and ask specific questions to determine how well an individual fits in a specific model of cancer risk. One of the best-known models is the Gail model, which predicts breast cancer risk based on race, current age, age when menstruation began, age of first live birth, number of close relatives with breast cancer, number of breast biopsies, and the presence or absence of changes called atypical hyperplasia on breast biopsies. Most of these models have limitations (for example, the Gail model does not ask about ovarian cancer history or breast cancer history in second-degree relatives such as aunts, cousins, or grandparents; it may also be less accurate in predicting risk in non-Caucasian women). Therefore, models should be selected based on each individual's situation in order to calculate risk as accurately as possible.

Several cancer risk assessment programs are available off the Internet. These programs may be less comprehensive than those available from cancer centers. Additionally, these programs cannot always answer questions you may have or individualize recommendations to your particular case. When using on-line programs, be sure to verify recommendations with your health care provider.

Hereditary Risk All cancers have a genetic component; the hallmark of all cancers is genetic instability. Although most cancers are sporadic (not inherited), about 10 percent occur because of hereditary predisposition. All men and women are born with cancer susceptibility genes, such as the breast cancer susceptibility genes BRCA1 and BRCA2. However, only people with alterations in cancer susceptibility genes are at higher genetic predisposition for cancer. Table 2 summarizes established risk factors for hereditary cancers and syndromes. Figure 3 illustrates a family pattern of breast cancer that is consistent with an inherited genetic predisposition.

Genetic alterations associated with inherited predisposition to cancer can be identified through analysis of a blood or tissue sample. At this time, genetic testing is recommended only for individuals who have a personal or family history suggestive of an inherited cancer syndrome. The most effective way to determine if a heritable genetic alteration is in a family is by testing the individual who has had the cancer that fits the hereditary pattern. If a genetic alteration is identified in the individual who has had cancer, other individuals in the family who are at risk can be tested for the mutation identified in their family member. Genetic analysis should always be preceded by careful genetic counseling, which continues after determining gene mutation status. Identification of a genetic alteration may change recommendations for cancer screening, and chemoprevention medications or surgery options may be appropriate for these individuals.

Some genetic testing kits have become directly available to consumers. However, the implications of finding or not finding a genetic mutation can be profound. We do not recommend undertaking such testing without appropriate counseling from a professional with training and expertise in this area.

Screening and Early-Detection Guidelines

Despite all the advances in cancer treatment, the approach most likely to

Table 2. Established Risk Factors for Hereditary Cancers and Cancer Syndromes

- Two or more first-degree relatives (parent, child, or siblings) with a specific cancer or cancers. These individuals can be on the mother's and/or father's side of the family.

- One first-degree and two or more second-degree relatives (grandparents, aunts, uncles, grandchildren) with a specific cancer or cancers.

- Evidence of transmission of cancer from generation to generation.

- Unusually early age of cancer onset.

- Clustering of the same types of cancers in close relatives.

- Family members with cancer in paired organs (both breasts, both kidneys, both eyes).

- Geographical heritage and ethnicity.

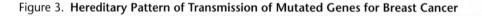

Figure 3. Hereditary Pattern of Transmission of Mutated Genes for Breast Cancer

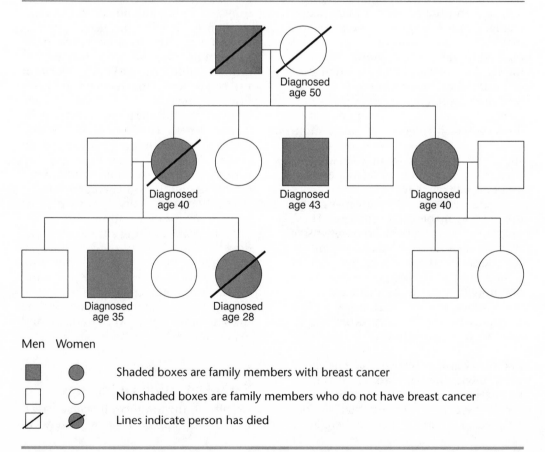

decrease cancer deaths is early detection. Catching cancer at its earliest stages can prevent spread to distant sites, which is the cause of most cancer deaths. Early detection depends on recognizing cancer's warning signals and receiving prompt medical attention when signs and symptoms appear. The cornerstones of early detection are self-examination, examination by a health professional, and screening tests.

Self-Examination Breast self-examination was previously recommended for all women by the American Cancer Society. The most recent recommendations state that the risks and benefits of self-examination should be discussed with women, and that performing self-examinations infrequently or not at all is acceptable. This recommendation has been changed due to research that demonstrated no decrease in breast cancer deaths in women who performed breast self-examinations compared to women who did not. However, many clinicians still recommend breast self-examination because it promotes awareness of the breast, helps find breast changes early on, and has no cost. Women who perform this examination should be trained by a health professional.

Likewise, testicular self-examination is not formally recommended by the American Cancer Society. However, it also promotes awareness, helps find changes early on, and has no cost. Although testicular cancer is uncommon overall, it is one of the most common cancers in men ages twenty to thirty-five. Testicular cancer is highly curable when detected early.

Skin self-examination is another important component of health that is often overlooked. Men and women are encouraged to become familiar with their skin, including any freckles or moles. A mole that is asymmetric, has an irregular border, is more than one color, or is larger than the size of a pencil eraser should be evaluated by a dermatologist. In addition, any new skin lesions or changes in an existing mole or freckle should also be reported right away.

Clinical Examinations and Screening Tests Screening guidelines for any type of cancer depend on two primary factors: the age of the individual undergoing screening, and the individual's risk factor profile. Risk factors can be due to lifestyle, family history, or other medical conditions. Table 3 summarizes the American Cancer Society recommendations for cancer screening for individuals at average risk of cancer. In the discussion below we will highlight some of the details behind the screening recommendations and note where controversies currently exist.

General Screening Regular health examinations should include inspection of the skin, mouth, lymph nodes, thyroid, testes, and ovaries for cancers and precancerous areas.

Breast Cancer Screening The American Cancer Society (ACS) recommends regular breast examinations by a clinician and mammography to detect breast cancer at early stages for women at average risk of this disease. For women between twenty and thirty-nine years old, examination should occur at least once every three years; for women over forty, clinical breast examination should take place annually.

Studies have shown that mammography, done on a regular basis, can decrease the number of deaths from breast cancer by as much as 30 percent. The ACS recommends that annual mammography should start at the age of forty for women at average risk. Although the appropriate starting age for mammography has been controversial in the past, more recent research has indicated that the benefit

Table 3. American Cancer Society Recommendations for the Early Detection of Cancer in Average-Risk Asymptomatic People

PROCEDURE	POPULATION	FREQUENCY
Breast self-examination	Women ages 20 and over	Every month*
Clinical breast examination	Women ages 20–39 Women ages 40 and over	Every 3 years Every year (to be done prior to mammogram)
Mammography	Women ages 40 and over	Every year
Pap smear	Women ages 18–30**	Every year (conventional Pap test) Every 2 years (liquid-based Pap test)
	Women ages 30 and over	If last 3 tests were normal: • Pap test every 2–3 years (either type) OR • Pap test + HPV (human papillomavirus) testing every 3 years If one or more of last 3 tests were not normal, follow guidelines for ages 18–30.
	Women who have had total hysterectomy	May choose to stop screening
	Women ages 70 and over	May choose to stop screening if 3 normal Pap tests and no abnormal tests in 10 years

(continues)

Table 3. American Cancer Society Recommendations for the Early Detection of Cancer in Average-Risk Asymptomatic People (continued)

PROCEDURE	POPULATION	FREQUENCY
Prostate-specific antigen (PSA) blood test and digital rectal examination	Men ages 50 and over with life expectancy of at least 10 years	Every year***
Colorectal cancer screening (any of the following procedures):	Men and women ages 50 and over	
• Fecal occult blood test**** or fecal immunochemical test, OR		
• Flexible sigmoidoscopy, OR		Every 5 years, starting at age 50
• Fecal occult blood test and flexible sigmoidoscopy, OR		Fecal occult blood testing every year with sigmoidoscopy every 5 years starting at age 50
• Double contrast barium enema, OR		Every 5 years, starting at age 50
• Colonoscopy		Every 10 years, starting at age 50

* Women should be informed of the benefits and limitations of breast self-examination (BSE). It is considered acceptable for women to choose not to do BSE or to perform BSE irregularly.

** Cervical cancer screening with the Pap smear should begin three years after starting vaginal intercourse but no later than twenty-one years of age.

*** Men should be informed of the benefits and limitations of PSA testing so that an informed decision can be made with the clinician.

**** Samples should be obtained at home from three consecutive specimens. A single sample obtained during digital rectal examination by a clinician is not adequate.

Source: American Cancer Society Guidelines for the Early Detection of Cancer, 2006

of mammography also applies to women between forty and fifty.

Use of digital mammography rather than film mammography may be beneficial for women who are under fifty, have dense breast tissue, or are premenopausal or perimenopausal. Increasing numbers of mammography units across the United States are adopting this technology. However, it is important to emphasize that no woman should defer screening with a mammogram due to a lack of access to digital mammography.

Several groups of women are considered to be at increased risk for breast cancer. Individuals with a history of radiation therapy to the chest, a strong family history of breast and/or ovarian cancer, or a known or suspected genetic predisposition to breast cancer are more likely to develop breast cancer than women in the general population. In addition, women with a personal history of breast cancer or breast lesions such as lobular carcinoma in situ (LCIS) and atypical hyperplasia also have a risk of having a second breast abnormality, which may be cancerous. Individuals in these groups may need to start breast cancer screening earlier, to have clinical breast examinations more often, or to have different screening procedures than women in the general population. In most cases, high-risk women should start screening when they are ten years younger than the age of diagnosis for their youngest relative with breast or ovarian cancer. Individuals who have a known genetic predisposition may require screening even earlier. These individuals may also be candidates for prophylactic surgery or chemoprevention to reduce their risk.

One newer screening procedure for breast cancer is breast magnetic resonance imaging (MRI). The primary use of breast MRI at this time is to assess women with a known genetic predisposition for breast cancer. Screening of these individuals must often start at a younger age, when the breasts are denser and harder to evaluate with mammography. Currently, breast MRI is not recommended for screening in the general population.

Cervical Cancer Screening Invasive cervical cancer is often preceded by precancerous changes in cervical tissue that can be identified with a Papanicolaou (Pap) smear. Screening for cervical cancer has been shown to reduce the number of deaths from this cancer. The ACS recommends that screening should start three years after a women starts having intercourse, or no later than age twenty-one. There are two types of Pap smears in current use, the conventional Pap smear and the liquid-based Pap smear. The conventional Pap smear should be performed on an annual basis, and the liquid-based Pap smear may be performed every two years. Once a woman has reached the age of thirty, less frequent screening can be considered if her last three Pap tests were normal. The Pap smear can be used alone or in combination with testing for human papillomavirus (HPV), the virus that causes cervical cancer. After the age of seventy, a woman may also consider stopping screening if she has recently had three consecutive negative Pap smears.

Women who have had a total hysterectomy for a noncancerous reason do not need to continue having Pap smears. However, if a woman has had a subtotal hysterectomy or has a history of cervical cancer or precancerous conditions, she should continue to have regular screening even after surgery.

Women who have a history of exposure to DES (diethylstilbestrol) are at increased risk of cervical and vaginal cancers. Continued screening with a Pap smear after hysterectomy is still recommended in this high-risk group. Other women who are at increased risk of cervical cancer include those who are immunocompromised due to organ transplant, chronic steroid use, chemotherapy, or infection with the human immunodeficiency virus (HIV). These individuals may require more frequent screening and do not have a designated age at which screening should stop.

Colon Cancer Screening Multiple procedures are currently in use for screening for colorectal cancer. For individuals at average risk for colon cancer, screening should start at age fifty. The ACS recommends any of the following options:

• Fecal occult blood test (FOBT) or fecal immunochemical testing (FIT) every year.
• Flexible sigmoidoscopy every five years.
• FOBT every year with flexible sigmoidoscopy every five years.
• Double-contrast barium enema every five years.
• Colonoscopy every ten years.

The option of combined FOBT with flexible sigmoidoscopy is preferred to either option alone. However, no one measure is preferred by the ACS for individuals at average risk of colon cancer. The National Comprehensive Cancer Network (NCCN) guidelines state that their preferred recommendation is colonoscopy, and that the barium enema is the least preferred option. The NCCN guidelines do not recommend use of FOBT or flexible sigmoidoscopy alone.

Individuals who choose to use FOBT for screening should perform at-home testing of three consecutive stool specimens. An FOBT of stool obtained during a rectal examination by a clinician is not considered sufficient for screening purposes. Also, dietary restrictions must be followed in order for this test to be interpreted accurately.

Fecal immunochemical tests (FIT) are also known as immunologic fecal occult blood tests or immunoassay fecal occult blood tests. Like the FOBT, this test assesses stool for the presence of a blood protein; however, it may be more accurate in determining if stool blood is present from the bowel rather than from another site higher in the gastrointestinal tract. The ACS has included this test as part of their screening recommendations, but the NCCN guidelines consider it an approach that is still under investigation at this time.

Other methods for screening the colon are under development. "Virtual colonoscopy," also known as computed tomography (CT) colonography, uses a CT scan to evaluate the colon for polyps or cancer. Like conventional colonoscopy, this test requires preparation of the bowel with a laxative regimen, and air is inserted in the bowel in order to improve viewing during the procedure. If polyps are found on this test, conventional colonoscopy is done to remove them. Another screening alternative currently under study involves testing of the stool for DNA changes associated with colon adenomas and cancers. Cells from the lining of the bowel are routinely sloughed off into the stool, and several different panels of genetic mutations have been proposed to look for cancer and precancerous changes in these cells. At this time, additional study is needed before these techniques can be used routinely for screening purposes in the general population.

Individuals who are considered to be at higher risk for colon cancer include those with inflammatory bowel disease, those who have previously had a colon cancer, and those who have had a type of colon polyp called an adenoma. Women who have had uterine or ovarian cancer prior to the age of sixty are also considered to be at increased risk for colon cancer. These individuals require earlier and more frequent colon screening, which should be done by colonoscopy.

Colonoscopy is also recommended for individuals who have a family history of colon cancer or a family history that suggests a genetic predisposition to colon cancer. The age to start screening depends on the age of the youngest individual in the family who has had colon cancer. In most cases, high-risk individuals should start screening when they are ten years younger than the age of diagnosis for their youngest relative with colon cancer or a related cancer.

Endometrial Cancer Screening At this time, the American Cancer Society does not recommend screening for endometrial cancer for women at average risk. The guidelines do suggest that all women should be informed of the symptoms of endometrial cancer and should report any unexpected vaginal bleeding to their health care provider promptly.

Women at high risk of endometrial cancer due to a possible genetic predisposition based on a strong family history may be recommended to have screening with transvaginal ultrasound and/or endometrial biopsy. However, these procedures are not recommended for screening women who are at average risk.

Lung Cancer Screening Screening for lung cancer is not currently recommended for individuals without symptoms, regardless of smoking history. However, studies are being conducted to determine if screening can decrease the number of deaths from this disease. The Prostate, Lung, Colorectal, and Ovarian (PLCO) Cancer Screening Trial is a 160,000-person study investigating whether chest X-rays can be used as a screening tool for smokers and non-smokers. Spiral computed tomography (CT) scanning is another new tool that is being assessed for early detection of lung cancer in smokers. Nearly 50,000 current and former smokers have been enrolled in the National Lung Cancer Screening Trial, which is evaluating chest X-rays and CT scans as screening strategies.

Ovarian Cancer Screening Currently, screening for ovarian cancer is not recommended in the general population. Tests that have been proposed for screening include transvaginal ultrasound and a blood test called CA-125. These tests are not in use in the general population at this time because they can be abnormal when no cancer is present, and they can be normal even in the setting of cancer. The high rate of false positive results may lead to unnecessary surgical procedures, particularly in women under fifty years of age. Transvaginal ultrasound and CA-125 are currently being evaluated as screening measures for the general population in the Prostate, Lung, Colorectal, and Ovarian (PLCO) Cancer Screening Trial.

Women who have a strong family history of breast or ovarian cancer are considered to be at increased risk of ovarian cancer. Screening with transvaginal ultrasound and CA-125 can be considered in these women, but the limitations of these tests should be discussed with a clinician before starting screening.

Prostate Cancer Screening Screening for prostate cancer remains a topic of considerable controversy. The American Cancer Society recommends that prostate cancer screening should be discussed with men ages fifty and over. Screening for prostate cancer consists of an examination of the prostate through the rectum and testing the blood for levels of prostate-specific antigen, or PSA. These tests should be performed on an annual basis for men who choose screening. However, men should also be informed of the limitations of PSA testing, since levels of the PSA protein can be elevated in conditions other than cancer and may be normal in the setting of cancer. Overall, about one-third of men with an elevated PSA level are found to have prostate cancer on biopsy.

Some groups have advocated starting screening with PSA testing in men at the age of forty and at average risk for prostate cancer. Men with a normal test at age forty would have the test repeated at age forty-five, and would start annual screening at age fifty. This approach is not universally accepted in average-risk men at the current time.

Two types of PSA tests exist, the complexed PSA and the total PSA. Either may be used, but it is important that the same test be used over time. Another test that can be helpful in assessing for prostate cancer is the PSA velocity, which is the average increase in PSA level in three measurements over eighteen months. Other forms of PSA testing are also in development but are not in current widespread clinical use.

Men who are considered at high risk for prostate cancer include African-Americans and those with a family history of prostate cancer. The ACS recommends starting screening at age forty-five in those of African-American descent and in those who have one close relative with a history of prostate cancer before the age of sixty-five. If an individual has more than one close relative with prostate cancer at an early age, screening should begin at age forty.

Preventing Cancer Through Lifestyle Choices and Clinical Trials

Studies are confirming what scientists, doctors, and many others have suspected for years—lifestyle does make a difference in our risk for developing cancer. As much as 60 percent of cancers may be the direct results of the lifestyle choices we make. Although many people have become more aware of cancer risk factors, many still resist changing their health habits. The success we can have in the fight against cancer hinges on two things that are within our power:

- increasing our understanding of the causes of cancer and cancer risk factors, and

- being willing to act upon that information to allow early detection of cancer and to implement lifestyle changes that reduce our chances of developing cancer.

Successful prevention and early detection require that we assume greater responsibility for our health. We also must work in partnership with health care professionals to make personal choices and risk-reducing decisions.

How Can You Reduce Cancer Risk?

Don't Smoke Smoking cessation is the single most important change you can make to improve your health. Nicotine is an addiction, perhaps the most deadly form of drug dependence, and it is a difficult habit to break. But quitting is possible, as over 46 million ex-smokers in the United States can confirm.

Quitting smoking reduces risk for heart disease and cancer and lengthens life. For former smokers who have quit for ten years, the risk of lung cancer is half that of current smokers. This risk falls to as low as 10 percent for ex-smokers who have quit for thirty years or more. The risk for cancers of the mouth, throat, and esophagus lessens significantly five years after quitting, and the risk of developing bladder or cervical cancer also decreases after just a few years of being nicotine-free.

Individual plans and group support programs can increase the success rate in the attempt to stop smoking. Many health care providers offer practical counseling, including problem-solving and skills training, social support as part of treatment, and social support outside of treatment. The National Cancer Institute (NCI) conducts research on smoking cessation and works with other government agencies and non-profit organizations to promote programs that reduce the rates of illness and death associated with smoking. Several NCI and American Cancer Society (ACS) publications provide tips on smoking cessation and dealing with secondhand smoke at work or in public places. These materials are available from the NCI-supported Cancer Information Service (CIS) at

800-4-CANCER (800-422-6237)
TTY (for deaf and hard-of-hearing callers): 800-332-8615
http://cis.nci.nih.gov

Another important resource is the National Network of Tobacco Cessation Quitlines, which can be reached at 800-QUITNOW (800-784-8669). This number will automatically route you to the quitline for your state or to the quitline for the National Cancer Institute if your state does not have a quitline.

Medications can also be used in combination with support and counseling. Nicotine replacement products deliver small, steady doses of nicotine into the body, which help to relieve nicotine withdrawal symptoms. These replacement products are available in a variety of forms, including patches, gum, nasal sprays, and inhalers. Bupropion (Zyban), a prescription drug approved by the FDA in 1997 to treat nicotine addiction, helps Wellbutrin to reduce nicotine withdrawal symptoms and the urge to smoke. This medication is generally well tolerated but should not be used by people with seizure conditions or eating disorders. Another newly approved medication for smoking cessation is Chantix, also known as varenicline tartiate. In addition to preventing cravings, this medication blocks the nicotine receptors in the brain to diminish satisfaction from nicotine. Your physician can help you determine if these medications are appropriate for you.

Finally, it's important not to become discouraged if your first attempt at quitting is not successful. Most people try to quit smoking five to seven times before they can eliminate nicotine from their lives. Consider each attempt a learning experience that will build toward success in a future attempt, and don't give up!

Watch Your Diet No diet is guaranteed to prevent cancer, but a diet low in fat with a wide variety of fruits, vegetables, and whole-grain products may reduce cancer risk. Table 1 lists the results of some major dietary studies in cancer prevention, and Table 4 summarizes cancer-risk-reducing dietary guidelines issued by the ACS and the American Institute for Cancer Research. Other dietary suggestions include using herbs and spices to season foods and limiting the consumption of salted foods and table salt, not eating food that has not been appropriately refrigerated, and not eating charred food. Studies from the NCI have documented that microwaving meats for two minutes and discarding the juices prior to cooking reduces the potential carcinogen content of these foods by as much as 90 percent. For people who follow the recommended dietary guidelines, supplements are not currently recommended for reducing cancer risk.

Exercise Regularly Increased physical activity helps maintain an ideal weight and prevent obesity, a cancer risk factor. Weight control can reduce excess hormone production that may promote cancer growth. Exercise may also reduce the production of tumor-promoting prostaglandins, boost the body's natural defenses, and strengthen the immune system to protect against cancer.

The American Cancer Society recommends that adults should engage in moderate exercise for at least thirty minutes a day, five or more days per week. Increasing the length of exercise to forty-five minutes or more may provide additional protection against breast and colon cancers. Children are recommended to exercise for at least sixty minutes per day for at least five days per week.

Ways to increase physical activity in daily life include using stairs instead of elevators, parking far away from your destination, and walking or riding a bike to work. Moderate exercise, such as brisk

Table 4. Dietary Guidelines for Reducing Cancer Risk

- Eat a variety of healthful foods, with an emphasis on plant sources.
  - Eat 5 or more servings of a variety of vegetables and fruits each day.
  - Choose whole grains in preference to processed (refined) grains and sugars.
  - Limit consumption of red meats, especially those high in fat and processed.
  - Choose foods that allow you to maintain a healthful weight.
- Adopt a physically active lifestyle.
  - Adults: Engage in at least moderate activity for 30 minutes or more on 5 or more days of the week. Moderate to vigorous activity lasting at least 45 minutes on 5 or more days per week may further enhance reductions in the risk of breast and colon cancers.
  - Children and adolescents: Engage in at least 60 minutes per day of moderate to vigorous physical activity at least 5 days per week.
- Maintain a healthful weight throughout life.
  - Balance caloric intake with physical activity.
  - Lose weight if you are currently overweight.
- Limit consumption of alcoholic beverages if you drink at all.

Source: American Cancer Society Guidelines on Nutrition and Physical Activity for Cancer Prevention, 2001

walking, helps burn fat, makes muscles firm, and builds bone strength.

Practice Safe Sex Use of condoms can prevent the transmission of human papillomavirus, the virus associated with cervical and other types of cancer. Know your partner's history of sexually transmitted diseases, such as AIDS and HIV, and avoid having sex with multiple partners.

Limit Consumption of Alcoholic Beverages Because of the increased risk of cancers that are associated with alcohol use, the American Cancer Society recommends limiting alcohol use to two drinks per day for men. Women should limit their intake of alcohol to one drink per day due to slower metabolism of alcohol. A drink is 12 ounces of beer, 5 ounces of wine, or 1.5 ounces of 80-proof liquor.

Avoid Excessive Exposure to the Sun's Rays Although existing damage cannot be reversed, we can limit further insult to

our skin by practicing sun safety. These safety measures include staying out of the sunshine during the peak hours of ten A.M. to four P.M., wearing protective clothing and hats, using sunscreen with a sun protection factor (SPF) of 30 or more, and avoiding artificial tanning devices. The higher the sunscreen's SPF number, the longer the protection period; however, all sunscreen should be reapplied periodically, and particularly after swimming or perspiring heavily. People with light complexions, blue eyes, blond or red hair, or a tendency to freckle easily, need to be especially vigilant because they don't have as much sun-protective melanin in their skin. Fundamental skin cancer prevention measures are summarized in Table 5.

Exercise Caution in Taking Hormone Replacements Women should talk with their health care providers so they can make an informed decision about using hormone replacement therapy (HRT).

Table 5. **Skin Cancer Prevention and Detection**

- Avoid the midday sun between ten A.M. and four P.M.
- Wear a sunscreen with SPF 30 or greater.
- Cover up with protective clothing and a hat.
- Avoid tanning booths.
- Know your moles.
- Bring any moles to the attention of your doctor if they have one or more of the "ABCDEs":

    A—asymmetry (one-half looks different from the other)

    B—border (irregular borders)

    C—color (different colors in the same mole)

    D—diameter (larger than a pencil eraser)

    E—evolving (a change in a mole)

HRT can be very effective in treating the symptoms of menopause and preventing bone loss, but other medications and habits may also be effective. For example, many women choose to reduce the risks of osteoporosis by exercising regularly, eating a balanced diet, and taking calcium supplementation and/or a bone-strengthening medication, such as raloxifene (Evista) or alendronate (Fosamax). Ultimately, each woman's decision about whether to take HRT and the duration of its use must be an individual one based on information she has received from her health care provider. This decision should also be based on the woman's personal and family history of cancer, heart disease, stroke, and osteoporosis. The current recommendation from the FDA is to use the lowest effective dose of hormone replacement therapy for the shortest duration of time.

Chemoprevention Chemoprevention involves the use of a dietary nutrient or drug to halt or reverse the process of carcinogenesis. At present, prescription chemoprevention medications are targeted only toward individuals with an increased risk of specific cancers. Several chemopreventive agents have been shown to be effective in large cancer prevention studies. Table 6 lists the results of some completed chemoprevention trials. These agents are not without side effects, so those taking them should receive close medical supervision.

One of the main examples of chemoprevention is the use of tamoxifen (Nolvadex) to prevent breast cancer. Based on a 50 percent risk reduction in the Breast Cancer Prevention Trial, tamoxifen has been approved by the Food and Drug Administration (FDA) to reduce the risk of breast cancer in women who are at high risk. This drug can be a valuable tool for reducing breast cancer risk in women who have a strong family history of breast cancer or have a personal history of premalignant breast conditions; however, it is not recommended for women at average risk of breast cancer due to uncommon but serious side effects, including increased risk of blood clots, stroke, and uterine cancer.

More recently, results of the Study of Tamoxifen and Raloxifene (STAR) trial have shown that raloxifene (Evista) is another drug that can be used for breast cancer prevention. Both raloxifene and

Table 6. Results of Selected Completed Large Chemoprevention Trials

STUDY NAME	PREVENTION TARGET	CHEMOPREVENTIVE AGENTS	NUMBER OF PARTICIPANTS	RESULTS
Alpha-Tocopherol, Beta-Carotene Lung Cancer Prevention Study (ATBC)	Lung cancer in male cigarette smokers	Oral alpha-tocopherol (vitamin E) and beta-carotene	29,000	Alpha-tocopherol did not reduce lung cancer incidence; 18% higher incidence of lung cancer with beta-carotene and 8% more deaths.
	Secondary target: prostate cancer in male cigarette smokers			Alpha-tocopherol reduced prostate cancer incidence in men ages 50 to 69 by 32% and prostate cancer deaths by 41%.
Breast Cancer Prevention Trial (BCPT)	Breast cancer in high-risk women	Oral tamoxifen (Nolvadex) versus placebo	13,400	Tamoxifen reduced incidence of invasive breast cancer by 49%; similar reduction in noninvasive breast cancer. Approximately 50% increase in curable uterine cancer with tamoxifen.
Beta-Carotene and Retinole Efficacy Trial (CARET)	Lung cancer in heavy smokers and asbestos workers	Oral beta-carotene and retinol (vitamin A) versus placebo	18,300	Beta-carotene and retinol groups had 28% more lung cancers diagnosed and 17% more deaths than in placebo group.
Nutritional Prevention of Cancer (NPC) Chemoprevention Trial	Secondary cancers in people with a history of skin cancer	Oral selenium (in yeast) versus placebo	1,300	Prostate, lung, and colorectal cancers were lower in selenium group; selenium group had 17% fewer cancers overall and fewer deaths from lung cancer.
Physician's Health Study	All cancers in male physicians	Beta-carotene versus placebo	22,000	Beta-carotene produced neither benefit nor harm for cancer incidence or deaths, but only 11% of physicians were current smokers.
Prostate Cancer Prevention Trial (PCPT)	Prostate cancer	Finasteride (Proscar) versus placebo	9,060	Finasteride reduced prevalence of prostate cancer by 25%; higher-grade prostate cancers were more likely in finasteride group.

(continues)

Table 6. Results of Selected Completed Large Chemoprevention Trials (*continued*)

STUDY NAME	PREVENTION TARGET	CHEMOPREVENTIVE AGENTS	NUMBER OF PARTICIPANTS	RESULTS
Women's Health Study	All cancers in female health professionals	Aspirin and vitamin E	39,876	Low-dose aspirin did not reduce risk of cancers, with possible exception of lung cancer. Vitamin E did not reduce cancer incidence or overall deaths.
Study of Tamoxifen and Raloxifene (STAR)	Breast cancer in postmenopausal women at increased risk	Tamoxifen (Nolvadex) versus raloxifene (Evista)	19,471	Tamoxifen and raloxifene groups had similar rates of invasive breast cancer; noninvasive breast cancer was increased and uterine cancer was decreased in raloxifene group.
Physicians Health Study II	All cancers and prostate cancer in male physicians. Secondary target: colon cancer	Vitamin E, vitamin C, beta-carotene, and multivitamin versus placebos	15,000	Results anticipated in 2008.
Selenium and Vitamin E Cancer Prevention Trial (SELECT)	Prostate cancer	Oral selenium, vitamin E, or both, versus placebo	32,400	Recruitment closed 2004. Results anticipated in 2011.

tamoxifen reduced the risk of breast cancer in postmenopausal, high-risk women by about 50 percent. In addition, both medications are highly successful strategies for reducing the risk of bone fractures in women. Women in the raloxifene group had fewer blood clots and fewer uterine cancers than those in the tamoxifen group. However, the women taking raloxifene had more noninvasive cancers, or carcinomas in situ, than the women taking tamoxifen. Although in situ cancers cannot spread to other parts of the body, it is uncertain why these lesions were more frequent in this group. These results suggest that raloxifene is a second option for risk reduction in postmenopausal women. The STAR trial did not include premenopausal women, so additional studies will need to be done to determine if raloxifene is also beneficial in women who have not yet undergone menopause.

Another important area of investigation in chemoprevention is the use of nonsteroidal anti-inflammatory drugs to prevent colon, breast, and other types of cancer in high-risk individuals. Regular use of these medications may decrease the risk of premalignant colon adenomas by as much as 45 percent in individuals who have already had a colon adenoma. Due to the cardiovascular effects associated with COX-2 inhibitors (types of nonsteroidal anti-inflammatory drugs), routine use of these medications for the prevention of cancer is not currently recommended outside of a clinical trial.

Human Papillomavirus Vaccine The human papillomavirus is an important cause of many cases of cervical cancer. Most women are exposed to this virus only for a brief period of time, but some women have persistent infection that can lead to cervical cancer. Gardasil, a vaccination against human papillomavirus, has recently been approved by the FDA. This vaccination is targeted toward girls ages eleven to twelve, but it may be administered to girls as young as nine and women as old as twenty-six. The vaccination consists of three shots given over a six-month period. Although this vaccination is highly effective in preventing most cervical cancers, women who have been vaccinated should still have regular screening with Pap smears (see also the chapter on cervical cancer).

Joining the National Fight Against Cancer

Community-Based Cancer Prevention and Control Initiatives The National Cancer Institute, the Centers for Disease Control and Prevention, and the American Cancer Society have launched large cancer prevention research studies and programs. These community-based efforts are designed to further our understanding of ways to prevent, detect, and control cancer.

Ongoing cancer prevention trials offer the public a way to participate in research, and advance the science of cancer prevention. These studies and programs target common cancer sites, such as the breast, lung, prostate, and colon. Listed below are examples of several ongoing cancer prevention studies taking place in multiple areas across the United States. If you are interested in participating in a cancer screening or cancer prevention trial, your physician may be able to provide you with information about studies in your area.

Vitamin D/Calcium Polyp Prevention Study This study will assess the effects of calcium and/or vitamin D supplementation on recurrence of colon adenomas. Individuals who have recently had a colon adenoma removed are eligible for participation, and approximately 2,500 participants will be enrolled in centers across the country. The prevention target is new colon adenomas seen on follow-up colonoscopy, which is done three to five years later.

Study of Selenium in Patients with Adenomatous Colorectal Polyps This trial is studying the micronutrient selenium to determine if it can effectively prevent the recurrence of colon adenomas in individuals with a history of adenomas. In order to participate, individuals must have a history of having a colon adenoma removed within the last six months. Approximately 1,600 participants will randomly be assigned to selenium or placebo, and the primary assessment will be the rate of adenoma recurrence after 2.5 to 5 years.

Computed Tomographic Colonography (Virtual Colonoscopy) Screening for Colon Cancer This study will investigate the use of computed tomography (CT) scans in screening for colon cancer. Participants must be at least fifty years old and due for a screening colonoscopy. Colonoscopy will also be performed for participants as part of the study. Multiple sites are participating in this study across the United States.

Cancer Control Advocacy Legislative action and public policy can complement research and education to reduce cancer incidence and deaths. To accomplish this goal, people need to speak out and demand action from Congress and from state and municipal bodies. Such public advocacy has already been successful. For example, mammography facilities in the United States are now required to meet strict accreditation and inspection guidelines. Smoke-free public buildings and work sites are commonplace. The government budget for breast cancer research has increased, largely from results of demands by grassroots organizations. Medicare now reimburses for screening mammography.

Additional public advocacy is warranted for prohibiting sales of tobacco products to youth and increasing penalties to vendors who sell to minors. Increasing access to and insurance coverage for early-detection and screening procedures is still on the horizon.

Advocacy is taken seriously by the NCI. The Director's Consumer Liaison Group advises and makes recommendations to the NCI director from the perspective and viewpoint of cancer consumer advocates on a wide variety of issues, programs, and research priorities. The committee serves as a channel for consumer advocates to voice their views and concerns.

Resources on the Internet

American Cancer Society:
www.cancer.org/docroot/home/index.asp

Cancer Research and Prevention Foundation:
www.preventcancer.org/index.cfm

National Cancer Institute (Information on clinical trials):
www.cancer.gov/clinicaltrials

My Pyramid (Information for a healthy diet):
www.mypyramid.gov

Smoking Cessation Information:
www.smokefree.gov

— 44 —

Investigational Anticancer Drugs

Franco M. Muggia, M.D., and Boris Kobrinsky, M.D.

■ ■ ■ ■

"Targeted Drugs"

New Era Begets New Language New advances in molecular biology introduce new words to our lexicon. As has happened in the past with words such as *engine, battery, atom,* and *rocket,* new medical terms such as *monoclonal antibody, targeted drugs,* and *tyrosine kinase inhibitors* are entering the common language of clinical oncology.

Historical Perspective "Targeted drugs" are not a new concept. Historically, the first anticancer drug—nitrogen mustard, an analogue of mustard gas that had been used as a chemical weapon during World War I—was noted to cause the death of human white blood cells and was subsequently successfully utilized to fight blood malignancies in 1943. As it turned out many years later, the drug "targeted" or "alkylated" cell DNA by making chemical cross-links with it. However, DNA was unknown in 1943 and the initial goal of using nitrogen mustard was simply to kill the "whole cancer cell." Thus, nitrogen mustard was the first of a class of drugs known as alkylating agents that belong to a large family of cytotoxic drugs, or "cell killers."

In contrast to nitrogen mustard, methotrexate (1948) and 5-fluorouracil (1956) were designed to "target" specific enzymes—dihydrofolate reductase and thymidylate synthase, which are important for constructing the building blocks of DNA. These drugs were the first

in a new class of drugs known as antimetabolites that also fell under the larger umbrella of cytotoxic agents. Multiple other cytotoxic drugs followed whose targets became known only years later. For example, camptothecin sodium, introduced in 1968, was found several years later to work by inhibiting topoisomerase I, a newly discovered enzyme helpful in unwinding DNA.

New Targeted Drugs A new generation of drugs, sometimes referred broadly as targeted agents, rely on the following principles: (1) our increasing understanding of a variety of other intracellular molecular targets besides tumor DNA—such as receptors, tyrosine kinases, proteins, and specific genes involved in tumor biology; (2) increased precision of targeting with the goal of a "bull's-eye" hit to specific cancer cells, organelles, or pathways (rather than their normal counterparts), in order to greatly decrease toxicity of the drug; (3) targeting of the important elements of the cancer cell environment, such as growth factors, to deprive cancer cells of growth signals and/or to induce them to commit suicide by going into apoptosis (programmed cell death); and (4) targeting of the "tumor as an organ"—to prevent cancer cells from forming a new tumor or forming new tumors at distant sites (the process called metastasis)—by interrupting tumor blood supply and/or targeting the stroma (the infrastructure surrounding the tumor).

New Cellular Targets: Receptors, Ligands, Tyrosine Kinases, Nucleic Acids, and Proteins Cell surface receptors are highly specialized molecular structures embedded in the cell membrane. The external part of the receptor outside the cell serves as an antenna that accepts chemical signals from the blood by interacting with blood-soluble substances called ligands. Some of these ligands are growth factors that stimulate cancer cell growth or growth of blood vessels supplying nutrients to the tumor. After a chemical signal is triggered by a receptor, it is transmitted down a chain of other molecular transmitting machines called tyrosine kinases (see chapter 42, "The Impact of Research on the Cancer Problem"). Tyrosine kinases are mostly located in the cell cytoplasm, and ultimately this signaling system controls the expression of genes in the nucleus. Alterations in gene expression affect protein production in the cytoplasm that eventually can lead to a change in cell behavior such as increased growth, immortalization, and propensity for invasion, among others; all are the hallmarks of cancer. All the above-mentioned receptors, ligands, tyrosine kinases, nucleic acids, and proteins can be attacked by a new generation of targeted drugs matching our advances in biology.

New Means to Attack Cellular Targets: Monoclonal Antibodies, Small Molecules, and Antisense Nucleotides Antibodies are molecules produced by animal or human white blood cells (B lymphocytes) to attack other molecules, called antigens, that are present on microbes, viruses, or other cells, including cancer cells. *Monoclonal* antibodies are produced by lymphocytes that originate from the same ancestor lymphocyte (clone). A given monoclonal antibody targets one specific antigen, such as a growth factor in the blood or a receptor on the surface of a cancer cell. In the suffix of the drug's name, *mab* means "monoclonal antibody." In addition, the letter or letters preceding the suffix signify the antibody origin: *o* means "fully mouse antibody," *xi* means "chimeric" (human portion fused with mouse portion), *zu* means "humanized" (very small portion of mouse antibody, while the rest is human), and *u* means "fully human antibody." For example, ibritum*o*mab (Zevalin) is a monoclonal mouse antibody, bevaci*zu*mab (Avastin) is a monoclonal humanized antibody, cetu*xi*mab (Erbitux) is a monoclonal chimeric antibody, and panitum*u*mab (Vectibix) is a monoclonal fully human antibody (for more information on all these examples, see below).

Small molecules are chemical substances that target important specific parts of bigger molecules such as tyrosine kinases and, by doing so, interfere with transduction of chemical signals within the cancer cell.

In addition to antibodies and small molecules, other classes of targeted agents are in development. For example, antisense nucleotides are molecules that interact with messenger ribonucleic acid (RNA) or deoxyribonucleic acid (DNA) to block their translation of gene action.

Targeting Specific Pathways

Targeting Angiogenesis Single tumor cells do not need a blood supply, as they are able to get their nutrients and oxygen through diffusion from the environment. But after tumor cells multiply and become a small ball of about 2 mm, they are not able to get their nutrients and oxygen by diffusion, and need a blood supply. They achieve this through multiple mechanisms, primarily leading to overproduction of a substance called vascular endothelial growth factor (VEGF). VEGF stimulates normal endothelial cells to proliferate and form new blood vessels—a process known as angiogenesis. Targeting tumor angiogenesis has become one new method for restraining cancer growth (see chapter 14, "Antiangiogenesis").

Bevacizumab (Avastin) is an antibody that interacts with VEGF and prevents it from stimulating new blood vessel production for the tumor. Bevacizumab showed its activity as an adjunct to cytotoxic drug combination in metastatic colon cancer and is approved by the FDA for that cancer as well as certain forms of lung cancer. It has also shown beneficial effects in clinical trials of breast, kidney, and ovarian cancers. Sunitinib (Sutent) is a recently approved small molecule inhibitor that includes as one of its targets the receptor of VEGF (VEGFR); it has demonstrated activity in kidney cancer and a rare type of gastrointestinal tumor.

Multiple other new drugs target tumor angiogenesis in different ways and are currently under investigation in clinical trials. Among them are PTK/ZK (vatalanib; a VEGFR kinase inhibitor), ABT-510 (a thrombospondin mimetic), ABT-828 (recombinant human plasminogen kringle 5), and VEGF Trap (targets VEGF).

Targeting EGFR and Cell Growth The key role of the epidermal growth factor receptor (EGFR) family in many cancers has been identified. The epidermal growth factor (EGF) and related molecules act on receptors in a complex multistep pathway that eventually leads to cancer cell growth and escape from programmed death. Therefore, targeting the EGFR pathway on different levels has become a major goal for new drug developers.

Cetuximab (Erbitux) is a partially human antibody that interacts with EGFR, blocking the EGFR pathway by binding to the receptors and presumably inducing their degradation as well as preventing binding by EGF. It demonstrates activity with radiation therapy in head and neck cancers, as well as a single agent and in combination with chemotherapy in metastatic colon cancer. Multiple trials are ongoing for other cancers.

Panitumumab (Vectibix) is a first fully human antibody against EGFR that has been approved for use in metastatic colon cancer refractory to other treatments. It may have an advantage over cetuximab in eliciting fewer allergic reactions that are common when foreign proteins are given.

Erlotinib (Tarceva) is an oral small molecule that targets an intracellular tyrosine kinase responsible for activating the signal receptor induced when EGF binds to EGFR. Erlotinib and a related oral drug, gefitinib (Iressa), both interrupt the EGFR pathway on a different level than cetuximab and, curiously, have a different spectrum of activity. Erlotinib has been shown to have activity in nonsmall cell adenocarcinoma of the lung as well as in pancreatic cancer. Multiple trials are ongoing for other cancers as well.

Targeting HER-2/neu Receptors HER-2/*neu* receptors are special receptors that are overexpressed on the surface of about 25 percent of breast cancer tumors, leading to a more aggressive tumor behavior. Trastuzumab (Herceptin), an anti-HER-2/*neu* monoclonal antibody, selectively binds the HER-2/*neu* receptor. It was shown to decrease the risk of death by 33 percent at three years of follow-up when used in combination with chemotherapy. It showed activity by itself and has more recently yielded striking results in preventing recurrences when used after surgery (adjuvant therapy).

Lapatinib (Tykerb) is a small molecule and a HER-2/*neu* tyrosine kinase inhibitor (TKI). This oral agent targets both EGFR and HER-2/*neu*, thus possibly having a "dual benefit." Activity has been seen primarily in HER-2–positive breast cancer. In a recent Phase III study of women with locally advanced or metastatic HER-2–positive breast cancer, the drug improved the results achievable with capecitabine (Xeloda). Also, it appears to decrease the size of brain metastases and is active in women with HER-2–positive inflammatory breast cancer as well.

Targeting BCR/ABL Kinase The BCR/ABL mutation is important for the growth of chronic myelogenous leukemia (CML) cells, by giving these cells a competitive advantage over normal bone marrow cells for survival and also arresting the development of white cells at a more primitive step in differentiating pathways.

Imatinib mesylate (Gleevec) is a small molecule that binds BCR/ABL tyrosine kinase and by doing so inhibits leukemia cell growth and triggers programmed cell death (apoptosis). This drug has become a major success story in modern oncology by revolutionizing our treatment of CML and paving the way for other "targeted agents." This was the first successful target of tyrosine kinase inhibitors and stimulated other drug discoveries.

There are multiple mutations that may render BCR/ABL-positive leukemic cells resistant to imatinib. Understanding of these has led to insight into how resistance to these molecules arises.

Dasatinib (Sprycel) has more than 300 times the potency of imatinib against BCR/ABL-positive CML cells. In ongoing clinical trials, it shows activity in CML patients resistant to Gleevec. The drug has just been approved by the FDA for this indication. Nilotinib (AMN 107, Tasigna) is another novel inhibitor of BCR/ABL. In a recent Phase II clinical trial, it showed activity in accelerated (most difficult to treat) phase CML.

Targeting Tumor Stroma *Stroma* is a term used to refer to the supportive structures around a tumor vital for tumor survival. Thalidomide (Thalomid), while not killing cancer cells directly, works on tumor stroma in the bone marrow, ultimately causing tumor cells to die through apoptosis. The drug is effective in multiple myeloma. Lenalidomide (Revlimid) is a recently approved thalidomide analogue

that is effective in multiple myeloma that is resistant to thalidomide.

Targeting mTOR Kinase PTEN is an important tumor suppression gene whose inactivation can trigger overactivation of a kinase called mTOR (mammalian *target of r*apamycin), which can then render a tumor cell to be resistant to the above-mentioned EGFR inhibitors and other drugs.

Temsirolimus (Torisel) is an mTOR kinase inhibitor that was approved by the FDA in 2006 for use in kidney cancer. Everolimus (RAD 001, Certican) and AP 23573 are two other mTOR inhibitors in clinical trials. Understanding what leads to sensitivity to these drugs may lead to expanded indications, since PTEN mutations are seen in breast, kidney, brain, endometrial, and other cancers.

Targeting Multiple Pathways The more knowledge of the molecular biology of cancer we obtain, the clearer it becomes that multiple molecular pathways are involved in cancer. In addition to the above-mentioned EGFR pathway, other pathways involving different receptors and kinases interact with each other in a complex way, creating a constant flow of molecular information within cancer cells. To add to the complexity, this information superhighway within a cancer cell is not a static but a dynamic system with ever-changing interactions between its players. Therefore, the idea of targeting multiple pathways at the same time, perhaps with a single agent (to avoid the extra toxicity of multiple agents), was born. Currently, numerous new drugs that target multiple pathways are either in development, in clinical trials, or have recently been approved:

• Lapatinib (Tykerb) targets both EGFR and HER-2/*neu* as discussed above.
• Sorafenib (Nexavar), initially introduced as an inhibitor to another kinase

called Raf kinase, is in fact a multitarget kinase inhibitor that works on VEGFR as well as Raf, platelet-derived growth factor receptor (PDGFR), c-Kit, and FLT3 kinases. This drug has been approved for use in metastatic kidney cancer. Numerous other trials are in progress to see if it will work in other cancers.

• Sunitinib (Sutent) is a small molecule approved by the FDA for treatment of metastatic kidney cancer and gastrointestinal stromal tumors (GISTs) resistant to imatinib mesylate (Gleevec). It works on VEGFR, PDGFR, c-Kit, and FLT-3 kinases. Likewise, numerous trials are in progress to see if it will work in other cancers.

• A number of other multitargeting receptor and kinase inhibitors such as GW 786034 (pazopanib), ABT-869, RAF 265, and TKI-258, just to name a few, are in clinical trials.

Other Novel Classes of Drugs

A variety of other drugs based on novel principles to fight cancer cells are currently in development. Highlighted here are only a few examples:

Proteasome Inhibitors Proteasomes are molecular structures that are used by cancer cells to degrade certain proteins. By interrupting this process, proteosome inhibitors decrease cancer cell proliferation and induce apoptosis.

Bortezomib (Velcade, produced by Millennium), a proteasome inhibitor, has been approved for use in patients with multiple myeloma. It is being tested in many other cancers as well.

Texaphyrins Texaphyrins are a new class of drugs currently in development. They act by generating what are called highly reactive oxygen species (ROS) specifically inside cancer cells, and thus can induce cell death by apoptosis. One texaphyrin, motexafin gadolinium (Xcytrin, produced by Pharmacyclics), has shown promise in patients with nonsmall cell lung cancer and brain metastases.

Glutathione Analogues Cells use glutathione for protection against a great number of toxins, including chemotherapeutic drugs such as platinums and alkylating agents. Many cancers overexpress an enzyme important to glutathione metabolism, called glutathione S-transferase P1-1 (GST P1-1). This led to the idea of using a toxin coupled with glutathione as a sort of "Trojan horse" for cancer cells.

Canfosfamide HCL (also known as TLK-286 or Telcyta, produced by Telik) is a prodrug, meaning an inactive precursor of a drug that is activated by normal metabolic processes of the body. It consists of two portions: a glutathione analogue, and a cytotoxic component. Once it is preferentially taken up into cancer cells, the drug is split into its two fragments, with the cytotoxic component responsible for killing the cell. The drug is currently in Phase II and III trials for ovarian and lung cancers resistant to platinums (a mechanism of resistance to platinums is an increase in glutathione production).

Apoptosis Inducers One of the mechanisms to escape programmed cell death, or apoptosis, is through the antiapoptotic *bcl-2* gene family. G3139 (produced by Genta) is a drug belonging to a class of antisense nucleotides that bind to RNA derived from *bcl-2* gene action. By doing so, the antisense nucleotides prevent the production of antiapoptotic proteins. Lack of antiapoptotic proteins, in turn, causes induction of apoptosis, and cancer cell death. The drug is in phase III of clinical trials.

ABT-737 (produced by Abbott) is another inhibitor of the *bcl-2* family that is in clinical trials.

Radioimmunoconjugates Ibritumomab tiuxetan (Zevalin, produced by Biogen

Idec) is a mouse antibody attached (conjugated) to radioisotope 90 Y. Tositumomab (Bexxar, produced by GlaxoSmithKline) is also a mouse antibody, this one conjugated to radioisotope I 131. Both of these antibodies target the CD20 antigen located on non-Hodgkin's lymphoma cells and are approved for use in low-grade follicular or transformed non-Hodgkin's lymphomas.

Poly (ADP-Ribose) Polymerase (PARP) Inhibitors ABT-888 (produced by Abbott) inhibits an enzyme called PARP that is involved in recognizing DNA damage and facilitating DNA repair. Thus, it may be useful in enhancing the effect of DNA-damaging agents, including both chemotherapy and radiation.

Deacetylase (DAC) Inhibitors Cancer cells use a special enzyme called deacetylase to remove acetyl groups normally present on proteins called histones, which are bound to DNA. This removal leads to a shutdown of important genes that normally prevent development of cancer. LBH589 (produced by Novartis) uses the novel approach of deacetylase inhibition within the nucleus.

Radiation Sensitizer IPdR IPdR (ropidoxuridine, produced by Hana Biosciences) is a novel oral prodrug designed as a radiation sensitizer.

Cytotoxics: Still Alive and Important

New targeted therapies, with the notable exception of imatinib mesylate (Gleevec), rarely cause tumors to disappear completely. Therefore, traditional as well as novel cancer-cell-killing drugs, or cytotoxics, remain the backbone of tumor therapy. The three major directions in the modern development of cytotoxics are (1) optimization of drug delivery to the tumor, (2) development of the new drugs

from the same class of drugs to improve efficacy and safety, and (3) development of novel classes of drugs.

Optimization of Drug Delivery to the Tumor

Liposomal Technology Liposomal technology uses a lipid bilayer, referred to as a liposome, to encapsulate a drug. This changes the pharmacology of the drug and potentially leads to an improved therapeutic index (i.e., higher, potentially more effective doses can be given without an increase in side effects).

Doxorubicin in pegylated liposome (Doxil) is an example of a well-established drug, doxorubicin (Adriamycin), encapsulated into a liposome. Liposomes with prolonged circulation in the blood and with preferential tumor distribution help make Doxil more effective and less toxic, particularly for the heart, which has been a problem with doxorubicin. Initially approved for AIDS-related Kaposi's sarcoma, and subsequently for ovarian cancer, doxorubicin liposomal is now being explored against other tumors to replace the more toxic-"free" drug.

Cytarabine liposomal (DepoCyt) is another example of a well-known antimetabolite drug, cytarabine (Cytosar), encapsulated in a special kind of liposome using DepoFoam technology. This leads to a slow release of the drug into the central nervous fluid of a patient suffering from meningitis caused by malignant lymphoma. Among new drugs that are optimized using liposomal-related technology are antimicrotubular agents vincristine sulfate liposomal, sphingosome encapsulated vinorelbine, and the topoisomerase inhibitor sphingosome encapsulated topotecan (all produced by Hana Biosciences).

Nanoparticle Technology Albumin-bound paclitaxel (Abraxane) is a different example of drug-delivery optimization. Using albumin (one of the common blood proteins) nanoparticles (size of 130 nm) bound to the well-known and broadly used antimicrotubular agent paclitaxel (Taxol), the result is an improved product that is now approved for use in breast cancer. Other indications are being sought.

Analogue Development

Antitubulin Drugs Tubulin is a key protein for cell division, and several classes of drugs have their main effect on stopping mitosis (the part of the cell cycle when a cell separates its chromosomes to produce two daughter cells). To separate chromosomes, cells use small protein-made tubes called microtubules. Several classes of anticancer drugs interrupt this process either by disrupting the microtubules (vinca alkaloid drugs such as vincristine [Oncovin] and vinorelbine [Navelbine], as mentioned above) or by stabilizing tubules not to be broken down at the right time (taxane drugs such as paclitaxel, which was mentioned above, and docetaxel [Taxotere]).

New drugs are still being developed to maximize this effect. For example:

- EPO906 (also called patupilone or epothilone B, produced by Novartis) is in Phase III trials (for solid tumors).
- BMS-247550 (ixabepilone, produced by Bristol-Myers Squibb) is in metastatic breast cancer Phase II trials.
- KOS-862 (epothilone D, produced by Kosan Biosciences) is in Phase II trials for solid tumors.
- ABT-751 (produced by Abbott) is an oral antimitotic agent currently being tested in Phase II studies.
- Halichondrin and vinflunine bind to tubulin dimers and also inhibit mitosis. They are currently in Phase II studies.

Topoisomerase I Inhibitors Cellular DNA is a complex double-helical structure and needs unwinding before it can be reproduced. Cells use a special enzyme called topoisomerase I that makes specific and temporary breaks in the DNA helical structure to help it unwind. Topoisomerase I inhibitors make these breaks permanent, leading to programmed cell death (apoptosis).

LBQ707 (gimatecan, produced by Novartis) is a new topoisomerase inhibitor that is designed to avoid mechanisms of resistance related to export of these molecules out of the cell. It is orally active and currently in Phase II trials for solid tumors.

Platinums Satraplatin, an oral platinum with unusual chemistry differing from other platinums, is currently being studied for use in prostate cancer. Other studies will be forthcoming if efficacy in prostate cancer is established.

Alkylating Agents Cloretazine is a new alkylating drug that selectively cross-links DNA at a specific site (O-6 position of guanine). It has shown activity and acceptable toxicity in elderly patients with poor risk acute myeloid leukemia (AML). It is being studied in clinical trials.

Antimetabolites Clofarabine, a novel antimetabolite that mimics a purine nucleoside (one of the building blocks of DNA), has shown activity in elderly patients with poor risk acute myelogenous leukemia. Triapene is a ribonucleotide reductase inhibitor. Both drugs are being studied in clinical trials.

General Issues Related to New Drug Development

Preclinical (Laboratory) Testing In the past, cancer drugs were discovered through drug-screening programs that measured the drugs' effects on small animals with experimental cancers, such as leukemic mice. More recently, the NCI has sought to minimize unnecessary experimentation on laboratory animals by first developing a profile measuring how actively a drug kills cells from different types of cancers growing in laboratory cultures. This profile is compared to the profile of established drugs. If the new drug seems promising, its effects against tumors in animals are studied, including human cancers transplanted into mice.

Most new drugs continue to be introduced because of knowledge acquired through the study of established agents. More and more, however, new compounds are being designed by computers to attack certain biochemical targets known to be more common in cancer cells than in normal cells.

Drugs of interest undergo preclinical testing. At this stage, they are characterized according to their stability and purity and their toxicity in animals. This testing ends with the development of a pure and stable preparation for administration to humans.

Clinical (Human) Testing Drugs going on to clinical testing are classified according to definitions introduced by the Cancer Therapy Evaluation Program of the NCI in the late 1970s:

• Group A drugs are at the earliest stage of development (Phase I).
• Group B drugs are in widespread testing by cancer centers and cooperative groups or by industry.
• Group C drugs are in routine use by qualified oncologists before commercialization.
• Miscellaneous drugs are given together with chemotherapy, either to protect against toxicity or to enhance antitumor activity.

Phase I Studies This is when clinical study begins. Phase I studies are most concerned with establishing the safety profile of the drug: what dose can be given safely and what are the side effects that should be expected. Studies are performed in facilities with experienced physician-investigators and the tools for accurate data collection. This minimizes risks to patients by quickly indicating if unusual toxicities or drug interactions are occurring. A starting dose level (based on a fraction of the dose that produces an effect on mice and other laboratory animals) is given to small groups of patients who volunteer for a clinical trial because their standard treatments have not been effective. In Phase I studies, blood samples are taken to assess how the drug is eliminated from the body (known as drug metabolism and pharmacology). The dose is then gradually increased in subsequent groups of patients until side effects start to occur.

When significant side effects do occur, they are very carefully documented and promptly treated. The dosage is not increased any more and the recommended dose of the drug is defined. The dose chosen for Phase II studies is that which produces drug concentrations in the blood that are in the range for antitumor effects found in preclinical research, without causing excessive side effects. For chemotherapy drugs, this is usually the highest dose tolerable to patients. It is particularly encouraging if patients are seen to benefit at doses below the recommended dose, as most patients have tumors that have been resistant to standard treatments.

Phase II Studies Phase II studies are the earliest studies that try to define the effectiveness of the drug. With the dose and side effects already established from the Phase I studies, the drug is tested in a limited number of patients who meet very specific requirements. The majority of Phase II studies are designed to primarily assess response rate (the percentage of patients whose tumor size is significantly decreased by therapy), and the results of these studies can make or break a drug. Paclitaxel, for example, was registered by the FDA for use in both ovarian and breast cancers on the basis of Phase II data alone. Another example is capecitabine (Xeloda), which was registered by the FDA for patients with metastatic breast cancer resistant to both anthracycline and taxanes without Phase III evaluation. Topotecan, however, followed the more standard procedure for registration. Like paclitaxel, it was initially studied in women with ovarian cancers that were resistant to the established drug cisplatin. It went on to be registered for this indication on the basis of the results of Phase II studies that were subsequently supported by randomized Phase III data demonstrating comparable activity of topotecan and paclitaxel. A myriad of other agents have been dropped from development when Phase II studies failed to demonstrate response rates that were competitive with standard therapies for the tumor being studied.

Phase III Studies Phase III studies are the definitive studies that assess the efficacy of the drug and are only performed when the Phase II results look promising. Phase III studies usually aim to show an improvement in survival or quality of life, as these are the main criteria used by the FDA to decide whether to register a drug. A randomized study is usually necessary to demonstrate that the new drug is better than the current standard. In a randomized study, half the patients receive the current standard therapy and the other half the new therapy, and the decision of which treatment to receive is decided by chance (e.g., flip of a coin, computer-generated random numbers). An example of a recently FDA approved drug based on this trial design is irinotecan (Camptosar, CPT-11), which showed significant benefit (extended survival and better quality of life) against refractory colorectal cancer when compared to retreatment with 5-fluorouracil in one study, and best supportive care in another

study. Many other agents have been dropped from development when Phase III studies failed to show any advantage for the new agent.

Studies of Drug Combinations These are often referred to as pilot studies and are based on experimental or early clinical observations. These are most logical when the two agents are synergistic (i.e., the anticancer activity of the combination is greater than the sum of the two single agents) in laboratory models, but also make sense when two agents are both very active in the same type of tumor and the side effects of the two drugs are different. Patients enrolled in Phase I trials of combinations often benefit from such study treatment, as Phase II and III data of the single agents is often already available to guide patient selection.

Expanded Access (Compassionate Use) Studies Group C drugs are most commonly available on expanded access programs. These "studies" register and monitor toxicities of all patients receiving the unregistered drug until the drug can be made commercially available. These drugs have shown definite antitumor activity but are still classified as investigational for a variety of reasons:

- The trials seeking FDA approval may be incomplete or currently inconclusive.
- A drug sponsor has not been identified or is under negotiation.
- The circumstances in which the drug has been shown to be useful do not easily lend themselves to the drug approval process, so approval is no longer being sought.

For oncologists registered in good standing as clinical investigators, drugs in the last two categories are often obtainable through the NCI. Drugs are also occasionally available from industry sponsors for "compassionate" use. With industrial sponsors, the label "group C" is not usually used, but such drugs may be available by concurrence of the sponsors and physicians seeking compassionate approvals from the FDA.

Approved Uses for Drugs

The FDA approves chemotherapeutic drugs for one or more specific indications. For example, paclitaxel (Taxol) was first approved only for treating ovarian cancers resistant to cisplatin or carboplatin. Subsequently, the indications have been extended to breast cancer, nonsmall cell lung cancer, and Kaposi's sarcoma. Once a drug is approved, the FDA does not prohibit its use for nonapproved situations. Such use, usually based on medical reports or the personal experiences of oncologists, have become a community standard for some cancers. For example, the use of carboplatin for treatment of nonsmall cell lung cancer is now routine based on extensive Phase II and III data that have not been submitted to the FDA.

When a drug is first released, insurance companies in particular tend to regard nonapproved uses as "experimental." But distinctions between "established" and "investigational" or "experimental" uses are often blurred. Drugs under investigation have often become therapeutic alternatives for patients who have failed standard treatments or have cancers with no known life-prolonging therapies. Many patients in the United States demand that everything possible be done to treat their disease and are therefore, rightly or wrongly, prescribed therapy "off-label," ahead of the availability of results of clinical studies that may or may not support this indication.

The FDA may accept tumor regression and improvement in quality of life as criteria for approval but will usually require evidence of prolongation of survival to approve a new drug in situations where other drugs are already available.

Conclusions

While the development of a new drug appears slow, a rigorous process is necessary to ensure that the side effects and activity of the new drug can be reasonably predicted for patients once it is registered. There are an enormous number of new agents currently in development, with only a few selected ones highlighted in this chapter. Hormonal therapy, radiosensitizers, modulators of chemotherapy activity, gene therapies, monoclonal antibodies, small molecule inhibitors, new cytotoxic drugs—all are under active investigation for a variety of different cancer types.

Clinical trials offer patients with resistant tumors access to untried therapies with novel mechanisms of action, and are the only way that we can objectively assess how new agents work in people with cancer. Currently available cancer trials are listed on the NCI's Web site at *http://cancertrials.nci.nih.gov.*

— 45 —

Advances in Cancer Biology

John W. Park, M.D.

■ ■ ■ ■

Dedicated research in cancer biology over a number of years has now produced a detailed picture of the cancer cell. While investigation is still not complete, many of the molecular and cellular events involved in cancer have now been uncovered. An important challenge has been to translate this revolution in biological insight into actual improvements in the diagnosis and treatment of cancer. In a number of areas, these new insights have already impacted cancer therapy. The future of cancer treatment will continue to be profoundly shaped by these new advances.

One of the central principles in cancer biology is that cancer involves changes or defects in our genes. Genes, which are composed of DNA, contain the key information for each cell in our body. There are an estimated 20,000 to 25,000 genes within each human cell, and this collection of genes is referred to as the genome. In most cells in our bodies, all of this genetic information is packaged in forty-six chromosomes, twenty-three inherited from each parent. A single chromosome therefore contains many thousands of genes, each of which directs the production of proteins such as receptors, enzymes, and structural proteins. Important milestones in the history of science include the demonstration that genes are composed of DNA (1944); the discovery that the structure of DNA is a double helix (1953); and the sequencing or deciphering of the entire human genome (2000).

It is important to distinguish between changes in our genes that are *acquired* in the course of living and those changes that are *inherited* at birth from either or both parents. Changes in genes are referred to as mutations. Only a small minority of cancers are predominantly due to mutant genes that are inherited, and these are referred to as familial or hereditary cancers. The majority of cancers develop following a series of mutations in genes at various times after birth or are due to a complex interplay between inherited genes that predispose to cancer and genes with mutations that are acquired during one's lifetime.

Tumor-Causing and Tumor-Suppressing Genes

Mutations that can lead to cancer typically do so because they increase the function of genes that stimulate cell growth or decrease the function of genes that suppress cell growth. Both types of genes are likely to be important contributors during normal human growth and development. But mutation of these genes can cause otherwise well-regulated processes within a cell to become uncontrolled. If a sufficient number of these changes occur, the cell can become malignant.

Oncogenes One of the seminal discoveries in the field of cancer research is that some of our normal genes can become abnormally activated in various ways, resulting in genes capable of transforming a normal cell into a cancer cell. These activated and cancer-causing genes are called oncogenes (i.e., associated with cancer). The proteins produced by oncogenes are sometimes called oncoproteins.

We carry normal, nonmutated forms of these oncogenes in our chromosomes. In their unaltered, normal state, these genes are referred to as proto-oncogenes and perform useful functions in the cell. However, if they become mutated or overactive ("overexpressed"), the oncogene versions can work with other oncogenes to hijack a normal cell and turn it into a cancer cell.

There are many known oncogenes. They are often named for the types of cancers they first caused in animals when discovered, such as *ras* for rat sarcoma and *neu* for neuroblastoma. The mechanisms by which oncogenes, once mutated and activated, cause cancer are diverse. One frequent theme involves oncogenes that produce abnormal amounts of growth factors (molecules that stimulate growth) or growth factor receptors (the partners of growth factors), leading to excessive cell growth and multiplication. Some oncogenes are part of the signaling machinery inside the cell. Activation of these oncogenes also leads to excessive stimulation and uncontrolled growth. Still other oncogenes help cancer cells become immortal; they resist the signal to die by what is called apoptosis, the natural dying process of cells.

There is usually more than one oncogene activated in any given tumor, and these oncogenes may coordinate with each other and with the loss of tumor suppressors to produce cancer.

Tumor Suppressor Genes As their name implies, tumor suppressor genes are normally protective, acting to regulate normal cell growth and multiplication. By doing this, they prevent the unregulated growth that is characteristic of a cancer cell. These genes can sometimes counteract the cancer-predisposing effect of an activated oncogene. If one of these genes is absent or its protein product is unable to work properly, the cancer-producing action of an oncogene may not be completely suppressed and a tumor may then develop.

A number of tumor suppressor genes have been identified. Some are referred to by their biological properties—p53, for example—while others are named for the cancer in which they were first discovered, as in RB (retinoblastoma) and BRCA1 and 2 (breast cancer).

Many tumor suppressor genes were discovered by studying inherited cancers, since abnormal forms of these genes can be transmitted from parents to offspring by either egg or sperm. But they also play important roles in noninherited cancers. Almost all cancers are believed to have a defect in one or more tumor-suppressor genes. A typical colon cancer, for example, may have at least four inactivated tumor-suppressor genes (APC, DCC, MCC, and p53).

The RB gene was the first tumor suppressor gene to be discovered, and retinoblastoma remains a model of a cancer caused by inactivation of tumor-suppressor genes. Retinoblastoma is a rare and sometimes fatal eye cancer occurring mainly in children. There is an inherited form that runs in families as well as a sporadic form that does not have a family connection. In the inherited form, one RB gene derived from one of the parents is defective. Sometime during childhood, the remaining "good" RB gene from the other parent becomes lost or mutated in a retinal cell. Then, because the cell no longer has any functioning RB, it becomes a cancerous retinoblastoma. In the sporadic form, all of the original RB genes were normal at birth. However, if a retinal cell sustains mutations in both genes, then a retinoblastoma can arise.

If detected early, both inherited and spontaneous forms of retinoblastoma

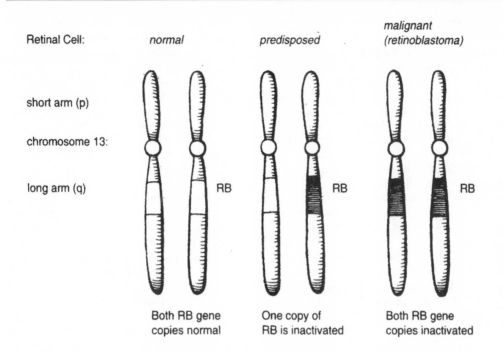

Retinal Cell: normal predisposed malignant (retinoblastoma)

short arm (p)

chromosome 13:

long arm (q) RB RB RB

Both RB gene copies normal

One copy of RB is inactivated

Both RB gene copies inactivated

Retinoblastoma occurs when a retinal cell has lost the tumor-suppressing function of both RB genes on chromosome 13. With the inherited form, retinal cells are predisposed at birth, since an inactivating mutation was transmitted by either sperm or egg. In the sporadic form, both genetic defects occur in the retinal cell during development but are not passed on to offspring.

are curable with radiotherapy, and vision can be preserved. Genetic probes can detect the abnormal RB gene, identifying children at risk. These children need careful clinical monitoring and frequent eye examinations.

"Multistep" Pathway to Cancer The processes by which proto-oncogenes are activated and tumor suppressor genes are inactivated involve changes to the DNA structure of these genes. As discussed above, abnormal genes can be inherited, such as defective tumor suppressor genes in familial cancers. More frequently, these changes or mutations may arise by exposure to a physical or chemical agent (a carcinogen) that can damage chromosomes

or DNA. Radiation in the form of sunlight or X-rays, certain toxic chemicals, and other environmental factors such as cigarette smoke and asbestos are all examples of carcinogens that are known to cause cancers with excessive exposure. Some viruses contain oncogenes that they introduce when they infect cells; an example of this is human papillomavirus, which can cause cervical cancer. Other viruses can also cause DNA damage indirectly, such as by incorporating into chromosomes.

Fortunately, our cells have many safety mechanisms to protect them from becoming malignant despite the mutations that they might sustain. For example, the cell can repair mutations after they occur. However, as we age, the number of mutations that we have accumulated may exceed the cell's capacity for repair. Also, mutations can occur in the very genes that control DNA repair, thus incapacitating this important function and leading to an accelerated rate of mutation throughout the genome. An example of this is inactivation of the DNA repair gene hMSH2 in colorectal and other cancers. The persistence of activated oncogenes or inactivated tumor suppressor genes that are not repaired will predispose a person to develop cancer in the tissue containing that abnormal cell.

Another safety feature in cells is that there are multiple mechanisms to control cell growth, ensuring that there are backup systems when one mechanism breaks down. Thus, cancer usually does not occur until a series of changes have accumulated, thereby defeating even the backup systems for proper regulation of the cell. In other words, multiple genetic mutations, or accumulated hits, are usually necessary to cause cancer. This is referred to as the multistep model of cancer. As we have seen, these hits would involve activation of oncogenes combined with inactivation of tumor suppressor genes. These genetic hits may accumulate over many months or years because of the effects of various environmental carcinogens on top of inherited susceptibilities. Eventually, if enough oncogene and tumor suppressor gene functions have been altered, this will allow a full-fledged cancer cell to emerge. Additional changes will then allow the cancer cell to gain further abilities that promote the cancer's effect on the body, such as migrating through tissue, attracting new blood vessels (angiogenesis), resisting the immune system, and other cancer behaviors.

Tests Based on Tumor-Causing and Tumor-Suppressing Genes

Based on this knowledge of the genes that can go awry in the development of a cancer, it has been possible to devise tests that can detect these changes in tumors. This can potentially provide useful information about the future behavior of a particular cancer, including guiding the selection of the most appropriate treatments for that cancer. The following examples illustrate this principle:

Gene Mutation For breast and ovarian cancers that run in families, it is frequently possible to detect the mutant gene responsible. The BRCA1 and BRCA2 genes are tumor suppressor genes that can become mutated; when a mutation is passed from parent to offspring, this leads to an inherited predisposition to these cancers. DNA-based testing to detect mutation of these genes can be performed, which can alert gene carriers that they have inherited this risk. For positively identified gene carriers, close monitoring and/or preventive measures can be implemented.

Gene Amplification Some breast and other cancers are associated with amplification and overexpression of the proto-oncogene called HER-2/*neu* (also called c-*erb*B-2). Normally, cells will have two copies of the gene (one copy inherited from each parent). Twenty to 30 percent of breast cancers acquire many additional copies of this oncogene via a process called gene amplification. These cancers have much higher than normal levels of the HER-2 protein, a growth factor receptor, leading to a more aggressive pattern of growth. On the other hand, HER-2–positive cancers can benefit from specific therapies that have been developed to target this oncoprotein (discussed below).

Targeted Therapies

Our understanding of cancer biology has led to a new generation of "targeted therapies" that are designed to counteract the effects of oncogenes or to restore or correct defective tumor suppressor genes. These approaches have already made a significant impact against many cancers. Many additional approaches are being investigated, and this field of targeted therapies has the potential to greatly enhance cancer treatment.

Anti-Oncogene Therapies One example is the use of artificial antibodies (monoclonal antibodies) directed against oncoproteins such as HER-2 and EGFR (epidermal growth factor receptor). For example, trastuzumab (Herceptin), a monoclonal antibody against HER-2/*neu,* has proven to be useful in the treatment of advanced breast cancers with high levels of HER-2. Newer types of antibody-based therapy include antibodies linked to chemotherapy drugs, radioactive atoms, toxins, and submicroscopic particles containing drugs. These approaches use the antibody portion to deliver potent anticancer agents right to the cancer cell. In addition to antibodies and antibody-based therapies, researchers are pursuing vaccines designed to stimulate the immune system to reject cancer cells containing oncoproteins. These approaches are discussed further in chapter 9, "What Happens in Biological Therapy and Immunotherapy."

A related approach involves chemical drugs that can inhibit oncoproteins/growth factor receptors such as HER-2/*neu* and EGFR. These drugs are designed to bind to important sites on these oncoproteins in order to "turn off" their functions. For example, a chromosomal translocation (a form of mutation involving rearrangement of chromosome sections) can create an oncogene known as BCR/ABL, which is an enzyme that leads directly to chronic myelogenous leukemia (CML). A recently developed drug, imatinib mesylate, inhibits the activity of the BCR/ABL enzyme and has proven useful in CML treatment. (See the chapter on the leukemias.)

Another strategy involves inhibiting the new blood vessel growth (angiogenesis) that tumors establish for themselves. These "antiangiogenic therapies" can block this process, thereby starving tumor cells and stopping tumor growth. (For an in-depth discussion of antiangiogenic therapies, refer to chapter 14.)

Tumor-Suppressor Therapies Restoring the activity of tumor suppressors in cancer cells is a rational but difficult strategy. Researchers are attempting to develop drugs that may help to regulate the cell cycle, the process that governs cell growth and multiplication. Other efforts involve replacing the tumor suppressor genes themselves by gene therapy.

Gene Therapy

Gene therapy involves insertion of new genes into cells, thus altering the genetic composition and biological properties of the recipient cells. The first serious attempts at gene therapy for cancer were undertaken in the early 1990s. Now, there are many ways in which gene therapy is being pursued, and many clinical trials around the world are testing these new treatments. The potential for gene therapy is great. Since cancer is generally caused by genes that become mutated and therefore defective, gene therapy can provide a direct "fix" of the problem by replacing the faulty genes with correct versions.

However, there are a number of major technical challenges that must be overcome before gene therapy can be routinely applied to the treatment of cancer. Gene therapy requires a vehicle to deliver the gene to its intended target cell. Delivery systems for genes include modified viruses such as adenovirus, which is one of the viruses responsible for the common cold. Another delivery system involves synthetic particles called liposomes. These systems are still being perfected for gene delivery. Researchers are attempting to improve these delivery systems so that they are safer, more efficient, and capable of "targeted delivery" so that they go to the tumor cells but not normal cells. Meanwhile, clinical studies of gene therapy are focusing on treatment of particular sites in the body, such as confined areas where genes can be delivered more efficiently.

— 46 —

Genetic Risk Assessment and Counseling

Amie M. Blanco, M.S., C.G.C., and Beth B. Crawford, M.S.

■ ■ ■ ■

The field of genetics is in the news daily, with researchers mapping the human genome, cloning animals, and identifying new disease genes. Among those members of the population who have a family history of cancer, researchers have identified inherited alterations in the genetic code (gene mutations) that increase the likelihood of developing cancer. Some of these mutations increase risk only slightly, and others make an eventual diagnosis of cancer nearly inevitable. These latter types of mutations are said to cause hereditary cancer syndromes, the most common of which are Lynch syndrome, also called hereditary nonpolyposis colorectal cancer (HNPCC); familial adenomatous polyposis (FAP); and hereditary breast and ovarian cancer syndrome (HBOC).

The main objective of genetic risk assessment and counseling is to prevent cancers from occurring (or at least to discover them at their earliest stages, when they are most curable) by identifying individuals and families at increased risk. This is a multifaceted process by which physicians, genetic counselors, and nurses determine the likelihood of inherited disease in a family, provide education about cancer risks for patients and other members of the family, facilitate genetic testing when appropriate, provide recommendations for cancer screening and prevention, and offer psychological support.

Overview of Genetics and Inheritance

It is worthwhile to review some basic genetic definitions and principles before discussing the relationship of inherited gene mutations to cancer. The human genetic code is contained in a long molecule called DNA, and virtually every cell in the human body has this molecule of DNA. The DNA is arranged in forty-six chromosomes and holds approximately 20,000–25,000 genes. Prior to conception, the sperm and the egg cells, also called germ cells, each carry twenty-three chromosomes. Upon fertilization, the sperm and egg cell fuse, resulting in an embryo with a total of forty-six chromosomes. Of these, forty-four are identical in men and women—these are called autosomes. The remaining two chromosomes are called sex chromosomes, which are designated X and Y. Women inherit two X chromosomes, one from their mother and one from their father; whereas men inherit one X chromosome from their mother and one Y chromosome from their father. Because of the way chromosomes are inherited, every person has two copies of each gene: one copy from your father and one copy from your mother. When the genes from your parents are combined to make a child, the DNA is "shuffled." This shuffling produces a brand-new, unique individual. The human genetic code is so complex that each person's combination of their father's and mother's genes is unique. That is why, except for identical twins, none of the 6.5 billion residents of planet Earth is the same as any other.

Genes determine all physical characteristics, such as skin and eye color, and all bodily functions, such as metabolism and growth. In scientific terms, a gene is a segment of DNA that codes for the production of a specific protein. The DNA code is much like a recipe made up of only four letters: *A, C, G,* and *T.* These letters, called bases, are the individual chemical units that "spell" out the protein recipe. Any change in the sequence of bases is called a mutation. Just like changing a letter in a word can change the word's meaning, a mutation can change the instruction contained in the gene. Proteins are responsible for carrying out all of the functions that keep cells alive and healthy, thus the accurate production of proteins depends on having normal genes.

When discussing inheritance of a disease, there are two genetic scenarios: monogenic inheritance, where there is only one gene responsible for the disease, and polygenic inheritance, where many genes contribute. Hereditary cancer predisposition syndromes are all examples of monogenic inheritance. There are two main types of monogenic inheritance: dominant and recessive. Dominant inheritance defines a situation where only one copy of a gene mutation needs to be inherited for the person to develop the disease—that is, either the mother's copy or the father's copy, but not both. Recessive inheritance, on the other hand, means that two copies of a mutant gene must be inherited for the disease to develop—one from each parent.

When a disease is dominantly inherited, each child of an affected parent has a 50 percent chance of inheriting the disease, because the affected parent has two copies of the gene, one normal and the other with a mutation. It is a matter of equal chance which copy from the affected parent goes into the sperm or the egg cell that produces a child. Familial adenomatous polyposis (FAP) is an example of a dominantly inherited cancer predisposition syndrome.

When a disease is recessively inherited, each parent must have at least one copy of the predisposing gene mutation and the child must inherit the gene mutation from both parents for the disease to occur. An individual with just one gene mutation is called a carrier and does not show the disease him- or herself. Each child of parents who are both carriers for a recessive gene mutation has a 25 percent chance of inheriting the disease. An example of recessively inherited cancer predisposition is MYH-associated polyposis (MAP), in which the inheritance of two copies of a gene mutation increases the risk for multiple colorectal polyps and colorectal cancer.

Gene Mutations and Cancer

Everyone acquires some mutations in their DNA during the course of their lives. These mutations occur in a number of ways. Sometimes there are simple copying errors that are introduced when DNA replicates itself. As our cells age and die, new cells must be made to replace them. For this to happen, each of the 3 billion letters of DNA that are found within every cell has to be copied, one letter at a time. Not surprisingly, mistakes sometimes occur. Other mutations are introduced as a result of DNA damage through environmental agents such as sunlight, cigarette smoke, and radiation. Cells have built-in mechanisms that catch and repair most of the changes that occur during DNA replication or from environmental damage. However, as the human body ages, DNA repair does not work as effectively, resulting in the accumulation of gene mutations.

The most important thing for the cell to do is to stop damaged DNA from

Figure 1A **Autosomal Dominant Inheritance**

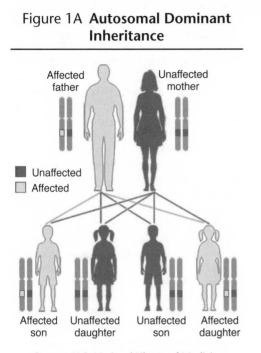

Source: U.S. National Library of Medicine

Figure 1B **Autosomal Recessive Inheritance**

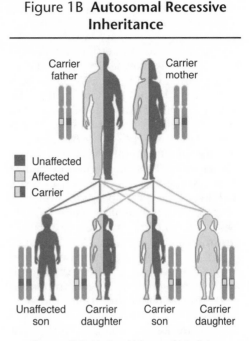

Source: U.S. National Library of Medicine

being passed on to the next generation of cells. If genetic damage is not too bad, it is repaired. If the damage cannot be repaired, typically the cell dies. However, sometimes genetic damage results in the inability of a cell to control its own growth and death. After accumulated damage to both copies of multiple genes in charge of cell growth and death, a cell can no longer be controlled and the result is cancer.

Hereditary Cancer Syndromes

In hereditary cancer predisposition syndromes, a gene mutation exists in one of the germ cells (egg or sperm) at the time of conception. This is called a germ line mutation.

Most of the time, the mutation is in the germ cell because the parent received it from one of his or her parents.

Sometimes it is a new mutation, meaning that the change in the gene occurred during the production of that germ cell and neither parent has the mutation in their other body cells. In both cases, the mutation will be copied during the development of the new individual, so that it will be present in every cell of the body. A germ cell mutation in a gene controlling cell growth or DNA repair is the first in the sequence of mutations leading to the development of cancer.

Since multiple mutations within successive generations of a cell are required for cancer to appear, most of the hereditary cancers occur in the adult years. On average, hereditary forms of cancer occur about ten to twenty years earlier than nonhereditary cancers because of the first critical mutation in each cell.

Hereditary cancer syndromes have specific patterns of cancer occurrences within the family. In Lynch syndrome, one or more members of the family may have multiple primary cancers such as colon and endometrial cancers. In HBOC, there is an excess of bilateral cancer in paired organs such as the breasts and ovaries. Within the same family, the expression of the cancer gene can vary in terms of the age of onset and the organs affected. The risk of cancer for a person with a germ line mutation is high but not 100 percent. This phenomenon of less than 100 percent risk of cancer in those with hereditary predisposition is referred to as the penetrance of the gene.

In the majority of hereditary cancer syndromes, the pattern of inheritance is dominant. The one known exception to this rule is MAP, in which the inheritance of two copies of a gene mutation increases the risk for multiple colorectal polyps and colorectal cancer. Some syndromes are heterogeneic, meaning that they can be the result of a mutation in more than one gene. Lynch syndrome can be caused by a germ line mutation in the MLH1, MSH2, MSH6, or PMS2 gene. Likewise, hereditary breast and ovarian cancer is caused by a germ line mutation in either the BRCA1 or BRCA2 gene.

The table on the following page lists some of the more common hereditary colon and breast cancer syndromes, the genes associated with them, and the clinical features of each.

Cancer Risk Assessment

Cancer is very common throughout the world. One out of three Americans will develop the disease at some point, so it should not be surprising that most people have a history of one or more cancer occurrences within a three-generation history of their families.

Most of these cancers will be sporadic or chance occurrences posing only a slight increased risk for cancer to those individuals' closest relatives. In some families, the cancer may be familial; multiple genes (polygenic) and/or common environmental exposures are believed to be the cause of these cancers. Family members who are closely related to an affected individual have about two to three times the risk for the same cancer that the general population has. Only 5 to 10 percent of all cancers are truly hereditary.

The case of Mrs. B (page 406) will be used as an example to illustrate the clinical services provided during cancer risk evaluation, genetic counseling, and predictive testing.

Family History Mrs. B was a twenty-eight-year-old female who sought cancer risk assessment and genetic counseling services because of her concern about multiple occurrences of colon cancer in her family. Mrs. B's mother (Mrs. H) had a history of colon cancer and her aunt had just died with colon cancer after surviving uterine cancer for ten years. Mrs. B's maternal grandmother and a maternal uncle had also both died with cancer, but she didn't know their ages or the sites of their cancers.

Gathering Information To determine the significance of the cancer occurrences in Mrs. B's family, it was essential to gather the history on her parents, brothers, sisters, children, nieces, nephews, aunts, uncles, cousins, grandparents, and any other relatives for whom medical information was available. The information required for a genetic evaluation includes any significant health problems, the primary site of all cancer occurrences, the age of diagnosis, current age or age at death, and cause of death, and exposures to carcinogens such as high-fat diets or tobacco.

Since Mrs. B did not know the medical history for all of these relatives, she was encouraged to ask her mother and her maternal uncle's widow to fill in the gaps. In many families, there is a "family historian" who can provide information

Common Hereditary Colon and Breast Cancer Syndromes

SYNDROME	GENE(S)	CLINICAL FEATURES
Lynch syndrome (HNPCC)	MLH1, MSH2, MSH6, or PMS2	Up to 80% lifetime risk for colorectal cancer in males, somewhat less in females, and 20–60% lifetime risk for endometrial (uterine) cancer. In some families, the risks for cancers of the stomach, ovary, urinary tract, kidney, hepatobiliary tract, skin, and brain are increased.
HBOC	BRCA1	50–85% lifetime risk for breast cancer in women, and 20–50% risk for ovarian cancer. An increased risk for male breast cancer and prostate cancer also exists.
	BRCA2	50–85% lifetime risk for breast cancer in women, 6% risk for male breast cancer, and 10–30% risk for ovarian cancer. The risks for melanoma and prostate and pancreatic cancers are also increased in some families.
FAP	APC	Hundreds to thousands of colonic adenomas develop at a young age. Without treatment, the lifetime risk for colorectal cancer is close to 100%. Risks for cancers of the stomach, small bowel, and thyroid are also increased. Some families have an increased risk for benign tumors in the abdomen (desmoid), bony growths (osteomas), epidermoid cysts, extra teeth, and extra pigment in the retina of the eye (CHRPE).

about previous generations. In others, information may have been recorded in the family Bible or a genealogy.

Families vary in how open they are to discussing health issues. Some individuals in Mrs. B's family were very reluctant to share information with her, possibly because of an inclination for privacy, a distrust of medical professionals, an avoidance of the emotional context of the family's history, or a fear of what might be learned from the evaluation.

Documenting the History Medical records, especially pathology reports for all reported cancers, are essential for iden-

tifying or verifying the primary site of the cancer. In addition, there are specific pathologic features of some tumors that are more frequently found in hereditary cancers.

Mrs. B, therefore, was asked to request a release of medical records from her mother, who had a history of cancer. Mrs. B asked her mother, cousin, and aunt (her maternal uncle's widow), as the nearest surviving relatives, to sign the release forms for her grandmother's, aunt's, and uncle's records. Unfortunately, the hospital where her grandmother was treated had destroyed the records and a death certificate was requested in hopes of

Mrs. B's Pedigree

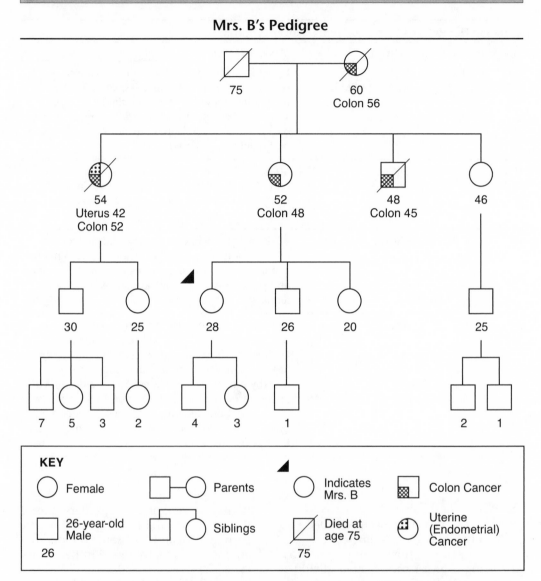

identifying the primary site of her cancer. Mrs. B's aunt declined the release of her husband's records.

Clinical Evaluation The clinical evaluation of the significance of the family history usually consists of a review of the individual's medical history and the family history and a physical examination. It's often helpful for the individual seeking the evaluation to bring someone along to provide emotional support or help clarify the family history. Several family members may choose to come together so they can provide and receive information at the same time. Mrs. B brought her husband and her mother with her for the evaluation.

While reviewing the history with the family, the genetic counselor also assessed their level of knowledge about cancer, the impact of early cancers and deaths in the family, and their perception of Mrs. B's risk for cancer. The information they had gathered about the family history and the information obtained in the medical records were recorded in a pedigree, which made it possible to visualize the history and determine if there was a pattern to the cancer occurrences consistent with a hereditary syndrome.

Diagnosis A diagnosis of Lynch syndrome was suspected based on the pedigree analysis, medical history, and physical examination.

While the records on all family members were important because they provided information about the primary sites of cancers, the records of Mrs. B's aunt's first cancer occurrence were especially helpful because they provided documentation about the primary site of her uterine cancer (endometrium), and endometrial cancer is a common site in Lynch Syndrome.

Genetic Counseling

Genetic counseling has been defined as a communication process related to either a medical condition or the risk of its recurrence in which information about the medical and genetic facts is provided and assistance is offered with decision making and adapting to the situation.

Mrs. B was told that the colon and endometrial cancers in her family were most likely due to a mutation in one of the genes known to cause Lynch syndrome. The family was informed that genetic testing might provide the possibility of identifying gene carriers before they were affected with cancer.

Predictive Testing Because of the potential repercussions, DNA testing for a hereditary cancer syndrome is not like most other blood tests. It requires careful consideration by the individual to be tested. Testing is not offered for minors unless there is some definite benefit to be derived, such as in FAP, where there is an increased risk for cancer in childhood.

Another unique aspect about DNA testing is that it is best initiated by a family member who is affected with cancer. While genetic testing for hereditary cancer predisposition is quite accurate, it will not always be informative. This is because of limitations in genetic testing technology, or because a mutation exists in a cancer predisposing gene for which a genetic test is not yet available. This type of testing can help to pinpoint the gene mutation that is responsible for the cancer in the person who has a diagnosis of cancer. Without knowledge of the mutation in the family, a negative result for an unaffected member could mean that the individual did not inherit the mutation, but it could also mean that the mutated gene in the family was beyond the scope of the testing and that the individual is still at high risk of cancer. Figure 3 shows the process of predictive testing.

Informed Consent To ensure the informed consent of the person to be tested, the counselor discusses all aspects of the testing process and the potential impact of the results.

The individual is informed about the test and the limitations of the knowledge that may be derived from the result. For example, a negative result does not equate with no risk because the individual still has the same risk for cancer as the general population. A positive result does not provide any indication of when cancer will occur, if it does. And, although there are laboratory safeguards, there is a chance of technical or human error during the testing. There also is the chance that the result will be inconclusive if the

Figure 3. **Flow Diagram of Predictive Testing**

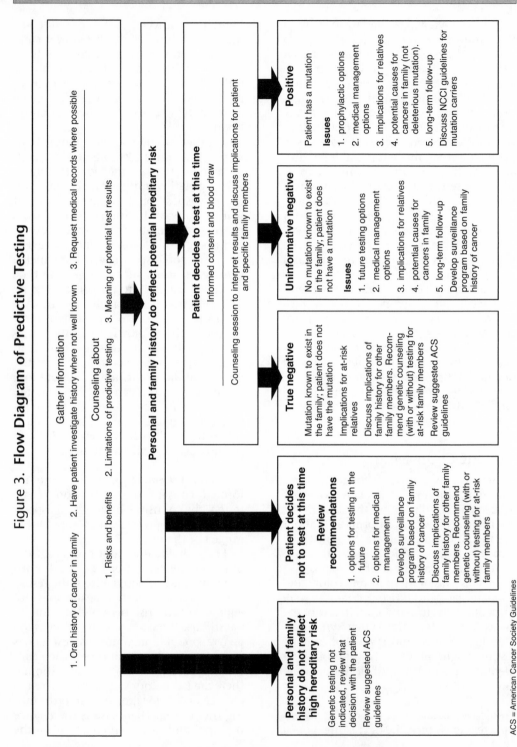

ACS = American Cancer Society Guidelines

family has a mutation that cannot be identified with the test performed.

The counselor will support the individual's right to make the best decision for him- or herself, although there may be pressure from one or more family members to do the opposite of what that individual wishes. A difficult dilemma may arise if a parent without a history of cancer does not want to know his or her status, but an offspring wants to know his or hers. A positive result for the offspring would reveal the parent's status as a gene carrier. In such a situation, family members are encouraged to discuss their positions and come to a mutually satisfying decision.

Costs DNA testing is expensive, often costing $3,000 or more for testing to identify the mutation in the family. Once the mutation is identified, other people in the family can usually be tested for $500 or less. Most insurance companies cover the expense of DNA testing.

Some individuals have questions about health insurance discrimination. To date, there have been no well-documented cases of health insurance discrimination based on results from hereditary cancer genetic testing. The Health Insurance Portability and Accountability Act (HIPAA) protects individuals in group health insurance plans by prohibiting the use of genetic test results to determine eligibility for or rates/cost of health insurance. Most states have additional laws that protect patients from genetic discrimination. Concerns about the potential for genetic discrimination and the use of the results should be discussed as part of the informed consent process.

The potential risks and benefits of both positive and negative results are also part of the informed consent discussion.

Making the Decision Mrs. B and her mother were encouraged to anticipate the impact of a positive result, a negative result, and a decision not to be tested and, in the process, to consider a number of questions:

• Do I cope better with a degree of uncertainty or with all the knowledge available to me?
• If my result is negative, will I feel guilty that others in the family have not been as fortunate?
• If my result is negative, will I feel left out because of the family focus on the risk or occurrence of cancer?
• If my result is positive, will I be able to deal with any sadness or depression?
• If my result is positive, will the fear of cancer interfere with my ability to follow through with the recommended surveillance plan?
• What impact will my results have on the important relationships in my life?
• Will the information gained allow me to consider medical options that are not available or relevant now?

Mrs. H wanted to proceed with the testing for the benefit of her children and her unaffected sister, nieces, and nephews.

After the Results For someone with a history of cancer, receiving a positive result may have different implications than for a family member without such a history. When informed that her test result identified a gene mutation, Mrs. H said she was relieved there would be a better chance for early identification of cancers in the next generation and also talked of her fears for her children who may have received the mutation from her. She then made plans for informing her family.

Genetic counseling includes working toward the best possible adjustment to each situation. For the genetic counselor, this aspect of the counseling process may include providing a supportive presence when times are difficult, helping to negotiate and resolve diverse opinions within a family, and providing referrals to social

Factors in the Informed Consent Decision

	BENEFITS	POTENTIAL RISKS
Negative Results	Relief from anxiety and fear of increased risk of cancer	Regret about decisions made based on the assumption of increased risk
	Avoidance of cost and discomfort of unnecessary surveillance	Survivor guilt
		Changes in family relationships
	Knowledge for making plans for the future	Feelings of alienation from the family
Positive Results	Targeted surveillance recommendations leading to early detection and treatment	Negative psychological impact (depression, anxiety, fear)
		Changes in personal relationships
	Information for making decisions about chemoprevention or preventive surgery options	Worry and guilt about potentially passing the mutation to one's children
	Improved opportunity to plan for the future	
	Increased compliance with surveillance	
	Relief from uncertainty	

workers, psychologists, or support groups. For the patient, it may mean an explanation for the personal and family history, and assistance with understanding and coming to grips with the implications of the test result.

For others, there may not be an answer, but by working together, there may be additional testing or new information that will provide answers for these other high-risk families in the future.

Recommendations for High-Risk Individuals

The ultimate goal of risk assessment and predictive testing is to reduce the morbidity and mortality of cancer in high-risk families. Most of the interventions recommended for this purpose are known to reduce cancer morbidity and mortality. However, a few are unproven at this time, and studies of their effectiveness are under way.

HBOC The current breast cancer screening recommendations for females at risk or known to have a BRCA1 or BRCA2 mutation include breast self-examination every month starting in the late teens and clinical breast examination by a health care provider twice a year. Annual mammography is recommended starting at age twenty-five and alternating with breast MRI, so that one type of scan is completed every six months.

Risk-reducing mastectomy is an option for the woman who considers the breast cancer risk to be too high to consider surveillance alone. Other women consider risk-reducing mastectomies if cancer risk is interfering with quality of life or if they have breasts that are difficult to evaluate by exam or mammography. Studies indicate there is a 90 percent reduction in breast cancer risk among women with a BRCA1 or BRCA2 mutation who have risk-reducing mastectomies. There are also chemoprevention trials using various agents such as tamoxifen (Nolvadex) and raloxifene (Evista) for women at high risk for breast cancer.

Ovarian cancer screening includes twice-yearly transvaginal ultrasound and cancer antigen 125 (CA-125) screening starting at age twenty-five. This screening is not as effective as breast cancer screening in detecting early-stage cancer, so mutation carriers are counseled to consider risk-reducing removal of the ovaries (oophorectomy) and fallopian tubes at age thirty-five or after they have had their children. It is recommended that the risk-reducing salpingo-oophorectomy surgery include a protocol of washings and fine sectioning of all of the tissue in the ovaries and fallopian tubes to rule out the possibility of a microscopic cancer.

Lynch Syndrome It is currently recommended that men and women at risk for Lynch syndrome have their first colonoscopy at age twenty (or ten years younger than the earliest colon cancer in the family, whichever is sooner), then repeat it every one to two years. Over the age of forty, annual colonoscopy is advised. Numerous studies have shown that regular colonoscopy can prevent colorectal cancer. Individuals with Lynch syndrome who are diagnosed with colorectal cancer are encouraged to consider colectomy (removal of the entire colon) when they undergo colon cancer surgery. For some individuals in whom colonoscopy is burdensome, removal of the colon prior to a diagnosis of cancer (called prophylactic colectomy) may be considered.

Women with Lynch syndrome also require annual screening for gynecologic cancers. While these gynecologic screening tests are not proven to prevent cancer, it is hoped that they will help identify cancers when they are at their earliest stages and therefore most curable. Gynecologic cancer screening includes annual biopsy of the endometrium, transvaginal ultrasound, and CA-125 blood tests beginning at twenty-five to thirty years of age. Women who are finished with childbearing are encouraged to consider surgical removal of the uterus and ovaries to prevent gynecologic cancers. Women with Lynch syndrome who are diagnosed with colorectal cancer may also consider hysterectomy and oophorectomy at the time of their colon cancer surgery.

Surveillance for other cancers that occur in Lynch syndrome are not routinely recommended unless there is a known family history of that type of cancer. For example, upper endoscopy is recommended if there is a family member with stomach or small intestine cancer. Chemoprevention trials utilizing agents such as aspirin and celecoxib (Celebrex) have shown mixed results in patients with Lynch syndrome. There is an active effort to identify additional chemopreventive agents for both colon and gynecologic cancers.

Familial Adenomatous Polyposis (FAP) Screening for FAP is initiated with annual colonoscopy by ten to twelve years of age. Upper endoscopy for polyps in the stomach and small intestine is performed every one to three years once colon polyps begin to develop. Prophylactic total colectomy (removal of the colon prior to a diagnosis of cancer) should be performed in all patients when the number and pathology of the polyps becomes unmanageable by colonoscopy. Most patients undergoing total colectomy are able to maintain normal bowel function through either preservation of the rectum or creation of a J-pouch (ileal pouch reconstruction), where the small intestine is used to create an internal reservoir for collecting stool. Following surgery, individuals with FAP still require surveillance of the rectum or pouch, stomach, and duodenum.

Individuals with FAP should also have annual thyroid exams. Chemoprevention trials with sulindac (Clinoril) have shown some promise of preventing the development of polyps, and additional trials with celecoxib are ongoing.

Patient and Professional Responsibilities

Throughout cancer risk assessment, counseling, and predictive testing, the patient and the professional share responsibility for both the process and the outcome.

Patient Responsibilities

• Gather the family-history information.
• Assist in the collection of medical records.
• Ask for clarification or for information to be repeated as necessary.
• Weigh the options and make decisions about genetic testing, use of the genetic knowledge, prophylactic surgeries, etc.
• Share experiences and responses, and allow others to provide support.
• Communicate with family members about the outcome of genetic risk assessment.

Professional Responsibilities

• Listen and hear what the patient is saying and asking.
• Take the time required to give both information and anticipatory guidance about risk reduction and surveillance.
• Present information in understandable terms.
• Provide a balanced view of options, pros, and cons, when the patient has a choice to make.
• Support the decision of the patient.

• Preserve and protect privacy and confidentiality.
• Discuss the implications for other family members and facilitate family communication.
• Provide referrals when the patient's needs are beyond the professional's realm of practice.

Future Directions

The genetic advances of the last twenty years have provided the ability to predict accurately the risk of cancer for members of families with hereditary cancer. Genetic counseling is an integral part of the testing process to reduce the risk of harm and enhance the potential for benefit. It is also instrumental in facilitating the assessment of cancer risk and developing recommendations for other family members.

Further research is needed to improve the genetic risk assessment and counseling process, identify cancer risks associated with specific mutations, and identify the effectiveness of some surveillance and prevention measures as well as develop new ones. The results of a few studies indicate that some high-risk individuals are not following through with the recommendations for cancer screening. Research is needed to identify the most effective ways of overcoming the barriers to screening for these individuals

More must also be done to assure affordable access to counseling, DNA testing, risk reduction, surveillance, and treatment measures for high-risk individuals. Without access for all, there will be no hope of reaching the ultimate goal of cancer prevention through the identification of all families at increased risk for cancer.

— 47 —

Cancer Information

Gail Sorrough, M.L.I.S., and
Gloria Won, M.L.I.S.

■ ■ ■ ■

Information can be a powerful ally in all aspects of cancer prevention, diagnosis, treatment, and supportive care. The development of health and medical information as a consumer commodity combined with the Internet has generated a vast amount of potential resources for retrieving cancer information. The challenges for anyone seeking information about cancer are deciding where to start and sorting out the reliable resources. The objective here is to introduce authoritative, distinguished organizations that have established records of reliability in providing comprehensive cancer information to patients, their loved ones, and the public at large.

Among the oldest and most reliable resources for comprehensive cancer information and support are the American Cancer Society and the National Cancer Institute.

American Cancer Society (ACS)
800-ACS-2345
TTY: 866-228-4327
www.cancer.org

Founded in 1913 as the American Society for the Control of Cancer, this organization became a pioneer in cancer education and information at a time when cancer was not discussed in public or in the media. Today, it has thirteen divisions spread throughout the United States and more than 3,400 local offices charged with providing information about cancer prevention, detection, treatment, and support. The ACS also supports research and is the largest nonprofit source for funding cancer research, second only to the federal government.

The Web site for the ACS is an excellent place to begin looking for answers to your questions about cancer. At this site, you can find information about cancer in general, treatment and treatment decision tools, support groups and services, special health needs of patients and survivors, and clinical trials, as well as information on how to locate a local ACS office in your area. The site also provides links to other reliable resources for cancer information on the Internet.

The ACS facilitates access to cancer information in languages other than English. All of the general cancer information at its site is available in Spanish. In conjunction with the Asian American Network for Cancer Awareness, Research, and Training (*www.aancart.org*), the ACS launched a Web site in 2006 designed to help Asians and Pacific Islanders with limited English skills to access cancer information. The Web site is accessible from the ACS home page at "Asian and Pacific Islander Materials," where users will find information in Chinese, Korean, and Vietnamese, plus links to more Asian language cancer information sources.

National Cancer Institute (NCI) and NCI's Cancer Information Service (CIS)
800-4-CANCER (800-422-6237)
TTY: 800-332-8615
www.cancer.gov
http://cis.nci.nih.gov

The National Cancer Institute, created in 1937, was given new responsibilities and requirements with the National Cancer Act of 1971. The law required that the NCI expand its research program and translate its research findings for use by health professionals, patients, and the general public. Acting on this mandate, the NCI developed the Cancer Information Service, and it has evolved into a comprehensive resource for providing access to information specialists and information on cancer treatments, supportive care, and clinical trials. Through its network of regional offices, CIS now serves the United States, Puerto Rico, and the U.S. Virgin Islands. A list of the regional offices with local information is available at the CIS Web site *http://cis.nci.nih.gov.*

Information Specialists The CIS information specialists answer questions about cancer, providing the most recent and accurate information in easy-to-understand language. These specialists are knowledgeable and experienced at explaining medical information; the service is confidential and a specialist will spend as much time as necessary to provide a thorough response. The specialists can also help you find out about clinical trials, cancer-related services, and other cancer organizations. They cannot provide personal medical consultation and they cannot make referrals to specific physicians.

There are three ways to contact a CIS information specialist:

• Telephone: 800-4-CANCER (800-422-6237; calls answered in English or Spanish from 9:00 A.M. to 4:30 P.M. local time).
• TTY: 800-332-8615 (calls answered in English from 9:00 A.M. to 4:30 P.M. Eastern time).
• Via the Internet: At the *cancer.gov* Web site, click on "Need Help?" and connect to the "LiveHelp" instant-messaging service. This service is available in English, Monday through Friday, from 9:00 A.M. to 11:00 P.M. Eastern time.

The NCI also collaborates with other federal agencies to disseminate information about cancer:

• The Veterans Administration and the NCI provide information on their inter-agency-partnership agreement in clinical trials for cancer: *www1.va.gov/cancer.*
• The FDA Cancer Liaison Program, Office of Special Health Issues, in collaboration with the NCI, answers questions directed to the FDA by participants, their families, and participant advocates about therapies for life-threatening diseases: *www.fda.gov/oashi/cancer/cancer.html.*

Cancer Information—PDQ (Physician Data Query) In fulfilling legislative mandates to disseminate cancer information, the National Cancer Institute has embraced the power of the Internet to provide access to its huge repository of resources on all aspects of cancer. The NCI Web site, *www.cancer.gov,* is essentially a "one-stop" resource for cancer information. A core component of *cancer.gov* is the PDQ database.

The following information about PDQ is directly from the Web site at *www.cancer.gov/cancertopics/pdq/cancerdatabase:* "PDQ is NCI's comprehensive cancer database. It contains peer-reviewed summaries on cancer treatment, screening, prevention, genetics and supportive care, and complementary and alternative medicine; a registry of approximately 5,000 open and 16,000 closed cancer clinical trials from around the world; and directories of physicians, professionals who provide genetics services, and organizations that provide cancer care."

Cancer Information Summaries The PDQ cancer information summaries are peer reviewed and updated monthly by six editorial boards comprised of specialists in adult treatment, pediatric treatment, supportive care, screening/detection, prevention, genetics, and complementary and alternative medicine. The boards review current literature from more than seventy biomedical journals, evaluate its relevance, and synthesize it into clear summaries. Many of the summaries are also available in Spanish.

• *Adult Treatment Summaries* PDQ contains evidence-based summaries that provide prognostic and treatment information on the major types of cancer in adults. Summaries are available for over seventy types of cancer, including a number of brief summaries on less common cancers. Health professional versions of the summaries provide detailed information on prognosis, staging, and treatment for each disease; refer to key citations in the literature; and link to abstracts for the citations. The PDQ adult treatment summaries are also available in patient versions, written in easy-to-understand, nontechnical language.

• *Pediatric Treatment Summaries* PDQ contains prognostic and treatment information on the major types of cancer in children, as well as information on unusual childhood cancers. Health professional versions of the summaries provide detailed information on prognosis, staging, and treatment for each disease; refer to key citations in the literature; and link to abstracts for the citations. All of the PDQ pediatric treatment summaries are also available in patient versions,

written in easy-to-understand, nontechnical language.

• *Supportive Care Summaries* The PDQ supportive care summaries provide descriptions of the pathophysiology and treatment of common physical and psychosocial complications of cancer and its treatment, such as pain, hypercalcemia, and nausea and vomiting. Each health professional version generally contains an overview; information on etiology, assessment, and management; and references to the current literature. Most of the supportive care summaries are also available in patient versions, written in easy-to-understand, nontechnical language.

• *Screening/Detection Summaries* Summaries on screening/detection for many of the common cancers such as lung, colorectal, breast, and prostate, as well as other cancers, are available. The health-professional-oriented summaries contain current data concerning screening/detection for particular disease sites, the levels of evidence for those statements, and the significance and evidence of benefit for the statements, which include supporting references to current literature. Most of the screening/detection summaries are also available in patient versions, written in easy-to-understand, nontechnical language.

• *Prevention Summaries* Summaries on prevention for many of the common cancers such as lung, colorectal, breast, and prostate, as well as other cancers, are available. Health professional versions of the summaries contain current data concerning prevention for particular disease sites, the levels of evidence for those statements, and the significance and evidence of benefit for the statements. Supporting references to current literature are included. Most of the prevention summaries are also available in patient versions, written in easy-to-understand, nontechnical language.

• *Genetics Summaries* The PDQ genetics summaries provide evidence-based information about the genetic basis of certain cancers. Information is given about risk factors related to family history; major genes and syndromes associated with the disease; interventions specific to individuals at high risk; and the ethical, legal, and social issues related to cancer risk counseling and gene testing. An overview of cancer genetics and summaries on the genetics of breast and ovarian cancer, colorectal cancer, medullary thyroid cancer, and prostate cancer are currently available. A summary covering the elements of cancer risk assessment and counseling is also available.

• *Complementary and Alternative Medicine Summaries* The treatments described in these summaries are generally not disease specific. The health professional versions of the summaries contain background information about the treatments; a brief history of their development; information about their proposed mechanism(s) of action; and information about relevant laboratory, animal, and clinical studies. They are also written using language for nonexperts and include glossary links to scientific terms. Most of the summaries are also available in patient versions that are written in question-and-answer formats and include links to definitions of scientific terms. In the future, summaries will be written on complementary and alternative medicine approaches to cancer prevention.

Clinical Trials The National Cancer Institute is the U.S. government's primary agency for managing cancer clinical trials. The following information is produced by the NCI:

The PDQ contains the world's most comprehensive cancer clinical trials database. It includes approximately 2,600 abstracts of trials that are open and approved for accepting patients, including trials for cancer treatment, genetics, diagnosis, supportive care, screening, and prevention. In addition, there is access to approximately 16,000 abstracts of closed clinical trials that have been completed or are no longer accepting patients. Abstracts are written in two formats, the health professional abstract (uses technical terminology) and the patient abstract (uses nontechnical language). However, some trials (obtained from the ClinicalTrials.gov database) contain the same text in both the patient and health professional abstracts.

The NCI's clinical trials database can be searched using a basic search form that allows selection of a type of cancer, stage/subtype, type of trial, and location. It is also possible to search for trials using additional criteria such as type of treatment or intervention, drug name, and phase of trial, or a combination of these, and other variables by using an advanced search form. Help links at the top of each clinical trials search form lead to more information and tips about searching for clinical trials.

In addition to the PDQ clinical trials, the NCI also supports the Clinical Trials Education Series. This series provides self-paced workbooks, slide programs, booklets, and videos to help individuals and health care professionals understand clinical trials. More information about this series may be found at the NCI Web site: *http://nci.nih.gov/clinicaltrials/ resources/clinical-trials-education-series.*

More Information on Finding Clinical Trials

Finding information about all cancer clinical trials requires going beyond the National Cancer Institute's resources. Two other reliable resources on the Internet are ClinicalTrials.gov and the

CenterWatch Clinical Trials Listing Service. In addition to cancer clinical trials, both ClinicalTrials.gov and CenterWatch Clinical Trials Listing Service include a wide range of diseases and conditions.

ClinicalTrials.gov
http://clinicaltrials.gov

The Food and Drug Administration Modernization Act of 1997 triggered creation of the ClinicalTrials.gov Web site. This legislation required establishment of a registry for both federally and privately funded clinical trials concerning serious or life-threatening diseases or conditions. The National Library of Medicine of the National Institutes of Health (NIH) developed the site in collaboration with all NIH institutes and the Food and Drug Administration. The site was launched in February 2000.

Today, ClinicalTrials.gov includes thousands of trials sponsored by NIH, other government agencies, the pharmaceutical industry, national and international universities, foundations, and other organizations. The site provides details about purpose and design of the study, trial phase, the recruitment status, criteria for participation, trial location, and specific contact information.

All of the NCI clinical trials should be accessible via ClinicalTrials.gov; however, the user interface for each database is different. The NCI advises exploring all clinical trials lists to ensure that you retrieve all relevant information.

CenterWatch Clinical Trials Listing Service
http://centerwatch.com

CenterWatch Clinical Trials Listing Service, founded in 1994 by the Thompson Corporation, focuses on the clinical trials industry and provides information services and educational materials on clinical research to patients.

At its Internet site, you can find "Clinical Trials Listings by Medical Areas," which leads you to "Clinical Trials in Oncology." In addition, there is a separate, extensive, regularly updated list of trials being conducted outside the United States. It is called the "International Clinical Trial Listings"; there is a section specific to oncology, and trials are organized by country.

In addition to the lists of trials, CenterWatch also has other clinical-trial-related services and resources for patients. These resources include an e-mail notification service to alert subscribers to new trials or new drugs when they are listed; drug directories that include recent FDA-approved drugs and results of recently completed and ongoing clinical trials; a section about clinical research that provides background on the clinical trials process; links to other relevant Web sites; and a patient bookstore.

Other Major Resources

National Institutes of Health—Health Information
http://health.nih.gov

The Web site of the National Institutes of Health devotes a section to health information that facilitates access to the health information resources of its various institutes. By accessing "Cancer" under "Health Topics A–Z" or "Browse Categories—Conditions/Diseases," you will be linked to cancer information at institutes that have data on your specific cancer topic. For example, selecting "Brain Tumors" from "Health Topics A–Z" leads you to information at the National Cancer Institute, the National Institute of Neurological Disorders and Stroke, the National Library of Medicine, the NIH Clinical Center, and MedlinePlus (NIH's premier consumer health Web site).

National Comprehensive Cancer Network (NCCN)
888-909-NCCN (888-909-6226) for Patient Guidelines
www.nccn.org

The National Comprehensive Cancer Network (NCCN), established in 1995, is a nonprofit alliance of leading cancer centers. Clinical professionals at NCCN member institutions pool their collective expertise to develop and disseminate clinical practice guidelines. A section of their Web site is devoted to information for patients and includes guidelines for treatment by type of cancer and guidelines for supportive care (both of these are available in English and Spanish). Other features for patients include finding NCCN clinical trials, finding physicians at NCCN institutions according to their specialties, and links to other reliable cancer information resources on the Internet.

PubMed
888-FIND-NLM (888-346-3656)
www.pubmed.gov

PubMed is a service of the National Library of Medicine (NLM) that contains over 16 million citations to the professional biomedical literature. PubMed is available to anyone anywhere in the world who has access to the Internet. PubMed also supports free access to many full-text journal articles on-line. The peer-reviewed journal citations accessed through PubMed represent the latest in published biomedical research, including all aspects of cancer. PubMed has a menu-driven interface to guide users through retrieving relevant citations and ultimately the full-text of journal articles. It is highly recommended that novice searchers read the on-line tutorials at the Web site and/or consult a professional medical librarian for assistance.

PART FIVE

Treating the Common Cancers

Adrenal Gland

Orlo H. Clark, M.D., and Malin Dollinger, M.D.

■ ■ ■ ■

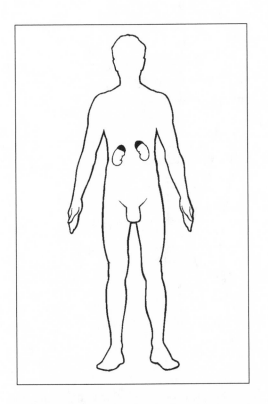

Functioning and malignant tumors of the adrenal gland are rare, but tumors involving the adrenal gland are discovered by CT scanning usually done for another purpose ("incidentaloma") in 1.5 to 8 percent of patients.

The adrenal glands, located just above each kidney, produce a variety of hormones that are essential for life. The central part of the gland—the medulla—produces norepinephrine (noradrenalin), a substance necessary for the transmission of nerve impulses, and epinephrine (adrenaline). The outer part—the cortex—produces four hormones: aldosterone, which regulates salt and water balance; hydrocortisone, which is essential for body metabolism; and both androgens and estrogens, which are the sex hormones in males and females respectively.

When excessive amounts of these hormones are produced, a variety of clinical symptoms can result, including feminization in men, masculinization in women, and the signs of excessive hydrocortisone production (Cushing's syndrome). Tumors of the cortex (aldosteronoma) or of the medulla (pheochromocytoma) produce excessive amounts of aldosterone or norepinephrine/epinephrine respectively, causing sustained or intermittent hypertension. Tumors that produce more than one hormone are frequently malignant.

The vast majority of adrenal tumors are benign, being discovered incidentally either when abdominal ultrasound, CT, or MRI scans are done or because of the effects of hormone overproduction. Malignant adrenal tumors are rare and are usually large ($\geq 2\frac{1}{2}$ inches [6 cm]) but are often treatable and curable when still confined to the gland.

Types Primary tumors of the adrenal gland include a benign tumor (cortical adenoma), which may develop in up to 8 percent of people, often without any symptoms or clinical findings. Other types include adrenocortical carcinoma, pheochromocytoma, neuroblastoma, and ganglioneuroma, as well as a variety of other benign tumors. The adrenal gland is also a common site for metastatic cancer,

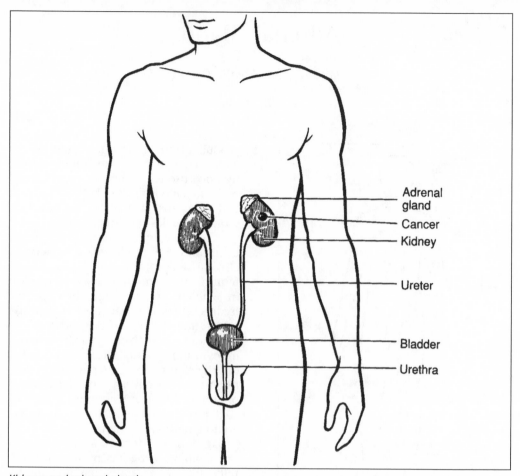

Kidneys and adrenal glands

particularly lung and breast cancers and melanomas.

Benign adrenocortical adenomas are generally less than 2 inches (5 cm) in diameter and, if functional, usually secrete a single hormone, such as hydrocortisone, which causes Cushing's syndrome. The most common malignant tumors, adrenocortical carcinomas, tend to be large and to secrete several hormones. About 30 percent of these are nonfunctioning, meaning that they do not produce hormones. These tumors are usually recognized only after they have grown to a considerable size.

Pheochromocytomas, which are tumors of the adrenal medulla (center), can be either benign (90 percent) or malignant (10 percent). Either type can produce hormones or other substances that may cause headaches and excessive perspiration along with significant health problems and sometimes fatal hypertension, but only the malignant tumors spread to other places. Benign tumors, however, can be bilateral and multifocal.

How It Spreads Adrenal tumors can directly invade nearby tissues and spread to regional lymph nodes. The most common sites for metastases are the lungs, liver, bone, and the other adrenal gland.

What Causes It Unknown.

Risk Factors

People with neurofibromatosis and the von Hippel-Lindau syndrome as well as the multiple endocrine neoplasia, type 2 (MEN-2), syndrome are prone to develop pheochromocytoma. Patients with MEN-1 may develop adrenocortical tumors, which are usually benign. No specific preventive measures exist.

Screening

Because these tumors are so rare, there are no specific screening measures. A physician should suspect some type of adrenal tumor, however, if there are signs of Cushing's syndrome or high blood pressure in the presence of a low blood potassium level, as well as unexplained hypertension, especially if it is severe or difficult to control medically and in patients with a family history of the above risk factors.

Patients with medullary thyroid cancer, von Hipple-Lindau, MEN-2, neurofibromatosis, and hypertension should always be screened for pheochromocytoma prior to stressful procedures. Patients with MEN-2 can also be diagnosed by a blood test for a RET point mutation.

Common Signs and Symptoms

Nonfunctioning tumors—those that don't produce hormones—are frequently discovered by CT or MRI. Patients may also have abdominal masses, often with pain, weight loss, or evidence of metastasis.

The hormonally active tumors produce a variety of symptoms. Women may have signs of masculinization (virilization) such as excess body and facial hair, a decrease in menstrual periods, and enlargement of the clitoris. Breasts can become enlarged in men. Puberty may come early to children. The signs of Cushing's syndrome include swelling of the face, shoulders, and back of the neck, along with bruising and purple lines over the abdomen. Hypertension and signs of diabetes may appear, and osteoporosis and kidney stones are more common.

People with a pheochromocytoma typically have headaches, excessive sweating, attacks of anxiety, and marked or sustained high blood pressure. Hypertensive crises may occur during minor operations or after trauma or exercise. The blood pressure often falls when the person rises from a sitting position. Other symptoms include palpitations and a rapid heartbeat.

Pheochromocytomas can produce other hormones besides norepinephrine, including epinephrine and dopamine, and rarely adrenocorticotropin hormone (ACTH) and corticotropin-releasing factor (CRF), so that some patients may also have Cushing's syndrome. If these tumors occur in both adrenal glands, this may represent a component of multiple endocrine neoplasia (MEN-2), which includes medullary carcinoma of the thyroid gland (see the chapter, "Thyroid") and in some patients (approximately 20 percent) multiple abnormal parathyroid glands.

Diagnosis

With the use of ultrasound, CT, and MRI scanning, adrenal tumors are now being discovered at an earlier stage. In fact, a diagnostic dilemma occurs when an adrenal mass is discovered on routine scanning. Most of these masses are fortunately benign adenomas, but a diagnostic work-up should be done to discover whether the mass produces hormones or is a metastatic or primary cancer.

Pheochromocytomas can occur outside the adrenal gland and may be difficult to find. An extensive search is appropriate for anyone with typical signs and symptoms, even if scans of the adrenals are negative. Most of these tumors can be identified by I-131-MIBG scans, and more than 90 percent are situated in the abdomen or pelvis.

Blood and Other Tests

- Endocrine studies (blood and urine tests)
- Serum chemistry profile

Imaging

- CT, MRI, I-131-MIBG, or ultrasound scan
- Chest X-ray or a bone scan to detect metastatic lesions

Biopsy

- A metabolic work-up must be done before a biopsy to rule out a pheochromocytoma.
- A biopsy cannot distinguish between a benign and a malignant adrenocortical tumor. It is most useful for patients with suspected metastatic disease.
- Alternatively, an accessible metastasis in the lymph nodes or liver, if present, can be biopsied.

Staging

Adrenocortical carcinoma is staged according to the TNM classification indicating the size of the tumor, the degree of invasion into adjacent tissues, and whether it has spread to regional lymph nodes or distant sites.

There is no acceptable staging system for pheochromocytoma other than localized and benign versus malignant and metastatic.

Treatment Overview

Adrenocortical carcinomas are curable if the diagnosis can be made before the tumor is larger than 2 inches (5 cm) and has not spread outside the adrenal gland. At the time of diagnosis, however, most people with adrenocortical carcinomas (70 percent) have Stage III or Stage IV disease. The initial treatment for all stages, even Stage IV, is to surgically remove the entire tumor and adjacent tissues, sometimes including the adjacent kidney. Radiation and chemotherapy may be used as adjuvant treatment after surgery.

The 70 percent of these cancers that produce hormones have a better prognosis than those that don't, but this is probably because the symptoms of excess hormone production lead to an earlier diagnosis. The 20 percent of patients who respond to the drug mitotane also have a better prognosis.

Surgery Removal of the entire tumor is the only treatment that can lead to a cure. This may sometimes also require the removal of the adjacent kidney. As much of the primary tumor as possible is removed, even if all of it can't be, to decrease the amount of hormones produced.

Prolonged remissions have been reported after the removal of metastatic disease in the liver, lung, and brain. As with the primary tumor, even if all the metastases cannot be removed, it may still be beneficial to remove most of them, for this will remove the source of the hormones and these cancers may grow slowly.

Surgery to remove pheochromocytomas requires specific preparation and management before, during, and after the operation. The management of patients with these tumors is complex, and the surgical and medical teams have to be familiar with the specific medical and pharmacologic measures needed to minimize the risk to the patient and control the anticipated complications. The blood pressure may rise significantly during anesthesia or surgery, causing a life-threatening crisis. Laparoscopic adrenalectomy is very effective for removing most adrenal tumors under 2 inches (5 cm), with less blood loss and more rapid recovery.

Radiation There may be an adjuvant role for radiation therapy after an early-stage tumor is removed, although this is still investigational. In more advanced disease, radiation therapy may shrink bone metastases.

Chemotherapy The drug mitotane (Lysodren) is the only chemotherapeutic agent known to be effective in some patients with adrenocortical carcinoma. Monitoring of blood levels is recommended for best results. Combination chemotherapy may also be helpful for patients with Stage IV disease. A recent research study showed that mitotane given in the adjuvant setting (after an operation to remove an adrenocortical carcinoma) results in a significant increase in recurrence-free survival. The lower dose used in this setting was much less likely to produce troublesome toxicity.

Treatment by Stage and Type

Adrenocortical Carcinoma

■ *Stage I*
TNM T1, N0, M0
The tumor is less than 2 inches (5 cm) and does not invade other tissues.

Standard Treatment Complete surgical removal of the tumor

Five-Year Survival 50 percent

Investigational
- Adjuvant radiation therapy
- Adjuvant chemotherapy with mitotane

■ *Stage II*
TNM T2, N0, M0
The tumor is larger than 2 inches (5 cm) but is still not invasive.

Standard Treatment Complete surgical removal, similar to Stage I

Five-Year Survival 30 percent

Investigational Clinical trials of new treatment combinations, especially with radiation therapy and mitotane, are appropriate for some patients.

■ *Stage III*
TNM T1–2, N1, M0 or T3, N0, M0
The tumor has invaded outside the adrenal gland into fat but does not involve adjacent organs (T3), or the regional lymph nodes have become involved (N1).

Standard Treatment The tumor is completely removed, along with any enlarged lymph nodes.

Five-Year Survival 20 percent

Investigational
- Radiation therapy if the tumor cannot be removed but remains localized.
- Chemotherapy with mitotane reduces hormone production and tumor growth and/or recurrence in some patients.
- Clinical trials of new treatment combinations of chemotherapy and radiation therapy may be helpful.

■ *Stage IV*
TNM Any T, any N, M1 or T3–4, N1, M0

Standard Treatment The goal of treatment for an adrenocortical carcinoma that has spread to adjacent organs (a T4 tumor) or has metastasized to distant sites is palliation rather than cure.

Chemotherapy with mitotane and other agents may lead to partial or complete remissions. Other treatment options are radiation therapy to bone metastases and/or the surgical removal of localized metastases, particularly those that produce hormones.

Five-Year Survival Less than 1 percent

Investigational

• Clinical trials are appropriate for patients with metastatic disease or with recurrent cancer.

• Cisplatin seems to benefit some patients with metastases and is being clinically evaluated.

Pheochromocytoma

■ *Localized*
Localized benign pheochromocytoma may be confined to one or both adrenal glands or situated in other (ectopic) locations.

Standard Treatment Before definitive treatment, phenoxybenzamine (Dibenzyline) is given for at least one week to block the action of the hormones produced by the tumor. During this time, the patient should be vigorously hydrated. Treatment with beta-blockers is used for patients with tachycardia after phenoxybenzamine and hydration. Because rather specific, specialized, and vital medical management is essential before surgery or any other treatment is given, an endocrinologist should be involved and surgery done in a major medical center with expertise in endocrine and laparoscopic surgery.

The standard treatment is removal of the tumor (adrenalectomy). Besides the essential preoperative management, blood pressure has to be controlled with specific drugs during surgery and patients must be kept well hydrated to avoid hypotension (low blood pressure) once the tumor is removed. Laparoscopic adrenalectomy is indicated for non-invasive tumors less than $2\frac{1}{2}$ inches (6 cm).

Five-Year Survival Over 95 percent

■ *Metastatic*
The pheochromocytoma has spread to nearby lymph nodes, to adjacent tissues, or to distant sites.

Standard Treatment If the pheochromocytoma has spread, it is still treated with aggressive surgery to remove all visible evidence of disease. This is to reduce the excess hormone production that causes many of the clinical problems these patients have. Long-term medical treatment decreases symptoms due to excess hormones. The same medical preparation used for patients with localized tumors is essential.

A variety of chemotherapy combinations have been used, including cyclophosphamide (Cytoxin) + vincristine (Oncovin) + dacarbazine (DTIC-Dome), which may produce tumor regression and improve symptoms, biochemical markers, and hypertension.

Radiation therapy may improve or palliate local complications caused by metastases.

Five-Year Survival 40 to 45 percent

Investigational

• Clinical trials are under way to find more effective chemotherapy treatments.

• One therapeutic approach for patients whose tumors cannot be removed, have recurred, or have metastasized is targeted radiation therapy with I-131-MIBG. This treatment has resulted in the shrinkage of tumors and a reduction in symptoms in some patients. Unfortunately, it is rarely curative.

Treatment Follow-Up

For adrenocortical carcinomas, treatment follow-up should include

• repeat CT, MRI, or MIBG scanning to assess possible local recurrence or metastases;

• measurement of specific hormones produced by the tumor; and

• studies—such as liver function tests, chest X-rays—to document the status of metastases.

Follow-up for pheochromocytomas should include

• measurements of hormones produced by the tumor by urine tests (VMA, catecholamines, metanephrines);

• abdominal CT or MRI scans to assess the status of the sites of primary tumor;

• bone scans, chest X-rays, and liver function tests to evaluate the status of metastases; and

• routine and regular blood pressure determinations to assess the effects of the hormones produced by the tumor.

Recurrent Cancer

The treatment for recurrent tumors depends on which therapy was initially used and the site of recurrence. Reresection for local recurrence is recommended when possible. Clinical trials evaluating new chemotherapy drugs should be considered for recurrent adrenocortical carcinoma. Recurrent pheochromocytoma is managed in the same way as metastatic disease.

The Most Important Questions You Can Ask

• What hormones are being produced by my tumor?

• Should an endocrinologist be involved in my care?

• Should I be receiving antihypertensive therapy?

• Should my tumor be removed by a laparoscope or by an open approach?

• If the tumor cannot be completely removed, would radiation therapy and/or chemotherapy be helpful?

• What is the role of mitotane and other chemotherapy in my treatment and what are the side effects?

• Can I live for a long time even if the tumor can't be completely removed?

Anus

J. Michael Berry, M.D., Barbara Klencke, M.D.,
and Mark Welton, M.D.

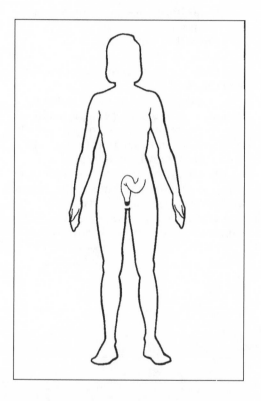

The anus is the external opening farthest from the mouth at the end of the alimentary canal. Composed of skin or squamous cells, it is only one to two inches long and connects to the rectum. The junction of the rectum and the anus is known as the dentate line. The anal canal is lined by an internal sphincter muscle, which opens during defecation. Beneath the skin surrounding the outside of the anus is the external sphincter muscle. Cancer of the anus is much less common than other bowel or colorectal cancers and accounts for only 1 to 2 percent of all cancers of the large bowel and its outlet. The American Cancer Society estimates that 4,650 new cases of anal cancer will occur in the United States in 2007, 1,900 in men and 2,750 in women. However, the rate of anal cancer has steadily been climbing in recent decades, probably related to changes in sexual behavior. The rate of anal cancer is markedly higher in men who have sex with men (MSM) and particularly in people who are immunocompromised, such as those infected with HIV, but in others as well, such as organ transplant recipients.

Anal cancer is highly treatable and often curable, especially in the early stages. The first sign of the cancer is often bleeding, which may be mistaken for hemorrhoids or benign anal disease. Others may report a mass, an ulcer, or pain. But it is also quite common to have no particular symptoms at all; the cancer can be discovered when the doctor or other health care provider carefully examines the inside of the anus, feeling for abnormal lumps or hard areas in patients at risk or experiencing symptoms. Anal cancer may be discovered accidentally when the pathologist routinely examines a specimen from a surgical operation done for apparently benign disease, such as removal of hemorrhoids.

Types The vast majority of all primary cancers of the anus are called squamous cell (epidermoid) carcinomas. These cancers may arise in an area that is visible such as at the anal opening (anal verge) or in the skin around the anus (anal margin), but they most often arise inside the anal canal. In fact, most arise one to two inches internally near the border between the anus and the rectum at the anal transition zone. Squamous cell cancers include a subset of tumors that lack the microscopic features of classic squamous cells. These tumors, known as cloacogenic or basaloid cancers, arise in the anal lining at this transition zone. The biology and prognosis of these tumors appear to be similar to classic epidermoid carcinomas and are currently classified as squamous cell cancers. Well-differentiated tumors have a more favorable prognosis than poorly differentiated tumors.

Other cancer types that may be found in the anus include adenocarcinoma, small cell carcinoma, lymphoma, sarcoma, melanoma, and Paget's disease of the mucous or sweat glands. Adenocarcinoma of the anal canal behaves like and is treated as rectal cancer.

How It Spreads Anal tumors remain confined to the pelvis throughout the disease course in over 80 percent of patients. As the tumor grows, it can extend directly into adjacent tissues, including the skin and sphincter muscle, or may involve adjacent organs such as the prostate, bladder, and vagina. Tumor cells can spread via the lymph system to lymph nodes in the groin (if the tumor is below the dentate line) or to pelvic lymph nodes (if the tumor is above the dentate line). Less commonly, tumor cells can also travel through the bloodstream (metastasize) to other locations in the body such as the lungs, liver, or bone.

What Causes It Human papillomavirus (HPV) causes the majority of anal cancers. HPV is also known to cause cervical, vaginal, vulvar, and penile cancers. HPV is the most common sexually transmitted infection, and up to 75 percent of sexually active adults have been exposed, but most are completely asymptomatic. Many women appear to clear the HPV infection from the cervix, but when it persists, it can lead to abnormal cellular changes known as dysplasia. Cancer develops only in a small proportion of those infected, and it can take years, generally decades, before cancer develops. Formerly, it was believed that cancers were due to chronic irritation of the anus (fistulas, fissures, and inflamed hemorrhoids). There is evidence for an increased risk of anal cancer in patients who have been treated for anal fistulas, fissures, and abscesses. Chronic inflammation and irritation may allow infection with HPV, which then leads to precancerous changes and to anal cancer.

There are many types of HPV. Types 6 and 11 do not cause cancer, but rather cause warts. Genital warts themselves are not dangerous, but they might indicate exposure to other HPV types, such as 16 and 18, which can cause cancer in some people. In June 2006, the FDA approved a vaccine that protects nearly 100 percent of women against cervical infection and dysplasia due to types 6, 11, 16, and 18. The ability of this vaccine to protect against anal infection and prevent anal cancer is being investigated, but is not known at this time.

Anal and cervical cancers are preceded by dysplasia, the result of persistent infection by the same high-risk types of HPV. Dysplasia simply means the growth or presence of abnormal cells that have the potential to progress to cancer in some persons. Cervical dysplasia can be detected by a cervical Pap smear, in which cells are gently scraped off the surface of the cervix as part of the routine annual pelvic exam. The cells are examined by the pathologist and classified as normal, atypical, low-grade or high-grade squamous intraepithelial lesions, or cancer. Low-grade lesions or mild dysplasia include warts and may often go away without treatment. High-grade dysplasia (HGD) is also known as moderate or severe dysplasia or cervical or anal intraepithelial neoplasia (CIN or AIN) 2 or 3. HGD is considered potentially precancerous. Detecting and removing high-grade CIN has dramatically reduced the incidence of cervical cancer. In parts of the world where women do not have access to cervical Pap smears and treatment, many more women die of cervical cancer than those in countries with good screening programs. Sometimes another term, known as carcinoma in situ, is used to describe CIN 3 or AIN 3; this is not cancer and is the same thing as severe dysplasia. Another term used to describe external or perianal high-grade dysplasia (HGD) is *Bowen's disease.*

HGD is a proliferation of abnormal cells infected by HPV that have the potential to progress to cancer in some people. A cancer develops in these vulnerable cells when other genetic changes develop, either serendipitously or as a result of exposure to a noxious agent in the environment, such as tobacco smoke. The lesions consist of abnormal cells, but these cells are not cancer cells and do not invade through the lower membrane that separates the lining cells of the skin or mucous membrane from the muscle and soft tissues underneath. The lesions are often flat and invisible to the naked eye and can be found next to an invasive cancer or within genital warts. When a woman has an abnormal Pap smear, she is referred for colposcopy. Applying vinegar or acetic acid to the cervix makes the lesions appear white so they stand out from the normal tissue and can be detected by using a microscope known as a colposcope. Commonly, a small piece of tissue is removed, which is known as a biopsy. The Pap smear may underestimate the severity of dysplasia present, so the biopsy is the best way to establish a diagnosis. In the same way, the anus can be examined in a procedure known as high-resolution anoscopy (HRA). Far fewer providers are experienced in performing HRA. This procedure was pioneered at the University of California, San Francisco, in the UCSF Anal Neoplasia and Natural History Study.

Anal Pap smears, more appropriately known as anal cytology, have recently been promoted by some as a possible way to screen people at risk for anal cancer. This has yet to become standard practice even for high-risk individuals such as gay men infected with HIV, primarily due to a lack of experienced clinicians and because studies have yet to be performed demonstrating that treatment of anal HGD can prevent anal cancer. There is no treatment for HPV infection, although vaccination at a young age prior to onset of sexual activity may drastically reduce HPV infection and its sequelae.

MSM have a risk for developing anal cancer that is thirty-five-fold higher then expected. Those who are infected with HIV (human immunodeficiency virus), especially those with low immune systems, are at more than twice the risk. Anyone who has anal intercourse may be at slightly higher risk than average for anal cancer, although, by far, most people who develop anal cancer do not report high-risk sexual behavior. HPV is transmitted pretty easily from one person to another and there is likely some degree of self-inoculation. It is thought that HPV probably first infects another part of the genital tract such as the cervix and then migrates to the anus. Thus anal intercourse or other high-risk sexual behavior is not required. In a study from Scandinavia, men whose wives had cervical cancer or cervical HGD had a small but statistically significant increased risk of anal cancer.

Risk Factors

At Significantly Higher Risk

• Anyone infected with the human papillomavirus (HPV), especially the high-risk types such as 16 and 18, or, less commonly, 31, 33, 45, and others, may be at higher risk.

- All HIV-positive persons are felt to be at higher risk. The immunosuppression of HIV may allow the HPV virus to be more active.

- Men who have sex with men are at higher risk through acquisition of HPV through receptive anal intercourse and have a prevalence of anal HPV infection of 60 percent.

- Anal cancer is more common in women over forty and in African-American women.

- Anal margin cancer (cancer involving the tissue encircling the anus) is more common in men.

- There is a possible increased incidence of anal cancer in cigarette smokers.

- The association with a history of chronic anal irritation that was felt for decades to be the primary cause of anal cancer may still be true for some who develop anal cancer. For instance, chronic inflammation and irritation related to fistulas, fissures, and abscesses might allow entry of HPV into the deeper layers of the epithelium. Anal cancer is associated with benign anal disease. Thus, a history of genital warts, also known as condyloma; chlamydia; trichomoniasis; genital herpes; gonorrhea; or anal abscess, fistula, or fissure are all risk factors, but rather than directly causing anal cancer, they suggest that one may have been exposed to HPV.

- Women who have already had an HPV-related problem, such as cervical, vaginal, or vulvar dysplasia or cancer are at higher risk for anal cancer.

- Immunosuppressed individuals such as those with an organ transplant (kidney, liver) and patients who receive chronic immunosuppression or corticosteroids for autoimmune disorders are probably at higher risk in a manner similar to HIV-positive patients.

Screening

Although anal cancer is close to the surface, it is not as easy to detect as one might imagine. A careful anal exam is an important part of a yearly physical. A digital rectal examination and anoscopy should be performed whenever there are rectal symptoms such as pain, bleeding, and itching and hemorrhoidal complaints. A physician with a special interest in anal or rectal disease should examine all patients with hemorrhoids, inflammation, and local anal symptoms. A biopsy should be obtained of any suspicious or persistent lesions in this area.

Given the similarities in this cancer to cervical cancer, anal Pap smears (or anal cytology screening) are proposed as a possible way to screen those without symptoms who may have precancerous lesions. Standards have been established for specimen adequacy. More pathologists, particularly in large urban centers, are becoming experienced at interpreting anal cytology. For the anal Pap test, a moistened Dacron or polyester swab is placed just inside the anus and rotated as it is withdrawn to obtain samples of cells for analysis. Any level of abnormality is considered an indication for referral for high-resolution anoscopy (HRA). In fact, screening is not recommended unless someone experienced in HRA is available to follow up on the results.

A colposcope is a microscope that is used to examine the anal canal and surrounding tissue after applying acetic acid. While there are many doctors in gynecology who are expert in the recognition of cervical dysplasia (found during colposcopy as opposed to high resolution anoscopy), there are few doctors expert in the recognition of anal dysplasia, but more are being trained. Without the use of vinegar or acetic acid to highlight abnormal cells, an inexperienced health care provider may notice nothing unusual in the exam even when severe dysplasia is present. If anal dysplasia is recognized, a biopsy will be taken and examined by a pathologist to confirm the presence of dysplasia, to exclude the presence of an early invasive cancer, and to grade any dysplasia as mild, moderate, or severe.

If moderate or severe dysplasia is confirmed, the area can be ablated in a simple office procedure using infrared coagulation. The IRC2100 infrared coagulator (Redfield Corporation, Rochelle Park, N.J.) has been used extensively since 2002 to treat anal HGD and condyloma. Historically, patients were treated with radical excisions requiring skin grafts and often developed recurrences. Using HRA, destruction of the abnormal lesions can be targeted and the areas most worrisome for cancer can be biopsied. Although anal surgery is often difficult and painful, patients recover within a few weeks. And although recurrences may occur, they can often be managed in the office. In fact, the recovery after office-based infrared coagulation is much easier and there is increasing evidence regarding the effectiveness of infrared coagulation in treating anal HGD. Current techniques have begun to make the prevention of anal cancer a reality, but formal large randomized studies demonstrating the effectiveness of this approach in preventing anal cancer have yet to be performed. Patients who have been diagnosed with anal HGD should be monitored with careful exams every three to four months by clinicians experienced in managing anal dysplasia.

One might wonder if there is a way to test for the presence of the human papillomavirus, particularly the higher-risk HPV types. HPV testing is currently available, but its usefulness in managing anal dysplasia is not clear. In risk groups with a high prevalence of HPV infection such as HIV-positive MSM, it probably is not helpful. However, in patient groups who do not have a high prevalence, but who may be at increased risk, a negative HPV test combined with a negative

anal cytology may indicate an individual who does not need to be seen as frequently. The vaccine that has recently been approved for prevention of cervical cancer may help to prevent anal cancer as well, but the studies demonstrating effectiveness will not be completed until 2008 or 2009.

Common Signs and Symptoms

There are often no symptoms of anal cancer in its early stages. But there may be bleeding, discomfort or pressure, pain, itching, or a palpable anal mass. There may also be local pain or pressure that is not relieved by a bowel movement. Small amounts of anal bleeding not associated with anemia are often attributed to hemorrhoids, and thus the recognition of the cancer is often delayed. If the tumor enlarges enough, eventually a change in bowel habits such as constipation or alternating diarrhea and constipation may be noted. In rare cases, a complete obstruction of the bowel might develop.

Diagnosis

Physical Examination

• Digital rectal exam is important to document the size and location of the tumor. An exam with local or general anesthesia may be necessary. Virtually all patients diagnosed with anal cancer have an abnormality that can easily be felt, which makes the digital exam the best way to detect anal cancer.

• A small anal mass, often like hemorrhoids, may be found. Sometimes the mass protrudes and reaches a significant size. The mass is generally firm and can even feel rock hard.

• Physical examination will attempt to determine if there has been local invasion into the muscle sphincter. The exam may reveal firmness or immobility of structures.

• Enlarged lymph nodes in the groin may indicate metastases. This is a finding that suggests very advanced anal cancer and is associated with a poor prognosis.

Blood and Other Tests

• Complete blood count.
• Liver function chemistries (alkaline phosphatase, LDH, AST).
• CEA (carcinoembryonic antigen), elevated in colon and rectal cancers, is normal in anal tumors. There is no comparable blood test that is useful as a tumor marker for anal cancer.
• Tests of kidney function (creatinine).
• An HPV test for the human papillomavirus, even if available, does not change the prognosis or management and thus is not routinely performed.
• Test for hidden blood in the stools.
• Anal Pap smears can be performed any time that anal cancer is suspected, but often do not detect the presence of cancer. If cancer has already been diagnosed with a biopsy, anal cytology does not provide any additional information.

Imaging

• CT and MRI scans of the pelvis to assess local invasion and whether the iliac and groin (inguinal) lymph nodes are involved (30 percent of patients have inguinal metastases).
• Endoanal ultrasound may help assess the size of the tumor, the extent of invasion into the sphincter muscle, and whether lymph nodes surrounding the rectum have been involved. This is a specialized procedure that is becoming more widely used. The lymph nodes in the pelvis need to be evaluated nonetheless and thus the CT or MRI of the pelvis is necessary.
• New data suggests that a positron-emission tomography (PET)/CT scan may be useful for evaluating the tumor and lymph nodes. In this study, sugar that is bound to a radioactive tag is injected and concentrates in tissues that are metabolically more active, such as cancer cells.
• Abdominal CT scan or ultrasound, especially if the liver is enlarged or if liver function tests are abnormal. However, less than 10 percent will have liver metastases at the time of diagnosis.
• Chest X-ray in order to screen for pulmonary metastases.

Anoscopy and Biopsy A biopsy of the abnormal area is mandatory to establish the diagnosis and verify the type of cancer before treatment is begun. If this cannot be done in the office, then an examination under anesthesia may be necessary. The tumor size is best determined by a physical examination rather than a scan.

Staging

The stage of anal cancer describes whether the cancer has remained within the anus, has spread to lymph nodes near the anus, or has spread to other sites, usually within the abdomen or other organs. The stage as defined by the TNM (tumor, node, metastases) classification is important in determining the initial treatment options, prognosis, and the probability of cure.

T represents the size of the tumor and whether it has invaded adjacent organs; involvement of the sphincter muscle without invasion of adjacent organs does not classify the tumor as a T4 or more advanced tumor, nor does invasion of the rectal wall, perianal skin, or subcutaneous tissue.

Tumor size is described in the following manner:

Tx: Tumor size cannot be determined.
T0: No evidence of tumor.
Tis: Carcinoma in situ (no evidence of invasion, a potentially precancerous lesion).
T1: Tumor is less than ¾ inch (2 cm).
T2: Tumor is greater than than ¾ inch (2 cm) but less than 2 inches (5 cm).

T3: Tumor is greater than 2 inches (5 cm).

T4: Tumor of any size that invades adjacent organs such as the vagina, urethra, and bladder.

N indicates whether the cancer has spread to any of the nearby lymph nodes and is described in a similar fashion:

Nx: Lymph nodes cannot be assessed.

N0: No involvement of any lymph nodes.

N1: Spread to perirectal lymph nodes (located around the rectum in the pelvis).

N2: Spread to unilateral internal iliac or inguinal lymph nodes (located only on one side of the body [unilateral] either next to the main blood vessel deep in the pelvis [iliac] or in the groin or crease of the leg [inguinal]).

N3: Spread to perirectal and inguinal lymph nodes or to bilateral internal iliac or inguinal lymph nodes (involving both left and right sides of the body).

M indicates whether the cancer has spread to other organs such as the liver, lungs, or bone:

Mx: Spread of the cancer cannot be assessed.

M0: No evidence of spread to distant organs.

M1: Spread to distant organs.

The *T, N,* and *M* are combined to determine the stage of the cancer:

STAGE	T	N	M
0	Tis	N0	M0
I	T1	N0	M0
II	T2 or T3	N0	M0
IIIA	T1–T3	N1	M0
	T4	N0	M0
IIIB	T4	N1	M0
	Any T	N2 or N3	M0
IV	Any T	Any N	M1

Treatment Overview

Surgery, radiotherapy, and chemotherapy have all been used to treat anal cancer. More than thirty years ago, it was first noted that chemotherapy and radiation therapy might work so well that radical and extensive surgery could be avoided. This has since become the standard treatment approach for most patients. A major mechanism of chemotherapy is to sensitize the tissues to the effects of radiation therapy and improve the effect of the radiation. The chemotherapy also has an effect on any cancer cells that might have spread but were still too small to be detected by common imaging tests. Therefore, patients treated with the combination of radiation and chemotherapy generally do better than patients treated with surgery or radiation alone.

The prognosis depends on the size and location of the tumor. The outlook is more favorable if the tumors are small (less than 2 inches [5 cm]) and there is no lymph node involvement or invasion into adjacent organs. The prognosis may be better if the primary tumor is in the anal margin (skin around the anal opening) rather than the anal canal. Primary tumors less than $3/4$ inch (2 cm) in size have an even better prognosis, as do tumors that are well differentiated (more mature) rather than undifferentiated or poorly differentiated.

Large studies have shown that chemotherapy added to radiation therapy provides a higher chance of cure than radiation therapy alone. Similarly, when one receives combination chemotherapy (administering two or more drugs) as opposed to single agent chemotherapy, again in combination with radiation, the effect is better. However, there is a fair amount of acute toxicity associated with this therapy. As the intensity of therapy increases, the cure rate increases—but so does the toxicity. The most difficult and common problem is the painful radiation burns of the genital skin and anus. While these generally heal well, patients are occasionally left with a chronic anal injury known as radiation proctitis or an ulcer that never heals. In studies, 6 to 12 percent of patients will require a colostomy (the bowel is diverted through the abdominal wall and empties into a bag) in order to manage the chronic toxicity. Even in the absence of severe injury like this, most subjects will have some mild impairment of anal function or overall quality of life in the years following this treatment, yet patients overwhelmingly prefer this to the idea of losing their anus. The tolerability of the therapy is even less in those who are infected with the human papillomavirus, especially in those with low immune systems such as those with a CD4 lymphocyte count of less than 200, but radiation and chemotherapy remain the standard of care for HIV-positive patients with invasive anal cancer.

A new way of delivering radiation that is becoming increasingly used is known as intensity-modulated radiation therapy (IMRT). This technique uses sophisticated modeling techniques guided by CT scan images of the patient to design a unique treatment regimen for each patient. The theoretical advantage is that a higher dose of radiation can be delivered to the tumor, while the normal tissues surrounding the cancer are spared from the effects of the radiation, therefore minimizing some of the side effects and toxicity.

Prior to the discovery that combined modality therapy was an effective treatment for anal cancer and was able to preserve the function of the anus, the standard of care was a radical operation known as an abdominoperineal resection (APR), with removal of the anus and placement of a colostomy. For patients who do not respond to combined modality therapy or who develop local recurrences, an APR provides a chance for cure in 40 to 50 percent of patients. An APR will result in a loss of anal function, a colostomy, and possibly urinary and/or sexual malfunction. An APR may be performed for those who are not likely to tolerate combined modality therapy such as the elderly, the infirm, or those with advanced HIV infection.

Following complete eradication of the tumor by radiation and chemotherapy, careful follow-up is vital. The lymph nodes in the groin have to be watched carefully, since the most common site of local recurrence is in the pelvis and lymph nodes. If the tumor recurs, salvage surgery may be needed.

Treatment of the less common adenocarcinoma involving the upper portion of the anus (near the rectum) differs from treatment of squamous carcinoma. Treatment recommendations should follow the recommendations for rectal cancer.

Options by Size of Tumor The success of combined modality therapy (CMT) for anal cancer (meaning radiation combined with chemotherapy) depends on the size of the tumor, the degree of local invasion, and the presence or absence of lymph node involvement. Some recommend less intensive treatment for those with smaller tumors because the cure rate can be fairly good without risking the added toxicity. While cure rates in the range of 70 to 90 percent are achievable with radiation therapy alone for very small tumors, the cure rate is even greater when combined modality therapy is used.

• Carcinoma in situ is not invasive cancer and should not be treated with radiation and chemotherapy. The treatment of choice for carcinoma in situ, also known as a high-grade dysplasia (HGD) or severe dysplasia, is excision and fulguration guided by high-resolution anoscopy or ablation using infrared coagulation for small lesions that are not suspicious for invasive cancer.

• Superficially invasive cancers are tumors in which the depth of invasion is very shallow—less than 3 mm. These early cancers may be treated with excision and fulguration in selected patients. Patients must be followed closely and are at high risk for recurrent HGD or precancerous lesions and for recurrent or second cancers. If recurrent cancer cannot easily be removed without compromising sphincter function, then patients should be referred for CMT.

• Small tumors—those that measure less than $3/4$ inch (2 cm) and that are not deeply invasive into the sphincter muscle—*can* be treated with local excision or radiotherapy alone. A risk of local surgery alone is that microscopic involvement of lymph nodes may be present. Left untreated, they might be hard to detect until they are advanced. Removing the groin lymph nodes as a prophylactic measure does not improve these results and often contributes to lymphedema. If radiation alone (without chemotherapy) were used, and if the cancer were to relapse, a major surgery (APR) would then be required. Therefore many doctors recommend combined modality therapy even for small tumors so as to provide the very best treatment up front. If more conservative treatment is to be used, it may be best reserved for those with well-differentiated tumors or tumors in the anal margin and for patients who are likely to return regularly for close follow-up.

• Tumors measuring $3/4$ to 2 inches (2 to 5 cm) are *best* treated by chemotherapy (5-fluorouracil + mitomycin, or 5-FU + cisplatin) plus radiotherapy, leaving surgery for "salvage" therapy. This is the standard of care for anal cancer.

• Tumors larger than 2 inches (5 cm) are treated similarly, using combined modality therapy. Investigational studies are under way with the goal of improving outcome in these patients with a poorer prognosis. Although treatment with chemotherapy prior to starting radiation had seemed successful by adding two cycles of chemotherapy (using 5-FU + cisplatin) before the start of combined therapy, recent data suggest that this is not helpful. There was no improvement using this approach compared with the standard 5-FU + mitomycin combined with radiation therapy.

Options by Lymph Node Status The lymph nodes in the groin (inguinal), pelvis, and perirectal area may become involved by anal cancer.

• Usually the inguinal lymph nodes are treated prophylactically for a portion of the radiation, even for small tumors less than $3/4$ inch (2 cm).

• When lymph nodes can be felt, a higher dose of radiation is delivered to the involved lymph nodes along with chemotherapy. Palpable groin node involvement suggests advanced disease, and involvement by cancer can be verified by performing a fine needle aspiration of the lymph node. Patients with involved lymph nodes are less likely to be cured with CMT, but some patients do quite well.

• Surgical removal of groin nodes (lymph node dissection) can be done for palliation of local symptoms.

Treatment by Stage

■ Stage 0
TNM Tis, N0, M0
Carcinoma in situ—a very early, microscopic, noninvasive cancer that has not spread below the basement membrane, or the bottom layer of anal epithelium. This is also known as severe dysplasia or anal intraepithelial neoplasia 3.

Standard Treatment Surgical removal of the tumor or lesion and treatment of any other areas of HGD.

Five-Year Survival 100 percent

Stage I
TNM T1, N0, M0
A tumor less than $\frac{3}{4}$ inch (2 cm) that may invade the sphincter muscle, but with no evidence of spread to lymph nodes or other organs.

Standard Treatment Small tumors of the skin around the anus and of the anal margin are treated by chemotherapy and radiation, with a 95 percent or higher success rate. Occasionally, if the tumor can be removed without compromising the sphincter and getting a margin of normal tissue around the cancer, surgery may be an acceptable option. Patients must be followed very carefully for evidence of recurrence.

Occasionally, radiation therapy is used alone for small lesions, particularly if there is a contraindication to chemotherapy.

Combination chemotherapy with 5-fluorouracil + mitomycin with primary radiation therapy (CMT) is considered the standard of care. CMT is more effective for larger lesions than radiation therapy alone, and patients are less likely to need surgery and a colostomy and more likely to be cured. 5-FU + cisplatin is an alternative chemotherapy combination with radiotherapy, though the role of cisplatin is less established than that of mitomycin. Both combinations seem to be equally effective. There may be less hematologic toxicity using cisplatin. A recent study evaluated the role of giving chemotherapy before the radiation as a form of induction therapy to shrink the tumor, thinking that this might improve the effectiveness of the radiation. This study used 5-FU + cisplatin for two cycles before the radiation and then repeated it with the radiation. This regimen was compared to the standard of 5-FU + mitomycin given with radiation. The induction therapy with 5-FU + cisplatin was not better than just giving 5-FU + mitomycin with the radiation. Patients treated with the induction chemotherapy required more colostomies than those treated with the standard therapy, although the proportion of patients who were alive five years after therapy was similar in both groups.

The standard approach prior to thirty years ago—an abdominoperineal resection (APR), which involves removal of the anus and rectum and requires a colostomy—is now rarely used except for recurrent disease. If there is still tumor in the anal canal after chemotherapy and radiation, then surgical removal may be necessary, ranging from simple excision with sphincter preservation for very small recurrences to a complete APR with colostomy.

Five-Year Survival Over 95 percent

Stage II
TNM T2–3, N0, M0
T2 tumors are larger than $\frac{3}{4}$ inch (2 cm) but less than 2 inches (5 cm). T3 tumors are ones that measure more than 2 inches (5 cm), but do not involve adjacent organs.

Standard Treatment Current treatment is combination chemotherapy with 5-FU + mitomycin or 5-FU + cisplatin plus radiation therapy. Depending on how much the tumor shrinks once the minimum radiation dose has been given, which is usually 45 Gy, a boost dose directly to the cancer or involved nodes of 10 to 14.4 Gy may be given. Usually higher doses are used for T3 tumors.

Five-Year Survival 79 percent for T2 and 53 percent for T3

Stage IIIA
TNM T1–3, N1, M0 or T4, N0, M0
The cancer has spread to nearby lymph nodes or has invaded nearby organs such as the vagina, urethra, or bladder (it is often hard to determine Stage IIIA, since many patients clinically appear to be Stage II).

■ *Stage IIIB*

TNM T4, N1, M0 or any T, N2–N3, M0

The cancer has spread to the internal iliac and/or groin lymph nodes on one or both sides or has spread to adjacent organs such as the vagina, urethra, and bladder. Metastatic disease to the groin (inguinal) nodes is a poor prognostic sign and markedly reduces the chance for cure, although cure is still possible.

Standard Treatment Current treatment is combination chemotherapy with 5-FU + mitomycin or 5-FU + cisplatin plus radiation therapy. Usually higher doses of radiation are used to treat these tumors. The involved lymph nodes also receive a higher dose of radiation. Once treatment is completed, patients are followed carefully every few months. In some cases, the tumor will continue to shrink after the radiation and chemotherapy have finished. Previously, biopsies were done to document response at the end of treatment, but in some cases there was poor healing after these biopsies. Today, most people only biopsy if the tumor begins to grow or if there is some reason to think that it did not completely respond to the treatment.

Five-Year Survival 20 to 60 percent (Stage IIIA)

Five-Year Survival 20 percent (Stage IIIB)

Investigational for Stages I–III Currently there is a trial enrolling patients with anal cancer in Europe that seeks to compare four different treatment strategies: radiation combined with 5-FU + mitomycin versus 5-FU + cisplatin versus the same two strategies followed by two cycles of maintenance chemotherapy with 5-FU + cisplatin. This study may help to answer the question of which is better: mitomycin or cisplatin. Another multisite study in the United States is evaluating the addition of cetuximab (Erbitux) to cisplatin, 5-FU, and radiation. Cetuximab is a monoclonal antibody directed against a protein known as epidermal growth factor

receptor (EGFR) that is found on the surface of some cells. Inhibiting EGFR may help cancer cells to stop growing. This monoclonal antibody has been approved for treatment of colorectal cancer, and some studies have demonstrated improvement in patients with squamous cell cancers of the head and neck. Another trial is recruiting HIV-positive patients with anal cancer and is evaluating cetuximab combined with cisplatin, 5-FU, and radiation.

For locally advanced cancers (large T2, T3, or T4), investigators are comparing radiation combined with traditional 5-FU + mitomycin to the combination of mitomycin + cisplatin given with radiation. Another study is evaluating an oral drug known as capecitabine (Xeloda) that is converted by the body to 5-FU along with a drug related to cisplatin known as oxaliplatin (Eloxatin) combined with radiation in patients with locally advanced anal cancer.

For current information on available clinical trials, please check *www. clinicaltrials.gov.*

■ *Stage IV*

TNM Any T, any N, M1

The cancer has spread to the tailbone (sacrum), to distant lymph nodes within the abdomen far from the original cancer site, or to other organs in the body such as the lungs, liver, and/or bone.

Standard Treatment There is no standard treatment for patients with metastatic anal carcinoma. Relieving the symptoms produced by the primary cancer is the major consideration because this is generally not a curable condition.

Palliation Treatment options include palliative surgery, palliative radiation, and palliative combined chemotherapy and radiation.

• Abdominoperineal resection is sometimes needed to control pain, bleeding, or infection caused by tumor breakdown.

• Radiation has helped control pain and bleeding. The use of radiosensitizing chemotherapy such as 5-FU may improve local control.

• Endoscopic laser treatment has been used to reduce local tumor obstruction and also, sometimes, to control bleeding.

• Combination chemoradiotherapy with 5-FU + mitomycin or 5-FU + cisplatin as well as investigational combinations can be considered.

Five-Year Survival Unusual

Investigational This is an uncommon disease and one for which the initial therapy is fairly successful, thus there are few trials looking at new agents specifically for this disease. Investigational agents that are being tested for advanced cancer are probably one's best choice for experimental therapy.

Treatment Follow-Up

Careful follow-up is essential. This includes a history and physical examination every two to three months for three years after treatment, then every three to six months for the next three to five years.

• A digital rectal exam to feel for evidence of the tumor returning is the most important part of the exam. A recurrence of the cancer in the same location is known as a local relapse. The majority of recurrences occur within the first two years. An abdominoperineal resection (APR) or removal of the anus may cure about half of patients.

• Careful observation for signs of enlarged inguinal lymph nodes.

• Chest X-rays and liver blood tests (alkaline phosphatase, SGOT) at intermittent follow-up visits. This is less important, as there is little benefit to early recognition of metastatic disease.

• CT scans of the abdomen and pelvis are often performed every six months for the first five years, particularly in patients with T3 or T4 tumors.

Recurrent Cancer

There are two reasons for aggressive treatment of a tumor that recurs after nonsurgical therapy: cure and palliation. Repeat staging studies to determine the extent of the cancer are required to help define the expectations of treatment. Cure is the goal whenever possible, but this is in general limited to situations when the recurrent tumor is amenable to surgical removal. In part, this is because resistance to chemotherapy and radiation therapy may now be present. Occasionally, but not very often, radiation therapy can be delivered to a previously treated area. If one has previously received 5-FU or 5-FU + mitomycin, then 5-FU + cisplatin can be tried along with a small boost of radiation therapy whenever possible. This may be successful enough to spare surgery in some cases. However, more often an APR is required. Even if distant metastatic disease is present, the same approach may be used to palliate symptoms related to recurrent tumor within the pelvis. If the tumor is not removable, then a variety of approaches may be considered, but none offer long-term control. Options may include endoscopic laser treatments, hyperthermia, radiation implants, the addition of various chemotherapy drugs, and intraoperative radiation therapy combined with an attempt at surgical resection.

The Most Important Questions You Can Ask

• Are we certain that I have anal cancer? Is it a squamous cell cancer?

• How should the anal cancer be further evaluated?

• What is the stage of my cancer and how does it affect my prognosis?

• For women, are there any signs of other HPV-related lesions in the cervix, vagina, or vulva?

• What are the side effects of radiotherapy and of chemotherapy?

• Is intensity-modulated radiation therapy (IMRT) appropriate for my cancer?

• Is there a clinical trial that I should consider?

• What new advances in therapy are being used to reduce the need for a colostomy?

• How will this treatment affect my long-term quality of life and sexuality?

Bile Duct

Alan P. Venook, M.D.

■ ■ ■ ■

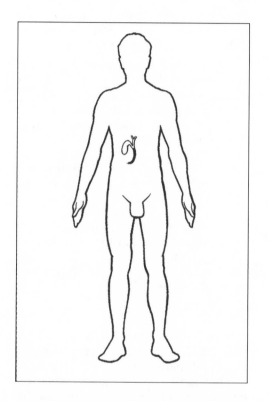

Bile duct cancer—also called cholangio-carcinoma—is a rare cancer. Bile is manu-factured in the liver and helps the body digest fats. The bile ducts course through-out the liver collecting bile, then travel beyond the liver to connect with the gall-bladder and small intestine (see page 599). Bile duct cancers may, therefore, arise in many locations in and around the liver.

A patient's prognosis depends largely on where the tumor begins and how large it has grown by the time of diagno-sis. The only definitive treatment is the complete surgical removal of the tumor, which is not often possible. If the cancer cannot be entirely removed, the princi-pal goals of therapy become the relief of symptoms caused by the accumulation of bile, and relief from pain.

Types The vast majority of these tumors develop in glandular tissue within the bile duct (adenocarcinoma). Other tissue types include squamous carcinomas and sarcomas. The therapy for all types of bile duct cancer is the same, depending on the extent of the tumor at the time of diagnosis.

How It Spreads Bile duct cancer tends to spread into the adjacent liver, along the bile duct surface, and through the lymph system to lymph nodes in the region of the liver (porta hepatis). Tumors in the bile duct leading from the gallbladder to the common bile duct (cystic duct) can spread to involve the gallbladder. Ultimately, other lymph nodes may become involved, as well as other organs within the abdomen.

What Causes It The cause is unknown. People with chronic inflammatory pro-cesses, such as ulcerative colitis and parasitic infections of the bile ducts, are at higher risk for developing this cancer. But no one cause has been clearly demonstrated.

Risk Factors

At Significantly Higher Risk

• People chronically infected with the liver fluke *Clonorchis sinensis*, which is prevalent in parts of Southeast Asia, may develop bile duct cancer. People may become infected with this parasite by eating raw or pickled freshwater fish from this region. Most people with this infection do not develop cancer.

• People with chronic ulcerative colitis have a higher incidence of both benign inflammatory processes of the bile ducts (sclerosing cholangitis) and bile duct cancer.

• People with congenital abnormalities of the bile ducts (choledochal cysts) are more likely to develop bile duct cancer.

Screening

There are no screening methods to detect bile duct cancer at an early stage.

Common Signs and Symptoms

There are no signs or symptoms unique to bile duct cancer. It usually develops slowly and the symptoms are often very subtle. Jaundice (the skin turning yellow) and itching are the most common signs. Jaundice is caused by the accumulation in the skin of a component of bile (bilirubin) that normally empties into the intestines after traveling through the bile ducts.

Bloating, weight loss, decreased appetite, fever, nausea, or an enlarging abdominal mass are all signs that may be attributable to bile duct cancer. Pain usually signifies advanced disease.

Diagnosis

Physical Examination There are no specific findings on physical examination. Even if the findings associated with bile duct cancer are present, other explanations are far more likely. Findings may include

• jaundice,
• fever,
• a tender mass below the ribs on the right side of the abdomen,

• enlarged, hard lymph nodes, and
• swelling of the legs (edema) and fluid in the abdomen (ascites).

Blood and Other Tests Diagnostic tests are usually done to determine the cause of jaundice. These tests may lead to the diagnosis of bile duct cancer, but a simple gallstone or other illnesses can cause the same problems and are much more likely to be the cause of the jaundice.

• A complete blood count may reveal a decrease in hemoglobin (anemia). A normal white blood cell count makes an infection in the bile duct (cholangitis) less likely, but an increased white count raises the likelihood of infection or cancer.

• Liver function tests may be abnormal, with the likeliest abnormalities being in the serum bilirubin and alkaline phosphatase, reflecting a blockage of flow within the bile duct.

• PT and PTT (prothrombin time and partial thromboplastin time) are tests of clotting that may reveal a disorder in patients with poor liver function caused by an obstructed bile duct.

Imaging

• Abdominal ultrasound images of the gallbladder and bile ducts may reveal an enlargement of the bile ducts behind the blockage, since these channels will enlarge (dilate) when the pressure within the drainage system increases.

• PTC (percutaneous transhepatic cholangiography) involves taking an X-ray after a dye has been injected through the skin into the bile ducts. This can make a "road map" of the bile ducts within and outside the liver and may establish the site of the blockage.

• ERCP (endoscopic retrograde cholangiopancreatography) may be done to investigate the cause of an elevated bilirubin. This technically difficult procedure involves passing an endoscope through the mouth and into the small intestine. The physician operating this scope (endoscopist) identifies the site within the intestines where the bile and pancreatic ducts empty their contents. By injecting dye into this opening and doing an X-ray, a "road map" of the bile ducts may be made. PTC and ERCP may both be necessary to completely define the site and cause of an obstruction and will correctly predict the presence of a cancer about 90 percent of the time.

• MRCP (magnetic resonance cholangiopancreatography) is a newer radiologic technique that, in some centers, may replace ERCP as a means of imaging the bile ducts. MRI (magnetic resonance imaging) may be helpful in determining if the bile duct cancer can be surgically removed.

• CT scanning assesses the extent of the tumor within the bile duct and its extension into the adjacent liver, the lymph nodes, or other structures within the abdomen. Often, bile duct cancer is not seen on a CT scan.

• If the diagnosis of cancer is confirmed or suspected, a chest X-ray should be done to look for tumor nodules in the lungs that would confirm the distant spread of the cancer.

Endoscopy and Biopsy Biopsy, either with a fine needle (FNA) or a regular needle, can be done through the skin without significant danger or through the scope when ERCP is done. The tumor cells may also be found in the bile. They are characteristic, and their presence may help decide whether surgery should be performed if the other studies also suggest the tumor has spread. It can be difficult to obtain an adequate biopsy sample because the tumors are often small and lie within normal liver tissue.

Staging

A TNM staging system is used for bile duct cancer, but when deciding which treatment option to use, there are really only two stages—localized and unresectable disease.

Treatment Overview

The optimal treatment for bile duct cancer is surgery. Unfortunately, by the time symptoms develop, the cancer has usually spread throughout the bile ducts and into the liver, meaning that the tumor cannot be entirely removed.

Chemotherapy and radiation therapy are occasionally useful to relieve symptoms. Although they have not been shown to be effective in curing the cancer, these measures can be taken to maintain the quality of life.

 Surgery The decision to take a surgical approach depends on the overall health of the patient and on the location of the tumor. If a patient is ill from complications of the cancer—jaundice or infection, for example—a drainage tube (stent) should be placed in the bile ducts to treat the complications. The patient then has to be allowed to recover before an operation is attempted.

If the tumor is in either the left or the right bile duct and has not spread to the lymph nodes, it may be possible to remove the tumor with its accompanying lobe of the liver because people with normal liver function do not need both lobes.

Tumors involving the junction of the right and left bile ducts (Klatskin tumor) create more problems. The tumor may not have spread, but its removal requires rebuilding the bile ducts. This can be done by removing the entire tumor and attaching a loop of intestine to the liver where the cut ends of the bile ducts are draining (called a Roux-en-Y). This is a difficult operation and the overall health of the patient is an important factor in deciding whether to perform it.

Bile duct cancers can also occur at the far end of the duct, near where it empties into the intestine. Removing these tumors may also require a Roux-en-Y, as well as removal of parts of the intestines and pancreas (called a Whipple procedure). This extensive surgery is extremely complicated and has many side effects. It should be done only when a tumor has not spread beyond the local area.

 Chemotherapy Studies have not shown that chemotherapy can prolong survival, but the standard drugs used (gemcitabine [Gemzar], capecitabine [Xeloda], and 5-fluorouracil) may cause tumors to shrink and help 20 to 25 percent of patients. Even with tumor shrinkage, however, patients may not be better off after chemotherapy. The treatment has side effects and the tumor ultimately regrows.

There may be a role for chemotherapy after surgery, although this has not been studied systematically. In the hope of finding a better chemotherapy treatment and improving survival, patients should be considered for clinical trials if chemotherapy is planned.

Radiation Radiation is effective against bile duct cancers and may play a significant role. If the tumor is fairly small, it may be treated with radiation without causing much damage to the surrounding noncancerous liver tissue. A newer computer-directed radiation technique called conformal radiation may allow for the radiation beam to pinpoint the tumor and spare the surrounding uninvolved liver, although it is often difficult to define the actual extent of bile duct tumors.

Treatment may include placing a radiation-containing probe in the bile duct (brachytherapy). This therapy may also apply to patients with a small bit of

tumor left after surgery or as a supplemental (adjuvant) therapy when the surgery is thought to have been complete but there is a suspicion that microscopic deposits of tumor are still present. Studies evaluating the role of radiation therapy are ongoing.

Combined Therapy The combination of radiation and chemotherapy may play a role as adjuvant therapy. This treatment, which should be done as part of a clinical trial, may delay any recurrence of the cancer or even cure people who have already had surgery.

Treatment by Stage

◼ Localized
At this stage, the cancer is confined to the bile duct. It is quite rare to find a bile duct cancer at this limited stage, for it would be unlikely to cause an obstruction of the bile flow when it is very small.

Standard Treatment Surgery can be done with hopes of a cure. The extent of surgery necessary depends on the tumor's location and size. It may be possible to remove a tumor limited to a small portion of either the right or the left bile duct with its surrounding liver in a routine operation. But cancers involving the bile ducts at their junction within the liver require removal of liver tissue and then the complicated reconstruction of the bile drainage system. Tumors close to the intestine and pancreas may demand even more difficult surgery.

Whatever the extent of the surgery, tubes may have to be left within the bile duct system for a time to ensure against bile leakage or the formation of scar tissue within the bile ducts.

It is not known whether drainage tubes should be placed through the bile duct blockage before surgery. If patients are ill because of the obstruction—the bile has become infected, for example— then a stent should be inserted to enable the patient to be in better condition for the surgery. Radiation to the tumor site is an alternative if patients are too sick to have surgery.

Unfortunately, even with meticulous surgery and careful screening, the majority of tumors will regrow within the bile ducts, in the nearby liver tissue, or elsewhere in the body. So it is generally agreed that treating the surgical area with radiation after the tumor has been removed is useful in that it may help to destroy any remaining tumor cells.

The chemotherapy drug 5-fluorouracil or capecitabine is often given at the same time as the radiation in an effort to improve the effectiveness of treatment. This combination therapy is felt to be better than other treatments.

Five-Year Survival Up to 25 percent

Investigational Various combinations of surgery, radiation, and chemotherapy may be considered. The most extreme approach involves pretreating localized tumors with chemotherapy and radiation, then performing a liver transplant. There is some evidence that this aggressive approach can eradicate the cancer in highly selected patients.

■ *Unresectable*
The tumor cannot be removed because it has spread to local lymph nodes, liver tissue, or elsewhere in the body.

Standard Treatment There is no standard treatment, so chemotherapy and/or radiation therapy clinical trials should be considered.

Significant relief of symptoms may be achieved. Patients with symptoms such as itching or infection may benefit from a procedure to create a bypass system for the bile. Such a bypass tube (stem) can be placed through the skin during percutaneous transhepatic cholangiography or through a scope during ERCP.

With the ERCP stent placement, the tube may drain into the intestines and a collecting bag may not be needed. Occasionally, neither of these methods drains the bile successfully. In that case, surgery designed to create a bypass channel may be done.

Two-Year Survival Less than 1 percent

Investigational
• Clinical protocols designed to test the additive benefit of radiation and chemotherapy are ongoing.
• Patients who wish to try chemotherapy may be offered new drugs.

Treatment Follow-Up

Careful follow-up is important after the surgical removal of a localized cancer because once a recurrent tumor is large enough to be seen on X-ray, it is probably too large to be cured.

CT scans should be done every two to three months for the first year after curative surgery, since an early recurrence may still be removed if it is small enough at the time of diagnosis.

Supportive Therapy

• Problems associated with jaundice can include severe itching and infections in the bile. If the drainage procedures described above are not effective, itching will often be relieved by Benadryl, Atarax, or cholestyramine (Questian). For unexplained reasons, the antibiotic rifampin may also alleviate the itching associated with jaundice.
• Large doses of narcotics may be needed to relieve pain. Such drugs may have excessive side effects, since they are eliminated by the liver, which may not be functioning properly.
• Nonsteroidal anti-inflammatory drugs may be surprisingly effective even against

the pain associated with bile duct cancer.

• Frequent small meals may be necessary to get enough nutrition, since an abdominal mass may reduce the size of the stomach.

• Water pills (diuretics) can reduce fluid in the abdomen or legs. They may cause significant imbalance in kidney function, however, and can create problems if not carefully monitored and adjusted.

• Nausea will often be relieved by standard medications, including suppositories.

• Loss of appetite may be helped by megestial (Megace).

• Sleep disturbances are common, but most sleeping pills are broken down by the liver, so they should be used carefully.

The Most Important Questions You Can Ask

• Should I see another physician to confirm that this tumor can or cannot be removed?

• Can the drainage of the bile ducts be done through the intestines so I won't have to have a tube coming out through my skin?

• Am I a candidate for an investigational therapy at another medical center?

• How sick will radiation and/or chemotherapy make me, and does the potential benefit make it worthwhile?

• Can anything be done to improve the quality of my life?

• Is the treatment worthwhile if the tumor is too advanced for surgery?

Bladder

Jonathan E. Rosenberg, M.D., Badrinath Konety, M.D., M.B.A., and Eric J. Small, M.D.

■ ■ ■ ■

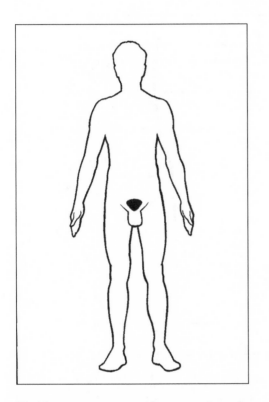

Bladder tumors account for approximately 4 percent of new cancers (61,000 cases) in the United States. Bladder cancer ranks as the fourth most common cause of cancer in men and eighth most common in women, and causes about 14,000 deaths (almost 3 percent of cancer deaths). It is the fourth leading cause of cancer deaths in patients over seventy-five. While the average age of people who get bladder cancer is sixty-eight, this tumor is found in people as young as forty years old.

Bladder cancer is three to four times more common in men than in women.

More than two-thirds of bladder cancers are limited to the surface lining of the bladder ("superficial"), and about one-third are invasive into the bladder wall or with regional or metastatic disease outside the bladder, at the time of diagnosis.

Five-year survival rates over the past thirty years have improved markedly. This is due to two important factors: (1) The disease is being found in earlier stages, when current therapies are more effective, and (2) treatments have become better at eradicating disease. Over 70 percent of cases are now being discovered with local tumors within the bladder. Only 20 percent have regional disease just outside the bladder, while 3 percent have distant metastases.

Types The urinary tract is lined with what are called transitional cells. More than 90 percent of bladder cancers, called transitional cell carcinomas, originate from these cells. While the vast majority of transitional cell carcinomas arise from the bladder, around 10 percent can arise from the cells lining the collecting system of the kidneys—the ureters that drain the kidneys and the urethra that drains the bladder.

The layer of three to four transitional cells lining the bladder can grow to six or more abnormal layers when they are irritated. Chemical carcinogens can accumulate in the urine and cause cellular changes that may eventually lead to cancer.

The superficial layer of transitional cells is separated from the bladder muscle (which contracts to expel urine) by

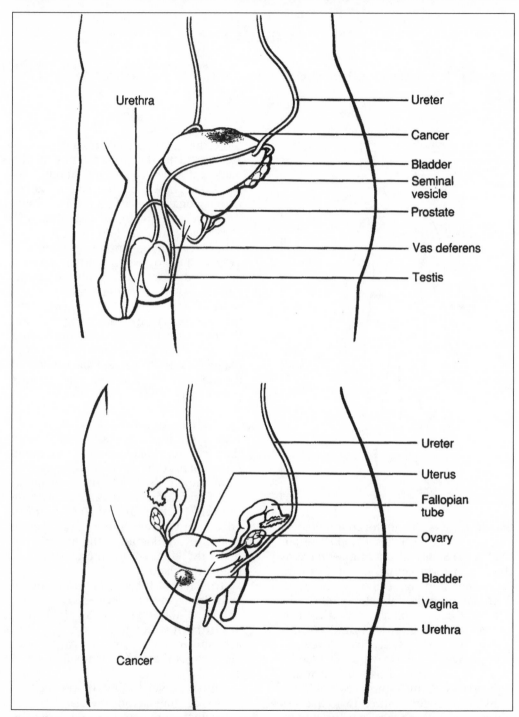

Overall view of pelvic organs showing bladder and surrounding structures

a thin, fibrous band called the lamina propria. Tumors that are superficial (non-invasive) do not penetrate through the lamina propria, while tumors that are invasive (invading into muscle) have pushed through the lamina propria into the muscle that lies underneath. Treatment options depend on the distinction between superficial and invasive cancer. Most bladder tumors are superficial and can be treated successfully while leaving the bladder in place.

Besides transitional cell carcinomas, other tumor types may be found in the bladder. These tumor types may exist either alone or combined with transitional cell carcinoma. Tumors may develop either in the glands of the bladder (adenocarcinoma) or in an embryonic remnant (urachal tumors). Most of the remaining bladder cancers are squamous cell carcinomas, which also are the most frequent type of urethral tumor in women. Such tumors may be caused by chronic bladder infections and chronic and repeated bladder trauma, such as repeated bladder catheterizations in paraplegics. Tumors also develop in the pelvis of the kidney, where urine is formed, and in the ureters, the tubes that carry urine to the bladder. About 7 percent of all kidney cancers originate in the renal pelvis. The majority of these tumors are transitional cell cancers, although the squamous cell type is noted more frequently in patients with a history of chronic stone problems.

Some bladder tumors possess a low probability of becoming malignant lesions requiring radical treatments. Such tumors, known as Ta, Grade 1 tumors, are very unlikely to progress to more worrisome malignant superficial tumors (carcinoma in situ, or Tis) or muscle-invasive tumors. Muscle-invasive cancers may go through a superficial phase (Tis) or may develop independently. Therefore, even though Tis does not invade muscle, risk of invasion is present. Unfortunately, Tis tends to recur again and again. Tis tumors, therefore, indicate an unstable bladder lining. However, only 25 percent of patients with muscle-invasive bladder cancer have had previously known superficial transitional cell carcinoma; the first time that bladder cancer is diagnosed in the other 75 percent, it has already invaded the muscle.

How It Spreads Tumors can grow through the bladder muscle directly into the surrounding tissue (perivesical fat) and/or into adjacent structures such as the prostate, vagina, rectum, and uterus. Bladder tumors can also enter into the small blood and lymph vessels that supply the normal bladder wall. When they enter these vessels, cancer cells can spread to local lymph nodes in the pelvis and to the lymph nodes higher in the abdomen, or they can be carried by the bloodstream to the lungs, bones, or liver.

Risk Factors

The United States and Europe have the highest incidence of transitional cell carcinoma. While the exact cause of bladder cancer remains unknown, the most commonly identified risk factor for bladder cancer in the United States is cigarette smoking. Cigarette smokers develop bladder cancers almost three times as often as nonsmokers. Smoking may be responsible for 50 percent of bladder cancers in men and 40 percent in women. Former smokers appear to have a risk of developing bladder cancer that lies somewhere between that of current smokers and nonsmokers. Interestingly, pipe and cigar smoke are only weakly associated with the development of bladder cancer. Smokeless tobacco is not associated with development of the disease.

The mechanism by which cigarette smoking leads to the development of bladder cancer is unclear, but it likely involves carcinogens that are present in cigarette smoke. These carcinogens, including the aromatic amines alpha- and beta-naphthylamine, appear in the urine of smokers. In addition, certain cyclic N-nitrosamines derived from tobacco smoke are known bladder-specific chemical carcinogens in animals.

Another risk factor for bladder cancer is occupational exposure to chemical carcinogens. Workers in the textile dye industry, rubber tire industry, and leather industry; hairdressers (from hair dyes); painters (from paint pigment); and metalworkers may potentially be exposed to chemical carcinogens that place them at risk for bladder cancer. Finally, some cancer therapy drugs (cyclophosphamide [Cytoxan]), local radiation therapy, various dyes and solvents, and chronic abuse of some pain medications such as phenacetin and possibly acetaminophen may also be risk factors for transitional cell carcinoma of the bladder. Whatever the cause of bladder cancer, it is clear that once one area of the urothelial tract has developed a transitional cell cancer, the whole urothelial tract is at risk for forming new tumors. Those with a renal pelvis cancer, for example, are twenty-one times more at risk to develop another urinary tract tumor compared with the general population. Approximately 4 percent of those with a bladder cancer have been found to develop a tumor in the renal pelvis or ureter. While a good deal of work is now being done to evaluate agents that can prevent the development of such tumors, at this point no such agent can be recommended.

Risk factors for squamous cell carcinoma include physical trauma to the bladder lining, such as chronic infection, prolonged catheterization, and bladder stones.

Screening

Several health care agencies have recommended against routine screening for bladder cancer in the general population. For asymptomatic patients at risk for the disease who wish to be evaluated, a urinalysis (urine dipstick and microscopic examination of the urine) is the best screening test. This test will determine whether or not there is microscopic blood in the urine. For patients who are symptomatic, as well as those who have experienced an episode of gross hematuria (bleeding in the urine that is noticed by the patient), urine cytology may be useful. Such an examination will often identify malignant transitional cells in the urine.

Newer diagnostic tests have recently been developed based on monoclonal antibodies that detect tumor-specific substances in a normal urine specimen. These tests are currently being evaluated, and their results with respect to bladder cancer detection are being compared with those of urinary cytology. One test, known as UroVysion FISH (fluorescence in situ hybridization), can detect abnormalities in chromosomes of transitional cells that are present in the urine. These chromosomal abnormalities are often associated with cancer. The clinical utility of these newer tests, however, has not yet been established, and it is not clear that any of these tests add useful information to a urinalysis and cytology.

Common Signs and Symptoms

Eighty percent of patients with bladder cancer first visit their doctor because of blood and/or clots in the urine. Other urinary signs include increased frequency of urination, the intense urge to urinate, bladder spasms, and pain or burning with urination (dysuria). It is important to emphasize that there are many more common reasons for these symptoms, such as an enlarged or inflamed prostate, urinary stones, injury, and various infections.

Symptoms of more advanced bladder cancer include loss of weight or appetite, fever, bone pain, and pain in the rectal, anal, or pelvic area.

Diagnosis

Physical Examination There are few physical findings indicative of early bladder cancer other than a bladder or pelvic mass discovered by abdominal or digital rectal examination. With more advanced disease, there may be enlarged lymph nodes in the groin, abdomen, or neck; a mass in the lower abdomen; or an enlarged liver. Examination of the bladder with both hands while the patient is under anesthesia is necessary to determine the depth and extent of tumor penetration.

Blood and Other Tests

- Urinalysis for blood in the urine (hematuria)
- Complete blood count (CBC) to evaluate anemia
- Chemistry profile to evaluate kidney, liver, and bone abnormalities
- Using urine or vigorous washing of the bladder for examination of the cells (cytology).

Cytology may detect the presence of cancer cells in the urine, especially in patients with carcinoma in situ or high-grade (aggressive) tumors. The disappearance of tumor cells after anticancer drugs are placed inside the bladder is associated with a good response to treatment.

When sufficient tumor tissue is obtained, it may be examined for alterations in the expression of genes that are involved in tumor progression. Increased expression of genes that promote tumor progression (oncogenes) or decreased expression of genes that slow tumor progression (tumor suppressor genes) may indicate a poor prognosis. A variety of genes and gene products have been examined in patients with bladder cancer, including p53 and RB. Although remarkable advances have been made in our understanding of tumor biology, further investigation is necessary before any of these genes can be used in routine clinical practice to determine the proper course of treatment for a given patient with bladder cancer.

Imaging It is essential that the "upper tracts" (kidneys and ureters) be visualized in a patient with a known bladder cancer. Intravenous pyelogram (IVP) can be used to image the kidneys, ureters, and bladder. Abdominal and pelvic CT is often used in place of IVP in the evaluation of patients with bladder cancer. In addition to imaging the kidneys, ureters, and bladder, CT scans can help find metastases to the lymph nodes, liver, and surrounding bladder structures. CT scan and MRI may help to establish the depth of invasion of the cancer, but they are not very accurate in this regard. MRIs may be used in patients who cannot tolerate intravenous contrast used for CT scans. Chest X-ray may be used to exclude metastasis to the lungs. Bone scans (and, rarely, bone X-rays) are used before surgery to exclude metastasis to the bones if there is concern regarding spread to the bones.

Endoscopy and Biopsy Cystoscopy is the direct visualization of the bladder by passing a small rigid or flexible telescope through the urethra into the bladder. This allows for examination of the entire lining of the urethra and bladder. Initial diagnostic cystoscopy is often performed in the office using local anesthesia. Biopsy and/or removal of tumor masses (transurethral resection of the bladder tumor, or TURBT) can also be done through the cystoscope. This is performed in the office in some instances, or in the operating room if general or spinal anesthesia is required. At times, random bladder biopsies may be done to exclude cancer or carcinoma in situ at areas distant from the primary tumor. A pathologist examines the tissue under a microscope. This examination allows for the determination of the presence or absence of bladder cancer, the type of bladder cancer, and the depth of invasion of the tumor into the bladder wall. In addition, the presence or absence of carcinoma in situ can be documented.

Staging

The TNM staging system is generally used for bladder cancer. This system allows for the independent determination of the extent of the primary tumor, the status of the lymph nodes, and the presence or absence of distant (metastatic) disease.

Clinical staging, or the determination of the depth of invasion and/or extent of cancer based on physical exam, X-rays, cystoscopy, and transurethral bladder tumor resection, is very useful in distinguishing superficial bladder cancer from muscle-invasive disease. However, a major problem in clinical staging of muscle-invasive disease is the inaccuracy rate of around 30 percent in precisely determining the extent of muscle and lymph node involvement when compared with surgical or pathological staging of a tissue specimen at the time of bladder removal.

Treatment Overview

Treatment of bladder cancer depends on the stage of disease. For superficial tumors that do not invade muscle, resection (cutting out), fulguration (burning out with heat or laser), and intravesical therapy (placing drugs directly in the bladder by a catheter inserted through the urethra) are the usual treatment options. Therapy for muscle-invasive lesions depends on the extent of invasion and the presence or absence of lymph node involvement, or metastatic (distant) disease in other parts of the body. It usually involves surgical removal of the bladder (cystectomy) with or without the addition of chemotherapy (either before or after cystectomy).

 Surgery Surgical removal of the bladder can often lead to cure of muscle-invasive bladder cancer.

Radical cystectomy involves removal of the anterior pelvic organs. In men, this includes removal of the bladder with its surrounding fat, the prostate, and the seminal vesicles. In women, the bladder with its surrounding fat and the cervix, uterus, anterior vagina, urethra, ovaries, and fallopian tubes are removed. In addition, this treatment option may be chosen for patients with high-risk superficial tumors. Patients with persistent carcinoma in situ despite other therapies, invasion into the lamina propria, or high-grade tumors should be considered for cystectomy if other treatments have failed.

In most cases, the entire bladder must be removed. However, in selected patients with a single tumor in the dome of the bladder and with no evidence of carcinoma in situ, removal of the tumor along with the adjacent portion of the bladder wall that guarantees an adequate margin of normal tissue (partial cystectomy) is appropriate. This is not a common situation and only select patients are eligible for this type of treatment.

Previously, cystectomy raised many quality-of-life issues, especially concerning its effect on sexual function. Nerves controlling penile erection were cut and an ileal conduit (a piece of the gut or small bowel) leading to a large plastic bag outside the body to collect urine was mandatory. However, both problems have now been addressed, and the various alternatives must be discussed with a urologist. For instance, "orthotopic urinary diversion" is now the procedure of choice for both men and women undergoing radical cystectomy. During this procedure, a portion of the intestine is used to make an internal urinary reservoir (neobladder) that can be connected to the urethra. The patient can then urinate through the urethra in normal fashion, without a need for an external bag or catheterization. An alternative approach uses a small tube of intestine or appendix made into a pouch connected to the belly button or the abdominal wall. A catheter is placed through this narrow tube into the pouch four to five times a day to drain the urine. There is no need to wear a bag, and the dime-sized opening of the tube of intestine/appendix can easily be covered over with a Band-Aid on the skin.

Sexual function in males may also be maintained in well-selected patients by sparing the nerves needed for erection. In addition, erections may be obtained through the use of medication (oral medication such as sildenafil [Viagra] or medications injected into the penis or inserted into the urethra before sex) or by implantation of a penile prosthesis (implant).

Radiation External radiation can be used for more advanced stages of bladder cancer, although as a single treatment, it is less effective than surgery. In some circumstances, it can be combined with chemotherapy as a means of avoiding surgical removal of the bladder. Patients who are ideal candidates for chemoradiation include those with an absence of carcinoma in situ; with no hydronephrosis (blockage of the ureters draining the kidneys); and with a solitary tumor site.

Chemotherapy When superficial tumors constantly recur, intravesical treatment is used. This therapy permits direct contact of high concentrations of chemotherapy or immunologic drugs in the bladder, which bathe the superficial cancer cells for one or two hours. Patients with renal pelvis, ureteral, and urethral cancers are usually not good candidates for intravesical therapy, although some reports have now described success (see chapter 9, "What Happens in Biological Therapy and Immunotherapy"). Many times, these drugs are placed in the bladder after a TURBT is performed.

There have been studies of chemotherapy with single and combination drug regimens for patients with muscle-invasive disease given intravenously before and/or after surgery. If used before surgery (neoadjuvant), the aim is to decrease tumor size, to destroy any tiny (microscopic) metastases that may later grow but cannot be seen on X-rays or other imaging studies at the time of surgery, to predict good-risk versus poor-risk cases, to lead eventually to bladder preservation (no need for the removal of the bladder), and, more important, to increase survival. Adjuvant therapy is chemotherapy used after surgery to reduce the risk of relapse by destroying microscopic residual disease. Although neoadjuvant therapy has been shown to improve survival, adjuvant therapy may be used in patients who after surgery have characteristics associated with increased risk of relapse (penetration of the tumor through the bladder wall, lymph node involvement, and invasion of cancer cells into the blood and lymph vessels).

Laser Therapy Superficial cancers can be treated by laser vaporization-coagulation with Nd:YAG or carbon dioxide (CO_2) lasers. Such treatment is rarely used.

Biological Therapy The best immunological drug is BCG vaccine (used for tuberculosis vaccination) given by catheter inside the bladder (intravesical) weekly for six consecutive weeks. Cystoscopy and urine cytology at six weeks after the last dose are used to evaluate effectiveness. If a partial response is seen—that is, fewer lesions are found than previously—another course may be given. BCG is completely effective in more than 70 percent of cases of superficial bladder cancer or carcinoma in situ and has been proven to be better than no therapy or cytotoxic drugs. People who respond completely to BCG not only have fewer superficial tumor recurrences, but also develop fewer muscle-invasive cancers requiring surgery.

BCG toxicity includes temporary local bladder irritation, fever, and, in very rare cases, a type of tuberculosis infection that can be treated successfully with antituberculous drugs. BCG + interferon-alpha is sometimes used for patients who have failed BCG treatment if they do not necessarily require cystectomy.

Treatment by Stage

■ Stage 0
TNM Ta, N0, M0

Stage 0 means the tumor is very superficial and does not even invade the lamina propria. It has not spread to lymph nodes, and there are no metastases. Tumors are a papillary exophytic mass (like a bunch of grapes on a thin stalk [Ta]).

The behavior of Ta tumors is determined, at least in part, by tumor grade. It is highly unlikely that a Grade 1 (very well differentiated) Ta lesion will progress, since the potential for spreading into the muscle or lymph nodes or metastasizing to other organs is almost nonexistent. In contrast, Grades 2 and 3 Ta lesions are true cancers having the potential to invade their stalk and travel down into the lamina propria and then into muscle. Overall, patients who develop superficial Ta tumors have a 50 to 70 percent chance of recurrence.

Standard Treatment Transurethral resection of the bladder tumor (TURBT) or removal of the tumor through a cystoscope is the treatment of choice and is generally curative. There is almost never a requirement for a total cystectomy for Ta tumors. In selected cases, however, a segmental or partial cystectomy may be appropriate.

■ Stage 0 Tis
TNM Tis, N0, M0

In contrast to Ta tumors, all flat Tis lesions should be considered aggressive, regardless of grade. These lesions usually demonstrate many of the same genetic changes that are evident in muscle-invasive cancers.

Standard Treatment For patients with Tis, the first step is biopsy of the tumor through a cystoscope. This is usually done as part of the diagnostic evaluation. Intravesical therapy with cytotoxic agents or BCG may be used mostly as a preventive agent. Effective anticancer drugs include thiotepa, doxorubicin (Adriamycin), mitomycin, and, in Europe, ethoglucid (Epodyl) and epirubicin. Complete tumor prevention succeeds in 20 to 45 percent of cases given cytotoxic drugs after resection and in 65 percent of cases given BCG. More important, none of these drugs seem to be cross-resistant with each other or with immunological drugs. BCG should be considered the standard of care.

Tis should be treated with intravesical BCG as weekly treatments over six weeks. Follow-up cystoscopy and cytology should then be repeated six weeks following the last treatment. Some patients may be treated with "maintenance" BCG over a prolonged time period. Surveillance cystoscopy should be performed every three months for the first two years following treatment.

Patients with diffuse recurrent Tis or who fail one or more trials of intravesical therapy should be considered for cystectomy. External radiation, radiation seeds or needles, and intraoperative radiation therapy have not yet been proven effective in controlling or in preventing Ta or Tis. Systemic chemotherapy cannot control Tis either.

Five-Year Survival Over 90 percent

Investigational New immunological drugs including interleukin-2, interferon-alpha, tumor necrosis factor, and keyhole-limpet extract are being evaluated. Chemopreventive agents that are designed to prevent tumor recurrence are also being tested.

■ *Stage I*
TNM T1, N0, M0
The tumor is superficial, but it does invade into the lamina propria. There is no spread to lymph nodes and no metastases.

Standard Treatment The same as for Stage 0 Tis. Patients may initially be treated with TURBT, followed by a course of intravesical BCG. Patients who fail this regimen are at high risk for disease progression and should be considered for cystectomy.

Five-Year Survival Over 75 percent

Investigational See the section for Stage 0 Tis.

■ *Stage II*
TNM T2, N0, M0
The tumor invades through the lamina propria into the muscle wall of the bladder. Using two hands, the physician can often feel the tumor before surgery.

Standard Treatment Surgery (radical cystectomy) is the standard of care. Repeat transurethral resection or a partial or segmental cystectomy when the bladder is otherwise normal can also be curative in very select patients. A repeat TURBT as the only therapy may be performed in patients with only minimally invasive bladder tumors. When TURBT alone is chosen as local therapy for invasive bladder cancer, an extensive or "radical" TURBT is performed by an experienced urologist. Follow-up must be vigilant due to the high risk of local recurrence.

Patients who are potential candidates for partial cystectomy must have a single tumor in a location amenable to obtaining negative surgical margins (i.e., no cancer cells at the edge of the surgical specimen), have tumor within a diverticulum (abnormal outpouching of the bladder wall), or be considered to be poor surgical risk secondary to other medical conditions or advanced age. Given these indications and contraindications, no more than 5 to 10 percent of all patients with muscle-invasive bladder cancer are considered appropriate candidates for partial cystectomy.

In summary, radical cystectomy should be considered as the standard of treatment for patients with muscle-invasive bladder cancer. It is only a very select population of patients who should be considered for other treatment options. Five-year survival is 55 to 90 percent, depending on tumor grade and extent of muscle wall invasion.

"Bladder sparing" treatment consisting of radiation plus chemotherapy is promising, with 30 to 50 percent of patients being rendered free of disease and finishing therapy with a functional bladder. Patients with T4 tumors (into adjacent organs) or with kidney obstruction (hydronephrosis) are not good candidates for this approach.

■ *Stage III*
TNM T3, N0, M0
In Stage III bladder cancer, the tumor invades deeply through the muscle wall of the bladder and into perivesical fat (fat surrounding the bladder).

Standard Treatment Cystectomy. For those patients with T3 tumors but lymph nodes without tumor, five-year survival ranges from 40 to 60 percent, depending on the extent of disease outside the bladder. Patients with Stage III tumors have such a high risk of microscopic metastatic disease that many specialists feel that chemotherapy either before or after cystectomy is warranted.

Chemotherapy given in addition to surgery is termed either neoadjuvant or adjuvant chemotherapy. Neoadjuvant chemotherapy is chemotherapy given *prior* to surgery. Potential advantages of this approach are (1) the immediate treatment of micrometastases (and therefore, hopefully, a decrease in the relapse rate), (2) reduction of tumor size to make surgery more feasible, and (3) provision of information about prognosis (if subsequent surgery reveals no residual disease, outcome is clearly better than if there is residual disease). Two large trials have shown a modest improvement in survival for patients receiving neoadjuvant chemotherapy. As a result, neoadjuvant chemotherapy should be considered in every patient undergoing radical cystectomy.

Adjuvant therapy is chemotherapy given *after* surgery. The advantages to this approach are (1) pathologic evaluation of the surgical specimen to distinguish patients who may be at high risk of relapse and who would benefit more from chemotherapy from lower-risk patients who may not require chemotherapy, and (2) treatment of micrometastases. Several small trials have suggested that adjuvant therapy reduces the risk of relapse substantially in high-risk patients, although definitive proof is still lacking. In addition, if the cancer is destined to return, relapse may be delayed for months to years by adjuvant chemotherapy.

Investigational Investigational treatment for this stage is controversial. There are no large studies under way in the United States for neoadjuvant or adjuvant chemotherapy at this time. Many small studies are piloting the idea of bladder preservation strategies with chemoradiation in this patient population.

▪ *Stage IV*

TNM T4, N0, M0 or any T, N1–3, M0 or any T, any N, M1

The tumor invades adjacent organs such as the prostate, uterus, and vagina alone (T4a, N0, M0), or it spreads to the pelvic bone and abdominal wall (T4b, N0, M0), to pelvic lymph nodes (any T, N1–3, M0), to abdominal lymph nodes (any T, N4, M0), or to other organs (any T, any N, M1). While these patients are grouped together, it is quite clear that patients without metastatic spread to other organs, as a group, do far better than patients whose disease has spread to other organs (any T, any N, M1). Common sites of metastases for bladder cancer are the lungs, lymph nodes in the abdomen, and bone. Somewhat less common is liver involvement.

Standard Treatment Patients with extensive nodal disease should first be treated with chemotherapy. Only if the tumor outside the bladder completely disappears should cystectomy be considered. Cystectomy can be beneficial in a very limited number of T4a, N0–1, M0 cases, but if more than microscopic nodal involvement is found, adjuvant chemotherapy should probably be used, as discussed above. Types of chemotherapy are discussed below.

Five-Year Survival While the average survival for patients with node involvement only can exceed two to three years, approximately 50 percent of patients with metastases to other organs die within one year, over 80 percent within two years, and less than 5 percent survive five years.

Recurrent or Metastatic Bladder Cancer

Combination chemotherapy has been shown to be effective in prolonging life in patients with recurrent or metastatic bladder cancer. In addition, the regimens described below are used in patients with muscle-invasive disease either before or after cystectomy.

• **MVAC** Methotrexate, vinblastine (Velban), doxorubicin (Adriamycin), and cisplatin are active single chemotherapy agents and have been combined in a four-drug regimen. Studies have proven that MVAC is better than cisplatin alone or cisplatin + doxorubicin and cyclophosphamide (Cytoxan), and until recently MVAC was the treatment of choice for patients with metastatic disease. Thirty-five to 70 percent of patients will respond, with 15 to 35 percent having a complete tumor regression. Complete remissions lasting more than five years occur in 10 to 15 percent of patients.

The use of MVAC is limited, however, by the need to maintain good kidney function (cisplatin and methotrexate are both excreted by the kidneys) and the requirement that the patients cannot have significant cardiac abnormalities because of doxorubicin cardiac toxicity. In addition, there is a significant risk of infection and death associated with MVAC chemotherapy due to low blood counts and inflammation of the mucous membranes of the body (mouth, esophagus, intestines).

• **Gemcitabine (Gemzar) + Cisplatin** After many recent trials showed gemcitabine and cisplatin to be a promising combination for the treatment of advanced bladder cancer, a randomized study was performed comparing this new regimen to the previous standard treatment, MVAC. The proportion of patients responding to treatment and the overall survival was nearly identical in the two groups. However, the gemcitabine-cisplatin regimen had significantly fewer side effects. Therefore, this two-drug combination is becoming the new standard chemotherapy treatment for advanced bladder cancer. As with MVAC, its use is limited by the need to have and maintain good kidney function.

• **New Agents** New agents that show great promise include ifosfamide (Ifex), paclitaxel (Taxol), docetaxel (Taxotere), pemetrexed (Alimta), and vinflunine (experimental at this time).

Not every patient is a candidate for cisplatin chemotherapy, due to other illness or poor kidney function. Cisplatin can cause kidney damage, hearing loss, and nerve damage (neuropathy). As a result, many other chemotherapy regimens are used. However, there is no standard treatment for patients who cannot tolerate cisplatin chemotherapy. Some regimens that are commonly used in that situation include gemcitabine + carboplatin (Paraplatin), paclitaxel + carboplatin, and gemcitabine alone.

Radiation therapy may relieve symptoms of bone and brain metastases and may be required at some point.

If first-line chemotherapy fails and the cancer returns and grows, there is no standard second-line chemotherapy. Many of the drugs listed above may be tried, either alone or in combination with other drugs. In this setting, participation in investigational therapy (clinical trials) is appropriate. Rarely, patients with an isolated site of tumor metastasis, without any other evidence of cancer in their bodies, may undergo surgery to remove that site.

The Most Important Questions You Can Ask

• Is my bladder cancer superficial or muscle invasive?
• What stage is my cancer?

• What grade is my cancer?

• If my cancer is superficial, will I require intravesical therapy [drugs placed into the bladder]? If so, with what agents, and for how long? How often will I need cystoscopy?

• Do I need surgery, and how extensive would it be?

• If surgery to remove my bladder is planned, will I have a neobladder constructed? If not, why not?

• How can I control my urine after my bladder is removed?

• How can I function sexually after my bladder is removed?

• Is there a role for chemotherapy either before or after surgery? Why or why not?

• What are the chemotherapy options available to me?

• What is my kidney function and how might that affect which chemotherapy I receive?

• How long will I receive chemotherapy, and how will its anticancer activity be measured?

Brain

Nicholas A. Butowski, M.D., Michael D. Prados, M.D.,
Michael W. McDermott, M.D., and Susan M. Chang, M.D.

■ ■ ■ ■

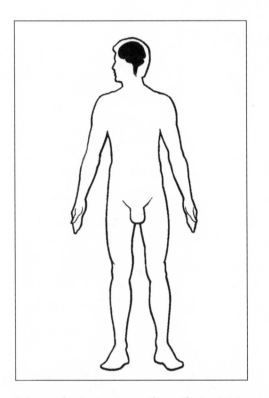

Primary brain tumors—those that arise in the brain itself—account for 1 percent of all cancers. Approximately 14 per 100,000 people in the United States are diagnosed with primary brain tumors each year. Out of these, roughly 7 per 100,000 are diagnosed with a primary malignant brain tumor and will account for approximately 2 percent of all cancer-related deaths. Brain tumors most commonly occur in the fifth and sixth decades of life but are the second most common form of cancer in childhood, next to leukemia.

Tumors arising in some other part of the body may also spread to the brain and are called metastases or metastatic tumors; these most commonly come from cancers of the lung, breast, kidney, and skin (malignant melanoma). Metastatic tumors to the brain are usually multiple, although a solitary metastasis can mimic a primary brain tumor. Metastases occur at some point in 10 to 15 percent of persons with cancer and are the most common type of tumor in the brain.

Types Brain tumors may develop from any of the different types of cells found within the brain. Tumors may originate from nerve cells, or neurons; however, tumors of the supporting cells, known as glial cells (including astrocytes, oligodendrocytes, and ependymal cells), are more common. A tumor is generally named after the cell from which it develops. Thus, a tumor derived from glial cells is known as a glioma. To be more specific, a tumor from astrocytic cells is called an astrocytoma and a tumor from ependymal cells is called an ependymoma. Tumors of the neurons include neuroblastomas, neurocytomas, and ganglioneuromas. Meningiomas are tumors that originate from cells in the meninges, a system of membranes that cover and surround the brain. Other tumors include those derived from specialized brain structures such as the pineal gland, pituitary gland, and choroid plexus (which makes cerebrospinal fluid).

Normally, primary brain tumors are graded pathologically on the basis of

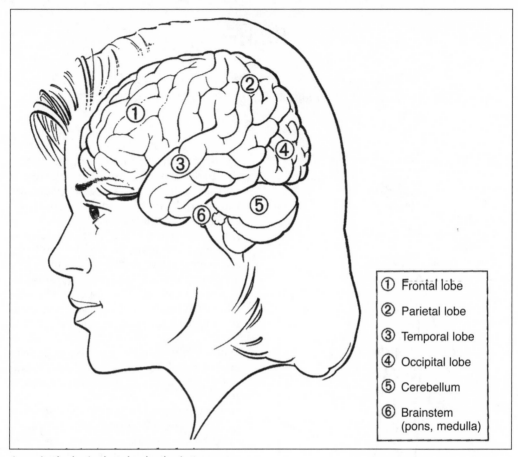

1 Frontal lobe

2 Parietal lobe

3 Temporal lobe

4 Occipital lobe

5 Cerebellum

6 Brainstem
(pons, medulla)

Areas in the brain that develop brain tumors

the most malignant or aggressive area identified according to the World Health Organization grading system. The pathologist is a physician who determines the grade of the tumor by examining tissue removed during surgery. The grade of a tumor refers to how abnormal the cancer cells look under a microscope and how quickly the tumor is likely to grow and thus influence the prognosis of the patient. For example, astrocytomas are graded on a scale of 1 to 4, with Grade 1 being the slowest growing and Grade 4 being the most rapidly growing and malignant lesions.

What Causes It Research into the causes of brain tumors is complicated by many factors, including the relative rarity of the disease and the swift death of patients with aggressive subtypes. Most brain tumors have no known cause, and to date, studies have revealed little with regard to specific causes. Nevertheless, research continues, and advances in the fields of genetics and epidemiology may lead to the discovery of not only why brain tumors occur, but how to better treat them.

The field of molecular genetics is devoted to understanding the changes that transpire in cells that allow them to acquire characteristics of cancer cells and form tumors. Many of these cell alterations have been identified, although the process of how these changes lead to the development of tumors still requires further investigation. The field of epidemiology is dedicated to understanding the potential relationships of environmental or acquired events that may either cause or predispose a person to develop a brain tumor. A variety of statistical and environmental associations have been made, but no chemical or environmental agent has been shown to cause brain tumors.

Some inherited conditions do predispose a person to the development of brain tumors. For instance, patients with neurofibromatosis type I (NF-1), tuberous sclerosis, and familial polyposis have a tendency to develop astrocytomas. However, these syndromes explain less than 5 percent of brain tumor cases.

Viruses are known to produce genetic changes in cells that in laboratory animals can induce the formation of a tumor. There is an association in people infected with the Epstein-Barr virus and primary central nervous system lymphoma (lymphoma is a cancerous tumor of the lymph cells, which are part of the body's immune system and help to fight infection), although a definite causal relationship remains to be established. Central nervous system lymphoma frequently develops in people whose immune system is not working properly, such as those patients who have received an organ transplant or those who have AIDS.

Radiation can produce genetic damage in cells and induce tumors. It was once standard medical practice to use low doses of radiation to treat ringworm of the scalp in children. Years later, it was found that children treated this way had an increased chance of developing tumors of the scalp, skull, and brain, particularly meningiomas. These radiation-associated tumors have a much greater likelihood of being malignant than those that occur spontaneously.

Screening

There are no useful screening measures to detect a brain tumor in otherwise healthy people. If your physician suspects a brain tumor on the basis of your clinical history and examination, a careful neurological evaluation as well as an MRI or CT scan of the brain will lead to an earlier diagnosis and the best chance for successful treatment.

Common Signs and Symptoms

Symptoms of brain tumors are produced by the tumor mass, the nearby brain swelling, and the damage of normal tissue caused by tumor infiltration. Brain tumors can cause either "generalized" or "focal" neurological symptoms.

Included within the generalized grouping are those symptoms related to increased intracranial pressure (ICP), and seizures. As a tumor grows, it occupies space and causes swelling in the surrounding brain. Since the brain is housed within a rigid and unyielding skull, only a limited amount of tumor mass and swelling is tolerated before symptoms are produced by increased pressure from the tumor. The symptoms produced by increased intracranial pressure include headache, nausea, vomiting, exhaustion, imbalance, and blurred or double vision.

Headache occurs in approximately 50 percent of patients with brain tumors. The headaches usually are not severe and are classically more noticeable in the morning, tend to improve later in the day, and worsen with coughing or straining. Of course, headache is a nonspecific symptom occurring in most people as the result of many causes other than a brain tumor. A physician should always consider other possible reasons why a patient may experience a headache. Furthermore, remember that the most distinguishing feature of a brain tumor headache is its association with other neurological symptoms such as personality changes, weakness, and seizures.

Approximately 30 percent of patients with any sort of brain tumor will experience a seizure, which is why many patients are prophylactically treated with antiseizure medicine. Seizures happen when the brain is irritated, producing abnormal electrical activity locally and in the surrounding brain tissue. If this activity remains confined to a small area of the brain, the result is a focal seizure. During this type of seizure, a patient remains conscious and may experience a strange sensation, such as an unusual smell or taste, or have a brief episode of uncharacteristic behavior. Another common type of focal seizure includes the uncontrolled movement of an arm or leg. These seizures usually last from seconds to minutes, and a complete recovery occurs within the same time period. A generalized seizure occurs when the electrical activity spreads throughout the brain. When this happens, the patient loses consciousness, falls to the ground, and may have uncontrolled movements of the body, arms, and legs. Control over the bowel and bladder may be lost. The seizure can go on for several minutes, and it may take several hours for the person to recover.

When a seizure occurs for the first time in an adult, a thorough evaluation, which includes a neurological examination and a diagnostic brain scan, should be done. It is important to remember, however, that not everyone with a seizure will have a brain tumor, and not everyone with a brain tumor will have a seizure. Daily medication may be administered to prevent further seizures. Blood tests may be performed to monitor the antiseizure medicine drug level in the blood to make sure that it remains within the therapeutic range. Several commonly used antiseizure medicines, including phenytoin (Dilantin), carbamazepine (Tegretol), and topiramate (Topomax), may affect chemotherapy drugs, and you should ask your treating doctor whether you should be changed to a seizure medicine that does not do so.

The second category of symptoms occurs because of focal, or localized, brain dysfunction. A tumor may invade or compress the surrounding brain. Depending on the extent or location of the tumor, the normal function of the brain at that location may be impaired. This loss of function may be noticed as numbness or weakness of an arm or a leg, loss of vision, difficulties with speech, and impaired memory and judgment. A brief location-specific discussion of symptoms follows:

• *Frontal Lobes of the Brain* A tumor in the frontal lobe often causes changes in decision-making ability or changes in mood. If the left frontal lobe is involved, the patient may experience difficulty talking.

• *Temporal Lobes of the Brain* A tumor in the left temporal lobe may lead to difficulty understanding speech, while a right-sided lesion may disturb the perception of musical notes or quality of speech. Temporal lobe involvement may also cause olfactory or gustatory seizures, where the patient experiences odd smells or tastes; these events may be accompanied by lip-smacking or -licking movements and an impaired level of alertness. More generalized involvement of the temporal lobe may lead to emotional changes, behavioral difficulties, and auditory hallucinations.

• *Parietal Lobes of the Brain* A tumor of the parietal lobe may cause loss of sensation or sensory seizures. Sensory loss may result in a feeling of numbness on one side of the body or an inability to detect where your limbs are without looking at them with your eyes. If the left parietal lobe is affected, the patient may experience difficulty with reading or writing.

• *Occipital Lobes of the Brain* A tumor of the occipital lobe (the visual center of the brain) generally produces partial or total loss of vision. Involvement of the left occipital lobe can result in an inability to recognize colors.

• *Cerebellum* In the case of a cerebellar tumor, if the middle of the cerebellum is affected, the patient will experience difficulty with balance while standing. If the sides of the cerebellum are affected, the patient will experience incoordination of the arms and legs.

• *Brain Stem* A tumor affecting the brain stem generally manifests itself with double vision, difficulty with swallowing, or weakness of the arms and legs.

• *Spinal Cord* Patients with primary spinal tumors generally present with pain in a portion of the body or in an arm or leg. The onset of symptoms may be gradual or fast, and generally one side of the body is more affected than the other. The exact set of symptoms depends on which spinal cord level is affected. In general, cervical spinal cord tumors affect the arms, shoulders, and neck. Thoracic, or truncal, tumors affect the abdominal muscles and region. Lumbosacral tumors may affect the legs, pelvic region, and bladder.

Physical Examination As well as a complete neurological and physical examination, specific tests such as visual field determinations and hearing tests are sometimes useful.

Blood and Other Tests
• Routine blood tests are performed as a baseline and followed as treatment is given.
• Some tumors secrete substances that can be measured in the blood and cerebrospinal fluid (CSF). This fluid is removed by lumbar puncture (spinal tap), a procedure similar to spinal anesthesia. CSF may also be examined for malignant cells from tumors that have a tendency to spread from the brain into the spinal cord or its covering. A lumbar puncture may be risky when there is increased intracranial pressure. This risk has largely been removed now that CT or MRI scan can determine if there is enlargement of the fluid cavities within the brain (ventricles) or major pressure shifts within the brain.

Diagnosis

Imaging When a brain tumor is suspected, the initial step in evaluation is brain imaging with CT or MRI scan. These images will assist the neurosurgeon in determining the location and size of the tumor and whether a biopsy or surgical resection should be performed. The images will also likely be used by the radiation oncologist to develop a precise treatment plan of radiation to the specific area of the tumor. These scans are repeated during the course of treatment to determine how the tumor is responding. The exact type of imaging study chosen will depend upon the preferences of the treating physicians and may be influenced by the results of an initial scan.

• MRI is generally the preferred study, as it provides a more accurate three-dimensional reconstruction of the tumor and thus can better guide surgical resection or biopsy. MRI images also provide the best definition between normal brain and tumors and can best depict the swelling associated with these tumors. During the MRI, the patient must hold very still in a tight space, which some find uncomfortable and confining. A new type of MRI allows the procedure to be completed in a more "open" scan area. Although there may be some loss of detail in the scan, for many patients who are claustrophobic, these scanners may be a solution.

• A CT scan takes only minutes to complete, but does not provide images with as much detail as an MRI. In some cases, CT scans may provide superior images of calcified tumors and the skull. Contrast substances injected into a vein just before the MRI or CT scan is performed will cause some tumors to be enhanced so that they can be better defined. When a tumor is suspected, scans are usually performed both before and after contrast has been given.

• A tumor may be found near important blood vessels or have characteristics that suggest that it could be derived from a blood vessel. In these circumstances, a blood vessel study (angiogram) is performed. Dye is injected into the major feeding arteries of the brain and X-rays are taken.

• Newer types of images are being investigated using the MRI scanner, such as MR spectroscopy, MR angiography, and blood flow and perfusion studies that may aid in the diagnosis and monitoring of disease. Another type of scan, called a positron-emission tomography (PET) scan, is used to assess the metabolic activity of a tumor and is sometimes helpful in distinguishing treatment-related side effects from actual tumor growth.

Biopsy

• The diagnosis can be suggested by the above tests, but tumor tissue must be obtained by biopsy or surgery to confirm the tumor type and grade.

• Sometimes the tumor is small or in an area of the brain where it cannot easily be approached or safely be removed. In such cases, a special procedure called a stereotactic biopsy can be performed. A computer is used to plot a pathway to the tumor based upon a CT or MRI image. A small-caliber needle is then passed through the brain to the site of the tumor and a biopsy is obtained. This approach has proved to be very safe and effective in establishing a tissue diagnosis.

In many cases, it can be performed under local anesthesia. Patients can usually be discharged from the hospital the following day.

• If the tumor is surgically accessible, a neurosurgeon may recommend an operation (craniotomy) to attempt to remove some or nearly all of the tissue. Tumor samples will be sent for diagnosis at the time of the craniotomy.

Staging

It is rare for primary brain tumors to spread outside the nervous system (brain and spinal cord), so staging procedures of organs in the rest of the body are not routinely performed. Certain brain tumors do have a tendency to spread not only in the brain, but also into the spinal cord. These tumors include primary central nervous system lymphomas, medulloblastomas, pineoblastomas, germ cell tumors, and ependymomas. When these kinds of tumors are diagnosed, staging of the spinal cord is also required. This staging process typically includes MRI scans of both the brain and spine and a lumbar puncture (spinal tap) to obtain cerebrospinal fluid for microscopic evaluation.

When a metastatic tumor of the brain is discovered, a thorough staging of the rest of the body should be performed, typically with CT scans of the chest and abdomen. Treatment for a patient with a metastatic brain tumor will depend on the extent of spread of the primary tumor.

Treatment Overview

Treatment for most brain tumors is complex and will involve multiple medical personnel. A neuro-oncologist is a physician who specializes in taking care of patients with brain tumors and can help coordinate your care among your neurosurgeon, radiation oncologist, medical oncologist, and neurologist. Most neuro-oncologists are located at academic or university hospitals. Your primary care physician or consulting physician should be able to tell you where the nearest neuro-oncology center is to you. Neuro-oncologists also specialize in conducting clinical trials that involve experimental or new medicines or treatments for brain tumors. Depending on your tumor type and health status, you may be able to participate in some of these clinical trials and receive novel treatments.

Before proceeding with a general discussion of how brain tumors are treated, it is useful to review several characteristics of brain tumors that distinguish them from other types of tumors.

• Most brain tumors range from a low- to high-grade type (the grade of each tumor is based on its microscopic features and determines the type of treatment and prognosis).
• Even the most aggressive or malignant brain tumors rarely metastasize outside the nervous system.
• The location of a tumor often determines whether a neurological deficit occurs.
• Even tumors regarded as slow growing or more benign can produce symptoms as severe and life-threatening as malignant tumors. This is because they may occur in a vital area of the brain or because when they reach a critical size, there is no room for them to expand within the surrounding skull, which puts significant pressure on key structures.
• The brain has no lymphatic vessels to remove the treated or dead tumor, so the tumor may not appear to shrink on CT or MRI scans even if treatment is successful.
• Treatment of a tumor can result in a new neurological deficit. For example, a temporary or permanent loss of function can occur after surgery and problems of brain swelling can occur during radiation treatments.

• Unless a dramatic, early, and sustained improvement occurs after therapy, it may be difficult to determine the response to treatment. Treatments may themselves produce temporary neurological deterioration that might take weeks or months to improve.

Surgery Surgery is the initial treatment for primary brain tumors. The goal of surgery is to determine the type and grade of tumor and to remove as much of the tumor as possible without causing a loss of neurological function. A few types of brain tumors may be completely removed and the patients cured, but surgery alone is not sufficient to cure a patient with a higher-grade or malignant tumor, and other forms of treatment will be required. Surgically reducing the size of the tumor may improve the effectiveness of other therapies.

Surgical removal of the tumor may improve a patient's neurological condition. Surgical removal will reduce intracranial pressure, and a focal neurological deficit may improve or resolve. The frequency of seizures may also be reduced by surgery. Tumors can block the fluid pathways in the brain, leading to buildup of fluid, called hydrocephalus, which can be associated with symptoms of increased intracranial pressure. To relieve these symptoms, it is sometimes necessary to place a permanent shunt device in the fluid cavities to divert the fluid to another part of the body, where it can be absorbed.

Specialized equipment used during surgery includes a microscope to magnify the area of interest, an ultrasonic aspirator that helps break up the tumor, lasers that vaporize tumor tissue, ultrasound localizing equipment, and computer-based navigational equipment to help the surgeon define the tumor boundaries.

Specialized techniques also are used to remove a tumor located near speech or motor brain regions. The surface of the brain can be stimulated with an electrical current to obtain clues about the function of a particular part of the brain. This is referred to as speech or motor "mapping." The process is painless and produces a temporary mild speech disturbance or twitching of the part of the body served by that area of the brain. A decision can then be made about whether it is safe to remove that part of the tumor. Speech mapping is done under sedation and local anesthesia and requires a cooperative patient. Motor mapping can be performed under general anesthesia.

 Radiation Radiation therapy is commonly used in the treatment of both primary and metastatic brain tumors. The treatments are designed to maximize the lethal effects of radiation on the tumor and to minimize the harmful effects to the surrounding brain. Whole brain radiation is rarely given for primary brain tumors. Instead, computer-generated models are used to plan the dose and area of irradiation in a pattern that is "conformal" to any residual tumor not removed during surgery and to a small area surrounding the tumor and surgical cavity. Radiation treatments are generally given once a day, five days a week, for up to six weeks. A patient then generally receives a two- to three-week break from any type of therapy before subsequent imaging studies (MRI) are performed to assess whether the tumor responded to radiation. Some patients may experience fatigue during radiation therapy; others may develop neurological problems such as headaches or weakness related to radiation-induced brain swelling. If such swelling occurs, the problem is usually brief and may be treated with steroid medication to alleviate the swelling.

A full course of conventional or conformal radiation is usually administered only once. Exposing the brain to further radiation could produce brain injury and create a disabling or life-threatening problem. However, new methods of delivering additional radiation to brain tumors are being used in special scenarios. For example, stereotactic radiosurgery ("Gamma Knife" or "cyber knife") may be used to deliver precisely focused radiation beams to a small area of residual or recurrent tumor, while the surrounding brain is spared the adverse effects. These approaches require that the tumor be small to medium-sized and in an area of the brain that could tolerate a radiation injury without causing the loss of an important function.

 Chemotherapy Chemotherapy may be effective and is frequently used before, during, or after surgery and radiation. It can also be used at the time of diagnosis and for a recurrence. Some tumors in the brain can be exquisitely sensitive to chemotherapy, including germ cell tumors, lymphomas, and some oligodendrogliomas. One difficulty in treating brain tumors with chemotherapy is that the drugs do not easily pass through the blood vessels in the brain into the brain substance where the tumor is located. Some experimental approaches have investigated ways to open this blood-brain barrier with drugs, while others have attempted to directly inject drugs into the major arteries feeding a tumor. Additional research is ongoing in developing strategies for injecting antitumor agents directly into the brain.

Biological Therapy There are many novel biological drugs in development that are not necessarily designed to kill tumor cells like older or traditional chemotherapy drugs. Instead, they are designed to prevent further tumor growth. For example, gene therapy is a new approach to treating brain tumors and relies on the transfer of a new gene into tumor cells. The tumor then receives a new set of instructions. One approach uses a virus to infect the tumor and insert a gene into the cancer cells. This technique has shown promise in laboratory experiments, and initial efforts have begun treating humans with a variety of gene-transfer strategies. Advances in the field of immunology have also led to important work in using the immune system to fight tumors. Methods have been developed to insert new genes or toxins into immune cells that will improve their tumor-fighting ability. In addition, vaccines are being developed and have also begun research testing. The hope of these approaches is that the treatment will affect only the tumor cell, sparing the rest of the body or brain of any toxic effects. Most of these agents are available only at research hospitals, and you should ask your treating physician whether you should investigate being evaluated at such a place.

Treatment by Tumor Type

Astrocytoma

Astrocytomas are categorized by their grade of malignancy. Most classification schemes include low-grade astrocytoma (Grade 1/2), anaplastic astrocytoma (Grade 3), and glioblastoma multiforme (Grade 4).

Standard Treatment Low-grade astrocytomas are sometimes treated only with complete surgical removal. However, even these patients must obtain serial MRI scans to make sure that the tumor does not recur. When surgery is not possible, or unable to completely remove a low-grade astrocytoma, radiation or chemotherapy may be considered. You should have a careful discussion regarding whether your doctor feels that chemotherapy or radiation is best suited to your tumor and general health. At the present time, there is no consensus as to whether low-grade astrocytomas are better treated with chemotherapy or radiation. In children, low-grade astrocytomas are more frequently treated with chemotherapy as the initial approach if complete surgical removal is not possible. Radiation would then be reserved if the tumor grew back. In both children and adults, tumors that recur despite either chemotherapy or radiation therapy may show more aggressive behavior and quicker rate of growth. The exception to this rule is a tumor frequently seen in children called juvenile pilocytic astrocytoma. These tumors can be cured if completely removed by surgery. Even if such a tumor grows back after incomplete resection, the tumor almost always continues to grow very slowly and will respond well to either further surgery, or radiation or chemotherapy.

Treatment for anaplastic astrocytoma includes surgery, radiation, and chemotherapy. Glioblastoma multiforme is a very aggressive tumor that grows quickly and invades into the surrounding brain. Complete surgical removal is uncommon. Surgery, radiation, and chemotherapy are used but are rarely curative.

Five-Year Survival Five-year survival is greater than 70 percent for younger patients with low-grade astrocytomas. For the anaplastic astrocytoma, the five-year life expectancy can be as high as 50 percent. For glioblastoma multiforme, the average life expectancy is approximately one year, with fewer than 5 percent of patients living five years. In each of these tumors, various patient variables or prognostic factors can improve life expectancy. The most important variable is the age of the patient when the tumor is diagnosed. For instance, a patient younger than forty-five with glioblastoma multiforme may have an average life expectancy of eighteen months, compared with a patient over the age of seventy, who has an average life expectancy of only nine months. Another important variable for low-grade astrocytoma may be the size of the tumor remaining after surgery.

Oligodendroglioma

Oligodendrogliomas also are categorized by their grade of malignancy. Most classification schemes include low-grade oligodendroglioma (Grade 2) and anaplastic oligodendroglioma (Grade 3). These tumors tend to present with a history of seizures and are frequently calcified on scans. Minor bleeding is more frequently noted in these tumors than in astrocytomas.

Standard Treatment Low-grade oligodendrogliomas are treated in a similar manner to low-grade astrocytomas, with surgery followed by radiation or chemotherapy. You should have a careful discussion regarding whether your doctor feels that chemotherapy or radiation is best suited to your tumor and general health. Like astrocytomas, the higher-grade anaplastic oligodendrogliomas have a worse prognosis than lower-grade tumors and are treated with both radiation and chemotherapy. However, higher-grade oligodendrogliomas tend to have a better prognosis than higher-grade astrocytomas, and respond to chemotherapy more frequently than anaplastic astrocytomas. Your doctor may order genetic tests to look for chromosome deletion (1p19q deletion studies) to determine whether your oligodendroglioma has a higher likelihood of being sensitive to chemotherapy.

Five-Year Survival Seventy-six percent for patients with oligodendroglioma Grade 2 and 50 percent for patients with oligodendroglioma Grade 3.

Brain Stem Glioma

This tumor is an astrocytoma (of any grade) that occurs in the brain stem (which connects the brain to the spinal cord) and is more frequent in children than in adults. Brain stem gliomas can cause incapacitating neurological deficits. They have a very characteristic appearance on MRI scan, and treatment is often performed without first obtaining a tissue diagnosis, since surgery in this area is very dangerous, making a large resection of the tumor impossible.

Standard Treatment These tumors are treated with radiation and sometimes chemotherapy. Surgery is rarely useful except for a minority of tumors that are found in more favorable locations in the brain stem.

Five-Year Survival Patient survival is dependent upon the grade of the tumor as well as the location of the tumor within the brain stem. High-grade tumors that involve most of the brain stem have an average life expectancy of one year or less despite treatment; tumors that are restricted in location are often low-grade astrocytomas and have a five-year survival of greater than 30 percent.

Medulloblastoma

This brain tumor occurs more often in children than in adults. Most cases occur in those under sixteen years of age, and the tumors are typically located in the cerebellum of the brain.

Standard Treatment Surgery is done to remove as much tumor as is safely possible, followed by irradiation to the brain and spine. Chemotherapy is used in most cases after radiation therapy. Chemotherapy may be the first treatment given following surgery in children too young to undergo irradiation or used in cases where tumor remains after surgery and irradiation. Medulloblastoma tends to spread throughout the central nervous system. Scans of the brain and spine, along with cerebrospinal fluid cytology, are used to follow the condition of the tumor. Survival depends on whether it has already spread when diagnosed.

Five-Year Survival Five-year survival is 70 to 80 percent when the tumor can be completely removed and there is no residual tumor in the brain or spine; five-year survival is less than 70 percent if there is residual tumor and disease has spread beyond the primary tumor area.

Meningioma

Meningioma is a tumor from the meninges, the membranous layers that surround the brain. Most meningiomas are benign lesions. Only a few have malignant features and behave aggressively. Meningiomas produce symptoms by compression of the surrounding brain and by the swelling that they incite.

Standard Treatment Meningioma can be cured by surgical removal alone, and when possible, surgery is the treatment of choice. Radiation can be an effective treatment for incompletely removed meningiomas and for malignant or recurrent forms, but repeated surgical resections are sometimes required. Meningiomas that grow along the skull base are very difficult to remove and often require a combination of surgery and radiation to control the tumor.

Pituitary Adenoma

The great majority of pituitary tumors are benign. They generally present with visual loss (which may occur when the tumor compresses the nearby optic nerves) or hormone-related problems caused by an excessive amount of pituitary hormones in the bloodstream. The most common hormonal problems include

• an excess of prolactin hormone, leading to impotence in men and excessive lactation in women;
• an excess of growth hormone that can lead to an enlarged heart, growth of

the hands and feet, and a change in facial features; and
• an excess of cortisol, which can lead to weight gain, diabetes, and high blood pressure.

Standard Treatment The drug bromocriptine (Parlodel) can successfully treat a prolactin-hormone-producing pituitary tumor. Treatment of other pituitary tumors involves a surgery known as a transphenoidal hypophysectomy; in this procedure, the tumor is removed through the sphenoid sinus at the back of the nasal cavity so the skull does not have to be opened (craniotomy). Some tumors can be cured with surgery alone. Others require postoperative treatment with medication and irradiation. If visual loss has been present only for a short time, some recovery of vision can occur after surgery relieves the pressure on the optic nerves.

Primary Central Nervous System Lymphoma

Lymphoma is a cancerous tumor of the lymph cells, which are part of the body's immune system and help to fight infection. Primary central nervous system lymphoma (PCNSL) occurs in the brain preferentially in patients whose immune systems have been suppressed, and in older patients without a known underlying cause. However, it is found in other patients as well. Those cases of PCNSL associated with immunosuppression may be due to inherited diseases, drug therapy for organ transplantation, or other acquired conditions that suppress the immune system. PCNSL was a common manifestation of HIV/AIDS before the introduction of more effective drug therapy for this disease. PCNSL may be present in the cerebrospinal fluid, in the vitreous (a jellylike substance in the center of the eye), and in multiple locations throughout the brain and spinal cord. As such, your doctor should perform an

MRI of the brain and spine, a spinal tap to examine spinal fluid, and an ophthalmologic evaluation of the eyes.

Standard Treatment Since PCNSL usually manifests itself as multiple lesions in locations in the brain that are inaccessible with surgery, only a small biopsy is performed in order to establish a tissue diagnosis. Methotrexate (Mexate)–based, multiagent chemotherapy currently is the treatment of choice, especially in elderly patients who are at highest risk of developing radiation-related neurotoxicity. Whole brain radiation is often used as well, but the optimal role and timing of such radiation has yet to be established.

Five-Year Survival It is unusual for patients older than sixty or seventy or patients with severely altered immunity to survive longer than two to four years. Otherwise healthy younger patients may have a chance of much longer survival, particularly if treated with chemotherapy.

Metastatic Cancer to the Central Nervous System

The number of patients with metastatic intracranial tumors exceeds the number of those with primary brain tumors by a factor of 10. Brain metastasis can occur in as high as 25 percent of all patients with cancer. Since cancer patients now live longer, it is expected that the number of people with metastatic tumors will continue to increase. The finding of brain metastases will radically change the intent and direction of therapy for the primary tumor and will generally take precedence over almost any other complication.

When someone with cancer develops headaches, drowsiness, personality changes, or problems with speech, strength, or balance, a brain metastasis should be suspected. Although a single metastasis can occur, it is more common for there to be multiple tumors. MRI scans are best able to detect multiple metastases, especially small ones.

If there are multiple brain lesions, there is a greater chance that they are metastatic rather than primary. A screening evaluation may then be performed to look for other tumors in the body. This evaluation includes blood tests, a chest X-ray, and CT scans of the chest and abdomen. Initial therapy for the brain lesions usually includes steroid hormones such as dexamethasone (Decadron) to reduce the pressure in the brain and thereby relieve symptoms.

Standard Treatment Surgery is generally reserved for a single metastatic tumor and for symptomatic lesions, if multiple tumors are present. Occasionally, a single lesion that is presumed to be metastatic will be found to be a primary brain cancer instead. Radiation is used after surgery. If there are multiple tumors, surgery is deferred and the treatment is irradiation. Even when small, these tumors can cause considerable swelling. In most cases, radiation is given to the entire brain with the hope of eliminating any small tumor deposits not yet seen on a scan. This can lead to memory loss and a decline in intelligence, so in most patients the highest radiation dose is limited to the tumor site. Avoiding these side effects is important for those with tumors with a fairly good prognosis, such as breast cancer. The treatment of brain metastasis with stereotactic radiosurgery has shown great promise. This focused radiation can successfully control local tumor growth. It offers the advantage of being able to treat multiple tumors at one time and can be repeated if new lesions develop.

Metastatic tumor cells can also line the fluid cavities and surface of the brain. This condition is called carcinomatous meningitis. It can be disabling and is treated by instilling chemotherapy into the spinal fluid. This can be done by lumbar puncture, or a specialized catheter can be placed in the ventricle of the brain and then connected to a small plastic reservoir placed under the skin. Drugs can then be injected into the reservoir to circulate throughout the spinal fluid.

Tumors of the Spinal Cord

Tumors can develop in the spinal cord just like in the brain. The most common types of primary spinal cord tumors are astrocytomas, ependymomas, and meningiomas. In general, primary spinal cord tumors are low grade rather than high grade. These tumors cause neurological deficits when they invade or compress the spinal cord. MRI imaging is more valuable for accurately evaluating spinal cord tumors than any other diagnostic test. These tumors are usually slow growing, and the problems they cause develop over months or years. These problems include sensory loss and pain, paralysis, incontinence of the bowel and bladder, and impotence in males.

Cancers arising elsewhere can metastasize to the spine or spinal cord and produce pressure symptoms such as pain, weakness, and loss of sensation (numbness). Diagnostic methods are similar to those for primary spinal cord tumors.

Standard Treatment Surgery is the preferred method of treatment. Ependymomas can often be completely removed. Radiation is used if there is residual tumor. Astrocytomas have infiltrating margins and usually cannot be completely removed. They are biopsied or the solid component is removed, and radiation is given after surgery. Meningiomas can often be completely removed. If there is residual tumor and it is benign, a series of clinical and radiographic evaluations will be performed. A repeat operation is performed or radiation is used if the tumor grows and causes new problems.

A fluid-filled cavity can develop within the spinal cord near a tumor. This is called a syrinx, and it can grow to a large size and cause pain and loss of spinal cord function. It can also lead to wasting of the affected muscles. An operation to shunt the fluid from this cavity can improve the neurological condition and alleviate symptoms.

Treatment Follow-Up

The response of a brain or spinal cord tumor to treatment may not be immediately apparent. A series of scans may be required to determine whether the tumor is growing or responding well to treatment. The changes that are seen on a brain scan after surgery can resemble residual tumor, and the swelling that occurs in response to the surgery can be identical in appearance to that caused by a tumor. Serial scans are performed at regular intervals with the goal of detecting a recurrent tumor early.

Supportive Therapy

• Swelling of the brain can persist after treatments have been completed. Swelling also often accompanies recurrent tumors. It can cause neurological deficits and create symptoms of increased intracranial pressure. The steroid medication dexamethasone (Decadron) is used to decrease this swelling. However, you should be aware of the potential side effects of dexamethasone: electrolyte mineral disturbance, high blood pressure, elevated blood sugar, infection, osteoporosis, leg edema, glaucoma, gastrointestinal pain, weight gain, skin changes, impaired healing, and acne. Corticosteroids can also cause a variety of neurological toxicities. The most common is proximal myopathy, weakness of the thigh and shoulder muscles. Central nervous system side effects of corticosteroids include mood alteration, insomnia, psychosis, and tremor. Most of these side effects are reversible with reduction of the steroid dose, which must be tapered slowly to prevent steroid withdrawal symptoms.

• A few patients require a very low maintenance dose of steroids even if the tumor is not active or has been controlled. In such cases, some of the original symptoms, such as headache, nausea, and neurological abnormalities, may recur if the steroid hormones are discontinued altogether.

• Medications are sometimes needed to eliminate nausea and relieve pain.

• A risk of seizures can persist over the patient's lifetime. Medications are given to prevent this from happening. The drugs used most often include phenytoin (Dilantin), carbamazepine (Tegretol), and levetiracetam (Keppra). Blood tests can be performed to measure the amount of some of these drugs in the blood. The dose required to control seizures varies from patient to patient. Sometimes two different drugs have to be used.

• Neurological status may change or deteriorate because of the secondary effects of treatment on the brain rather than because of tumor growth. Factors causing apparent neurological deterioration may include lowering the steroid dosage too rapidly, mineral or electrolyte imbalance, complications such as infections or metabolic problems, other medications (particularly for pain), and the effects of radiation and chemotherapy. Tumor destruction from radiation or chemotherapy may produce waste products that may irritate the brain. Because the brain lacks lymphatic blood vessels, there is no efficient method of removing the waste materials, which is why tumors responding to treatment may not appear to change in size for a long time.

• Tumors cause neurological problems that can persist well after all treatments have been completed. The speed and extent of any recovery will depend on how severe the deficits are. Rehabilitative therapies can speed the recovery along, improve overall endurance, and maintain muscle tone and strength. Children, young adults, and the elderly can all benefit from rehabilitative therapies.

Recurrent Cancer

The earlier a recurrent tumor is found, the more options there are for treatment and the greater the chance that treatment will be successful. Health permitting, surgery is the most effective treatment for a recurrent tumor. A focal boost of radiation to the recurrent tumor using stereotactic radiosurgery may be used. Chemotherapy is often used to treat recurrent tumors.

The Most Important Questions You Can Ask

• What type of brain cancer do I have?
• How does it usually behave?
• Is it possible that my life is going to be shortened?
• What type of surgery is most useful and what are the risks?
• Will I need radiation afterward?
• Is there a role for chemotherapy?
• What are the side effects of treatment?
• Will my symptoms go away?
• What medications do I need?
• How functional can I expect to be?
• Are experimental treatments available?
• Do research centers exist that I may contact?
• Where can I obtain more information about treatment?
• Are there patient and family support groups available?

Breast

Debu Tripathy, M.D., Loren B. Eskenazi, M.D.,
William H. Goodson, III, M.D., Britt-Marie Ljung, M.D.,
Beth B. Crawford, M.S., Malin Dollinger, M.D., Ernest H. Rosenbaum, M.D.,
Edward A. Sickles, M.D., Lawrence W. Margolis, M.D.,
and Hope S. Rugo, M.D.

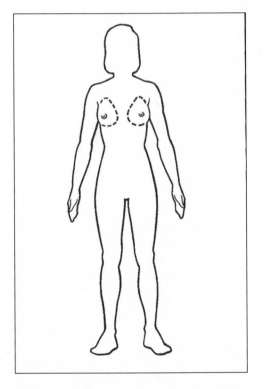

Breast cancer is the most common malignancy in women in the Western world, affecting about one woman in eight over their lifetime. About 215,000 women will develop breast cancer in the United States every year, and about 41,000 die of it. Breast cancer is most treatable when detected in its earliest stages, and there is great interest in screening healthy women—beginning when they are between forty and fifty years old—with mammography and periodic physical examinations. These measures will help detect breast cancers at an earlier stage, resulting in earlier treatment and a better chance for cure. The proper instruction in breast self-examination beginning at an even earlier age may also help with early detection, although this has not been proven in clinical studies. In the United States and western Europe, breast cancer is most often diagnosed at an early stage due to increased awareness and availability of screening and treatment, and hence is most often cured with surgery. The incidence of breast cancer has been rising in industrialized countries for reasons that are still not fully understood. In the United States, this rise has finally leveled off for the last few years, while the death rate due to breast cancer has begun to fall somewhat, due to both screening and improvements in treatment.

Advances in operative techniques and radiation therapy have led to less invasive surgery. Newer medical treatments following surgery for early-stage breast cancer and the wider application of these have led to improvement in curability and survival. The spread of breast cancer, which happens to a minority of breast cancer patients in the United States, still remains incurable, but newer therapies have begun to emerge that can

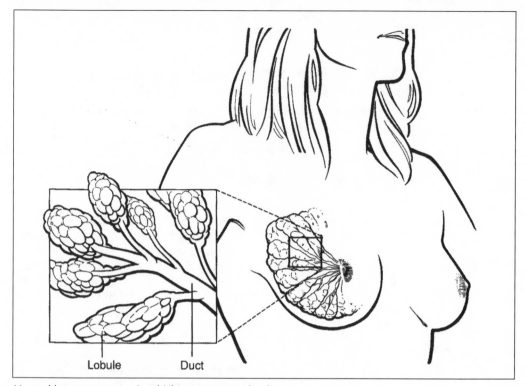

Normal breast structures in which cancers may develop

prolong life and improve the quality of life. Revolutions in the biological sciences have the potential to further this trend and also to be used for new strategies in earlier detection and better individualization of treatment.

What Causes It No definite cause has been established, although genetic factors, lifestyle, and diet all play a role. Most women with breast cancer do not have a clear risk factor and in any given case of breast cancer, it is not possible to pinpoint a specific cause.

Types Breast cancers are divided generally into two types: invasive cancers and noninvasive (or in situ) cancers. Invasive cancers have the capacity to spread to lymph nodes under the arm or to distant sites such as the lungs and bone, whereas in situ cancers rarely spread even though they can return both as in situ or invasive cancers within the breast after they are removed. Invasive cancers are generally divided into lobular and ductal cancers. Lobular cancers start in the many small sacs in the breast that produce milk. The much more common ductal cancers start in the tubes that carry milk from the lobules to the nipple. Within these broad categories, there are over thirty histologic types as seen under the microscope. About half are infiltrating ductal cancers, meaning that they spread through the duct wall. Another 28 percent are combinations of infiltrating ductal cancers and other types, including mucinous, papillary, and lobular. For the most part, these different types of invasive cancers

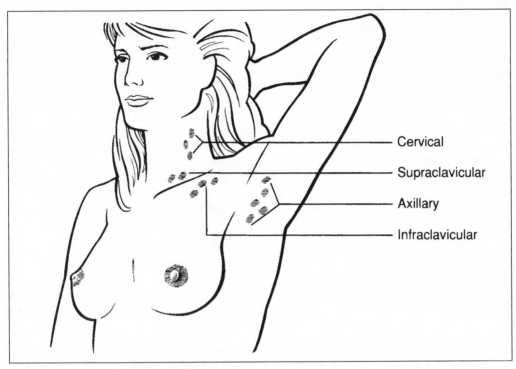

Cervical

Supraclavicular

Axillary

Infraclavicular

Regional lymph nodes important in breast cancer

are treated similarly, as outlined later in this chapter.

Infiltrating lobular carcinoma (5 to 10 percent of breast cancers), which is often detected as a thickening of the breast tissue rather than as a lump, can sometimes involve several areas throughout the breast. Other infiltrating cancers include Paget's disease, a cancer that begins in the area of the nipple and is associated with bleeding, redness, itching, and burning (this is not the same as Paget's disease of the bone, which is a chronic benign process); and inflammatory breast cancer, which shows up as a hot, red, swollen area having the appearance of an infection or inflammation. This subtype has a worse prognosis, because the red color and warmth of the skin indicate that tumor cells have already spread into many lymphatic vessels.

In situ cancers are confined within the lining of the ducts or lobules. These are early cancers or precancerous lesions that have not developed the ability to spread beyond the breast. They are generally of two types:

• Ductal in situ carcinomas (also called intraductal or ductal carcinoma in situ [DCIS]) do have the ability over a long period to lead to invasive cancer if untreated, so these tumors are treated with complete surgical removal. In many cases, radiation therapy and hormonal therapy (tamoxifen [Nolvadex] for five years) are used to lower the risk of the cancer returning in the breast when breast-conserving surgery (like a lumpectomy) is used. Even without these treatments, the risks of spread of DCIS and death due to breast cancer are very remote.

• In situ lobular cancers (also called lobular carcinoma in situ [LCIS]) are best understood as markers for the risk of developing cancer. Since LCIS tends to reflect risk in both breasts, it is not usually possible to remove all lobular carcinomas in situ without removing all of both breasts. This is excessive treatment in most situations, although it is sometimes considered in younger patients who have many years of risk ahead. Careful follow-up is recommended (see "Screening," in this chapter) when this diagnosis is made. In a similar vein, the entity of atypical ductal hyperplasia is sometimes found on pathology after a biopsy of a lump or an abnormal finding on a mammogram. This is also a marker of higher risk, especially if accompanied by a family history of breast cancer, and may therefore warrant closer surveillance.

Nearly all breast cancers arise from glandular tissue (adenocarcinomas), although other types also occur, including squamous cell carcinomas, sarcomas, carcinosarcomas, phyllodes tumor, sweat gland carcinomas, and lymphomas, and these are treated differently. There are several less common types, which have a generally better prognosis than infiltrating ductal cancer, such as medullary carcinoma (6 percent of cases), mucinous (2.5 percent), and tubular (1 percent). Each type has prognostic and therapeutic implications.

How It Spreads After cancer starts, it may be several years before a lump appears. It may remain confined to the breast for a long time, or, in other cases, spread to nearby lymph nodes and distant organs early in the disease. In general, more aggressive cancers tend to spread to lymph nodes more readily and this is also an indicator of a higher chance of spread to a distant site. Very little is known about the mechanisms that a cancer cell uses to facilitate spread. Cancer cells are known to be less "sticky" to one another than normal cells, and also to make enzymes that can help dissolve tissue barriers. Oftentimes, spread can occur years after the initial diagnosis of localized cancer. Much less commonly, distant spread is found at the time that a breast cancer is initially diagnosed, but in less developed countries where patients present later in the course of their disease, such a presentation is more common. As will be discussed later, several medical therapies can be used to lower the risk of spread after surgery for early-stage breast cancer.

Risk Factors

At Higher Risk

• Increasing age. Breast cancer is uncommon under the age of forty and increases in frequency after the age of fifty.

• Family history of breast or ovarian cancer, primarily in parents, daughters, and sisters. This is true for relatives on the father's side as well as on the mother's. The risk is higher if there are multiple family members and cancer(s) at a younger age. This is due to the fact that this increases the chances that there may be an inherited genetic predisposition for breast and ovarian cancer. Several genes, including BRCA1 and BRCA2, have been identified that can contain mutations and confer a risk for these and other cancers. This is discussed later in this chapter and in more detail in chapter 43, "Cancer Risk Assessment, Screening, and Prevention."

• History of previous cancer in one breast, especially if it occurred before menopause.

• Some noncancerous or precancerous lesions of the breast may be associated with development of breast cancer, including multiple papillomatosis, atypical hyperplasia, and lobular carcinoma in situ (LCIS).

• Excessive radiation, with an increased risk for women who were given radiation for postpartum mastitis, received prolonged fluoroscopic X-ray evaluations for tuberculosis, or were exposed to therapeutic radiation therapy for other cancers before the age of thirty. Mammography does *not* expose the breasts to excessive radiation, and to date, there is no evidence that mammography or periodic diagnostic X-rays increase the risk of breast cancer.

At Slightly Higher Risk
• Family history of breast cancer in more distant relatives, such as aunts, grandmothers, and cousins.
• Women with a family history of cancer of the uterus or colon have a slightly increased risk of developing breast cancer (with multiple family members or if of Jewish background, the risk may even be higher).
• Some large breast cysts, especially if accompanied by early atypical hyperplasia (not the more common fibrocystic condition).
• Taking postmenopausal estrogens with progesterone for more than ten years. In general, taking estrogen replacement after menopause remains an individual decision, since there are benefits in terms of lowering osteoporosis risks and improving symptoms of menopause. It may be best, however, to limit exposure to brief durations (less than five years) in women at higher-than-average risk for breast cancer. Also, recent studies have shown that estrogen and progesterone replacement increase the risk of heart attacks and stroke. Of note, oral contraceptives at today's doses do not appear to elevate breast cancer risk.
• Never having carried a term pregnancy or first pregnancy after age thirty.
• Use of alcohol, with a slight increase in risk with even moderate use (one to two drinks per day) and increasing risk with higher alcohol use.
• Early onset of menstruation and late onset of menopause.

• Individuals of European Jewish background have a higher-than-normal risk.
• Higher body weight increases the risk, especially among postmenopausal women.

At Lower Risk
• Term pregnancy under age eighteen.
• Early menopause.
• Surgical removal of the ovaries before age thirty-five.
• Asian ancestry (but not if born in America and adopting American dietary habits).
• Exercise and physical activity at a younger age.

Factors That May Affect Risk, but Whose Role Is Unclear
• A low-calorie, low-fat (especially animal fat), high-fiber or Asian-style diet may decrease risk. This may pertain mostly to the diet early in life, since the majority of studies on adult diet have not uncovered consistent associations with breast cancer risk. There have been numerous studies examining diet and breast cancer risk, and most have been inconclusive. The most definitive study to date shows a slight decrease with a low-fat, high-vegetable/fruit diet, but as of yet, the difference is not statistically significant.
• Controversy continues regarding breast-feeding. Some studies suggest that breast-feeding may reduce the risk of breast cancer, particularly in cultures where prolonged breast-feeding (several years for each child) is the norm.

Factors Not Related to Breast Cancer
• Fibrocystic breasts.
• Multiple pregnancies.
• Coffee or caffeine intake.

Screening

A thorough breast examination should be part of every routine physical and be included with a yearly gynecologic checkup. There are three well-accepted methods for detecting early breast cancer.

• **Mammography for Apparently Healthy Women** There is now widespread agreement that mammography (low-dose X-ray imaging of the breasts) can discover some cancers at least a year before—and sometimes as much as four years before—they can be felt. The scientific evidence that this earlier detection translates to a reduction in the death rate from breast cancer is most convincing for screening women ages fifty and older, but there is evidence that it is also beneficial for women in their forties, although to a somewhat lesser degree. Still, mammography does not detect all cancers, and a positive mammography test does not always mean a cancer is present. Digital mammography may provide clearer images and allows for computer enhancement for detection as well as for sending the images long distance for expert reading. Currently, it appears to be a little more effective for younger (less than age fifty) or premenopausal women and those whose breasts appear more dense on mammogram.

• Many health organizations recommend that women have mammography every year beginning at age forty. There is some controversy as to whether mammograms are not as accurate in younger women, since the breast is denser and may make a lump harder to discern on film. Since younger women have a lower chance of having breast cancer in the first place, they are more likely to have a higher number of benign biopsies for every cancer detected when they undergo screening mammograms. Yearly mammograms are recommended beginning at age thirty or perhaps even earlier when the risk of breast cancer is very high (because of prior breast cancer, very strong family history, hereditary predisposition, or a breast biopsy showing atypical hyperplasia or LCIS).

• The smallest lump usually felt is about $\frac{1}{2}$ inch (1 cm) and contains about 1 billion cancer cells. Routine mammography can detect smaller cancers, some even less than $\frac{1}{4}$ inch (0.5 cm). It is estimated that five-year survival is 20 to 25 percent better for cancers detected by mammography than for those diagnosed after a lump has appeared. Women screened regularly with modern mammography (after 1985) have only a 10 to 30 percent rate of axillary node metastasis, compared to 50 percent for women who do not undergo screening.

• Some concern has been expressed about the risk of frequent X-ray imaging, but the benefits far outweigh any potential risks. The X-ray dose of a mammogram today is considered to be negligible. It is about one-tenth that of twenty-five years ago and is about the same as the cosmic radiation received during a transcontinental airplane flight. However, it is true that most biopsies (about two in three) done because of abnormal mammograms end up being negative for cancer.

• Magnetic resonance imaging (MRI) has gained much attention as a screening tool, but it is currently recommended only in patients with very high risk, such as those who carry a BRCA1 or BRCA2 mutation. It is sometimes also used in individuals who have breast implants or those who are higher risk but have dense breasts that are harder to screen by mammogram. Even with MRI, mammography should also be done, since some cancers may be seen only by one of the tests. Because it can pick up so many benign changes, ultrasound for screening is still being studied and is currently recommended only to pursue a specific area that may be abnormal on mammogram or MRI or on physical examination.

• **Breast Self-Examination** Monthly breast self-examination (BSE) is widely advocated and taught, although studies have not shown that this actually lowers the breast cancer death rate. BSE can be taught by trained physicians and nurses, and most communities have centers to teach women how to perform this examination. BSE also identifies a large number of breast lumps that are not cancer, more so than either mammography or physical examination. Even though formal studies are negative, it makes sense that women should be familiar with the nature of their breasts so that they can report any changes to their doctor.

• **Breast Examination by a Physician or Trained Health Care Provider** Examination of the breasts is a component of routine physical checkups. Benign lumps and masses as well as areas of thickening occur from time to time in most women, and repeated examinations by a physician may call attention to areas that deserve further testing. Physicians often draw in their records diagrams of areas of change or concern, which makes it easier to detect small changes at the next examination.

Although mammography is the most effective screening method, 10 to 15 percent of cancers will be missed by mammography yet found by physical examination, including BSE. Complete breast cancer screening involves all three methods.

Common Signs and Symptoms

A breast lump, usually discovered by the individual, is the most common presenting sign. Sometimes, a mass or speckles of calcium seen on a mammogram may appear suspicious for a cancer but no lump can be felt. When felt, the cancer is often hard and irregular and may feel different from the rest of the breast. There may also be a persistent lump in the armpit (axilla), a symptom of enlarged lymph glands. Pain in the breast is more often due to a benign condition, but medical evaluation is advised, since 5 to 10 percent of breast cancers can also present as pain.

Spontaneous discharge from the nipple of one breast may indicate breast cancer, but most discharges are from benign conditions and most cancers do not have a discharge. Discharges that contain blood or greenish fluid are of more concern. There may be irregularity or retraction of the breast skin or nipple. Scaling of the nipple may indicate Paget's disease, a form of breast cancer that starts in the nipple.

In advanced cases, there may be significant swelling or distortion of the skin or breast. Skin pores may be accentuated because of lymphatic involvement, creating an appearance resembling the skin of an orange, known medically as *peau d'orange*. This may indicate a rare type of cancer termed inflammatory breast carcinoma, which may also be signaled by redness, swelling, or increased heat in the skin.

Breast cancer may occasionally first appear as metastatic disease, with signs or symptoms related to whatever other organ is involved—pain in an area of bony metastasis, swelling in the neck, lung nodules seen on chest X-rays, or liver enlargement.

Breast Cancer Prevention

In earlier trials of the hormonal therapy tamoxifen (Nolvadex) used for early-stage breast cancer, it was noted that fewer new cancers in the other breast developed in women taking tamoxifen. Therefore, a large trial was initiated to compare five years of tamoxifen to a placebo (an inactive drug) in preventing the development of breast cancer in women who were at higher risk based on their age, family history, and other factors. This trial showed that in the short term (about five years), the number of breast cancer cases was cut in half by the use of tamoxifen. In terms of actual numbers, this translated into going from 40 cases of breast cancer for every 1,000 women over five years to 20 cases with the use of tamoxifen. Complications of tamoxifen, which include the risk of blood clots, stroke, and uterine cancer, are more prevalent in older women and the benefits of tamoxifen are greater in women at high risk of getting breast cancer. A balanced decision of risks and benefits must therefore be undertaken in considering the use of tamoxifen in women at higher breast cancer risk. Raloxifene (Evista), another drug in the same class as tamoxifen, is used to prevent osteoporosis and may have a lower risk of uterine cancer induction (a known side effect of tamoxifen). Preliminary evidence supports that raloxifene may also reduce breast cancer risk and have fewer side effects, particularly less clotting and uterine cancer risk.

Inherited Risk of Breast Cancer

About 5 to 10 percent of all breast cancer cases are associated with a familial inherited predisposition. In these cases, there is usually a strong family history of breast or ovarian cancer and it can be either on the father's or the mother's side. The probability of carrying an inherited predisposition is higher in women with a family history of cancer. You can ask yourself the following questions: Do I have a paternal or maternal family history that includes

• two or more female relatives diagnosed with breast cancer before they reached menopause (or before the age of fifty)?
• any family member diagnosed with bilateral breast cancer, or breast cancer in both breasts?
• any family member diagnosed with ovarian cancer at any age?
• any family member with breast and ovarian cancers or more than one primary cancer (e.g., prostate and colon, or breast and pancreatic cancers)?
• a pattern of certain types of cancers among close relatives? (In addition

to breast and ovarian cancers, there are other types of cancers that may suggest the presence of a hereditary cancer syndrome; for example, colon, uterine [endometrial], and ovarian cancers diagnosed before age fifty may suggest hereditary nonpolyposis colorectal cancer [HNPCC]).

There are several known genes that increase risk for breast cancer, but a majority of women with inherited susceptibility to breast cancer have mutations in the BRCA1 or BRCA2 gene. Tests for mutations in these genes are now available. If an individual carries a BRCA1 or BRCA2 mutation, he or she has a 50 percent chance of passing it to each offspring or sharing it with a sibling. There are still many unanswered questions about the risks associated with a positive test.

Not every woman who carries a mutation in the BRCA1 or BRCA2 gene will develop breast and/or ovarian cancer, but the risk is high for these women. A female carrier of a BRCA1 mutation has a 55 to 85 percent lifetime risk of developing breast cancer, a 20 to 40 percent lifetime risk of developing ovarian cancer, and a 6 percent risk of developing colon cancer, by age seventy. This is compared to the 10 to 12 percent lifetime risk of developing breast cancer and the 1 to 2 percent risk of developing ovarian cancer in the general population. The lifetime risk for breast cancer in the second breast, after cancer has developed on one side, is 40 to 60 percent. Males who carry a mutation in BRCA1 are at higher risk of developing prostate and colon cancer.

Women who carry a mutation in the BRCA2 gene have the same risk of developing breast cancer as women who carry a BRCA1 mutation, 55 to 85 percent by age seventy. However, they have a slightly lower risk of developing ovarian cancer, 15 to 30 percent risk by age seventy. Males who carry a mutation in the BRCA2 gene have a 5 to 10 percent risk of developing breast cancer in their lifetime and a risk of prostate cancer of 20 percent by age eighty. The pattern of cancers seen with BRCA2 can also include pancreatic, fallopian tube, and laryngeal (throat) cancers.

This risk may vary somewhat depending on other inherited factors or on lifestyle factors. Furthermore, there is very little information on how closer monitoring or even preventive surgery in BRCA1 and BRCA2 mutation carriers will affect the risk of developing cancer or dying of cancer.

There are other genes that can be involved in the predisposition to breast cancer and other cancers; these include Chk 1, p53, PTEN (Cowden syndrome), and p16.

When there is a strong family history suggestive of the possibility of an inherited predisposition, a session with a genetic counselor or an appropriately trained specialist should occur prior to any testing. This session is designed to verify the family history and then see if the risk of carrying a BRCA1 or BRCA2 mutation or other gene mutation is in the range of warranting genetic testing. A balanced discussion that covers the accuracy of the test, the meaning of the test results, and the options for surveillance, prophylactic surgery, and other risk-reduction strategies needs to be held prior to a decision to proceed with testing.

Individual initiation is an important aspect of genetic testing, and a cancer risk assessment and genetic counseling provide vital information and support to address decisions such as genetic testing, treatment, drug therapy for prevention (such as tamoxifen [Nolvadex] therapy), and surveillance. The information from genetic counseling and gene-testing results has implications for the individual and for many other at-risk family members. Often one family member takes on the task of searching out this information for the rest of the family. The individual

who is seeking BRCA1 and BRCA2 testing may or may not have a personal history of breast or ovarian cancer. It is always more informative to first test a family member who has cancer.

If no one in the family has yet been tested, the initial genetic testing should ideally be done on the individual that already has (or had) cancer. In some cases, other cancers in the family, such as colon cancer, may prompt the testing for other genes that confer risk for other cancers. If the results of genetic testing are negative in the presence of a very strong family history, it is possible that there is still a familial risk that is carried on a gene other than BRCA1 and BRCA2. There is still active research to discover other cancer susceptibility genes. In individuals of Jewish background, 90 to 95 percent of the mutations are clustered within two sites on the BRCA1 gene and one site on the BRCA2 gene. Testing for only three mutations is cheaper and less time-consuming. Otherwise full sequencing of the BRCA1 and BRCA2 genes, a more laborious test, is necessary. If one family member is known to carry a mutation, then only that specific site of the BRCA1 or BRCA2 gene needs to be tested in other family members. Direct relatives of the involved person (parent, child, or sibling) will have a 50 percent chance of having the same mutation.

For individuals testing positive for BRCA1 or BRCA2 mutations, the options are as follows:

• Frequent surveillance: mammograms yearly beginning at age twenty-five to thirty. Breast exams every six months. For ovarian cancer, a bimanual pelvic exam, transvaginal ultrasound with color-flow Doppler ultrasound, and CA-125 serum marker blood tests are recommended every six months.
• Prophylactic (preventive) surgery. Because these surgeries do not completely remove breast or ovarian tissue, there is

still a small risk of developing cancer. Prophylactic mastectomy is estimated to lower the risk by 90 percent (that is, from 60 to 85 percent lifetime to 6 to 10 percent). Prophylactic oophorectomy, or removal of the ovaries, at age thirty-five or when childbearing is complete, can also be considered. This is estimated to cut the risk of ovarian cancer significantly and can also reduce the risk of breast cancer in premenopausal women because estrogen levels are lowered.

Numerous uncertainties still exist in the field of cancer genetics and genetic testing. Over time, better estimates of the benefits of surveillance, prophylactic surgery, and new experimental screening and prevention options will be available. Ethical issues such as protection against insurance discrimination and confidentiality of records are still not completely resolved and will need special policies and laws.

Diagnosis

It may be difficult to clinically distinguish malignant from benign breast masses such as fibrous tumors (fibroadenomas), fatty collections, inflammatory masses, infections, and cysts. In premenopausal patients, it is common for benign lesions to enlarge just before menstrual periods and then shrink.

It is often helpful for the physician to draw an exact diagram with a description of a newly detected mass. Mammography and/or biopsy may be useful, but if these are not done, the mass should be reexamined one or two months later if there is any suspicion that it might be cancer. If the mass persists, mammography and biopsy should be considered as outlined below.

Physical Examination

• Physical examination of the breast is conducted with the patient in various positions and with careful recording of any suspicious masses or abnormal findings.

• This should be accompanied by a complete physical, including a pelvic examination and evaluation for signs of cancer in other locations such as the skin, lymph nodes, and liver.

Blood and Other Tests

The following tests are commonly done as part of the evaluation before or after biopsy or surgical treatment. Not all tests need to be done in all situations, since the results may sometimes not be needed to make optimal treatment decisions (this process is outlined in "How Prognostic Factors Affect Treatment Choices," in this chapter).

• Blood counts and a chemistry panel to determine organ function and detect metastases, including liver function and bone enzyme (alkaline phosphatase, LDH, SGOT, and SGPT) tests.

• Tumor marker blood tests— including serum carcinoembryonic antigen (CEA), CA 15-3, and CA 27-29—may be performed to help determine prognosis and response to therapy. The use of these markers in treatment decisions still remains controversial. In patients with advanced metastatic breast cancer, these markers may help determine response (or lack of response) to treatment.

• Tumor tissue tests, including hormone receptors (estrogen and progesterone receptors), DNA, and other protein markers with potential diagnostic and prognostic value.

• Chest X-rays will assess lungs, ribs, and the spine for metastases. Specialized X-rays of other areas may be done if there are specific bodily complaints.

• A bone scan will help exclude bone metastases. This is often not necessary with small cancers but should be done if there is new bone or joint pain.

• An abdominal CT scan may be done to evaluate the liver, especially if the serum alkaline phosphatase (a bone and liver enzyme) is elevated. This test is not done routinely in someone without symptoms or with normal blood tests, unless the cancer is of very high risk (such as many positive lymph nodes).

Imaging

• Mammography is helpful in evaluating a suspicious mass, especially if it is new or persistent. It is also useful in women whose breasts are large and difficult to examine or who have had implants. Mammography is also used to locate precisely the position and extent of a known tumor. A standard two-view mammogram and specialized views, including magnified images, can provide vital information, but mammography is not a definitive diagnostic test, since 10 to 15 percent of cancers are not detectable by this technique. A biopsy should be done of any suspicious palpable (able to be felt) mass even if mammography does not suggest the presence of cancer.

• Mammograms may detect an abnormality elsewhere in the same or opposite breast. These images may show microcalcifications suspicious for cancer (even if no mass is palpable) or a smaller, nonpalpable but still suspicious mass. In this situation, a biopsy must be done, usually guided by mammography, to determine whether the lesion is cancer.

• Mammography may also be used to evaluate women with precancerous breast conditions, to evaluate yearly the opposite breasts of women with known breast cancer (as there is a higher risk of developing cancer there), and to evaluate women with metastatic adenocarcinoma of an unknown primary site. Sometimes the primary site is a hidden breast cancer. This last point is especially important because breast cancer may respond to chemotherapy or hormonal therapy not used to treat other forms of metastatic cancer.

• Ultrasound evaluation (breast ultrasonography) may be used to diagnose cysts. Ultrasonography is fairly accurate in determining whether a mass is cystic (containing fluid) or solid. This may eliminate the need for more complex procedures, including needle aspiration and biopsy. Some physicians prefer to withdraw the fluid from some cysts with a simple needle and syringe (aspiration), especially if the cysts are painful. If nonbloody fluid is removed and the mass completely disappears, no further treatment or evaluation is needed. Solid masses are more suspicious for cancer and therefore will usually be evaluated with a biopsy.

• Ultrasound imaging, like mammography, can also be used to locate precisely the position of a known but nonpalpable tumor to guide biopsy.

• Tissue should be removed by biopsy for microscopic examination if a mass is still present after fluid is removed, if blood is removed, if abnormal cells are found in the fluid, if no fluid can be aspirated, or if the mass returns two weeks later.

• Magnetic resonance imaging (MRI) may be done to evaluate breast implants if there are signs or symptoms suggestive of implant rupture. MRI may also help determine the extent of cancer or DCIS once a diagnosis is made, to help better plan for surgery. Since cancer may rarely be found in a completely different area of the breast or in the opposite breast when a known cancer is diagnosed, MRI is being studied to see if diagnosing and treating "incidentally detected" breast cancer will improve a patient's chances of remaining free of recurrence over time.

Biopsy Almost all biopsies of suspicious breast masses used to be open surgical biopsies—removing a lump or part of a lump after cutting through the skin. This typically left behind a scar and a defect of varying size in the breast tissue. Now more options are available. Fine needle aspiration (FNA) biopsy is frequently used and entails placing a very thin needle inside the mass and extracting cells for microscopic evaluation. The procedure itself takes only seconds and the discomfort is comparable to a blood test. In order to make FNA reliable, it is important that the sampling as well as the interpretation of the specimens is done by specially trained physicians who use the procedure frequently.

Another option is a core needle biopsy, which uses a larger bore needle that extracts a thin core of tissue. This latter procedure requires local anesthesia and is more likely than FNA to be associated with significant bruising of the area. Bruising may be associated with temporary soreness in the breast but subsides gradually on its own.

In cases where a mass lesion is not palpable but can be seen by imaging studies such as mammography, ultrasound, or MRI, any one of these three imaging techniques can be used to guide fine needle aspiration or core needle biopsy. Generally, if ultrasound is able to visualize the target, it is the preferred method, because of ease of use and minimized discomfort for the patient.

If a fine needle aspirate or a core needle aspirate is nondiagnostic (does not contain enough material for the diagnosis) or indeterminate (does not allow a definitive benign or malignant diagnosis), then either a repeat attempt at needle biopsy is done or an open surgical biopsy is carried out.

The accuracies of FNA and core biopsies are similar when carried out by specifically trained practitioners. In large studies, two to five palpable breast cancers in one hundred are not identified as cancers. Because of this limitation, biopsy results are looked at in combination with palpation (what the mass feels like) and any image study, including mammogram and ultrasound. This is called the triple test. If any of the three indicate a high degree of concern for cancer, then an open biopsy is carried out. By using this combination, the frequency of missed cancers can be brought to 1 percent or less, which is comparable to the miss rate when using open biopsy alone.

Mammography may help guide the surgeon to do an open biopsy of the correct area. This is especially important for nonpalpable lesions. A needle is placed within or adjacent to the lesion under X-ray guidance (needle localization). An X-ray of the removed specimen (mass) is done during the surgery to be certain all the abnormal findings, including calcifications if present, seen on the mammogram have been removed.

Staging and Prognosis

Once a diagnosis of cancer is made, it is important to know the exact location and the extent of cancer and any possible sites of spread—this is referred to as the tumor stage. Some of this information comes from the surgical treatment itself and examination of the tissue removed, while other information is gathered from X-ray and blood tests. Stage is directly related to prognosis and determines the type of treatment to be offered, especially when several therapies are available. The main aspects of prognosis include the risk of recurrence and death due to breast cancer. There are two general types of recurrences. Local recurrences are those that occur in the same breast, in the chest wall at or near the surgical incision, or in the remaining lymph nodes under the arm of the involved side. These are considered curable with surgery, sometimes with radiation, although this usually does portend a higher later risk of recurrence. Distant recurrences (also called metastases) refer to the spread of tumor to distant organs, most commonly the bone, lungs, and liver, or to nodes other than those under the same arm. Distant recurrences are generally not curable and account for most of the deaths due to breast cancer, even though some individuals can live a normal life for a long time with metastases.

The TNM classification system is used to stage breast cancer according to the size of the primary tumor (T), the involvement of the lymph nodes in the armpit (axillary nodes) next to the affected breast (N), and the presence or absence of metastasis to distant organs or nodes other than the same side axilla (M). The clinical stages range from Stage I to IV. Stage 0 (or Tis) is in situ cancer, which is still localized to the point of origin and has not yet begun to invade outward or spread. TNM staging and treatment for breast cancer is shown on pages 508–512. The presence of axillary nodal involvement with tumor and the number of nodes involved constitute the most powerful prognostic factor. Tumor size, along with several other features, can also predict risk, but to a lesser extent. The appearance of the tumor under the microscope can also help determine prognosis. Tumor grade refers to several qualities of the cancer cells, such as the amount of glandular formation, the size of the cell nucleus (center of the cell, where the genes and cell division functions reside), and the fraction of cells that are actively dividing (referred to as the mitotic index). A higher grade is associated with a higher risk of both local and distant recurrence, and other microscopic features such as the presence of tumor cells in the lymphatic and blood vessels of the tumor itself.

How Prognostic Factors Affect Treatment Choices

Most treatments like chemotherapy and hormonal therapy tend to have a greater effect when the risk of recurrence is higher. If the risk of recurrence is very low, such as would be seen in a small tumor of low grade with negative nodes, then the amount by which the risk could be further reduced would be very small indeed. For this reason, staging and analysis of the above-mentioned prognostic factors is important. Also, some tumor tissue tests can help determine which type of treatment would be most effective. In addition to lymph node status, tumor size, and grade, other factors can help in determining prognosis and deciding what treatments are most important following surgery. It is important to remember that none of the markers listed below should be looked at singly, but rather should be put together with all the prognostic factors. For example, someone with a small node-negative tumor has a low risk of recurrence, and even though one of the markers below may indicate higher levels of aggressiveness, this may raise the risk of recurrence only by a small amount. These tumor tissue tests include the following:

• The measurement of protein receptors for two types of female hormones that affect breast cancer tissue—estrogen and progesterone receptors. The tumor content of these receptors—positive or negative—correlates with prognosis and response to hormonal therapy. Therefore, most patients with either estrogen- or progesterone-receptor-positive (ER or PR) tumors will derive a reduction in the future risk of recurrence with the use of the hormonal therapy tamoxifen (Nolvadex; covered in more detail in "Hormonal Therapy for Early-Stage Breast Cancer," in this chapter).

• Cell cycle analysis. Both normal and malignant cells go through a complete cell cycle known as mitosis. During one phase of the cycle (the S-phase), new DNA is synthesized in preparation for the division of one cell into two. Flow cytometry as well as other techniques is used to measure the S-phase fraction, or growth rate. The percentage of tumor cells in this S-phase is an indication of how rapidly a tumor is dividing. As might be expected, tumors with a high S-phase fraction are more aggressive and have a less favorable prognosis. Ki-67 (or MIB-1) correlates with the S-phase and the growth rate, and high levels of staining for this protein also indicate a higher risk of recurrence.

• Immunohistochemical detection of abnormal tumor proteins, including secreted enzymes and stress proteins, are under investigation. Lower levels of the enzyme cathepsin-D or specific "heat-shock" proteins, for example, are associated with better survival in some studies.

• There are also abnormal oncogene and growth-factor-related products. The product of the HER-2/*neu* oncogene, a growth factor receptor protein, is overproduced in about one-quarter of breast cancers. The overproduction appears to be associated with earlier tumor relapses and lower survival rates. There is preliminary evidence that this marker may also influence the degree of benefit that might be seen with certain chemotherapy and hormonal drugs. There is preliminary evidence that overexpression of HER-2/*neu* may render cancer more sensitive to doxorubicin (Adriamycin)–based therapy (see "Adjuvant Chemotherapy for Early-Stage Breast Cancer," in this chapter). Most important, it has been shown that patients with HER-2–positive tumors can derive a significant benefit from therapy with an antibody against HER-2 (trastuzumab [Herceptin]) and this is discussed further in the section on adjuvant chemotherapy.

• More recently, multigene assays, or tests that look at many genes at a time, have been able to use the patterns of actively expressed genes to predict how well someone might respond to chemotherapy. These tests have been applied primarily in situations where the average benefit of chemotherapy might be very small and possibly confined to a subgroup of patients that could be identified by multigene analysis. In the future, this approach may also help determine which of several treatment options would be ideal for a specific patient and allow for tailored therapy based on individual tumor and "host" characteristics.

Further clinical testing will be needed to confirm how many of these tests add to our ability to identify individuals with a higher risk of relapse and to better individualize therapy. It is expected, however, that during the next few years, many additional tests will be discovered and routinely performed on all breast tumors. At the current time, the most important markers that are used in treatment decisions are nodal status, tumor size, tumor grade, estrogen/progesterone receptor, and HER-2/*neu* receptor.

Treatment Overview

It is now standard practice for primary physicians, surgeons, radiation oncologists, and medical oncologists to work together to plan and carry out each patient's treatment. Any one of these physicians can assume the role of "quarterback," serving as the leader for decision making and conveying information to the patient and family and other members of the medical team.

Surgery The basic principle of breast cancer treatment is to remove the identifiable cancer and a rim of surrounding normal tissue to make sure that there is a "margin" of safety around the tumor. The degree of excision depends on the individual. The surgeon and the pathologist evaluate the extent of the cancer and its location within the tissue that has been removed. Fortunately, most cases of breast cancer, especially those detected

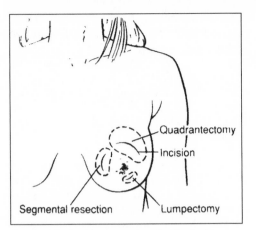

Types of limited surgery, showing typical incisions and amount of tissue removed

on a mammogram, can be treated with breast-conserving surgery.

Smaller tumors can be treated with lumpectomy, which consists of removal of the lump and a surrounding normal rim of tissue (in this case, radiation to the breast is recommended). Only larger tumors require a quadrantectomy. If a tumor is advanced or has spread throughout the breast, complete removal of the cancer will remove a large portion of the breast itself and it may be advisable to proceed with a mastectomy. The judgment as to the amount of tissue that can be removed before it is wiser to do a mastectomy must be discussed between a patient and her surgeon. Radical operations such as the Halsted radical mastectomy (which removes muscles on the chest wall) should be used only in very advanced situations where a cancer is attached to the muscle. In some cases where the tumor is large, or in those that might require a mastectomy instead of a lumpectomy, chemotherapy may be given before surgery to shrink the tumor and improve the chances of being able to perform breast-conserving surgery.

Lymph nodes are generally removed as part of the surgical procedure to determine the extent of the cancer, although it is possible that their removal can also contribute to lowering the risk of subsequent recurrence. Cancer present in the lymph nodes indicates a significant risk of microscopic (and therefore undetectable) metastases outside the breast and the axillary (armpit) area, possibly in the lungs, liver, or bone. The finding of positive lymph nodes usually means that additional adjuvant therapy—hormonal or chemotherapy following surgery—will be recommended to lower the risk of spread. If the lymph nodes do not contain cancer, the likelihood of distant metastases is lower. Removal of the lymph nodes per se does not seem to make a difference to survival. Following lymph node dissection, there may be a small risk of lymphedema, or chronic swelling of the arm, that can develop after surgery—sometimes even many years later (see chapter 20, "Coping with the Side Effects of Chemotherapy"). This risk is higher if nodes in the upper part of the axilla are removed or if radiation to the upper lymph nodes is used (sometimes these procedures are necessary because of suspicious changes noted at the time of surgery or the finding of multiple lymph nodes involved with tumor).

It is now also recognized that axillary lymph nodes are not an effective barrier to tumor spread. The nodes are removed not as a curative measure, but mainly to provide information about the risk of recurrence and metastasis and to better define the need for adjuvant therapy. In the past, most women with invasive cancer underwent removal of many lymph nodes at the time of their surgery, a procedure termed axillary lymph node dissection. Today, for patients who do not have nodes that are suspicious for containing cancer, either on physical examination or on an imaging test, a sentinel lymph node biopsy is done. In this procedure, the surgeon uses a blue dye, sometimes with a radioactive tracer, to mark the first axillary node that may receive cancer cells. The blue dye and/or tracer are injected into the breast beside the tumor. They then travel through normal lymphatic channels to one or more sentinel nodes, which are identified by the surgeon visually and, if applicable, with a radioactive probe. The surgeon may also remove additional nodes that feel hardened or enlarged at the time of surgery. If the sentinel node or nodes have no cancer, it is unlikely that other nodes contain cancer. If the sentinel node contains cancer, there is concern that other nodes may also contain cancer and this is usually followed by a full lymph node dissection. Surgery to find the sentinel node is 90 percent successful, and its ability to predict if any nodes contain cancer is 90 to 95 percent accurate. This means there are three possible outcomes of the procedure. You should discuss the plan for each outcome with your surgeon. The three possibilities are as follows:

1. Your surgeon finds the sentinel node, and a pathologist examines the node during your surgery. If it does not contain cancer, there is a 90 to 95 percent chance that you do not have cancer in the remaining nodes, and no further surgery may be needed. The final pathology analysis, which sometimes includes the use of antibodies to help detect cancer cells in the nodes, is available a few days after surgery.

2. Your surgeon finds the sentinel node, the node is evaluated by a pathologist during surgery, and the node contains cancer. This happens 20 to 30 percent of the time and may not be evident until the final pathologic examination after surgery. Because of the possible spread of cancer from a positive sentinel node to other nodes, the usual plan is to remove additional nodes, which converts the operation to a standard node dissection or is done as a separate surgery later.

Studies are currently under way to determine whether it is necessary to remove additional nodes when the sentinel node contains cancer. Sometimes the specific situation involves a detailed discussion with your surgeon and others on your team as to exactly what findings should form the basis for the need of a follow-up axillary node dissection.

3. Your surgeon may not be able to identify the sentinel node. This happens less than 10 percent of the time. In this situation, the usual plan is to remove the lymph nodes as would be done in a standard axillary dissection.

When a very small amount of cancer (less than 2 mm) is found in the sentinel or other nodes, it is called a micrometastasis (not to be confused with distant metastasis) and is still considered a marker of higher risk. However, if the amount of tumor is less than 0.2 mm, this is at the current time considered to portend the same risk as negative nodes and also may not require subsequent axillary nodal dissection.

If only the sentinel node—and possibly a few additional nodes—are removed, there is less chance of long-term lymphedema, nerve injury, or loss of motion in the shoulder after surgery. Sentinel node removal is a relatively new procedure, and information changes frequently. Ask your surgeon for a time to discuss the plan for *your* surgery.

Breast Reconstruction Another role for surgery is reconstructing a breast after one has been removed. This is being done more often than it used to be. It is also being done earlier and with techniques that produce a more cosmetically acceptable result. An experienced plastic or reconstructive surgeon may see the patient before primary surgery to give advice and assistance but is more often consulted near the end of therapy if the patient wants her breast reconstructed.

Postmastectomy Breast Reconstruction

Women who have had a mastectomy have a number of options to restore their normal physical appearance, including wearing a breast prosthesis. In many cases, however, breast reconstruction greatly improves an overall feeling of wholeness, elevating a sense of well-being and body image. This also eliminates the need for an external prosthesis and decreases the number of clothing restrictions. Reconstruction almost never interferes with monitoring for recurrence, and also can be coordinated around other needed treatments such as chemotherapy.

Postmastectomy breast reconstruction is one of the most significant advances in plastic surgery over the past two decades. There are now several ways to reconstruct the breast, each with its advantages and disadvantages. Improved techniques are now also available for reconstructing the nipple. The opposite breast may have to be reshaped or have its size altered to provide the best symmetry. A team approach in which the plastic surgeon works with the primary care physician, general surgeon, and radiation and/or medical oncologist generally leads to the most satisfactory result.

The first question to be decided is whether to reconstruct the breast immediately, at the time of the mastectomy, or to delay the procedure. The immediate approach of creating a breast mound at the same time as the mastectomy has the advantage of being less psychologically disruptive ("mourning" for the lost breast) and has a superior aesthetic result to delayed reconstruction. Immediate reconstruction is appropriate for women with smaller cancers or for those women with tumors that do not closely approach the chest wall or skin of the breast. If the tumor is larger than 2 inches (5 cm), or if the general surgeon is not confident that the cancer can be removed with clear margins, reconstruction of the breast is usually delayed. The primary goal is always curing the cancer. Breast reconstruction is always a secondary goal and should not interfere with the cancer treatment.

The delayed approach has few advantages. It allows the surgical wound to heal completely, so the reconstruction does not compound possible postmastectomy healing problems in those women who are at high risk for complications (diabetics, smokers, and those who have had previous radiation to the breast). These days, an experienced reconstructive surgeon can perform a successful reconstruction in most patients, even those at high risk. There will always be some women who do not want their breasts reconstructed or who are unable to decide whether they want reconstruction prior to their mastectomies. For these women, it is better to leave the decision to a later date.

Some consideration should be given to the timing of radiation therapy when it is needed. For example, this may affect the cosmetic outcome when using implants, due to increased fibrosis (scarring). For patients that need radiation to the chest wall, it may be best to avoid using implants immediately after surgery and to consider other reconstructive options.

In the early 1990s, isolated cases of possible reaction to silicone gel leading to autoimmune disease received a great deal of attention. Scientific studies were launched and the routine use of silicone gel for breast augmentation was suspended until more was known about this. However, the use of silicone implants for breast-reconstruction patients was never suspended. Now that the scientific studies have been done showing "no link" between silicone and autoimmune disease, silicone implants are being reintroduced rapidly into the marketplace for both reconstructive and cosmetic patients. In addition, alternative materials are being studied that may have advantages over both silicone and saline. These new materials are undergoing rigorous investigation, and it will be several more years before they are available in the United States.

The most common complication following silicone breast implantation has historically been capsular contracture. In up to half of women, the normally thin layer of scar tissue surrounding the smooth surface of the implant thickens and contracts. This creates an abnormal firmness and sometimes pain and/or distortion of the breast. Capsular contracture can often be corrected with additional surgery.

One-Stage Implant Breast Reconstruction

After a "skin-sparing mastectomy," in which the breast tissue is most commonly removed along with the nipple and biopsy site, there is usually enough skin left on the chest to reconstruct the breast mound with an implant in "one stage." In the case of immediate reconstruction, postoperatively adjustable implants are commonly being employed instead of tissue expanders. These implants do not need to be replaced at a later date like tissue expanders. The implant is inserted at the time of the mastectomy under general anesthesia. Minor adjustments in the volume of the implant may be made in the doctor's office following this surgery. A few months later, a small injection dome is removed and the nipple is made with local anesthesia. It is also possible in some patients to achieve excellent results by preserving the nipple and entire skin envelope, reconstructing the breast with an adjustable implant with only a scar under the breast.

Advantages

• Reestablishes the completed breast mound with minimal additional surgery.

• Patients may also be less psychologically stressed, since they have an immediately visible result of the reconstruction procedure rather than the absence of a breast. Some studies have shown this leads to faster recovery and return to work.

• This may also be done in the delayed situation, occasionally using a permanent, nonadjustable implant for small-breasted women.

Disadvantages

• The general and plastic surgeons must schedule the surgery together in the case of immediate reconstruction. This can be logistically challenging in some cases.

• The opposite breast generally needs a small procedure (such as a breast reduction or a breast lift) at the same time to provide symmetry. (Many surgeons are able to accomplish this in the initial operation.)

• As with any implant, there is a low but definite risk of complications, which could lead to further surgery.

• There is a higher risk of complications with this procedure if the patient has undergone prior radiation therapy.

• If radiation is needed at a later date, the implant may become hard and uncomfortable.

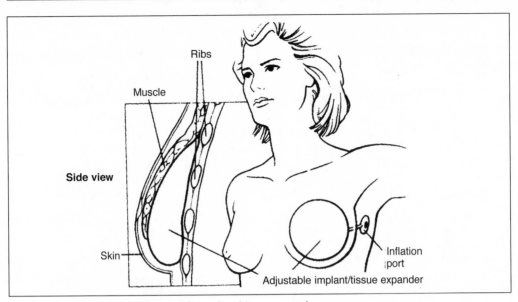

Breast reconstruction using adjustable implant/tissue expander

Tissue Expansion Technique

When there is not enough skin available on the chest wall, or in the case of delayed reconstruction, an inflatable prosthesis is placed under the skin and sometimes the muscles of the chest wall and is gradually inflated with saline. This is usually done weekly in the doctor's office. Several months are generally required before the breast reaches the size needed to match the opposite breast. The expander is then exchanged for a permanent prosthesis in an additional operation. A postoperatively adjustable implant may also be used instead of a tissue expander. This implant does not need to be replaced at a later date.

Advantages

• As a delayed procedure (done after the mastectomy has healed), this technique is simple and can be done on an outpatient basis under local or general anesthesia.
• This technique may afford the shortest recovery and time off work when done after the mastectomy has healed.

Disadvantages

• This is a multistaged procedure and often requires many months to complete.
• The opposite breast generally needs a small procedure (such as a breast reduction or a breast lift) at the same time to provide symmetry.
• As with any implant, there is a low but definite risk of complications, which could lead to further surgery.
• There is a higher risk of complications with this procedure if the patient has undergone prior radiation therapy.
• If radiation is needed at a later date, the implant may become hard and uncomfortable.

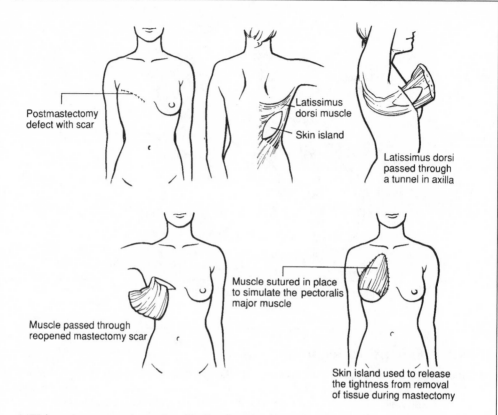

LATS breast reconstruction, using skin flap from back muscle

Latissimus (LATS) Flap Technique

This technique became very popular in the late 1970s and early 1980s. Today, it is most useful when the TRAM or DIEP flap (see page 493) is not an option or when an implant/expander alone does not suffice (e.g., when there has been localized radiation damage after the mastectomy). A breast implant is generally used along with the broad, fan-shaped back muscle (latissimus dorsi) and a segment of overlying skin, which is rotated around to the chest wall to replace tissue removed during the mastectomy.

Advantages

• Adds fullness to the lower portion of the breast, where it is most needed to produce a natural-looking breast.

• Offers an option for additional healthy skin if the skin on the chest wall has been irradiated.

Disadvantages

- An implant is needed as well as the flap in most cases.
- Creates an additional chest scar and a visible scar on the back.
- Transferring this back muscle may impair muscle power for some athletic activities.
- Skin from the back may be a different shade or texture.

TRAM (Transverse Rectus Abdominus Myocutaneous) Flap Technique

This is one of the more complex of the commonly used techniques and is not appropriate for all patients. A portion of one or both of the vertical muscles in the center of the abdomen (rectus abdominus) and a large ellipse of skin and fat from the lower abdomen are transferred through a subcutaneous tunnel onto the chest wall and shaped into the form of a breast.

In some areas of the country, this technique is currently being replaced by the DIEP flap, which does not harvest the muscle for blood supply. The TRAM is still an excellent option and in skilled hands is a shorter, less complex operation with a lower complication rate.

DIEP and Microsurgical Free-Flap Technique

Just as with the standard TRAM flap, this technique uses a similar skin and fat ellipse from the lower abdomen transferred to the chest wall and shaped into a breast mound. When the free flap is transferred to the chest wall, the divided blood vessel ends are joined directly to an appropriate chest wall artery and vein by microsurgical technique. This eliminates the need for the full length of rectus muscle (which surrounds the nourishing vessels) to be twisted and turned upward as the flap is repositioned onto the chest wall. The free (microsurgical) TRAM surgery is a longer operation than the standard TRAM. The added advantage of the DIEP (deep inferior epigastric perforator flap) is that the muscles of the abdomen remain intact; thus there is in the majority of cases no loss of abdominal function. Today it is the microsurgical flap of choice and, in experienced hands, has a relatively low complication rate and equal or better cosmetic outcomes.

Patients who have had their abdominal muscles cut during previous surgery (a gallbladder operation, for example) would not be acceptable candidates for a standard TRAM flap, but a DIEP or a free TRAM flap could safely be used in such cases.

The DIEP flap is the most complex of the commonly used techniques and is not appropriate for all patients. Other microsurgical flaps, such as the TUG (inner thigh) flap or gluteal (buttock) flap, may be used if the DIEP or TRAM are not available, but because of donor site issues should not be the first choice for breast reconstruction.

Advantages

- Cosmetic results are usually more natural than implants and more often match the opposite breast in and out of clothing.

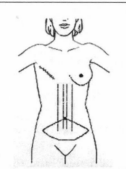

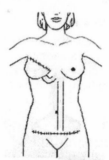

1. Delayed TRAM: *After mastectomy, the abdominal skin and underlying fat are isolated along with a segment of muscle that maintains the blood supply of the elliptical skin island.*

2. *The tissue (including skin, fat, blood vessels, and one or both of the abdominal muscles) is tunneled up beneath the upper abdominal skin and shaped into a breast. In the case of a free (microsurgical) TRAM, there is no tunneling, as the vessels of the flap are sewn to other vessels in the armpit area.*

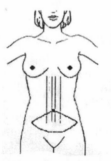

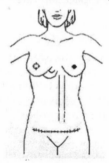

3. Immediate TRAM: *The procedure is the same as above. After a skin-sparing mastectomy, only a small circle of abdominal skin is needed to replace the nipple and biopsy site. The abdominal fat and muscle are buried under the breast skin.*

4. *For both immediate and delayed TRAM flaps, the nipple is made at a later date using tattoo and small local flaps. Skin grafts may also be used. The resulting abdominal incision is similar to that from a "tummy tuck."*

• No further maintenance surgery on the breast is needed at a later date as in the case of implant reconstruction.

• An implant is not required.

• In the case of a TRAM flap, a "tummy tuck" follows the transfer of skin and fat from the lower abdomen. A patient must request that the DIEP surgeon repair her muscles if necessary.

• Sparing the rectus muscles in the case of the DIEP flap.

Disadvantages

- Possible weakness or hernia of the abdominal wall.
- Additional scar across the lower abdomen.
- Involves a lengthy surgical procedure under general anesthesia.
- A plastic surgeon with microsurgery skills is required for the free-flap technique.
Always ask your surgeon how many DIEP flaps he/she has personally done.
- There may be a higher risk of complications.

Radiation Radiotherapy is often part of standard treatment for early-stage breast cancer to treat the remaining breast tissue after the primary tumor has been removed as part of breast-conserving surgery (such as a lumpectomy). This is based on the frequent risk of microscopic (and undetectable) cancer cells remaining in the breast. For smaller breast cancers, the combined treatment of surgery (lumpectomy or segmental resection) and subsequent radiotherapy has been shown to be equivalent to the modified radical mastectomy.

Another use of radiation therapy as primary treatment is in postmastectomy radiation to the chest wall. This may be done if the tumor was found at surgery or after tissue examination to invade the skin or chest wall muscles, if it was very large, or if many lymph nodes were involved. The assumption is that there may be hidden tumor cells in the chest wall or armpit (axilla) after surgery that can be eradicated effectively by radiation. In addition to the chest wall, the area treated (the radiation field or port) sometimes includes the lymph nodes in the armpit or over the collarbone (supraclavicular nodes). If chemotherapy is being used for early-stage breast cancer (see section below), then radiation is usually given after all of the chemotherapy.

In patients who later develop chest wall recurrence, radiation therapy is often used (if the area was not previously treated with radiation), usually with a wide margin to kill the presumed microscopic tumor implants that could also be nearby. This therapy to localized recurrences may achieve permanent control over the cancer in up to half of patients.

Radiation is given daily, usually five days a week, over about six weeks. The usual technique involves external-beam radiation to the entire involved breast, sometimes with an additional booster dose to the tumor area. This boost may be given by an external beam or with radiation seeds surgically implanted directly into the tumor area (brachytherapy). There is no increased risk of a secondary malignancy or a breast cancer on the opposite side as a result of radiotherapy. Radiation is also used in certain situations for advanced metastatic breast cancer, and this is further described in the section on treatment for advanced breast cancer.

More recently, partial breast irradiation has been given in certain cases of smaller, node-negative tumors, and this technique spares the whole breast from radiation and can be given over a small period of time, typically a few days, or even less. Different techniques for partial breast irradiation include brachytherapy as described above but given without whole breast radiation, the use of a balloon that is inflated inside the tumor cavity and filled with a radioactive material and then deflated and removed after your last radiation session (MammoSite balloon), and the use of focused and tailored radiation beams (conformal radiation). These techniques are currently being tested in higher-risk cancer, such as cases with positive nodes, and being compared to standard radiation.

Systemic or Medical Therapy Systemic therapy refers to drugs that circulate throughout the body and include chemotherapy, hormonal therapy, and, more recently, biological therapy such as antibodies as well as a combination of these types of therapies. These can be given as adjuvant therapy, which refers to therapy after surgery for early-stage breast cancer and which is designed to lower the future risk of distant recurrences (metastases) and thereby improve survival. It can also be given to patients with metastatic advanced breast cancer to shrink or prevent growth of cancer and to improve the quality of life, but generally is not curative in this situation.

Adjuvant Systemic Therapy for Early-Stage Breast Cancer Adjuvant or prophylactic chemotherapy, hormonal therapy, and antibody therapy, are now given to many patients after surgery for early-stage breast cancer (Stages I, II, and III) to try to prevent or minimize the growth of microscopic deposits of tumor cells that might grow into a recurrent tumor. It is believed that recurrence of breast cancer in the years following initial surgery is due to growth of these microscopic deposits of breast cancer cells that are undetectable by current standard tests. Treating some patients who have no obvious metastases at the time of surgery, but who are at high risk for recurrence or spread due to the size of the tumor, the presence of metastases in axillary lymph nodes, and other factors, has been shown to result in improvements in long-term survival without cancer. Although in the past, chemotherapy was primarily used to treat cancers in premenopausal women, and hormonal therapy to treat cancers in postmenopausal women, there is growing evidence that both types of treatment are effective regardless of menopausal status (see Table 1 below). Chemotherapy appears to be most effective in premenopausal women; however, chemotherapy may still be quite effective for treating postmenopausal women at higher risk of recurrence, for example, those with positive nodes. In some cases, such as larger tumors or Stage III breast cancer, chemotherapy or hormonal therapy may be given before surgery. A rough approximation as to how much chemotherapy and hormonal therapy can reduce the risk of breast cancer recurring in the future is shown below.

Therefore, one can estimate the benefit for a specific case depending on what the recurrence would be in the first place. For example, a sixty-year-old woman with a ¾-inch (2 cm) breast cancer with negative nodes would have about a 25 percent (one in four) chance of developing metastases over the next five years without any systemic adjuvant therapy. With

Table 1. **Benefits of Adjuvant Therapy**

Chemotherapy in women under age 50	Lowers the risk by about one-third
Chemotherapy in women over age 50	Lowers the risk by about one-fifth
Hormonal therapy for estrogen-receptor or progesterone-receptor-positive breast cancer	Lowers the risk by about one-half

tamoxifen (Nolvadex), this would be cut in half, to about 12 or 13 percent (one in eight). Chemotherapy would then lower the remaining risk by another 2 to 3 percent (one-fifth of the remaining 12 to 13 percent risk) to 10 percent (1 in 10). A general schematic that outlines the types of adjuvant systemic therapy used based on the overall risk of the cancer is shown in Table 2, "Types of Adjuvant Systemic Therapy."

Adjuvant Chemotherapy for Early-Stage Breast Cancer Chemotherapy for early-stage breast cancer is usually given in combination, rather than as a single drug, in order to overcome any resistance the cancer cells may have to a specific agent. Details on commonly used regimens are provided in Table 2. Common drug combinations include the following:

• Cyclophosphamide (Cytoxan) + methotrexate + 5-fluorouracil (5-FU). This regimen is abbreviated CMF and is given on an outpatient basis over six months, requiring twelve visits to the clinic. Common side effects include nausea, vomiting, fatigue, moderate to complete hair loss, mouth sores, diarrhea, and lowering of the white blood cell count with a small risk of infection. This is an older regimen not used much today, but it is not associated with the small risk of heart problems as described with the regimens below.

• Doxorubicin (Adriamycin) + cyclophosphamide (this is abbreviated AC) given on an outpatient basis over three months, requiring four treatment visits to the clinic. Common side effects include nausea, vomiting, fatigue, complete hair loss, mouth sores, diarrhea, and lowering of the white blood cell count with a small risk of infection. Doxorubicin can on rare occasions cause weakness of the heart muscle (cardiomyopathy).

• Cyclophosphamide + doxorubicin + 5-fluorouracil (this is abbreviated CAF). This regimen is given over four to six months and has the same side effects as AC chemotherapy listed above, with perhaps more chance of mouth sores and diarrhea.

• Taxane drugs, which include paclitaxel (Taxol) and docetaxel (Taxotere), are increasingly used in combination with doxorubicin or following AC to treat higher-risk cancers, particularly with positive lymph nodes. These are given every three weeks for four cycles. Common side effects include fatigue, moderate to complete hair loss, numbness and tingling of hands and feet, mouth sores, diarrhea, allergic reactions, and lowering of the white blood cell count with a small risk of infection. For higher-risk cancers such as node-positive, higher grade, or hormone receptor–negative, therapy should include an anthracycline drug (doxorubicin or epirubicin [Ellence]) and a taxane (paclitaxel or docetaxel) in patients who are in good enough health to receive these drugs.

Ideally, chemotherapy is given within three to twelve weeks following the final surgery, provided all healing from surgery is nearly complete. If doxorubicin (Adriamycin) is going to be used, a scan of the heart (either a multiple gated acquistion [MUGA] scan or an echocardiogram) is first done to make sure there is no preexisting heart muscle weakness. Blood counts are also checked before each cycle of chemotherapy to make sure they have adequately recovered from the prior cycle. Many of the side effects listed above affect different individuals to different extents. Newer drugs can help minimize these side effects. For example, newer antinausea drugs can cut down on the chance of nausea and vomiting from the AC regimen from 80 percent to 20 percent. These drugs are often given preventively before chemotherapy to avoid nausea altogether. If recovery of the white blood cell counts delays the next cycle of chemotherapy, or if an infection or fever develops due to low

Table 2. **Types of Adjuvant Systemic Therapy**

REGIMEN NAME	RISK SETTING USED	AGENTS USED	NUMBER OF CYCLES	FREQUENCY OF CYCLES	TOTAL DURATION
CMF	Low to moderate	Cyclophosphamide (Cytoxan), methotrexate (Mexate), and 5-fluorouracil (5-FU)	6	4 weeks	6 months
AC	Low to moderate	Doxorubicin (Adriamycin) and cyclophosphamide (Cytoxan)	4	3 weeks	3 months
TC	Low to moderate	Docetaxel (Taxotere) and cyclophosphamide (Cytoxan)	4	3 weeks	3 months
FAC	Moderate	5-Fluorouracil (5-FU), doxorubicin (Adriamycin), and cyclophosphamide (Cytoxan)	6	3 weeks	4½ months
FEC	Moderate	5-Fluorouracil (5-FU), epirubicin (Ellence), and cyclophosphamide (Cytoxan)	6	3 weeks	4½ months
AC Taxol	Moderate to high	Doxorubicin (Adriamycin), cyclophosphamide (Cytoxan), and paclitaxel (Taxol)	8 (4 of AC, 4 of paclitaxel [Taxol])	2 weeks	4 months
AC Taxotere	Moderate to high	Doxorubicin (Adriamycin), cyclophosphamide (Cytoxan), and docetaxel (Taxotere)	8 (4 of AC, 4 of docetaxel [Taxotere])	3 weeks	6 months
TAC	Moderate to high	Docetaxel (Taxotere), doxorubicin (Adriamycin), and cyclophosphamide (Cytoxan)	6	3 weeks	4½ months
FEC Taxotere	Moderate to high	FEC as described above followed by either taxane or Taxol*	6 (3 of FEC, 3 of taxane)	3 weeks	4½ months

* Both docetaxel (Taxotere) and paclitaxel (Taxol) are classified as taxanes.

white cell counts, then a self-injectable drug called a granulocyte colony-stimulating factor, or G-CSF (filgrastim [Neupogen] or pegfilgrastim [Neulasta]), is given with subsequent chemotherapy cycles. Also, drugs including epoetin alfa (Procrit) and darbepoetin alfa (Aranesp) can be given to help minimize drops in the red blood count and to lower the rare need for blood transfusions. Most side effects resolve after completing chemotherapy but can sometimes linger for several months. However, some effects are permanent, such as transition into menopause and loss of ovarian function and fertility. This is more likely in women who are closer to menopausal age. Long-term side effects of chemotherapy rarely cause major problems that interfere with life or normal activities. However, there are reports of changes in cognitive function (ability to think, remember, and reason) in women who have received chemotherapy for early-stage breast cancer. There is also an increase in the chance of developing leukemia, although this is very rare, about 1 in 300 or 400.

High-dose chemotherapy with bone marrow or stem cell transplant is being investigated for high-risk patients. Currently, this approach has not been proven to be superior to the standard chemotherapy regimens described above, but clinical trials to address this are still ongoing.

Hormonal Therapy The lining of the ducts and lobules in the breast change under the influence of hormones, and breast cancer cells also can be responsive to hormones. It has been known for some time that removing the ovaries can sometimes make breast cancers regress. In many cases, breast cancer treatment today includes drugs that affect the ovaries, otherwise affect production of estrogen, or interfere with the way that estrogen stimulates cancer cells. These treatments are used when the tumor cells test positive for the presence of the estrogen receptor (ER) or progesterone receptor (PR). ER and PR are proteins that bind to hormones like estrogen and progesterone and are present not only in some breast cancers but also in normal breast and many other tissues such as the lining of the vagina, uterus, liver, and bone. When estrogen binds to ER, it causes many different cellular activities depending on the type of cell as well as the presence of other hormones and factors. Tamoxifen (Nolvadex) is the most widely used hormonal drug and works by binding to the estrogen receptor and interfering with its function. Short-term side effects of tamoxifen include hot flashes, mild nausea, occasional changes in mood, and slight weight gain. These side effects usually improve or resolve over one to three months after starting therapy. Other side effects include an increased risk of blood clots, thickening of the lining of the uterus, and an increased risk of developing cancer of the lining of the uterus (endometrial cancer), about 1 in 100 over five years. The risk of blood clots is similar to the risk of blood clots caused by estrogen use, or during pregnancy. Regular gynecologic examinations are recommended for women taking tamoxifen, and a biopsy of the lining of the uterus (done in the office) should be performed if vaginal bleeding develops.

Other hormonal treatments involve removing the function of the ovaries, since in women who are still menstruating, removing the ovarian source of estrogen can have an impact both in early-stage and advanced breast cancer. This can be done by surgical removal of the ovaries (oophorectomy) or by using an injectable monthly drug that stops the ovaries from cycling and producing estrogen (sometimes termed chemical or medical oophorectomy).

A newer form of hormonal therapy, aromatase inhibitors (AIs), are now commonly used for postmenopausal women. After menopause, when the ovaries no longer make estrogen, the only source of estrogen is what is converted from androgens by a chemical reaction mediated by an enzyme termed aromatase. AIs lower the already low estrogen levels but work only after the ovaries have stopped making estrogen and should not be used in premenopausal women or immediately after periods have stopped. AIs have been shown to be slightly better than tamoxifen and in addition do not have the side effects of increasing the risk of uterine cancer or blood clots. However, they can sometimes cause joint and muscle pains and can also accelerate bone loss and osteoporosis over time.

Hormonal Therapy for Early-Stage Breast Cancer Some form of hormonal therapy is recommended for all patients with ER- or PR-positive breast cancer unless medically contraindicated. This can be omitted altogether in very low risk cancers, such as those that are node-negative, low grade, and less than $\frac{1}{4}$ to $\frac{1}{2}$ inch (0.5 to 1 cm), if the risk-benefit ratio favors no therapy. In patients who also receive chemotherapy, recent studies indicate that the best outcomes are obtained when hormonal therapy is given after all the chemotherapy.

For premenopausal women, tamoxifen (Nolvadex) is given daily for five years to most women whose tumors are positive for estrogen or progesterone receptors, whether chemotherapy is added or not. It can be begun either during chemotherapy (if given) or following chemotherapy, or following radiation therapy (if given). The use of tamoxifen for more than five years is being studied in clinical trials. Even though tamoxifen is discontinued after five years, the effect on lowering mortality persists for at least ten years.

Medical or surgical oophorectomy (described above) can also be effective in lowering the risk of recurrence for premenopausal women with estrogen-receptor-positive tumors. Prior to the advent of chemotherapy and tamoxifen, it was used fairly commonly. It appears to be as effective as chemotherapy but has never been compared alone to chemotherapy plus tamoxifen. Furthermore, it is not clear if oophorectomy adds to the effect of tamoxifen (in the absence or presence of chemotherapy). For these reasons, it is not commonly used in routine practice, but results of ongoing studies may in the future resurrect the use of this treatment.

Aromatase inhibitors (AIs) are slightly better than tamoxifen for postmenopausal women in lowering recurrence risk and are generally favored, although sometimes tamoxifen is used if significant side effects are seen with these drugs. The approved AIs include anastrozole (Arimidex), letrozole (Femara), and exemestane (Aromasin). Studies have also shown that two to five years of an AI following two to five years of tamoxifen is slightly more effective than tamoxifen for five years, so sequential therapy is also being used, especially in women who have just undergone menopause, or do so slightly after beginning tamoxifen. For premenopausal women who have contraindications to tamoxifen, such as a history of a blood clot, oophorectomy (either medical or surgical) along with an AI can be considered, but this is not a routine recommendation and this approach is still being studied in clinical trials.

HER-2 Antibody Therapy for Early-Stage Breast Cancer The antibody trastuzumab (Herceptin) works against breast cancer cells that make high levels of the HER-2 protein or that make extra copies of the HER-2 gene. Tumor tissue is tested for HER-2 and if the test is positive, then trastuzumab is added to the therapy, especially for higher-risk breast cancer. So far, all the studies have used trastuzumab either after chemotherapy or with overlap with the taxane part of the chemotherapy regimen, and the overall duration of treatment is currently recommended for one year. If radiation and/or hormonal therapy is used, trastuzumab can overlap with this treatment. Trastuzumab can cause heart muscle weakness (cardiomyopathy), which is usually temporary and responds to cardiac medication. Heart function needs to be tested before and periodically during trastuzumab therapy. As with other therapies, your doctor will need to balance the benefits and risks of trastuzumab for your specific case prior to making this decision.

Follow-Up After Treatment for Early-Stage Breast Cancer

Monitoring for Recurrence Following therapy for early-stage breast cancer, there remains a risk for recurrence. Local recurrences refer to those in the breast or in the remaining lymph nodes under the arm that are still curable (see "Recurrent Cancer," in this chapter), hence follow-up with physical examinations every six months (or more frequently in the first year after treatment) as well as mammograms is recommended. In some centers, a recommendation is given for mammograms every six months for five years on the side of the involved breast if breast-conserving surgery was used, since most recurrences in the breast tend to happen in this frame of time. Annual mammograms on the other breast should continue, since there is a higher chance of a new cancer in the other breast (10 to 20 percent lifetime risk) compared to women who have never had a diagnosis of breast cancer.

Monitoring for distant recurrences (metastases) is primarily done by evaluating new symptoms or findings on physical examination that could be indicative of recurrence. These include an enlarged lymph node, new unexplained bone pain (such as in the back, hips, or ribs), chest tightness, shortness of breath, and headaches. Such signs should be investigated by the appropriate X-rays and biopsies depending on the findings.

In patients with no symptoms or abnormalities on physical examination, it is controversial whether or not routine blood tests or X-rays are useful in detecting metastases. Blood tests such as chemistry panels (especially liver function tests) and tumor marker tests (e.g., CEA, CA 15-3, CA 27-29) can oftentimes detect a distant recurrence months or even years before it may cause symptoms. However, even when detected very early, advanced metastatic breast cancer cannot be cured, even though some patients can respond to treatment and live a very long time. Therefore, it is not clear that such testing is really beneficial. In fact, serum markers are not always accurate and can lead to a false alarm and numerous tests and biopsies. Therefore, most expert organizations do not recommend the use of serum markers or routine X-rays or scans for follow-up after treatment of early-stage breast cancer if there are no symptoms or abnormalities on physical examination. On the other hand, these tests are used by many oncologists, and many patients feel a sense of reassurance when these are negative. There always remains the possible scenario of detecting a resectable recurrence even though it is not clear that this would be curative or affect long-term survival. This controversial area is best addressed by discussing the pros and cons with your oncologist.

Postmenopausal Symptoms and Health Maintenance Many women go through menopause after chemotherapy. Estrogen replacement is generally avoided in women with a history of breast cancer or those who are at increased risk for breast cancer because of the theoretical increase in the risk of cancer recurrence. Some studies have actually demonstrated a higher recurrence risk in patients with hormone-receptor-positive breast cancer who take estrogen replacement therapy.

Hot flashes can be a problem with menopause or when women who are already postmenopausal and on estrogen replacement discontinue estrogen when they are diagnosed with breast cancer. Hot flashes can also be a problem with taking tamoxifen (Nolvadex) even in premenopausal women. There has been interest in the use of soy (found in tofu, soybeans, and tempeh) to treat hot flashes, although a recent study did not find it to be helpful in this regard. Antidepressants like venlafaxine (Effexor) have also been found to be helpful, although they may have side effects such as dry mouth and loss of appetite. The progesterone drug megestrol acetate (Megace) at low doses also helps with hot flashes but can be accompanied by weight gain.

Vaginal dryness and thinning of the vaginal wall can sometimes be a problem. Local preparations such as testosterone and vaginal estrogens can help even though there is a potential that these treatments could affect the risk of recurrence. This has not been studied extensively in women with breast cancer; however, a local slow-release estrogen (estradiol) ring (Estring) has been shown not to result in estrogen entering into the bloodstream.

Osteopenia (thinning of the bone mineral) can occur after menopause and may be more of a problem in women who enter early menopause due to chemotherapy or loss of ovary function. Postmenopausal women on tamoxifen may actually have less bone loss. Periodic measurement of bone mineral density can be done with a simple test. If bone mineral density is well below normal, nonestrogen drug treatment options to prevent osteoporosis are alendronate (Fosamax), risedronate (Actonel), ibandronate (Boniva), and raloxifene (Evista). Since raloxifene is similar to tamoxifen, these drugs would not be used together or sequentially.

Recurrent Cancer

Local or Locoregional Recurrences Recurrent breast cancer can be classified as a local recurrence if it occurs in the same breast after breast-conserving surgery, in the skin or chest wall near the breast, or in the axillary nodes on the same side. This is usually treated with mastectomy, resection of the skin/chest wall tumor, or lymph node excision. It is controversial as to whether further hormonal therapy, chemotherapy, or radiation therapy can influence the risk of another local recurrence or distant recurrence. If several years have

passed since chemotherapy was used for the original cancer, a different chemotherapy regimen may be considered, but clinical trials have not been done to show that this is effective. Alternatively, if the tumor is hormone receptor–positive, changing hormone therapy from tamoxifen (Nolvadex) to an aromatase inhibitor (or initiating tamoxifen if it was not used initially) may also be an option. These types of local recurrences may portend a higher risk of later recurrence. When local recurrences involve the chest wall, skin, or muscle, this tends to be a more ominous sign of future risk for distant recurrence. If surgically removable, these recurrences are excised with attempts to obtain clear surgical margins (no tumor cells seen microscopically at the edges of the specimen). Radiation therapy to the area may also be used. If local recurrences cannot be removed surgically or are not amenable to treatment with radiation due to their extent, location, or prior radiation (which usually precludes further radiation), then systemic therapy (hormonal, chemotherapy, or biological therapy) can be used as described in "Systemic Medical Therapy for Advanced Breast Cancer," in this chapter. Recurrences should be evaluated with X-rays to check for the possibility of distant recurrences (CT scan of the chest and abdomen and bone scan, or PET scan).

Distant Recurrences Distant recurrences, or metastases, refer to the spread of tumor to sites beyond the breast and lymph nodes under the arm (to the bone, liver, or lungs, for example) or to skin and chest wall involvement beyond the breast area. This can either be the initial presentation of the cancer or be a recurrence that can develop even years after early-stage breast cancer. Upon diagnosis of Stage IV breast cancer, a biopsy (either with a needle or a surgical excision) may be needed to confirm that the metastases seen on X-rays or on examination is indeed a recurrence of breast cancer. For example, a single spot seen on a chest X-ray could be a scar from an old infection, or a primary lung cancer, in which case the treatment may be different. In addition, it is important to know if the cancer is positive for the estrogen or progesterone receptor as well as HER-2/*neu* in order to choose the proper therapy (discussed in the following sections). Full-staging X-rays are done at the time of diagnosis of Stage IV breast cancer, and this usually includes a CT scan of the chest and abdomen and a bone scan. A brain scan may be performed if there are signs of possible brain metastases, such as headaches, visual changes, weakness, numbness, and dizziness. In rare cases, such as a single metastasis to the lung, liver, or brain, surgical removal can be contemplated, since occasionally this will result in long-term cure with no further metastases developing. However, in almost all cases, there is likely to be progression or new sites of involvement over time. Therefore, advanced metastatic breast cancer is generally not considered to be curable. However, systemic therapy (discussed in the next sections) can be effective in controlling cancer progression and maintaining normal or near-normal quality of life for some period of time. In contrast to treatment for early-stage breast cancer, the choice of drugs and length of treatment depend on the individual case. Decisions need to be made on an ongoing basis depending on the response of the cancer to treatment and the side effects of both the cancer and the treatment.

Systemic Therapy for Advanced Breast Cancer Advanced metastatic breast cancer cannot be cured, although cancer shrinkage, or remissions, can be seen with therapy. It is very difficult to predict if a remission will be seen at all, or how long it will last before the cancer becomes resistant to therapy. Treatment of advanced breast cancer is felt to have only a modest impact on the length of life on the average, but when used appropriately, it can improve symptoms or delay the onset of symptoms, and thereby improve the quality of life. The subset of patients who are very sensitive to treatment and have long remissions are those that get a better-than-average prolongation of life—on the order of months or even many years in some cases.

An examination and X-rays or scans that assess known areas of tumor are repeated periodically during therapy; the interval of these assessments depends on the rapidity of growth and the type of treatment used. Response (shrinkage of cancer) is usually associated with an improvement in symptoms and quality of life. Responses can last from a few months to several years, with the average being around one year (perhaps longer in the case of hormonal therapy). The goals of treating advanced metastatic breast cancer are different from those for early stage. The type and length of therapy depends on how the tumor is responding to treatment, what effect this is having on symptoms and quality of life, and how the therapy itself may be adversely affecting quality of life. In general, treatment is continued as long as there is regression of cancer and the side effects appear to be acceptable, such that the improvement in symptoms (or the calculated prevention of the onset of symptoms) outweighs the side effects of therapy. If there is progression (growth) of cancer, then another therapy can be tried. In hormone-receptor-positive cancer, hormonal therapies are tried first (this is described in more detail in the next section). If there was initially a response to the first hormonal therapy before the cancer progressed, then there is a better chance that the second hormonal approach will temporarily shrink the cancer or prevent growth. Using combinations of two or more hormonal therapies at the same time has not generally been shown to be better than using these drugs alone.

Chemotherapy is generally used if it is felt further hormonal treatment is not likely to work. If chemotherapy is being used, treatment can be stopped when it is felt the best response has been attained as opposed to simply continuing indefinitely, since there has not been shown to be a difference in survival from either approach. Decisions about changing chemotherapy are made when there is progression of cancer. This is discussed further in "Chemotherapy for Advanced Breast Cancer," in this chapter.

Hormonal Therapy for Advanced Breast Cancer Hormonal therapy is typically used as a first option for treatment of metastatic advanced breast cancer if the cancer is positive for either the estrogen or progesterone receptor. In some cases, if there is organ involvement (like lungs or liver) that is extensive and appears to be rapidly growing, then chemotherapy might be used initially. Hormonal therapy is continued until there is progression of cancer or intolerable side effects of treatment. Tamoxifen (Nolvadex) is often used in patients who did not receive this drug as part of adjuvant therapy for early-stage breast cancer. In this case, tamoxifen is continued until the cancer shows signs of growing. A newer class of hormonal agents, called aromatase inhibitors or inactivators, block the production of estrogen in postmenopausal women. Three agents are currently approved for use in advanced cancer: anastrozole (Arimidex), letrozole (Femara), and exemestane (Aromasin). It now appears that anastrozole and letrozole may be as effective as or even more effective than tamoxifen when used as the first hormonal treatment for advanced disease. Aromatase inhibitors have few side effects, primarily hot flashes and joint aching. For premenopausal women, oophorectomy can also be used, either as first hormonal therapy or after progression on tamoxifen. This can be accomplished by surgical removal of the ovaries or by medical (or chemical) oophorectomy using drugs called gonadotropin-releasing hormone analogues (e.g., goserelin [Zoladex]), which are given by injection once a month or once every three months. Patients whose tumors lack both estrogen and progesterone receptors are not candidates for hormonal therapy.

Chemotherapy for Advanced Breast Cancer Several chemotherapeutic agents are used for advanced breast cancer. The most common of these are doxorubicin (Adriamycin), paclitaxel (Taxol), and docetaxel (Taxotere). Sometimes these drugs are used as combinations (e.g., doxorubicin + cyclophosphamide [Cytoxan], or paclitaxel + doxorubicin). Other chemotherapy drugs with activity against breast cancer include capecitabine (Xeloda), vinorelbine (Navelbine), gemcitabine (Gemzar), and doxorubicin liposomal (Doxil). Table 3 outlines the dosing schedule and some of the side effects of these drugs.

Of the numerous chemotherapy agents available, it is not clear that a particular sequence of which drug is used first is better than any other. There is still controversy as to whether it is better to use combinations of chemotherapy agents or to use these drugs one at a time. There are also conflicting results as to whether combinations of certain chemotherapies are better than using them as single drugs in sequence as needed at the time of progression. While combinations may increase the chance of a response compared to single drugs, they have not always been shown to improve survival time and are also accompanied by more side effects. Some combinations such as docetaxel + capecitabine and paclitaxel + gemcitabine have actually shown slightly improved survival times, but it is still not clear if it is better to use these drugs in sequence (switch from one to the other if the cancer grows) than to use them in

Table 3. Commonly Used Chemotherapy Agents for Advanced Breast Cancer

DRUG	SCHEDULE	SIDE EFFECTS
Doxorubicin (Adriamycin)	Every 3 weeks or weekly by vein	Hair loss, nausea, vomiting, low white count/risk of infection, mouth sores, diarrhea
Paclitaxel (Taxol)	Every 3 weeks or weekly by vein	Hair loss, numbness/tingling, low white count/risk of infection, mouth sores, diarrhea
Docetaxel (Taxotere)	Every 3 weeks or weekly by vein	Hair loss, low white count/risk of infection, swelling, mouth sores, diarrhea
Capecitabine (Xeloda)	Pill by mouth twice a day for 2 weeks, every 3 weeks	Diarrhea, redness and peeling of the palms of the hands and soles of the feet, mouth sores
Vinorelbine (Navelbine)	Every 1–2 weeks by vein	Low white and red cell count, fatigue, numbness/tingling, constipation, muscle pain
Gemcitabine (Gemzar)	Every 1–2 weeks by vein	Low white and red cell count, fatigue
Doxorubicin Liposomal (Doxil)	Every 3–4 weeks by vein	Redness and peeling of the palms of the hands and soles of the feet, mouth sores

combination. High-dose chemotherapy with bone marrow or stem cell transplant currently does not appear to be better than standard-dose therapy. In patients who have already shown resistance (growth of cancer while on treatment) to several chemotherapy drugs, the chance of responding becomes less, as does the expected length of the remission.

The difficult choice of stopping all therapy and focusing on end-of-life care (see chapter 31, "Palliative Care") needs to be addressed when it is very unlikely that the treatment will result in a response and an improvement in the quality of life and will only cause toxic side effects.

Trastuzumab (Herceptin) for Advanced Breast Cancer New biological agents are more fully discussed in "Investigational Agents," in this chapter. Many of these are being tested to see if they are effective in ongoing trials. The only currently

approved biological agent for breast cancer is trastuzumab (Herceptin), which is useful both as a single drug and in combination with chemotherapy. This drug is an antibody to the HER-2/*neu* protein. It is effective only in patients whose tumors are positive for HER-2/*neu* (at a level of 3+ by an antibody, or immunohistochemistry, test; or when positive by a gene test called fluorescence in situ hybridization, or FISH). Trastuzumab has actually been shown to improve survival when added to chemotherapy. Although it is not a curative drug, some patients have had long responses. Side effects of trastuzumab are a chance of a reaction (usually to the first dose only) that includes fevers and chills as well as uncommon mild diarrhea, cough, and a small chance of weakness of the heart muscle (cardiomyopathy). When given in combination with chemotherapy (usually paclitaxel [Taxol]), it is common practice to give the two together until after the best response has been seen and then to continue trastuzumab alone as long as there is no progression. Trastuzumab is also effective with other chemotherapy drugs such as vinorelbine (Navelbine), docetaxel (Taxotere), carboplatin (Paraplatin), cisplatin (Platinol), gemcitabine (Gemzar), and capecitabine (Xeloda).

Newer Biological Drugs for Advanced Breast Cancer Two drugs are in the process of being approved for breast cancer in combination with chemotherapy. An antibody against tumor-associated blood vessels, bevacizumab (Avastin) has been shown to delay progression of tumor growth when added to chemotherapy. For HER-2/*neu*–positive advanced breast cancer that has progressed on trastuzumab (Herceptin), a new drug that blocks the enzyme activity of the HER-2/*neu* receptor, lapatinib (Tykerb), has also been shown to delay progression when added to the chemotherapy capecitabine (Xeloda). Many newer drugs are being tested in clinical trials and even before this latest edition of *Everyone's Guide to Cancer Therapy* is out, it is likely that newer drugs will be approved for specific biological subtypes of breast cancer, in many cases combined with standard or with other biological agents.

Radiation Therapy for Advanced Breast Cancer Radiation is often used in treating metastatic disease, both to shrink tumors and to relieve local symptoms such as pressure and pain. If metastatic bone lesions occur in a weight-bearing bone such as the leg, for example, the bone may fracture with very little provocation. This is called a pathologic fracture. Such areas are usually given radiation to help heal the bone (usually after being surgically repaired), decrease pain, and control local spread of the tumor. If a bone lesion is extensive, there may be a significant risk of pathologic fracture during the next several months it might take to complete radiation therapy and healing.

An orthopedic surgeon is often called in to determine if a fixation device—such as a rod or plate surgically placed over the cancerous bone to stabilize it—should be used to minimize the risk of fracture during this time.

Similarly, pain in the spine or spinal lesions seen on a bone scan or X-ray should be promptly investigated. If a metastatic tumor is present, there may be a risk of compression fractures of the vertebrae (even on simple walking) or of pressure on the spinal cord by the tumor, which can result in paralysis. Tumors that spread to the neck are especially worrisome because compression and fractures there can lead to paralysis of both arms and legs (quadriplegia) as well as loss of bladder and bowel control (incontinence).

Pain is often produced by tumors pressing on nerves, and radiation may help relieve the pain by shrinking these tumors. As is true in other types of cancer, the radiation dosage has to be kept low in some locations because of the limited tolerance of normal tissues.

Side effects of radiotherapy may include tiredness and skin changes, but with modern techniques major complications are infrequent (see chapter 6, "What Happens in Surgery," and chapter 16, "Integrative Oncology: Complementary Therapies in Cancer Care").

Other Treatments Used in Advanced Breast Cancer Patients with bone metastases may benefit from treatment with the bisphosphonate pamidronate (Aredia) or zoledronic acid (Zometa), which may reduce pain, the need for radiation to control pain, and the risk of fractures and other complications. Bisphosphonates are given intravenously every month for two hours. Sometimes fever and bone pain can be seen after the treatment, but this usually becomes less of a problem or disappears altogether upon subsequent doses. Rarely, drops in calcium levels or interference with kidney function can be a problem. Monitoring of kidney function and calcium levels should be done periodically. Very rare problems with damage to the jawbone have been reported and it is recommended any needed dental procedures be done before starting these drugs.

G-CSF (filgrastim [Neupogen]), long-acting pegylated G-CSF (pegfilgratim [Neulasta]), and granulocyte macrophage–colony-stimulating factor, or GM-CSF (sargramostim [Leukine]), are growth factors that stimulate the white blood cells to grow. These medications are given by injection under the skin and are used to either prevent or minimize low white blood counts, which can result in serious infections or delays in chemotherapy. These growth factors stimulate the rapid production of blood cells (see chapter 8, "What Happens in Chemotherapy") and can lower the risk and duration of serious infections associated with chemotherapy. Rather than using these factors, sometimes a reduction in the dose of chemotherapy may be more prudent, since there is little evidence to suggest that attempting to maintain higher doses of chemotherapy is more effective in delaying progression or improving the length or quality of life.

Another significant side effect from chemotherapy, especially for metastatic cancer, is anemia (lowering of the red blood cell count) and can be associated with fatigue. The growth factor erythropoietin and synthetic derivatives (epoetin alfa [Procrit] and darbepoetin [Aranesp]) are given by injection under the skin every one to three weeks and can improve a low red blood cell count, resulting in less need for transfusions, less fatigue, and an improved quality of life. The use of these drugs is reserved for anemia associated with chemotherapy use. It is important to make sure that there is enough iron in the body to make red blood cells when erythropoietin is used.

Monitoring Response to Treatment For either recurrent or metastatic disease, appropriate studies are done to determine response to treatment. Before any significant change in therapy—a new chemotherapy program, for example—it is essential to establish baseline information, documenting current status by examinations, tumor measurements, X-rays (including CT scans and sometimes MRI and/or PET scans), and blood tests. Any abnormal studies, such as bone scans, X-rays (including CT), and blood tests, are repeated at appropriate intervals. Tumor markers such as carcinoembryonic antigen (CEA), CA 15-3, and CA 27-29 can be used when scans or physical examinations are not reliable in assessing tumor response.

Objective clinical response (partial remission, or PR) is ordinarily defined as at least a 30 percent shrinkage in the greatest diameter of a metastatic lesion or the sum of these measurements—this classification is more important to define response for clinical trials than in clinical management of patients. A metastatic tumor in the lung $1\frac{1}{4}$ inches (3 cm) in diameter would have to shrink to about $\frac{3}{4}$ inch (2 cm) for this to be called a significant response, with such shrinkage being classified as a partial response. A complete response or remission occurs when all visible and detectable disease disappears. Disease progression means that measurable tumors increase in size during treatment by more than 20 percent or new tumors appear. "Stable disease" suggests disease that does not grow in any area and that does not meet the definition of response or progression.

It is easier to assess metastases in certain areas such as lymph nodes and the lung. Measurements can be made with a ruler held against a chest X-ray. Smaller, multiple lung metastases must be visualized by CT scan. Tumors in the liver can be monitored by liver function tests, especially the alkaline phosphatase, but also by direct measurement of metastatic tumors seen on abdominal CT, MRI, or ultrasound images. Measuring response in bone lesions is more difficult. Most metastatic breast cancers produce a softening or dissolving of the bone with the appearance of a "lytic" spot that looks like a hole. If treatment is successful, the lytic lesion will fill in with new bone, but this takes many months. Other cancers cause an increase in the density of the affected bone (blastic lesion) that may not be visible on bone scan and may require both CT scans and plain bone X-rays to be seen.

For determining the response to chemotherapy or hormonal therapy, a bone lesion that has not received radiation therapy has to be chosen as a marker. Obviously, if a lesion given radiation heals and chemotherapy or hormonal therapy is also being given, it would be impossible to know which treatment brought about the healing.

Bone lesions seen on bone scan sometimes require that an X-ray be done before treatment and another as soon as the treatment has been given an adequate trial. Following bone scans for evidence of response to treatment may not be as useful as conventional X-rays of lytic bone lesions. Scans may show "hot spots" in any abnormal area, and these spots may also indicate healing. They may also be produced by inflammation, metabolic diseases, or severe arthritis. The area could remain positive for months or a few years with successful therapy. Other types of bone lesions may not be visible on bone scan (see above). In a few patients with positive bone scans but without any lesions on X-rays, response may be signified by no new lesions developing. If the bone scan is unchanged after six months, especially if pain lessens, the positive areas can be presumed to indicate healing.

Positron-emission tomography (PET) scans are being increasingly utilized to assess the extent of metastatic disease and to follow the status following cancer therapy. Sometimes if something is seen on a CT scan but it is not definitive for cancer, a PET scan might help determine if it is likely to be cancer. Not all breast cancers can be seen on a PET scan, and sometimes a finding on a PET scan might be a "false alarm" and not represent cancer. It is important that this scan be used by knowledgeable physicians and in the right setting.

The "Flare" Response Hormone treatment and also chemotherapy can sometimes produce worse bone pain during the first few weeks of therapy, and the serum calcium level may also rise. This endocrine "flare" may be early evidence that the cancer is responding to the hormone treatments. If possible, pain medication is given to allow therapy to continue while the elevated calcium level is evaluated and treated. Usually the calcium returns to normal and the pain decreases, confirming a response.

Similarly, the bone scan sometimes becomes temporarily worse in a patient who is clinically improving. The increased uptake on the scan may represent healing of the destroyed bone. The X-ray appearance may not change for several months even in patients with a good response to treatment and whose pain has decreased. Likewise, blood tumor markers (see "Monitoring Response to Treatment," above) may rise temporarily in patients whose cancers are responding to treatment.

Treatment by Stage

■ Stage 0 (Carcinoma In Situ)
TNM Tis, N0, M0
Noninvasive or in situ cancers consist of lobular carcinoma in situ (LCIS) and ductal carcinoma in situ (intraductal carcinoma, or DCIS). These cancers are often small and may be discovered incidentally by mammography before a mass can be

felt. They may also be in several locations in one or both breasts. In situ cancer can also be found in the presence of invasive cancer, in which case the cancer is staged and treated according to the invasive cancer.

Standard Treatment

• For DCIS, conventional therapy is a wide excision of the tumor. It is critical to remove an additional area around the initial biopsy if the edges of the biopsy showed tumor cells. Axillary lymph nodes do not need to be removed in most cases, as the risk of positive nodes is quite low in most situations. Axillary sampling may occasionally be performed when the intraductal carcinoma is very aggressive (high grade) and extensively involves the breast. Following surgical excision of the tumor, radiation therapy is given to the remaining breast tissue, since this significantly reduces the chances of additional cancer developing in the same breast. Another option is to remove the entire breast tissue (total mastectomy). This is done if the intraductal carcinoma is very large or involves several different areas of the breast or when it is desirable to avoid radiation. It has also been shown that treatment with tamoxifen (Nolvadex) following surgery and radiation can further reduce the risk of recurrence of both intraductal and invasive cancers. The use of tamoxifen is generally reserved for cancers with a high risk of recurrence. Studies are ongoing to see if radiation can be omitted when the intraductal carcinoma is small and low grade and there is a wide area of normal breast tissue around the cancer removed at the time of surgery.

• In situ lobular cancer—a form that more commonly occurs in both breasts—is thought by some to be less malignant. However, patients with this lesion have a 25 percent risk of developing some form of invasive cancer in either breast over many years. There are some differences of opinion about management of patients with LCIS. Standard treatment can include periodic examinations (including mammography) and follow-up without any additional therapy. This may be adequate if the patient is aware of the long-term risk of developing invasive cancer and will participate in the frequent evaluations. Axillary lymph node sampling is not necessary. A very aggressive alternative is total mastectomy on both sides. This choice may be appealing to women who don't want to have examinations several times a year, mammograms once or twice a year, and the constant worry that invasive cancer may be found during their next visit to the doctor. Also, tamoxifen can be used to lower the risk of breast cancer development in patients who have LCIS.

Five-Year Survival 98 to 100 percent*

■ *Stage I*
TNM T1, N0, M0
The tumor is ¾ inch (2 cm) or less in size, without any evidence of spread to nearby lymph nodes or distant sites.

Standard Treatment This stage is most often curable with surgery. The treatment plan may use radiotherapy (if breast-conserving surgery is done) and chemotherapy or hormone therapy as well as surgery and has to be tailored to the individual, taking the risks and benefits of each plan into account. (See "Surgery" and "Adjuvant Systemic Therapy for Early-Stage Breast Cancer," earlier in this chapter.) For many years, it was not customary to treat Stage I breast

---

* Survival times listed are averages from large population studies and significant variability exists in these estimates.

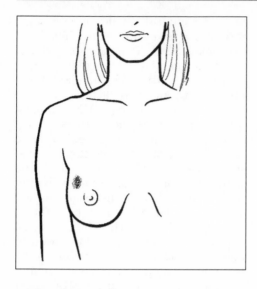

cancer with chemotherapy or hormone therapy. These patients generally have a good prognosis, with only about one chance in four of developing recurrent cancer. For most cancers smaller than $\frac{1}{2}$ inch (1 cm) in diameter, the chance of recurrence is less than 10 to 20 percent within ten years of diagnosis. Studies now have proven that there is a small benefit from the use of hormonal therapy and chemotherapy for Stage I breast cancer. A careful discussion with each patient regarding these issues is very important. For example, a premenopausal woman with a 1.9 cm aggressive HER-2/*neu*–positive, ER-positive cancer might have a five- to ten-year risk of recurrence of 20 percent or higher. Chemotherapy might reduce her risk of recurrence by as much as 5 to 6 percent, and hormonal therapy by about 8 percent. In this situation, chemotherapy may add a significant benefit to hormonal therapy. In contrast, a postmenopausal woman with a 0.8 cm slow-growing cancer that is HER-2/*neu*–negative and ER-positive might have a five- to ten-year risk of recurrence of less than 10 percent. Tamoxifen (Nolvadex) could reduce this risk further to less than 5 percent, but chemotherapy would be

expected to provide only a 2 percent reduction in risk of recurrence. In this situation, tamoxifen (or no therapy for older women at higher risk for tamoxifen-related side effects) would be the appropriate choice of adjuvant therapy.

Five-Year Survival 85 to 97 percent

■ *Stage II*
TNM T0, N1, M0 or T1, N1, M0 or T2, N0, M0 (IIA)
T2, N1, M0 or T3, N0, M0 (IIB)
Stage IIA consists of a small primary lesion (less than $\frac{3}{4}$ inch [2 cm]) and positive axillary lymph nodes, or a larger primary lesion between $\frac{3}{4}$ inch and 2 inches (2 to 5 cm) without positive nodes.

Stage IIB consists of a primary lesion between $\frac{3}{4}$ inch and 2 inches (2 to 5 cm) and positive axillary nodes, or a very large tumor (greater than 2 inches [5 cm]) with no axillary nodes involved.

Standard Treatment Stage IIA and IIB cancers are treated with a combination of surgery and systemic therapy. Conservative surgery that removes only a portion of the breast, followed by radiation therapy, has

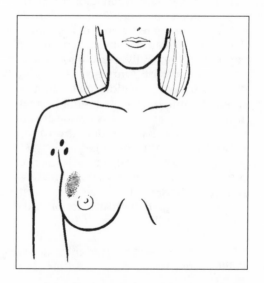

been shown to be equivalent to more radical surgery for tumor control. The same considerations for selection of the surgical procedure apply as in Stage I, including the size of the cancer, the size of the breast, and concerns about breast preservation. The indications for axillary dissection are similar to those in Stage I. Surgical options are also similar (see "Surgery," earlier in this chapter). Hormonal therapy in the form of tamoxifen (Nolvadex) for five years as well as chemotherapy is usually recommended (see "Adjuvant Systemic Therapy for Early-Stage Breast Cancer," earlier in this chapter).

Five-Year Survival 70 to 90 percent

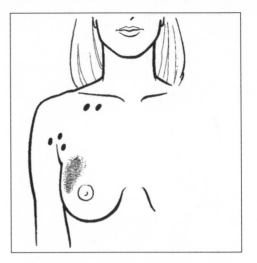

■ *Stage III*
TNM Any T, N3, M0 or T4, any N, M0

Standard Treatment This stage includes patients with large tumors that may be more difficult to treat with surgery first. Studies have shown that using neoadjuvant (preoperative) chemotherapy will yield equal results compared to chemotherapy after surgery, but more patients can have breast-conserving surgery. This stage also includes inflammatory carcinoma (Stage T4d), which is generally regarded as inoperable. The breast is usually enlarged and may be red and warm. Surgery is usually limited to the initial diagnostic biopsy, with treatment of the local tumor by chemotherapy or radiation. Neoadjuvant chemotherapy is often given first. If a good response is obtained with chemotherapy and/or radiation, surgery may be helpful to remove residual tumor. Chemotherapy regimens may include any of those listed in "Adjuvant Chemotherapy for Early-Stage Breast Cancer," earlier in this chapter. It is becoming increasingly common to give all the chemotherapy prior to surgery.

Because all three therapies are used, but their best sequence has not yet been determined, newly diagnosed patients with Stage IIIB cancer should be considered for clinical trials. Complex treatment programs involving integrated chemotherapy and radiotherapy followed by surgery are under study. If a clinical trial is not available, consideration should be given to one of the commonly used aggressive combined treatment plans.

Five-Year Survival 40 to 70 percent

■ *Stage IV*
TNM Any T, any N, M1
This stage applies to the presence of any distant metastases (to the bone, liver, or lungs, for example) or skin and chest wall involvement beyond the breast area. This can either be the initial presentation of the cancer or be a recurrence. Upon diagnosis of Stage IV breast cancer, a biopsy (either with a needle or a surgical excision) may be needed to confirm that the metastases seen on X-rays or on examination are indeed a recurrence of breast cancer. For example, a single spot seen on a chest X-ray could be a scar from an old infection, or a primary lung cancer, in which case, the treatment may be different. In addition, it is important to know if the cancer is positive for estrogen and progesterone receptor as well as

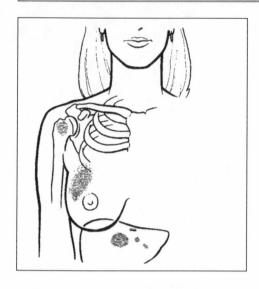

HER-2/*neu* in order to choose the proper therapy. Full-staging X-rays are done at the time of diagnosis of Stage IV breast cancer, and this usually includes a CT scan of the chest and abdomen and a bone scan, or a PET scan. If there are signs of possible brain metastases, such as headaches, visual changes, weakness, numbness, or dizziness, then a CT scan or MRI of the brain should be done to exclude metastases to the brain. Once information about the tumor markers (estrogen/progesterone receptors, HER-2/*neu*) and X-rays/scans is complete, decisions can be made about starting the treatment plan as outlined in the sections on therapy for advanced breast cancer, earlier in this chapter.

Five-Year Survival 5 to 20 percent

Breast Cancer In Men

Male breast cancer is rare, but 1 out of every 125 cases of breast cancer involves a man, usually one over sixty years old. There is a higher frequency of Stage III disease, principally because of skin involvement by the tumor. Although a painless breast lump is the most common sign, most breast lumps in men are benign and are related to some other cause, such as medications or liver disease. Sometimes there is delay in seeking therapy, which is perhaps due to low awareness by the public and doctors of the possibility of this diagnosis.

Standard Treatment Both simple and radical mastectomies have been done, but no statement can be made about a standard method. Skin grafting may be required for advanced disease. Radiation therapy is sometimes used postoperatively to decrease the risk of local recurrence. Treatment with chemotherapy, hormonal therapy, and/or biological therapy is used following the same criteria discussed in prior sections of this chapter.

Investigational Agents

Patients with advanced or metastatic breast cancer (Stage IV) are often eligible for clinical trials involving newly developed agents not yet approved for breast cancer treatment. These new agents span all of the types of treatments used for breast cancer and include new chemotherapies, new hormonal therapies, and new biological or immunological therapies. By definition, investigational agents are not yet proven to be effective for the particular clinical situation in which they are being tested, and that is why a clinical trial has been organized.

New chemotherapies include drugs that are similar to existing chemotherapies but are potentially improved in terms of effectiveness, side effects, and/or convenience. These drugs usually affect how cancer cells divide, so can have many side effects on normal cells. Examples include versions that can be taken as a pill at home rather than requiring intravenous infusion. Other investigational chemotherapies are completely new and include drugs that are designed to attack particular aspects of cancer cells. In this respect, they are similar to many of the biological agents (see below), in that they are designed using our improved understanding of how cancer develops.

New hormonal or endocrine therapies include drugs that block the effects of estrogen, since estrogen can stimulate breast cancer growth. Examples include drugs that are "pure antiestrogens," which always block estrogen throughout the body. Tamoxifen (Nolvadex), the most commonly used hormonal therapy, blocks estrogen in many but not all tissues. It is possible that these new versions may be more effective in some patients, and are also likely to avoid the important but rare side effect of increased uterine cancer risk. Others may work in situations where other hormonal agents are no longer effective.

Biological agents comprise the largest group of new agents in clinical trials and include new monoclonal antibodies and antibody-based agents; cancer vaccines; inhibitors of tumor invasion; and inhibitors of tumor angiogenesis (blood vessel formation that is necessary for tumor growth). A milestone in breast cancer therapy was the approval of trastuzumab (Herceptin) as the first monoclonal antibody treatment for breast cancer with high levels of HER-2/*neu*. Newer types of monoclonal antibodies and antibody-based agents are in development and include antibodies linked to drugs and other toxins for greater potency against cancer cells, as well as antibodies against other molecular targets besides HER-2/*neu*. Several drugs called kinase inhibitors are being tested in many types of cancers, as these drugs inhibit enzymes called kinases, which propagate several signaling pathways that mediate important cancer cell activities such as growth and development. One such drug, lapatinib (Tykerb), has just been approved in HER-2/*neu*–positive breast cancer that has progressed on trastuzumab. Vaccines against cancer have been studied for many years and with recent improvements in design may become useful in breast cancer treatment. A number of cancer vaccines are in clinical trials for breast cancer at advanced and even early stages.

Alternative Medicine for Breast Cancer

Alternative medicine refers to approaches that are not mainstream and sometimes not accepted by the conventional medical community. These include mind-body techniques, herbal medicine, nutritional therapy, megavitamin supplementation, homeopathy, prayer, and many other modalities. Very little information exists from well-done clinical trials to make definitive recommendations in this area. Some studies have shown that vitamin C or E as well as an antioxidant like selenium might be associated with a lower risk of cancer, but none have shown that these can actually treat cancer. Herbal therapies are often used for side effects, cancer treatment, and improving the immune system. While some studies have shown these effects in the laboratory, no clear conclusions can be made about how effective these might be in actual practice. Acupuncture can be helpful in some cases of pain and nausea that may not respond to other treatments. The National Institutes of Health issued a consensus statement supporting acupuncture for these indications. The use of megavitamins and antioxidants during radiation therapy or chemotherapy to alleviate side effects remains very controversial. Proponents say that this can help with symptoms and even effectiveness, while detractors state that this could diminish the effect of treatment. Certainly, there is a need to perform serious research in the area of alternative medicine, since there is the potential to uncover therapies of use as well as to dispel useless treatments that could be harmful or expensive. For individuals interested in seeking alternative medicine, it is recommended that an experienced practitioner be sought who can clearly articulate the reasons for the therapy and give a balanced assessment of the pros and cons and of the information upon which this is based. Careful attention to possible improvements or side effects should be tracked, and all the information should be shared with both practitioner and physician.

The Most Important Questions You Can Ask

• Can I save my breast? Is this wise?

• When can I have breast reconstruction done and what are my choices? What will I look like afterward?

• Will I need radiation therapy?

• Will the radiation therapy produce any damage to the skin or any deformity? What are the other side effects?

• If I need chemotherapy, what are the choices? How long will it last and what are the side effects (both short-term and long-term)? By how much will it lower my risk of recurrence and risk of dying of breast cancer? Is there a role for hormonal therapy or biological therapy?

• Why do I have to stop taking female hormones?

• What can you give me to help me with my hot flashes?

• Will I lose my hair? When will I start losing it and how long will it take to come back?

• How often do I need to be examined afterward? What tests will I have?

• How often should I have a mammogram?

• When will I be sure that my cancer will not come back?

• If I have advanced, or metastatic, breast cancer, what are the expectations of therapy?

• How will the treatment regimen be chosen, how will I be monitored, and what adjustments or changes will be made over time?

Cancer of an Unknown Primary Site (CUPS)

John D. Hainsworth, M.D., and F. Anthony Greco, M.D.

■ ■ ■ ■

Cancer of an unknown primary site (CUPS) is a metastatic tumor with no obvious source. It is detected by a biopsy that shows cancer from a part of the body that does not produce that type of malignancy, and no site of origin is identified despite a thorough physical examination, blood tests, X-rays, and other imaging studies.

No primary site of origin can be identified in 2 to 5 percent of patients diagnosed with metastatic cancer. This is often because the primary tumor is so small that it is undetectable or the primary site is difficult to see directly or by using imaging techniques.

Since by definition the disease is diagnosed at a metastatic stage, the prognosis is generally poor. A significant percentage of patients, however, can have symptoms relieved and can occasionally be cured. For example, germ cell tumors, choriocarcinomas, lymphomas, and certain sarcomas are potentially curable even in their metastatic stages. Other tumors such as prostate cancer, breast cancer, and endometrial carcinomas are amenable to hormonal therapy.

Unfortunately, many of the cancers that can present as CUPS are relatively resistant to treatment when they are advanced. Examples of such tumor types include lung cancer and tumors originating in the gastrointestinal tract (particularly the pancreas). Although there has been modest recent improvement in the treatment of these cancers, they remain incurable when advanced. Most patients with CUPS are also incurable, with an average survival of six to eight months. However, there is an extremely wide range of treatment outcomes, and identification of subgroups of patients for specific treatments is very important.

Finding the Primary Site

In trying to discover the primary site, there are two important considerations:

1. Some primary cancers are much more treatable than others. These include cancers of the breast, prostate, thyroid, and ovary; lymphomas (including Hodgkin's disease); and germ cell tumors similar to those that develop in the testes. Great efforts are made to determine if one of these is the primary site. Not only is the prognosis much better with these types of cancer, but the treatment has to be specific for that cancer.

2. There are important clues your doctor can use to discover the primary site:

• One clue is the location of the metastases. A woman with a tumor that develops in glands (adenocarcinoma) and is found in the lymph nodes of the armpit, for example, is more likely to have carcinoma of the breast. A woman who develops fluid in the abdomen (ascites) or has a tumor involving the lining of the abdominal cavity (peritoneum) should be suspected of having ovarian cancer.

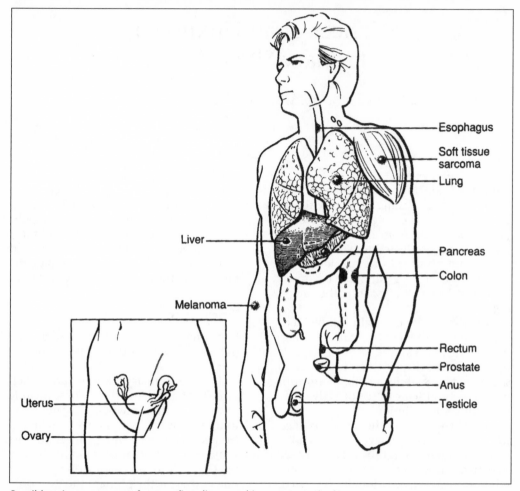

Possible primary sources of cancer first diagnosed in a metastatic site

• The most common sites of CUPS are metastases to the lung(s), lymph nodes, bone, and liver. When CUPS is found in the upper part of the body (above the diaphragm), the most common source is the lung. When it appears in the liver, the usual primary site is the gastrointestinal tract, including the pancreas.

• Another clue is the type of pathology. If a person has epidermoid (squamous) carcinoma in lymph glands high in the neck, for example, the primary site is most often in the nasopharynx, the throat, or the tonsils. Special endoscopic procedures and biopsies can be used to look for the primary site, and even if it is not found, such people should be treated using guidelines for head and neck cancer. Epidermoid cancer involving lymph nodes in the lower neck is usually of lung origin. Cervical lymph nodes with metastases of other pathological appearance may represent breast cancer, lymphoma, melanoma, or other tumors (see also "Special Pathologic Methods," in this chapter).

Table 1. **Treatable Cancers That May Present as CUPS**

POTENTIALLY CURABLE	CHANCE OF SIGNIFICANT REMISSION
Germ cell tumors	Breast cancer
Hodgkin's disease	Some lymphomas
Lymphoma	Small cell lung cancer
Trophoblastic tumors	Prostate cancer
Thyroid cancer	Sarcoma
Ovarian cancer	Bladder cancer
Head and neck cancer	

Diagnosis

People with CUPS undergo certain standard methods of medical evaluation to discover the primary site (if possible) and other potential areas of spread. Evaluation will include a history as well as a specific work-up for the major potential sites of the cancer's origin that can be treated—breast cancer, germ cell tumors, lymphomas, and cancers of the head and neck, lung (especially small cell), prostate, thyroid, and ovary. A consensus about the minimal investigation that has to be performed includes the following.

Physical Examination

• When CUPS is found in high cervical (neck) lymph nodes, a thorough examination of the nasopharynx, throat, and upper respiratory tract should be done, usually by an ear, nose, and throat specialist.

• A gynecological examination, including a rectal examination, a Pap smear, and a pelvic ultrasound or CT, should be done for any woman with CUPS, especially if the inguinal (groin) lymph nodes

are enlarged or there is fluid in the abdomen (ascites).

Blood and Other Tests

• Complete blood counts.

• Urinalysis to check for blood.

• Test for hidden (occult) blood in the stool.

• Blood chemistry tests to assess liver and kidney function.

• Tests for serum tumor markers that may be elevated with specific cancers, such as prostate-specific antigen (prostate), alpha-fetoprotein (hepatomas, germ cell tumors), HCG (choriocarcinomas, germ cell tumors), and thyroglobulin and calcitonin (thyroid gland). Other commonly used serum tumor markers (e.g., CEA, CA-125, CA 15-3, CA 19-9) are frequently elevated but nonspecific. However, they may be useful in following response to treatment.

Imaging

• Chest X-ray may reveal the most common tumor origin, carcinoma of the lung. It is often impossible, however, to distinguish between a primary lung cancer and a metastatic lesion within the lung. Sometimes chest CT is also helpful.

• Mammograms for all women diagnosed with CUPS. For women with clinical features suggesting breast cancer, a breast MRI scan should also be performed. For example, over half of the women with isolated metastases in the lymph nodes in the armpit will have a primary breast cancer. However, this will not always be seen even with a mammogram and a breast MRI (false negative results).

• Abdominal CT scan sometimes identifies a primary site in the abdomen, particularly in the pancreas, and frequently provides additional information regarding the location of metastases.

• PET scanning is a new technique that is sometimes successful in detecting cancers not evident on the CT scan. When used in conjunction with CT scanning, the PET scan can detect a primary site in 20 to 30 percent of patients.

• It is not helpful to do extensive X-rays—bowel X-rays, for example—to look for a primary site unless there is a specific complaint in that area, such as constipation or gastrointestinal bleeding.

The following imaging studies are occasionally done:

• CT, MRI, and ultrasound studies of the area of known tumor and likely primary sites.
• Nuclear scans of bone, liver, and thyroid.

Endoscopy and Biopsy
• Endoscopic evaluation of the colon, urinary tract, or lung is performed when indicated either by symptoms or by results of the previous studies.
• Biopsy of suspicious lesions identified by X-rays may establish a primary site; breast, prostate, and pancreas may need special studies on biopsy; hormone-receptor, DNA, and other studies may also be performed.

Special Pathologic Methods

The pathologist has a crucial role in the diagnosis, evaluating the biopsy specimen and determining not only if it is malignant, but, on the basis of his or her experience and the tissue's appearance under the microscope, the most likely source.

The pathologist is often consulted before the biopsy is done because some special immunohistochemistry studies require frozen tissue, or tissue may have to be specially prepared for examination by an electron microscope. These methods offer a significant advantage in obtaining an accurate diagnosis, particularly when tumors appear "poorly differentiated" under the regular microscope. The limited material obtained with a needle biopsy may not be adequate for specialized pathologic studies. In such cases, a larger biopsy, obtained surgically, is recommended.

Immunohistochemistry Along with the usual tissue stains used to examine the tumor tissue under the microscope, special stains using monoclonal antibodies are directed against specific tumor antigens. These can reliably identify several treatable types, particularly lymphoma, thereby allowing therapy to be more specific and improving the chance of remission or even cure.

Electron Microscopy (EM) Regular microscopes magnify tissues up to 1,000 times. The electron microscope can magnify tissues 50,000 to 100,000 times. Very small structures inside and on the surfaces of cells, often characteristic of certain types of cancer cells, can be seen. There are structures characteristic of squamous cell cancers, cancers of neuroendocrine origin, muscle tumors, and most melanomas. Besides suggesting likely sites, EM studies are useful in eliminating certain tumor types.

Polymerase Chain Reaction (PCR) This new method detects minute amounts of genetic material (DNA or RNA). PCR may detect abnormal DNA or RNA structures in the biopsy specimen. A few of these abnormalities are specific for certain cancers and, thus, will suggest the origin of the tumor.

Tissue Stains Many new tissue stains are being developed and are rapidly enlarging the diagnostic capability of the modern pathologist (see Table 2).

Staging

The actual tumor origin is the most important thing in planning treatment and assessing the prognosis. By definition, all

Table 2. **Special Stains Used for Specific Tissues**

- The presence of keratin, a protein found in epithelium (surface tissue), indicates the tumor is a carcinoma rather than a sarcoma or lymphoma.

- S-100 and HMB-45 are useful in the diagnosis of melanomas.

- Chromogranin and synaptophysin are positive in small cell (oat cell) lung cancer and other neuroendocrine tumors.

- Leukocyte-common antigen, found on the surface of leukocytes, is positive in leukemia and lymphoma.

- Prostate-specific antigen (PSA) is positive in prostate cancer.

- Alpha-fetoprotein (AFP) is present in primary liver cancer and certain germ cell tumors.

- Estrogen receptors are present in breast cancer and cancer of the lining of the uterus (endometrial cancer). Finding estrogen receptors not only helps in the diagnosis, but suggests that hormonal therapy may be useful.

CUPS are in an advanced stage because the cancer has already metastasized. It has been suggested that doctors caring for patients with CUPS should refrain from extensive investigations, since the cost of the evaluation financially and with respect to time and discomfort is not worth the results and may not affect survival anyway.

The results of exhaustive tests are also sometimes misleading. The tests may sometimes seem to show a positive finding when none is really there (false positive) or may instead fail to show an abnormality that is present, but not detectable (false negative).

Treatment Overview

There is no generally recommended treatment for *all* patients with CUPS. Whenever there is a likely primary origin, based on the opinion of the pathologist as well as the clinical, laboratory, and imaging studies, the treatment will be given according to that probable diagnosis.

The prognosis for people with CUPS is highly variable because so many different tumors may be involved. However, a number of subgroups recognized by typical clinical or pathologic features are now known to benefit from specific treatments. Some of the patients who do not fit into any of these subgroups can benefit from empiric combination chemotherapy treatment.

Treatment for Specific Presentations

Certain rules have been recommended for a number of specific presentations of CUPS.

"Midline" Tumors

These tumors originate in the middle part of the body such as the mediastinum (chest) or midabdominal lymph nodes. Some people with these tumors who are under fifty years of age, have lung and lymph node metastases, and have a poorly differentiated histology respond well to combination chemotherapy that contains cisplatin and etoposide.

Sixty percent of the patients in one such group had a significant response to therapy and 15 percent were apparently cured. Some of these patients had blood markers (HCG or AFP) suggesting that they had a germ cell tumor.

CUPS in the Neck Lymph Nodes

When epidermoid (squamous) carcinoma is found in the neck (upper cervical) lymph nodes, patients should be treated as if they had a tumor of the upper respiratory area even though a thorough ear, nose, and throat evaluation—including blind biopsies of the base of the tongue and the nasopharynx—may have been negative.

Treatment is potentially curative and may include

• Chemotherapy combined with radical radiotherapy to the cervical lymph nodes and pharyngeal areas or
• a combination of surgery (to remove lymph nodes in the neck) and radiotherapy.

CUPS in the Armpit Lymph Nodes

Women with this site of involvement are frequently curable if no other sites are involved. Over half of such women actually have breast cancer, with an undetectable primary site. Treatment will emphasize

• surgery, including removal of all axillary nodes in the involved site;
• total mastectomy or radiation to the breast;
• hormonal therapy, especially if hormone receptors are present in tumor tissue; and/or
• chemotherapy, sometimes with trastuzumab (Herceptin) added, as recommended for treatment of Stage II breast cancer.

CUPS Involving the Peritoneum

In women, CUPS involving the lining of the abdominal cavity should be treated following the recommendations for ovarian cancer, even if the ovaries are normal or have been removed. Treatment will include

• initial exploratory surgery with removal of all tumor possible, and

• chemotherapy, usually with a taxane (paclitaxel [Taxol] or docetaxel [Taxotere]) and carboplatin [Paraplatin].

CUPS Presenting with a Single Metastasis

Occasionally, only one metastasis is found, even after complete evaluation. A variety of such presentations have been described, including isolated involvement of lymph nodes, lung, brain, adrenal gland, and liver. Involvement of a single lymph node is one of the more common of these presentations. Special care should be made to rule out other types of tumors (lymphoma, melanoma) that frequently involve lymph nodes. When metastatic carcinoma involves a single site, surgical excision is the treatment of choice if possible. Usually other metastases will eventually appear but sometimes after a long delay.

Neuroendocrine CUPS

Neuroendocrine carcinomas are a family of tumors identifiable by the pathologist. The most common neuroendocrine carcinoma in adults is small cell lung cancer. Occasionally, neuroendocrine carcinomas present with unknown primary sites. Most are rapidly growing tumors. It is important to identify these cancers, since they respond well to chemotherapy. About two-thirds of patients have major tumor shrinkage following treatment with paclitaxel (Taxol) and carboplatin (Paraplatin); a few patients have long-term remissions.

Multiple Skeletal Lesions

In males, a prostatic cancer should be suspected. This diagnosis can usually be confirmed by detecting elevated blood levels of PSA or by detecting PSA in the tumor biopsy of special stains. Hormonal therapy is usually of benefit and should be given if prostate cancer is suspected.

In females, breast cancer is a possibility.

In both sexes, a thyroid cancer should be kept in mind, since both tumors may be treated effectively even in the metastatic stage (with hormonal therapy and chemotherapy for breast cancer and with radioiodine for thyroid cancer). Metastatic thyroid cancer that does not resemble normal thyroid tissue (poorly differentiated or undifferentiated), however, seldom responds to treatment with radioactive iodine.

Empiric Chemotherapy

Patients who do not fit into any of the above subgroups should receive a trial of combination therapy unless they are already very ill (confined to bed) as a result of their cancer. Regimens containing new drugs such as paclitaxel (Taxol),

docetaxel (Taxotere), and gemcitabine (Gemzar) have produced substantial tumor shrinkage in 40 to 50 percent of patients, with improved survival. New chemotherapy programs and several of the new targeted agents are being evaluated in clinical trials.

The Most Important Questions You Can Ask

• How much investigation is really needed to increase my chance of survival or to improve my quality of life?

• Has the pathologist used any of the special studies described here?

• What is the most probable diagnosis?

• Can I benefit from surgery, radiotherapy, chemotherapy, or hormonal therapy?

Carcinoids of the Gastrointestinal Tract

Nancy M. Gardner, Ph.D., A.R.N.P., Larry K. Kvols, M.D.,
Malin Dollinger, M.D., and Ernest H. Rosenbaum, M.D.

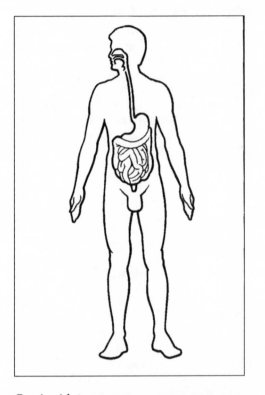

Carcinoid tumors are uncommon cancers. Although they can develop in other organs, especially the lung, they generally arise in the intestinal tract, including the stomach, pancreas, small bowel, appendix, and rectum. They are the most common tumors of the appendix, occurring in 1 out of every 300 appendectomies. They make up 30 percent of small bowel tumors but less than 2 percent of all gastrointestinal malignancies.

In their early stages, carcinoid tumors are highly treatable and often curable.

They are usually slow growing, and the risk of metastasis is related to the size of the primary tumor. Because these tumors are indolent in their behavior and the patient is usually asymptomatic early in the disease, the tumor often goes undetected for many years. Consequently, the disease is often in a more advanced stage at the time of diagnosis.

Small bowel carcinoids may occur in multiple sites (about 25 percent of patients have multiple tumors) and, except for those of rectal origin, may produce biologically active hormones and peptides. In many cases, there are no symptoms, so some carcinoid tumors are discovered incidentally during abdominal operations performed for other reasons. The survival of most people with carcinoid tumors is quite good, although symptoms may develop when the tumor cannot be removed, when it recurs after treatment, or when there is metastatic disease.

Types There are no meaningful cell type (histologic) variations that help predict the clinical course of these tumors. Carcinoids are broadly defined as neuroendocrine or APUD (amine precursor uptake and decarboxylation) tumors. They are classified as foregut, midgut, or hindgut, according to site of primary tumor. Foregut tumors include lung, gastric, duodenal, and pancreatic tumors; midgut tumors include those in the small bowel, appendix, and the first portion of the large intestine; and hindgut tumors are from the remainder of the large intestine and the rectum. Each classification

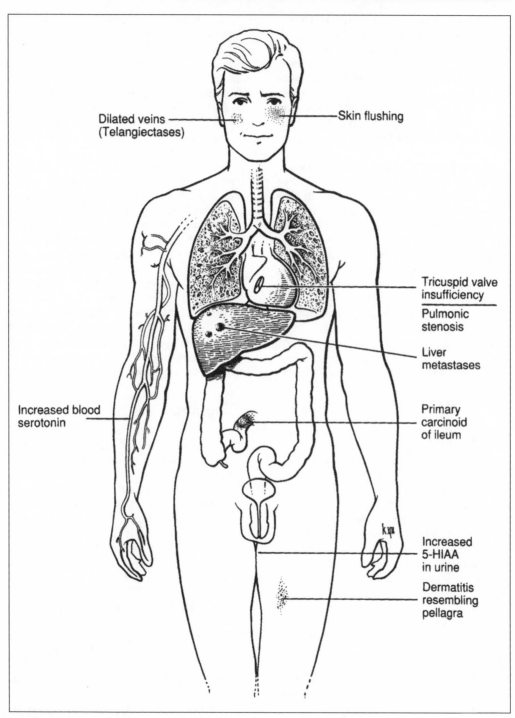

Manifestations of the carcinoid syndrome

of carcinoid tumors represents not only differences in location of the primary tumor, but also where the tumor is likely to spread and differences in hormone production. Malignant midgut carcinoids may produce at least two hormones, serotonin and substance P, but some carcinoid tumors are nonfunctional and do not release any substances.

How It Spreads Carcinoid tumors spread by direct invasion of the underlying layers of tissue (submucosally). They can also spread via lymphatics to regional lymph nodes and through the bloodstream to the liver, lung(s), bones, or other organs.

The site of origin and size of the primary tumor are important in determining whether the carcinoid tumor is likely to spread. A tumor less than ½ inch (1 cm) rarely metastasizes. But 88 percent of patients with tumors larger than ¾ inch (2 cm) have metastases, and 18 percent of these develop the carcinoid syndrome (see "Common Signs and Symptoms," below).

What Causes It Unknown

Risk Factors

Factors that put an individual at risk have not been identified. It is exceedingly rare for carcinoids to be hereditary. However, there are certain genetic mutations found to be associated with the development of the disease. The majority of mutations associated with carcinoid tumors appear to be spontaneous mutations rather than a result of an inherent risk.

Screening

There are no effective screening methods.

Common Signs and Symptoms

Symptoms are unusual in the early stages. The tumors are small and grow slowly and the symptoms so vague, any changes noticed are considered normal. When pronounced symptoms do occur, the tumor has already spread in 90 percent of patients. The most common symptoms associated with gastrointestinal tumors are periodic abdominal pain, intermittent intestinal obstruction, and kinking of the bowel. Gastrointestinal bleeding is uncommon and ulcerations of the tumor are rare.

In addition to the symptoms caused by the tumor, there may be symptoms of the carcinoid syndrome. This is characterized by facial flushing, wheezing, diarrhea, and cardiac valvular disease. Midgut carcinoid tumors are more likely to be associated with the syndrome compared to foregut tumors. Hindgut tumors are usually asymptomatic. The syndrome is associated with abnormal amounts of the two hormones produced by malignant carcinoids, serotonin and substance P. The syndrome occurs in approximately 10 percent of patients with carcinoid tumors, almost always because of carcinoid metastases in the liver.

Diagnosis

Physical Examination
• Palpating the abdomen to identify an abdominal mass and/or an enlarged liver.
• Examination of the facial skin to identify prominent skin veins (telangiectasis) and flushing.
• Listening with a stethoscope for signs that may be associated with carcinoid syndrome—heart murmur and wheezing on expiration.

Blood and Other Tests
• Chromogranin A (CgA) is a general biochemical marker for neuroendocrine tumors. Not all carcinoid tumors overproduce and secrete measurable CgA, but most do. If levels are abnormal, it provides a marker for the disease.
• Metastatic carcinoid tumors may be diagnosed by the twenty-four-hour urine

5-hydroxyindoleacetic acid (5-HIAA) test, which detects elevated levels of 5-HIAA, a metabolic product of the serotonin produced by the tumor. Plasma serotonin levels represent only the level at the time of blood sampling, but the 5-HIAA urine sample provides a twenty-four-hour picture of the serotonin levels, thus providing a more accurate measure for abnormal serotonin production. False positive 5-HIAA tests can be caused by foods such as bananas, avocados, and pineapple and by certain drugs. The laboratory should provide a complete list of foods to be avoided during urine collection.

Imaging

• X-rays of the chest and gastrointestinal tract (small bowel and barium enema).

• Endoscopic evaluation of the stomach may include endoscopic ultrasound (EUS), bronchoscopy for lung tumors, enteroclysis (small bowel enema) for tumors of the small intestine, and colonoscopy to detect large intestinal or rectal tumors.

• CT or MRI scans (with contrast) of the abdomen to detect primary tumors and liver metastases.

• Octreoscan is a nuclear medicine test to determine where the tumor has spread. This test uses a radio-labeled somatostatin analogue that binds to receptors in a lock-and-key fashion. These receptors are located on the tumor cell surface and allow the tumor to be detected through imaging by a nuclear medicine camera. This imaging is used for initial staging of disease and restaging when disease progression is suspected. Since this test reveals somatostatin receptors, it also provides a means for evaluation if the tumor cells would be responsive to somatostatin analogue therapy.

Biopsy Tissue biopsy is the most definitive means of diagnosing the disease. Biopsies may be done of the primary tumor and/or the metastatic lesions.

Staging

There are no specific staging criteria for carcinoids. The tumors are usually referred to as local, local/regional, or metastatic, with emphasis on the extent and location of metastatic disease.

Treatment Overview

Surgery is the standard therapy. The extent of disease spread is important in deciding treatment options.

Surgery Surgical removal of the tumor is the standard treatment for cure. If the primary tumor is localized and can be removed, the five-year survival rate is in the range of 70 to 90 percent. Since carcinoid tumors are usually slow growing, even patients with tumors that can't be removed have an average survival of several years. Surgery often offers excellent relief from symptoms—for example, by removing the liver metastases causing the carcinoid syndrome or by resecting or bypassing intestinal obstructions. Such surgery may add years to a patient's life, an uncommon result of surgery for other types of liver metastases.

Radiation Radiation therapy may be used for symptomatic treatment of bone metastases.

Chemotherapy There has been modest success with chemotherapy. Drug combinations of 5-fluorouracil and streptozocin (Zanosar) have had responses of 10 to 30 percent. Clinical trials evaluating newer drugs are preferable.

Palliation Drugs such as Periactin (cyproheptadine), alpha- and beta adrenergic blockers, chlorpromazine (Thorazine), and corticosteroids may be used to alleviate the symptoms related to the carcinoid syndrome.

Octreotide (Sandostatin), a somatostatin analogue, is very effective in decreasing the secretion of serotonin and can help relieve symptoms of the carcinoid syndrome such as flushing, diarrhea, and wheezing. Interferon-alpha may alleviate symptoms and arrest tumor growth.

Treatment of Localized Tumors by Site

Appendiceal Carcinoids

Appendiceal tumors account for 22 percent of all carcinoids. They are treated by appendectomy and, in fact, are usually diagnosed for the first time at surgery. Lesions less than ¾ inch (2 cm) in diameter are essentially 100 percent curable.

Appendiceal tumors larger than ¾ inch (2 cm) are rare and treated like a carcinoma of the colon. For these larger tumors, removal of the right side of the colon and the lymphatics is recommended.

Five-Year Survival 99 to 100 percent

Rectal Carcinoids

These account for a quarter of all carcinoids. Rectal carcinoids less than ½ inch (1 cm) can be treated adequately by local excision (fulguration), with cure rates approaching 100 percent.

Carcinoid lesions larger than ¾ inch (2 cm) are treated surgically. As with carcinoma, an abdominal-perineal resection may be necessary, but sphincter-preserving surgery may be performed in some cases.

Lesions between ½ and ¾ inch (1 to 2 cm) are in a "gray zone" and receive individualized treatment depending on age, operative risk, and acceptability of a colostomy. The cure rate is excellent.

Five-Year Survival 76 to 83 percent

Small Bowel Carcinoids

Small bowel tumors make up 28 percent of all carcinoids. Conservative local excision is sufficient for tumors less than ½ inch (1 cm) in diameter. For larger tumors, a wedge of the tissues supporting the bowel (mesentery) containing the regional lymph nodes should also be removed.

Anyone with a tumor larger than ¾ inch (2 cm) should be followed closely for a minimum of ten years. The follow-up program should include quarterly or semiannual CT scan of the abdomen and measurements of CgA and urinary 5-HIAA levels.

Five-Year Survival 54 to 67 percent

Treatment of Invasive and Metastatic Carcinoids

Regional Gastrointestinal Carcinoids

Carcinoid tumors with regional metastasis or local extension should be treated by aggressive surgery. If all visible malignant disease can be removed, long-term survival rates will be excellent.

No surgical adjuvant treatment is known to be helpful.

If the regional disease cannot be removed, palliative surgery—to remove all the accessible disease, for example—should be carried out.

Chemotherapy is not required; these patients frequently have many months or even years of comfortable life without further treatment.

Metastatic Carcinoid Tumors

A number of standard treatment options are available for metastatic carcinoid tumors.

 Surgery This has considerable value when there are large liver metastases involving surgically accessible areas of the liver. Liver metastases that recur after surgery should be considered for another resection if they are in an area where the operation can be done with minimal complications. Since these tumors are often slow growing, such surgery may result in significant improvement in life span.

• Radiofrequency ablation of liver metastasis is an option for multiple smaller tumors (less than $2\frac{3}{4}$ inches [7 cm]) and it is often used in conjunction with surgical removal of larger liver tumors. A needle is placed in the tumor, and radiofrequency current is transmitted. This current heats the tumor tissue, causing tumor cell death. The heat also closes up small blood vessels, thereby minimizing the risk of bleeding.

• For very carefully selected patients with slowly progressive disease and symptomatic carcinoid heart disease, heart valve replacement may be indicated.

Hepatic Artery Embolization This is an option for bulky or symptomatic liver metastases that are not surgically resectable. Hepatic artery embolization is used to reduce the blood flow through the hepatic artery, the artery that feeds most liver cancer cells. A material that can plug up the artery is injected. Most of the healthy liver cells will be unaffected because they get their blood supply from the portal vein. A catheter is inserted into an artery in the groin area and threaded up into the liver. A dye is usually injected into the bloodstream at this time to allow the doctor to see the path of the catheter by a special type of X-ray called angiography. Once the catheter is in place and it is confirmed that the portal vein is not blocked, small particles are injected into the artery, cutting off the blood supply to the tumor cells.

Embolization may be done with or without chemotherapy. This can lead to substantial tumor regression. It can also cause significant side effects—abdominal pain, fever, nausea, and a short-term worsening of the syndrome—but many patients do experience substantial relief from symptoms.

Embolizations are often performed over several procedures until the desired effect is appreciated, usually one month apart. This procedure can be repeated years later in the course of disease management.

Radiation The role of radiation therapy in managing carcinoid tumors with distant metastasis is restricted to relief of symptoms, most commonly from bone involvement. However, localized metastasis will occasionally respond to radiation therapy.

Supportive Therapy There are a number of ways to manage symptoms from metastatic disease with medication:

• Diarrhea, if not severe, will frequently respond to standard antidiarrheal medications such as Lomotil, Imodium, or tincture of opium and to dietary changes such as restricting consumption of foods high in fat.

• The somatostatin analogue octreotide (Sandostatin) has been shown to be useful in improving symptoms of the carcinoid syndrome and may be life saving in carcinoid crisis (sudden exacerbation of symptoms). It targets the cell receptors that control the abnormal production and release of the hormones that cause the syndrome and carcinoid heart disease. This method of therapy is the standard for reducing elevated levels of 5-HIAA.

• Interferon-alpha preparations may have a role in controlling symptoms of the carcinoid syndrome and/or in arresting tumor growth.

• Acute symptoms—carcinoid crisis—may be prevented by pretreatment, and an active crisis can be reversed with short-acting octreotide. Some specific drugs are to be avoided in these patients because of the risk of causing the release of vasoactive substances. This is especially true during surgery and in the treatment of low blood pressure.

Chemotherapy Although activity with a variety of single agents and drug combinations has been reported—5-fluorouracil (5-FU), doxorubicin (Adriamycin), and dacarbazine (DTIC) or 5-FU + streptozocin—response rates seldom exceed 30 percent. Complete responses are uncommon, and the duration of the response may be short, if chemotherapy is used alone.

Chemotherapy should be used for palliation in patients with symptoms and in the case of liver metastases, after blocking the hepatic (liver) artery and then giving chemotherapy (chemoembolization) (see the chapter "Metastatic Cancer").

Investigational A novel approach has been introduced recently where octreotide is tagged with a radionuclide that kills tumor cells. This is given intravenously and targets tumor cells with somatostatin receptors. Newer drugs that target other molecular pathways are also being investigated.

Treatment Follow-Up

Patients should be evaluated every three to twelve months. The evaluation should include

- physical examination;
- twenty-four-hour urine 5-HIAA levels;
- chromogranin A;
- octreoscan, if required;
- chest X-ray, if required; and
- abdominal MRI or CT scan, if required. If a CT scan is used, it is preferable to use a three-phase scan.

Recurrent Cancer

The selection of further treatment depends on many factors, including the therapy initially used, the site of the recurrence, and individual considerations.

Since some tumors grow rather slowly, attempts to remove them again or multiple operations to remove liver metastases are worthy of consideration. Reducing tumor volume may provide long-term relief of symptoms.

Investigational treatments are appropriate and should be considered when standard treatment fails.

The Most Important Questions You Can Ask

- How are carcinoids different from the usual cancers of the bowel?
- What tests are needed to follow my progress after surgery?
- What does a rising urine 5-HIAA mean?
- What are the toxic side effects of chemotherapy?
- What is the role of repeated surgeries for recurrent carcinoid cancers?
- Am I eligible for any research or investigational protocols?

Cervix

Jeffrey L. Stern, M.D.

■ ■ ■ ■

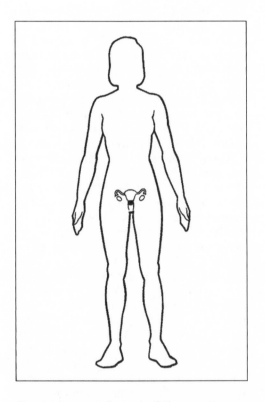

Cervical cancer is one of the most common cancers worldwide, especially in poor countries, with approximately 260,000 deaths annually. Invasive cervical cancer accounts for 6 percent of all cancers that afflict women in the United States. About 10,400 cases of invasive carcinoma of the cervix are diagnosed in the United States each year, while there are at least 500,000 new cases of a preinvasive cervical cancer—known as a squamous intraepithelial lesion—where the cancer cells are confined to the surface skin of the cervix.

Since 1940, there has been a steady decrease in the yearly incidence of carcinoma of the cervix because many women have been screened with Pap smears, detecting cancer before it becomes invasive. It is estimated that over half the women diagnosed with cancer of the cervix have never been screened for cervical cancer, and an additional 10 percent have not been screened within the past five years.

Types Over 90 percent of cervical carcinomas start in the surface cells on the cervix and are known as squamous cell carcinomas. Five to 9 percent start in endocervical glandular tissue (adenocarcinoma). There are several types of adenocarcinomas. Sixty percent are the endocervical cell type, 20 percent are also endometrioid or clear cell carcinomas, and 20 percent are adenosquamous carcinomas. Adenocarcinomas are more difficult to diagnose but are treated the same way as squamous cell carcinomas, with a similar survival rate, stage for stage.

There are two rare types of cervical cancers, known as small cell carcinoma and cervical sarcoma, both of which have a poor prognosis.

There are two categories of preinvasive squamous lesions: The first is known as a low-grade squamous intraepithelial lesion (LGSIL). It was also known in the past as mild dysplasia or cervical intraepithelial neoplasia (CIN-1). Most cases of LGSIL do not progress to invasive cancer. The second category is known as a high-grade squamous intraepithelial lesion (HGSIL), which in the past was also known as moderate dysplasia (CIN-2), or severe dysplasia (carcinoma in situ, or CIN-3). Most physicians believe that about two-thirds of all cases of HGSIL progress to invasive cancer if left untreated. This transformation takes anywhere from two to thirty years, with about five to ten years on the average.

How It Spreads Once the cervical cancer becomes invasive, it can spread locally to the upper vagina and into the tissues surrounding the upper vagina and the cervix (the parametrium). Eventually it grows toward the pelvic sidewall, obstructing the ureters (tubes that drain urine from the kidney to the bladder). It can also spread directly into the bladder and rectum.

Cervical cancer cells can also invade the lymphatic system and spread to the lymph nodes around the vessels on the pelvic walls. Eventually they may spread to the lymph nodes higher in the pelvis, the aortic lymph nodes, the nodes above the collarbone, and even occasionally to the groin nodes.

Distant metastases can also occur through the bloodstream to the lower vagina, vulva, lung, liver, and brain. Distant metastases are more common in women with cancer spread to the lymph nodes or higher-stage cancer. Invasion of the pelvic nerves is common in advanced cases. There may also be spread within the abdomen when the tumor penetrates the full thickness of the cervix.

What Causes It Most scientists believe that the human papillomavirus (HPV) causes preinvasive and invasive cervical cancer. Preinvasive cervical cancer is thought to develop within six months to five years after exposure to HPV, while invasive cancer is thought to develop within one to ten years after exposure. The human papillomavirus is the most common sexually transmitted illness in the United States, with approximately 20 million men and women currently infected. It is estimated that as many as 6 million people become

infected every year. The Centers for Disease Control and Prevention (CDC) has estimated that 50 percent of sexually active people will be exposed to the human papillomavirus in their lifetime. Over forty types of HPV exclusively infect the genital skin of the cervix, vulva, vagina, urethra, anus, and penis.

There are two general groups of human papillomavirus: the low-risk group for causing cancer, with HPV types 6 and 11 being the most common, and the high-risk group for developing cancer, with HPV types 16 and 18. The low-risk types usually result in genital warts, low-grade squamous intraepithelial lesions (LGSIL), and on very rare occasions respiratory tract warts in children exposed during birth.

Genital warts most often appear on the external genitalia or near the anus. However, warts can also occur on the cervix and the vagina. It is estimated that genital warts may occur within weeks, months, or years after exposure, or not at all. Genital warts are usually not symptomatic, although they may cause itching, burning, or occasional bleeding. They are treated after careful evaluation with cryotherapy (freezing), laser, topical medications, or topical anticancer drugs.

The high-risk HPV types are responsible for most cases of high-grade squamous intraepithelial lesions (HGSIL), adenocarcinoma in situ, and cancer (both squamous cell and adenocarcinoma).

Exposure to HPV does not necessarily result in warts, precancerous changes, or cancer (either squamous cell or adenocarcinoma). Similarly, most people do not have symptoms after exposure to the virus. It is not clear how long the infection with HPV lasts either with or without treatment.

Risk Factors

The risk factors for preinvasive cervical cancer and cervical cancer are the same. The average age of women with invasive

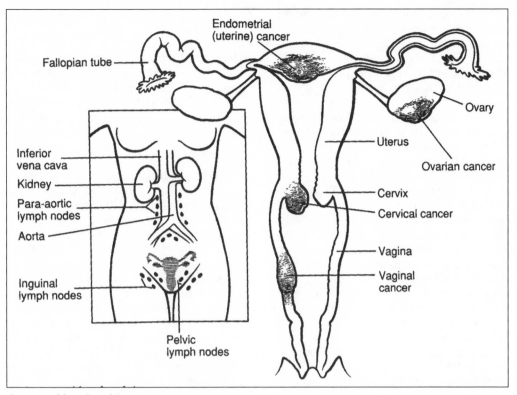

Cancers of female pelvic organs

cervical cancer in the United States is between thirty-five and fifty-five, while the average age of women with HGSIL is between twenty-five and thirty-five. The difference is attributed to the long latent period of progression of a precancerous lesion confined to the cervical skin to an invasive cervical cancer.

Circumcision is no longer believed to lower the risk of cervical carcinoma.

At Significantly Higher Risk

• Anything that results in an increased risk of exposure to genital HPV

• A history of genital HPV (warts, pre-invasive lesions)

• Suppression of the immune system from corticosteroids, organ transplants, therapy for other cancers, or HIV

• A history of herpes simplex virus infection

• Early age at first intercourse

• Multiple sexual partners

• Cigarette smoking

• Women whose male partners either have had penile warts, have had multiple sexual partners, or have had previous partners with cervical cancer

Screening

Liquid-based cytology and HPV DNA testing is now widely performed in the United States. It has resulted in an increased accuracy in the diagnosis of both pre-malignant and malignant changes in the female lower genital tract. The abnormal findings on physical exam, Pap smear, or colposcopy (magnification 7.5 to 15 times) are confirmed with a biopsy.

The American College of Obstetricians and Gynecologists recommends that a Pap smear be performed on all women by age eighteen or who are sexually active, regardless of age. Women who have multiple sexual partners should be screened annually, but those in long-term, stable relationships who have had three consecutive negative yearly Pap smears may be screened less often.

A major problem with the Pap smear is that it is often thought to be normal when it is actually abnormal. The estimated false negative rate is about 10 percent, half of which can be attributed to faulty sampling techniques. The pathologist examining the cells can make an error, or the health care provider may not sample the cervix adequately. It is important to have both the squamous cell component and the endocervical component present on the Pap (in women with a cervix) in order to have a reliable Pap smear. Sometimes women are asked to return for another Pap smear if they lack the endocervical component. Testing for HPV can help triage women with a mildly abnormal Pap smear, or atypical squamous cell of undetermined significance (ASCUS).

Unfortunately, adenocarcinomas and adenosquamous carcinomas are more difficult to detect on Pap smears, since they start higher up in the cervical canal and may not be sampled by the Pap smear.

Pap Smear Diagnoses

• Normal
• Atypical squamous cell of undetermined significance (ASCUS)
• Low-grade squamous intraepithelial lesion (LGSIL)
• High-grade squamous intraepithelial lesion (HGSIL)
• Atypical glandular cells of undetermined significance (AGUS)
• Adenocarcinoma in situ (ACIS)

• Cancer-type specific
• Other

Partners Partners of women with an HPV infection, warts, squamous intraepithelial lesions (SIL), or cancer should be carefully examined as well for genital warts, precancerous skin changes, and cancer.

Prevention and Vaccination

Recently, a human papillomavirus recombinant vaccine known as Gardasil has been developed and approved for use. Gardasil is quadrivalent, which means it can protect against infection with human papillomavirus types 6, 11, 16, and 18. Gardasil will not protect against HPV types other than types 6, 11, 16, and 18. It will, however, prevent approximately 70 percent of the cervical cancers and 90 percent of the cases of genital warts. The vaccine also does not protect against HPV types that an individual has already been exposed to. It will not protect against other sexually transmitted illnesses.

Currently, it is recommended that women ages nine through twenty-six be vaccinated. Three injections of the vaccine are required. The second injection is given two months after the first dose, and the third dose is given six months after the first dose.

All three doses are required for significant protection, although there may be some benefit from only one or two injections of the vaccine. Side effects, generally mild and uncommon, include pain, swelling, itching, redness, fever, nausea, and dizziness.

The vaccine will not substitute for routine cervical screening, a careful pelvic exam, and a Pap smear. It is not recommended in those women infected with HIV or who are pregnant.

Common Signs and Symptoms

In many cases of cervical cancer, and in almost all cases of preinvasive cancer, there are no symptoms. The most common symptoms in women with cancer include abnormal vaginal bleeding or discharge, bleeding after intercourse, and back, pelvic, or leg pain.

Diagnosis

Physical Examination

• Most women with cervical cancer will have a normal general physical examination.

• Careful evaluation of the external genitalia.

• Lymph nodes in the groin and above the collarbone should be examined to detect any enlargement.

• A pelvic and rectal examination is important to detect disease in the tissue surrounding the cervix and vagina.

Blood and Other Tests

• Complete blood count.

• Liver function chemistries.

• Kidney function chemistries.

• The levels of the serum carcinoembryonic antigen (CEA) in the blood should be measured in women with advanced cancer. CEA is elevated in about 20 percent of all women with cervical carcinomas. Although CEA is not accurate enough to use for screening, it is useful to monitor the response to treatment and for follow-up to detect recurrent disease.

Imaging

• Chest X-ray.

• CT or MRI scan of the chest, abdomen, and pelvis.

• PET/CT scan in advanced cases.

Endoscopy and Biopsy

• Cystoscopy in advanced cases of cancer.

• Sigmoidoscopy in advanced cases of cancer.

• All women with an abnormal Pap smear or cervical lesions should undergo an office colposcopic examination. A colposcope is an instrument that can magnify the cervix from 7.5 to 15 times. Usually 3 to 5 percent acetic acid is applied to the cervix and/or vagina to facilitate detection of abnormal changes.

• The definitive diagnosis of an adenocarcinoma or squamous intraepithelial lesion (SIL) is made on a single biopsy, usually performed in the office. Early cancers are occasionally diagnosed on a large biopsy of the cervix, either with a LEEP (loop electrosurgical excision procedure) or a cold-knife cone biopsy. A cervical LEEP is a biopsy performed in the office with an anesthetic or in the operating room. A LEEP is used for diagnosis and/or treatment of SIL. A cervical LEEP or conization is performed when (1) colposcopy cannot determine if there is an invasive cancer; (2) when there are no obvious lesions on the cervix, and the Pap smear is consistently abnormal; (3) when a colposcopically directed biopsy does not adequately account for abnormal cells found on a Pap smear; (4) when a diagnosis of microinvasion (early invasion) is found on the biopsy; (5) when an SIL is identified by a scraping from the cervical canal (endocervical curettage); or (6) when there is a diagnosis of adenocarcinoma in situ of the cervix.

Staging

Most gynecologic oncologists use the FIGO (International Federation of Gynecologists and Obstetricians) classification, which divides cervical cancer into five stages, with further divisions in each stage. HGSIL on biopsy or carcinoma in situ is Stage 0. A cancer confined to the cervix is Stage I. In Stage II, the disease either extends beyond the cervix but not to the pelvic sidewall, or involves the vagina but not the lower third. A Stage III carcinoma extends to the pelvic sidewall, involves the lower third of the vagina, or obstructs one or both of the ureters. In Stage IV, the cancer has spread to distant organs beyond the true pelvis or involves the lining of the bladder or rectum.

Treatment Overview

Squamous cell carcinoma and adenocarcinoma are generally treated similarly. Radical surgery and radiation therapy are equally effective treatments for early-stage disease (Stage IB and a small IIA). For carcinomas more advanced than Stage IIA, treatment is with radiation therapy and chemotherapy. Higher stages are generally treated with higher doses of radiation therapy as well.

Surgery For younger women, surgery is usually recommended because one can preserve the ovaries, thereby preventing premature menopause. It also avoids the vaginal scarring that can result from radiation. Lastly, there is a small chance that women who survive many years after radiation therapy will develop a second malignancy in the radiated area.

Radical exenterative surgery—removal of the rectum and/or bladder and the cervix, uterus, and vagina—is usually reserved for recurrent carcinoma confined to the central pelvis.

Surgery may also be used to stage cervical cancer, since other methods, even CT, MRI, and PET scans, are notoriously inaccurate in detecting lymph node metastasis and intra-abdominal spread in the more advanced stages. Unfortunately, there is no reliable way to diagnose microscopic metastases to the pelvic and para-aortic nodes without removing them, so many gynecologic oncologists recommend a surgical staging procedure before radiation therapy to evaluate the intra-abdominal surfaces and the status of the pelvic and aortic lymph nodes.

Surgical staging is done, if possible, through an approach outside the lining of the abdominal cavity (extraperitoneal). This avoids the manipulation of the intra-abdominal organs as much as possible (as in an intra-abdominal operation) and results in fewer complications following radiation therapy.

The incidence of cancerous pelvic and para-aortic nodes increases with more advanced disease, and there may be a survival advantage to removing the involved nodes. Women with microscopic metastases to the pelvic and aortic nodes can be cured if the nodes are removed. Usually radiation therapy and chemotherapy is given postoperatively to improve the cure rate. Generally, two-thirds of women with pelvic node metastases are cured, while only one-third of women are cured if the aortic nodes are positive.

Women with positive para-aortic nodes may have distant metastases to the lymph nodes above the collarbone (10 percent of cases). If the neck nodes are positive, then only palliative therapy is warranted.

Radiation Several radiation modalities may be used depending on the stage of the disease—usually a combination of external-beam therapy and intracavitary therapy (the insertion of radioactive substances around the tumor or into the tumor [interstitial radiation]). Intracavitary radiation may be of two types—low-dose-rate and high-dose-rate (see chapter 7, "What Happens in Radiation Therapy").

Chemotherapy It is now standard therapy to give chemotherapy simultaneously with radiation therapy in women with advanced cervical cancers. Chemotherapy is also being actively investigated for women at high risk for recurrent disease, regardless of the stage (i.e., for those with multiple pelvic lymph node or aortic lymph node metastases).

Treatment by Stage

▣ Stage 0 (Squamous Cell Carcinoma)
Carcinoma in situ (intraepithelial carcinoma). High-grade squamous intraepithelial lesion.

Standard Treatment There are four treatment options for this early-stage tumor:

1. A LEEP (loop electrosurgical excision procedure) is similar to a cone biopsy and is for both diagnostic and therapeutic indications. It is usually performed in the office with a local anesthetic with only rare side effects. A portion of the face and canal of the cervix is removed.
2. A cervical cold-knife conization is performed when a LEEP is not appropriate—usually for recurrent disease or difficult anatomy.
3. Laser vaporization therapy may be recommended for larger lesions.
4. Freezing the cervix (cryotherapy) can be performed in the doctor's office and has a negligible complication rate. It is used less frequently nowadays.

Occasionally a hysterectomy may be recommended.

Five-Year Survival 100 percent

▣ Stage 0 (Adenocarcinoma)

Standard Treatment Adenocarcinoma in situ (confined to the surface of the cervix) is often difficult to diagnose. The diagnosis is usually made with a cervical biopsy or an endocervical curettage. In all cases, a conization is required to rule out a truly invasive lesion.

For women who may want to have children, a LEEP or cone biopsy may cure the disease if the surgical margins (or edges) do not show any evidence of disease. Even so, adenocarcinoma in situ or an invasive adenocarcinoma is occasionally found in the residual cervix even if the cone biopsy has negative margins.

For those who have completed childbearing, the treatment of choice is a simple vaginal or abdominal hysterectomy.

Five-Year Survival 100 percent

▣ Stage I
Stage I is cancer confined to the cervix. Stage IA involves a carcinoma of the cervix diagnosed only microscopically. All visible lesions, even those with minimal invasion, are Stage IB. Stage IA is further divided into two stages based on the depth of invasion of the cervix.

▣ Stage IA1
In Stage IA1, there is less than 3 mm of invasion and the invasion is less than 7 mm wide.

Standard Treatment When the depth of invasion is less than 3 mm from the surface and there is no vascular space involvement, a total vaginal or abdominal hysterectomy with or without removal of the tubes and ovaries is usually recommended. However, a cervical LEEP or conization may be curative if the edges (margins) of the biopsy are free of disease and if there is no vascular space involvement. This may be the appropriate therapy for those women who want to preserve their fertility or who want to avoid a hysterectomy.

Five-Year Survival 100 percent

▣ Stage IA2
The depth of stromal invasion is greater than 3 mm and less than 5 mm from the surface of the cervix. It must also be less than 7 mm wide.

Standard Treatment In the United States, women with cancer invading greater than 3 mm into the cervix or those with invasive cancer less than that, but with blood vessel involvement, are treated like those women with Stage IB1 disease.

Five-Year Survival 85 to 95 percent

■ Stage IB
Lesions are larger than Stage IA2 but are still confined to the cervix.

■ Stage IB1
Cervical cancer confined to the cervix but no greater than $1\frac{1}{2}$ inches (4 cm) in size.

■ Stage IB2
Cervical cancer confined to the cervix but greater than $1\frac{1}{2}$ inches (4 cm) in size.

Standard Treatment There are two options for treatment. A radical hysterectomy may be done, with removal of the lymph nodes from the blood vessels from both sides of the pelvis and from around the aorta. An alternative is external-beam radiation (given in divided doses five days a week for five weeks) followed two weeks later by intracavitary or interstitial radiation (low-dose- or high-dose-rate). Both options result in an equal rate of cure. The choice depends on available local expertise, the age of the patient, and the patient's medical condition. Small lesions (Stage IB1) are usually operated on, while large ones are often treated with surgery or radiation. Women who have metastatic disease in the removed lymph nodes are frequently treated with external-beam radiation therapy with concurrent chemotherapy to the affected area following surgery.

A radical abdominal hysterectomy and a bilateral pelvic and aortic lymph node dissection is usually performed through either a midline incision or a large lower transverse abdominal incision.

Investigational Recently, a procedure known as a radical trachelectomy has been performed for Stage IA2 and early small IB1 cancers. A large portion of the cervix and a portion of the vagina and surrounding tissues are removed and a pelvic/aortic lymph node dissection is performed. This allows preservation of the cervix and uterus. There are a small series of patients in the literature with encouraging results.

However, more recently, a number of gynecologic oncologists have been performing the same operation using a minimally invasive surgical technique (known as laparoscopy). The entire procedure is performed through four to five small incisions in the abdominal wall. One just below the navel, the second above, the third just above the pubic bone, and the other two on opposite sides of the pelvis. Although this procedure is still investigational, as the technique is learned by more laparoscopists, it will become more widely available. Its limitations are primarily based on the patient's weight, as obese women are not good candidates. There are also a number of gynecologic oncologists who believe that the lymph nodes should be removed laparoscopically and the radical hysterectomy performed through the vagina. Generally, the complication rate of these techniques is higher than that of an open incision.

Stage IB2 cervical cancers (greater than $1\frac{1}{2}$ inches [4 cm]) confined to the cervix may be treated with surgery alone, radiation therapy followed by surgery six weeks later, radiation therapy and concurrent chemotherapy alone, or chemotherapy followed by radical hysterectomy.

Five-Year Survival 70 to 95 percent

■ Stage II
The cancer is one that either extends beyond the cervix (but not to the pelvic sidewall) or involves the vagina (but not the lower third).

■ Stage IIA
In Stage IIA, there is no obvious involvement of the tissue surrounding the cervix

(parametrium), but there is involvement of up to the inner two-thirds of the vagina.

Standard Treatment Treatment with either a radical hysterectomy and removal of the lymph nodes or external-beam radiation therapy followed by intracavitary or interstitial radiation given with concurrent chemotherapy is standard.

Women with large lesions of the cervix are sometimes managed with preoperative radiation therapy with concurrent chemotherapy, followed by a hysterectomy and lymph node dissection.

Women who have metastatic disease in the lymph nodes are usually given external-beam radiation therapy to the pelvis and sometimes the para-aortic region with concurrent chemotherapy after surgery.

Five-Year Survival Approaching 70 to 95 percent

■ *Stage IIB*
There is obvious parametrial involvement but no extension to the pelvic sidewall.

Standard Treatment Concurrent chemotherapy and external-beam radiation therapy are given in divided doses over five weeks, followed by intracavitary or interstitial radiation.

Five-Year Survival 65 to 80 percent

Investigational
• High-dose-rate brachytherapy, which allows for shorter treatment times in an outpatient or office setting.
• Various types, doses, and timing of chemotherapy.

■ *Stage III*
The cancer extends to the pelvic sidewall, involves the lower third of the vagina, or obstructs one or both ureters or there is a nonfunctioning kidney.

■ *Stage IIIA*
Stage IIIA is defined as having no extension to the pelvic sidewall, but the tumor involves the lower third of the vagina.

■ *Stage IIIB*
There is extension to the pelvic sidewall or obstruction of one or both ureters (the tubes that connect the kidney to the bladder), or there is a nonfunctioning kidney.

Standard Treatment External-beam radiation therapy followed by intracavitary or interstitial radiation therapy with chemotherapy is standard.

Five-Year Survival 40 to 60 percent

Investigational Same as for Stage IIB.

■ *Stage IV*
Stage IV is defined as cancer that has spread to distant organs beyond the true pelvis or involves the lining of the bladder or rectum.

■ *Stage IVA*
In Stage IVA, a biopsy has shown that either the lining of the bladder or the rectum is involved with cancer.

Standard Treatment This stage is usually treated with radiation therapy and chemotherapy or by the surgical removal of the uterus, the vagina, and the bladder and/or rectum (pelvic exenteration).

Five-Year Survival 20 to 30 percent

■ *Stage IVB*
In Stage IVB, there is spread to distant organs.

Standard Treatment Radiation may be used to relieve the symptoms of pelvic disease or isolated distant metastases. A number of chemotherapeutic drugs are useful for treating metastatic cervical cancer, but they are rarely curative. They include cisplatin or carboplatin, which has a response rate of 15 to 25 percent, and ifosfamide, which has a response rate of 30 percent. Other drugs such as paclitaxel (Taxol), doxorubicin (Adriamycin), cyclophosphamide (Cytoxan), and 5-fluorouracil may be recommended.

Combination chemotherapy, including cisplatin + etoposide + bleomycin, has a response rate of about 50 percent. Other drug combinations that have been used in women with metastatic disease include mitomycin-C + bleomycin + cisplatin, carboplatin + ifosfamide, and cisplatin + ifosfamide with or without bleomycin.

Investigational Many of the drugs used in the standard treatment are being tested in different combinations and doses.

Treatment Follow-Up

A Pap smear and careful examination of the pelvis, abdomen, and lymph nodes are performed every three months for the first two years after treatment, and then every six months for three more years.

• Routine chest X-rays and pelvic and abdominal CT scans or PET scans are often performed even in the absence of symptoms.
• The serum levels of carcinoembryonic antigen may be measured at each visit if they were elevated prior to treatment.

Recurrent Cancer

Symptoms of recurrent cervical carcinoma may include vaginal bleeding or discharge; pain in the pelvis, back, or legs; leg swelling (edema); chronic cough; and weight loss.

• Cervical cancer can recur in the vagina, pelvis, lymph nodes, lung, or liver.

• If radiation was not given previously, recurrences that are confined to the pelvis may be treated with external-beam radiation and intracavitary or interstitial radiation therapy with concurrent chemotherapy.
• In selected cases with a recurrent cancer in the vagina, bladder, or rectum in which radiation therapy was already given, the only option is to remove the vagina, uterus, and bladder and/or rectum with the creation of an artificial bladder (pelvic exenteration). The five-year survival rate after a pelvic exenteration is about 50 percent.
• Women with recurrent tumors that cannot be surgically removed or with metastatic disease are usually treated with chemotherapy. Commonly used drugs include single-agent cisplatin or carboplatin. Other regimens include cisplatin or carboplatin + ifosfamide, vincristine + mitomycin-C + bleomycin + cisplatin, and bleomycin + mitomycin-C + 5-fluorouracil, (paclitaxol) Taxol, etoposide, cyclophosphamide (Cytoxan), gemcitabine (Gemzar), or doxorubicin liposomal (Doxil).
• Those with unresectable pelvic disease may be reirradiated with interstitial radiation or given pelvic arterial chemotherapy.

The Most Important Questions You Can Ask

• What qualifications do you have for treating cancer? Will a specialist in gynecologic oncology be involved in my care?
• What is the advantage of surgery versus radiation therapy?
• If the cancer is advanced, will a staging surgery be performed?
• Is the HPV vaccine appropriate for me?

Childhood Cancers

Ramesh Patel, M.D., and Jerry Z. Finklestein, M.D.

■ ■ ■ ■

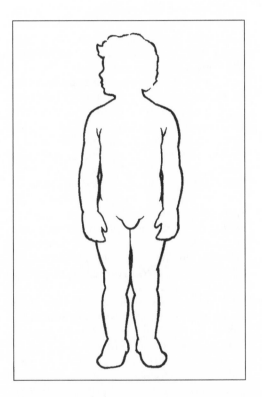

Cancer in children is a rare disease. For every 120 adults who develop cancer, there is 1 child. Yet next to accidents, cancer is the second most common cause of death in children between the ages of one and fourteen. In the United States, about 12,400 children and adolescents younger than twenty years will be diagnosed with cancer each year, and 1,400 will die of cancer. Recent evidence suggests that the incidence of cancer in children has increased approximately 1 percent per year during the past twenty-five years. However, the overall mortality rate in children younger than fifteen has decreased by 38 percent.

Childhood cancers are different from those in adults. The growth pattern is different and tumors react differently to treatment. Most important, the problems seen in a child differ from those of an adult.

Fortunately, with the development of new drugs, new treatment methods, and better diagnostic tools and the involvement of multidisciplinary medical teams, the outlook for childhood cancers has improved dramatically over the past few decades. Currently, the overall cure rate for the United States for children and adolescents with cancer has exceeded 75 percent.

Types The most common childhood cancer is leukemia, accounting for about one-third of all cancers seen. The most common types in children are acute lymphoblastic leukemia and less frequently, acute nonlymphocytic leukemia. A smaller number of children may develop chronic granulocytic leukemia.

Brain tumors—gliomas, medulloblastomas, and ependymomas—are the second most common type of cancer in children. A new term has recently been designated for certain types of brain tumors—*PNET*, which stands for primitive neuroectodermal tumors.

Some cancers seen in children are rare in adults. A cancer of the sympathetic nervous system known as neuroblastoma may occur in the adrenal glands located on top of the kidneys or may originate anywhere there is a particular kind of nerve ending—in the chest, the abdomen, the pelvis, and, rarely, other sites. A cancer of the kidney known as Wilms' tumor is also particular to children, occurring most commonly in children two to four years of age and rarely in those over sixteen. It may occur in one or both kidneys.

Other childhood tumors that are uncommon in adults are a tumor of the membrane at the back of the eye, the retina, called retinoblastoma; a muscle tumor called rhabdomyosarcoma; teratomas, which are tumors of young cells known as germ cells; and a tumor of the liver known as hepatoblastoma.

Bone tumors such as osteogenic sarcoma, Ewing's sarcoma, and chondrosarcoma occur in children, particularly in teenagers. Histiocytosis X, or Langerhans cell histiocytosis, is not a malignancy but is often cared for by physicians who specialize in pediatric cancer therapy.

Children, like adults, develop lymphomas known as Hodgkin's disease and non-Hodgkin's lymphoma. They may also have tumors of the liver (hepatomas), skin cancer (melanoma, which is rare), and cancers of the thyroid and adrenal glands and blood vessels.

Over 80 percent of cancers in adults develop in the glands or lining tissues of the breast, lung, or intestinal or urinary tract and are called carcinomas. Leukemias, central nervous system tumors, and lymphomas account for over 60 percent of all the cancers diagnosed in children. About 15 percent of cancers of children are malignancies of muscle, bone, supporting tissues, or blood vessels and are called sarcomas. The types of cancers seen in children, therefore, differ from those in adults not only in name, but in their microscopic appearance.

What Causes It We do not know why children develop cancer. Occasionally there are clues from the environment or from a genetic inheritance pattern that a child may be at risk. But specific causes have not been identified. However, children with certain diseases do have an increased incidence of cancer (see "Risk Factors," in this chapter).

For more than thirty years, there have been reports of "clusters," or concentrations, of childhood cancer developing in certain geographic areas. There were clusters of children with leukemia in Niles, Illinois, in 1963; in Woburn, Massachusetts, in 1979; and in central California in the early 1990s. But physicians have not been able to determine the significance of these clusters.

It is believed that children are more likely than adults to develop leukemia as a result of exposure to radiation. Children exposed to the radiation of the atomic bomb blasts in Japan had an increased risk of acute leukemia in childhood, with the peak occurring about five years after exposure. A higher incidence of leukemia in children exposed to radiation after the accident in Chernobyl, Ukraine, has occurred. Radiation therapy is useful in the treatment of many cancers in children, but there is a risk that children cured of their first cancer may develop a second one partly related to the use of radiation therapy.

A number of cancer-causing chemicals and industrial processes are all around us. Their role in causing childhood cancers is the subject of ongoing research.

There has also been publicity about electromagnetic waves produced by high-tension power lines as a possible cause of cancer in children. Recent reports have refuted the claim. In recent years, new information has been released about causation with discoveries in the field of molecular genetics. Oncogenes (tumor-promoting genes) have been found in certain childhood cancers. Anti-oncogenes (tumor-suppressing genes) have been found in association with other childhood tumors.

For parents, it is frustrating to acknowledge that there is very little they can do to protect their children from environmental or genetic factors. Research is continuing, however, and one day, we may have better means of protection.

Risk Factors

The cancer rate for African-American children in the United States is about 80 percent of that seen in white children; children who are black do not have the same incidence of common cancers such as acute lymphocytic leukemia and lymphomas as children who are white. Black children rarely have Ewing's sarcoma, but there is a suggestion that they have a higher incidence of Wilms' tumor, retinoblastoma, and the bone tumor known as osteogenic sarcoma.

Several cancers in children—leukemia and Wilms' tumor, for example—peak in incidence between the ages of two and four years. Others, such as lymphoma and bone cancer, have a peak incidence in older children.

At Significantly Higher Risk

- Previous exposure to radiation.
- Children who do not have an iris—the colored circle in the eye—have a higher incidence of developing the kidney cancer called Wilms' tumor.
- Children whose bodies are bigger on one side than the other (hemihypertrophy) have a higher incidence of Wilms' tumor.
- Males with an undescended testicle (cryptorchidism) are at higher risk for testicular cancer.
- Children with the skin disease xeroderma pigmentosum have a higher risk of developing skin cancer.
- Children with the immune disorder ataxia telangiectasia, Down's syndrome, Fanconi's anemia, and Bloom's syndrome are at higher risk for developing leukemia.

Screening

A number of tests screen for cancer in adults, but very few such tests exist for children. In Japan, Quebec, and some other parts of North America, there is an attempt to screen the urine of very young children to detect the presence of abnormal amounts of the chemical group known as catecholamines in the hope that earlier detection of neuroblastoma will result in an improved cure rate.

The child with a risk factor for developing cancer should be evaluated carefully by his or her physician. The screening may be as simple as a blood test in an identical twin of a child with leukemia or a series of ultrasound examinations of the abdomen for many years in a child with hemihypertrophy.

Common Signs and Symptoms

Many of the symptoms and signs of childhood cancers are very common to other illnesses, and only health professionals with sufficient training will be able to tell whether a complaint is due to a normal childhood disease or a rare disease such as cancer.

Tiredness and paleness are usually the result of nothing more than the flu but could also signal the onset of leukemia. Fever is often noted in a child with infection, but recurrent fever, especially with bone pain, may be a symptom of leukemia or a bone tumor.

Children who have headaches with vomiting may have nothing more than an upset stomach, but recurrent headaches with vomiting that do not go away with time require a physician to make sure there isn't a brain tumor.

Children who have a mass in their abdomen are probably just constipated, but the mass could be Wilms' tumor, neuroblastoma, lymphoma, or a liver tumor. Lumps in the neck are usually due to an infection, but if they don't respond to antibiotics, a lymphoma is a possibility. Drainage from the ear is usually due to an ear infection and only rarely due to some tumor.

Weight loss is rare in a young child, although it is something teenagers often desire. If the weight loss is not controlled, however, there may be psychological reasons involved or a lymphoma such as Hodgkin's disease.

Obviously, children's complaints are usually the result of normal childhood ailments. But when parents are concerned that their child has a persistent problem, they should take him or her to the doctor. The findings of a physical examination may suggest that special tests are necessary to discover whether the child does in fact have a cancer.

Some signs and symptoms are not common. Any newborn child with a cat's eye—a white dot in the center of the eye—should be seen by a physician, since the dot may indicate a retinoblastoma. It is also very rare for children to have blood in their urine, so any child with this complaint should be seen by a physician. Blood in the urine may be the result of an infection but may also be caused by Wilms' tumor.

Diagnosis

Physical Examination

• A complete physical examination should include the groin area, the testicles, the skin, and the nervous system. A rectal examination may also be performed to rule out a tumor in that area.

• An enlarged liver and/or spleen or a mass in the abdomen may indicate a tumor.

• Lumps in the neck that are firm, nonmovable, and have not responded to antibiotics may be due to lymphoma, leukemia, and other cancers.

• The eyes may be examined, a procedure that requires the child's cooperation. A special instrument for looking into the eyes (ophthalmoscope) lets the physician see if there is increased pressure in the brain, which is often due to a brain tumor.

Blood and Other Tests

• A simple blood test examining the red cells, white cells, and platelets will usually let the doctor decide whether acute leukemia is a serious possibility.

• A special type of urine test will be helpful in cases of suspected neuroblastoma.

Imaging X-rays and CT and MRI scans help the physician decide whether there are tumors in the brain, chest, abdomen, or extremities.

Endoscopy and Biopsy Some suspected tumors might have to be biopsied for a definitive diagnosis.

Staging

Many so-called solid tumors of childhood—those that do not develop in the blood—are often staged by a system that classifies the disease by whether the tumor can be completely removed surgically. The involvement of lymph nodes and spread to distant sites are also considered. Greatly simplified, Stage I usually refers to local disease that can be entirely removed by the surgeon. Stage II could still be a local disease that may also be removed but has extended beyond the immediate area of the tumor. Stage III disease tends to be more extensive but localized in a particular region of the body, and Stage IV disease is widespread, having spread through the blood or lymphatic system to produce new tumors (metastases) in other organs.

Acute lymphoblastic leukemia (ALL) is categorized as standard (low) risk and high risk, according to its potential risk of recurrence (relapse). Two major factors—age at diagnosis and white blood cell (WBC) count—are used for staging of ALL. The child with low-risk leukemia has an excellent chance of responding to therapy in the long term and the best chance of being cured. On the other hand, a child with high-risk leukemia may still respond to therapy and may still have a good chance of being cured, although he or she may need more intensive treatment.

Treatment Overview

The treatment of a child's cancer may involve surgery, chemotherapy, radiation therapy, immunotherapy, and various supportive measures.

The special problems seen with childhood cancers mean that a child should not be treated only by a single physician. A team approach is required, with physicians assisted by many specialists, including psychologists and experts in nursing, social services, nutrition, physical therapy, occupational therapy, pharmacy, child life, and other fields. They should all be involved in designing the appropriate treatment and support program for the child and his or her family.

This kind of multidisciplinary approach can be accomplished only in a "center of excellence," an approved pediatric cancer specialty unit. In the United States and Canada, various cooperative groups have merged to form a single Children's Oncology Group (COG). Nearly 95 percent of children younger than fifteen with cancer receive their care at institutions affiliated with COG. Families of adolescents and young adults between sixteen and twenty-one are encouraged to seek a referral to one of these centers.

When a child is diagnosed with cancer in most of these centers, his or her case is presented to a tumor board, a meeting of physician specialists, subspecialists, and other members of the treatment team who evaluate the child, discuss the options, and agree to a proposed treatment plan.

Clinical Trials Cancer in children is rare. Each year in the United States, slightly over 3,000 children develop leukemia, and 2,000 develop various kinds of brain and nervous system tumors.

Approximately 500 children develop Wilms' tumor. Rhabdomyosarcoma, retinoblastoma, osteosarcoma, and Ewing's sarcoma are less common. Obviously, if progress is to be made on more effective treatment methods, physicians throughout the nation have to work closely together in designing therapies.

Accordingly, all children with cancer who are treated in a center of excellence are asked to participate in a clinical research program. It is because of these programs that we have made such gratifying progress in the treatment of childhood cancers over the past few decades. Parents and their children are encouraged to participate in them.

Phase III Trials A child may be a candidate for a research program known as a clinical protocol, which will compare one form of treatment to another. The research protocol will be explained, and parents will be asked to agree to participate with their child in the program.

The program may involve "randomization," meaning that which one of the several potentially effective treatments the child receives will be decided by chance. Parents are often upset when they learn that if they participate in a research program, the decision about which treatment their child will receive will not be chosen by their child's physician. But parents should understand that their child's physician would not participate in the program unless he or she were comfortable that *all* the various treatment choices were reasonable and appropriate and offered the child an excellent chance of attaining a response.

The initial treatment programs designed to answer which treatment program is best are often known as Phase III studies. Sometimes a research protocol is not available, and then the physician chooses the best-known effective treatment available for the disease and presents it as the proposed treatment plan.

Most children respond very well to the initial treatment of their cancer. The opportunity to cure a child with cancer may be as great as 80 to 90 percent for some children with acute lymphoblastic leukemia and Wilms' tumor, but unfortunately less in most other tumors. The patient's physician will be able to describe in detail the treatment being proposed and the chances of the child being cured.

Phase II Trials Unfortunately, not all children respond to therapy. Even those who do may relapse. These children may still have their disease controlled or cured.

Children with recurrent disease or with an extraordinarily challenging cancer may be candidates for Phase II protocols, treatment programs in which the dose and many of the side effects of a particular drug or treatment are unknown. The goal of treatment is to determine how effective the therapy is for certain kinds of childhood cancer.

If this kind of study is available and the child and parents are asked to participate, the physician will describe in detail the proposed treatment, the risks involved, and the possible advantages of the child's working with the physician in this research approach.

Phase I Trials Occasionally, there are drugs to be tested in children for the first time. Research protocols involving new drugs are called Phase I studies. The goal is to find the appropriate dose to be used, with the hope that the children will respond to the treatment.

Investigational Treatments There is a long list of investigational protocols for most childhood cancers. These protocols are devised after close cooperation and collaboration among investigators working in specific centers of excellence affiliated with the Children's Oncology Group.

The protocols may involve new drugs that have rarely been used in children or

they may involve new types of radiation therapy such as high-dose radiation given in a series of small doses (fractionated radiotherapy) or Proton irradiation—a high-energy radiation given to discrete tumors, thus sparing the surrounding normal tissues.

Most pediatric cancer experts do not consider such programs experimental but rather investigational. They consider these protocols an opportunity for the child and his or her family to participate on the frontier of medicine. A child with cancer should be treated with the methods being devised today that will possibly improve the chances for a cure tomorrow.

Bone Marrow Transplantation Several treatment programs for childhood cancers use the concept of bone marrow transplantation, although with many concerns, as it is still considered an investigational treatment under evaluation (see chapter 15, "Bone Marrow and Blood Stem Cell Transplantation").

Allogeneic bone marrow transplantation—which involves giving the child who has cancer bone marrow taken from a donor, ideally a close relative such as a brother or a sister—is being used very often in children with acute nonlymphocytic (granulocytic) leukemia. It is also used quite frequently in children with acute lymphoblastic leukemia who have had a relapse.

In autologous bone marrow transplantation, the patient's own bone marrow is used. A portion of the bone marrow is stored in the laboratory while the patient receives treatment, and then returned in the form of an intravenous infusion of bone marrow cells. These cells circulate throughout the body and settle into the bone marrow compartment from which they came. They subsequently grow and regenerate the bone marrow.

Newer approaches have also recently been devised. It is now known that bone marrow cells may circulate through-out the blood, and machines that can remove some of the circulating cells are being developed, raising the possibility of removing bone marrow cells from a vein rather than by drawing them out of bones through a needle.

In high-dose rescue therapy—also called autologous rescue—the patient's bone marrow cells are stored while high-dose chemotherapy is given. The cells are then reinfused. The higher doses of chemotherapy may kill cancer cells more effectively but might also seriously damage the bone marrow if rescue therapy were not performed.

Supportive Therapy

Throughout the course of the child's treatment, there will be a need for many kinds of support therapies:

• Transfusions of blood products, plate-lets, and white cells may be needed.

• Infections are common in children and may require specific antibiotics. Exposure to contagious disease is likely to occur, so the child may require specific gamma globulin.

• Supportive measures can include nutritional support such as artificial feed-ings through a vein (hyperalimentation) or enteral feedings through nasogastric or nasojejunal tubes. Access to a vein may be a problem, so central venous catheters are often used, such as the Broviac or Hickman catheters or the Port-a-Cath.

• Drugs, other agents, and psychologi-cal support techniques may be necessary to help children with anticipatory nau-sea, or nausea and vomiting after radia-tion or chemotherapy treatments.

Treatment Follow-Up

Whatever the treatment a child with can-cer is receiving, he or she will be followed closely by the pediatric oncologist, other physician specialists, and the multidis-ciplinary team assembled to work with both the child and the family.

Since the child will be on a research protocol in most cases, the physician will be able to outline for the parents an organized plan for follow-up evaluations. These may include specific liver function tests, urine tests for children with neuro-blastoma, specific X-rays, psychological testing, and other tests that can help fol-low the progress and effects of the disease and the response to treatment.

Even when a child finishes a course of treatment, he or she will require long-term follow-up by a pediatric cancer expert. This is not only because some treatments have long-term side effects, but also because children who are cured of a first cancer do have a small risk of developing a second one. So even the child who finishes therapy and is appar-ently cured should be followed by a spe-cialist for the rest of his or her life.

Some of the Most Important Questions (and Answers) for You and Your Child

For the Child

What do I have?

It is now known that children do bet-ter when they are told the truth about their illness. We no longer hide from them the fact that they have cancer. We explain the nature of their disease, tell them about the therapy, and ask them to work with physicians and other experts to help them attain a cure. Honesty is the best way to help a child face the serious problems of the disease.

Why did this happen?

We do not know why children develop cancer. Although there are some environ-mental or genetic clues that a child may be at risk, specific causes have not been found in the same way that streptococcus bacteria causes a sore throat.

It is important for the child—and the parents—to realize that having cancer is not a punishment. Cancer occurs in children throughout the world. Parents should not feel guilty. Their strength and optimism is needed by their child, who is facing a serious disease and requires their support to conquer the cancer and win the battle for his or her life.

Will my hair grow back?

Most children lose their hair temporarily after chemotherapy. In rare cases, such as when very intensive radiation treatments are used, hair may not grow back. But in most cases, the child develops a beautiful head of hair after the temporary period of baldness. Many children use wigs to help them with their self-image during these periods.

What will happen with the acne and chubby face I have when I'm getting prednisone treatment?

Steroids such as prednisone and dexamethasone (Decadron) do cause a temporary gain in weight and may cause facial acne. Once these drugs are stopped, the weight gain and the puffiness of the face disappear and the skin improves dramatically. There are very few if any permanent side effects of these treatments. Occasionally, stretch marks may be seen in the abdomen, but otherwise the child's complexion and facial configuration do return to normal.

For the Parent

When will I get my child back?

When a child is diagnosed as having cancer, he or she may experience a change in personality. The child's spirit, temperament, and behavior pattern may change substantially. The initial treatment may require a long period of hospitalization, and even if the child is seen as an outpatient, there are frequent visits that may include uncomfortable injections. It may take a while before the family pattern gets back to normal. Parents have to be patient. It may take several months before their child's behavior returns to what it was before the illness.

How about school?

For a child, school is the normal working environment. Just as an adult wishes to return to work and continue his or her normal activities, so does the child wish to get back to the normal routine. Multidisciplinary programs will offer the family support to work with the school system so that the child with cancer can reenter his or her normal environment. School administrators, teachers, and others are becoming more familiar with the fact that children in their classrooms may be undergoing cancer therapy. For the most part, school personnel are understanding. They can develop flexible schedules that permit the child to take advantage of the maximum number of educational opportunities while continuing with treatment programs.

How can we help relieve the nausea, vomiting, and other side effects of chemotherapy?

Unfortunately, many cancer chemotherapy drugs cause nausea, vomiting, mouth sores, constipation, skin rashes, sore eyes, and generally a lower resistance to infection. Prompt attention should be given to the constipation caused by vincristine (Oncovin).

Medications are available to help the child tolerate these side effects. Occasionally, the medications themselves will cause tiredness.

What are the long-term effects of therapy?

A number of long-term effects of childhood cancer therapy are currently being studied. Radiation therapy to the brain may leave some children with certain deficits in intellectual or motor development, which is why psychometric testing is so important as part of the general treatment follow-up.

Some children may have growth problems. Some may have an organ abnormality because of the effects of radiation therapy or surgery. Rehabilitation may be necessary, such as a new bladder to urinate or an artificial limb. Some drugs also affect the way organs such as the lungs and heart work. Children with cancer may have to be followed for many years to discover whether some of the treatments used to cure the disease will result in organ problems later on in life.

What are the chances of my child being cured?

A physician will be able to explain to the child and the parents the chances of attaining not only remission—control of the disease—but actual cure. These "chances" are statistical averages, however, and children are not statistics. A family can concentrate on the negative or on the positive. As long as there is an opportunity for a cure, it makes more sense to concentrate on the positive and focus the family's energy on the possibility that their child will be cured and will grow up and live a normal life span. Most children with cancer are cured and become healthy adults, parents, and productive members of society.

What happens if my child does not respond?

There are children who do not respond to treatment and unfortunately the disease may take their lives. If it appears that this is going to happen, the child's physician will be the first to explain to the parents the nature of the problem and the reason why it looks as though the child is not going to have his or her life saved.

The health care team will make sure that the child is comfortable and treated in a kind, caring manner. The physician and other members of the multidisciplinary team will work with the family to provide emotional, psychological, and spiritual support.

"Climbing the Mountain"

For the child with cancer and his or her parents, there are two basic choices: They can choose the pessimistic road, which goes downhill with the expectation that the cancer will cause the child to die. Or they can choose the optimistic road, an admittedly uphill road leading to the top of a mountain.

The curves in the mountain road are many. They represent problems that may occur during treatment, such as

• recurrent admission to the hospital for fevers and infections requiring intravenous antibiotics;
• side effects of chemotherapy, including hair loss, nausea, vomiting, mouth ulcers, stomach ulcers, blood in the urine, and rectal ulcers;
• side effects of radiation therapy, including hair loss, skin irritation, nausea, vomiting, and fatigue;
• side effects of surgery, including discomfort and organs that do not work in a normal way;
• allergic reactions to blood, blood products, or antibiotics;
• changes in plans to attend school or social functions or to go on family trips;
• therapies that are only partially successful; and
• special kinds of treatment, including investigational protocols and bone marrow transplantation.

Each and every one of these problems or curves can be difficult to manage. But each and every one has been managed successfully by other children and other families of children who have cancer. Sometimes, a curve can't be maneuvered and it is necessary to move onto the pessimistic road. But for most children with cancer, the curves can be managed and the climb up the mountain is successful. Treatment may last for six months or a year, or even two, three, or more years, but the top of the mountain can be reached.

The goal for all children with cancer is that they will be cured. More and more children with cancer are attaining this goal and are growing up to be healthy adults. So children and their parents should be optimistic. Knowing that cure is a possibility, each child and his or her family should plan on climbing the mountain and reaching the top. On the top, the sky is blue and the sun is shining.

Childhood Cancers: Brain Tumors

Ramesh Patel, M.D., Malin Dollinger, M.D., and Mark L. Greenberg, M.B., Ch.B.

■ ■ ■ ■

Primary brain tumors—those that start in the brain rather than spread there from other parts of the body—are the most common "solid" tumors children get and are second only to leukemia in their overall incidence. They pose a major treatment challenge that has to be met by the coordinated efforts of a variety of health care professionals, including specialists in pediatric neurosurgery, radiation therapy, and oncology, as well as neuroradiologists and neuropathologists. Significant emotional stresses and problems may occur, requiring intervention by specialized health care professionals.

Every year, about 3,100 children in the United States are diagnosed as having brain or spinal cord tumors. Many tumors are controllable or curable with treatment, and over half of the children diagnosed with brain tumors will live more than five years. Every child's therapy should be aggressively planned with the intent to cure if possible. This is true even in situations where the same tumor occurring in an adult would not likely be cured.

As is true of all pediatric cancers, but especially with brain tumors, most advances in treatment have been produced by clinical trials of new therapies. The National Cancer Institute (NCI) oversees a large cooperative group of almost all the children's hospitals in the country—the Children's Oncology Group (COG)—which develops new treatment protocols for children with brain tumors. These protocols generally represent the most advanced and promising methods of treatment.

Types Brain tumors are classified by the appearance of their cells under the microscope (histopathology) and their location in the brain. The types that occur in children are generally similar to those seen in adults, although there are a few types that are much more common in children.

There is a structure in the back part of the brain, a rooflike membrane called the tentorium. This is just above the cerebellum (the portion of the brain having to do with balance and coordination) and the brain stem. There are significant differences in the types of tumors occurring above and below this membrane, as well as in the methods used to make a diagnosis and follow the results of therapy.

About half the brain tumors in children occur below the tentorium, most being in the cerebellum or the nearby cavity called the fourth ventricle. This area of the skull cavity is the posterior fossa. Tumors in this region include astrocytomas, medulloblastomas, ependymomas, and brain stem gliomas.

The area above the tentorium, which makes up most of the brain, is called the supratentorial region. Tumors in this area include astrocytomas, cerebral neuroblastomas (primitive neuroectodermal tumors [PNET]), ependymomas, craniopharyngiomas, meningiomas, germ cell tumors, optic nerve gliomas, pineal tumors, and choroid plexus tumors.

There may be many different names for these tumors, especially as newer classification systems are more descriptive or accurate.

How It Spreads Brain tumors rarely spread outside the central nervous system but can spread within the brain and the spinal cord.

What Causes It Unknown, although some genetic disorders have been associated with an increased risk.

Screening

There are no effective screening measures.

Common Signs and Symptoms

Brain tumors are often difficult to diagnose because their signs and symptoms may mimic those of other common childhood disorders. Symptoms related to the increased pressure in the brain as the tumor expands include irritability, failure to thrive, headache, nausea, vomiting (which may or may not accompany nausea), and seizures. Symptoms related to the tumor's location and the pressure it puts on nearby structures include weakness or changes in sensation in various parts of the body, difficulties in coordination or balance, vision and speech problems, and seizures.

Diagnosis

Physical Examination

• Complete neurologic examination.

• Evaluation for optic tract glioma includes neuro-ophthalmological testing, including visual fields. Subtle changes in the tumor that may not be apparent with CT or MRI scanning can be measured in this way. Young children may have a test called visual-evoked response for diagnosis and follow-up.

Blood and Other Tests

• Bone marrow may be analyzed for tumors that spread outside the central nervous system (medulloblastomas).

• For tumors that may spread to the spinal cord or through the cerebrospinal fluid (medulloblastomas, ependymomas, intracranial germ cell tumors, pineal tumors, cerebral neuroblastomas, or primitive neuroectodermal tumors [PNET]), spinal fluid is examined for malignant cells.

• For intracranial germ cell tumors, tumor markers including alpha-fetoprotein (AFP) and human chorionic gonadotropin (HCG) are measured in the blood and cerebrospinal fluid. The same markers are also measured in pineal tumors to exclude the possibility of a malignant germ cell tumor.

Imaging

• Imaging has conventionally been done by CT scan for the brain and myelography for the spinal cord. Recently, MRI imaging with gadolinium enhancement has been shown to be extremely sensitive, useful, and simpler for both the brain and spinal cord.

• Images of the entire brain and spinal cord should be done for tumors that may spread to the spinal cord (medulloblastomas, ependymomas, intracranial germ cell tumors, pineal tumors, cerebral neuroblastomas, PNET).

• Bone scans and bone marrow examinations are sometimes done in medulloblastoma because this tumor may spread outside the central nervous system, especially to bone and bone marrow.

Biopsy

• Tumors of the brain stem, the medulla, and the pons (brain stem glioma) may be biopsied. The procedure is risky. They cannot be removed surgically (radiation therapy is the standard treatment). Stereotactic needle biopsy techniques may enable biopsy to be done when it could have an effect on treatment—for example, if it is not certain that a mass in this area is malignant, if the tumor grows outward and protrudes into the ventricles, or if there is a need to remove part of the tumor because of pressure symptoms.

• Biopsy of optic tract glioma is not always possible because it is difficult to expose the area surgically.

Staging

There are no generally useful staging systems for most brain tumors, although some are classified according to grade. With brain stem glioma, for example, tumors in the higher region—the midbrain—are more likely to be lower grade and have a higher chance of long-term survival than tumors lower down in the pons and the medulla (40 percent versus less than 20 percent).

A variety of staging systems have been used for medulloblastoma. The Children's Oncology Group has divided this tumor into low and high stages groups. Essentially, *low stage* implies smaller tumors without metastases, in which the tumor remaining after surgery is smaller than 1.5 cubic cm. *High stage* refers to larger tumors with evidence of metastatic spread or brain stem involvement, and tumors larger than 1.5 cubic cm remaining after surgery.

Treatment Overview

Treatment includes surgery, with or without radiation therapy, and for some tumors, chemotherapy. Radiation therapy of pediatric brain tumors is very complex and should be carried out in facilities with extensive experience.

Chemotherapy has recently shown some activity in children with brain tumors. Children with high-stage medulloblastoma are treated with maximal surgical resection followed by radiation therapy and chemotherapy to prevent relapse. There is great interest in using chemotherapy after surgery as the only therapy in children under age three,

since radiation therapy to the brain in this age group may seriously impair brain development.

Clinical Trials All children with brain tumors should be considered for entry into clinical trials. This form of cancer is rare in children, and trials offer the advantage of the pooled experience of pediatric cancer centers around the country.

Pediatric clinical trials are designed in two ways. One method divides the children into two groups, with one receiving the best currently accepted standard treatment and the other receiving the new therapy that appears promising. The other method is to evaluate a single new treatment in all patients and then compare the results with those obtained with existing therapy, often in the same institution.

Treatment by Tumor Type
Medulloblastoma

Medulloblastoma is the most common malignant brain tumor of childhood, accounting for approximately 20 percent of all primary childhood central nervous system tumors. It arises in the cerebellum and may spread to adjacent tissues. It can also spread via the cerebrospinal fluid to the rest of the brain or to the spinal cord and very rarely to sites outside the nervous system. If it occurs elsewhere in the brain, it is called primitive neuroectodermal tumor (PNET).

Standard Treatment An attempt is made to surgically remove as much tumor as possible. Studies are done during and after the operation to define the risk of relapse, and treatment is given according to the best estimate of low-stage or high-stage disease.

For low-stage disease, standard therapy after surgery is a high dose of radiation to the tumor area and a lower dose to the entire brain and spine. Lowering the dosage of radiation to reduce problems with nervous system development reduces the chance for cure. Children under three should be entered in studies that use chemotherapy and probably delayed or modified radiation therapy.

Treatment of high-stage disease involves chemotherapy in addition to surgery and radiation therapy similar to that given in low-stage disease.

These patients should be considered for entry into clinical trials to establish the best combination and sequence of chemotherapy.

Five-Year Survival About 60 percent

Recurrent Cancer Medulloblastoma that recurs after radiotherapy should be considered for treatment with investigational protocols using new agents. Fewer than one-third of those patients respond, and long-term control of disease is unusual.

Cerebellar Astrocytoma
These are generally low-grade tumors occurring in the cerebellum. Spread is unusual.

Standard Treatment The primary treatment is surgical removal of the tumor, which is successful in removing the entire tumor in most cases. In contrast to most other brain tumors, some patients with microscopic and even larger residual tumor after surgery may survive a long time without any symptoms or tumor growth even without postoperative therapy. This may be significant because a second operation may produce neurological problems.

The use of radiation therapy for patients with astrocytoma depends on the anatomic location and extent of tumor and whether it is resectable or not. Radiation therapy is indicated for unresectable tumors (midbrain and thalamic lesions).

Ten-Year Survival About 80 percent

Recurrent Cancer Cerebellar astrocytoma that recurs is treated, if possible, with another surgery. If this is not possible, local radiation is used. If it recurs in an area where it can't be removed and has already received maximum radiation, chemotherapy should be considered. Since there is little information available about the role of chemotherapy, Phase I and Phase II clinical studies should be considered.

Infratentorial Ependymoma
These tumors arise from the cells lining the fourth ventricle (a cavity within the brain), as well as those lining a cavity in the center of the spinal cord. They can occur anywhere in the brain or spinal cord, but 60 percent of them start in the part of the brain in the back of the skull, the posterior fossa. The prognosis depends on the grade and size of the tumor and the degree of spread. These tumors may spread via the spinal fluid pathways.

Standard Treatment Surgical excision followed by high-dose radiation to the back part of the brain is the usual treatment. The tumor can be completely removed surgically in about 30 percent of cases. Radiotherapy to the entire brain and spinal cord is controversial, being used most commonly in high-grade tumors.

There is no clear benefit for adjuvant chemotherapy, although consideration should be given to using chemotherapy to delay or modify radiation therapy in very young children.

Five-Year Survival 25 to 60 percent

Recurrent Cancer This tumor is seldom controlled permanently if it recurs after surgery and radiotherapy. About one-third of patients respond to cisplatin, so Phase I and II clinical trials should be considered.

Brain Stem Glioma

Tumors arising in the brain stem are often astrocytomas, tumors of neuron-support cells. These are also referred to as brain stem gliomas. They may be low, intermediate, or high grade. The majority of these tumors growing in the brain stem cannot be removed surgically.

Standard Treatment The usual treatment is high-dose radiation therapy (over 5,500 cGy). Higher doses may be possible using twice-daily (hyperfractionated) treatment.

The role of chemotherapy is not well defined. Occasionally, patients may be candidates for surgical removal. Children younger than three may be given chemotherapy to delay or modify radiation therapy to reduce the risk of neurologic impairment.

Two-Year Survival Varies with site and grade of tumor

Investigational Chemotherapy before the standard radiotherapy treatment

Recurrent Cancer There is no standard therapy for recurrent brain stem glioma. These children cannot have surgery and have already received maximum radiation therapy, and there are no standard chemotherapy drugs that have significant results. They should be entered in a Phase I or Phase II clinical drug trial.

Cerebral Astrocytoma
■ *Low Grade*

These tumors may sometimes be completely removed surgically, in which case they have a favorable prognosis. These tumors spread by extension to the adjacent brain and sometimes occur in multiple sites.

Standard Treatment The treatment for low-grade supratentorial astrocytoma is surgery. If the tumor cannot be completely removed, radiotherapy is given after the operation. In some centers, radiotherapy is withheld until progression of disease is shown. The role of chemotherapy is not defined, but initial results are promising.

Five-Year Survival 50 to 80 percent

Recurrent Cancer Patients may benefit from chemotherapy if tumors recur after maximum surgery and radiation therapy. No standard agents have a high degree of response, although cyclophosphamide (Cytoxan), cisplatin (Platinol), and the nitrosoureas may be useful. Carboplatin (Paraplatin) has shown promise. Consideration should be given to clinical trials.

Cerebral Astrocytoma
■ *High Grade*

Sometimes called anaplastic astrocytoma or glioblastoma multiforme, these tumors often grow rapidly and involve portions of the brain that cause major neurological problems.

Standard Treatment Treatment includes surgery, radiation therapy, and chemotherapy. Radiation is given after as complete a surgical resection as possible to an area that encompasses the entire tumor and sometimes the whole brain.

A Children's Cancer Group (CCG) study with radiation therapy and three chemotherapy agents (vincristine [Oncovin] + lomustine [CeeNU] + prednisone) produced a 46 percent survival of five years compared with 18 percent for children treated with radiation therapy alone. Again, children under the age of three may receive chemotherapy to delay or modify radiotherapy. A number of clinical trials are evaluating the role of newer chemotherapeutic agents.

Two-Year Survival Less than 25 percent. The prognosis may be better if the tumor can be totally removed. Younger patients and those with lower-grade tumors may do better.

Recurrent Cancer Chemotherapy is given if relapse occurs after radiation therapy. Since no standard agents have a high degree of activity, entry in a clinical trial should be considered.

Supratentorial Ependymoma
These ependymomas arise outside the posterior fossa (back of the skull), usually within and adjacent to the ventricles.

Standard Treatment Surgery followed by radiation therapy is the usual treatment. In low-grade tumors, the primary tumor area is given radiation. With high-grade tumors, the entire brain and spinal cord are treated.

Adjuvant chemotherapy is under evaluation. Consideration should be given to its use in very young children to delay or modify radiation therapy.

Two-Year Survival About 40 percent

Investigational Various radiotherapy trials, with and without chemotherapy

Recurrent Cancer This tumor is seldom controlled if it recurs after surgery and radiation therapy, although one-third of patients respond to cisplatin. Phase I and II clinical studies should be considered.

Craniopharyngioma
These benign tumors arise in the central portion of the brain and produce problems primarily because of their location. Since they are benign, metastasis is unknown.

Standard Treatment Surgery is the treatment of choice and produces a high rate of control in most patients. For recurrent unresectable tumors, radiotherapy is recommended. There is no reported role for chemotherapy.

Ten-Year Survival About 80 percent

Intracranial Germ Cell Tumor
Germ cell brain tumors—there are a number of subtypes—usually arise in the central portion of the brain. Under the microscope, they resemble more common germ cell tumors of the testis and ovary. The prognosis relates to the cell type and is especially favorable in patients with germinoma.

Standard Treatment The role of surgery is usually a biopsy to establish the diagnosis, since the location of these tumors usually prevents complete removal. Germinoma may be treated with radiation therapy to the brain and spinal cord, with high doses to the tumor and somewhat lower doses to the rest of the nerve tissue. There is emerging evidence that local radiation therapy plus chemotherapy produces equivalent cure rates.

Advanced or disseminated germinomas, as well as the various germ cell tumors other than germinomas, are usually treated with radiation to the brain and spinal cord. There are several views about the dosage and areas that should be treated.

Nongerminoma germ cell tumors may respond to a variety of chemotherapeutic agents, including bleomycin, cisplatin, etoposide, cyclophosphamide, and vincristine. The role of adjuvant chemotherapy, in addition to radiation, is not yet determined for these tumors that arise within the brain, although chemotherapy is extremely effective in these tumors elsewhere in the body.

Survival Variable

Recurrent Cancer Intracerebral germ cell tumors may be responsive to the same type of chemotherapy combinations used against germ cell tumors in other locations—PVB (cisplatin + vinblastine + bleomycin) and VAC (vincristine + dactinomycin + cyclophosphamide).

If the tumor recurs after treatment with these programs, Phase I and II clinical studies should be used to try to find agents that may be useful in treating this tumor, which is often responsive to chemotherapy.

Pineal Region Tumors

Three principal groups of tumors—germ cell tumors, pineal parenchymal tumors, and astrocytomas—account for tumors in this region. The pineal parenchymal tumor resembles medulloblastoma, but it develops in the region of the pineal gland in the center of the brain. The prognosis depends upon the size of the tumor and its degree of spread.

Standard Treatment The usual treatment is radiation therapy. There is some controversy about the possibility of surgical removal, although biopsy is recommended whenever possible to establish a diagnosis. A high dose of radiation is given to the tumor, with a lower dose to the brain and spinal cord.

Studies are exploring the role of chemotherapy for poorly differentiated pineal tumors, although well-differentiated tumors may be treated with simple local radiation therapy. Young children may be given chemotherapy to delay or modify the radiation treatments.

Two-Year Survival Less than 50 percent

Optic Tract Glioma

These tumors grow along the optic tracts of the brain that carry visual impulses. They are low-grade and slow-growing astrocytomas that produce visual symptoms.

Standard Treatment Radiation therapy is the usual treatment for optic tract gliomas that are growing. Some tumors that do not appear to be growing and have no symptoms may be carefully observed without treatment as long as they are stable.

Chemotherapy has not been used as an adjuvant to radiation therapy as part of standard treatment, but the previous considerations about the risks of radiation in children under the age of three apply. The use of vincristine and other drugs of relatively low toxicity has enabled radiation therapy to be delayed in more than 80 percent of children and is being further evaluated.

Five-Year Survival Over 75 percent

Cerebral Neuroblastoma (Supratentorial Primitive Neuroectodermal Tumor, or PNET)

There are a variety of names for these tumors. They are poorly differentiated tumors, which microscopically may have features of various primitive tumors of other cell types. Prognosis depends upon the extent of disease.

Standard Treatment The usual treatment is high-dose radiation therapy. Many radiation oncologists also radiate the entire brain and spinal cord because of this tumor's tendency to spread to the rest of the central nervous system through the cerebrospinal fluid. Chemotherapy has been used in several clinical trials, especially in younger children. It appears to produce good control and has particular value in younger children to delay or avoid the use of radiation therapy and its consequences. Carboplatin may be a particularly useful drug.

Two-Year Survival 30 to 50 percent

Treatment Follow-Up

• Repeated clinical evaluation, emphasizing initial neurologic signs and symptoms.

• Repeated CT or MRI scanning.

• Repeated studies of any other abnormal tests, such as cerebrospinal fluid and visual fields.

• Since radiotherapy can affect growth hormone production and brain development, careful endocrine and neurologic follow-up is very important.

The Most Important Questions You Can Ask

• What type of brain tumor does my child have?

• How does it usually behave?

• What is the chance of cure?

• What is the standard treatment and how successful is it?

• Should radiotherapy be used? When?

• Should chemotherapy be used? When?

• If the treatment is not completely effective or my child relapses later, what else can be done?

Childhood Cancers: Retinoblastoma

Ramesh Patel, M.D., and Jerry Z. Finklestein, M.D.

■ ■ ■ ■

Retinoblastoma is the most common childhood malignant tumor of the retina, the membrane at the back of the eyeball. About 300 children in the United States develop this cancer each year. The vast majority of retinoblastoma cases occur in very young children: 66 percent occurring before age two and 95 percent before age five. In some instances, retinoblastoma is diagnosed at birth. The tumor may occur in one eye (75 percent) or both eyes (25 percent).

How It Spreads The tumor may be confined to the retina or extend directly to other parts of the eye (commonly the optic nerve). In its later stages, it may spread to the central nervous system or other parts of the body.

What Causes It There are hereditary (40 percent) and nonhereditary (60 percent) forms of retinoblastoma. The hereditary form may be unilateral (one eye) but more typically is bilateral (both eyes). When there is disease in both eyes, it is almost always the hereditary form. There is no racial or gender predilection. The retinoblastoma (RB) gene has been identified on chromosome 13. Retinoblastoma is the best example of a genetic predisposition to cancer. Children who inherit defects in the RB gene have a 90 percent chance of developing retinoblastoma. The incidence of retinoblastoma is increasing because survivors of childhood retinoblastoma are now of an age to have their own children. Families of children with retinoblastoma should have genetic counseling.

Diagnosis

Most children in the United States are diagnosed while the tumor remains within the eye. The tumor is detected by shining a light into the child's eye and looking for what is called a cat's eye—a white spot in place of the dark pupil. There may also be symptoms such as poor vision and strabismus (squinting).

It is important for children with retinoblastoma to be seen in a specialized center where physicians have experience in evaluating the size of the tumor and the extent of the disease.

Staging

Several staging systems are used, but for purposes of treatment, retinoblastoma is divided into intraocular (within the eye) and extraocular (spread beyond the eye) disease.

Treatment Overview

Standard Treatment In some cases, it may be possible to destroy the tumor within the eye by using light (laser) treatment (photocoagulation), freezing (cryotherapy), or heat treatment (thermotherapy). Other options include enucleation (removal of the diseased eye), with eventual replacement with an artificial eye, and radiation therapy (brachytherapy or external-beam).

Which of these procedures is used depends on the size of the tumor and whether the child has potentially useful vision.

The use of chemotherapy requires additional investigation, although tumors generally respond in a satisfactory manner to a number of chemotherapy drugs.

Five-Year Survival Over 90 percent if disease is confined to the eye; less than 10 percent if it has spread beyond the eye

Treatment Follow-Up

Children with retinoblastoma, especially the hereditary form, have an increased risk for developing other malignancies later in life and so should be followed closely. Up to 8 percent, for example, may develop bone tumors after eighteen years, and the percentage may be higher with longer follow-up. Second cancers may develop spontaneously or be the result of treatment.

Childhood Cancers:
Soft-Tissue and Bone Sarcomas

Robert E. Goldsby, M.D., Malin Dollinger, M.D., and Arthur R. Ablin, M.D.

■ ■ ■ ■

Cancers involving muscle, bone, blood vessels, and other supporting tissues in the body are termed sarcomas. They are different from carcinomas, which are malignancies of the tissues that line or cover the body's internal organs and passageways. Of all the cancers of solid tissues, children most frequently have sarcomas. Carcinomas are much more frequent in adults.

Types Rhabdomyosarcoma of muscle is the most common soft-tissue sarcoma in children, accounting for slightly more than half of all soft-tissue sarcomas. Many different tissue types account for the rest. They may be located in nerves or their covering sheaths (e.g., malignant peripheral nerve sheath tumors), blood vessel walls (e.g., angiosarcomas), joint linings (e.g., synovial sarcomas), or fatty tissues (e.g., liposarcomas).

Other sarcomas in children occur in or around bone. The most common is osteogenic sarcoma, which is a cancer of the bone tissue itself. The second most common is Ewing's sarcoma. Although Ewing's sarcoma occurs in or around bone, this tumor probably originates from the nerve tissue in these locations.

In the United States, an estimated 500 to 700 children under eighteen are diagnosed with rhabdomyosarcoma each year. Osteosarcoma strikes 450 to 600 young people, and Ewing's sarcoma affects 350 to 400.

The rarity of sarcomas in children and adolescents emphasizes the need for treatment by a small number of physicians in a limited number of children's cancer centers so that the most experienced physicians and expert care can be available. This also allows the most rapid accumulation of knowledge about treatment, since it facilitates cooperative studies between institutions. The great progress made in treating these tumors over the past two to three decades has in large part been due to cooperative clinical studies designed to find the most effective treatments.

What Causes It Examination of some types of sarcoma cancer cells has shown that a transfer of genetic material has taken place from one chromosome to another within the cell; this is called a translocation. We do not know why this transfer occurs, but it most probably results in the cancer. Other sarcomas may have genetic changes, called mutations, that drive the cell to grow and spread. All of the genetic alterations associated with sarcomas are seldom inherited.

Rhabdomyosarcoma

This tumor is almost always found in muscle areas that can be controlled voluntarily, such as the eye, bladder, arms, and legs. (Involuntary muscles are those that work automatically, such as the heart and the wall of the intestinal tract.) The head and neck area is the most common site, followed by the genitourinary area—the vagina in girls, near the testes or prostate in boys, and the bladder. The trunk, chest, and back of the abdomen are less frequently involved.

How It Spreads The tumor can spread directly into surrounding tissues, through the lymphatic vessels to regional lymph nodes, or through the bloodstream to the lungs, bone, bone marrow, and central nervous system.

Symptoms Symptoms vary according to the location. The tumor is often painless but produces symptoms when it impinges on nearby nerves or tissues. The first sign may be a painless lump in or around the eye, on a limb, or in the abdomen. A small mass may extrude from the vagina. When the tumor is in the bladder, there may be difficulty urinating or blood in the urine. Back or abdominal pain or jaundice can develop when the tumor is large enough to cause pressure or obstruction of abdominal organs.

Diagnosis and Staging Other entities can produce the same physical signs and symptoms as rhabdomyosarcoma, so a biopsy is always necessary to establish the diagnosis with certainty. X-rays, CT and/or MRI scanning, and bone marrow examinations are used to determine the extent of the disease.

Treatment Overview Surgery, radiation, and chemotherapy are combined in the treatment of this diverse tumor. The order in which they are given, which combination of drugs is used, and how much radiation is delivered vary according to the location, tissue type, and extent of the disease. Putting together the many variables about each tumor—tissue subtype, surgical result (Group) and location (Stage)—allows a specific treatment plan based on risk and the most accurate estimate about outcome to be formulated.

Treatment by Risk

■ *Low-Risk Patients*
No evidence of tumor remaining after surgery, favorable tissue subtype, and favorable location.

Standard Treatment Surgery, followed by chemotherapy and, possibly, radiation. The tumors with the best outlook are those around the eye or testes that can be completely removed and have no evidence of spread. Patients are usually treated with vincristine (Oncovin) and dactinomycin (Cosmegen).

The next best outlook is for tumors in the head and neck and pelvic areas, other than the bladder and prostate, that can be completely removed. Chemotherapy with agents such as vincristine, dactinomycin, and cyclophosphamide (Cytoxan) may be used and radiation may also be used.

Five-Year Survival 75 to 95 percent

■ *Intermediate-Risk Patients*
Tumor remaining after surgery and/or unfavorable tissue type and/or unfavorable location, but not spread to other sites.

Standard Treatment These tumors are treated with a combination of chemotherapy and radiation therapy.

Five-Year Survival 70 percent

■ *High-Risk Patients*
The tumor has spread to distant sites at the time of diagnosis.

Standard Treatment New combinations of drugs are used in the hope of finding effective agents that are then combined with standard combinations of vincristine (Oncovin), dactinomycin (Cosmegen), and cyclophosphamide (Cytoxan) and radiation.

Five-Year Survival 20 percent

Other Soft-Tissue Sarcomas

There are many types of sarcomas, and any single one occurs very rarely. Treatment varies from one patient to the next and can range from simple surgical excision alone to extensive surgery and aggressive chemotherapy, with or without radiation. In general, staging and treatment are similar to those for rhabdomyosarcoma. Treatment can be somewhat less aggressive for small, completely excised tumors.

MOST USUAL TYPES	MOST COMMON LOCATIONS
Fibrosarcoma	
• Congenital	• Extremity and trunk
• Adult form	• Thigh and knee
Neurofibrosarcoma	Extremity, back of abdomen, trunk
Synovial sarcoma	Around but not in joints
Hemangiopericytoma	Head, neck, back of abdomen
Malignant peripheral nerve sheath tumor	Extremity
Malignant fibrous histiocytoma	Extremity
Liposarcoma	Extremity, back of abdomen

Recurrent Cancer

Several options are available if there is a relapse or inadequate response to initial therapy. Intensive treatment with radiation and chemotherapy can be considered. Alternatively, investigational drugs or biological agents are often available for trial at children's cancer centers. Supportive treatments are always available, especially for dying patients, who should never be allowed to feel that treatment is stopping.

Osteogenic Sarcomas

These highly malignant tumors are composed of abnormal cancerous bone cells. They can spread throughout the body, producing new masses, called metastases.

Osteogenic sarcomas occur most commonly during or just after the years of rapid growth, in the teens and early twenties.

Symptoms There is usually swelling and persistent pain in the involved bone, which is most commonly just above or below the knee, in the hip, or in the arm at the shoulder. Any bone may be involved, however. Because of the weakening of the bone by the tumor, there may be a fracture at the cancer site.

Diagnosis and Staging An X-ray may lead to suspicion of an osteogenic sarcoma, but a biopsy is needed for a diagnosis. Determining the extent of disease—staging—is done by looking at the most likely areas of spread with CT, MRI, and bone scans. These areas include the lungs and other bones.

Treatment by Stage

■ Localized

This stage of the disease is highly treatable and often curable. The surgeon, radiation oncologist, and pediatric oncologist, along with the pathologist and radiologist, should meet at a tumor board to plan the overall approach to therapy.

Standard Treatment Some years ago, it was customary to recommend amputation for bone sarcomas involving the arms or legs. Nowadays, it may be possible to save the extremity (limb salvage) by the use of a combination of several treatment methods, often including a prosthesis, which is surgically inserted to replace the bone that must be removed. Often the first intervention is chemotherapy using drugs such as cisplatin, doxorubicin (Adriamycin), and methotrexate (Amethopterin, Folex) in an attempt to shrink the tumor. Whether a limb-saving surgery or an amputation is performed depends on many factors, including the location of the tumor, the response to chemotherapy, the age of the patient, and the wishes of the patient and family. Further chemotherapy is given after surgery, sometimes with the same drugs used preoperatively.

Five-Year Survival 60 to 70 percent

■ *Metastatic*
When the tumor has spread through the blood, the disease is still treatable and occasionally curable.

Standard Treatment The most aggressive chemotherapy approaches are used. More intense chemotherapy, made possible by the use of bone-marrow-stimulating factors and optimum supportive care measures for complications such as infections and bleeding, may improve survival. Best results are achieved when all sites of disease can be surgically removed. Radiation may occasionally be given to sites of metastases, but radiation is not particularly effective.

Five-Year Survival 10 to 20 percent

Recurrent Cancer

When osteogenic sarcomas recur, optimal results are achieved if it is possible to surgically remove all sites of disease. Chemotherapy may or may not be necessary. Consideration for investigational

or palliative therapy is very reasonable if the disease is not surgically resectable.

Ewing's Sarcoma

This is the second most common bone cancer in adolescents and young adults, occurring usually in those between five and twenty years of age. It may also occur in soft tissue (extraosseous Ewing's sarcoma). A more differentiated or mature form of this tumor can develop in either bone or soft tissue, especially in the chest wall, and this form was previously called a peripheral primitive neuroectodermal tumor (pPNET).

Symptoms The most typical sign of the disease is persistent bone pain in one place, most commonly in an extremity, the pelvis, or a rib.

Diagnosis and Staging Bone X-rays and CT or MRI scans can strongly suggest a diagnosis of Ewing's sarcoma, but definitive diagnosis depends on a biopsy. Chromosome analysis of tumor tissues is often helpful in establishing the diagnosis.

A bone scan, a bone marrow analysis, a CT scan of the chest, and an MRI scan of the primary site are necessary to determine the extent of the disease.

Treatment by Stage
■ *Localized*
The tumor has not spread beyond the site of origin.

Standard Treatment When the tumor is in a bone that can be removed without causing a significant physical handicap, the bone is surgically removed. Unlike treatment for osteogenic sarcomas, major bones are not removed and amputations are not generally recommended because the tumor is sensitive to radiation therapy.

Chemotherapy is usually given before local control (surgery and/or radiation) to shrink the original tumor and treat microscopic spread that does not show up on imaging studies. Combinations of vincristine, doxorubicin (Adriamycin), cyclophosphamide (Cytoxan) and/or ifosfamide, and etoposide are used.

Five-Year Survival 70 to 80 percent

▨ *Metastatic*
The tumor has spread, usually to the lungs, other bones, and the bone marrow.

Standard Treatment The initial treatment is similar to that for localized disease, but more aggressive chemotherapy and radiation are used. Some patients may even be treated with higher doses of therapy and bone marrow transplant.

Supportive care measures, such as administering bone marrow growth factors, preventing infections, and intensively treating fever, are important parts of the treatment plan.

Five-Year Survival 20 to 45 percent

Recurrent Cancer

This serious complication is even worse if it occurs while the initial treatment is being given. If combination chemotherapy causes the tumor to shrink, consideration should be given to very high dose chemotherapy combined with radiation therapy. This would require a subsequent bone marrow transplant to replace the bone marrow destroyed by these treatments. No reliable figures are yet available to predict the outcome of this approach. Investigational therapy is an alternative, as is palliative treatment.

The Most Important Questions You Can Ask

• What are the details of treatment that will allow my child to receive optimum care?

• Is my child being treated at a medical center that specializes in cancer in children and adolescents?

• What can I do to minimize side effects of chemotherapy or radiation?

• How can I help my child [especially teenagers] cooperate with the treatment program?

• Is a limb-salvage operation or an amputation for osteogenic sarcoma the best procedure and how will each affect quality of life and survival?

• Are further surgical procedures likely if a limb-salvage procedure is done?

• Does my child understand that the disease is not his or her fault and that no one else can catch it?

Colon and Rectum

Emily K. Bergsland, M.D., Alan P. Venook, M.D., Jonathan P. Terdiman, M.D., Andrew H. Ko, M.D., Malin Dollinger, M.D., and Robert S. Warren, M.D.

■ ■ ■ ■

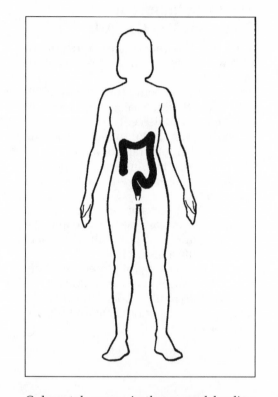

Colorectal cancer is the second leading cause of cancer deaths in the United States and the third leading cause of cancer deaths worldwide. Cancer of the large bowel, or colon and rectum—the last 4 to 6 feet (1 to 2 m) of the intestine—is a highly treatable and often curable disease when it is localized and diagnosed in its early stages. But when it spreads through the bowel wall to lymph nodes or nearby organs, the chances for cure are reduced.

Ten percent of all cancers in the United States involve either the colon or the rectum, which accounts for an overall lifetime risk for this cancer of 6 percent (one out of every seventeen Americans). An estimated 153,760 colorectal cancers will be diagnosed in 2007, 112,340 in the colon and 41,420 in the rectum. Colorectal cancer is the third most common cancer in both men and women and is second only to lung cancer as a cause of cancer deaths in the United States (accounting for 10 percent of all cancer deaths, with 55,170 deaths per year). Worldwide, approximately 1 million new cases of colorectal cancer are diagnosed each year.

These tumors may be common because about half the population over forty are thought to have clumps of tissues protruding from the inner layer (mucosa) of the colon or rectum. These mushroom-like growths are called polyps, and while most are benign, at least one type—adenomatous polyps—may be a precursor to cancer. About 90 percent of colorectal cancers are thought to arise from these polyps, and a person with a colorectal adenoma runs a threefold risk of developing colorectal cancer.

The rectum is the final 5 inches (12 cm) of the colon above the anus. However, while the colon and the rectum look similar and are connected to each other, there are major differences in the way colon and rectal tumors are treated.

Colorectal cancer is primarily a surgical disease; almost 50 percent of all patients can be cured with resection alone. In addition, long-term survival can be improved by using adjuvant chemotherapy in patients with colon cancer and chemoradiation in patients with cancer of the rectum. The chance for cure and the role of adjuvant therapy after resection is related to how far the tumor has invaded through the bowel wall and to whether or not it has spread to the nearby lymph nodes. For patients whose lymph nodes are invaded by cancer, tumor recurrence after surgery is a significant problem. Recurrent cancer is the ultimate cause of death in one-third of cases.

Types Most colorectal cancers develop in the glands of the inner lining, or mucosa, and are called adenocarcinomas. Other kinds of tumors, such as lymphomas, melanomas, squamous cell carcinomas, sarcomas, and carcinoids, occur much less frequently (less than 5 percent).

How It Spreads Colorectal cancer spreads directly from the mucosa, or inner lining, through the muscle wall of the bowel and into adjacent tissues. The tumor may metastasize through the lymphatic system to nearby lymph nodes, to the liver through the portal vein, and, less frequently, via the bloodstream to the bones or lungs.

What Causes It Environmental factors thought to contribute to the development of colorectal cancer include diet (high in saturated fat, low in fiber, and possibly low in calcium) and lack of exercise. It is most common in industrialized countries with high standards of living. It is becoming more common in Japan as consumption of fat increases. Recent data suggest that aspirin and nonsteroidal anti-inflammatory drugs (NSAIDs) may reduce colorectal cancer (possibly by reducing the incidence of colorectal adenomatous polyps). This has led to interest in using these agents to prevent colon cancer.

About 10 percent of all colorectal cancers can be attributed to an inherited cancer syndrome. One percent of colorectal cancers is related to an inherited condition called familial polyposis, in which multiple polyps begin to appear in childhood and adolescence. Given enough time, most affected individuals will develop cancer.

Several genetic factors linked to colorectal cancer have been found. *Ras* gene mutations, largely in the k-*ras* gene resulting from environmental causes rather than being passed on genetically, are found in half of all people with colorectal adenomas and cancers. The tumor-suppressor gene p53 on chromosome 17 seems to be inactivated in most cases. A second tumor-suppressor gene has been found on chromosome 18, and other genetic abnormalities have been found on chromosome 5. These may be important for tumor suppression. Once a colon cell has one of these chromosome changes, other "hits" to the cell may cause polyps and then cancers to develop. Defective mismatch repair genes, MLH1, MSH2, and MSH6, which are responsible for repairing errors that occur during DNA replication, are responsible for up to two-thirds of the inherited forms of colon cancer. When these genetic defects are identified in a patient with cancer, family members can be screened and tested to determine if they are at increased risk for the disease and are therefore in need of more intensive cancer screening.

Risk Factors

At Significantly Higher Risk

• Advanced age. 90 percent of colorectal cancers occur in people over the age of fifty.

• Male sex. Men are more likely to develop colorectal cancer than women, although the disease remains common in women, too. The risk of cancer in a fifty-year-old man equals the risk in a sixty-year-old woman.

• Family history of colorectal cancer, especially among first-degree relatives.

Patients with one affected first-degree relative have two to three times the risk of an average person.

- Inherited cancer syndromes, including
  - hereditary nonpolyposis colorectal cancer (HNPCC), or Lynch syndrome —patients in this group are also at increased risk for other tumors, such as adenocarcinomas of the ovary, endometrium, breast, and pancreas—and
  - familial adenomatous polyposis (FAP)—affected patients develop hundreds of intestinal polyps as early as age ten, and almost all patients will go on to develop invasive colorectal cancer unless a prophylactic colectomy is performed.
- Personal history of benign polyps of the colon or rectum. Personal history of cancer of the ovary, endometrium, or breast is also a risk factor.
- Personal history of inflammatory bowel disease (such as ulcerative colitis or Crohn's disease). Patients with ulcerative colitis have a risk of colon cancer that is about five times the average. Cancer may also develop in the flat surface of the mucosa rather than in polyps.
- Personal history of pelvic radiation.
- Diets high in fat and low in fiber and calcium. Animal rather than vegetable fat is believed responsible. One study indicated that women who eat red meat (beef, lamb, and pork) daily have $2\frac{1}{2}$ times the risk of those who eat red meat less than once a month. Those eating fish and chicken without the skin are at lesser risk.
- High consumption of charcoal-broiled foods; smoking; heavy alcohol consumption; and inadequate dietary intake of fruits and vegetables.
- Obesity and inactivity.
- African-Americans.
- Certain medical conditions, including non-insulin-dependent diabetes mellitus.

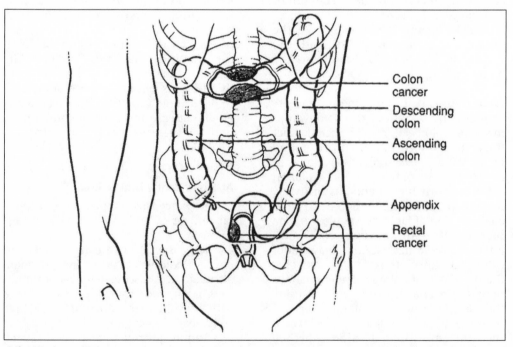

Colon and rectal cancers

At Lower Than Average Risk

• Seventh-Day Adventists, lacto-vegetarians who do not drink alcohol or smoke, and Mormons, who abstain from alcohol, tobacco, coffee, and tea and eat meat in moderation.

• Mediterraneans.

• Hispanics.

• People that regularly use aspirin or nonsteroidal anti-inflammatory drugs (NSAIDs).

• Regular intake of folic acid and calcium and hormone replacement in postmenopausal women may also be protective.

Screening

Death from colorectal cancer is highly preventable. Likely over 80 percent of colorectal cancers are preventable by use of screening tests. Screening has the capability of detecting precancerous polyps and removing them via a colonoscope before cancer ever occurs. Even if cancer does occur, colorectal cancer is highly curable in the early stages, and cancers detected at screening are much more likely to be in a curable stage. Several techniques for prevention/early detection are recommended and are widely available. These apply to the general population but are especially recommended for people at high risk (patients with first-degree relatives with colorectal cancer or other high-risk features). Several large studies have conclusively shown that screening decreases the mortality from colorectal cancer. However, only a minority of the population is undergoing regular colorectal cancer screening.

The American Cancer Society recommends that average-risk adults begin colorectal cancer screening at age fifty, with one of the following options: (1) annual fecal occult blood test (FOBT) or fecal immunochemical test (FIT); (2) flexible sigmoidoscopy every five years; (3) annual FOBT or FIT, plus flexible sigmoidoscopy every five years (this option is preferred over either procedure alone); (4) double-contrast barium enema (DCBE) every five years; (5) colonoscopy every ten years. Emerging data suggest that a special computerized tomography (CT) scan of the colon (CT colonography or virtual colonoscopy) may be an adequate or even superior replacement for the DCBE.

About 4 percent will have a positive hidden-blood test (FOBT or FIT), and anywhere from 20 to 50 percent of these will be positive for polyps or cancer (10 percent will have cancer, and 20 to 30 percent will have adenomas). The likelihood that a single use of the test will be positive in a patient with a large polyp or cancer is only 20 to 40 percent. False negatives are high because colorectal cancers bleed intermittently and the test may be done between bleedings. The chance of a false negative test can be reduced by repeating the test regularly (every year or every other year). A false positive test is common, with only 5 to 10 percent of individuals with a positive test being found to have a cancer or very large polyp. The false positive rate can be reduced by not consuming red meat and avoiding foods high in vitamin C and iron—cantaloupe, broccoli, parsnips, cauliflower, mushrooms, potatoes, cucumbers, red radishes, and horseradish—for twenty-four hours before the test. Immunochemical tests for occult blood (FIT) have fewer false positive and negative results, but they are more expensive and not widely used. Many physicians take the opportunity to do a FOBT on stool obtained during a routine digital rectal exam. However, studies have shown that the likelihood of one-time testing identifying a colorectal cancer is very low. Therefore, while convenient, one sample, in-office FOBT is not recommended for colorectal cancer screening. Any one positive test (FOBT or FIT) should be followed up with a full colonoscopy.

The sigmoid colon and rectum should be examined with a flexible or rigid tube (sigmoidoscopy) every five years after age fifty. Alternatively, one can undergo a colonoscopy to examine the entire colon every ten years or a double-contrast barium enema every five years starting at the age of fifty. It takes about ten years for an adenomatous polyp to grow to the size where a cancerous change may occur. Both fecal occult blood tests and flexible sigmoidoscopy (combined with endoscopic or surgical removal of polyps) have been shown to substantially decrease colon cancer mortality in large studies. The National Polyp Study showed that colonoscopy and removal of polyps reduces the incidence of colorectal cancer by 76 to 90 percent. Measuring the level of the carcinoembryonic antigen (CEA) in the blood can sometimes detect an early recurrence after removal of a tumor, but it is not a good test for screening.

When the family history suggests the presence of a hereditary syndrome, genetic studies can be used to screen for people at high risk for developing colorectal cancer in selected cases. Other tests currently under investigation include stool DNA testing, but this test is not routinely recommended for screening at this time

Screening is costly but may be effective. Finding colorectal cancer before it invades tissues or spreads to lymph nodes will improve the cure rate. The American death rate from this cancer fell 5.5 percent from 1973 to 1985, but there are still 54,900 deaths per year.

Early Detection

Each person should be aware of the cancer early-detection guidelines that pertain to him or her. To understand the role of the cancer-related checkup, the American Cancer Society has adopted the following definitions: *Screening* is the search for disease in persons without symptoms.

Once a person has had a positive screening test, or once signs or symptoms have been identified, further tests are considered diagnostic. *Detection* is the discovery of an abnormality in a person with or without symptoms. *Diagnostic evaluation* is the evaluation of a patient who has signs or symptoms suggestive of disease to determine the actual existence and nature of the disease.

Common Signs and Symptoms

Colon cancer symptoms depend on the location of the tumor. Cancers of the larger and more pliable right colon frequently bleed, causing anemia, but do not usually block the colon because the stool is still liquid in the right side of the colon. Cancers in the left colon may obstruct the bowel, causing a change in bowel habits (including diarrhea and constipation) and in stool size. There may be dark red rectal bleeding, or stools that are long and narrow.

Cancers in the rectum often cause an obstruction, causing a change in bowel habits (including constipation and a feeling that the bowel does not empty completely) and in the size of stools, which may also become long and narrow. There may also be rectal bleeding. Other symptoms include abdominal or pelvic pain, gas, bloating, vomiting, persistent constipation or diarrhea, weight loss, and weakness. Pain is a worrisome problem with rectal cancer, since it often means the tumor is growing into nerves.

Diagnosis

The evaluation of someone suspected of having colorectal cancer is variable but generally includes a physical examination, blood work, and radiographic imaging to assess the extent of disease.

Physical Examination

• General survey of the body.

American Cancer Society Colorectal Cancer Screening Guidelines

Beginning at age fifty, both men and women should follow one of these five testing schedules:

- Yearly fecal occult blood test (FOBT)* or fecal immunochemical test (FIT)
   or
- Flexible sigmoidoscopy every five years
   or
- Yearly FOBT or FIT, plus flexible sigmoidoscopy every five years**
   or
- Double-contrast barium enema every five years
   or
- Colonoscopy every 10 years

People should talk to their doctors about starting colorectal cancer screening earlier and/or undergoing screening more often if they have any of the following colorectal cancer risk factors:

- A personal history of colorectal cancer or adenomatous polyps
- A strong family history of colorectal cancer or polyps (cancer or polyps in a first-degree relative [parent, sibling, or child] younger than sixty)
- A personal history of chronic inflammatory bowel disease
- A family history or genetic testing indicating the presence of a hereditary colorectal cancer syndrome (e.g., familial adenomatous polyposis or hereditary nonpolyposis colon cancer)

*For FOBT, the take-home multiple sample method should be used.

**The combination of yearly FOBT or FIT and flexible sigmoidoscopy every five years is preferred over either of these options alone. All positive tests should be followed up with colonoscopy.

- Digital rectal examination to feel for lumps.
- Abdominal exam to check for a mass or an enlarged liver (hepatomegaly).
- Exam to rule out enlarged lymph nodes over the left collarbone and in the groin (inguinal) area.

Blood and Other Tests

- Test for hidden blood in the stools (stool tests for bleeding may be negative in half of colorectal cancer cases).
- Complete blood count (CBC) to check for anemia.
- Blood chemistry tests to evaluate the liver enzymes (often elevated in the setting of liver metastases).
- Blood test for carcinoembryonic antigen (CEA), a serum tumor marker that may be elevated with primary or recurrent colorectal cancer. Very high levels of CEA may indicate more advanced disease. The CEA level should be measured before surgery and, if elevated, periodically (every three to six months) after surgery.
- Other laboratory tests may include creatinine (to assess kidney function), albumin (to assess nutritional status), and serum iron studies (to evaluate for the presence of blood loss/anemia).

Imaging

- Barium enema X-ray (also called a lower GI series)—often done in combination with a flexible sigmoidoscopy.
- Ultrasound of the abdomen—sometimes done to assess for disease outside the colon or rectum.
- Endorectal ultrasonography and/or pelvic MRI scan—often performed to assess for local extension or lymph node involvement in patients with rectal cancer.

Ultrasound done via the rectum (endorectal) can accurately show tumor invasion and enlarged lymph nodes outside the rectum, but cannot indicate if enlarged lymph nodes actually contain metastatic tumor.

• Abdominal/pelvic computed tomography (CT) scan—to identify the extent of disease.

• Chest X-ray—to rule out lung metastases.

• PET (positron-emission tomography) scanning—can help identify possible tumor sites by measuring differences in sugar metabolism in different sites throughout the body. When a patient is suspected of having colorectal cancer, a PET scan can sometimes help differentiate between benign and malignant sites of disease. However, PET scans are not routinely performed in all patients. Instead, PET scans are more commonly used to identify occult metastases in patients previously treated for colorectal cancer in whom the CEA is elevated.

Endoscopy and Biopsy Colonoscopic examination of the entire colon with a biopsy of any suspicious mass. A biopsy is important to confirm the diagnosis of colorectal cancer. While most colorectal cancers are adenocarcinomas, other tumor types occasionally occur in the bowel. An examination of the entire colon is important because multiple cancers or polyps occur in a minority of patients. The surgeon needs this information to assist planning for surgical resection. (Note that if a patient presents with a complete obstruction, then a double-contrast barium enema [or computed tomography colonography/virtual colonoscopy] should be done preoperatively if possible, and a complete colonoscopy should be performed three to six months after surgery to rule out additional polyps or primary tumors.)

Other Cystoscopy (or IVP, intravenous pyelogram)—sometimes required preoperatively in patients with rectal cancer to rule out involvement of the bladder.

Staging

The stage of colorectal cancer reflects whether the cancer has remained within the bowel or has spread to other sites. As with all cancers, defining the exact stage of disease is an important step toward identifying the appropriate therapy.

A number of different staging systems for colorectal cancer have been employed over the past century. The original system developed by Dr. Dukes in 1932 has been modified several times. Since 1985, a staging system based on the tumor/nodes/metastasis (TNM) classification has been used. This staging system corresponds to the Dukes classification scheme but is thought to be more informative. The 1990 National Cancer Institute Consensus Panel recommended using the TNM system to identify people at high risk for recurrence because it incorporates the tumor size and degree of invasion, as well as the number of lymph nodes involved. The TNM staging system is described in more detail in the next section and was recently modified to subclassify traditional Stage II and III patients into distinct prognostic groups.

Treatment Overview

Colorectal cancers are primarily treated surgically, resulting in cures in 50 to 60 percent of patients. The type and extent of surgical resection are determined by the precise location of the tumor. In addition to surgery, depending on the stage of the tumor, adjuvant chemotherapy for colon cancers and chemoradiation therapy for rectal cancers increase survival. In patients with metastatic colorectal cancer, chemotherapy extends survival, radiation is used to palliate symptoms, and the utility of several new biologically based agents (targeting specific properties of cancer cells or tumors in general) has been established.

The approach to treatment is different in patients with rectal cancer compared to patients with colon cancer. This relates to the location of the rectum in the pelvis and the fact that the rectum lacks the covering layer present in the colon (the serosa), both of which factors contribute to a higher rate of local recurrence. Most researchers believe that adjuvant radiotherapy alone decreases the risk of local recurrence in patients with rectal cancer without improving survival. In contrast, combined radiotherapy and chemotherapy increases the disease-free survival in patients with rectal cancer more than radiation alone and improves long-term survival as well. The prognosis of rectal cancer depends on how far the tumor has penetrated through the bowel wall or into adjacent structures and on whether the cancer has spread to local lymph nodes. After surgery alone in node-negative patients with rectal cancer, local recurrence is 5 to 10 percent for Stage I patients and 25 to 30 percent for patients with Stage II disease.

Recent studies indicate that the *number* of local lymph nodes involved is important. When one to four nodes are involved, survival is significantly better than if more than four nodes are involved.

Additional poor prognostic factors for both colon and rectal cancers include

- penetration through the bowel wall,
- perforation or obstruction,

- high histologic grade under the microscope,
- mucinous (colloid) histologic subtype,
- invasion of the blood vessels, lymphatics, or nerves under the microscope, and
- high DNA content or aneuploidy.

Several features suggest an unfavorable outcome in patients with rectal cancer:

- Fixed, nonmobile tumor or invasion of or adherence to other parts of the pelvis or adjacent tissues.
- Deep ulceration.
- The tumor penetrates through the bowel wall or encircles the rectal wall.
- The radial margin is positive after resection.
- The tumor is larger than 2 1/2 inches (6 cm).

Other features portend a poor prognosis in patients with colon cancer:

- Involvement of abdominal nodes.
- Involvement of adjacent organs.
- The level of carcinoembryonic antigen (CEA) in the blood is high before surgery.

Thus, the prognosis (chance of recovery) in a given patient depends on multiple factors, including the stage of the tumor, whether the cancer has blocked or created a hole in the colon or rectum, the blood levels of carcinoembryonic antigen before treatment begins, whether the cancer has recurred, and the patient's general health. In each case, all of these factors are integrated to determine the final treatment plan.

Colon

 Surgery Tumors of the colon should be removed whenever practical in an effort to prevent complications such as blockage of the bowel and bleeding from developing. Because of the potential problems related to leaving the primary tumor in place, surgery should even be considered in patients with metastatic disease. However, recent advances in the treatments available for patients with distant spread have reduced the imperative to remove the primary tumor in asymptomatic individuals.

The standard operation is designed to remove the affected portion of the bowel along with the entire lymph node drainage. This requires removing the vessels that supply blood to a considerable portion of the bowel, so most of the time about one-third to one-half of the colon is removed even if the tumor itself is relatively small. After removal of the cancer and a length of normal tissue on either side of the tumor, the remaining sections of the colon are reconnected (anastomosis). Recent data suggest that in some cases, a laparoscopically assisted (minimally invasive) colectomy may be an acceptable alternative to an open surgery for colon cancer when performed by a qualified surgeon. A laparoscopically assisted procedure should not be considered in the setting of acute obstruction or perforation, rectal or transverse colon tumor, prohibitive abdominal adhesions, or locally advanced disease.

Sometimes reconnecting the bowel is not possible after tumor resection because there is too much stool or contamination in the area. This occurs most commonly in patients who have tumors in the left side of the colon and who presented with a partial or complete obstruction. These patients receive a temporary colostomy, which can be reversed as soon as six to ten weeks later (see chapter 26, "Living with an Ostomy").

Local excision may be used for the removal of polyps in most cases.

 Radiation Therapy Radiation therapy has a limited role in the treatment of colon cancer. In selected cases, radiotherapy may help reduce local recurrences. Palliative radiation is primarily used for localized metastatic tumors.

Chemotherapy More than 50 percent of patients with colon cancer have tumors that penetrate the serosa (T3) or have positive lymph nodes (N1–3). Interest in adjuvant therapy stems from the fact that roughly 20 to 25 percent of those with Stage II disease and 50 percent of those with Stage III cancer have recurrences if treated with surgery alone.

Adjuvant therapy is controversial in patients with Stage II disease, as randomized clinical trials have failed to establish a clear benefit. While routinely offered to individuals perceived to be at relatively high risk for recurrence, participation in clinical trials should be encouraged for patients with Stage II disease. In contrast, adjuvant chemotherapy is of proven value in patients with Stage III colon cancer (positive lymph nodes), decreasing both the risk of recurrence and death. Fluorouracil (5-FU)–based chemotherapy (often in combination with oxaliplatin [Eloxatin]) has emerged as the standard therapy in this setting and is generally given for a total of six months. While it has no direct antitumor activity, leucovorin (LV) is often added to 5-FU–based chemotherapy because it increases the activity of 5-FU. Clinical trials exploring additional regimens are ongoing.

Patients with metastatic disease limited to the liver, pelvis, or lungs should be evaluated for resection. In general, metastatic colon cancer is incurable unless resected completely, in which case the five-year survival approaches 30 percent. For decades, 5-FU combined with leucovorin was the mainstay of therapy for patients with unresectable metastatic disease in spite of limited response rates (15 to 20 percent) and the lack of a significant impact on survival.

The results of several recent studies have changed our approach to the treatment of patients with advanced disease. Infusional 5-FU is better tolerated than bolus 5-FU and is somewhat more efficacious. Capecitabine (Xeloda), an oral 5-FU prodrug, is associated with continuous infusion-type pharmacokinetics and is likely to replace infusional 5-FU in the future. Treatment is associated with less diarrhea and bone marrow suppression than bolus 5-FU, but palmar-plantar-erythrodysesthesia is more common (hand-foot syndrome) and consists of pain, redness, and rash involving the hands and feet. Furthermore, the addition of irinotecan (Camptosar, CPT-11), oxaliplatin, and/or bevacizumab (Avastin; an antiangiogenic agent) increases the chance of tumor shrinkage (response rate) and prolongs overall survival compared to 5-FU/leucovorin alone. Combination chemotherapy is associated with increased toxicity, however, and the optimal drug sequence and regimens have not yet been defined. Thus, the current approach to the treatment of patients with advanced disease involves individualizing therapy after integrating symptoms (e.g., from primary tumor versus metastases), other medical conditions, and patient/physician preference. Participation in clinical trials should be encouraged.

Depending on the choice of agent in the first-line setting, oxaliplatin or irinotecan can be used in patients with 5-FU–refractory disease. Biologically based agents like the antiangiogenic agent bevacizumab and the epidermal growth factor inhibitors cetuximab (Erbitux) and panitumumab (Vectibix), also play a role in the treatment of patients with chemotherapy-refractory disease.

Colon Cancer Treatment by Stage

■ *Stage 0*
TNM Tis (tumor or carcinoma in situ), N0, M0
This is a very early cancer that is found only in the innermost lining of the colon; it has not spread below the limiting membrane of the first layer of colon tissue (mucosa).

Standard Treatment Local excision of the tumor or polyp is sometimes sufficient. Standard surgery, however, involves removing the tumor along with at least 2 inches (5 cm) of normal colon on either side of the tumor site, and the nearby lymph nodes and veins. Because of the way blood is supplied to the colon, it is usually necessary to remove either the entire right side or the entire left side of the colon. This decreases the chance for local recurrence and increases the safety of the operation.

Five-Year Survival 95 percent

■ *Stage I (Dukes' A, B1)*
TNM T1–2, N0, M0
The cancer has spread beyond the innermost tissue layer of the colon to the middle layers; it is confined to the lining or muscular wall of the colon and has not yet spread anywhere else.

Standard Treatment This stage is highly curable. Radical surgery is the primary treatment and results in a high cure rate. No adjuvant therapy is warranted for this stage because of the low risk for recurrence.

Five-Year Survival 90 to 95 percent

■ *Stage II (Dukes' B2, B3)*

TNM T3–4, N0, M0 (IIA and IIB)

The cancer has spread through the muscular wall of the intestine (T3, N0 [IIA]) and possibly extended to adjacent organs and/or through the peritoneum (T4, N0 [IIB]), but has not spread to lymph nodes. (Note that at least twelve lymph nodes should be examined to establish node-negative disease according to the American Joint Committee on Cancer and a National Cancer Institute–sponsored panel.)

Standard Treatment Surgical removal of the primary tumor, with or without adjuvant chemotherapy, is standard. Adjuvant therapy is controversial in patients with Stage II colon cancer (i.e., no lymphatic spread). On average, there is a 20 to 25 percent chance of recurrence in these patients (a range of 15 to 30 percent in recent studies). Randomized trials have failed to establish a consistent benefit (the improvement in disease-free survival at five years is thought to be less than 5 percent). As a result, 5-FU–based adjuvant chemotherapy is not routinely recommended outside of a clinical trial in the absence of high-risk features. In every patient, the potential benefit of chemotherapy needs to be weighed against the potential for toxicity (including a 0.5 to 1.0 percent risk of treatment-related death).

Note that some patients with Stage II colon cancer are at relatively high risk for recurrence and may be particularly likely to benefit from adjuvant chemotherapy (although this has not been proven in randomized controlled trials). Potential high-risk features include complete obstruction or perforation (e.g., five-year survival 60 to 70 percent), invasion of adjacent organs, inadequate lymph node sampling, and poorly differentiated histology.

A number of molecular markers also hold promise in predicting the outcome of patients with Stage II disease. Patients with tumors containing loss of heterozygosity at chromosome 18q may be at a greater risk of recurrence. In contrast, patients with tumors associated with evidence

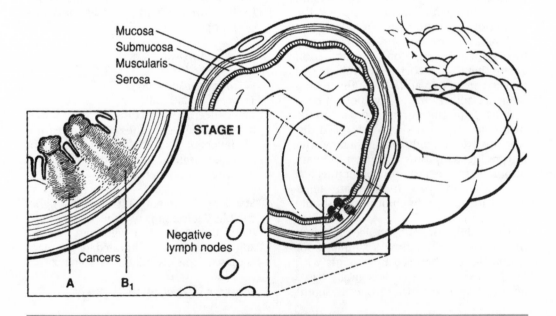

Mucosa
Submucosa
Muscularis
Serosa

STAGE I

Negative lymph nodes

Cancers

A   B₁

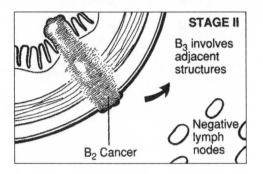

STAGE II

B₃ involves adjacent structures

B₂ Cancer

Negative lymph nodes

for microsatellite instability may have a relatively good outcome. While not yet routinely incorporated into practice, the utility of such tumor-associated molecular markers for guiding therapy in patients with Stage II disease is currently under investigation. Participation in clinical trials is encouraged.

Five-Year Survival 70 to 85 percent (lower if the tumor invades adjacent organs or causes complete obstruction or perforation)

Investigational
• Clinical trials of chemotherapy, radiation therapy, and/or biological therapy after surgery
• Adjuvant chemotherapy with capecitabine (Xeloda)-based regimens
• Adjuvant therapy incorporating the antiangiogenic agent bevacizumab (Avastin) or epidermal growth factor inhibitors (e.g., cetuximab [Erbitux] and panitumumab [Vectibix])
• Postoperative local radiation therapy (may help control tumors that have perforated or spread to tissues adjacent to the colon)
• Identification of molecular markers with prognostic significance

■ *Stage III (Dukes' C)*
TNM Any T, N1–2, M0 (IIIA, IIIB, and IIIC)
The cancer has spread outside the intestine to one or more lymph nodes near the bowel. N1 is three or fewer lymph

nodes involved. N2 is four or more lymph nodes involved.

The cancer is Stage IIIA if it invades the lining or muscular wall of the bowel (T1/T2) and up to three lymph nodes are involved (N1). The cancer is considered Stage IIIB if the tumor has invaded through the bowel wall or to nearby tissues (T3), or involves adjacent organs and/or is through the peritoneum (T4), and up to three lymph nodes are involved (N1). The cancer is considered Stage IIIC, regardless of how much it extends through the bowel wall, if four or more lymph nodes are involved (any T, N2).

Standard Treatment All patients with Stage III colon cancer should be considered for adjuvant chemotherapy, as only about 50 percent of patients are cured by surgical resection alone. Treatment with adjuvant 5-FU/leucovorin (LV) chemotherapy improves the five-year survival to 65 percent. Thus, the standard treatment is removal of a wide section of the colon and rejoining the remaining ends (creating an anastomosis), followed by six months of 5-FU–based adjuvant chemotherapy. Recent findings suggest that the addition of oxaliplatin (Eloxatin) improves three-year disease-free survival (77.8 percent versus 72.9 percent, a statistically significant difference) based on pooled data from patients with resected Stage II and III colon cancer compared to treatment with 5-FU/LV alone (the incremental benefit was statistically

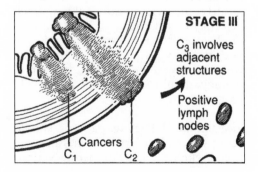

STAGE III

C₃ involves adjacent structures

Positive lymph nodes

Cancers
C₁ C₂

significant in Stage III, but not Stage II, patients). Final data related to overall five-year survival are still pending. The addition of oxaliplatin was associated with increased toxicity (low white blood cell counts and peripheral neuropathy). Nevertheless, oxaliplatin + 5-FU + LV (FOLFOX) was approved by the FDA for the treatment of Stage III colon cancer in 2005; the regimen has since become a standard option for patients who are candidates for combination chemotherapy. For patients with Stage III colon cancer in whom treatment with only 5-FU and leucovorin is planned, capecitabine (Xeloda) (an oral fluoropyrimidine that undergoes a three-step enzymatic conversion to 5-FU) is an equivalent alternative. In the absence of residual disease, radiation therapy has no current standard role in the treatment of patients with completely resected colon cancer. Participation in clinical trials is also appropriate.

Five-Year Survival 50 percent overall with surgery alone (a range of 25 to 60 percent depending on the extent to which the tumor penetrates the bowel wall and the number of lymph nodes involved); 40 to 60 percent when the tumor is within the bowel wall (T1–2, Dukes' C1); 20 to 40 percent when the tumor extends through the bowel wall (T3, Dukes' C2); 30 percent or less when adjacent structures are involved (T4, Dukes' C3). These data do not reflect adjuvant therapy programs.

The 1990 NCI Consensus Conference used positive lymph nodes for determining prognosis. If one to four nodes are positive, the five-year survival is 55 to 60 percent in the absence of adjuvant chemotherapy. When five or more nodes are positive, only 33 percent will be cured with surgery alone. Adjuvant chemotherapy should improve all of the old prognostic figures.

Investigational Eligible patients should be considered for entry into carefully controlled clinical trials comparing various

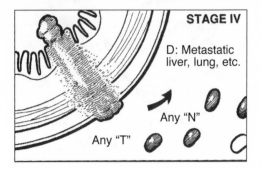

postoperative chemotherapy regimens, radiation, or biological therapy alone or in combination.

• Adjuvant chemotherapy with capecitabine (Xeloda)-based combination chemotherapy regimens
• Adjuvant therapy incorporating the antiangiogenic agent bevacizumab (Avastin) or epidermal growth factor inhibitors (e.g., cetuximab [Erbitux] and panitumumab [Vectibix])
• Postoperative local radiation therapy (may help control tumors that have perforated or spread to tissues adjacent to the colon)
• Identification of molecular markers with prognostic significance

■ *Stage IV (Dukes' D)*
TNM Any T, any N, M1
Patients with Stage IV disease have cancer that has spread beyond the colon to distant sites or organs, possibly including the liver or lungs.

Standard Treatment
Surgical Options Cancer at this stage is not usually curable, but removal of a large section of the colon and reconnection of the bowel is still considered so complications such as obstruction, bleeding, and bowel perforation can be avoided. Tumors that are blocking the colon may be surgically bypassed (diverting colostomy), leaving the tumor in place. Importantly, recent

advances in the treatments available for patients with distant spread have reduced the imperative to remove the primary tumor in asymptomatic individuals.

The liver is the most common site of metastases in colorectal cancer. As such, 80 percent of colon cancer patients ultimately die of liver failure. If the metastases are resectable, surgical removal of the metastases can cure 20 to 30 percent of patients. The prognosis is better if there are fewer lesions—one lesion is better than three—and there is no survival benefit unless all lesions are removed. Noncurative surgery has the same prognosis as no surgery at all. In selected cases, both the colon cancer and the liver metastases (if there are three or fewer) can be removed at the same surgery. For selected patients with unresectable disease isolated to the liver, ablative therapies such as cryotherapy and radiofrequency ablation represent alternatives to resection, although their long-term benefits have not been clearly defined. In addition, use of preoperative chemotherapy to convert initially unresectable liver metastases to tumors that can be removed surgically should be considered; the long-term outcome of such patients appears to approach that of patients with initially resectable disease. Resection should also be considered in rare cases of isolated lung or pelvic metastases, as up to 25 percent of patients may be cured if all tumors can be removed.

The risk of recurrence after resection of liver metastases may be reduced if 5-FUDR chemotherapy (floxuridine) is delivered by infusion pump through the main hepatic artery after surgical resection of all known liver metastases (see chapter 6, "What Happens in Surgery"). Clinical trials are ongoing, however, and the precise role of adjuvant systemic or liver-directed chemotherapy after liver resection remains ill-defined.

Chemotherapy For decades, 5-FU (+/- leucovorin) has been the mainstay of therapy for patients with unresectable metastatic disease in spite of limited response rates and the lack of a significant impact on survival (a median survival of around twelve months). Capecitabine (Xeloda), an oral 5-FU prodrug, is associated with continuous infusion-type pharmacokinetics and is likely to replace infusional 5-FU in the future. Treatment is associated with less diarrhea and bone marrow suppression than bolus 5-FU, but palmar-plantar-erythrodysesthesia (hand-foot syndrome) is more common and consists of pain, redness, and rash involving the hands and feet. Recent studies suggest that the addition of irinotecan (Camptosar, CPT-11; a topoisomerase-1 inhibitor) or oxaliplatin (Eloxatin; a DNA-damaging agent) to 5-FU–based chemotherapy increases the response rate in previously untreated patients (35 to 50 percent). Furthermore, the addition of oxaliplatin and irinotecan to our armamentarium has translated into a dramatic improvement in the median of survival of patients with metastatic colorectal cancer (now eighteen to twenty-one months). The data suggest that the order in which patients receive specific agents may be less important than the availability of all three drugs (e.g., irinotecan, oxaliplatin, and a fluoropyrimidine [5-FU or capecitabine]). As such, second-line therapy has become routine but varies depending on the patient's prior treatment. In general, therapy must be individualized according to comorbidities, performance status, and kidney and liver function.

Targeted Agents Recent results suggest that the addition of agents designed to block tumor blood vessel growth (angiogenesis) or growth factor signaling (e.g., the epidermal growth factor receptor (EGFR) inhibitor) may enhance the activity of chemotherapy alone in Stage IV disease. There is an expanding body of evidence suggesting that tumors need to grow new blood vessels (angiogenesis) in order to grow and metastasize. This information has translated into an entirely new approach to the treatment of cancer, in which surrounding normal cells are the target of the therapy as opposed to the tumor cells themselves. A number of approaches are in development and more than twenty agents are already being tested in clinical trials (see chapter 14, "Antiangiogenesis").

Bevacizumab (Avastin), a humanized monoclonal antibody directed against the angiogenesis regulator vascular endothelial growth factor (VEGF), has been shown to enhance the activity of chemotherapy for metastatic colorectal cancer (and was approved for use in this setting in 2004). Unlike traditional cytotoxic agents, the use of bevacizumab is associated with hypertension, proteinuria, arterial thromboembolic events, bleeding, and gastrointestinal perforations. Cetuximab (Erbitux), a chimeric antibody targeting the epidermal growth factor receptor, is indicated in combination with irinotecan (Camptosar, CPT-11)–based therapy for patients refractory to irinotecan-based chemotherapy (roughly 20 percent response rate) or as single-agent therapy for patients intolerant to irinotecan (10 percent response rate). The main side effect of an EGFR inhibitor like cetuximab is an acneiform rash. Panitumumab (Vectibix), another recently approved EGFR inhibitor, is associated with an 8 percent response rate as a single agent in patients with chemotherapy-refractory disease. Its relative efficacy compared to cetuximab is unknown. Both cetuximab and panitumumab have been and are being explored as components of first-line treatment, in combination with chemotherapy and/or bevacizumab (Avastin), but neither of these EGFR inhibitors is specifically approved for this setting at this time.

Hepatic Arterial Therapy Treatment of unresectable liver metastases with intraarterial chemotherapy (floxuridine [5-FUDR]) by an infusion pump or a hepatic artery catheter is associated with a response rate of over 50 percent, although a definitive increase in survival has not been shown. While convenient and generally well tolerated, liver-directed chemotherapy requires that a pump (connected to the hepatic artery) be placed surgically. Treatment-related toxicity can be seen, including liver toxicity, scarring of the bile duct (biliary sclerosis), gastritis, diarrhea, and pain, requiring dose reductions in 40 to 50 percent of patients (see the chapter "Metastatic Cancer"). 5-FUDR intra-arterial therapy may also benefit patients who have failed systemic treatment with 5-FU. Approximately 30 percent of these patients will respond to liver-directed therapy, although a clear increase in survival has not been shown. The utility of this approach after failure of or in combination with a modern irinotecan (Camptosar, CPT-11)– or oxaliplatin (Eloxatin)-based chemotherapy regimen is under investigation.

Radiation Radiation therapy may be given to help control tumor-associated symptoms and may be given in combination with continuous-infusion 5-FU. Radiation is most frequently used to control bony metastases or recurrent disease in the pelvis.

Individualizing Care Patients with metastatic disease should be considered for clinical trials with novel agents and/or combinations. Since chemotherapy for metastatic colorectal cancer is not curative, however, one needs to compare the potential risks and benefits in every individual case. Some patients are not optimal candidates for systemic chemotherapy due to personal preference or debilitation from concomitant medical illness, the cancer itself, or the development of treatment-related toxicity. In these patients, supportive care may be the best option. Alternatively, treatment with infusional 5-FU (with or without bevacizumab [Avastin]) or single-agent capecitabine (Xeloda), or an EGFR inhibitor may be feasible.

Five-Year Survival Less than 10 percent, rising to 20 to 30 percent if liver or lung metastases can be removed surgically

Investigational
- Adjuvant therapy after resection of metastatic disease.
- Preoperative (neoadjuvant) chemotherapy prior to resection of metastatic disease.
- Clinical trials are constantly being designed to develop better ways of delivering known chemotherapeutic agents (in an attempt to enhance efficacy and decrease toxicity) alone or in combination with other drugs, radiation, or surgery. In addition, novel chemotherapeutic agents continue to be developed and tested in the clinic. The most exciting new treatment strategies, however, are based on fundamental advances in our understanding of the molecular mechanisms underlying the development of colorectal cancer. While primarily being studied in the setting of advanced disease, many of these strategies may have the greatest promise in the adjuvant setting, when all obvious disease has been removed.

Treatment Follow-Up

After definitive treatment for a primary colon cancer (or curative resection of a metastatic site), patients should be followed regularly for evidence of recurrent disease. The interval between appointments generally increases after two years, but regular visits continue for five years.

- History and physical examination every three to four months for two years, then every six months.
- Obtaining a chest X-ray every twelve months for five years should be considered.

- Complete blood count and liver function tests every three to four months for two years, then every six months.
- Blood CEA level every three to four months for two years, then every six months. The CEA level may rise before other clinical, X-ray, or laboratory tests are suggestive of tumor recurrence. If the CEA rises above normal, about one-third of patients may have a recurrent tumor that can be totally removed with surgery and so may be cured.
- CT scans of the abdomen and pelvis if a patient's symptoms, physical examination, or laboratory studies suggest recurrent disease (alternatively, surveillance CT scans every six to twelve months in patients with resected Stage II-IV colon cancer should be considered).
- Colonoscopy every one to three years depending on whether or not additional polyps are discovered.

Recurrent Colon Cancer

Cancer may recur in the colon or any part of the body, including the liver and lungs.

Treatment for recurrent colon cancer is essentially the same as for Stage IV, although therapy also depends on the site of the recurrence.

- Resection should be considered if there is only one area of recurrence such as the liver or lung.
- Occasionally, the cancer will come back at the site of the original colon surgery (anastomotic recurrence), where sections of the bowel have been sewn together. These local suture-line recurrences can be removed surgically with a reasonable chance for cure.
- Chemotherapy with single drugs (10 to 20 percent response rate), combinations (30 to 45 percent response rate), and investigational drugs have been used for palliation. The specific chemotherapy employed depends on the time interval between prior adjuvant

therapy and tumor recurrence. Tumors that recur within one year of adjuvant chemotherapy are generally considered 5-FU–resistant. In contrast, 5-FU–based chemotherapy is often used as first-line therapy in chemo-naive patients or patients whose tumors recur more than one year after adjuvant therapy.

Rectum

Surgery Surgery is the primary treatment for rectal cancer and results in cure in approximately 45 percent of all patients. The prognosis of rectal cancer is clearly related to the degree of penetration of the tumor through the bowel wall and the presence or absence of nodal involvement. Preoperative clinical staging plays a critical role in determining which patients are candidates for local excision rather than a more extensive surgery and which patients may benefit from preoperative chemotherapy and radiation therapy in an attempt to maximize the chance of a curative resection.

State-of-the-art treatment for localized rectal cancer involves removing the tumor, at least $\frac{3}{4}$ inch (2 cm) of normal tissue on either side of it, and the regional lymph nodes. The precise surgical procedure performed depends on the size and location of the tumor. In general, a major limitation of surgery for the treatment of rectal cancer is the inability to obtain wide radial margins because of the presence of the bony pelvis. As a result, several different operations are considered when a patient presents with rectal cancer. Most frequently, the surgeon does an excision via the anus (transanal excision), a low-anterior resection (LAR) of the involved portion of bowel allowing preservation of the sphincter (coloanal anastomosis), or an abdominoperineal resection (APR) of the entire rectum and sphincter, resulting in permanent colostomy placement. A key principle underlying the transabdominal approaches to removing rectal cancers (LAR and APR, coloanal anastomosis) is incorporation of a total mesorectal excision, whereby the tissue surrounding the rectum is also removed, thus decreasing the chance of incomplete resection. Furthermore, unlike in transanal excisions, the draining lymph nodes are removed during transabdominal resections of rectal cancers. The final treatment plan also takes into account the relative merits of chemotherapy and radiation and depends on the clinical stage of the tumor, its location in the rectum, and what percentage of the circumference of the rectum is involved.

Most rectal tumors can be resected without impairing sphincter function (transanal resection or LAR). Noninvasive tumors that appear to be confined to the top layers of the rectal lining (mucosa and submucosa) can sometimes be treated with endocavitary radiation or removed from below, entering through the anus and using a cold probe (cryotherapy), electrofulguration, or simple excision without removing part of the bowel. Transanal excision can also be considered in the setting of an invasive cancer, but only if it is small (less that $1\frac{1}{4}$ inches [3 cm]), well-differentiated, and without evidence of involvement of the local lymph nodes or adjacent structures. If the margins are negative and there is no evidence of gross pelvic disease after local excision, adjuvant pelvic radiation is often employed to reduce the risk of local recurrence as an alternative to an APR.

Cancers in the upper part of the rectum, close to where it connects to the sigmoid colon, are removed by a low-anterior resection. The remaining colon is attached to the anus (coloanal anastomosis), thus allowing preservation of sphincter function. Very low lying rectal tumors (within 2 to 2½ inches [5 to 6 cm] of the anus), however, require removal of the entire rectum and anus, leaving the patient with a permanent colostomy (abdominoperineal resection) (see chapter 26, "Living with an Ostomy").

In some patients with a tumor that is low in the rectum, radiation given before the operation may reduce the size of the tumor, allowing it to be removed while still leaving enough bowel below the tumor site for the surgeon to sew the bowel back together. This will spare the rectum and the sphincter muscle, thereby avoiding the need for a colostomy in up to 85 percent of patients with rectal cancer. Since the type of operation performed affects the risk of local recurrence, a sphincter-sparing procedure should be pursued *only* if a curative resection (with negative margins) can be achieved. About 10 to 15 percent of patients have a late local recurrence of cancer in the pelvis, particularly when sphincter-preserving operations have been used for low-lying tumors.

 Adjuvant Radiation Therapy Because of an increased tendency for first failure in locoregional sites, the impact of perioperative irradiation is greater in rectal cancer than in colon cancer. Radiation given before or after surgery decreases local failure, although most clinical trials have failed to show a significant impact on survival with radiation therapy alone.

Placing the radiation source inside the rectum (intraluminal radiation therapy) may result in a high cure rate in some cases, such as a small, well-differentiated tumor above the sphincter. This may preserve the sphincter.

Combined Modality Therapy In contrast to treatment with radiation alone, 5-FU–based chemotherapy combined with radiation is associated with a decrease in locoregional failures *and* a small increase in survival. Furthermore, protracted continuous infusion is superior to bolus infusion (daily injections of chemotherapy for several days in a row) of 5-FU in combination with radiation therapy and has become the standard of care in patients receiving chemoradiation. The use of capecitabine (Xeloda) instead of infusional 5-FU is an area of intense interest.

Stage I (Dukes' A, B1, and Tis, T1–2) tumors have a high cure rate with definitive surgery alone, and there is no need for adjuvant chemotherapy for these stages, unless the patient had a T2 lesion treated with transanal excision (the risk of local recurrence is 25 percent without radiation). Stage II and III tumors (Dukes' B2, C, and T3–4, N1–2) are characterized by penetration of the tumor through the bowel wall and/or spread into lymph nodes at the time of diagnosis. Because of the relatively poor prognosis and high risk of local recurrence, patients with Stage II and III tumors of the mid to low rectum should be considered for adjuvant chemoradiation using 5-FU–based chemotherapy plus radiation. This has historically involved 5-FU plus radiation, sandwiched between 5-FU–based chemotherapy.. Cancers that develop high in the rectum (above the peritoneal reflection) behave and are treated like colon cancers, and radiation is not usually used. The relative importance of chemotherapy and radiation is an area of intense interest in the face of evolving surgical techniques. Similarly, extrapolating from colon cancer, the use of capecitabine and/or oxaliplatin (Eloxatin) in the treatment of rectal cancer is the focus of several ongoing clinical trials.

Neoadjuvant Therapy The optimal timing of adjuvant therapy for rectal cancer is controversial. Neoadjuvant therapy (delivered before surgical resection) harbors the promise of preoperative tumor regression, leading to a higher chance of curative resection and a sphincter-sparing procedure. On the other hand, neoadjuvant therapy can be associated with toxicity and resultant delays in a potentially curative resection. In addition, by definition, neoadjuvant therapy limits our ability to accurately stage the cancer at surgery. Consequently, we may overtreat patients who receive neoadjuvant therapy, since the exact stage at presentation can't be determined.

The decision to use neoadjuvant therapy is based on preoperative staging with ultrasound, CT, and MRI, techniques that are relatively imprecise. However, pathological staging, from the surgical resection specimen, remains the gold standard. Since neoadjuvant therapy has the potential to "downstage" the tumor by changing the histopathological findings, it can be impossible to know the true stage at diagnosis based on a sample collected intraoperatively after neoadjuvant therapy (in 15 to 25 percent of cases, there is evidence for a complete response—i.e., no residual tumor seen in the operative sample). Thus, because the true initial stage is unknown, patients treated with neoadjuvant chemoradiation typically receive 5-FU–based chemotherapy after surgical resection regardless of the pathological findings at surgery. For patients with bulky tumors or tumors adherent to local structures (e.g., vagina, bladder, or pelvic sidewall), neoadjuvant therapy is routine. It is also frequently recommended for Stage II and III disease characterized by tethering and circumferential involvement. In addition, long-term bowel function may be superior after neoadjuvant chemoradiation compared to postoperative treatment, hence a trend toward preoperative treatment in any patient with evidence for probable T3–4 or lymph node–positive disease.

In general, as in the adjuvant setting, cancers that develop very high in the rectum (near the junction with the colon) behave and are treated like colon cancers. As such, the role of neoadjuvant radiation is very limited in this setting.

 Palliation As with metastatic colon cancer, resection should always be considered in patients with metastatic rectal cancer, as there is the potential for long-term cure in up to 30 percent of patients with resectable liver or lung metastases. In general, patients with advanced rectal cancer are treated in the same way as patients with metastatic colon cancer; recent advances in treatment options using combination chemotherapy and biologically based agents have led to significant improvements in overall survival.

Pelvic radiation therapy (with or without 5-FU chemotherapy) may be used for palliation of symptoms or to prevent a local recurrence in patients who were not previously irradiated.

Laser therapy may be a very effective way to relieve an obstruction or control localized bleeding (see chapter 10).

Rectal Cancer Treatment by Stage

▓ Stage 0 (Dukes' A)
TNM Tis (tumor or carcinoma in situ), NO, MO
This superficial, noninvasive carcinoma in situ is a very early cancer that has not spread below the mucosa (first layer of rectal tissue).

Standard Treatment Because of its superficial nature, limited rather than radical surgery, as well as other procedures, may be used. Surgery may involve cutting out only the tumor itself (enucleation) or the tumor and a small wedge of tissue.

Other options include electrocoagulation and external or internal (inside the rectum) radiation therapy for rectal sphincter preservation.

Five-Year Survival Over 95 percent

■ *Stage I (Dukes' B1)*
TNM T1–2, N0, M0
Stage I rectal cancers are confined to the lining or muscular wall of the rectum and have not yet spread outside the rectum. In T1–2 tumors, the cancer is limited to the bowel wall.

Standard Treatment Surgery will generally result in a cure. There is a 5 to 10 percent chance of a local recurrence with this stage of cancer. When the tumor is in the upper rectum, a wide margin of tissue may be removed and the bowel reconnected (low-anterior resection [LAR]). When the tumor is near the anus, an abdominoperineal resection (APR) and colostomy is the standard treatment.

Local transanal resection (i.e., removal of the tumor via the anus with no abdominal incision) can be done in selected patients with small (less that 1½ inches [4 cm]), well- to moderately differentiated tumors that are mobile, completely resectable, noncircumferential, and without evidence for involvement of local lymph nodes or adjacent structures. Adjuvant pelvic radiation is often employed to reduce the risk of local recurrence (especially for T2 lesions, which have a more than 20 percent chance of lymph node involvement and require adjuvant chemoradiation or a more extensive surgical resection). Tumors excised transanally and found to have high-risk features like positive margins, lymphovascular invasion, and/or poor differentiation require additional, definitive surgery (and postoperative chemoradiation therapy, depending on the surgical staging).

Radiation inside the bowel (intraluminal) may be used in selected patients. This technique requires special equipment and experience, but the results are equivalent to surgery and can preserve the sphincter muscle.

Five-Year Survival 85 to 95 percent

Investigational
• Use of oral 5-FU prodrugs and/or oxaliplatin (Eloxatin) in combination with radiation
• Novel surgical techniques

■ *Stage II (Dukes' B2, B3)*
TNM T3–4, N0, M0
A Stage II cancer has penetrated all layers of the bowel wall with or without extension to adjacent tissues (uterus, ovaries, or prostate), but has not spread to lymph nodes. T3 tumors extend through the bowel wall; T4 tumors involve adjacent structures such as the uterus, ovaries, bladder, and prostate.

Standard Treatment Stage II rectal cancer is highly treatable and often curable. There are several options for treatment:

• Wide surgical excision with abdominoperineal resection or low-anterior resection followed by adjuvant chemoradiation therapy.
• Bulky tumors or tumors near the anus are generally treated with preoperative (neoadjuvant) chemoradiation followed by surgical resection in an attempt to preserve sphincter function. In addition, long-term bowel function may be superior after neoadjuvant chemoradiation compared to postoperative treatment, hence a trend toward preoperative treatment in any patient with evidence for probable T3–4 or lymph node–positive disease. Since accurate pathological staging is difficult after neoadjuvant therapy, most patients also receive additional 5-FU–based chemotherapy postoperatively.

Five-Year Survival 30 to 70 percent (50 to 70 percent for T3, N0; 30 percent for T4, N0)

Investigational
- Neoadjuvant hyperfractionated radiotherapy.
- Radiation during surgery (intraoperative radiation therapy) is being evaluated for locally advanced disease.
- Identification of molecular markers with prognostic significance.
- A novel stapling device to join the ends of the bowel may allow the surgeon to perform a low-anterior resection in some patients with low rectal cancers (sphincter-sparing).
- Laparoscopic surgery and other novel surgical techniques.
- Studies exploring the relative contributions of systemic chemotherapy and chemoradiation in the treatment of patients with completely resected rectal cancer (margins negative).
- Use of oxaliplatin (Eloxatin), irinotecan (Camptosar, CPT-11), and/or oral fluoropyrimidines (capecitabine [Xeloda]), alone or in combination with radiation, in the adjuvant or neoadjuvant setting.
- Use of biologically based therapies such as bevacizumab (Avastin) and EGFR inhibitors in the adjuvant or neoadjuvant setting.
- Studies exploring the optimal timing of resection after neoadjuvant chemoradiation.

■ *Stage III (Dukes' C1, 2, 3)*
TNM Any T, N1–2, M0
The cancer has spread within or outside the rectum and one or more lymph nodes are involved. N1 means that up to three lymph nodes are involved; N2 means that four or more lymph nodes are positive.

Standard Treatment The number of lymph nodes that are involved has prognostic significance in rectal cancer. Overall, there is a 50 percent chance of recurrence with this stage of disease. The 1990 Consensus Conference on Colon and Rectal Cancer noted that if one to four lymph nodes are positive, 55 to 60 percent of patients will be cured with surgery alone; if five or more nodes are positive, only 33 percent will be cured with surgery alone. Based on these data, adjuvant/neoadjuvant chemoradiation and adjuvant 5-FU–based chemotherapy is standard for this stage of disease.

Standard treatment for rectal cancer involves surgical resection plus adjuvant chemotherapy and radiation. Chemoradiation may be given either pre- or postoperatively. There is a trend to treat patients with fixed or bulky tumors with neoadjuvant (preoperative) chemoradiation. For tumors near the anus, chemoradiation therapy followed by surgery may allow the sphincter function to be preserved. In general, patients with rectal cancer involving the lymph nodes are also offered several additional cycles of 5-FU–based chemotherapy after recovering from surgery and radiation.

Removal of rectal cancer near the anus requires an APR and permanent colostomy. In contrast, tumors in the upper rectum can often be resected without compromising sphincter function (LAR); the proximal bowel is reconnected to the anus (coloanal anastomosis). When adjacent organs are involved, removal of the pelvic organs (pelvic exenteration) may be necessary to completely remove all of the cancer.

Five-Year Survival 30 to 70 percent (depending on the number of lymph nodes involved and the extent of invasion through the bowel wall)

Investigational See Stage II Rectal Cancer.

■ *Stage IV (Dukes' D)*
TNM Any T, any N, M1
The cancer has spread outside the rectum to distant areas, including organs such as the liver and lungs. The approach to treatment in patients with metastatic rectal cancer is very similar to that of patients with advanced colon cancer (see Stage IV colon cancer).

Standard Treatment Treatment is basically directed toward palliation, although there can be long-term disease-free survival if isolated metastases in the liver or lung can be removed.

Surgical Options Even in the setting of metastatic disease, palliative resection of the primary tumor should be considered in order to treat or prevent complications such as pain, obstruction, and bleeding. In addition to systemic chemotherapy, radiation is an option for treatment of local disease that can't be removed. The relative benefits need to be compared to the potential impact on quality of life in the face of incurable distant disease. In some cases, obstructing tumors may be bypassed instead of removed (diverting colostomy).

Resection of isolated liver, ovary, or lung metastases should be entertained and can lead to a long-term cure in roughly 25 to 30 percent of patients. Liver metastases can be removed or ablated at the same time the primary rectal cancer is resected in selected cases.

Chemotherapy See Stage IV colon cancer.

Five-Year Survival 5 percent, rising to 20 to 30 percent if liver or lung metastases can be removed surgically

Investigational See Stage IV colon cancer.

Treatment Follow-Up

Rectal cancer has a much higher rate of local recurrence than colon cancer. Close follow-up may lead to the earlier diagnosis of recurrent disease and improved treatment. After definitive treatment for rectal cancer, patients should be followed regularly for evidence of recurrent disease. The interval between appointments gradually increases after two years, but regularly scheduled visits should continue for at least five years.

• History and physical examination every three to four months initially.

• Obtaining a chest X-ray every six to twelve months for five years should be considered. Isolated lung metastases are much more likely to occur in patients with rectal cancer than in patients with colon cancer.

• Complete blood count and liver function tests every three months.

• Blood CEA level every three to four months, since the CEA level may rise before other clinical, X-ray, or laboratory tests are suggestive of tumor recurrence. If the CEA rises above normal, about one-third of patients may have a recurrent tumor that can be totally removed with surgery and so may be cured.

• CT scans of the abdomen and pelvis if a patient's symptoms, physical examination, or laboratory studies suggest recurrent disease (surveillance CT scans every six to twelve months in the case of Stage II rectal cancer or greater should be considered).

• Colonoscopy every one to three years depending on whether or not additional polyps are discovered.

Recurrent Rectal Cancer

Rectal cancer can recur locally or often in the liver or lungs, and it is important to determine if the recurrence is only local or metastatic. Treatment depends on the site of recurrence as defined by physical and X-ray examinations and scans.

• Local recurrence in the rectum or isolated metastases to the liver or lung can sometimes be surgically removed, possibly leading to a cure or significantly prolonged survival.

• Patients who develop recurrent disease more than six months after completion of adjuvant chemotherapy are often treated with the same 5-FU–based regimen again. Recurrent disease that occurs less than six months after adjuvant therapy is generally considered chemotherapy-resistant and an alternative regimen is employed.

Standard Treatment Removal of isolated lung or liver metastases may be done in selected cases. The five-year survival rate for patients with solitary metastases exceeds 20 percent. The chances for cure are improved when there are only two or three metastases to be removed. Noncurative removal provides no benefits to patients who have no symptoms, since survival is not affected.

Both palliative radiation therapy and palliative chemotherapy may be given for recurrent disease (see Stage IV colon cancer).

Investigational See Stage IV colon cancer.

The Most Important Questions You Can Ask If You Have Colorectal Cancer

- What is the stage of my cancer?
- What is my prognosis?
- Do I need surgery? How extensive does my surgery need to be? Will I need a colostomy? Will it be permanent?
- Will I need adjuvant or neoadjuvant chemotherapy?
- Do I need radiation? Should it be delivered before or after surgery? Will it be combined with chemotherapy?
- Will adjuvant chemotherapy or radiation increase my chance of being cured?
- What treatment-related side effects am I likely to experience?
- Will there be any long-term side effects from my treatment (surgery, chemotherapy, or radiation)?
- Are my children or other relatives at higher risk for colorectal cancer?
- How will I know if I am cured? What kind of follow-up will you be doing after my therapy?
- How are chemotherapy, surgery, and radiation used in the setting of metastatic disease? What are the goals of therapy?
- What clinical trials might be appropriate?
- What will happen if I don't have the suggested treatment?

Summary: Treatment of Colorectal Cancer

1. Stage I Colon and Rectal Cancer

No adjuvant therapy is warranted, since there is a low risk of recurrence (except in the setting of a transanal excision for T2, N0 rectal cancer).

2. Stage II Colon Cancer

Specific adjuvant therapy cannot be recommended routinely for low-risk tumors outside a clinical trial. Patients whose tumors have poor prognostic features are often considered candidates for adjuvant chemotherapy. All patients should consider enrollment in a clinical trial.

3. Stage III Colon Cancer

There is a high risk for recurrence, and treatment with 5-FU–based chemotherapy is recommended (alone or in combination with oxaliplatin [Eloxatin]). Capecitabine (Xeloda) is an acceptable alternative to 5-FU/LV alone. Enrollment in clinical trials is encouraged.

4. Stages II and III Rectal Cancer

Adjuvant or neoadjuvant radiotherapy and chemotherapy (chemoradiation) is recommended to improve local control and survival. Systemic 5-FU–based chemotherapy (outside the context of radiation) is also recommended. Enrollment in clinical trials is encouraged.

5. Stage IV Colorectal Cancer

Resection of metastatic deposits can be curative in selected cases. In the absence of resectable disease, treatment with palliative chemotherapy with or without bevacizumab (Avastin) should be considered. Use of an EGFR inhibitor should be considered in patients with chemotherapy-refractory disease. Participation in clinical trials is appropriate. Radiation is used to control local symptoms (e.g., those related to pelvic disease or bone metastases). Because of the potential problems related to leaving the primary tumor in place (including bleeding, obstruction, and perforation), resection of the affected segment of bowel should be considered even in patients with metastatic disease. The relative benefits need to be weighed against the potential impact on quality of life in the face of incurable distant disease. In some cases, obstructing tumors may be bypassed instead of removed (diverting colostomy).

A Prevention Program for Colorectal Cancer

Seven Steps to Lowering Your Risk of Colorectal Cancer

1. Get regular colorectal cancer screening tests beginning at age fifty. If you have a personal or family history of colorectal cancer or colorectal polyps, or a personal history of another cancer or inflammatory bowel disease, talk to your health care provider about earlier screening tests. Based on the available data, many health care providers consider colonoscopy the preferred screening test because of its accuracy in detecting polyps and its ability to remove polyps before cancer occurs.

2. Eat a diet rich in fruits and vegetables and whole grains from breads, cereals, nuts, and beans. Include sources of calcium such as low-fat milk products. Although the data on adding fiber supplements to the diet to prevent colon cancer or polyps has been disappointing, there remains suggestive data that dietary fiber may be protective over the long term.

3. Eat a diet low in red or prepared meats and fat.

4. Eat foods containing folate such as leafy green vegetables.

5. If you use alcohol, drink only in moderation. Alcohol and tobacco in combination are linked to colorectal cancer and other gastrointestinal cancers.

6. If you use tobacco, quit. If you don't use tobacco, don't start.

7. Exercise for at least twenty minutes, three to four days each week. Moderate exercise such as walking, gardening, and climbing steps may help you reduce your risk.

Additional Points to Discuss with Your Health Care Provider

- Consider supplements of vitamins and minerals such as folate and calcium, which may regulate the growth rate of the cells that line the colon.

- Consider the use of daily aspirin, especially if you have already had polyps or colorectal cancer.

Esophagus

Andrew H. Ko, M.D., Kevin G. Billingsley, M.D., David R. Byrd, M.D.,
Ernest H. Rosenbaum, M.D., Carlos A. Pellegrini, M.D.,
Malin Dollinger, M.D., and Daphne A. Haas-Kogan, M.D.

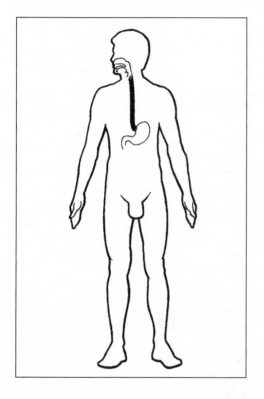

The first recorded case of esophageal cancer was described in China 2,000 years ago. It was called *ye ge*, which seems to have been a polite way of referring to difficult swallowing (dysphagia) and belching. It is a treatable and sometimes curable cancer, although most patients have a poor prognosis because the cancer is usually advanced by the time symptoms appear.

Special attention to good nutrition is an important part of treatment, especially since people in good physical condition with minimal weight loss have a better prognosis. Overall five-year survival for cases amenable to surgery is in the range of 15 to 25 percent; however, only 25 to 40 percent of cases are amenable to surgery. Earlier diagnosis and treatment can improve survival. Recent improvements in radiation therapy and chemotherapy results are somewhat encouraging.

Esophageal cancer is relatively uncommon in the United States, with an estimated 15,560 new cases in 2007, and approximately 13,940 deaths. It is responsible for less than 1 percent of all cancers and for 6 percent of gastrointestinal cancers.

Types Fifty percent of esophageal cancers appear in the cells lining the esophageal tube (squamous cells), usually in the upper two-thirds of the esophagus. About 50 percent develop in the glands (adenocarcinoma) in the lower third. One to 2 percent are relatively rare tumors, such as melanomas, primary lymphomas, and tumors in the smooth muscles, among others.

Whereas the incidence of squamous cell cancer has been declining in the United States, the number of patients with esophageal adenocarcinomas has been increasing over the past several decades. In particular, cancers located at the bottom end of the esophagus, right at the junction between the esophagus and the stomach, have become much more frequent. These cancers, known as GE (gastroesophageal) junction cancers, are sometimes classified as esophageal cancers, sometimes as gastric cancers, and sometimes as their own unique entity. Reasons for this trend may include the increased incidence of obesity and reflux disease (heartburn), which predispose individuals to a precancerous condition called Barrett's esophagus.

How It Spreads Carcinoma of the esophagus usually starts on the surface layer, invades the surrounding tissue, and grows to cause an obstruction that makes swallowing difficult. It spreads through the lymph system to lymph nodes. The most common sites for metastases are the lymph nodes, lungs, liver, brain, adrenal glands, and bone.

What Causes It Alcohol and tobacco abuse are the most common causes of esophageal squamous cell cancer in North America. Contributing factors in other parts of the world include exposure to environmental carcinogens such as nitrosamines and diets deficient in riboflavin, magnesium, nicotinic acid, and zinc. Betel nut chewing and *bidi* smoking are major factors in India.

For esophageal adenocarcinomas, the primary cause is inflammation of the lower portion of the esophagus related to a chronic backup (reflux) of stomach acid with bile (gastric reflux) causing

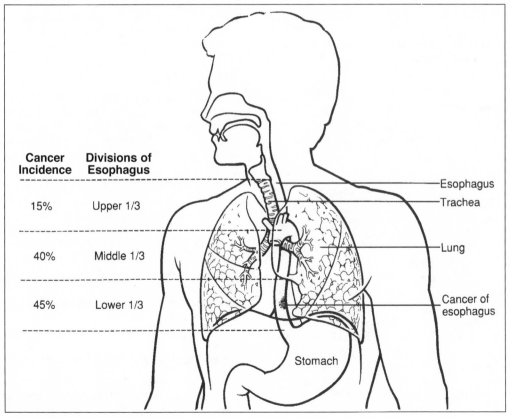

The esophagus and nearby organs

"heartburn." This may also develop from a malfunction of the gastroesophageal valve. The cellular changes (called metaplasia) that result from long-term bathing of the esophageal lining with stomach acid is referred to as Barrett's esophagus. Barrett's is a precancerous condition in which the normal squamous lining of the esophagus is replaced by glandular (columnar) epithelium resembling the intestines.

Who Gets It Esophageal cancer is much more prevalent in China, Singapore, Iran, Puerto Rico, Switzerland, and France than in North America. On this continent, it is most prevalent among men over sixty, smokers, drinkers, and blacks. In the United States, men with esophageal cancer outnumber women by more than 3 to 1. The incidence of squamous cell cancers is higher in blacks than in whites, while the reverse is true for adenocarcinomas.

Risk Factors

At Significantly Higher Risk for Squamous Cell Cancers of the Esophagus

- Men over sixty.
- Long-term drinkers, especially in whites.
- Long-term smokers (more common in blacks than in whites).
- Smokers who drink alcohol (more common in blacks than in whites).
- Other causes of esophageal injury, such as lye ingestion and, possibly, long-term consumption of very hot beverages.
- Diets low in fruits, vegetables, and certain vitamins and minerals (vitamin E, beta-carotene, selenium).
- Individuals with esophageal muscle spasm (achalasia) or chronic stricture.
- Human papillomavirus (HPV) in certain parts of the world, such as Asia and South Africa.

At Significantly Higher Risk for Adenocarcinomas of the Esophagus

- A known diagnosis of Barrett's esophagus. Individuals with Barrett's esophagus confirmed by endoscopy have a 30- to 125-fold increased risk of developing esophageal adenocarcinoma compared to the general population at large.
- Obesity. According to one study, the risk of developing esophageal adenocarcinoma was almost three times higher for individuals in the highest 25 percent of body mass index compared to those in the lowest 25 percent.
- Long-standing gastroesophageal reflux disease (GERD), especially manifested by reflux/heartburn symptoms at least once a week and occurring at night.
- Poor diet (similar to that seen in esophageal squamous cell cancers).

Screening

Screening is not routinely performed in North America because of the low incidence of esophageal cancer. But high-risk individuals (such as those with Barrett's esophagus) should undergo regular screening by upper endoscopy (also called esophagogastroduodenoscopy, or EGD for short). This procedure should be performed anywhere from once every three to six months to once every two to three years, depending on the severity of the Barrett's. Patients with Barrett's esophagus may be cured if treated when premalignant (high-grade dysplasia) or mucosal (noninvasive) malignant changes are detected.

Common Signs and Symptoms

The most common symptom of esophageal cancer—occurring in 90 percent of patients—is difficulty or pain in swallowing foods and liquids (dysphagia). Other symptoms include weight loss, which can be severe (cachexia), heartburn, hoarseness, pain in the throat or back, vocal cord paralysis, pneumonia, and coughing up blood.

Diagnosis

Physical Examination

• Enlarged lymph nodes, particularly over the left collarbone.
• The vocal cords may be less mobile or paralyzed.
• Tapping the spinal area may cause pain in the vertebrae.
• Rarely, thickening and scaling of the palms and soles.

Blood and Other Tests

• Cells for analysis similar to a Pap smear cytology may be scraped off a swallowed balloon or obtained with a brush inserted through an endoscope or a nasogastric tube.
• Blood counts and serum chemistry profile.
• Serum liver function tests to measure alkaline phosphatase, bilirubin, transaminases, and LDH. Elevated levels may suggest metastases to the liver or bone.
• An elevated CEA (carcinoembryonic antigen) may indicate liver metastases.
• Analysis of cell DNA and DNA histograms (flow cytometry) as well as molecular biological alterations are under evaluation as investigational diagnostic tools and may help identify patients with Barrett's esophagus who are about to develop cancer. Preliminary data suggest that a tumor with abnormal chromosomes has a poorer prognosis.

Imaging

• A barium swallow and X-ray of the esophagus may reveal abnormalities suggestive of an esophageal tumor.
• A chest X-ray can detect masses in the midchest area and the lungs.

• CT scans of the chest and abdomen can often identify the location, size, and depth of penetration of the tumor through the wall of the esophagus (T stage), as well as surrounding lymph nodes (N stage). However, endoscopic ultrasound (below) is a more accurate tool to assess T and N staging. CT scans can also evaluate for the presence or absence of metastatic lesions (e.g., in the liver or lungs).
• Endoscopic ultrasound (EUS) is a specialized procedure in which a gastroenterologist places a long flexible tube down the patient's throat, similar to a regular upper endoscopy. However, in EUS, an ultrasound probe is present on the end of the tube, which allows for visualization and accurate assessment of the size and depth of the tumor's invasion of the esophagus, as well as evaluation of the status of nearby lymph nodes.
• Positron-emission tomography (PET) scans are often used as part of the staging evaluation, especially to look for the presence of metastases.

Endoscopy and Biopsy

• Upper endoscopy is the key test because it allows both visualization and biopsy. A flexible fiber-optic tube is passed through the mouth and down the esophagus. A piece of tissue may be removed with forceps (punch biopsy and cytology). Twenty-five to 40 percent of patients have a narrowing of the esophagus, which does not permit an endoscope to be passed, so an esophageal dilation may be needed.
• For tumors near the place where the trachea (central air passage) divides into the right and left bronchi, it is advisable to include bronchoscopy to evaluate whether the tumor has eroded through the esophagus into the airway.
• A mediastinoscopy (inspection of the center of the chest through a thin telescope) may be needed occasionally to assist in staging, for biopsy, and to help decide on surgery.

Staging

The TNM classification system is used to describe the stage, referring to the depth of penetration through the esophageal wall (T stage), the involvement of lymph nodes near the esophagus (N stage), and the presence or absence of metastases (M stage). Clinical staging is typically arrived at through a combination of CT scanning, endoscopic ultrasound (if available), and sometimes PET scan. Laparoscopy (a minimally invasive surgical procedure in which a camera is placed in the abdomen to evaluate the abdominal contents) is used on the rare occasion. Precise staging can truly be made only from an operation in which the esophageal tumor and regional lymph nodes are removed.

Treatment Overview

The treatment of esophageal cancer typically involves a multimodality approach, in which any one or a combination of different strategies—radiation therapy, surgery, chemotherapy—are used.

Surgery Since most patients in North America have advanced (Stage III) esophageal cancer before diagnosis, only 25 to 40 percent have tumors that can be removed in an attempt at cure. Before surgery, an evaluation for metastases is performed.

Radical surgery for cure involves removing the entire esophagus (or a good part of it) and the surrounding tissues and lymph nodes. If the lesion is in the lower esophagus near the stomach, the top of the stomach has to be removed as well. Once the esophagus is removed, the stomach can be brought all the way up to bridge the gap (esophagogastrostomy). A portion of the colon may be used instead. This operation is rather demanding of both patient and surgeon. It should be performed only in major medical centers because complex care will be needed during and after surgery.

Mortality ranges from 5 to 10 percent, but the removal of the esophagus relieves swallowing problems in over 90 percent of patients and is imperative for a chance of cure.

Tumors in the upper half of the esophagus may have invaded the trachea or larynx, so reconstruction (with a high risk of complications) will be required.

In patients with Barrett's esophagus who appear to be at very high risk for development of cancer, the esophagus may be removed as a prophylactic (preventive) measure.

Radiation Therapy Radiation therapy is used in several different settings for esophageal cancer. It is typically used concurrently with chemotherapy, as the combination of chemotherapy and radiation produces higher rates of response and better patient outcomes than radiation alone. The settings in which radiation is used include (1) before a planned operation (in combination with chemotherapy), to shrink the cancer; (2) for the definitive treatment of esophageal cancer (also in combination with chemotherapy), in patients who are not good operative candidates; and (3) for palliation, in patients who have obstructive symptoms or active bleeding from their tumor that is difficult to control (either with or without concurrent chemotherapy). Side effects of radiation therapy can include a short-term inflammation of the esophagus and the development of a benign stricture (30 percent), which can be dilated.

Very precise treatment planning using an X-ray simulator is important for the best results, with CT scans used to plan treatments accurately. This involves lying on a flat table, similar to that of an actual radiation therapy machine, and drinking

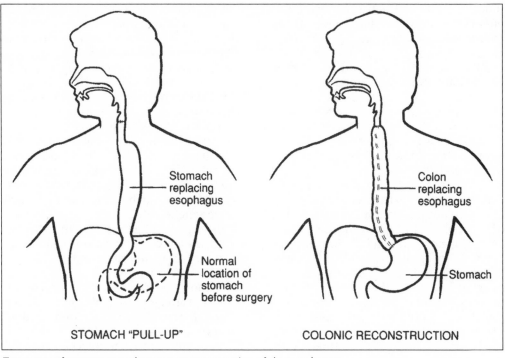

Two types of surgery to replace a cancerous portion of the esophagus

oral contrast (which may taste like a sour milkshake). The radiation oncologist will then take simulation films. He or she will transfer the tumor volume from the CT scans, endoscopic ultrasound, and oral contrast onto the simulation films in order to set up a daily treatment port. This will include the primary tumor, draining lymph nodes, and a margin of healthy tissue.

Intraluminal radiation using a radiation source placed inside the esophagus (intraluminal brachytherapy) may complement external radiation in some circumstances, typically as part of palliative treatment. A radiation source (iridium-192) is inserted into the esophagus and left at the tumor site for several hours. Side effects can include inflammation of the esophagus, bleeding, and a hole from the esophagus into the lungs (esophago-bronchial fistula).

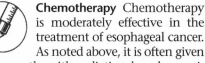 **Chemotherapy** Chemotherapy is moderately effective in the treatment of esophageal cancer.

As noted above, it is often given concurrently with radiation based on evidence that combined chemotherapy and radiation is superior to radiation by itself. The combination of two drugs, cisplatin (Platinol) and 5-fluorouracil, is the most commonly used chemotherapy regimen administered together with radiation; however, other chemotherapy agents and newer targeted therapies have also been looked at and are currently being evaluated.

Giving chemotherapy with or without radiation therapy prior to an operation for esophageal cancer (referred to as neoadjuvant therapy) remains a controversial issue. Many studies have examined this question, comparing preoperative chemotherapy and/or radiation followed by surgery, versus surgery alone. A few of these studies have shown a survival advantage by giving the preoperative treatment, but most of them have failed to demonstrate any difference. Thus, this remains an important study question. Tumors of the gastroesophageal junction are sometimes treated as esophageal cancers and sometimes as stomach cancers; in the latter case, surgery is often performed first, then chemotherapy and radiation are delivered after the patient has recovered from the operation (see the chapter "Stomach").

Chemotherapy is also given for individuals with more extensive, advanced disease, such as those with metastases. Many different chemotherapy agents have been used, alone and in combination, including platinum agents (cisplatin, carboplatin [Paraplatin], oxaliplatin [Eloxatin]), fluoropyrmidines (5-FU, capecitabine [Xeloda]), taxanes (paclitaxel [Taxol], docetaxel [Taxotere]), irinotecan (Camptosar, CPT-11), and epirubicin (Ellence), among others. In general, using two or three drugs in combination produces higher response rates than using single drugs, although this has not been definitively proven to translate into longer survival time. Furthermore, combination regimens, predictably, are associated with greater toxicities, and so quality-of-life issues need to be balanced out.

 Palliation Symptoms associated with the esophageal tumor, most commonly obstruction of the esophagus resulting in difficulty and discomfort with swallowing, can often be managed using the previously described modalities. For example, sometimes patients with moderate swallowing difficulties experience significant relief after starting chemotherapy, or with a short course of radiation. An aggressive operation purely for the goal of palliating symptoms (as opposed to trying to remove all disease) should be undertaken with caution, given that the other options available to patients are less invasive.

Mechanical dilation, most commonly using a balloon dilator, can be used to open up areas of esophageal narrowing due to tumor, or due to benign strictures that develop following an operation or postradiation. Esophageal rupture is an infrequent but serious complication of dilation. Esophageal stenting is another approach that can be used to palliate obstructive symptoms that develop from esophageal cancer. A stent is placed by a gastroenterologist (or, less commonly, by an interventional radiologist) via endoscopy. Stents may be either plastic (which have a higher rate of migrating to a wrong location after they are placed) or metallic; they are compressed onto a delivery catheter and then deployed (expanded) once in the correct location.

Endoscopic laser therapy (ELT), administered through a flexible tube inserted through the mouth, has been used to relieve swallowing problems. Lasers can vaporize the tumor and cut a hole through a blockage in the esophagus, although the hole will last only a few weeks to three months. The procedure can be repeated to keep the obstruction open, but repeated laser treatments may be more difficult. With laser therapy, there are dangers of perforation, bleeding, and fistula formation. Also, lasers can treat tumors only inside the esophagus, not tumors outside the esophageal wall (see chapter 10, "Laser Therapy"). More recently, a newer technique called photodynamic therapy incorporates the intravenous administration of hematoporphyrin derivatives (photosensitizing drugs) with laser therapy to palliate symptoms of dysphagia, as well as obliterate Barrett's esophagus and some early esophageal cancers.

Treatment by Stage

■ *Stage 0*
TNM Tis (tumor or carcinoma in situ)
This very early cancer has not spread below the lining of the first layer of esophageal

tissue. It is unusual for cancer to be found at this stage in Western countries, although it's not unusual in China, where esophageal cancer is seen frequently and screening programs are common.

Standard Treatment Early-stage esophageal cancer can be cured with surgery. Radiotherapy could be an option in poor-risk patients.

Five-Year Survival The prognosis is excellent if the tumor is treated surgically or with radiotherapy.

■ Stage I
TNM T1, N0, M0
The tumor does not penetrate the muscular wall, and there is no spread to lymph nodes, adjacent structures, or other organs. While patients may have some difficulty swallowing, there is usually no obstruction of the esophagus.

Standard Treatment Stage I esophageal cancer is treatable and often curable. Surgical removal of the tumor is the treatment of choice, with the highest success rate for cancer in the lower third of the esophagus. The diseased portion of the esophagus and the adjacent lymph nodes are removed. With surgery, there is a 5 to 10 percent mortality rate and a 15 to 30 percent complication rate.

For individuals who are not operative candidates for some reason, radiation therapy may effectively control and sometimes cure small tumors. As noted previously, the concurrent use of chemotherapy and radiation produces better outcomes than radiation therapy alone.

A newer approach, endoscopic mucosal resection, is being actively investigated as a less aggressive alternative to surgical resection for early-stage esophageal cancers. This is performed using a small cap with a wire loop that fits on the end of the endoscopy tube. The tumor is suctioned into the cap, and the wire loop is closed, snaring the tumor while the area is cauterized to minimize bleeding.

Five-Year Survival 40 to 80 percent

■ Stage IIA
TNM T2–3, N0, M0
■ Stage IIB
TNM T1–2, N1, M0
The cancer has not spread to adjacent organs, but may have spread to regional lymph nodes (Stage IIB).

Standard Treatment Surgery still represents the mainstay of treatment for patients with this stage of disease who are robust enough to sustain a major operation. Cure is still possible in some individuals. The potential for cure has to be counterbalanced by the significant operative risks and perioperative mortality and morbidity, including infection, leak at the surgical anastomosis site (the area where the organs are reattached), vocal cord paralysis, and stricture.

Combination therapy with chemotherapy and radiation is sometimes given prior to surgery, although, as noted above, the benefits of preoperative therapy remain controversial. The choice of chemotherapy agents that can be given in this context is expanding, with the most well-studied regimen being cisplatin and 5-fluorouracil. About 20 percent of patients treated with preoperative chemotherapy plus radiation have had a complete pathologic response at the time of surgery, meaning that no tumor was found at the time they went to operation. Patients who are found to have had a complete pathologic response have a better prognosis than those patients who have a lot of residual tumor at the time of surgery. For some individuals, especially those who are poor operative candidates, chemotherapy plus radiation, without surgery, may be the best option and may still offer the possibility of long-term survival.

Five-Year Survival 25 to 50 percent

■ Stage III

TNM T3–T4, N1, M0 or T4, any N, M0

The tumor has spread outside the esophagus and there is extensive lymph node involvement, but there are no metastases.

Standard Treatment The same treatment strategies apply here as discussed for Stage II disease, with the notable difference that fewer patients will be able to undergo a successful operation. Given the bulky tumor and the presence of multiple lymph nodes, there is usually more of an impetus to start with chemotherapy and radiation before attempting surgical resection, to debulk the tumor and try to eradicate as much of the cancer as possible. Prophylactic placement of a feeding tube for nutritional support is often necessary. For patients who are not appropriate surgical candidates, definitive chemotherapy and radiation is the most common approach and can sometimes produce long-term remissions.

Five-Year Survival 10 to 15 percent

■ Stage IV

TNM Any T, any N, M1

The tumor has spread to other organs (distant metastases).

Standard Treatment Chemotherapy represents the mainstay of care for patients with Stage IV esophageal cancer. As noted in the chemotherapy section above, a variety of chemotherapy agents have been tested in esophageal cancer, both alone and in various combinations, with varying degrees of success. Many of the combination regimens produce similar rates of response, in the range of 30 to 50 percent, each with its own unique schedule and side-effect profile. Regimens should be tailored according to a patient's functional status as well as his or her personal preference (in terms of schedule, intravenous versus oral admin-istration, willingness to accept particular side effects, etc.). For individuals with poorer functional status, single-agent therapy may be more appropriate.

All patients may be considered candidates for investigational protocols evaluating novel approaches to treatment, including promising chemotherapy combinations and new targeted agents in development.

While chemotherapy alone may palliate symptoms effectively, some patients may require other modalities as discussed above, such as radiation, stenting, dilation, and insertion of a feeding tube.

Five-Year Survival Less than 5 percent

Supportive Therapy

People with esophageal tumors often have a poor nutritional status. Attempts to correct weight loss may help reduce the complications of surgery, radiotherapy, chemotherapy, and combined treatments.

• A nasogastric feeding tube (if it can be passed through the obstruction) or a percutaneous (through the skin) feeding tube (gastrostomy or jejunostomy) may be used for enteral nutrition.

• Parenteral hyperalimentation (nutrition given intravenously) may be necessary for support during therapy.

• Esophageal dilation, stenting, or laser therapy to maintain an open esophagus may help maintain nutrition.

Treatment Follow-Up

Patients who have had treatment for cure should visit their physician every few months for close follow-up, including history and physical examination. Laboratory work, imaging studies (chest X-ray and CT scans), and endoscopies can be performed as indicated.

Recurrent Cancer

Depending on the location and extent of disease recurrence, chemotherapy, radiation, and local palliative procedures as described above may be considered in the treatment plan, although the likelihood of cure at this point is remote.

Prevention

• Avoid drinking alcohol and smoking.
• For Barrett's esophagus, it is important to try to heal the esophagitis and prevent the reflux of stomach acids.

Reflux may be managed by using H-2 blockers or proton pump inhibitors to relieve symptoms, by changing the pressure in the lower esophagus with metoclopramide (Reglan), and by not eating for several hours before sleep. Proton-pump inhibitors such as Prilosec (omeprazole), Prevacid (lansoprazole), and Nexium (esomeprazole) may not only help heal esophagitis, but also heal or normalize a Barrett's esophagus. Avoid being overweight and increase intake of fresh fruits and vegetables. Dietary restrictions—avoiding fats, caffeine (coffee), chocolate, and peppermint—and opiates, calcium-channel blockers, and anticholinergic drugs may also help control reflux.

The Most Important Questions You Can Ask

• Do I have squamous cell cancer or adenocarcinoma?
• Am I an appropriate candidate for surgery?
• What kind of surgery will be performed [remember, there are different types of operations for esophageal cancer]? How experienced is my surgeon in performing this type of operation?
• How does my stage of disease relate to the chance for cure?
• If I am being considered for surgery, would you recommend I receive chemotherapy and radiation beforehand?
• How can I obtain nutritional support?

Gallbladder

Alan P. Venook, M.D.

■ ■ ■ ■

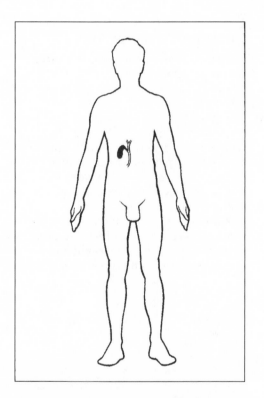

The gallbladder stores bile, which aids in the digestion of fat-containing foods. It is a nonessential organ and can be removed without significant consequences. Gallbladder cancer—also called carcinoma of the gallbladder—is extremely rare. And unless it is very small and found when the gallbladder is removed for other reasons, the treatment now available is not particularly effective.

Because it is so uncommon and because its symptoms mirror those of far more common ailments, cancer of the gallbladder is usually not found until it is at an advanced stage and cannot be surgically removed. In the advanced stages, pain relief and the restoration of normal bile flow from the liver into the intestines are the principal goals of therapy.

Types The majority of gallbladder tumors are found in glandular tissue within the gallbladder (adenocarcinoma). Others originate in the connective tissue (sarcoma) or other tissues (squamous carcinoma). The management for all gallbladder cancer types is the same, always depending upon the extent of the tumor at the time of diagnosis.

How It Spreads Gallbladder cancer tends to spread to nearby tissues and organs such as the liver and intestines. It also spreads through the lymph system to lymph nodes in the region of the liver (porta hepatis). Ultimately, other lymph nodes and organs can become involved.

What Causes It No one factor has been clearly shown to cause gallbladder cancer. Although it occurs most often in people with gallstone disease, it is extremely rare even in such patients. It is not known if bouts of gallstones predispose people to developing this cancer.

Risk Factors

At Significantly Higher Risk About 85 percent of people with gallbladder cancer have a history of gallstones (cholelithiasis). Sometimes, although not often, the

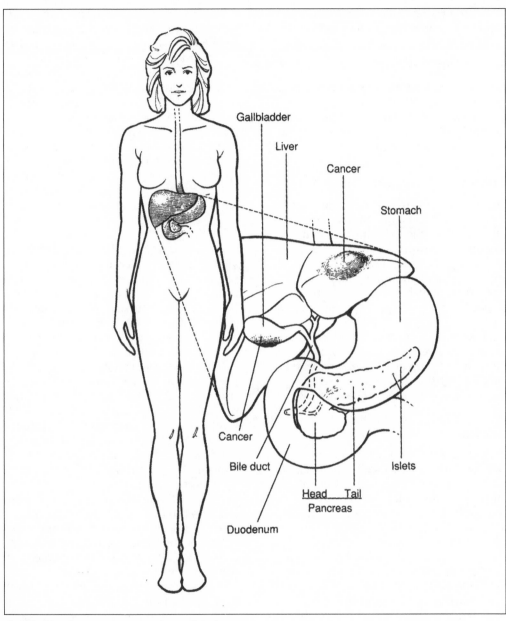

Gallbladder
Liver
Cancer
Stomach
Cancer
Bile duct
Islets
Head   Tail
Pancreas
Duodenum

Gallbladder, liver, pancreas, and associated organs

gallbladder becomes hardened (calcified) from repeated inflammation as gallstones are passed. People with this "porcelain gallbladder" have a higher risk of developing this cancer than do others. The typical patient with gallbladder cancer is an elderly woman with a history of gallbladder problems.

At Slightly Higher Risk Gallstone disease without a "porcelain gallbladder"

Screening

No screening tests are available to detect this cancer at an early stage. But, since the gallbladder isn't essential, people with a calcified gallbladder may consider having it removed as a preventive measure.

Common Signs and Symptoms

There are no clinical signs or symptoms characteristic of gallbladder cancer. Jaundice (the skin turning yellow), bloating, abdominal pain, weight loss, decreasing appetite, fever, nausea, and an enlarging abdominal mass are all signs that may be attributable to gallbladder cancer. Frequently, jaundice is a late development and the other symptoms have been present for a long time. Itching may result from the buildup in the skin of a derivative of bile, bilirubin, which turns the skin yellow. This symptom usually reflects advanced disease.

Diagnosis

Physical Examination There are no specific findings for gallbladder cancer on physical examination. Even if the following were found, gallbladder cancer would still not be the prime suspect because it is so uncommon:

- Fever.
- Tender mass below the ribs on the right side of the abdomen.
- Enlarged, hard lymph nodes.
- Jaundice (the skin turning yellow).
- Swelling of the legs (edema).

Blood and Other Tests Diagnostic tests are notoriously inaccurate in their ability to pinpoint gallbladder cancer before surgery. A standard evaluation, however, would include the following:

- A complete blood test, which may be normal or may reveal a decrease in hemoglobin (anemia). The white blood cell count may be normal or increased.
- Liver function tests may be abnormal. The most likely abnormalities are in the serum bilirubin and alkaline phosphatase, indicating a blockage in the bile duct leaving either the liver or the gallbladder.
- Prothrombin time and partial thromboplastin time (PT and PTT) are tests of clotting that may reveal a disorder in patients with poor liver function related to a blocked bile duct.

Imaging

- An abdominal ultrasound study to view the gallbladder area without exposure to X-rays can confirm that the gallbladder wall has thickened and provide information about the size and characteristics of any mass in the region.
- Swallowing pills with dye that travels to the gallbladder, enabling it to be seen on X-ray (oral cholecystography), or the injection of dye into the bile ducts through the skin followed by an X-ray of the area (percutaneous cholangiography) may be done because of symptoms or an elevated serum bilirubin level. While both studies may document an abnormality within the bile ducts or gallbladder, neither can reliably distinguish between inflammation of the gallbladder (cholecystitis) and gallbladder cancer.
- A CT scan may help determine the extent of the tumor within the gallbladder bed and the possible involvement of other organs.
- Magnetic resonance imaging (MRI) may be helpful in determining if the cancer can be surgically removed, but it is usually not necessary because the CT scan shows similar information.
- If the diagnosis of cancer is confirmed or suspected, a chest X-ray should be obtained. A finding of tumor nodules in the lungs would mean that the disease is already metastatic.

Biopsy If cancer is suspected in a situation not involving gallbladder surgery for other reasons, a biopsy, either with a fine needle (FNA) or regular needle, is always required. This can be done through the skin without significant danger. The tumor cells are characteristic and may enable evaluation of whether surgery should be performed if the other studies suggest that the tumor has spread.

Staging

A TNM staging system exists for gallbladder cancer, but for the purposes of deciding on which therapeutic option to use, there are only three stages—localized resectable, localized unresectable, and advanced disease.

Treatment Overview

Gallbladder cancer can be cured only when it is localized enough to be removed surgically. Unfortunately, virtually the only people with such localized disease are those whose cancer is found unexpectedly when the gallbladder is removed for other reasons.

The goal of the diagnostic work-up is to determine if the cancer can be entirely removed. This is rarely possible because the tumor usually spreads to local regions early in its course. More effective chemotherapy and radiation therapy than are available today are under investigation. These treatments are occasionally useful to relieve symptoms related to the cancer. Although patients with advanced gallbladder cancer have a poor prognosis, measures can be taken to maintain the quality of life.

 Surgery Surgery is the only possible cure. If there is no distant tumor spread, the gallbladder as well as the draining lymph nodes and a wedge of normal underlying liver tissue may be removed. This may cure a patient, can help relieve symptoms, and may improve the quality of life.

If a gallbladder cancer is found unexpectedly in the pathology specimen after surgery performed for problems not thought to involve cancer, a second operation may be required. If the tumor is limited to only the superficial layers of the gallbladder, observation may be adequate. If the cancer has spread into the surrounding tissues, lymph nodes, or blood vessels, however, a second operation may be performed to remove those other tissues.

When the tumor cannot fully be removed, it may still be necessary to create a drainage system for the bile from the obstructed gallbladder or bile ducts. This may require surgery, although draining the gallbladder by a tube placed through the skin by a radiologist or through a tube in the stomach and small intestine usually suffices.

The presence of tumor anywhere else in the body—in the lung(s), bone, or lymph nodes, for example—is a clear indication that surgery will not be curative. If the disease has already spread, there is rarely a need to remove a gallbladder cancer, for such surgery involves a difficult recovery period and so may be more damaging to the patient.

Chemotherapy Studies have not yet shown that chemotherapy can prolong the survival of patients with gallbladder cancer. The standard drugs used— 5-fluorouracil, capecitabine (Xeloda), and gemcitabine (Gemzar)—may cause tumor shrinkage in 20 to 25 percent of patients. Even with tumor shrinkage, however, patients may be in a worse condition afterward because the tumor usually regrows quickly and the treatments have some side effects.

There is no proven role for adjuvant chemotherapy after a cancerous gallbladder has been removed, but it is logical to consider chemotherapy. In the hope of finding drugs that may work better than the chemotherapy now used, patients should be entered into clinical trials if chemotherapy is planned.

Radiation The usefulness of radiation in gallbladder cancer is limited by the damage it causes to the surrounding noncancerous liver tissue. Radiation may help patients who have small bits of tumor remaining after surgery or those who have had large tumors removed.

Patients who are not candidates for surgery may also benefit from radiation to the gallbladder area, although they are still likely to have recurrent tumors. The toxicity of such radiation may also worsen existing symptoms such as nausea and loss of appetite.

Combined Therapy The combination of external-beam radiation and chemotherapy may play a role after surgery, perhaps prolonging the period before the cancer returns or even curing people who have undergone surgery without complete tumor removal. This treatment is still being studied.

Treatment by Stage

■ Localized Resectable
In this stage, the cancer is confined to the superficial layers (mucosa and submucosa) of the gallbladder. Cancers at this limited stage are generally found when the gallbladder is removed because of other problems.

Standard Treatment Experts disagree over the extent of surgery needed for a localized gallbladder cancer. Studies are ongoing, but most experts would recommend

- removal of the gallbladder,
- a lymph node dissection of all the draining lymphatic vessels in the region, and

- the removal of a wedge of about 1½ inches (4 cm) of apparently normal liver.

Such surgery is the most likely treatment to render a patient cancer-free. If the cancer is not recognized until after surgery, the need for a second operation is considered. A patient with a truly limited cancer (superficial) may just be observed closely, but because of the poor prognosis should the cancer recur, it is difficult to argue against the aggressive approach outlined above.

Five-Year Survival About 80 percent. Those with cancers that are still very small but cause symptoms have a somewhat lower five-year survival rate.

Investigational

- There is no certain role for adjuvant chemotherapy. Although chemotherapy such as 5-fluorouracil (5-FU) or mitomycin-C is often recommended, no studies have shown that the chance of cure can be increased.
- Radiation is often given to the liver area after surgery but has never been proven to be beneficial.
- The use of a combination of 5-FU and radiation therapy following complete removal of the cancer is now being studied.

■ Localized Unresectable
Despite being a localized mass, the tumor cannot be removed because of the particular way it has spread to local lymph nodes or adjacent liver tissue.

Standard Treatment There is no standard treatment. Patients should be considered for clinical trials aimed at prolonging survival and relieving the symptoms associated with the tumor.

Two-Year Survival Less than 5 percent

Investigational Protocols designed to test the additive benefit of combining radiation with chemotherapy are ongoing.

■ *Advanced*
The cancer has metastasized to distant sites.

Standard Treatment No standard therapy is known to prolong survival in patients with advanced gallbladder cancer. The usual approach is a trial of chemotherapy with a single agent such as 5-FU, capecitabine (Xeloda), or gemcitabine (Gemzar). Even if the tumor shrinks, patients may not benefit because of the side effects of the chemotherapy and because the tumor usually regrows very quickly.

Two-Year Survival Less than 1 percent

Investigational Combination chemotherapy or new drugs may prove to be better in the treatment of advanced gallbladder cancer than therapies now available. Because the side effects are likely to be greater than those caused by single-agent chemotherapy, such treatment should be done in a clinical protocol.

Treatment Follow-Up

Careful follow-up is important after the removal of a localized gallbladder cancer, although once a recurrent tumor is large enough to be seen on an X-ray, it is probably too large to be cured. Follow-up should include CT scans every two to three months for the first year after surgery, since another small tumor may still be resectable at the time of diagnosis.

Supportive Therapy

• Symptoms associated with jaundice can include severe itching and a general sense of poor health. These symptoms can usually be managed with a drainage procedure to bypass the blockage in the biliary tract. This procedure may include the placing of a tube through the skin or through the stomach. Surgery is rarely necessary to bypass an obstruction. If such drainage is ineffective, itching may be relieved by the use of Benadryl, Atarax, or cholestyramine (Questran). For unexplained reasons, the antibiotic rifampin may also alleviate the itching associated with high bilirubin.

• Pain relief may require large doses of medication. Narcotics must be used carefully, however, since they may have excessive side effects and are metabolized by the liver, which may not be working properly.

• Nonsteroidal anti-inflammatory drugs may be surprisingly effective even against the severe pain associated with gallbladder cancer.

• Water pills (diuretics) to reduce fluid in the abdomen or legs may be helpful but may cause significant imbalance in kidney function if not monitored carefully.

• Nausea can be treated with standard medications, including suppositories.

• Sleep disturbances are common, but sleeping pills should be used carefully, since most are metabolized by the liver.

• Frequent small meals may be necessary, since an abdominal mass may reduce the size of the stomach.

• Patients with severe loss of appetite may be helped by an appetite-stimulating drug called megestrol acetate (Megace).

The Most Important Questions You Can Ask

• Should I see another physician to confirm that this tumor can or cannot be removed for cure?

• Could I benefit from an investigational therapy available at another institution?

• How sick will the proposed chemotherapy make me relative to its potential benefit?

• Can anything be done to improve the quality of my life?

Gastrointestinal Stromal Tumor

Derrick Wong, M.D., and Andrew H. Ko, M.D.

■ ■ ■ ■

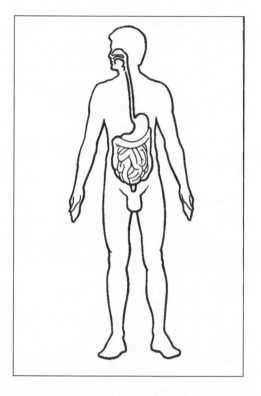

Gastrointestinal stromal tumor (GIST) is a rare malignancy of the gastrointestinal (GI) tract. Unlike the vast majority of GI cancers such as esophagus, stomach, and colon cancers, which come from epithelial cells (cells that form the inner lining of the GI tract), GIST derives from cells in the mesenchymal tissue (nonepithelial cells) and thus falls into the broad family of tumors called soft-tissue sarcomas.

GISTs represent less than 1 percent of all primary GI cancers. A study using the National Cancer Institute Surveillance,

Epidemiology, and End Results (SEER) registry reported less than one case (0.68 case) of GIST per 100,000 people, or about 4,500 to 6,000 total cases annually, in the United States between 1992 and 2000.

Prior to the 1990s, there was much debate as to the type of cell in the GI tract that gave rise to GISTs. In the early 1990s, a significant breakthrough was made when almost all GISTs were discovered to express a protein called c-Kit (also known as CD117). C-Kit belongs to a class of proteins known as kinases that perform crucial functions in regulating the growth of cells. The c-Kit protein is found on the surface of malignant cells that form GISTs. Furthermore, in 80 percent of GISTs, the c-Kit protein contains mutations that render it more active, ultimately resulting in the uncontrolled growth of the malignant cells. The recognition of c-Kit expression as a common feature of GISTs now allows these tumors to be more readily distinguished from other malignancies of the GI tract, such as leiomyosarcomas.

It is now believed that GIST originates from cells in the mesenchymal tissue of the GI tract known as the interstitial cells of Cajal. These cells, which also produce c-Kit, are sometimes described as the "pacemaker" cells of the gut. They have characteristics of both smooth muscle cells and nerve cells and are important in regulating gut contractility (peristalsis), which helps move food through the gastrointestinal tract.

How It Spreads GISTs most frequently occur in the stomach, followed by the small intestine, omentum or mesentery (lining of the abdomen), colon, and esophagus. GISTs usually start in the second layer of the bowel wall and may grow inward (toward the cavity, or lumen, of the bowel, where food passes through) or outward. GISTs typically invade the local surrounding tissues by extension of the primary tumor and metastasize (spread) to distant sites such as the liver and abdominal cavity. GISTs rarely metastasize to the lymph nodes.

What Causes It The exact cause of GIST is unknown. Almost all GISTs express (make) the c-Kit protein on the surface of their cells. In 80 percent of GISTs, a mutation is found in the c-Kit protein that makes it much more active than the normal c-Kit protein. Most often, a mutation is found in a position of the c-Kit gene known as exon 11; less often, a mutation is found in exon 9, 13, or 17. Although the exact mechanism is unknown, it is believed the widespread expression of c-Kit and the presence of c-Kit mutations play a large role in the pathogenesis of GISTs. In rare cases, GISTs do not express the c-Kit protein and instead make a protein called platelet-derived growth factor receptor (PDGFR).

Risk Factors

There are no known risk factors for GIST. The vast majority of GISTs are sporadic (no evidence of inheritance from one generation to the next). However, a few families whose members have a predisposition to developing multiple GISTs have been described. These families were found to have germ line mutations in the c-Kit gene, which get passed on from one generation to the next.

Screening

Due to the low incidence of the disease and the fact that there are no known risk factors, there are no screening programs or recommendations for GIST.

Common Signs and Symptoms

The most common symptom caused by GIST—occurring in 40 percent of cases—is gastrointestinal bleeding, which is manifested as vomiting blood, passage of black tarry stools, or passage of bloody stools, depending on whether the tumor is in the stomach or further down in the intestines. Gastrointestinal bleeding usually causes anemia. When GISTs are large, they can result in bowel obstruction, which causes nausea, vomiting, severe abdominal pain, and constipation.

Diagnosis

The diagnosis of GIST depends on where the tumor is located.

Physical Examination There are few findings on physical examination.

- Paleness, due to anemia.
- Abdominal tenderness, due to bowel obstruction.
- An abdominal mass that can be palpated (felt).
- An enlarged liver (hepatomegaly).
- Fluid in the abdominal cavity (ascites).

Blood and Other Tests

- Fecal occult blood test (test for hidden blood in the stool).
- Complete blood count, which may indicate anemia due to gastrointestinal bleeding.
- Liver function blood tests (transaminases, alkaline phosphatase, bilirubin, and LDH), which may indicate tumor in the liver.
- Levels of serum iron and ferritin, which may indicate anemia.

Imaging

- X-rays of the upper gastrointestinal tract (upper GI series) by standard and double-contrast methods may find GISTs in the esophagus, stomach, and small intestine.

• Chest X-ray can detect tumors that have metastasized to the lungs and the midchest area (mediastinum).

• CT scan of the abdomen detects tumors in the liver and abdominal cavity and, less often, in the stomach, small intestine, and colon. CT scan of the chest detects tumors in the lung and midchest. CT scans define the size and lateral extent of tumors.

• PET scan is a nuclear medicine study that can distinguish whether a mass seen on CT is a GIST, and can occasionally detect tumors that are missed by CT scan. Tumors appear as bright spots on PET scan because they take up the radioactive sugar that is injected into the vein.

• MRI of the abdomen is sometimes used when CT scan with contrast (dye) cannot be used because of allergy to contrast or kidney failure.

Endoscopy and Biopsy

• Esophagoduodenoscopy (EGD) is the key test in the diagnosis of GIST found in the stomach or esophagus. A flexible fiber-optic tube with a camera at the end is passed through the esophagus into the stomach. The entire esophagus and stomach can be visualized with this technique to look for a GIST. If a mass is found in the stomach or esophagus, a piece of tissue from the mass can be biopsied using forceps located at the end of the fiber-optic scope.

• Colonoscopy is similar to EGD except that the flexible fiber-optic scope is passed through the rectum into the colon and is used to visualize the entire colon to look for masses. As in the case of EGD, biopsy of any colonic masses can be obtained during colonoscopy.

• Endoscopic ultrasound is a newer technique that uses an ultrasound probe at the end of an endoscope (such as an EGD) to evaluate the extent of a mass in the stomach or esophagus and to evaluate for any abnormal lymph nodes that may be affected by cancer near the stomach or esophagus.

• CT-guided biopsy is a technique in which a CT scan is used to locate a mass in the chest or abdomen while a needle is simultaneously used to biopsy the mass under the guidance of the CT image. This technique can be used to biopsy a mass in the abdominal cavity that is suspicious for a GIST.

• Pathology review of the tumor samples obtained by biopsy is done by looking at thin sections of the tumor tissue under the microscope. Immunohistochemistry, wherein the tumor tissue is stained by an antibody that recognizes the c-Kit protein, is also performed. Since almost all GISTs express the c-Kit protein, positive staining of the tumor tissue for c-Kit confirms the diagnosis of GIST.

Staging

There is no current staging system for GIST. However, two parameters are often used after removal of a GIST by surgery to determine its aggressiveness and to predict how likely it is to recur. The two parameters are the size of the tumor and its mitotic rate (the number of dividing tumor cells seen under the microscope). Using these two parameters, GISTs are divided into very low risk, low risk, intermediate risk, and high risk.

Treatment Overview

The most important initial treatment decision for patients with GIST is to determine whether the tumor can be completely removed by surgery. If the GIST is not removable by surgery, other treatment options, including targeted therapy, may be considered.

Surgery Surgery is the only realistic means of cure in patients with GIST. Surgery is an option for patients with localized GISTs that have not metastasized to distant sites or invaded adjacent

GIST Risk

RISK	TUMOR SIZE	MITOTIC RATE
Very low risk	< ¾ inch (2 cm)	< 5 per 50 HPF*
Low risk	¾–2 inches (2–5 cm)	< 5 per 50 HPF
Intermediate risk	< 2 inches (5 cm)	6–10 per 50 HPF
High risk	> 2 inches (5 cm)	> 5 per 50 HPF
	> 4 inches (10 cm)	Any mitotic rate
	Any size	> 10 per 50 HPF

* HPF denotes high-powered field seen under the microscope.

organs or vital structures (such as major blood vessels). When the tumor originates from the omentum or mesentery (lining of the abdominal cavity), surgery may be difficult, since the tumor usually spreads to multiple places in the abdominal cavity. Other factors determine whether a patient with GIST is a candidate for surgery. These include the overall health of the patient and whether the patient can tolerate an extensive operation.

The goal of surgery is complete resection of the tumor, whether it is in the esophagus, stomach, colon, omentum, or mesentery. During surgery, the rest of the abdominal cavity and the liver are explored to make sure there are no residual tumors or occult tumors that were not seen on preoperative imaging studies. GIST is usually encased by a sheath of tissue called a pseudocapsule, so care is taken during surgery to ensure that the tumor does not rupture. Even when GISTs are extending into adjacent organs (for example, a GIST that arises in the stomach and extends to the pancreas), they usually only displace these organs and do not invade them. Therefore, it is often possible to lift the tumor off the adjacent organs during surgery. For tumors in the esophagus or colon, surgery usually involves removing the tumor and portions of the esophagus or colon. For tumors in the stomach, either the entire stomach or a part of it is removed, depending on the size of the tumor. In all cases, the goal is to obtain a negative resection margin—a border of normal tissue surrounding the tumor that does not contain any cancer.

Most GISTs that are localized to one area are removable by surgery. For example, in a large series of patients with GIST published by the Memorial Sloan-Kettering Cancer Center, 85 percent of patients with localized GIST were able to undergo complete resection. Nearly 45 percent of these patients remained free of disease recurrence five years after their surgery.

In general, the likelihood of recurrence after complete resection of a GIST depends on two factors: the size and the mitotic rate (number of dividing cells) of the original tumor. As described in the table above, tumors that are greater than 4 inches (10 cm) in dimension or have a mitotic rate greater than ten per fifty high-powered fields are at high risk of relapse (greater than 50 percent at five years). Tumors that are smaller than 2 inches (5 cm) and have a mitotic rate of less than ten per fifty high-powered fields have a less than 10 percent chance of recurrence at five years. Several studies are investigating the value of administering a drug called imatinib mesylate (Gleevec) following surgery to try to decrease the risk of tumor recurrence (see "Targeted Therapy," below). In some instances, patients may also receive this same drug prior to their planned surgery, with the goal of shrinking the tumor to allow for a safer operation.

Chemotherapy Traditional chemotherapy agents, in contrast to newer targeted therapies such as imatinib mesylate (Gleevec) and sunitinib (Sutent), are not effective in the treatment of GIST.

Targeted Therapy Metastatic GISTs or locally advanced GISTs that have invaded (grown into) adjacent organs are not resectable by surgery. Prior to the year 2000, there was no known effective treatment for patients with these unresectable tumors. However, the discovery in the late 1990s that almost all GISTs express the c-Kit protein and that the c-Kit protein is abnormally activated in the tumor cells led to the development of a very effective treatment for unresectable GIST.

In the early 2000s, imatinib mesylate (Gleevec) was discovered to specifically bind to (target) the c-Kit molecule and block its function. Imatinib is a small molecule that comes in the form of an oral pill and is easily absorbed by the bowel. It belongs to a new class of drugs called receptor tyrosine kinase inhibitors (RTKIs). Imatinib is a prototype of so-called targeted therapy, in which drugs are designed to specifically target and inactivate proteins (in this case, c-Kit) that are thought to be responsible for the uncontrolled growth of the cancer cells. Imatinib was originally approved for the treatment of chronic myelogenous leukemia (CML) when it was found to effectively block the activity of another protein, called BCR/ABL, which causes CML (see the chapter "The Leukemias"). In clinical trials, most patients with CML who took imatinib had complete remission of their disease.

Due to its ability to block the activity of c-Kit, imatinib was studied in patients with GIST. In a large multinational clinical trial comparing two doses of imatinib in patients with unresectable GIST, 66 percent of patients had marked shrinkage of their tumors, and another 16 percent had tumors that remained stable on treatment. The median duration of response was twenty-seven months. There was no difference in response rates between the two doses tested (400 mg and 600 mg daily). Based on these positive results, imatinib was approved by the FDA in 2002 for the treatment of unresectable or metastatic GIST.

Imatinib is generally very well tolerated by patients. Its most common side effects are swelling of the area around the eyes, generalized swelling, mild skin rash on the face, and mild decrease in blood counts (decreased red blood count, called anemia, and decreased platelet count). Other side effects include nausea, abdominal bloating and cramping, and diarrhea. All of these side effects are usually mild.

Interestingly, it appears that the type of c-Kit mutation found in a patient's GIST determines how well the patient responds to imatinib treatment. In a large clinical trial in which patients with unresectable GIST were treated with imatinib, patients whose GIST contained a c-Kit mutation at exon 11 did much better than patients whose tumor contained a c-Kit mutation at exon 9 or no c-Kit mutation at all. A higher percentage of patients with an exon 11 mutation had tumor shrinkage with imatinib treatment; these patients also lived longer than patients with an exon 9 mutation or no mutation. While these sorts of mutational analyses are useful, they are not a part of routine testing at most pathology laboratories.

Despite the effectiveness of imatinib, most advanced GISTs eventually become resistant to imatinib treatment. For patients whose GIST has progressed despite imatinib treatment, another drug, called sunitinib (Sutent), has been found to be effective. Similar to imatinib, sunitinib is a tyrosine kinase inhibitor that targets and blocks the c-Kit protein, in addition to other proteins. Sunitinib also comes in the form of a pill that is taken orally. In a clinical trial comparing sunitinib to placebo in patients whose GIST had progressed despite imatinib, patients who took sunitinib had a longer period of tumor control (shrinkage or stable tumor) compared to those who took placebo. Patients whose GIST contained an exon 9 mutation in c-Kit did much better on sunitinib than patients whose tumor contained an exon 11 mutation. This is opposite of the effect seen with imatinib.

Sunitinib is also generally well tolerated by patients. Its most common side effects include diarrhea, skin discoloration, mouth sores, fatigue, high blood pressure, and decreased blood counts (red blood count and platelet count). Based on its efficacy, sunitinib was approved by the FDA in January of 2006 for the treatment of patients with GIST after disease progression on, or intolerance to, imatinib.

Because of the effectiveness of imatinib in patients with advanced GIST, this agent is being studied in patients whose GIST has been completely removed by surgery, to determine if it can increase the chance of cure in these patients. This type of therapy given after surgery is called adjuvant treatment. Two large clinical trials, one in Europe and the other in the United States, are currently evaluating imatinib as adjuvant therapy for GIST. Both trials are comparing imatinib treatment to no adjuvant treatment in patients with intermediate or high-risk GIST (determined by tumor size and mitotic rate) that has been completely removed by surgery. Results from these studies are not yet available. Furthermore, potentially operable patients whose tumors are very large at the time of diagnosis, may initially start treatment with imatinib for a period of time, with the goal of shrinking the tumor to make eventual surgical resection safer and easier (referred to as neoadjuvant therapy).

Assessing Treatment Response

Two types of scans are usually used to determine whether a patient with GIST is responding to treatment with imatinib or sunitinib—CT and PET scans. Either scan is obtained every three to six months while the patient is on treatment. A CT scan often shows shrinkage of tumors if they are responding to therapy. However, GISTs can sometimes increase in size or remain the same size on the CT scan in early treatment, due to bleeding in the tumor or death and degeneration of tumor cells; thus, this is not indicative of treatment failure. Often, GISTs that are responding to treatment become less bright on CT scan (hypodense) and PET scan (decreased uptake).

Treatment by Stage

■ Localized

The standard for patients with localized GIST that has not metastasized to distant organs or invaded adjacent organs is surgery. For GISTs in the stomach, the tumor and either part of the stomach or the entire stomach are removed (gastrectomy). For tumors in the esophagus, small intestine, or colon, portions of the esophagus, intestine, or colon are removed along with the tumor. In all cases, the goal is to achieve a negative margin around the tumor.

Five-Year Survival 35 to 87 percent, depending on the size of the tumor and the mitotic rate

Investigational The adjuvant treatment of patients with completely resected GIST is currently being evaluated in two Phase III clinical trials, one in the United

States and the other in Europe. Both trials are comparing imatinib treatment to no adjuvant treatment in patients with intermediate or high-risk GIST (determined by tumor size and mitotic rate) that has been completely removed by surgery. The goal of adjuvant therapy is to reduce the risk of disease recurrence. Results from these studies are not yet available. As noted above, neoadjuvant therapy with imatinib is also a strategy frequently used for GISTs that are very large at initial presentation.

■ *Localized Advanced or Metastatic*

The standard treatment of patients with locally advanced or metastatic GIST is targeted therapy with imatinib. The rate of tumor shrinkage with imatinib is in the range of 60 to 70 percent. If patients progress on imatinib, the dose of imatinib is increased or the patients are switched to treatment with sunitinib (Sutent). Patients who exhibit an excellent response to treatment and have isolated sites of residual disease may benefit from surgical exploration to resect these areas, but the long-term advantages of such an approach have yet to be proven.

Five-Year Survival 10 to 20 percent

Investigational Other novel targeted-therapy agents are being evaluated in clinical trials in patients with unresectable GIST that is resistant to imatinib treatment. These include sorafenib (Nexavar) and PTK/ZK (vatalanib), both of which are tyrosine kinase inhibitors that block vascular endothelial growth factor (VEGF). VEGF plays a key role in tumor blood vessel formation, which in turn is important in tumor growth and

metastasis. Another clinical trial is evaluating the combination of imatinib and bevacizumab (Avastin), which is an antibody directed against VEGF.

Recurrent Cancer

Patients whose GIST recurs after surgery may undergo a repeat operation if the recurrence is localized and the individual is a good candidate for surgery. If the recurrent disease is more extensive, patients are typically treated with imatinib mesylate (Gleevec) and sunitinib (Sutent) as in the case of metastatic disease.

Prevention

Because GIST is so rare and is not associated with any known risk factors, there are no recommended preventive measures against GIST.

The Most Important Questions You Can Ask

• Is my GIST removable by surgery? If not, why not?

• Is there a role for imatinib either before or after my planned surgery to remove the tumor?

• Based on the pathology of the tumor, is my GIST high, low, or intermediate risk and what does that mean?

• Does my GIST express the c-Kit protein?

• Can the tumor be analyzed for its mutational status (e.g., exon 11 or 9 mutation)?

• If the tumor is not removable by surgery, can I take imatinib or sunitinib (Sutent)?

• Is there a clinical trial available for my condition?

Head and Neck

Steven J. Wang, M.D., James T. Helsper, M.D.,*
James A. Recabaren, M.D., and Malin Dollinger, M.D.

■ ■ ■ ■

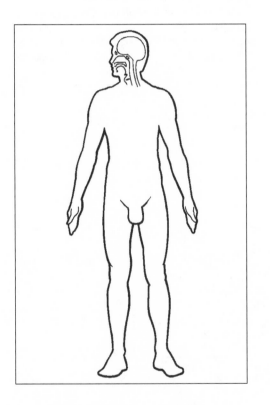

Head and neck cancers include cancers of the mucous membranes of the nose, sinuses, mouth, and throat, as well as cancers of the salivary glands. Taken together, head and neck cancers account for 5 to 10 percent of all malignancies. These cancers are more common in men by a ratio of 3 to 1 and are much more common in people over 50. Head and neck cancers are unique in a helpful way in that they often do not spread to the rest of the body until late in their course and have a longer time in which they are still curable. Thus, they have a good cure rate if found early, evaluated adequately, and treated with the best available therapy. All three main treatment methods—surgery, radiotherapy, and chemotherapy—are used.

There are about 50,000 new cases in the United States each year, and about one-third of head and neck cancer patients die of their disease. The most common locations for head and neck cancers are in the mouth and throat (oral cavity and oropharynx), which account for more than half of all cases. About one-third are in or around the voice box (larynx or hypopharynx).

One of the recent advances in head and neck cancer treatment is the use of chemotherapy (such as cisplatin [Platinol]) combined with radiotherapy for advanced-stage disease, which can offer similar cure rates to radical surgery with the possibility for better preservation of function. Active clinical trials of standard as well as new chemotherapy drugs are under way in an effort to provide a better cure rate for head and neck cancers in the future.

The broad category of head and neck cancers includes tumors in several areas:

• **Lip and Mouth (Oral Cavity)** This includes the lips, the tongue, the inside

---

*Dr. Helsper passed away this past year, and will be remembered for his expertise and devotion to head and neck cancer patients.

lining of the cheeks (buccal mucosa), the floor of the mouth, the gums (gingiva), and the hard palate.

• *Oropharynx* This is the upper part of the throat that can be seen when you say, "Ahhh." It also includes the tonsils.

• *Nasopharynx* The nasopharynx is behind the nose and above the oropharynx. It cannot be seen directly, but is viewed with a mirror or a scope.

• *Hypopharynx* This is the lower part of the throat (pharynx) where food goes just before we swallow it.

• *Larynx* The larynx (voice box) is in the front of the neck in the region of the Adam's apple.

• *Paranasal Sinuses and Nasal Cavity* Sinuses are found below and above the eyes and behind the nose.

• *Salivary Glands* These glands produce saliva to moisten our mouth and help us chew and swallow food.

• *Metastatic Squamous Cell Cancer to Cervical Lymph Nodes* If a cancer that is discovered in lymph nodes in the neck is squamous cell cancer, it is usually a metastasis

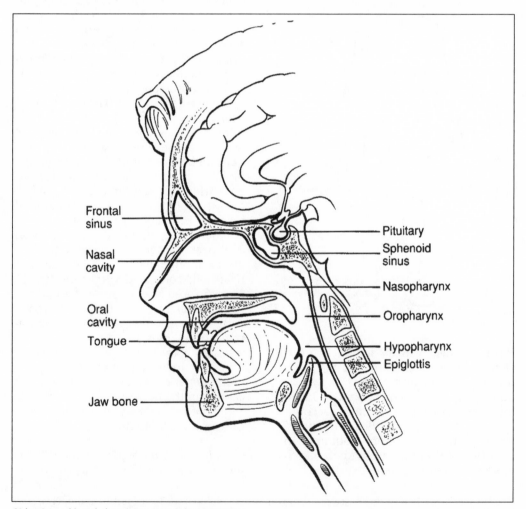

Side view of head showing potential cancer sites

from a head and neck cancer. Unless some other primary source can be found (such as lung cancer), this tumor is generally treated as a head and neck cancer. It is important to know that this type of metastatic cancer may be curable (discussed later in the chapter); see also the chapter "Cancer of an Unknown Primary Site [CUPS]").

Because of the involvement of the upper digestive and the upper respiratory tracts, head and neck cancers and their treatment can have a profound impact on some of the most fundamental functions of life. Patients with head and neck cancers frequently develop significant problems with eating, swallowing, speaking, and breathing. The importance of these affected functions on an individual's interaction with the outside world can lead to additional emotional challenges and psychological distress.

Successful treatment must, therefore, not only include an attempt to eradicate all the cancer, but also take into account

• the need for adequate function—swallowing, eating, speech—after treatment and
• a satisfactory cosmetic result. It is also important to consider what reconstruction, rehabilitation, and/or prosthetic options are available after surgical treatment.

Many health care specialists are essential to the successful treatment of head and neck cancers. This team should include, at the minimum, a surgeon specializing in the care of head and neck cancers—typically an otolaryngology (ear, nose, and throat) surgeon—a radiation oncologist, and a medical oncologist. Many centers also draw on the expertise of other specialists with an interest in head and neck cancers, such as plastic or head and neck reconstructive surgeons, dentists, pathologists, radiologists, various rehabilitation specialists, dietitians, oncology nurses, and social workers. The patient and his or her family, friends, and employer are all involved during the treatment and recovery process.

Risk Factors

The abuse of tobacco and alcohol are the most important risk factors for the development of most head and neck cancers. Smokers and drinkers who fail to stop after treatment for a primary head and neck cancer are at significantly higher risk of developing another cancer. Other risk factors include the following:

• Poor oral hygiene, poorly fitting dentures, or broken teeth cause chronic irritation of oral membranes.
• Wood dust inhalation (furniture workers) is related to nasal cavity cancer.
• Betel nut chewing (India) is related to cancer of the mouth (oral cavity).
• Increased carcinoma of the nasopharynx is seen among southern Chinese (environmental, not genetic).
• Epstein-Barr virus (EBV) infection is associated with nasopharyngeal cancer.
• Chronic iron deficiency in women is associated with tongue and hypopharynx carcinoma.
• Nickel exposure is associated with paranasal sinus cancer.

Screening

Screening is not generally practiced in North America. There are three approaches to early detection:

• Your awareness of typical signs and symptoms and your calling them to the attention of your physician.
• A careful examination of the head and neck by your doctor, including an examination of the throat with the aid of a mirror (indirect laryngoscopy) or a scope.
• Your dentist is in an excellent position to call your attention to suspicious lesions in the mouth such as the premalignant lesions called leukoplakia (white patches). Many oral cancers are discovered by dentists.

Common Signs and Symptoms

These tumors can appear as ulcerations of the mucous membranes with hard, rolled edges, or less commonly as protruding growths that look like small mushrooms. Specific symptoms depend on the location.

• *Lip and Mouth (Oral Cavity)* A swelling or ulcer that doesn't heal.

• *Oropharynx* Difficulty or pain on swallowing, ear pain, or development of an enlarged lymph node in the neck. May also have no symptoms.

• *Nasopharynx* Bloody nasal discharge or nasal obstruction, decreased hearing, nerve signs (double vision, pain, hoarseness), or enlarged lymph nodes in the neck.

• *Hypopharynx* Difficulty swallowing, ear pain, or enlarged lymph nodes in the neck. May have no symptoms.

• *Larynx* Persistent hoarseness, difficulty breathing or swallowing, or pain in the throat.

• *Paranasal Sinuses and Nasal Cavity* Pain, swelling, bloody nasal discharge, nasal obstruction, double vision, or chronic sinus trouble that does not respond to antibiotics.

• *Salivary Glands* Painless swelling and later paralysis of one side of the face.

• *Metastatic Squamous Cell Cancer to Cervical Lymph Nodes* Swollen, painless lymph nodes in the neck.

Diagnosis

Specific tests depend on the location of the cancer.

Physical Examination

• Inspection of the oral and nasal cavities, using mirrors and telescopes.

• Examination of suspicious lesions with the fingers (palpation), as well as examination of the back of the tongue.

Blood Tests Not typically performed

TNM Stage Grouping	
Stage I	T1, N0, M0
Stage II	T2, N0, M0
Stage III	T3, N0, M0
	T1–3, N1, M0
Stage IVa	T4a, N0–2, M0
	T1–3, N2, M0
Stage IVb	T4b, any N, M0
	Any T, N3, M0
Stage IVc	Any T, any N, M1

Imaging

• CT and MRI scans, barium esophogram, and Chest X-ray.

• PET scans may be useful to help identify the site of origin in cases of metastatic cancer of unknown primary sites, or for surveillance following treatment.

Biopsy

• Biopsy of any suspicious lesion. (This is most important.)

• In cases of metastatic cancer in neck lymph nodes, biopsy of apparently normal tissues in the tonsils, throat, and nasopharynx may be necessary to discover the site of origin.

Staging

Head and neck cancers are staged according to the TNM (tumor, node, metastasis) system. Accuracy of staging is especially critical, since a slight difference in the location and size of the tumor has a significant effect on the therapy chosen, the extent of surgery, and the prognosis.

Accurate staging requires visual inspection, palpation when possible, X-rays, appropriate biopsies, and careful measurement of enlarged lymph nodes. The mobility of enlarged nodes should be determined, since a lymph node that cannot be moved back and forth

Staging Outline

	PRIMARY TUMOR (T) *Oral Cavity, Oropharynx*	*Nasopharynx, Hypopharynx, Larynx*
Tx	Tumor cannot be assessed	Same
T0	No evidence of primary tumor	Same
Tis	Carcinoma in situ	Same
T1	Tumor no larger than $\frac{3}{4}$ inches (2 cm)	Tumor confined to one subsite
T2	Tumor $\frac{3}{4}$–$1\frac{1}{2}$ inches (2–4 cm)	Involves more than one subsite
T3	Tumor over $1\frac{1}{2}$ inches (4 cm)	Same
T4	Tumor invasion of adjacent structures	Same
T4a	Tumors involve invasion of structures that are still generally amenable to surgical cure.	
T4b	Tumors involve invasion of structures that generally preclude curative surgery. These tumors may still be treated with radiation and chemotherapy.	

	REGIONAL (NECK) LYMPH NODES (N)
Nx	Nodes cannot be assessed
N0	No involved lymph nodes
N1	Single involved node, same side, less than $1\frac{1}{4}$ inches (3 cm)
N2	Node(s), less than $2\frac{1}{2}$ inches (6 cm); divided into N2a, N2b, and N2c
N2a	Single involved node, same side, $1\frac{1}{4}$–$2\frac{1}{2}$ inches (3–6 cm)
N2b	Multiple nodes, same side, none greater than $2\frac{1}{2}$ inches (6 cm)
N2c	Nodes on opposite or both sides, none greater than $2\frac{1}{2}$ inches (6 cm)
N3	Any node over $2\frac{1}{2}$ inches (6 cm)

	DISTANT (BELOW THE COLLAR BONES) METASTASIS (M)
Mx	Distant metastasis cannot be assessed
M0	No distant metastasis
M1	Distant metastasis

may contain cancer that has spread to adjacent tissues. Typically, examination under anesthesia is required for accurate staging, especially for tumors of the larynx, nasopharynx, and oropharynx, as well as to perform necessary biopsies. Furthermore, the risk of having a simultaneous second primary head and neck cancer may be as high as 15 percent, so endoscopic examination of the entire upper aerodigestive tract is done to detect other cancers prior to starting treatment.

Sentinel Node Biopsy This is a new technique being performed in some centers, to sample the most likely lymph node to contain metastatic cancer. This node is selected by injecting a special blue dye or radioactive material near the cancer site, followed by removal of the node through a small incision in the neck. The "sentinel" node is then examined by a pathologist, and if negative, the neck dissection need not be done (see page 617). The patient is thus saved from more extensive surgery. This technique is commonly performed for melanomas, including those arising in the head and neck; however, sentinel node biopsy should be considered investigational for most other types of head and neck cancers.

Treatment of Head and Neck Cancers

The rest of this chapter discusses the treatment of various cancers of the head and neck, divided into different sites of origin. In each case, we discuss the roles of various treatment options, including surgery, radiation therapy, and chemotherapy. The relative role and importance of each type of therapy in the primary treatment of head and neck cancers may be different for each cancer site and for each stage.

The Expanding Role of Chemotherapy In the past, chemotherapy occupied a lesser role, often to assist in the treatment of recurrences or metastases. There has been great interest recently in the use of combinations of chemotherapy drugs and radiation therapy. Recent studies have demonstrated that combination chemotherapy and radiation therapy can provide equally effective cure rates for some types of advanced-stage head and neck cancers compared to radical surgery, resulting in better preservation of function. For example, it is now possible for some advanced larynx cancers to be treated successfully using chemotherapy and radiation therapy without the need for total surgical removal of the voice box.

Another promising area of research and clinical trials is the use of newer therapeutic agents that have potentially fewer side effects than standard drugs. For example, a new class of drugs, the EGFR inhibitors,

has recently been approved by the FDA for the treatment of advanced head and neck cancers. The prototype of this class of drugs is cetuximab (Erbitux), a monoclonal antibody. Cetuximab, when combined with radiation therapy, appear to improve cancer control rates without the dramatic increase in side effects typically associated with standard chemotherapy drugs. This is only one of many new and promising treatment strategies, and it may be very worthwhile for patients to investigate the possibility of participating in a clinical trial of one of these new methods of treatment.

Microvascular Free Flaps Head and neck cancer surgery can lead to disabling deformities. While small cancers can be removed and the site reconstructed with simple techniques, for larger defects, the new standard for reconstructive surgery utilizes microvascular free-tissue transfer (or free flaps). This technique involves transferring tissue from a distant site on the patient's body, together with its blood supply, to the site needing reconstruction and immediately reestablishing its blood supply by suturing the transferred tissue's blood vessels to nearby vessels. Microvascular free flaps allow three-dimensional reconstruction of complex head and neck defects, such as after removal of the jaw or tongue, providing better functional and cosmetic results.

Treatment Follow-Up

Because all patients with head and neck cancers are at risk for recurrence of their original cancer as well as development of a second cancer, follow-up is essential. A typical follow-up schedule for patients after treatment of head and neck cancers is monthly for one year, every two months for the next year, every three months the next year, and then every six months thereafter.

Lip and Mouth (Oral Cavity)

These cancers most commonly arise from the floor of the mouth and the tongue. They may be treated first with surgery or radiation therapy; however, surgery is generally the preferred initial treatment for most oral cavity cancers, followed, when indicated, by radiation therapy and sometimes chemotherapy, too. Reconstruction and rehabilitation are essential parts of the treatment plan. Patients who are not surgical candidates may be treated with radiation therapy.

Early cancers (Stages I and II) of the lip and oral cavity are often curable by surgery alone. Advanced cancers (Stages III and IV) are usually treated with a combination of surgery and radiotherapy. Patients with these advanced stages are at risk to develop recurrences after treatment, and the use of chemotherapy in addition to postoperative radiation should be considered. Patients whose tumors grow into nerves or blood vessels, or who have positive margins after surgery, have a worse prognosis.

Treatment Overview

• If surgery is the chosen method, the tumor must be removed completely along with a cuff of surrounding normal tissue to minimize the risk of leaving residual cancer cells. The impact on speech and swallowing function will depend on the location and size of the resulting defect after tumor removal. Various reconstructive options may be employed, and the method selected can influence the functional result. The reconstructive surgery may be performed by the same cancer surgeon or is sometimes done by a surgeon specializing in head and neck reconstructive surgery. A speech therapist is often helpful for successful rehabilitation.

• If the cervical nodes are involved and surgery is the chosen method for the primary tumor, all the lymph nodes on that side of the neck are usually removed at the same time in a procedure called a neck dissection. Even when there is no obvious involvement of lymph nodes, because many oral cavity cancers have a high risk for spreading to the neck lymph nodes, an "elective" neck dissection is often performed to remove the neck lymph nodes most likely to harbor cancer cells. In the past, neck dissections typically included removal of not only lymph nodes, but also other important structures such as the nerve to the shoulder and the major neck vein (called a radical neck dissection), which sometimes resulted in significant functional and cosmetic deficits. Recent studies have demonstrated that similar cancer control can be achieved when non–lymph node structures in the neck that are not directly involved with cancer are preserved (called a modified or selective neck dissection). Nowadays, patients can often undergo modified or selective neck dissections rather than radical neck dissections, with better functional and cosmetic results.

• Cancer of the space around the teeth usually requires the removal of some of the teeth as well as the primary cancer site in the gingiva (gums). A dental prosthodontist is needed to create a specialized plate for optimal rehabilitation.

• Occasionally, when the cancer involves the upper gums, it may be necessary to remove a portion of the sinus. A dental prosthodontist is needed to create an obturator for rehabilitation.

• For larger cancers that have a lower cure rate with surgery alone, combination treatment with surgery, radiation therapy, and/or chemotherapy may be indicated.

Treatment by Location and Stage

▓ Stage I
Standard Treatment

• **Lip** Surgery or radiotherapy, but surgery is generally preferred.

• **Front of Tongue** Surgery or radiotherapy, but surgery is generally preferred. Reconstruction may require a small skin graft.

• **Inside of Cheek** Surgery or radiotherapy, but surgery is generally preferred.

• **Floor of Mouth** Surgery or radiotherapy, but surgery is generally preferred. Reconstruction with a small skin graft may be required.

• **Lower Gums** Complete surgical removal is performed, possibly with removal of some bone. Radiotherapy results are usually not as good as surgery.

• **Behind Wisdom Teeth** (**Retromolar Trigone**) Surgery or radiotherapy, but surgery is generally preferred.

• **Upper Gums and Hard Palate** Complete surgical removal is performed. Radiotherapy results are usually not as good as surgery.

Five-Year Survival About 90 percent

▓ Stage II
Standard Treatment

• **Lip** Surgery is generally preferred. Larger or recurrent lesions may require more complex reconstructive surgery to achieve a satisfactory functional outcome.

• **Front of Tongue** Surgery is generally preferred. Reconstruction may require skin grafts or larger tissue flaps. An elective neck dissection on the same side as the tongue cancer should be performed.

• **Inside of Cheek** Small T2 lesions are treated typically with surgery. Larger T2 lesions are treated with surgery, radiotherapy, or both.

• **Floor of Mouth** Surgery is generally preferred. Reconstruction may require

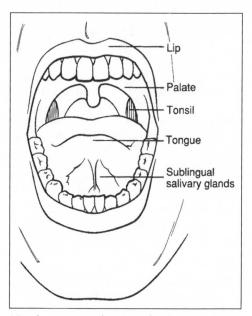

Mouth structures that may develop cancer

skin grafts or larger tissue flaps. An elective neck dissection on the same side as the floor-of-mouth cancer should be performed.

• **Lower Gums** Tumors are treated with surgery, sometimes requiring removal of some bone. Radiotherapy results are generally not as good. An elective neck dissection on the same side as the lower gums with cancer should be performed.

• **Retromolar Trigone** (**Behind Wisdom Teeth**) Surgical removal is performed, also sometimes including part of the jawbone. An elective neck dissection on the same side as the retromolar trigone cancer should be performed.

• **Upper Gums and Hard Palate** Complete surgical removal is performed. Radiotherapy results are usually not as good as surgery.

Five-Year Survival 70 to 90 percent (higher for lip, lower for tongue and floor of mouth)

■ *Stage III*

Standard Treatment Combination treatment with surgery followed by radiotherapy is generally used, depending on the location of the tumor. The neck lymph nodes must also be part of the treatment plan. Reconstructive surgery should be performed at the same time as the cancer removal and may be more complex with these larger defects. A common reconstructive surgical technique is to use a free flap from the forearm to rebuild the tongue or floor of the mouth.

• *Lip* Surgery followed by postoperative radiotherapy.

• *Front of Tongue* Surgery followed by postoperative radiotherapy. Reconstructive surgery may utilize free flaps. For patients who decline surgery or are not surgical candidates, radioactive implants may be used as an alternative.

• *Inside of Cheek* Surgery followed by postoperative radiotherapy.

• *Floor of Mouth* Surgery followed by postoperative radiotherapy. Reconstructive surgery may utilize free flaps.

• *Lower Gums* Surgery followed by postoperative radiotherapy.

• *Retromolar Trigone* (**Behind Wisdom Teeth**) Surgery followed by postoperative radiotherapy.

• *Upper Gums and Hard Palate* Surgery followed by postoperative radiotherapy.

Five-Year Survival 40 to 60 percent

■ *Stage IV*

Standard Treatment Stage IVa cancers are best treated with a combination of surgery followed by radiotherapy possibly with chemotherapy, too. Stage IVb cancers are generally not treatable by surgery; rather, consideration should be given to radiation therapy and/or chemotherapy. These cancers often invade the jawbone, requiring its partial removal. When surgery is performed for these tumors, the reconstructive surgery is often complex and free flaps are frequently used. For partial jawbone reconstruction, free flaps using bone from the lower leg (fibula) may be used.

Five-Year Survival Up to 40 percent

Recurrent Cancer

Treatment depends on the location and size of the recurrent tumor, as well as on the nature of the original treatment. If radiotherapy was used initially, surgery is preferred if possible. If surgery was used initially, additional surgery followed by radiotherapy possibly combined with chemotherapy may be indicated. When tumors cannot be completely removed with surgery, consideration of radiation therapy and/or chemotherapy for palliation is appropriate. Because results for recurrent cancer are often poor, clinical trials using new chemotherapy agents should be considered.

Oropharynx

The most common cancers in this area begin in the base of the tongue and the tonsils. The vast majority of cases of oropharyngeal cancer are related to cigarette smoking or other forms of tobacco use such as pipe smoking and tobacco chewing. Heavy alcohol consumption along with tobacco use further increases the risk. Most oropharyngeal cancers occur in men, although as more women are now smoking, their risk of developing these cancers has increased.

Treatment Overview

• Because these cancers are more hidden from view compared to oral cavity cancers, they are often not discovered until a more advanced stage. Commonly, the presenting symptom may be a metastasis to a neck lymph node.

• These cancers can be treated with either surgery or radiation (with or without chemotherapy). However, recently, many of these cancers have been treated using radiation therapy (with or without chemotherapy) with very good outcomes, but without many of the debilitating consequences of radical surgery. Surgery is then reserved for patients who fail to respond to their initial treatment, or who recur.

• Oropharyngeal cancers that invade bone, such as the jawbone, respond poorly to radiation therapy and require surgery, if possible, to maximize chances for cure.

Treatment by Stage

■ Stage I

Standard Treatment The choice is determined by the anticipated functional and cosmetic results. Radiation therapy is commonly used. Surgery is equally successful. Either might be used in a location such as the tonsil, where function is expected to be normal after surgery. In an area such as the base of the tongue, radiation may be preferred, since surgery could result in a worse functional outcome. However, if adequate surgical margins around the cancer can be achieved through a trans-oral approach, the functional results with surgery may compare favorably to radiation treatment.

Five-Year Survival 70 to 90 percent, depending on the site

■ Stage II

Standard Treatment If radiation is used, the technique is individualized by a radiation oncologist experienced in treatment of tumors of this area. Surgery is an alternative, and, as with Stage I, the anticipated functional outcome frequently determines whether surgery or radiotherapy is preferred.

Five-Year Survival 60 to 80 percent

■ Stage III

Standard Treatment Increasingly, many centers are treating Stage III oropharyngeal cancers using a combination of chemotherapy and radiation therapy, with surgery used only for treatment failure or recurrence, and the results reported have been quite favorable. When surgery is performed for these cancers, immediate reconstruction with flaps, often free flaps, is recommended. Postoperative radiation therapy is usually indicated. Patients in this stage may be candidates for various adjuvant chemotherapy clinical trials.

Five-Year Survival 50 to 60 percent

■ Stage IV

Standard Treatment Whether a combination of surgery followed by radiation therapy—or, alternatively, a combination of chemotherapy given simultaneously with radiation therapy—is recommended depends on the extent of the cancer and other factors. Cancers that involve the jawbone respond poorly to chemotherapy and radiation and should be treated initially with surgery if possible. As in Stage III disease, a multidisciplinary treatment approach by physicians experienced in treating this type of cancer is necessary. Patients in this stage may be candidates for various adjuvant chemotherapy clinical trials.

Five-Year Survival Up to 40 percent

Recurrent Cancer

If radiotherapy was not used originally, it can be used to treat recurrences.

Otherwise, surgery is recommended, if possible. Chemotherapy can be used in combination with surgery or radiotherapy. Chemotherapy is also used for metastatic disease and for recurrences that can no longer be treated with surgery or radiation.

Supportive Therapy

Appropriate rehabilitation is essential after aggressive surgery and/or radiation. Cosmetic appearance, swallowing, speech, chewing, and psychological functioning may require attention. The patient must be motivated, and successful rehabilitation requires a team approach, with speech therapists, social workers, physical therapists, prosthodontists, occupational therapists, and nurses all playing important roles. The family is also extremely important in supporting the patient during and after therapy.

Nasopharynx

The nasopharynx is right behind the nose and above the oropharynx. It cannot be seen directly. It is shaped somewhat like a box. On the sides are the eustachian tubes that adjust the air pressure in our middle ears. At the top is the sphenoid sinus.

Cancers of the nasopharynx are different from other head and neck cancers in that there does not appear to be a link with alcohol and tobacco use. These cancers may also occur at a younger age. While relatively rare among native-born residents of the United States, nasopharynx cancer is very common in certain geographic regions of the world, including parts of southeastern China. The Epstein-Barr virus (EBV) has been implicated in some patients.

Common early signs include nasal obstruction or nosebleeds, inability to equalize the air pressure between the ears, hearing loss or signs of middle ear infection, and cranial nerve problems. There may be no symptoms related to the primary tumor, and patients may first present with a mass in the neck (a lymph node metastasis). Around 80 percent of patients will have some evidence of spread to these lymph nodes, some only microscopically.

Evaluation of patients includes a very careful physical examination and endoscopic examinations of the nose and throat. Most of these cancers are the squamous cell type. The diagnosis is best made by biopsy of the primary site in the nasopharynx and a needle biopsy of any enlarged lymph nodes in the neck.

Once the diagnosis has been made by biopsy, CT and MRI scans are essential for determining tumor extent and stage. A chest X-ray and PET scans may also be used to evaluate for metastases. Various factors appear to affect prognosis, including bone invasion, the involvement of cranial nerves, and the presence of lymph nodes involved by tumor. Patients who have evidence of EBV infection (as shown by a blood test) have a poorer prognosis after treatment.

Treatment Overview

The initial treatment for most cancers of the nasopharynx is combined chemotherapy and radiation therapy. Small cancers of the nasopharynx are curable by radiotherapy in 80 to 90 percent of cases. Moderately advanced tumors can be cured in 50 to 70 percent of cases. Advanced tumors, especially with extension to other structures such as bone and cranial nerves, are difficult to control.

• In patients with extension of tumor into the skull bones or involving cranial nerves, the use of surgery is rarely of help and is seldom attempted.

• Radiotherapy is used for treatment of neck metastases. Surgery is usually used only for lymph nodes that do not disappear after radiotherapy.

• Once treatment is completed, extensive follow-up is essential. This includes physical examination, X-rays and scans, blood tests, attention to dental and oral hygiene, jaw exercises, and evaluation of vision and hearing.

Treatment by Stage

■ Stage I
Standard Treatment High-dose radiotherapy is used.

Five-Year Survival 65 to 95 percent

■ Stages II and III
Standard Treatment Combined chemotherapy and radiotherapy is used. Surgical neck dissection may be needed if enlarged lymph nodes in the neck do not completely disappear after radiotherapy or recur.

Five-Year Survival 50 to 65 percent (Stage II); 30 to 60 percent (Stage III)

■ Stage IV
Standard Treatment Combined chemotherapy and radiotherapy is used. Surgical neck dissection is done for persistent or recurrent enlarged lymph nodes.

Five-Year Survival 5 to 40 percent

Recurrent Cancer

Select patients may be given additional radiotherapy and chemotherapy. Some may be candidates for surgical removal of recurrent tumors.

Metastatic disease and local recurrences not treatable by surgery or radiation may be treated with chemotherapy.

Hypopharynx

The hypopharynx is below the oropharynx. It is the place the food first passes through when we swallow. There are three areas in the hypopharynx:

• the postcricoid area (junction of pharynx and esophagus),
• the pyriform sinus, and
• the posterior (back) pharyngeal wall.

The hypopharynx is best examined with mirrors or scopes that can be passed into the mouth or nose. Almost all of the cancers in this area are squamous cancers arising in the mucous membranes. A few cancers are of minor salivary gland origin.

Other cancers may occur elsewhere in the head and neck at the same time or later, so the entire larynx, oropharynx, nasopharynx, and oral cavity should be searched. The esophagus should also be evaluated. CT and MRI scans are useful in establishing the extent of the disease. Since treatment will vary depending on the stage and spread of disease, it is very important to establish the stage precisely before therapy is begun.

Symptoms generally occur late and spread tends to occur early, so the survival rates for cancers in this area are lower than for other sites in the head and neck.

Because hypopharyngeal cancers tend to present at an advanced stage, combined treatment (surgery plus radiation therapy or chemotherapy plus radiation therapy) is usually indicated. Choice of treatment depends on a careful review of each case, with attention to the stage, the physical condition of the patient, the experience of the physicians, and the treatment facilities available.

Treatment by Stage

■ *Stage I*
Standard Treatment It is unusual for hypopharyngeal cancers to present at this stage; however, these tumors can be treated with equal efficacy with either radiation therapy or surgery. In some centers, surgical excision using lasers and scopes placed through the mouth may be performed, avoiding the need for external neck incisions.

Five-Year Survival 70 to 90 percent

■ *Stage II*
Standard Treatment Treatment can be with either radiation therapy or surgery. Anticipated functional outcome and other factors, including patient preference, determine the treatment choice. The risk of microscopic lymph node metastasis is also increased, so elective treatment of the neck is indicated.

Five-Year Survival 50 to 70 percent

■ *Stage III*
Standard Treatment These cancers generally require combined treatment with either surgery followed by radiation therapy or chemotherapy given at the same time as radiation therapy. The surgery necessary for these cancers often requires total removal of the voice box.

Anticipated functional outcome and other factors, including patient preference, determine the treatment choice. Patients should be managed by head and neck surgeons and radiation oncologists experienced in the complex treatment protocols for these tumors.

Patients may be considered for clinical trials evaluating standard or new chemotherapy agents or investigational radiotherapy protocols.

Five-Year Survival 40 to 60 percent

■ *Stage IV*
Standard Treatment For Stage IVa tumors, the treatment options are similar to those for Stage III. However, the factors favoring either an initial surgical approach or an initial chemotherapy and radiation therapy approach are complex and require a careful assessment and discussion among an experienced team of doctors and the patient. For tumors that cannot safely be removed surgically (Stage IVb), chemotherapy and/or radiation therapy is given.

Patients may be considered for clinical trials evaluating standard or new chemotherapy agents or investigational radiotherapy protocols.

Five-Year Survival 15 to 25 percent

Recurrent Cancer

If radiotherapy was not used originally, it can be used to treat recurrences. Otherwise, surgery is recommended, if possible. Chemotherapy can be used in combination with surgery or radiotherapy. Chemotherapy is also used for metastatic disease or for recurrences that can no longer be treated with surgery or radiation.

Larynx

The larynx, or voice box, is divided into three regions. From the top down, these are as follows:

• *Supraglottis* This includes the epiglottis (a flap that keeps food from going into the lungs), the false vocal cords, the ventricles, the aryepiglottic folds, and the arytenoids. Tumors of this area cause sore throat, painful swallowing, and sometimes a change in voice quality.

• *Glottis* This includes the true vocal cords and the anterior (front) and posterior (back) commissures. Tumors here may involve one or both vocal cords or may extend out on either side of them. Tumors are usually detected early because they cause hoarseness. Because of these early symptoms and the lack of lymphatic channels where cancer can spread, the cure rate here is better than for supraglottic or subglottic cancer.

• *Subglottis* This area is below the true vocal cords and extends downward to about the first tracheal ring (cartilage ring around the trachea). Tumors here are rare.

Almost all cancers of the larynx arise from the lining membrane (mucosa) and are called squamous cell cancers. Salivary gland cancers and other types can also occur in this area.

Common symptoms can include persistent sore throat or hoarseness, difficulty in swallowing, the feeling of something in the throat, a change in voice quality, and the appearance of a lump in the neck.

A complete diagnostic work-up includes a thorough head and neck physical examination with mirrors and scopes, CT or MRI scan to outline the tumor and show its extent, and chest X-ray to rule out spread to the lungs. Finally, it is necessary for the larynx to be examined under anesthesia with the aid of a laryngoscope. Biopsies of the cancer as well as any other suspicious lesions are performed, and the entire area is carefully examined to establish the extent of tumor involvement.

Treatment Overview

• Small cancers of the larynx have a good prognosis. If there is no spread to lymph nodes, the cure rate is 75 to 95 percent. Although most early lesions can be cured by radiotherapy or surgery, radiotherapy is often chosen as the initial treatment in an attempt to preserve a better voice. Surgery is used later if the tumor recurs. Laser excision surgery, through scopes placed in the mouth and throat, is also sometimes used, especially if the tumor is limited to one vocal cord.

• Locally advanced lesions, especially with invasion into and beyond the cartilage framework of the larynx, are poorly controlled by either radiation therapy or surgery alone, so both methods may be used together.

• Recent studies of patients with advanced laryngeal cancer have demonstrated that combination treatment with chemotherapy and radiotherapy can allow preservation of the larynx and provide cure rates equal to those of total laryngectomy (total voice box removal).

• Intermediate-sized cancers require individual decision making about the most appropriate treatment. Factors such as the site, stage, degree of lymph node involvement, and general status of the patient will influence the type of therapy chosen.

• Most recurrences occur in the first two to three years, and close follow-up, especially in patients who undergo primary radiation therapy or partial laryngectomy surgery, is essential so that cure may still be possible. Examinations are repeated to document the progress of treatment and detect recurrence.

Treatment by Stage

■ Stages I and II
Standard Treatment

• **Supraglottis** External-beam radiotherapy alone or surgery. Surgery for these cancers is a partial removal of the voice box (supraglottic laryngectomy) that is performed either with an external approach through incisions in the neck or with lasers and scopes passed through the mouth. Patients must be healthy enough to undergo this type of surgery, which does impair the functioning of the larynx, primarily increasing aspiration. Radiotherapy offers the advantage of better preserving the function of the larynx; however, once used, it cannot be used again for larynx cancer recurrence. Supraglottic cancers have a high risk for microscopic cancer spread to lymph nodes, so elective treatment of the neck is indicated.

• **Glottis** External-beam radiotherapy alone or surgery. Surgery for these cancers is a partial removal of the voice box (vertical partial laryngectomy) that is performed either with an external approach through incisions in the neck or with lasers and scopes passed through the mouth. Patients must be healthy enough to undergo this type of surgery, which does impair the functioning of the larynx, primarily increasing aspiration. Radiotherapy results in better voice quality in most patients; however, once used, it cannot be used again for larynx cancer recurrence.

• **Subglottis** Radiotherapy alone, with surgery used for recurrence.

Five-Year Survival Stage I: 75 to 95 percent. Stage II: 60 to 80 percent (supraglottis); 70 to 90 percent (glottis).

■ Stage III
Standard Treatment

• **Supraglottis** Radiation therapy combined with chemotherapy, or surgery followed by radiation therapy. For most cancers of this stage, the surgery necessary is total voice box removal (total laryngectomy). Patients who are treated with radiation and chemotherapy, and who fail to respond to treatment or recur, can still undergo surgery (salvage total laryngectomy). Treatment of the neck lymph nodes is necessary.

• **Glottis** Radiation therapy combined with chemotherapy, or surgery followed by radiation therapy. For most cancers of this stage, the surgery necessary is total voice box removal (total laryngectomy). Patients who are treated with radiation and chemotherapy, and who fail to respond to treatment or recur, can still undergo surgery (salvage total laryngectomy). Treatment of the neck lymph nodes is necessary.

• **Subglottis** Very rare for this stage, but should be treated similarly to Stage III glottic and supraglottic tumors.

Five-Year Survival 45 to 65 percent (supraglottis); 55 to 70 percent (glottis)

■ Stage IV
Standard Treatment

• **Supraglottis** For Stage IVa tumors, the treatment options are similar to those for Stage III. However, the factors favoring either an initial total laryngectomy or combination chemotherapy and radiation therapy are complex and require a careful assessment and discussion among an experienced team of doctors and the patient. For tumors that cannot safely be removed surgically (Stage IVb), chemotherapy and/or radiation therapy is given. Patients may be considered for clinical trials evaluating standard or new chemotherapy agents or investigational radiotherapy protocols.

• **Glottis** For Stage IVa tumors, the treatment options are similar to those for Stage III. However, the factors favoring either an initial total laryngectomy or combination chemotherapy and radiation therapy are complex and require a careful assessment and discussion among an experienced team of doctors and the patient. For tumors that cannot safely be removed surgically (Stage IVb), chemotherapy and/or radiation therapy is given. Patients may be considered for clinical trials evaluating standard or new chemotherapy agents or investigational radiotherapy protocols.

• *Subglottis* Total laryngectomy, including thyroidectomy and tracheoesophageal lymph node dissection, followed by radiotherapy. Patients who are not candidates for surgery are treated with chemotherapy and/or radiotherapy.

Five-Year Survival 10 to 40 percent

Recurrent Cancer

If initial treatment was with radiation therapy or partial laryngectomy, patients may be candidates for further surgery, which is usually a total laryngectomy. Select patients who recur after total laryngectomy may be candidates for further surgery, but prognosis is generally quite poor. Patients with recurrent larynx cancers who are not surgical candidates may respond to palliative chemotherapy.

Supportive Therapy

Patients who have had their voice box (larynx) removed need supportive treatment to help them to learn to speak again. There are three methods:

• An electronic larynx—a buzzerlike battery-operated unit—may be pressed against the neck while the mouth and tongue form the words. Another version of the electronic larynx uses a unit that looks like a pipe that is placed in the mouth.

• Another method involves learning the technique of esophageal voice, where the patient is taught to swallow air and bring it back up to speak.

• A third method requires a surgical procedure (tracheoesophageal puncture) to create a connection between the airway and the esophagus to insert a voice prosthesis ("button") and breathing valve.

Paranasal Sinus and Nasal Cavity

These cancers are often diagnosed late because they may have no symptoms in early stages and symptoms may resemble chronic sinusitis. These cancers can easily spread throughout the sinus area. Local growth into adjacent vital areas is a more common cause of death than metastases.

There are six sinuses, two just below the eyes (maxillary), two above the eyes (frontal), and two in the center, behind the nose (ethmoid and sphenoid). The maxillary sinus is the one most commonly involved, and cancer there can be difficult to diagnose.

The most common type of cancer of the paranasal sinus and nasal cavity is squamous cell cancer. Other cancer types include adenocarcinoma, esthesioneuroblastoma (also called olfactory neuroblastoma), minor salivary gland cancers, and occasionally melanoma and lymphoma.

Risks factors for squamous cell cancer and adenocarcinoma of the paranasal sinuses and nasal cavity include smoking and certain environmental exposures associated with workers involved in wood, leather, or nickel.

Treatment Overview

Treatment of these tumors is very complex and requires precise pretreatment evaluation and planning. Most patients require a combination of surgery and radiotherapy.

• Since lymph nodes are involved in only about 20 percent of cases, surgery or radiotherapy to the lymph nodes in the neck is used only if these nodes contain tumor.

• The proximity of the eye socket to the paranasal sinuses puts the eye at risk for invasion by these cancers. In some centers, paranasal sinus cancers with possible eye socket invasion on preliminary imaging scans are treated with initial radiation therapy, followed by surgery, in order to increase the chances of saving the eye.

• Paranasal sinus and nasal cavity cancers with invasion superiorly into the skull base and brain have a poor prognosis; select cases may still be surgically removed with a combined neurosurgery and head and neck surgery procedure.

• Esthesioneuroblastoma, melanoma, and lymphoma are staged differently from squamous cell carcinoma and adenocarcinoma, and their treatment may differ from that described below. Patients with these rare cancers should consult carefully with their doctors regarding treatment options.

Treatment by Stage

■ Stages I and II
Standard Treatment Surgery with wide surgical margins is typically indicated for these cancers. If the tumor extends near the surgical margin or if the tumor specimen is found to contain certain worrisome pathologic characteristics, postoperative radiotherapy is given.

The standard surgical approach is through a small incision along the side of the nose or between the nose and eye. Some centers offer surgical excision of tumors using scopes and instruments passed through the nose, avoiding the need for external facial incisions. Preliminary reports suggest that for select cases, the more minimally invasive approach can offer similar treatment outcomes.

Five-Year Survival 60 to 90 percent

■ Stage III
Standard Treatment Combined surgery with radiation therapy. Typically surgery is performed first. However, if there is a question of cancer involving the eye, some centers prefer to use radiotherapy first in order to increase the chance that the eye can be saved in the subsequent surgery. Rehabilitation with immediate reconstructive surgery, often with free flaps or use of prosthetic devices, may be needed following cancer-removal surgery.

Clinical trials using chemotherapy combinations in addition to radiotherapy and/or surgery may also be considered.

Five-Year Survival 35 to 50 percent

■ Stage IV
Standard Treatment When possible, surgery to widely excise the cancer is performed. This surgery may involve removal of the eye socket and/or require surgical access to the brain (by a neurosurgeon, called a craniofacial resection) to completely clear the cancer. Rehabilitation with immediate free flap reconstructive surgery or use of prosthetic devices may be needed following cancer-removal surgery. Following surgery, radiotherapy with or without chemotherapy is given. When surgery is not possible, radiotherapy with or without chemotherapy may be given for palliation.

Clinical trials for paranasal sinus and nasal cavity tumors evaluating chemotherapy combinations in addition to radiotherapy and/or surgery should be considered.

Five-Year Survival Up to 25 percent

Recurrent Cancer

Recurrent cancer of the paranasal sinuses and nasal cavity carries a poor prognosis.

If the initial treatment was a limited surgery or did not include radiotherapy, the patient may be a candidate for a more radical surgery and postoperative radiotherapy. If the patient is no longer a candidate for surgery or radiotherapy, chemotherapy may be given for palliation, improved quality of life, and in some cases improved survival.

Salivary Glands

There are three major paired salivary glands. The parotid glands are in front of each ear (enlarged during mumps), the submandibular glands are just below the jawbone, and the sublingual glands are under the tongue. In addition, there are many small, minor salivary glands that line the mouth, nose, and throat.

There are both benign and malignant tumors of these glands, although the term *benign* may be misleading. These "benign" tumors rarely if ever metastasize, but their growth can be fairly aggressive and the surgery needed to control them may resemble that needed for malignant tumors of the same gland.

There are multiple kinds of malignant and benign tumors. The more common malignant salivary gland tumors include mucoepidermoid carcinoma, adenoid cystic carcinoma, adenocarcinoma, acinic cell carcinoma, and carcinoma expleomorphic adenoma. The more common benign salivary gland tumors include pleomorphic adenoma, Warthin's tumor, and lipoma. The treatment is different for each kind of tumor, so expert pathologic study is necessary.

Because there are lymph nodes within the parotid gland, cancers in the parotid gland may also represent metastasis or lymphoma. Primary skin cancer and melanoma of the head and neck frequently metastasize to the parotid gland.

Twenty-five percent of parotid tumors, 40 percent of submandibular gland tumors, 95 percent of sublingual gland tumors, and 50 percent of minor salivary gland tumors are malignant.

We don't know the exact cause of most salivary gland cancers. However, increased incidence of some salivary gland cancers appears associated with heavy tobacco use, certain workplace environmental exposures, and previous radiation exposure to the head and neck. Radiotherapy was used to treat acne during the 1930s, 1940s, and 1950s, with a resulting significantly higher risk of developing cancer of adjacent salivary glands.

Treatment Overview

The size of the tumor, the degree of invasion, and the presence of regional or distant metastasis determine the stage of these cancers. For salivary gland cancers, unlike most other head and neck cancers, the pathologic type and grade, in addition to the stage, are critical factors that determine the appropriate treatment as well as prognosis.

• If possible, the initial treatment of most salivary gland cancers is complete

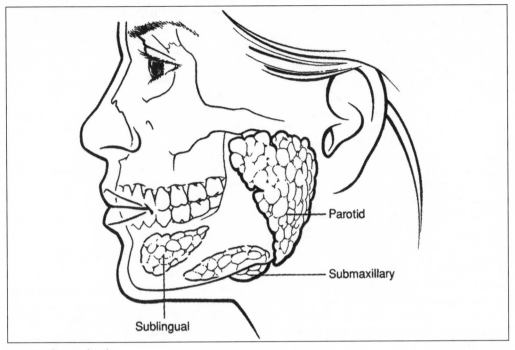

Major salivary glands

surgical resection. The need for additional treatment with radiation therapy is determined by the factors listed above.

• For cancers involving the parotid gland, treatment decisions must be made regarding the facial nerve. This nerve runs through the middle of the parotid gland and controls the muscles of facial expression. In general, this nerve can be preserved unless it is invaded by cancer. More advanced cancers of the parotid gland can involve not only the facial nerve, but also the overlying facial skin, the ear, and the bones around the ear.

• Adenoid cystic carcinoma is a somewhat unique salivary gland malignancy that is characterized by slow growth, a propensity to invade nerves, and a progressive relentless course. While these cancers are difficult to cure, patients tend to live with their cancer, sometimes even with distant metastasis, for many years.

• Early-stage, low-grade salivary gland tumors, especially tumors of the parotid gland, are usually curable by surgery. Large, bulky, or high-grade tumors have a poorer prognosis and often require postoperative radiotherapy.

• The minimum therapy for low-grade malignancies of a portion of the parotid gland is superficial parotidectomy. Great care is taken to preserve the facial nerve that goes through the middle of this gland and controls the muscles on that side of the face. For other kinds of parotid tumors, total parotidectomy is needed to obtain a safe margin around the tumor because the tumor frequently grows microscopically far beyond where it is grossly visible.

• Postoperative radiotherapy is indicated for lesions that are high grade or have close surgical margins.

• There is no established role for chemotherapy, but it is sometimes used in special circumstances when radiation or surgery is not possible or refused, or for recurrent or unresponsive tumors.

• When the tumor has spread to lymph nodes in the neck, a neck dissection should be performed. Sometimes radiotherapy is also used to treat the neck.

• There are several investigational protocols that are sometimes used, including chemotherapy and radiation therapy with fast neutron beams. Neutron-beam radiation therapy—available in a limited number of centers—has been effective in the treatment of inoperable and/or recurrent tumors and may be more effective than conventional radiation therapy.

Treatment by Location

Parotid Gland Cancers

Standard Treatment

• For low-grade tumors, surgery alone, usually superficial parotidectomy. Radiotherapy is also used after surgery if the surgical margins are involved with cancer.

• For high-grade tumors, surgery (typically superficial or total parotidectomy) followed by radiotherapy. When there is invasion of the facial nerve by cancer, it must be removed. Various reconstructive surgeries to rehabilitate patients following facial nerve sacrifice are available. Tumors extending beyond the confines of the parotid gland may require resection of surrounding structures, including the skin, jawbone, and ear. If the tumor has spread to the neck lymph nodes, these nodes need to be removed. If the tumor cannot be removed, radiotherapy may be used for palliation.

• Local recurrence may be reduced by postoperative radiotherapy. Fast-neutron-

beam radiation is under clinical evaluation, and recent studies indicate that these tumors may occasionally respond to chemotherapy.

Submandibular Gland Cancers

Standard Treatment

• For low-grade tumors, surgery alone, usually a submandibular gland excision.

• For high-grade tumors, more extensive surgery to achieve a wider margin, followed by radiotherapy especially if the surgical margins are positive or the nerves or soft tissues of the neck are involved.

Sublingual Gland and Minor Salivary Gland Cancers

Standard Treatment

• For low-grade tumors, wide surgical excision.

• For high-grade tumors, wide surgical excision followed by radiotherapy.

Five-Year Survival Depends on stage, pathologic type, grade, and adequacy of treatment (surgery and/or radiotherapy). Adenoid cystic carcinomas tend to have good five-year survival rates but lower survival rates at ten or more years even with aggressive treatment.

Recurrent Cancer

Additional more extensive surgery when possible offers the best chance for salvage. When surgery is not possible, palliative radiotherapy or chemotherapy should be explored. The prognosis for recurrent salivary gland cancer is generally poor, although patients with recurrent or even metastatic adenoid cystic carcinoma may live with their disease for many years.

Metastatic Cancer to Cervical (Neck) Lymph Nodes (Unknown Primary)

Persistently enlarged neck lymph nodes in an adult, particularly if they are painless, may contain cancer and should always be evaluated. With the exception of lymphomas, which are primary cancers of the lymph nodes, cancers found in lymph nodes almost always begin elsewhere in the body and may be the first sign of a new cancer. Once a preliminary history and exam is performed, the initial diagnostic study of a persistently enlarged neck lymph node is a fine needle aspiration biopsy. The biopsy of the lymph node should always be done first by fine needle aspiration biopsy, never by an open lymph node biopsy. An open biopsy tends to spread tumor to the adjacent tissues, making cure more difficult. Once a diagnosis of metastatic cancer in a neck lymph node is made, a search is begun for the primary site, which is usually in the head and neck. If a cancer has previously been diagnosed elsewhere, it naturally is the likely source, especially if the pattern under the microscope is similar. A vital part of the solution to the puzzle is provided by pathologic examination of the biopsy specimen. Immunohistochemical studies and special stains can be applied to the tissue slides to help in diagnosis.

If repeated fine needle aspiration biopsies are not successful, the node may be excised under general anesthesia with a plan to go immediately to a neck dissection under the same anesthesia if it turns out to be a metastatic squamous cell cancer.

Metastatic cancers other than squamous cell can also be found in neck lymph nodes. Thyroid cancers may present with metastasis in a neck lymph node. Sometimes the lymph node biopsy will show another type of cancer such as an adenocarcinoma. In these cases, the primary site is less likely to be in the head and neck. For enlarged nodes containing squamous carcinoma in the lower half of the neck, the primary site may be in the head and neck but may also be in the esophagus, lung, or genitourinary tract. Most squamous cell carcinomas found in lymph nodes in the upper half of the neck are a result of spread from primary head and neck cancers.

The first step in the evaluation of a patient with squamous cell cancer in a neck lymph node from an unknown primary site is a very thorough head and neck examination to try to find the primary tumor. A careful head and neck exam with mirrors and scopes frequently turns up cancer in the nasopharynx, oropharynx, or hypopharynx. Next, imaging studies such as MRI, CT, and PET scans may be performed to search for a primary site and further assess the neck metastasis.

Finally, patients with squamous cell cancer in a neck lymph node from an unknown primary site should undergo examination under anesthesia of head and neck areas directly and with scopes. Suspicious areas are biopsied. If there are no suspicious areas, directed biopsies are done of the nasopharynx, base of the tongue, and pyriform sinus on the same side as the neck lesion. If the tonsil is present, it should be biopsied or removed. If a cancer originating in the head and neck is not found, other organs such as the lungs, colon, breast, and prostate should be evaluated. In about 90 percent of cases initially considered to be from an unknown primary site, a primary tumor is found.

Treatment Overview

Standard Treatment If a head and neck primary tumor is found with these studies, treatment is given as outlined previously.

Sometimes even after extensive work-up, a primary tumor is not found. In this case, it is usually assumed that the patient has a head and neck primary tumor that has escaped detection. The patient is treated with external-beam radiation therapy that targets the neck metastasis as well as the most likely sites of a head and neck primary tumor, including the nasopharynx, tonsil, base of the tongue, and pyriform sinus. The morbidity and side effects associated with such a wide field of radiation can obviously be quite significant, underlining the importance of identifying a primary site. Following radiation treatment, the patient is again examined carefully under anesthesia for a primary site, and a neck dissection is performed if there are any neck lymph nodes that remain enlarged. Alternatively, some centers perform a neck dissection as the initial treatment, followed by radiation therapy to the likely head and neck primary sites and the neck lymph node region. Chemotherapy given with radiation therapy may also be appropriate if the metastatic lymph nodes are large or extensive.

Five-Year Survival If a head and neck primary tumor is found, prognosis is as described previously. For patients with metastatic neck squamous cell cancer from an unknown primary site who undergo standard treatment, five-year survival rates are approximately as follows: 50 percent for Tx, N1 tumors, 35–50 percent for Tx, N2 tumors, and up to 20 percent for Tx, N3 tumors.

Recurrent Cancer

If the disease progresses, recurs, or relapses, the prognosis is poor. Further treatment depends on the type of cancer, what initial treatment was given, and the site of recurrence.

The Most Important Questions You Can Ask If You Have a Head and Neck Cancer

- What is the primary site or source of my cancer?
- What is the stage and what organs are involved?
- What tests are necessary to find this out? Are they uncomfortable?
- Is there a choice between surgery and radiation? Should I receive both?
- Is there a role for chemotherapy? When?
- What kind of functional disability might I have? Will I have trouble eating, swallowing, or speaking?
- How will I look after the treatments? Will I have a cosmetic disability?
- How much experience have the surgeon, radiation oncologist, and medical oncologist had with this type of tumor, and with what results?
- What complications can result from treatment?
- How long does it take to recover from the treatment?
- How often will you examine me afterward?
- When will I know I am safe?

Kaposi's Sarcoma

Susan E. Krown, M.D.

■ ■ ■ ■

Kaposi's sarcoma (KS) is a tumor that usually begins on the skin. Typically, the skin lesions are red or purple, but they may also be pink or dark brown. The typical red to purple color of the lesions is caused by the disorganized network of small blood vessels that is present within the tumors. These blood vessels allow red blood cells to leak out into the tumor tissue, giving the lesions their characteristic color. The lesions may be flat or raised up from the surface of the skin.

Several types of KS have been described that are distinguished from each other by the situations in which they are diagnosed. The "classic" form of KS was originally described in 1872 by Moritz Kaposi, a dermatologist in Vienna. This form most commonly occurs in older individuals of central and eastern European origin, particularly among those of Ashkenazic-Jewish descent, and also among individuals originating in Italy and the other countries of the Mediterranean basin. In Israel, KS is seen among both Ashkenazic and Sephardic Jews. The classic form of KS is relatively uncommon. It is found more often in men, but also occurs in women, and most commonly presents in older individuals (seventy and older), although younger people may be affected.

Before the AIDS epidemic, various forms of KS were also described in parts of Africa. These included an aggressive form seen in children (both boys and girls) that mainly involved the lymph nodes, as well as several forms that affected adults, mostly men. The African forms of KS that are not associated with acquired immunodeficiency syndrome (AIDS) are sometimes referred to as endemic KS.

KS is now also known to be associated with two types of decreased body immunity. The first occurs when certain drugs are given to suppress the immune system, such as after kidney transplantation. These drugs are given so that the foreign organ will not be rejected. KS may sometimes disappear when the drugs are stopped. The second circumstance in which immune suppression occurs is in association with AIDS. This form of KS, now the most common form of the disease, is referred to as epidemic KS.

How It Spreads Most malignancies begin in one area of the body, perhaps in one cell or a small group of cells. As the tumors grow, they can spread to other parts of the body by traveling through the blood or lymphatic system. Unlike most other tumors, KS often appears simultaneously in many sites. This suggests that there is a causal agent, possibly in the blood, that triggers the development of the lesions in several areas at the same time. In this, KS bears a strong resemblance to some viral "rash" diseases, like measles and chicken pox.

What Causes It The idea that KS resembled certain viral diseases was confirmed when a new virus, known as human herpesvirus 8 (HHV-8), or Kaposi's sarcoma-associated herpesvirus (KSHV), was discovered in 1994. Since then, scientists have studied this virus and found that it is present in all forms of KS. A person must be infected with this virus in order for KS to develop. However, other factors are required for the tumors to form, so not everyone who is infected with the virus will develop KS lesions. Although some factors (in addition to the virus) that predispose patients to the development of KS are known, others are not. Certain types of chemicals produced by the body that are required for the development of new blood vessels, and that are produced during inflammation, appear to be important additional factors involved in the development of KS lesions. There also appear to be certain inherited (genetic) factors that regulate susceptibility to infection with the virus that causes KS.

Who Gets It Classic KS is a disease of older adults, with an average age of onset of over seventy. The disease is diagnosed more frequently in people of Mediterranean background and in Jews but has been reported around the world. Men have a higher risk than women of developing all types of KS; the reasons for this gender disparity are unknown. Although marked immunosuppression has not been described in either the classic form or the endemic African forms of the disease, it is possible that declining immune function with age (in the case of classic KS) or caused by the presence of other infectious diseases (in endemic African KS) may contribute to susceptibility.

KS that develops following administration of immune-suppressing drugs accounts for about 3 percent of all tumors that occur in people who have had kidney transplants in the United States; this is about forty times higher than the rate of KS in the general population. In this group, the risk is higher in areas of the world where classic KS is more common. The age of occurrence depends on the age when the immune-suppressive treatment started.

Epidemic, or AIDS-related, KS can occur in all age and HIV risk groups but is most commonly diagnosed among HIV-infected gay men in their thirties and forties. When AIDS was first described in the early 1980s, about 40 percent of infected people developed KS as a complication. The proportion of HIV-positive people who develop KS has been declining in developed countries since the late 1980s. However, rates of KS in HIV-infected people are extremely high in parts of Africa. In some African countries in which HIV infection is prevalent, KS is the most common cancer diagnosed in men, is second only to cervical cancer in women, and has also become a common childhood cancer.

There may be several reasons for the decrease in rates of KS among HIV-infected patients in developed countries. The decrease may in part be traced to the introduction of better drugs to treat HIV infection. The use of drugs such as protease inhibitors became widespread in developed countries starting in 1996 and was associated not only with a decrease in new KS cases, but also, in some instances, with shrinkage or even disappearance of KS that was already present. However, the decrease in KS cases is not entirely because of better HIV treatments, since the decrease in the number of KS cases began before these drugs were available. Some people speculate that there was a decrease in KSHV infection rates by the late 1980s, possibly because of safer sexual practices. Also, better control of other infections associated with HIV may have decreased some of the inflammation that can contribute to KS development.

Although the number of patients with AIDS-associated KS has declined, new cases continue to be diagnosed despite treatment with multidrug regimens that effectively suppress HIV. Additionally, some patients with HIV do not respond to these regimens and have a higher risk of KS.

Risk Factors

The virus that causes KS is more common in certain parts of the world, so being from an area where the virus is more common, or a descendant of someone who is from such an area, is a risk factor. KS is more common among Jews of central and eastern Europe and among people from countries surrounding the Mediterranean, especially southern Italy. Nonetheless, this is an uncommon disease even among people from regions where the virus is more common. The virus is also more common in certain parts of central and east Africa. Taking immunosuppressive drugs increases the risk of developing KS, but these patients must also be infected with the KS virus for KS to develop.

At Significantly Higher Risk People who are infected with HIV. Although all HIV-infected people have an increased risk of developing KS, the highest risk is among men who have sex with men.

Screening

There are no standard screening tests for KS. Careful skin examination will usually detect lesions, which will then require biopsy for confirmation of the diagnosis. There are blood tests that can detect infection with the virus that causes KS, but these are nonstandard tests that are currently available only in research laboratories.

Common Signs and Symptoms

There are no general symptoms of early Kaposi's sarcoma. In the epidemic form, KS may be the first sign of AIDS, but the tumor often occurs after other symptoms of HIV infection have developed. In the classic form of KS, swelling of the feet and legs may precede the development of skin lesions. In a particular form of KS that occurs in African children, swollen glands may be the first sign of KS.

Once KS occurs, symptoms relate to the site of involvement. Early and even more advanced skin lesions are usually only mildly uncomfortable or may not cause any symptoms, although some lesions can be painful and develop ulcers. Swelling (edema) is a common complication and can affect any part of the body, but is most common in the feet and legs. Edema around the eyes can cause problems with vision. KS can occur in the mouth. When mouth lesions are small and flat, they cause no symptoms, but larger, raised lesions can cause problems with eating and speaking. Gastrointestinal lesions are common. They rarely cause significant symptoms but can sometimes be associated with bleeding or pain. Early lesions in the lung have no symptoms, but severe lung involvement will produce shortness of breath and sometimes coughing up blood. Most of these severe symptoms occur in people with epidemic KS and except for foot and leg edema are uncommon in people with other forms of KS.

Diagnosis

Careful physical examination of anyone suspected of having KS requires an evaluation of all organ systems. Physical findings relate to the site of involvement. The most common sign of the illness is the appearance of one or more of the characteristic skin lesions. Lesions may be found in many locations, although the characteristic finding in classic KS is a single flat or raised purple-red spot or a cluster of lesions in a single area of the body, most commonly on the feet or legs. Among patients with epidemic KS, the first lesions can appear anywhere on the body. In these patients, unusual sites of skin lesions include behind the ears and on the nose.

Physical Examination

• The skin must be carefully examined. Although the lesions of classic KS occur most commonly on the feet and legs, all forms of the disease can affect any area of the skin.

• Typical early skin lesions are flat or slightly raised above the surface of the skin; round, oval, or irregularly shaped; and pink, red, or purple in color. In darker-skinned individuals, the color may appear dark brown. Skin lesions can also first appear as lumps (nodules), and flatter lesions can grow into nodules over time.

• Many patients will have a yellow-brown pigment around the lesions. This bruiselike appearance is caused by blood cells leaking into the tissue around the lesion.

• As the disease progresses, the skin lesions may grow together, occupying large areas, blocking drainage from an extremity, causing swelling, and breaking down (ulcerating) in areas. Lesion breakdown can result in infection.

• Swelling (edema) is a common complication. This occurs most commonly in the feet and legs but may also affect the genitals, the area around the eyes, and other parts of the body.

• Lymph nodes may be enlarged. A biopsy is needed to distinguish KS in nodes from other causes of lymph node enlargement.

• Mucous membranes are often involved. In the mouth, the hard and soft palates are most frequently affected.

• The membrane covering the eye (conjunctiva) may be involved, or lesions may be seen beneath the white of the eye (sclera).

• Involvement of internal organs may be suspected by physical examination but cannot be proven without further testing. The physician will listen for abnormal sounds in the lungs and feel for enlargement of the liver or spleen and for abnormal masses.

Blood and Other Tests

• There are currently no standard blood tests for KS. If standard tests for the virus that causes KS (HHV-8/KSHV) become available, it may be possible to predict which patients are at risk for developing KS and to develop treatments to prevent it.

• Patients with epidemic (AIDS-associated) KS will have a positive blood test for HIV, but this does not predict the development of KS. However, if the HIV infection is found to be under poor control, treatments for HIV may help prevent KS from occurring or treat existing KS lesions.

Imaging KS may appear on a chest X-ray or CT scan but usually cannot be distinguished from infections or other tumors. A direct view of the lung (bronchoscopy) may be needed.

Endoscopy and Biopsy

• Careful rectal examination with an anoscope or proctoscope may reveal involvement.

• In patients who have symptoms suggestive of involvement of the gastro-intestinal tract such as pain or bleeding, upper gastrointestinal tract endoscopy can reveal KS lesions in the esophagus or stomach, and lower gastrointestinal tract endoscopy (colonoscopy) can reveal KS lesions in the lower intestine. If pigmented lesions resembling KS are seen, they can be biopsied during these endoscopy procedures.

• Although the only diagnostic test for KS in the gastrointestinal tract is a positive biopsy of a suspicious lesion, a presumptive diagnosis of KS can be made based solely on the appearance of the lesion, especially if a diagnosis of KS has been made on a biopsy elsewhere in the body.

Staging

There are several systems that have been designed to stage KS. Since KS differs from other solid cancers, such as lung or breast cancer, in that it can arise in several places at the same time, standard staging systems for cancer generally do not apply. The staging system most commonly adopted for the staging of epidemic (AIDS-associated) KS takes into consideration the location and extent of the KS lesions, the severity of immune system suppression, and the presence or absence of signs and symptoms of HIV-associated disease.

Treatment Overview

Because KS is caused by a virus that probably cannot be completely eradicated from the body with currently available medications, it is not considered curable by any current treatment. Neither surgical removal of the first-detected lesions nor obtaining a complete remission of multiple sites with chemotherapy or other techniques results in cure.

Nevertheless, treatment may cause shrinkage or disappearance of KS lesions that lasts for many years, and long-term survival can occur both with and without treatment. Survival with classic KS is usually years and sometimes decades; most patients with classic KS are elderly and die from causes other than KS. Some patients with AIDS-related KS have survived for more than ten years. It is likely that more patients with AIDS-related KS will have long survival because improved treatments for HIV are now available. Although it may not be possible to eliminate the cause of KS, many treatments are available that may control the lesions, and new treatments are being investigated. Patients should consider participating in clinical research programs in major medical centers and hospitals, such as those conducted by the AIDS Malignancy Consortium (*www.amcoperations.com*).

Treatment for HIV Infection For those patients with epidemic KS, treatment for the HIV infection with combinations of antiviral drugs appears to be critical to the success of KS treatment. In some cases, KS lesions may shrink or disappear with HIV treatment alone. For others, it appears to improve the response to chemotherapy and interferon, which are discussed below.

Surgery Surgical biopsy for microscopic examination of a suspicious lesion is needed to confirm the diagnosis of KS. Once the diagnosis is made, biopsy of other lesions is usually not needed except in cases where a deep lesion—a lung tumor, for example—has to be evaluated.

Other than for a biopsy, surgery is not commonly used to treat KS. In rare cases, lesions in the gastrointestinal tract may bleed or obstruct the passage of food and require surgical treatment. Conventional surgery and lasers have been used to remove bulky lesions in the mouth. Removal of multiple skin lesions does little to provide any meaningful relief of symptoms.

Radiation All forms of KS are sensitive to radiation therapy. Radiation may be useful for lesions that are cosmetically disturbing, painful, involve the mouth extensively, bleed, or protrude greatly from the skin. Response rates are high and treatment is usually well tolerated. However, since KS is caused by a viral infection that is not limited to the visible lesions, radiation given to local sites will not treat or prevent KS elsewhere in the body, and other forms of therapy may be more appropriate, especially when the lesions are widespread.

The tissues of the mouth are very sensitive to radiation in epidemic KS, resulting in poor tolerance to treatment. The surfaces of the mouth may become inflamed or ulcerated. Anesthetic mouthwashes can control pain and speed the healing, which may take days or weeks.

Different methods of radiation are used depending upon the number, size, and location of the lesions. The best methods to use for a given patient need to be individualized by the radiation therapist.

Chemotherapy Chemotherapy is usually reserved for treating individuals with widespread or rapidly progressive KS that is producing symptoms that have a negative effect on quality of life. Most of the recent experience with chemotherapy drugs for KS has been in patients with epidemic (AIDS-associated) KS. However, there is no reason to believe that others with advanced KS would respond differently to these drugs. Before the recognition of KS in association with AIDS in the early 1980s, most of the experience with chemotherapy for KS was in Africa, and the African studies provided the basis for the earliest studies of chemotherapy in AIDS-associated KS.

The chemotherapy drugs most commonly used to treat KS are doxorubicin liposomal (Doxil), daunorubicin liposomal (DaunoXome), and paclitaxel (Taxol). The first two drugs are made by enclosing two older drugs in a liposome, which is a type of lipid (fat) sphere. These liposomal preparations make the drugs concentrate in the tumor cells, while preventing them from accumulating in other tissues, such as heart muscle cells. These drugs have been shown to be more effective in treating KS and to be less toxic than some of the older drugs used to treat KS. The major side effect of all of these drugs is lowering of the white blood cell counts, which could make patients more susceptible to infections. Paclitaxel can also cause a condition called peripheral neuropathy, which causes numbness, tingling, and sometimes pain in the hands and feet; people with HIV infection may be particularly susceptible to this side effect. Nonetheless, these drugs

are usually quite well tolerated and lead to shrinkage of KS lesions and improvement of symptoms in a majority of patients.

In certain resource-poor countries where KS is common, such as in parts of Africa, these newer drugs are not available. In these places, some of the older drugs used to treat KS, such as doxorubicin (Adriamycin), bleomycin (Blenoxane), vincristine (Oncovin), vinblastine (Velban), and etoposide (Etopophos), may be used either as single drugs or as part of two- or three-drug combinations.

Chemotherapy treatments should always be given by a physician experienced in using these agents. This is usually a medical oncologist.

Local Therapy Chemotherapy drugs injected directly into KS lesions may lead to shrinkage of the tumors. This approach was more commonly used in the past but is now used relatively rarely. Another local treatment is freezing of the lesions with liquid nitrogen. This may lead to shrinkage or flattening of the lesions and a decrease in the color of the lesions, but can leave white spots on darker-colored skin. Neither of these approaches usually results in permanent disappearance of KS lesions.

Topical application of alitretinoin (Pararetin) gel has been shown in some cases to be effective in shrinking skin lesions. This approach works best in patients with limited numbers of small skin lesions. As with radiation therapy, these local approaches are effective only in the treated skin lesions and do not affect the development of new lesions or lead to shrinkage of untreated lesions.

 Biological Therapy The only biological therapy considered a standard therapy for KS is interferon-alpha. This agent has been studied most often in epidemic KS, but there are also some small studies indicating that it may also be useful for some patients with classic KS. The best responses of epidemic KS to interferon-alpha occur in patients who do not have very advanced HIV infection. Interferon-alpha is more likely to be effective against KS, and can be used at lower doses that cause fewer side effects, when it is used together with drugs used to treat HIV infection.

Drug-induced KS, especially KS that develops in patients who have received kidney transplants who are receiving certain standard drugs to prevent rejection of the transplanted kidney, may regress if the immunosuppressive drug therapy is stopped. Unfortunately, this often results in rejection of the transplanted organ. It has recently been described that switching kidney transplant patients with KS to a different drug, known as sirolimus (Rapamune), results in remission of the KS lesions without rejection of the kidney. Studies are being developed to see if this drug can also cause regression of KS lesions in other types of patients, such as those with epidemic KS.

Investigational A class of new drugs known as angiogenesis (blood vessel formation) inhibitors has been found to be useful for a number of cancers, including KS. Among the drugs that have shown some activity against KS in clinical trials are thalidomide (Thalomid) and imatinib mesylate (Gleevec), both of which are approved for use in other types of cancer. In addition, a variety of other investigational (nonapproved) drugs that inhibit angiogenesis have shown some evidence for activity in KS and are being studied in clinical trials.

In addition to drugs that may inhibit the new blood vessel growth seen in KS lesions, some studies are investigating whether the virus that causes KS can be inhibited. There are some data that indicate that drugs active in treating another viral infection, cytomegalovirus (CMV), may prevent the development of KS in HIV-infected people who do not already have KS, but there is not much evidence that these drugs can make KS lesions that are already present shrink or disappear. There is much current research on other types of drugs that can affect the KS virus and that may prove useful in KS treatment.

Whenever possible, patients should consider participating in a clinical trial with the hope of improved response and survival. A resource for identifying clinical trials for patients with KS can be found at *www.amcoperations.com*.

Treatment by Stage and Site

Decisions on whether, when, and how to treat patients with KS are based on factors such as the rate of growth of the lesions, the site of involvement, the general physical condition of the patient, and the severity of symptoms.

Among patients with epidemic KS, the extent of the tumor has been shown to affect survival. Patients with extensive involvement of internal organs, such as the lungs and gastrointestinal tract, or those with severe tumor-related swelling, have a shorter survival than those with less widespread tumors. Those with KS in the lung appear to have a particularly short survival if not treated. Such patients should be treated immediately with chemotherapy. While some feel that there is no reason to treat patients with very early KS (other than to treat their HIV infection), others have argued that early treatment, especially with drugs that may affect the KS virus or that can inhibit new blood vessel formation, might prevent progression to more advanced disease, which can be harder to treat.

For patients with classic KS, which usually progresses quite slowly, treatment is generally dictated by symptoms. Very early KS can often be left untreated. Localized areas of involvement may be successfully treated with radiation therapy.

Occasionally, patients with classic KS may develop more widespread, aggressive lesions, or may show recurrence of lesions after radiation therapy, and may require a systemic therapy such as chemotherapy.

For patients whose KS develops while receiving drugs that cause immunosuppression, if medically indicated, the drugs can be stopped or their doses reduced. This may not always be possible, and patients may require additional treatment for KS. A very promising development for those with transplant-associated KS is the finding that switching the drugs used to prevent graft rejection in kidney transplant recipients who developed KS led to regression of KS, without rejection of the kidney.

For patients with endemic, African KS, the therapeutic options available are often limited by the local treatment resources. In these patients, symptomatic lesions have successfully been treated with local radiation and standard chemotherapy; generally, the newer chemotherapy drugs used to treat KS in developed countries are not available in Africa.

Supportive Therapy

There are several common treatment-related problems with KS—especially depression of the bone marrow and nerve damage, which should be monitored carefully.

• In patients receiving chemotherapy, frequent checks of the blood counts help reduce the risk of serious bone marrow effects, especially a decrease in the white blood cell count, which could increase the risk of infection. Lowering of the white blood cell count is often treated with injections of granulocyte–colony-stimulating factor G-CSF; filgrastim [Neupogen]); lowering of the red blood cell count (anemia) is often treated with injections of erythropoietin (epoetin alfa [Procrit]; or darbepoetin alfa [Aranesp]).

• Nerve damage will regularly be checked in patients receiving chemotherapy, with changes in medicine as needed to minimize this problem.

• Patients often need emotional and psychological support. Physical appearance is an important part of self-image, and cosmetics may be needed to cover lesions (see chapter 27, "The Look Good . . . Feel Better Cosmetic Program"). Patients with KS and HIV infection may also need to deal with many psychosocial issues related to their underlying illness, including discrimination, job loss, loss of insurance, depression, and isolation. Help may be found from a variety of hospital-based, public, and private organizations devoted to these problems.

• Pain is not common with KS, but if it does occur, pain relievers may be needed.

• Fluid may build up in body tissues, especially the legs, because KS lesions can block drainage. This swelling often goes down when the legs are elevated but usually recurs once the patient is back on his or her feet. The use of diuretics (water pills) under close supervision is sometimes effective in relieving edema from KS, but the most effective treatment is to treat the KS, usually with chemotherapy.

• Loss of appetite and poor nutrition may occur as a complication of HIV infection but may be worse in KS patients who are receiving chemotherapy or who have KS lesions in their gastrointestinal tract. In patients with poor appetites, certain appetite stimulants may be useful. Some patients may also benefit from nutritional counseling.

Treatment Follow-Up

To discover whether the treatment is working, the physician will measure skin and oral lesions. Sometimes photographs of lesions are helpful in assessing the response to treatment, as is measurement of the size of swollen legs. Periodic examinations using X-rays and scans may also try to detect whether internal organ involvement is getting better or worse.

Recurrent Cancer

Because KS is not considered curable, the disappearance of detectable disease (clinical remission) means only that the presence of the disease cannot be demonstrated at a particular time. It is not known how long drug treatments should be continued once remission has been obtained.

In the past, it was often the case that patients with AIDS-associated KS in either complete or partial remission who stopped drug treatments for KS relapsed rapidly. Since the introduction of more effective drug regimens to treat HIV infection in the mid-1990s, KS remissions have tended to be longer lasting, even without continued KS treatment, if the HIV infection has been well controlled. However, even people with good control of their HIV infection may show recurrence if KS treatment is stopped, so the length of treatment needs to be individualized.

The Most Important Questions You Can Ask

- When should treatment begin?
- When is interferon treatment helpful?
- What types of chemotherapy treatment are available?
- When is radiation useful?
- How long will treatment last?
- Are there any new treatments available or clinical trials in which I can take part?
- What supportive services and treatments are available?

Kidney

Brian I. Rini, M.D.

■ ■ ■ ■

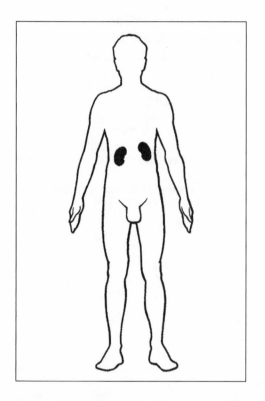

Cancer of the kidney—also called renal cell cancer (RCC), kidney adenocarcinoma, or hypernephroma—accounts for about 3 percent of new cancers in the United States, and an estimated 51,190 new cases in the year 2007. Almost 12,890 persons will die of kidney cancer in the year 2007.

The kidneys lie deep in the body between the lining of the abdominal cavity (peritoneum) and the back muscles at the level of the lowest two ribs. By the time symptoms such as back pain and bloody urine are noted, a kidney tumor

can often be large (average size is 3 inches [7.5 cm]) and have invaded lymph nodes and/or surrounding structures. RCC is very vascular because of certain inherent genetic changes. This increased vascularity soon leads to spread to the lung(s), liver, and bone. Five-year survival ranges from 50 to over 95 percent for small tumors within the kidney that can be completely removed by surgery. Advanced disease invading lymph nodes or the inferior vena cava has a five-year survival rate of about 35 percent; fewer than 5 percent of patients with metastatic disease will survive five years.

Types More than 90 percent of renal cancers develop in glandular tissue (and are called adenocarcinomas). Within the adenocarcinoma category, several subtypes can be defined by microscopic appearance. The clear cell variety is seen in 75 percent of cases, and the papillary histology in 10 percent. Less common subtypes include chromophobe, medullary, and unclassified renal cell carcinomas. *Sarcomatoid* refers to a specific pattern of appearance that can occur in any histologic subtype and is usually associated with more aggressive disease. Another renal cancer, Wilms' tumor, is found exclusively in children.

How It Spreads Kidney cancer cells frequently spread through the bloodstream by penetrating blood vessels within the tumor, then entering the renal vein and/or the inferior vena cava, the largest abdominal vein. Once cells have entered the bloodstream, they can travel to the lung(s), liver, brain, or bone and multiply at these sites, producing metastases.

Cells can also directly invade the abdominal lymph nodes that drain the kidney and extend into structures surrounding the kidney (perinephric tissues) such as fat, the adrenal gland, and the liver. This kind of invasion is found at diagnosis in about 45 percent of cases. Invasion of the inferior vena cava is found in 10 to 15 percent of cases, and invasion of local lymph nodes in 10 to 30 percent. In over half the cases with lymph node involvement, distant metastases are also found.

What Causes It Risk factors are poorly defined, although the incidence is twice as high for those using tobacco (cigars, chewing tobacco, and cigarettes). Renal cell cancers can develop in patients exposed to chemotherapy and radiation therapy five to ten years prior. Exposure to ionizing radiation at very high levels may also increase the risk.

Risk Factors

At Significantly Higher Risk

• Gender. This tumor is twice as frequent in men as in women, occurring mostly between the ages of thirty and seventy.

• Tobacco use.

• Dialysis. Patients on long-term dialysis acquire small, fluid-filled areas in their kidneys called cysts, which have an increased risk of developing cancer in them.

• Weak risk factors include obesity in women and a high-animal-fat diet.

• Genetic. Only 1 to 2 percent of all kidney cancers are inherited. The most common is clear cell RCC from von Hippel–Lindau (VHL) syndrome, which also causes blood vessel tumors of the eye, brain, and spinal cord. There are other very rare inherited syndromes that lead to different histologic subtypes of RCC.

Screening

The urine can be examined for blood (hematuria) to detect early lesions that can be surgically removed, although routine screening has not been shown to be of benefit. Ultrasound screening of the kidney, which is used in some countries, is more accurate, but is not cost-effective and is not routinely used. Intravenous pyelography (IVP) and CT scans are used only in the diagnostic work-up to discover the cause of persistent and unexplained symptoms such as abdominal or flank pain, anemia, blood in the urine, and fever. Better screening procedures will have to await a simplified and less expensive urine or blood test.

Common Signs and Symptoms

The most common symptom is blood in the urine (hematuria), which is present in up to 65 percent of cases. Abdominal pain is found in 40 percent of patients and an abdominal mass in 35 percent. Other common symptoms include anemia, bone pain, unexplained weight loss, low-grade fever, general weakness or loss of energy, and loss of appetite.

Unusual symptoms may include hypercalcemia (high blood calcium), high blood pressure, abnormal liver tests, and too many red cells in the blood (polycythemia). These symptoms develop because renal tumors can produce substances that indirectly affect other organs, producing conditions called paraneoplastic syndromes.

Diagnosis

A doctor may suspect kidney cancer if a patient complains of the common symptoms noted above.

Physical Examination

• An abdominal mass felt below the rib cage in the back or side area may be felt if a kidney has a large tumor in it.

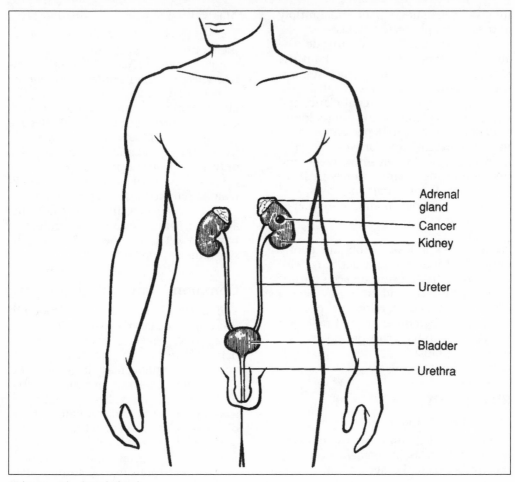

Kidneys and adrenal glands

• An abdominal bruit (a sound over the renal artery) can be heard if blood flow to a kidney with a tumor in it is altered.

Blood and Other Tests

• A urinalysis can detect blood in the urine; one cause of this is kidney cancer, although it is not the most common cause (kidney stones, infection, bladder cancer, and trauma would be other causes).

• Liver function tests can be abnormal if the cancer has spread to the liver.

• A complete blood count can show whether the red blood cell count (called the hemoglobin or hematocrit) is high or low.

• A blood calcium test can indicate a high calcium level. Kidney cancer releases certain substances that increase the calcium level.

Imaging

• An intravenous pyelogram (IVP), also called excretory urography, is a detailed X-ray of the kidney and suspected tumor after the injection of a relatively harmless contrast medium into the bloodstream that supplies the kidney. The material is concentrated in the urine and provides a silhouette of the kidney. This reveals any changes in the kidney's shape due to a tumor and gives information about the other normal kidney.

• Ultrasound is the most sensitive test, being able to find masses as small as ¾ inch (2 cm) in over 90 percent of cases. Sonograms can often distinguish between the more commonly occurring benign, or noncancerous, cyst and a solid tumor. When this test is combined with the intravenous pyelogram (IVP), the accuracy of a tumor diagnosis is over 90 percent. The sonogram can also be very helpful in determining whether the tumor has induced a clot in or invaded the renal vein or the inferior vena cava.

• CT with intravenous dye (the same dye used for intravenous pyelograms) will accurately diagnose renal tumors in 95 percent of cases and be falsely positive in fewer than 2 percent. This test may also show the tumor extension outside the kidney and can determine the extent of lymph node, liver, and blood vessel involvement.

• MRI is used for determining more clearly the extent of blood vessel involvement and involvement of adjacent structures. It is useful in obtaining preoperative information in some patients with particularly large tumors. It is not, however, routinely used for all patients.

• Selective renal arteriography is helpful in finding small tumors and providing information that may sometimes be needed at the time of surgery about uncommon blood vessel patterns and, in selected cases, in determining the possibility of a partial nephrectomy (removal of only a portion of the kidney) for small localized tumors.

• Other tests before surgery attempt to ensure that there are no distant metastases. These include chest X-rays or chest CT scans, bone scans or skeletal X-rays, and, occasionally, head CT.

Biopsy Ultimately, the diagnosis is made either by removing all or part of the kidney (nephrectomy) or by a biopsy of the kidney itself or of a tumor deposit in another organ. Looking for tumor cells in the urine is not useful.

Treatment Overview

Surgical removal of the kidney (simple nephrectomy) and the additional removal of the surrounding fat, the adrenal gland, and the lymph nodes (radical nephrectomy) can lead to a cure for Stages I and II and can even cure Stage III in a few cases. Advanced stages (III and IV) require surgery and systemic therapy.

Surgery Partial nephrectomy is usually performed for a tumor in patients with small (less than 3 inches [7 cm]) tumors and either one kidney or health conditions that could affect future kidney function. Radical nephrectomy is generally accepted as the standard treatment approach for cancer confined to the kidney.

No evidence exists that radiation therapy alone without surgery is of any benefit.

Adjuvant Therapy There is no evidence that routine preoperative (neoadjuvant) or postoperative (adjuvant) therapy (either radiation therapy, immunotherapy, or chemotherapy) can reduce the risk of relapse. Such approaches should be undertaken only as part of a clinical trial.

Embolization Embolization involves blocking off the blood supply to the kidney tumor. A catheter is temporarily placed in a blood vessel in the groin and pushed up through the major blood vessels until it is at the level of the kidney, at which point coils or other particles are used to block the blood supply to the kidney. Usually, embolization is done before a nephrectomy to facilitate surgery, although it can also be used instead of surgery to control pain and/or bleeding if surgery is not an option.

 Radiation Radiation therapy can be effective in controlling the pain from metastases to the bone. It is also used to control the growth of metastases to the brain. Its effectiveness in treating other areas or several places at one time is limited because of side effects.

Systemic Therapy Systemic therapy is given in the vein, under the skin, or by mouth and travels throughout the body to potentially treat any areas of metastatic deposits. Three forms of systemic therapy are used to treat renal cell carcinoma: antiangiogenic therapy (attacks blood vessels), chemotherapy, and biological therapy (also known as immunotherapy).

Antiangiogenic Therapy Kidney cancer produces a protein called vascular endothelial growth factor (VEGF), which causes new blood vessels to form and kidney cancer to get worse. Several treatments are now used that either bind this protein (bevacizumab [Avastin]) or block the action of this protein on blood vessel cells (sorafenib [Nexavar] and sunitinib [Sutent]). These drugs shrink tumors in up to 70 percent of patients, sometimes by a small amount and sometimes by a large amount. These drugs are relatively new in kidney cancer, so the durability of response and affect on survival is not yet known.

 Chemotherapy Chemotherapeutic agents have some activity against renal cell carcinoma, usually less than 20 percent, although two agents appear to be effective against this cancer: gemcitabine (Gemzar) and 5-fluorouracil (5-FU; and its derivative floxuridine [FUDR]). There is no standard chemotherapy program for renal cell carcinoma, although it is a viable option after biological therapy fails.

Biological Therapy Several proteins regulate the immune system and are normally produced by the body. These proteins (also called cytokines) can also be administered at higher doses to augment a patient's immune response against the cancer. Interferon-alpha appears to have a 15 to 20 percent response rate. Interleukin-2 (IL-2) is the only FDA-approved drug for the treatment of renal cell carcinoma, with a 20 percent response rate, including a small number of complete responses that are probably cures. The use of intravenous "high-dose" IL-2 (in the dosage in which it was approved by the FDA) is used by some investigators in younger, healthy patients. It requires a specialized medical center because of toxicity. It leads to a slightly higher overall and complete response rate and may be appropriate for some patients. Vaccines are being investigated but are as yet of unproven benefit.

Treatment by Stage

■ Stage I
TNM T1, N0, M0
Stage I means the tumor is confined within the renal capsule and is less than 3 inches (7 cm) with no lymph node or distant metastases. About one-third of cases are Stage I or II disease, many of which are Grade 1 (very well differentiated) to Grade 2 (moderately well differentiated).

Standard Treatment Radical nephrectomy. Partial nephrectomy can be performed in selected cases, for low-grade small masses less than 3 inches (7 cm) (ideally less than

1½ inches [4 cm]). A urologic surgeon will determine which surgery is appropriate. Radical nephrectomy involves tying the renal artery and vein, removing the surrounding fibrous layer (called Gerota's fascia), and thereby completely excising the kidney, the surrounding fat, the adrenal gland, the regional lymph nodes, and the ureter.

Five-Year Survival 60 to 90+ percent

Stage II
TNM T2, N0, M0
The tumor is larger than 3 inches (7 cm) without lymph node or distant metastases. The tumor invades the surrounding fat or the adrenal gland.

About 10 percent of cases are diagnosed in Stage II, and one-third of those patients will have micrometastases found at the time of surgery.

Standard Treatment Radical nephrectomy.

Five-Year Survival 50 to 65 percent

Stage III
TNM T1–2, N1, M0 or T3, N0–1, M0
The tumor invades the renal vein, the inferior vena cava, or the adrenal gland or spreads outside the kidney capsule (T3) or involves a single regional lymph node (N1).

Twenty-five to 35 percent of cases are found in Stage III.

Standard Treatment Radical nephrectomy may be possible, depending on the extent of local and/or lymph node invasion.

Five-Year Survival 20 to 40 percent

Stage IV
TNM T4, N0–1, M0 or any T, any N, M1
The tumor invades adjacent organs (T4) or nearby lymph nodes (N2) or has distant metastases (M1).

Approximately 30 percent of cases are diagnosed in Stage IV, with 10 percent low-grade tumors and more than 60 percent high-grade tumors.

Standard Treatment Two large studies have shown that patients undergoing radical nephrectomy before systemic biological therapy have an improved survival compared to those receiving only the systemic therapy. Thus, "debulking" nephrectomy is a standard of care for Stage IV RCC, but is not necessarily possible or appropriate for all patients. Nephrectomy for Stage IV cases should also be considered if there are symptoms attributable to the kidney tumor. Surgery can also be performed in select cases to remove metastatic disease when the cancer is limited to one site that can be safely and completely removed.

Antiangiogenic therapy and biological therapy are both standard for advanced disease. Further investigation will be needed to determine which is optimal for a given patient.

Five-Year Survival 5 percent

Treatment Follow-Up

- Regular physical examinations
- Blood chemistry panel
- Chest X-rays or chest CT (every three months) and abdominal CT scan (every three to six months)
- Bone scan (and specific bone X-rays) only if bone pain is present or serum alkaline phosphatase is elevated
- X-rays or imaging studies for specific areas only if symptoms are present (brain CT or MRI for persistent headaches; spine MRI for back pain with leg weakness or nerve symptoms)

These studies are done more frequently immediately after surgery and less often thereafter if there is no evidence the cancer has returned. They are done more frequently in patients with metastatic disease receiving treatment.

There is no routine role for PET scanning in RCC.

Recurrent Cancer

Investigational treatments should be explored as outlined for Stage IV disease. Patients with a single site of recurrent cancer, particularly if it has been more than two years since surgical removal of the primary tumor, may be candidates for surgery to remove the one site of cancer. Up to 30 percent of patients can obtain prolonged remissions and, possibly, cures in this fashion.

The Most Important Questions You Can Ask

• Has my cancer spread?

• What is the chance for cure with surgery alone?

• What are the complications of surgery?

• Is there any role for other treatments such as antiangiogenic or immunotherapy?

• What investigational approaches are available?

• What are the side effects of treatment; how common and how severe are they?

The Leukemias

Charles A. Linker, M.D., and Lloyd E. Damon, M.D.

■ ■ ■ ■

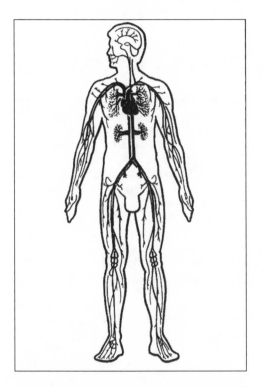

The leukemias are a group of cancers of cells of the blood and bone marrow. It is important to realize that the leukemias differ greatly in their levels of seriousness. Some leukemias (such as the acute leukemias) are aggressive and often life-threatening, requiring urgent treatment in order to avoid death. Other leukemias (e.g., chronic lymphocytic leukemia) may not cause problems or require any treatment for years or decades. Almost all the leukemias are treatable, and most are potentially curable.

Most leukemias arise in the bone marrow and cause problems by interfering with the function of the normal bone marrow. The bone marrow produces all the types of circulating blood cells, and deficiencies in these cell types result in problems according to the cell type involved. Red blood cells transport oxygen in the body, and when their level drops (called anemia), the person becomes tired and possibly short of breath. White blood cells (especially the type called neutrophils) fight infection, and low levels of these cells lead to a risk of infection. Some of these infections—especially bloodstream infections (sepsis) and pneumonia—can be rapidly progressive and life-threatening during a period of very low white blood cells (neutropenia) and are medical emergencies. Platelets are a type of blood cell that protects against bruising and bleeding. Low levels of platelets (thrombocytopenia) can lead to bruising and bleeding.

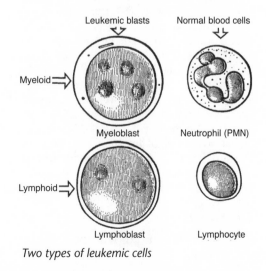

Two types of leukemic cells

Types   Leukemias are classified as "acute" or "chronic." The acute leukemias are more aggressive and cause major medical problems quickly. Without effective treatment, most patients will die within weeks. Chronic leukemias grow much more slowly. Some do not even require treatment for months or years, although some behave more aggressively.

Leukemias are also classified as "myeloid" or "lymphoid." This refers to the type of white blood cell that has become cancerous. Myeloid cells are the cells that give rise to neutrophils, the most important type of white blood cell for killing bacteria. Lymphoid cells give rise to lymphocytes, which protect against nonbacterial germs.

Acute Myeloid Leukemia (AML)

Acute myeloid leukemia (AML) is a cancer of primitive white blood cells in the bone marrow. It is the most common type of acute leukemia seen in adults, accounting for 80 percent of such cases. AML can occur in children and young adults but (as with almost all cancers) becomes more common later in life.

Common Signs and Symptoms

Typically, AML comes on suddenly—within days or weeks. Less often, a patient has been ill for a small number of months. AML makes people sick primarily by interfering with the normal functioning of the bone marrow. The bone marrow is the place in the body where all normal blood cells are produced, and when leukemia replaces the normal bone marrow, there is a lack of normal blood elements. The lack of red blood cells is called anemia and causes people to be tired and pale. A lack of platelets leads to vulnerability to bruising and bleeding, especially in the skin, nose, and gums. Lowered levels of normal white blood cells, especially neutrophils, lead to a risk of infection. Infections can be of any type, but pneumonia and infection of the bloodstream (called sepsis) are the most dangerous and can be rapidly life-threatening.

Diagnosis

The diagnosis of acute leukemia can be strongly suspected from abnormal blood counts (found on a CBC, complete blood count) and an abnormal appearance of the blood under the microscope. The leukemia cells (called blasts) are usually but not always visible in the blood. The diagnosis is established by examination of the bone marrow. Bone marrow biopsies are an indispensable part of the diagnosis and monitoring of treatment of AML. Bone marrow biopsy procedures are uncomfortable and sometimes painful for a very brief period of time, but with proper pain medication, they should not be a bad experience.

The bone marrow is initially examined under the microscope and this may be sufficient to give a diagnosis. At other times, additional laboratory studies such as peroxidase stains and immunophenotyping, looking for white blood cell markers, are important to establish a correct diagnosis. Usually the diagnosis of AML, or the alternative acute leukemia, acute lymphoblastic leukemia (ALL), can be made within a day after bone marrow examination. A very important part of the initial evaluation of AML is a chromosome analysis called cytogenetics. These results often take one to two weeks to be available and often do not influence the initial phase of treatment. However, they are often critical in determining the proper subsequent treatment.

There are several different subtypes of AML, but many types are treated in a similar fashion. One subtype, called acute promyelocytic leukemia (APL), has a unique biology and is treated differently.

Treatment Overview

Induction Chemotherapy Most patients with AML need to be treated in a short period of time, usually within days or weeks of diagnosis and sometimes the same day. For most cases of AML, the only effective treatment is with chemotherapy. The first phase of treatment, called induction chemotherapy, is done in the hospital and typically requires a hospitalization of four weeks or even longer. The most important chemotherapy drugs used are Ara-C (cytarabine) in combination with either daunorubicin or idarubicin. Additional chemotherapy drugs such as etoposide may also be used.

Chemotherapy is usually given over a period of seven days. During most of the time in the hospital, the patient needs to receive intensive supportive care to safeguard the patient during the period of very low blood counts. Most patients with AML have deficiencies in blood counts due to their leukemia before they start treatment, and chemotherapy temporarily takes away even the small number of normal cells present at that time. It usually takes at least three weeks for the normal blood counts to recover, and this is the major reason for the lengthy hospitalization. The support for low blood counts includes transfusions of red blood cells to correct anemia and transfusions of platelets to prevent bleeding. Antibiotics are usually used preventively to avoid bacterial and fungal infections during the period of high risk of infection; however, sometimes infections occur despite this and then antibiotics need to be changed to treat these "breakthrough" infections. In addition to transfusions and antibiotics, antinausea drugs are important and growth factors such as filgrastim (Neupogen) are helpful in bringing the white blood count back more quickly, thereby shortening the period of risk for infection.

In addition to effects on blood counts, the chemotherapy used for AML causes complete but temporary hair loss. Other common side effects include sores in the mouth and throat and disturbance of the intestinal tract including poor appetite, nausea, vomiting, and diarrhea.

After blood counts have returned to normal, it is important to have a repeat bone marrow biopsy to determine that chemotherapy has been successful and that the patient is in a "complete remission." A complete remission means that there is no visible leukemia in the blood or bone marrow and that bone marrow function has returned to normal as evidenced by the return of normal blood counts.

Acute promyelocytic leukemia (APL) is handled differently from other types of AML. Initial induction chemotherapy includes a combination of either idarubicin or daunorubicin and all-trans retinoic acid (ATRA, tretinoin), a derivative of vitamin A. The development of this highly effective vitamin as a part of the treatment of APL has led to major improvements in the results of treatment.

Postremission Therapy Once a patient is in complete remission, additional treatment is needed to give a chance at either a very long remission or a possibility of cure. This additional postremission treatment is necessary because in "remission," small numbers of leukemia cells can remain in the bone marrow but be below the level that can be detected with current methods. Without further treatment, these undetected leukemia cells will be able to grow back and cause a recurrence or "relapse." The best postremission treatment depends on a number of factors and should be done in a risk-adapted approach—that is, the intensity of the treatment should match the level of risk of the leukemia. The level of risk is determined primarily by cytogenetics (which is the most important risk factor in AML) and by the response of the leukemia to the treatment used.

Most patients with AML who are less than age sixty should be treated with the intent to produce a cure. This is not always achieved, but should be the goal. Acute promyelocytic leukemia (APL) is one of the "favorable" types of AML and is usually treated with repeated courses of chemotherapy plus ATRA, with cure rates of approximately 70 percent. If APL recurs after initial treatment, the recommended treatment is with arsenic trioxide (Trisenox), and this has a high chance (90 percent) of producing a second remission.

Other "favorable" subtypes of AML can be treated with follow-up chemotherapy, including high-doses of Ara-C (cytarabine) as the main component. Each of the two or more "consolidation" chemotherapy treatments given is similar in intensity to induction chemotherapy and requires a substantial hospitalization. With such treatment, the chance of cure is roughly 50 percent. Some doctors advocate more intensive treatment with autologous stem cell transplantation for "favorable" subtypes of AML, and the chance of cure is 70 percent or higher with this treatment. Alternatively, autologous transplant can be reserved for those patients whose leukemia recurs after less aggressive initial treatment.

For intermediate-risk AML, which accounts for two-thirds of all cases, consolidation chemotherapy with high-dose Ara-C produces a cure approximately 30 percent of the time. For that reason, more intensive treatment with stem cell transplantation (also called bone marrow transplantation) is often recommended. Autologous stem cell transplantation using cells collected from the patients themselves after they have achieved remission appears to produce a cure 40 to 50 percent of the time for intermediate-risk AML. Allogeneic transplantation, using stem cells (or bone marrow) from a matched (having the same bone marrow type or HLA type) sibling, produces a cure 50 to 60 percent of the time. However, allogeneic transplantation is significantly more difficult and dangerous than either chemotherapy or autologous transplantation, and 20 to 30 percent of patients do not survive the initial phases of treatment. For this reason, it is often reserved for more difficult cases.

Poor-risk AML is best treated with allogeneic transplant despite the difficulties and dangers of this treatment. Cure rates are 20 to 35 percent. For patients with poor-risk leukemia who do not have a matched sibling donor, it is appropriate to search for an unrelated donor through the National Marrow Donor Program (NMDP).

Patients who have relapsed after an initial remission can often be re-treated and can achieve a second complete remission. In order to have a chance of cure in second remission, intensive treatment with transplantation (either autologous or allogeneic) is needed.

Older adults with AML (between ages sixty and seventy-five) are more difficult to treat with curative intent. An attempt to produce an initial complete remission is almost always warranted unless the patient's general health is poor. Postremission treatment should be individualized according to a number of factors. It is very difficult to effectively treat AML in patients over age seventy-five because of the side effects of most treatments.

Investigational Femtzumab (Myelotarg) combines an antibody that specifically targets leukemia cells with a toxin that gets inserted directly into the leukemia cell once the antibody binds to it. This treatment has the advantage of not producing hair loss, mouth sores, or disturbance of the intestinal tract. However, it produces the same kind of long periods of low blood counts as standard chemotherapy, and the chance of reaching a remission is not as good as with chemotherapy. Further work needs to be done to determine the best role of this agent in the treatment of AML.

A type of arsenic called arsenic trioxide (Trisenox) is very useful in the treatment of acute promyelocytic leukemia (APL) and, despite the frightening name, is the best treatment for APL that has recurred after initial treatment. Clinical trials are studying whether it can increase the cure rate when used as part of initial treatment, but the results are not known at this time. Arsenic is not useful in forms of leukemia other than APL.

A very interesting development in the field of allogeneic stem cell transplantation is the so-called miniallogeneic transplant. It is a technique that makes allogeneic transplantation significantly less dangerous and more suitable to individuals who are older or have medical conditions that make full-dose transplants too dangerous. This approach is being studied in clinical trials to see if it can give more hope for cure in older adults with AML.

Nonchemotherapy agents such as tipifarnib (Zarnestra) are now being tested to see if they can be useful in the treatment of patients with AML for whom chemotherapy is not a good option. Many other such "targeted therapies" are being developed based on an increased understanding of the biology of leukemia cells.

Prognosis

For patients under age sixty, the chance of achieving initial complete remission is good, approximately 75 percent. Five to 10 percent of patients will die of treatment-related complications during initial treatment, and another 15 to 20 percent of patients will fail to enter complete remission. For the subtype of acute promyelocytic leukemia, initial remissions are achieved in 90 to 95 percent of patients.

The cure rates for patients in first remission depend on the risk type of the leukemia and the treatment used, as outlined above.

It is more difficult to treat AML in patients over age sixty and especially over age seventy-five. Initial complete remission rates are 50 to 60 percent. The risk of dying from treatment-related complications is higher than for younger adults, approximately 15 percent, and the leukemia fails to respond to chemotherapy in 30 percent of cases. Once in remission, less than 10 percent of these older adults are currently cured, but remissions typically last one to two years. The quality of life during remission time is usually normal.

Acute Lymphoblastic Leukemia (ALL)

Acute lymphoblastic leukemia (ALL) is a cancer of primitive lymphocytes that live in the bone marrow, lymph nodes, and spleen. ALL accounts for 20 percent of acute leukemia in adults but is the main type of acute leukemia in children.

Common Signs and Symptoms

As with AML, ALL usually causes illness suddenly, within days or weeks. Most problems are related to replacement of normal bone marrow and diminished normal blood counts. Anemia (low red blood cell counts) leads to tiredness, low platelet counts lead to vulnerability to bruising and bleeding, and low normal white blood cell counts lead to vulnerability to infections. In addition to these signs of bone marrow failure, ALL can sometimes cause enlarged lymph nodes or pain in the bones or joints.

Diagnosis

As with AML, the disease is usually suspected because of abnormal blood counts and the appearance of leukemic "blasts" in the blood. However, the diagnosis is established by examination of the bone marrow. It is usually difficult to be certain of a diagnosis of ALL (as opposed to AML) simply by the appearance of cells under the microscope, and additional laboratory tests are needed. One important test is immunophenotyping (also called flow cytometry), which will determine whether the cells are lymphoid (ALL) rather than myeloid (AML). Immunophenotyping will also determine whether these are T or B lymphocytes. These results are usually available within one day of bone marrow examination. As with AML, chromosome testing called cytogenetics is an important part of the initial evaluation, but these results may not be available for one to two weeks. One particular subtype of ALL, having the Philadelphia chromosome, requires special treatment. New molecular tests for the abnormal gene BCR/ABL may show this abnormality even when the standard cytogenetic test does not.

Treatment Overview

Induction Chemotherapy As with AML, treatment of ALL is usually urgent and needs to be given within days of diagnosis and sometimes the same day. Treatment is with chemotherapy. The first phase, induction chemotherapy, is done in the hospital, and most patients need to be in the hospital for approximately four weeks.

The most common drugs used in the treatment of ALL are daunorubicin, vincristine, prednisone, and asparaginase. Sometimes cyclophosphamide (Cytoxan) is used as well. For the subtype of Philadelphia-chromosome-positive ALL (Ph+ ALL), the addition of the nonchemotherapy drug imatinib mesylate (Gleevec) greatly improves the results. Induction treatment for ALL is somewhat more gentle than that for AML. Intensive supportive care is still needed, including transfusion of red blood cells and platelets. Antibiotics are needed both preventively and as treatment for bacterial and fungal infections. As with AML, the agent G-CSF (filgrastim [Neupogen]) can be useful in bringing the white cell count back sooner. Compared with treatment for AML, there is a lower incidence of mouth sores and disruption of the intestinal tract, but there is usually complete but temporary hair loss. Once blood counts have returned to normal, a repeat bone marrow biopsy and/or aspiration are performed to determine that the patient has entered complete remission. A complete remission is achieved when the blood and bone marrow show no evidence of persistent leukemia and blood counts have returned to normal.

Postremission Therapy Once a patient has achieved complete remission, further treatment is necessary. The earlier, more intensive parts of postremission chemotherapy are called consolidation treatment, and the more prolonged period of low-dose chemotherapy is called maintenance treatment. One difference between the treatment of ALL and AML is that patients with ALL require preventive treatment given to the spinal fluid and brain to prevent leukemia from invading this site. This is called central nervous system (CNS) prophylaxis and is performed with direct injections of chemotherapy into the spinal fluid (intrathecal chemotherapy) or sometimes a combination of intrathecal therapy and radiation to the brain.

As with AML, postremission treatment is given in a risk-adapted approach, with the intensity of treatment geared to the intensity of the leukemia. Most patients with ALL in first remission are treated with a chemotherapy program without bone marrow transplantation. The intensive part of chemotherapy usually takes approximately 6 months, and treatment programs vary in their details. Low-dose oral maintenance chemotherapy is typically given until a patient has been in remission for 2.5 years, at which point treatment is stopped. For patients with Ph+ ALL, imatinib mesylate (Gleevec) is also an important part of treatment.

High-risk types of ALL are best treated with allogeneic stem cell (or bone marrow) transplantation. A patient has high-risk ALL if he or she has high-risk cytogenetics such as the Philadelphia chromosome or if it takes extended treatment to achieve an initial remission. Young patients with very high risk ALL who need an allogeneic transplant but lack a matched sibling donor are sometimes appropriately treated with allogeneic transplant using a matched unrelated donor located though the National Marrow Donor Program (NMDP).

Patients who have relapsed after an initial remission can often be re-treated and can sometimes achieve a second complete remission. In order to have a chance of cure in second remission, intensive treatment with transplantation (either autologous or allogeneic) is needed.

Investigational Autologous stem cell transplantation is being actively studied and is promising as a form of treatment for patients with high-risk types of ALL who do not have matched sibling donors for allogeneic transplantation. It appears that autologous transplantation will be able to cure some of these patients, but its exact role in the treatment of adult ALL remains to be determined.

The drug nelarabine (Arranon) has recently been approved for the treatment of T-cell varieties of ALL. Its role in overall treatment remains to be determined.

Clofarabine (Clolar) is a new drug that has shown some effectiveness in children with ALL.

Prognosis

For patients under age sixty, ALL should be treated with a curative intent. Complete remission is achieved in approximately 90 percent of patients. Approximately 5 percent of patients die of treatment-related complications during initial induction therapy and another 5 percent fail to respond to chemotherapy. For patients with standard-risk ALL in first remission, chemotherapy treatment leads to cure in 40 to 50 percent of patients. Allogeneic stem cell transplantation leads to cure in 50 to 60 percent of patients, but there is a 20 to 30 percent chance of not surviving the treatment. Some "favorable" types of ALL have a 70 percent chance of cure with chemotherapy alone. For very high risk patients with ALL in first remission, allogeneic transplant leads to cure in 30 to 40 percent of patients, but may be the only potentially curative option.

Older adults over the age of sixty are more difficult to treat for cure. The chance of complete remission is approximately 70 percent. Most remissions will last one to two years, but less than 10 percent of these patients will be cured. It is difficult to perform transplant in this older age group.

Chronic Myelogenous Leukemia (CML)

Chronic myelogenous leukemia (CML) is one of the "myeloproliferative disorders." It is a chronic leukemia associated with a specific genetic abnormality in the leukemia cell called the Philadelphia chromosome, or t(9;22). This abnormal gene is produced by the displacement of genetic material called ABL from chromosome 9 replacing the normal part of chromosome 22 next to a region called BCR. The resulting fusion gene BCR/ABL causes abnormal function of the ABL gene, and this leads directly to the leukemia. The treatment and prognosis of CML has been completely transformed by the development of "targeted therapy" with the agent imatinib mesylate (Gleevec), which was approved by the FDA in 2001. This development is a milestone in medical history.

Common Signs and Symptoms

Many patients with CML come to medical attention because of fatigue, low-grade fevers or sweats, or fullness in the abdomen caused by an enlarged spleen. In other cases, the first finding is an abnormal blood count done for some other reason. The disease typically starts in the "chronic phase." In this early phase, the disease is usually easy to control with treatment, and patients can lead nearly normal lives. The disease can progress over time to the "accelerated phase." When this happens, the blood counts worsen and patients can experience high fever, bone pain, and painful enlargement of the spleen. The "blast phase" of CML is a form of acute leukemia that is very difficult to treat.

Diagnosis

CML is generally suspected by the finding of an elevated white blood cell count with immature "myeloid" cells in the blood. The diagnosis is then confirmed by the finding of the Philadelphia chromosome, formerly by chromosome analysis (cytogenetics) and more recently by molecular testing for the abnormal BCR/ABL gene. The BCR/ABL test on blood is sufficient to make the diagnosis of CML, and the diagnosis of AML cannot be made without this finding. A bone marrow biopsy is done to determine whether the CML is in an early or advanced stage.

Treatment Overview

As noted above, the treatment of CML has been transformed by the development of the nonchemotherapy drug imatinib mesylate (Gleevec), and the entire field of CML is now said to be in the "imatinib era." This drug was the first truly "targeted therapy," as it was designed to interfere with the function of the abnormal BCR/ABL gene, which causes the leukemia. It would be hard to overstate the impact of this drug on the disease CML. Imatinib is an oral drug that is usually taken once daily. It has very few serious side effects, and fewer than 5 percent of patients cannot take the drug because of toxic effects. Side effects are usually mild and include nausea, skin rashes, and swelling (edema) in the ankles or around the eyes. Approximately 97 percent of patients enter initial remission, usually within weeks of beginning therapy. Sometimes, if the starting white blood cell count is very high, the oral chemotherapy drug hydroxyurea is added for the first weeks of treatment. Hydroxyurea does not cause hair loss or serious side effects.

There are different levels of remission of CML. When the blood counts return to normal and the signs and symptoms of the disease disappear, the disease is said to be in "hematologic remission." As noted above, almost all patients reach this level of control, and this can be determined from blood tests. After several months of treatment, the bone marrow is tested to see if the Philadelphia chromosome is gone; when this is so, the disease is in "cytogenetic remission." The most accurate way to assess disease control is with blood tests for the BCR/ABL gene using a technique called quantitative PCR. This test measures the amount of the abnormal gene present and is very sensitive, able to detect one abnormal gene out of a million genes. The current goal of therapy is to get this PCR level down to less than 0.1 percent of the starting level, referred to as a 3-log reduction or a good molecular response. With this sensitive test, few patients have undetectable BCR/ABL levels ("complete molecular remission").

Because of the relatively recent introduction of imatinib (since 2001), the long-term results of this treatment cannot be known at this time. We do not know if this treatment has the potential to cure the disease. Currently, the most common treatment plan is to use imatinib and to assess the degree of remission. For the few patients who do not have a hematologic remission, an alternative treatment such as a stem cell transplant needs to be considered. Usually, the goal of treatment is to achieve at least a cytogenetic remission and a good molecular response. If this is accomplished and the side effects of imatinib are mild, the usual recommendation is to continue the drug and monitor the BCR/ABL level with blood tests every three months.

The only proven curative treatment for CML is an allogeneic stem cell (or bone marrow) transplant. It is common practice to test CML patients to see if one of their brothers or sisters is a match. This test is performed by a blood test called HLA typing. When allogeneic transplantation is performed using a matched sibling donor in the early chronic phase, the chance of long-term survival (and probably cure) is 80 percent or better. The disadvantage of transplantation is that 10 to 15 percent of patients will die of treatment-related complications. This is quite different from simply taking an oral medication. In the past, before imatinib, transplantation was recommended to all CML patients early in treatment. However, the role of transplant in this new era remains to be determined. If a matched unrelated donor is used because of the lack of a matched family donor, there are more complications and the cure rate falls to approximately 70 percent. In the past, delaying transplant for more than two years led to much poorer outcomes, but this may no longer be the case. Once CML has progressed to the accelerated or blast phase, results are much worse.

Reduced-intensity allogeneic (so-called miniallos) transplants are considerably less toxic and difficult than full-intensity transplants, but it remains to be seen if the long-term ability to cure is equal to that of the standard procedure.

When CML enters the blast phase, it becomes an acute leukemia and is extremely difficult to treat. One-third of patients will have a lymphoid blast crisis, which resembles acute lymphoblastic leukemia (ALL). This can be treated with ALL induction chemotherapy, and 70 percent of patients will enter a remission. Myeloid blast crisis is more common. It requires AML induction therapy and results are poor.

Investigational Dasatinib (Sprycel), a second-generation targeted agent similar to imatinib has just been approved and can be successful in controlling disease that has become resistant to imatinib. Other targeted agents, including AMN-107 (nilotinib [Tasigna]), are also being tested.

Prognosis

The outlook for CML patients has been transformed by recent developments in treatment. Before imatinib, the average survival without transplant was roughly five years, and CML invariably progressed to the accelerated and then the blast phase. Now, more than 90 percent of CML patients are alive beyond five years, and the long-term outlook is not yet known. For the 50 percent of patients who get good molecular response, there is almost no risk of the disease worsening in the first five years. For patients who do not get an optimal response, the dose of imatinib can be increased, or treatment switched to dasatinib (Sprycel). If the disease is still not well controlled, transplant needs to be considered.

The outcome of allogeneic transplantation depends on a number of factors. Young patients with matched sibling donors who get their transplant during the first years after diagnosis have an 80 percent chance of cure.

Myelodysplasia
(Myelodysplastic Syndromes)

The myelodysplastic syndromes (MDS) are a group of premalignant blood disorders that are related to the leukemias. They used to be called preleukemias. In MDS, the bone marrow is abnormal and the production of normal blood cells is decreased.

Common Signs and Symptoms

Most patients with myelodysplasia are over age sixty and come to medical attention because of fatigue related to anemia. The anemia may be severe and may require red blood cell transfusions. Some patients have bruising and bleeding due to a low platelet count. Other patients develop infections due to a low white blood cell count. MDS can cause fevers and sweats, fatigue, poor appetite, and weight loss.

MDS can worsen over time and change to an acute leukemia (AML).

Diagnosis

The diagnosis is suspected by abnormal results of blood tests (CBC, or complete blood count). Often there is an anemia that is otherwise unexplained. At other times, the white blood cell or platelet count is reduced. Often the appearance of the blood cells under the microscope is abnormal. The diagnosis is made by bone marrow biopsy, including a chromosome analysis. The appearance of the bone marrow cells is abnormal and an increased number of primitive cells (blasts) may be found. The finding of typical chromosomal abnormalities (cytogenetics) can help make the diagnosis more definite. In particular, one needs to look for abnormalities of chromosome 5 for the so-called 5q– (deletion of part of the long arm of chromosome 5) .

There are several types of MDS. The mildest form is refractory anemia (RA). When there are more blasts in the bone marrow, the diagnosis is refractory anemia with excess blasts (RAEB). Another serious type is chronic myelomonocytic leukemia (CMML).

Treatment Overview

Some patients with MDS do not need any initial treatment. In most cases, treatment is designed to make the patient feel better and not to cure, and patients who feel well can be monitored without intervention.

When anemia becomes a problem and affects the quality of life by causing fatigue, patients with MDS will benefit from transfusions of red blood cells. The medication erythropoetin (epoetin alfa [Procrit, Epogen], darbepoetin alfa [Aranesp]) given by injection under the skin every one to two weeks may be tried. Some patients (20 percent) will increase their production of red blood cells enough not to need transfusions. When low white blood cells lead to infections, G-CSF (filgrastim [Neupogen], pegfilgrastim [Neulasta]) can increase the white cells and decrease this risk. Platelet transfusions are sometimes given to reduce bleeding.

During the past year, the oral nonchemotherapy medication lenalidomide (Revlimid) has been approved for treatment of anemia due to MDS. This medicine has few side effects and is generally well tolerated, but can lower white blood cell and platelet blood counts. Patients with MDS and the chromosome abnormality 5q– have a 65 percent chance of responding well to this, and other MDS patients have a 30 percent chance of responding. Lenalidomide does not appear to benefit blood counts other than those of the red blood cells.

The drug 5-azacitidine (Vidaza) has been approved for treatment of MDS based on clinical trials, showing improved survival for patients with high-risk forms of MDS that appear to be heading toward transformation to leukemia. This medicine is given by injection under the skin for five to seven days and is repeated monthly. It can produce good responses in blood counts and can relieve symptoms of MDS.

A similar drug, decitabine (Dacogen), was recently approved for similar use, but this drug is given by vein and usually requires a hospital stay.

The only known curative treatment is allogeneic stem cell (or bone marrow) transplantation. However, most patients with MDS are too old to be candidates for this intensive treatment. Younger patients (under age sixty) with an HLA-matched sibling donor or a good matched unrelated donor should consider allogeneic transplant. Reduced-intensity transplants should make this procedure available to more MDS patients. Although 20 to 30 percent of patients will die early of treatment-related complications, long-term survival and cure can be achieved. Results are better when transplant is performed before the disease progresses to acute leukemia (AML).

When MDS transforms to AML, treatment similar to that given for AML may be used and remissions may be achieved. However, most patients with AML following MDS have a poor-risk type of leukemia and may be too old or sick to tolerate intensive chemotherapy.

Investigational Tipifarnib (Zarnestra) is being tested, along with other nonchemotherapy drugs.

Prognosis

Although not strictly a cancer, myelodysplasia is a serious condition. Patients with the mild form (RA) usually live five to ten years. Patients with more advanced forms usually live one to two years. Allogeneic transplant offers the possibility of cure.

Chronic Lymphocytic Leukemia (CLL)

Chronic lymphocytic leukemia (CLL) is a disorder in which the B lymphocytes lose their normal ability to die, and accumulate over time. At first, the cells increase only in the blood, but over years they also begin to increase in the lymph nodes, liver, spleen, and bone marrow.

Common Signs and Symptoms

Many patients have no symptoms at all at the time of diagnosis and are simply found to have an elevated white blood cell count. Some patients will notice fatigue or enlargement of lymph nodes or fullness in the abdomen due to an enlarged spleen.

When CLL becomes more advanced and replaces normal bone marrow, low blood counts can be a problem with anemia and infections. CLL also leads to a risk of infection because of low production of antibodies (gamma globulins) that help fight bacteria. In 5 to 10 percent of cases, CLL causes the destruction of the patient's own red blood cells or platelets (or both) through an "autoimmune" process. Destruction of platelets is called immune thrombocytopenia purpura (ITP), and destruction of red blood cells is called autoimmune hemolytic anemia (AHA).

CLL is the one type of leukemia for which there is a formal staging system. Early disease (Rai Stage 0–I) consists of an elevated lymphocyte count and enlarged lymph nodes. In intermediate stage (Rai Stage II), the spleen becomes enlarged. In advanced disease (Rai Stage III–IV), the bone marrow function is disturbed and there is significant decrease in red blood cell and platelet counts.

In 5 to 10 percent of cases, CLL can transform to an aggressive lymphoma. This is called Richter's syndrome.

Diagnosis

The diagnosis of CLL is made by finding a high white blood cell count composed primarily of small lymphocytes. The diagnosis is confirmed by immunophenotyping (flow cytometry) that shows coexpression of the markers CD19 and CD5. Recent advances in the understanding of CLL have led to several new tests that can help determine the level of aggressiveness of the disease. These include measurement of CD38 (part of the flow cytometry test) and ZAP-70.

Treatment Overview

Most patients with early-stage disease do not need any treatment when the disease is first diagnosed. These patients will live ten to fifteen years on the average and early treatment offers no proven advantage at this time. Treatment should start when the patient either has advanced disease based on falling normal blood counts or has intermediate stage with significant symptoms, very enlarged lymph nodes, or a rapid increase in the lymphocyte count (doubling in less than twelve months).

The treatment of choice for most patients with CLL is the chemotherapy drug fludarabine (Fludara) combined with the nonchemotherapy antibody rituximab (Rituxan). Fludarabine is given intravenously (IV) five days per week once monthly for six months. Fludarabine is thus inconvenient but causes only a modest side effect, fatigue. Rituximab is given by four to six hour IV infusion on the first day of each monthly treatment. Most patients will have a good response to this treatment and remain in remission without further treatment for three to seven years. Some doctors add a second chemotherapy drug, cyclophosphamide (Cytoxan), to the treatment.

This produces more infections and other side effects and is being tested to see if improved results justify these difficulties.

Alemtuzumab (Campath) is an antibody that has been approved for treatment of CLL that has not responded to fludarabine. It is given by either injection under the skin or IV. It causes many side effects and risk of infection and is usually used for difficult cases.

Chlorambucil (Leukeran), an oral chemotherapy drug, may be used instead of fludarabine, especially for elderly or frail patients. Although it is less effective than fludarabine, it is much more gentle and convenient than the latter. Fludarabine can then be reserved for the time when chlorambucil has lost its effectiveness.

Some patients with CLL who have low gamma globulin levels and recurrent infections can benefit from monthly infusions of gamma globulin. This is expensive and cumbersome but is worthwhile if the infection problem is serious. Patients with autoimmune problems such as ITP and AHA are treated with prednisone and sometimes with surgical removal of the spleen (splenectomy).

Allogeneic stem cell (or bone marrow) transplantation is a potentially curative therapy but is seldom used in CLL. However, the occasional young patient with aggressive CLL should be considered for this approach. A new variation of transplant, the "miniallogeneic" transplant, is a promising approach that increases the safety of the procedure and may come to play more of a role in the treatment of CLL.

Investigational Clinical trials will examine whether with improvements in treatment, some patients with CLL should start treatment when still in the early stages of disease. These decisions will be made based on measurement of biological features of the CLL cells such as genetic changes.

Prognosis

Patients with Rai Stage 0–I CLL typically live twelve to fifteen years. If they are elderly at the time of diagnosis, their CLL may not have an important effect on their health or survival. Survival decreases to an average of six to eight years for Stage II and two to four years for advanced disease. It is likely that the newer CLL treatments will lead to improved survival.

Hairy Cell Leukemia (HCL)

Common Signs and Symptoms

Hairy cell leukemia (HCL) is a rare type of chronic leukemia. Patients with HCL usually complain of fatigue, often as a consequence of anemia. They may also note an enlarged spleen, easy bruising or bleeding from low platelets, and occasionally an infection or fever because of a low white blood cell count.

Diagnosis

The diagnosis is made by bone marrow biopsy. Occasionally, abnormal hairy cells are seen in the peripheral blood. The diagnosis is confirmed by immunophenotyping (flow cytometry) because hairy cells have a characteristic pattern of proteins on the cell surface.

Treatment Overview

The treatment of choice is a single seven-day continuous intravenous (IV) course of the drug 2-chlorodeoxyadenosine (2-CdA, cladribine [Levstatin]). Almost all patients experience a fever on the last day of the infusion and most have low blood counts, which require antibiotics and observation to ensure that no serious infection has occurred. Patients often have low blood counts for several months after treatment. The response rate to 2-CdA is 85 percent. Most patients will have long remissions, often longer than ten years. It is not yet known if 2-CdA is curative or whether it simply produces prolonged remissions. For patients who do not respond to 2-CdA, deoxycoformycin (pentostatin [Nipent]) may be helpful.

Prognosis

The availability of effective treatment has dramatically changed the outlook for patients with HCL. Most patients will now live longer than ten years and may never have a recurrence.

Liver

Alan P. Venook, M.D.

■ ■ ■ ■

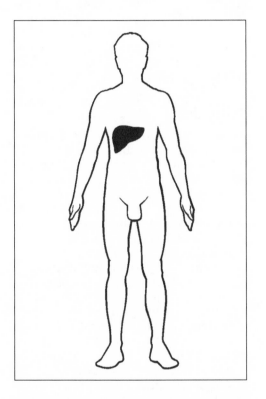

Primary liver cancer—also called hepatocellular carcinoma or hepatoma—may be the most common cancer worldwide. It occurs with great frequency in Asia and Africa, and is becoming more common in the United States as a complication of chronic hepatitis C viral infection. About 30,000 cases are diagnosed yearly in the United States.

Because it is so uncommon here, liver cancer is often not suspected and is at an advanced stage by the time it is diagnosed. Even when it is identified in its early stages, the coexistent liver damage that is almost always present may limit treatment options. Because the liver plays a vital role in removing toxins from the blood, cancer within it causes major metabolic problems. The treatment now available for advanced liver cancer is not particularly effective, and the principal goal of therapy is to relieve the symptoms related to the disease.

Types The most common type of cancer originating in the liver itself—referred to as primary liver cancer—develops in liver cells and is called hepatocellular carcinoma. Rarely, tumors arise from blood vessels in the liver (hemangioendothelioma), glands in the liver (adenocarcinoma), or connective tissue in the liver (sarcoma, angiosarcoma). An unusual type of hepatocellular carcinoma called fibrolamellar tends to occur in young women. Tumors that develop in the bile ducts are called cholangiocarcinomas (see the chapter "Bile Duct"). Most commonly, cancer in the liver has spread there from another organ and is therefore a type of metastatic cancer (see the chapter "Metastatic Cancer").

How It Spreads Liver cancers can spread to other areas through either the lymph system or the blood. Most often, the cancer first moves into the lymph nodes in the region of the liver (porta hepatis), then goes to other lymph nodes or into the lung or bone. Tumor cells can also spread into adjacent blood vessels and into the abdominal cavity, causing the accumulation of fluid (ascites) or masses elsewhere in the abdomen (see the illustration on page 599).

What Causes It Hepatocellular carcinoma most often develops in damaged livers. Long-standing infection with either the hepatitis B or the hepatitis C virus often precedes it and is therefore seen as a significant risk factor.

Cirrhosis of the liver (from, for example, a viral infection, alcohol, toxin exposure, or a genetic defect) also increases the likelihood of hepatocellular carcinoma, presumably because of chronic inflammation in the liver. In fact, an estimated 5 percent of people with cirrhosis will eventually develop liver cancer. Fifty to 80 percent of all people with liver cancer have cirrhosis.

Certain chemicals are associated with increased liver cancer, and a link has been established with a plant fungus (aflatoxin) that is ingested with the normal diet in a part of Africa. Oral steroid use may also increase the risk.

Risk Factors

At Significantly Higher Risk

• Worldwide, men are twice as likely as women to develop liver cancer.

• Chronic hepatitis B and/or hepatitis C virus infection, with or without cirrhosis of the liver. The usual route of transmission of hepatitis B and C is through blood transfusions or shared drug needles. Because hepatitis B may also be transmitted by a mother to her offspring during pregnancy or childbirth, or may be transmitted during sexual intercourse, it is not unusual for members of the same family to develop liver cancer after becoming infected with hepatitis B.

• Cirrhosis of the liver from any cause—alcohol damage or genetic errors of metabolism such as hemochromatosis and enzyme deficiencies.

• Exposure to aflatoxin, a fungus poison found in the soil in Africa.

• Exposure to the fumes of vinyl chloride or to Thorotrast (a contrast material no longer used for radiologic procedures) is associated with an increased risk of angiosarcoma of the liver and hepatocellular carcinoma.

At Slightly Higher Risk

• Anabolic steroid use, as by weight lifters and other athletes, is known to increase the risk of benign liver tumors and may cause an increase in liver cancer.

• Estrogen therapy, such as oral contraceptives, may increase the risk, although this has not been proven.

Screening

People with known chronic hepatitis and/or cirrhosis of the liver may benefit from screening tests to try to find the cancer before it has spread beyond the liver. Thorough screening includes frequent monitoring of serum alpha-fetoprotein (a product found in the blood of 30 to 50 percent of all hepatocellular carcinoma patients in the United States and more commonly worldwide) and ultrasound of the liver. These tests are not useful for identifying primary liver tumors other than hepatocellular carcinoma. Patients with specific serotypes of hepatitis C, particularly 1b, may be at great risk for hepatocellular carcinoma and may be good candidates for screening.

Although these screening methods may be useful in Asia and Africa, where liver cancer is very common, they are not routinely used in North America because of the rarity of this cancer. Screening of hepatitis B virus-infected Asian and African immigrants to the United States may be beneficial.

Common Signs and Symptoms

Common symptoms include bloating, abdominal pain, fever, weight loss, decreased appetite, and nausea. But because liver cancer is so rare, its symptoms are usually attributed to more common, benign conditions. Frequently, the diagnosis of cancer is not considered until these symptoms persist or until a person develops an enlarging abdominal mass or fluid in the abdomen. Jaundice (the skin turning yellow) and swelling in the legs are usually associated with more advanced tumors. Sometimes, people with liver cancer feel entirely well.

Diagnosis

Physical Examination

There are no findings specific to liver cancer on physical examination. Findings may include the following, all of which may have other explanations:

- Fever.
- Enlarged liver and spleen.
- Enlarged, hard lymph nodes.
- Swelling of the abdomen from fluid (ascites).
- Jaundice (the skin turning yellow).
- Swelling of the legs (edema).

Blood and Other Tests

- A complete blood count may be normal or may show a decrease (anemia) or increase in red blood cells.
- Routine liver function studies—blood tests measuring serum bilirubin and liver enzymes—may be abnormal but can be normal even in advanced stages of primary liver cancer.
- Prothrombin time and partial thromboplastin time (PT and PTT) tests of clotting—usually done if a liver problem is suspected—may be abnormal.
- The serum alpha-fetoprotein (AFP) is elevated in 30 to 50 percent of people in the United States with primary liver cancer. It may also be elevated in people with germ cell cancer, gastric cancer, or cirrhosis of the liver and in pregnant women.

Imaging

- Abdominal ultrasound can evaluate the density of the liver if a mass is suspected. It can reveal the presence of fluid in the abdomen and is particularly useful for distinguishing a solid mass from a noncancerous accumulation of fluid in the liver (benign cyst).
- A CT scan is useful for determining the extent of a tumor within the liver and evaluating the possible extension of tumor tissue into lymph nodes or to other structures within the abdomen.
- Magnetic resonance imaging (MRI) may help determine if the liver cancer can be surgically removed by revealing whether the tumor involves both lobes of the liver or is invading blood vessels. Usually, MRI is not necessary because the CT scan provides essentially the same information.
- An X-ray involving the injection of dye into the artery going to the liver (arteriography) may be necessary before any attempt is made to remove the tumor, since the surgeon needs to know exactly what the blood supply of the tumor is in order to remove it.
- If surgery is being considered, a chest X-ray should be done. If the cancer has spread to the lungs or any other organ, surgery should be reconsidered. PET scanning (positron-emission tomography) scanning is helpful for excluding the presence of cancer elsewhere in the body but is generally not helpful in determining the extent of the cancer in the liver.

Biopsy Biopsy, either by fine needle aspiration (FNA) or with a regular needle, is almost always necessary. This procedure can be done through the skin without significant danger. Because of the variation in the tumor cells of different types of cancers, the biopsy sample can be used to distinguish between a primary liver cancer and a cancer that has spread from another organ. Occasionally, if the AFP is extremely high and the tumor is very large, a biopsy may not be necessary.

Staging

Although a TNM staging system exists for hepatocellular carcinoma, for purposes of deciding about therapeutic options, there are only three stages—localized resectable, localized unresectable, and advanced disease.

Treatment Overview

Surgery is the only way to cure primary liver cancer, so the goal of the diagnostic work-up is to discover if all the cancerous tissue can be removed. Removal is often not possible, either because the tumor has already spread beyond the liver or because removal of the damaged liver tissue would leave a person without enough liver function to survive.

Chemotherapy and radiation therapy are occasionally helpful in relieving symptoms. Primary liver cancer may progress rapidly, but these and other measures can be taken to maintain the quality of life. Newer treatments, such as more effective chemotherapy and liver transplantation, may someday allow the surgical removal of cancers now felt to be inoperable.

Surgery Surgery can cure liver cancer if the entire tumor can be removed. The liver has two distinct lobes—right and left—and a tumor confined to one lobe can often be removed even if the patient has cirrhosis of the liver. If cirrhosis is only minimal or is not at all present, a tumor involving parts of both lobes of the liver can be removed with an extensive operation (trisegmentectomy). This surgery is potentially dangerous, however, and people with poor liver function may not survive it.

A liver transplant may be considered for someone whose cancer has not yet spread and who cannot tolerate the removal of part of the liver because of underlying liver disease or the size of the tumor. So far, this approach has been beneficial only in people with tumors less than 3 inches (7.5 cm), with no more than three tumors, and without hepatitis B. It may also be beneficial for patients with the fibrolamellar variant of hepatocellular carcinoma. Even if patients with hepatocellular carcinoma have no evidence of metastases, the tumor often redevelops after transplantation, perhaps because of the suppression of the immune system that allows the transplanted liver to function. Rarely, cancer is not found in the liver until after a person has had a transplant for another reason. Such patients may be cured because the cancer is in an earlier stage.

The presence of tumor anywhere else in the body—lung, bone, or lymph nodes, for example—means that removal of the liver tumor alone will not bring about a cure. If the disease has already metastasized, removing part of a liver tumor is not considered beneficial because of the side effects of surgery, including a long recuperation period.

Cryosurgery, which involves freezing the tumor tissue by placing a cold probe directly into it, may be useful in selected patients. Similarly, radiofrequency ablation, which applies a heated probe to the tumor, can be used. A tumor that cannot be removed because it is too close to blood vessels or because of extensive underlying liver disease may be "killed" by these techniques.

A number of other techniques whereby alcohol or other fluids are injected through the skin into the tumor have been shown to kill tumors less than $1\frac{1}{4}$ inches (3 cm) in size.

 Radiation The usefulness of radiation is limited in liver cancer because it is extremely damaging to noncancerous liver tissue. A technique called conformal radiation may be useful in selected patients with isolated liver tumors. Radiation is sometimes used to treat the liver area after a tumor has been removed, although this has not been shown to be of definite benefit. A new technique involving the administration of radio-active beads into the liver through the hepatic artery may benefit an occasional patient. The principal role for radiation is the management of painful liver masses or metastases.

Chemotherapy Chemotherapy may result in tumor shrinkage, but this does not necessarily prolong survival. The standard drug, doxorubicin (Adriamycin), may shrink tumors in 10 to 15 percent of patients and seems to help some. A combination of this drug with cisplatin (Platinol), 5-fluorouracil, and interferon-alpha may be effective in patients with hepatoma related to hepatitis B. But the side effects of these drugs, including nausea, vomiting, and hair loss, may leave patients in a worse condition even if the tumor shrinks, and does not clearly improve survival rates compared to doxorubicin alone. Other drugs that may shrink the tumor are capecitabine (Xeloda), etoposide (Etopophos), and mitoxantrone (Novantrone), although these have similar side effects to doxorubicin.

These drugs seem to shrink tumors more successfully when administered directly into the liver via the hepatic artery. Although tumors within the liver regress in about 50 percent of patients, the therapy is difficult to give and is extremely toxic to an already damaged liver. Because few patients feel better after such therapy and because distant metastases nearly always develop, it is generally not advisable to surgically implant an infusion device into the hepatic artery.

In 2007, results were presented of a large Phase III trial suggesting that a drug called sorafenib (Nexavar) improves survival in patients with advanced hepatoma and without severe liver cirrhosis, compared to patients receiving best supportive care only. This drug, which targets several enzymes, including those important in angiogenesis, may be approved for hepatoma in the United States within the next six to twelve months.

Investigational There is substantial experience in Asia and at some institutions in the United States with a process called chemoembolization. This involves administering a combination of chemotherapy and colloid particles directly into the liver tumor via its main (hepatic) artery.

Generally, it is performed as a single treatment and does not require surgery or prolonged bed rest. While results show that tumors will shrink in about 50 percent of patients, prolonged survival has not been proven. Since the tumor in the liver usually causes the most symptoms even if it has metastasized, chemoembolization may help relieve pain in someone with advanced disease.

There may also be a role for chemoembolization before the surgical removal of the liver tumor, since significant shrinkage may enable the removal of a previously unresectable tumor.

Treatment by Stage

■ Localized Resectable

The tumor is confined to a portion of the liver that allows for its complete surgical removal. The tumor may be localized to either the right lobe or the left lobe of the liver or possibly involve the right lobe and only a portion of the left lobe.

Standard Treatment Surgery is the standard therapy but depends on the relative health of the remaining underlying liver, since a person with cirrhosis of the liver may not be able to tolerate the removal of one-half or two-thirds of the liver tissue.

Surgery also depends on the presence of a clear zone between the tumor and the neighboring blood vessels. In some patients, radiofrequency ablation (RFA) can be done, wherein a heat probe is placed in the tumor (or tumors) and used to destroy the tumor. This can be done in selected patients whose tumors are localized but cannot be technically removed by the surgeon. Only a small percentage of people are candidates for surgery and, unfortunately, the majority experience a tumor recurrence.

Five-Year Survival 10 to 30 percent

Investigational

• The role for chemotherapy after surgery is unknown. Although doxorubicin (Adriamycin) is often recommended, no systematic studies have been done to see if it increases the chances of cure. One study in Japan suggests that a vitamin derivative called polyprenoic acid may diminish the risk of hepatocellular carcinoma recurrence after surgery, but this drug is not available in the United States.

• Radiation is often applied to the liver area after surgery but has never been proven to be beneficial. A novel method of delivering radiation into the artery going to the liver by employing radioactive materials has been demonstrated to be beneficial in one study from Hong Kong, but it is not available in the United States.

■ *Localized Unresectable*
Despite being a localized mass, the tumor may be unresectable because crucial blood vessel structures are involved or because the liver is impaired.

Standard Treatment There is no standard therapy, so patients should be considered for clinical trials.

Two-Year Survival Less than 5 percent

Investigational

• Liver transplantation may be attempted in patients who are deemed unresectable because of poor liver function and whose tumors are not intertwined with blood vessels in the abdomen. This seems to be of benefit in patients with the fibrolamellar variant of hepatocellular carcinoma as well as in those patients with no tumor larger than 2 inches (5 cm), with no more than three tumors, and without hepatitis B.

• Cryosurgery and radiofrequency ablation hold some promise to allow the removal of otherwise unresectable tumors, but these techniques are done only by a few specialized physicians.

■ *Advanced*
The tumor involves both lobes of the liver and/or has spread to involve other organs such as the lungs, intra-abdominal lymph nodes, or bone.

Standard Treatment Until recently, no standard therapy was known to prolong survival. The usual approach involved a trial of single-agent chemotherapy such as doxorubicin (Adriamycin) or 5-fluorouracil, or combinations also including cisplatin (Platinol) and interferon-alpha. However, as noted above, recent results from a large Phase III trial have shown a survival benefit with a new drug called sorafenib (Nexavar), which may soon gain approval in the United States for treatment of advanced hepatoma. Radiation to the tumor along with intravenous chemotherapy may relieve the pain of large liver masses, and radiation to painful bone or other metastases may also be appropriate.

Two-Year Survival Less than 5 percent

Investigational

• Combination chemotherapy or new drugs may prove to be better treatment than those currently available. These would best be administered in a clinical trial, rather than using random combinations.

• Chemoembolization may improve symptoms even if there is metastatic disease.

• Newer drugs, including derivatives of doxorubicin (Adriamycin) and 5-fluorouracil, are being studied.

Treating Other Primary Liver Tumors

The approach taken with other primary liver tumors is generally the same as for hepatocellular carcinoma. Patients with these other tumors are more likely to be candidates for surgery because they usually do not have underlying liver disease.

Angiosarcoma and Hemangioendothelioma

These diseases are less predictable than hepatocellular carcinoma and survival is variable.

• They may not have spread at the time of diagnosis and surgery should be considered.

• As in hepatocellular carcinoma, no systematic study of adjuvant chemotherapy or radiotherapy has been done.

• Localized unresectable disease may respond to the same intravenous chemotherapy used for sarcomas, and the tumors may occasionally shrink enough to allow the surgeon to remove them completely.

• Advanced disease is approached in the same way as a sarcoma.

Adenocarcinoma

This type of tumor is approached in the same way as hepatocellular carcinoma. Its prognosis is similar.

Supportive Therapy

• Problems associated with jaundice can include severe itching. Itching may be relieved by Benadryl, Atarax, or cholestyramine (Questran). For unexplained reasons, the antibiotic rifampin may also alleviate the itching associated with jaundice.

• Pain relievers are sometimes called for in liberal doses. Narcotics may have excessive side effects because they are metabolized by the liver, which may not be functioning properly.

• Nonsteroidal anti-inflammatory drugs (NSAIDs) may be surprisingly effective even against the severe pain associated with liver cancer and may also be helpful if patients are having fevers and sweats related to the cancer.

• Frequent small meals may be necessary to provide enough nutrition, since an enlarged liver might reduce the capacity of the stomach.

• The loss of appetite that frequently accompanies liver cancer may be relieved with megestrol acetate (Megace).

• Water pills (diuretics) to relieve fluid in the abdomen or legs may cause significant imbalance in kidney function if not carefully monitored.

• Nausea can be treated with standard medications, including suppositories.

• Sleep disturbances are common. Most sleeping pills are metabolized by the liver, however, so they should be used carefully.

Treatment Follow-Up

Careful follow-up is important after the removal of localized liver cancer because patients are at risk for a second occurrence as well as tumor metastases. Such monitoring should include the following:

• Serum alpha-fetoprotein (AFP) every two to three months. A rising AFP suggests tumor recurrence, which might still be curable with further surgery.

• CT scans should be done every two to three months for the first year after surgery. Tumors are most likely to grow again within the first year, and they may still be curable if caught in the early stages.

• The liver function of patients with underlying cirrhosis or hepatitis has to be closely monitored, since it may deteriorate after surgery.

The Most Important Questions You Can Ask

• Should I see another physician to confirm that this tumor can or cannot be removed for cure?

• Could I benefit from an investigational therapy available at another institution?

• How sick will the proposed chemotherapy or radiation treatment make me relative to the potential benefit?

• Should any tests be done on my spouse or children to see if they are at risk for developing this cancer?

• Is a liver transplant an option for me?

Lung: Nonsmall Cell

Thierry M. Jahan, M.D., Sarita Dubey, M.D., Alexander R. Gottschalk, M.D., Ph.D.,
Pierre Theodore, M.D., and David M. Jablons, M.D.

■ ■ ■ ■

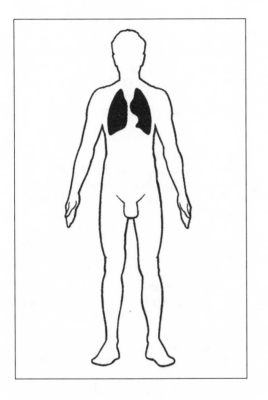

Lung cancer is the second most common cancer and the number one cause of cancer death in both men and women in the United States. Although there has always been a higher incidence in men, the incidence in women has risen rapidly in recent years. In fact, lung cancer has now surpassed breast cancer as the number one cancer killer of women, killing twice as many women as breast cancer. It has long been the leading cancer killer of men.

An estimated 213,380 people will develop lung cancer in the United States in 2007, and about 160,390 people will die of it. This is especially unfortunate because it is one of the most preventable cancers. The cause is well known. Before tobacco use became popular, lung cancer was a rare disease. Furthermore, it has been estimated that if all tobacco were removed from the earth, the number of all cancers would fall by 17 percent.

There are two general types of lung cancer—small cell and nonsmall cell. The nonsmall cell variety is much more common, accounting for 80 percent of all lung cancer cases. There has been slow but definite improvement in the survival rate over the past two decades. The slow rate of improvement is due to the fact that we lack a satisfactory, widely applicable screening test that could increase our ability to detect lung cancer at an early stage, when it has the best chance of being cured, and also to the fact that lung cancer is a biologically aggressive cancer. In addition, while there has been some progress in our ability to control lung cancer and extend the survival of some patients with advanced lung cancer, there is a continued need for more effective therapy.

Types There are at least four distinct types of nonsmall cell lung cancer—squamous cell carcinoma, adenocarcinoma, large cell carcinoma, and bronchoalveolar carcinoma—the treatment of all four subtypes is generally similar. Squamous cell carcinoma used to be the most common, but, for reasons that are poorly understood, adenocarcinoma has steadily increased in frequency and is now the most common type of nonsmall cell lung cancer, especially in women.

Squamous cell (also known as epidermoid) carcinoma of the lung is the microscopic type formerly most frequently related to smoking. Surgical removal of the tumor along with the nearby lymph nodes can produce a cure more often than with other types. Squamous cell tumors can cavitate (break up from the inside out) on their own and lead to coughing up blood. They account for only 30 percent of nonsmall cell lung cancer in the United States, but account for a higher percentage in western Europe and Asia.

Adenocarcinoma of the lung accounts for over 50 percent of all lung cancer cases in the United States. It is more common in women and is still the most frequent type seen in nonsmokers. However, it occurs frequently in smokers as well. It is more likely than other types to be in the peripheral portions of the lung (near the edge), and therefore may invade the lining of the chest and produce fluid in the chest cavity more commonly than in other types. It also has a tendency to spread early to other sites (metastasize) away from the primary, so that it is often diagnosed at a more advanced stage.

Large cell carcinoma, especially those tumors with neuroendocrine features, is commonly associated with spread of the tumor to the brain. It is arguably the most aggressive nonsmall cell subtype.

Bronchoalveolar carcinoma accounts for a minority of nonsmall cell lung cancers. It often presents with advanced stage, yet patients are likely to have very few symptoms because the rate at which the cancer grows may be slower than that of other subtypes. It is more difficult to diagnose microscopically, so its true incidence is probably higher than the 3 percent generally quoted in various lung cancer papers. It may develop more in women and in nonsmokers. It may also be more common in Asian patients, especially Asian women.

How It Spreads Nonsmall cell cancer can spread through the lymphatic system and through the blood. It can directly invade the center of the chest (mediastinum), the lining of the chest, the ribs, or, if it is in the top part of the lung, the nerves and blood vessels leading into the arm. If it invades the lymphatic system, it often spreads to the lymph nodes, either in the lung itself or in the mediastinum. When nonsmall cell lung cancer enters the bloodstream, it can spread to distant sites such as the liver, bone, brain, adrenal glands, and other places in the lung.

What Causes It Cigarette smoking has been a major factor in the development of both small cell and nonsmall cell lung cancers. The increase in cigarette smoking by men in the 1920s, apparently related to increased cigarette production, advertising, and marketing at that time, was followed in the 1940s by a dramatic increase in the incidence of lung cancer in men. The marked increase in cigarette smoking by women in the 1940s was unfortunately followed two decades later by a similar increase in the incidence of lung cancer among women, so that now, lung cancer has overtaken breast cancer as the leading cause of cancer-related death in women. It should be noted, however, that there has also been an increase in the rate of lung cancer among people who have never smoked, especially women. The reasons for this increase are not well understood, but may have something to do with secondhand smoke exposure or other as yet unidentified factors. Finally, while quitting smoking does reduce the risk of developing lung cancer, it does not remove it completely. The majority of patients diagnosed with lung cancer have effectively quit for quite some time prior to their diagnosis.

Lung tissue scarred by a connective tissue disease such as scleroderma may be associated with the development of bronchoalveolar carcinoma. Lung cancer may predispose a person to a higher incidence of developing another lung cancer later. Lung cancer may also occur at sites of old scars in the lung resulting from an infection (tuberculosis, for example) or an injury (scar carcinoma) or prior radiation.

Risk Factors

At Significantly Higher Risk

- Cigarette smokers.
- The male to female ratio remains 4 to 1. Peak incidence occurs between ages fifty and sixty, with less than a 1 percent incidence under the age of thirty and about a 10 percent incidence in people over seventy.
- Workers exposed to industrial substances such as asbestos, nickel, chromium, cadmium, uranium, radon compounds, and chloromethyl ether, especially those who smoke.
- Prior early-stage lung cancer or head and neck cancer.

At Slightly Higher Risk

- Patients with previous or preexisting lung disease, especially a type of lung disease leading to heavy scarring, such as interstitial lung disease.
- Former smokers.
- People exposed to secondhand smoke over many years.
- People exposed to radon.

Screening

Lung cancer is very difficult to detect at an early stage. Tests such as the examination of sputum (phlegm) for malignant cells and regular chest X-rays have not proven to be beneficial. Chest X-rays can detect lung cancer in smokers, but these findings may not always be early enough to improve the survival of patients. Other techniques such as fluorescence bronchoscopy and spiral-computed tomography are also in the process of being perfected with a goal to detect the cancer as early as possible. Recently, the use of spiral CT scanning in patients at high risk for developing lung cancer has shown promising preliminary results in detecting nonsmall cell lung cancer at a very early stage, when it may still be curable. Efforts are currently under way to confirm these promising results through a large national randomized clinical trial. Additionally, efforts are under way to develop tests that can detect very early molecular changes associated with nonsmall cell lung cancer in the bloodstream or the sputum. The goal of these efforts is to develop effective screening tests in order to increase the number of early-stage cancers that we can detect and treat.

Common Signs and Symptoms

A new or changing cough, the sputum sometimes containing blood, is a common symptom, along with hoarseness and shortness of breath or increased shortness of breath during exertion. There may also be an increase in the amount of sputum, recurrent episodes of lung infection (sometimes in the same lobe of the lung as the cancer), weight loss, and swelling of the face or arms. By far the most common symptom is fatigue.

If the tumor has spread, or metastasized, the symptoms can include severe headaches, double vision, and pain in the bones, chest, abdomen, and neck and down the arms.

Diagnosis

Physical Examination

- Lymph node enlargement in the neck or in the region above the collarbone.
- Enlarged liver or another mass in the abdomen.

• Signs of a mass in one lung, such as decreased breath sounds, noises in the lung that are not usually present, and areas of dullness when the chest is tapped with the fingers, indicating the presence of fluid in the lung.

Blood and Other Tests Sputum examination for malignant cells.

Imaging

• A chest X-ray that shows an abnormality does not establish a diagnosis until some tissue is obtained and examined under the microscope.

• CT scans of the chest and abdomen, to include the entire liver and the adrenal glands.

• PET scans can be helpful in staging the mediastinum (the area between both lungs where a lot of the lymph nodes that drain the lungs are located). A positive PET scan strongly suggests that cancer might be present. Lately, the use of simultaneous CT and PET scans, so-called CT-PET fusion scans, is increasing the accuracy and usefulness of preoperative scanning to stage patients prior to initiating treatment. CT-PET fusion scans generally include the brain, neck, chest, abdomen, and pelvis, all the way through the thighs.

• Sometimes PET, CT, or MRI scans of the brain can provide useful information.

Endoscopy and Biopsy

• Fiber-optic bronchoscopy with brushing, lavage, and/or biopsy.

• Mediastinoscopy with biopsies. In this procedure, a small incision is made at the base of the neck and a long, thin tube called a mediastinoscope is inserted down to the lymph nodes in the middle of the chest. Tissue can be obtained through this instrument. The procedure is usually safe and easy but does require general anesthesia and a short hospital stay.

• Needle aspiration through the chest wall (see the section on FNA biopsy in

chapter 2, "How Cancer Is Diagnosed") with a local anesthetic and often under CT guidance.

• Removal and analysis of fluid in the chest to detect tumor cells.

• Pleural (chest lining) biopsy.

• Lymph node biopsy.

• Bone biopsy.

• Liver biopsy.

• Biopsy of a nodule during surgery.

• DNA analysis. With the advent of genetic probe studies, certain genes appear to be more frequent in patients who develop lung cancer. Patients, women especially, with amplification of the k-*ras* oncogene, for example, may have a much worse prognosis. We are rapidly approaching the time when we can have our genes analyzed and we can be made aware of our risks, not only for lung cancer, but for other cancers as well. These types of genetic analyses will soon be carried out on a simple blood sample, thereby avoiding the need to obtain lung tissue and making it easy and safe to obtain these important answers.

Staging

Once a diagnosis of a malignant tumor is made, further staging studies are carried out to establish the stage of disease. More than any other factor, the stage helps determine the prognosis and helps guide the selection of treatment.

Stage is based on a combination of clinical findings (physical examination, chest X-ray, and lab studies) and pathologic findings (biopsy). The stages are now commonly defined according to the TNM classification.

Treatment Overview

Surgery Surgical treatment—removal of the tumor—remains the mainstay of curative treatment in early-stage (I, II) nonsmall cell lung cancer.

This will involve removing a lobe of the lung when a tumor is very central in the lung. When a tumor is small and located in the periphery of the lung, it can be removed by a smaller surgery, called a wedge resection. Whenever possible, though, the fuller lobectomy procedure should be employed, as it is usually more effective in improving the chance of survival. It should be stressed that surgery for lung cancer has evolved significantly over the past twenty years. Now patients can undergo resection with smaller, muscle-sparing incisions, which, with the use of epidural catheters, greatly improve the control of postoperative pain. When pain is better controlled, patients are more likely to be up and about faster, thus reducing the risk of major complications. Typically, the risk of serious complications for a routine lobectomy should be less than 1 to 2 percent.

In the last few years, the use of video-assisted surgery using special instruments called thorascopes have allowed a greater number of patients, who might otherwise not have been candidates for normal open surgery, to undergo removal of their primary lung cancer. It remains to be seen if the use of video-assisted surgery is as effective in controlling lung cancer as the more involved open procedures.

 Radiation Radiation is used in different scenarios. It is used as an addition to surgery if it appears that there might be some disease left after surgery. In cases where the lymph nodes in the mediastinum are involved and surgery might not be possible, radiation is used at the same time as chemotherapy to control and cure nonsmall cell lung cancer. Finally, in patients with lung cancer that has spread to organs like the bones or the brain, radiation is used to improve the symptoms caused by the involvement of these organs. In these cases, radiation is not felt to be curative, but instead felt to be palliative.

Chemotherapy The role of chemotherapy has evolved over the past number of years. Several recent analyses of multiple studies have led to the following conclusions:

1. While not a cure for advanced nonsmall cell lung cancer, chemotherapy can provide a significant survival benefit in selected patients.
2. Chemotherapy appears to be more effective than simple palliative care for patients with advanced nonsmall cell lung cancer.
3. Chemotherapy combined with surgery improves outcomes for patients with Stages II–IIIA nonsmall cell lung cancer that has been fully resected. At this time, it is not clear if the addition of chemotherapy to surgery for patients with Stage I disease yields a survival benefit.

When a platinum drug is combined with drugs such as paclitaxel (Taxol), docetaxel (Taxotere), gemcitabine (Gemzar), and vinorelbine (Navelbine), response rates of 30 to 40 percent can be observed in Stage IV cancer. All of these compounds have excellent activity in combination with the platinum compounds cisplatin (Platinol) and carboplatin (Paraplatin). Forty percent or more of patients receiving chemotherapy for advanced nonsmall cell lung cancer can expect to live at least one year. There is now consistent evidence of survival improvement through the use of these agents in Stage IV nonsmall cell lung cancer. In addition, these agents may give palliative benefit by reducing the size of the tumors and relieving symptoms. A large, randomized clinical trial comparing four different platinum and modern chemotherapy drug combinations confirmed the efficacy of the drugs, while demonstrating that the various combinations were essentially equivalent in terms of effectiveness and overall benefit.

The addition of the new drug bevacizumab (Avastin) to a platinum-based combination can yield further improvements in survival of patients with metastatic nonsmall cell lung cancer. Bevacizumab can, however, increase the risk of serious, life-threatening complications, so its use is limited to patients who do not have tumors located in the middle of their chest or in close proximity to large blood vessels. In addition, patients should not present with hemoptysis (coughing up blood) and should not have brain metastases, as the risk of life-threatening complications may be higher in these patients.

Improvements in the effectiveness and tolerability of chemotherapy have made it possible to go beyond first-line chemotherapy. Patients whose disease is stabilized by the first line of treatment are often candidates for further therapy with different treatment options. In the last few years, docetaxel, first, followed by pemetrexed (Alimta), has been approved by the FDA specifically as a treatment option for nonsmall cell lung cancer patients whose disease has progressed after first-line therapy.

A new class of drugs labeled targeted chemotherapy has emerged as an important option for patients with nonsmall cell lung cancer. The first drug to be approved in this class was gefitinib (Iressa). However, in the United States and Europe, gefitinib did not confirm its initial encouraging results. Gefitinib remains in use in Asia, where it appears to have excellent activity. The leading drug in nonsmall cell lung cancer to come from this class is erlotinib (Tarceva). The drugs from this class target a precise molecular event in the cancer cell. These drugs are inhibitors of the actions that occur when the epidermal growth factor receptor (EGFR) is stimulated by the epidermal growth factor (EGF). EGFR stimulation leads to a number of molecular signals that allow the cancer cell to survive and thrive. The EGFR is present in normal cells, like skin cells, but its actions are not crucial for normal cells. As a result, the side-effect profile of these drugs tends to be gentler for most patients than that seen with conventional chemotherapy. Patients taking erlotinib can expect a characteristic skin rash and occasionally diarrhea. Less often, the drug can cause fatigue and nausea. It can also cause the skin to crack, which can be quite uncomfortable. Very rarely and mostly in Asian patients or in patients who have received a great deal of radiation to their chest, erlotinib can cause a life-threatening inflammation of the lungs. The vast majority of patients treated with erlotinib have the gentler forms of the side effects mentioned above.

Erlotinib has been shown in clinical trials to be useful in patients whose disease is resistant to at least one prior chemotherapy treatment. It can reverse the disease dramatically in a few patients and less so in other patients. The majority of patients who respond to treatment with erlotinib experience stabilization of their disease with improvement in their symptoms. Certain groups of patients appear to have a higher chance of response to erlotinib—nonsmokers, women, and Asian patients have the best chance of response to treatment with erlotinib. These groups of patients are more likely to have a mutation on the EGFR, which is the target for erlotinib and which makes their cancer cells more vulnerable to treatment with this drug.

Advances in our understanding of the molecular biology of lung cancer have allowed us to identify targets for drugs like erlotinib. Many more possible targets and drugs are in development and we should have a whole new generation of safe and effective options in a few short years.

Neoadjuvant Chemotherapy and Radiation New protocols to explore curative strategies in lung cancer include using chemotherapy or radiation therapy, or both, before surgery, to try to convert some patients from an inoperable stage to one where the tumor can be removed. An example is the use of chemotherapy initially in Stages IB–IIIA lung cancer patients. Small studies have indicated that this approach may be beneficial, although it is too early to make any definite claims about this technique. Several larger studies in Europe and North America have been completed, and their results should be available in a few years, but for now the technique is best reserved for use in the setting of a clinical trial.

When one adds radiation to chemotherapy followed by surgery for Stage IIIA nonsmall cell lung cancer, there may be a benefit, but the risk of severe postoperative complications does exist. The decision to use these techniques prior to surgery must be carefully weighed against the chance of life-threatening complications.

 Laser Therapy Laser bronchoscopy with light sensitizers has been an interesting experimental technique to try to open the airways when they are blocked by a tumor (see chapter 10, "Laser Therapy").

Gene Therapy We are now beginning to understand precisely the molecular defects that lead to the transformation of a normal cell into a cancerous cell. The damage to some of the more crucial controlling steps can be repaired in cells in the lab. In those experiments, copies of the damaged gene are replaced with new copies, usually delivered by a virus. When a specially engineered virus carrying a copy of the desired gene infects an abnormal cell, it can restore the cell to a more normal state. The difficulty lies in being able to deliver the normal gene to all of the cancer cells or to as many as possible.

Preliminary studies have been carried out to prove the concept that replacing a damaged gene leads to improvement. To date, these initial efforts show that when the virus can be delivered to the cancer cells, the cancer cells can be controlled more easily. In order to achieve more significant improvements, the next step will be to successfully replace copies of the damaged gene in all of the cancer cells. Therein lies the great difficulty in establishing this option as a viable solution.

Vaccine Therapy Harnessing a patient's own immune system to fight cancer cells has been a strategy that can work for some cancers. To date, there have been attempts at making a vaccine by taking a patient's own cells and altering them to allow them to stimulate the patient's immune system more effectively. The approach has a great deal of scientific merit and has on occasion yielded provocative results. Unfortunately, it requires surgery to remove enough cancer cells to make the vaccine. Clinical trials performed with this approach have not shown strong enough results to make it a reasonable choice at this time. Other vaccine approaches try to stimulate the immune system to recognize a specific molecule associated with the cancer. Clinical trials are ongoing to see if this latest vaccine strategy is reasonable.

Treatment by Stage

■ Stage I
TNM T1–2, N0, M0
The tumor can be removed surgically and has not spread to involve the lymph nodes.

Standard Treatment If possible, the lobe of the involved lung with the tumor in place is removed along with the nearby lymph nodes. Sometimes the entire lung on one side needs to

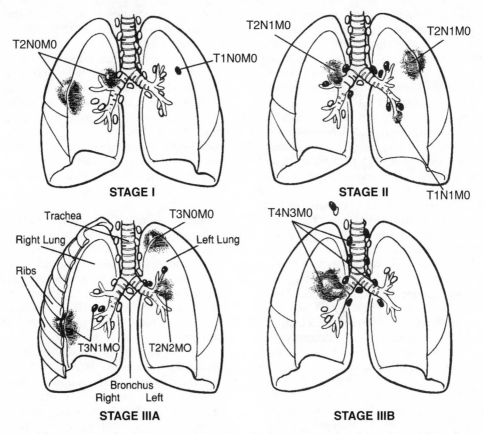

Stages of lung cancer, showing size and location of primary cancer, and lymph nodal involvement. (Based on drawings in *Contemporary Internal Medicine,* September 1990.)

be removed to ensure that the entire tumor is resected.

In patients with a small (T1) tumor, or in patients with impaired lung function, only a wedge segmental resection, which removes the tumor with a small amount of normal surrounding tissue, is done. The limited wedge resection is reserved for patients who are otherwise felt not to be able to tolerate the removal of standard amounts of lung tissue as necessitated by the removal of a lobe. Whenever possible, a lobectomy or a segmentectomy should be performed, as it has better success in preventing a local recurrence than

a wedge resection. Almost all patients can tolerate an upper lobectomy unless they have severely reduced pulmonary function.

In those patients with severe lung or heart disease who cannot tolerate surgery, limited radiation therapy is sometimes used, with much smaller survival benefits. In recent years, the use of advanced radiation techniques, including stereotactic radiosurgery (CyberKnife or Gamma Knife) have yielded promising results. Further clinical trials are needed to determine the true value of these newer techniques.

Chemotherapy after surgery has yet to be proven useful in patients with Stage IA disease and remains controversial for patients with Stage IB disease.

Five-Year Survival 50 to 80 percent

■ *Stage II*
TNM T1–2, N1, M0 or T3, N0, M0
The tumor has spread to the hilar (N1) nodes or the tumor invades the chest wall, mediastinum, or diaphragm (T3).

Standard Treatment This stage is likewise treated with surgery. Recently, several large-scale international clinical trials have shown that patients with Stage II nonsmall cell lung cancer may derive a survival benefit from the addition of platinum-based chemotherapy (cisplatin [Plantinol] or carboplatin [Paraplatin]) after they recover from their surgery. Patients who do not experience serious complications from their surgery can be considered for postoperative chemotherapy. The benefit from postoperative chemotherapy is on the order of a 5 to 15 percent improvement in overall survival.

Patients unable to withstand surgery may be candidates for radiation therapy with intent to cure, although the chance of cure is generally less than what is expected with surgery.

A special situation under Stage II is a superior sulcus tumor, which involves cancers in the top of the lung that invade local nerves and cause pain in the arm (they are often classified as T3, N0, M0). These tumors seem to have a reduced potential for distant metastases, so local radiation therapy is possible for cure. Surgery is frequently used after radiation. The results of a recently completed national clinical trial strongly supported adding chemotherapy to radiation, followed by surgery, to significantly increase the cure rate of these upper-lung tumors.

Five-Year Survival 30 to 50 percent

Investigational Trials are exploring whether the use of chemotherapy before surgery can improve the cure rate. Preliminary trial data suggest that preoperative chemotherapy is safe and well tolerated. Whether or not preoperative chemotherapy leads to improved survival remains to be determined.

■ *Stage IIIA*
TNM T1–2, N2, M0 or T3, N1–2, M0
Stage III is divided into IIIA and IIIB. Both show involvement of nodes in the center of the chest, but Stage IIIA tumors may be removed surgically under certain circumstances.

Standard Treatment These tumors are treated mainly with radiation therapy and chemotherapy, surgery, or all three, depending on the clinical circumstances.

Patients who undergo surgery should be considered for treatment with chemotherapy upon their recovery from surgery. Recently, several large-scale international clinical trials have shown that patients with Stage IIIA nonsmall cell lung cancer may derive a survival benefit from the addition of platinum-based chemotherapy after they recover from their surgery. This benefit is on the order of a 5 percent improvement in overall survival.

Radiation therapy is frequently given after surgery. Although there is no evidence that this improves survival, there can be a decrease in recurrences at the original tumor site.

For patients who are not felt to be surgical candidates, the use of chemotherapy concurrently with radiation is more effective than either treatment followed by the other.

Although most patients do not completely respond to radiation therapy alone, 15 to 20 percent do experience long-term survival benefit.

Patients whose tumors invade the chest wall or the upper portions of the lung or chest can often be treated with surgery, which may involve the removal of some of the chest wall, including ribs, and chest wall reconstruction. Radiation therapy is often used along with surgery.

Some patients with extensive metastatic disease in the center of the chest may develop what is called the superior vena cava syndrome, in which the great vessels in the chest are compressed by the tumor. When this involves the large vein that returns blood to the heart, the blood gets backed up into the tissues of the neck, head, and arms. This is an urgent situation and patients should be given prompt radiation therapy.

Five-Year Survival 10 to 30 percent

Investigational Treatment with radiation or chemotherapy or both before surgery (neoadjuvant) has been used on an investigational basis. Preliminary results suggest that there may be benefit by combining all three treatments in selected cases. Newer trials are giving cisplatin (Platinol) and docetaxel (Taxotere) by themselves or together with radiation, followed by surgery. T4 lesions can oftentimes be completely resected in centers with experienced general thoracic surgeons using induction chemotherapy and radiation followed by surgery; three-year survival of greater than 30 to 40 percent can be achieved using reduction chemotherapy and radiation.

■ *Stage IIIB*
TNM Any T, N3, M0 or T4 (noneffusion lesions), any N, M0
The tumor cannot be removed because of technical reasons or because there would be no benefit to the patient.

Standard Treatment These tumors are best managed with radiation therapy and chemotherapy. Recently completed clinical trials both in the United States and Japan and Europe strongly support the use of chemotherapy administered

concurrently with radiation therapy as a more effective approach than chemotherapy followed by radiation, or radiation without the use of chemotherapy. T4 (effusion) or N3 treatment predominately includes definitive chemoradiation or investigational treatment.

Five-Year Survival 5 to 20 percent

Investigational Trials are examining the effectiveness of chemotherapy and/or radiation therapy before surgery. These treatments have occasionally converted some patients to an operable stage, but it is too soon to know if using this aggressive approach will increase the rate of cure. Other trials are examining using newer chemotherapy agents at the same time as radiation.

■ *Stage IV*
TNM Any T, any N, M1
The cancer has spread to distant sites.

Standard Treatment Metastatic disease cannot be cured by surgery, so treatment for this stage is directed toward relieving symptoms with either radiation therapy or chemotherapy.

Radiation may relieve local symptoms such as tracheal, esophageal, or bronchial compression; bone or brain metastases; pain; vocal cord paralysis; coughing up blood (hemoptysis); and superior vena cava syndrome. Patients without symptoms should be kept under close observation. Sometimes treatment may appropriately be deferred until symptoms or signs of a progressive tumor develop.

Chemotherapy with a platinum compound combined with drugs such as paclitaxel (Taxol), docetaxel (Taxotere), irinotecan (Camptozar, CPT-11), gemcitabine (Gemzar), and vinorelbine (Navelbine) has response rates of 30 to 50 percent in Stage IV cases. Chemotherapy will give modest but consistent and significant improvements in survival. The new combinations are usually well tolerated; the more severe side effects deal mostly with suppression of the bone marrow. Nausea and vomiting are usually well controlled through the use of medications such as dexamethasone (Decadron), ondansetron (Zofran), granisetron (Kytril), dolasetron (Anzemet), and palonosetron (Aloxi). Newer antinausea drugs like aprepitant (Emend) have been very effective for patients who develop nausea and vomiting with drugs like cisplatin (Platinol). Loss of hair is mostly seen with the use of either paclitaxel, docetaxel, or irinotecan.

Recent trials using a cisplatin-based regimen of chemotherapy showed some survival benefit and give hope for more benefit in the future. Combinations currently in use include carboplatin (Paraplatin) or cisplatin + paclitaxel, cisplatin or carboplatin + vinorelbine, cisplatin or carboplatin + gemcitabine, cisplatin + docetaxel, and cisplatin + irinotecan. Recent studies with newer combinations such as docetaxel + gemcitabine suggest that cisplatin-containing regimens are probably more effective, even if the noncisplatin regimen may be better tolerated. The use of three conventional chemotherapy drugs has been abandoned as too toxic while not more effective.

For patients who progress after first-line chemotherapy, the use of second-line chemotherapy with either pemetrexed (Alimta), docetaxel, or erlotinib (Tarceva) is an excellent option.

Other potentially useful adjuncts to the treatment of advanced lung cancer include feeding gastrostomies when the esophagus is obstructed by the cancer, and the use of lasers to open up an airway obstructed by a tumor mass.

Occasionally, persons with excellent performance status and a limited metastatic disease (isolated from advanced metastases) can benefit (at 20 to 25 percent three- to five-year survival) with aggressive combined treatment, including chemotherapy, radiation, and resection or stereotactic radiotherapy of metastatases and the primary tumor.

Five-Year Survival Less than 5 percent

Investigational New drugs that target the growth of blood vessels (angiogenesis inhibitors) are in accelerated development. Drugs that target the internal communication system of the cancer cell (signal transduction inhibitors) are also receiving a great deal of attention. Combinations of these drugs, or drugs that affect multiple internal pathways, are being developed.

Supportive Therapy

The importance of supportive therapy in the treatment of lung cancer cannot be overemphasized.

• Psychosocial support to help maintain a positive attitude and the will to live and to aid in coping with cancer can help a patient survive the rigors of surgery, chemotherapy, and radiation therapy (see chapter 19, "Living with Cancer," and chapter 32, "The Will to Live").

• Quite clearly, malnutrition results in a bad outcome in patients with lung cancer. Patients must be served palatable meals and attempts must be made to work with patients to determine food preferences (see chapter 23, "Maintaining Good Nutrition").

• Pain control is of critical importance, and the tools to achieve control are available even for the most advanced cases. These include the use of pain-relieving (analgesic) drugs such as nonsteroidal anti-inflammatory agents, mild narcotics, strong narcotics, continuous narcotics, and narcotics delivered into the spinal canal (epidural). Pain control can generally be achieved without interfering with mental competence (see chapter 24, "Controlling Pain").

• Nausea can be controlled with a variety of drugs (see chapter 20, "Coping with the Side Effects of Chemotherapy").

• Physical therapy will help maintain muscle strength to keep life as normal as possible (see chapter 29 "Staying Physically Fit").

Maintaining Quality of Life In the management of lung cancer (as well as all other malignancies), it is critical that patients maintain as high a quality of life as possible. Patients must feel that they are contributing members of society. Certainly, this keeps them in a happier mental frame.

Being with family and friends, going out to meals and movies, and participating in enjoyable recreational events are all important parts of maintaining lifestyle. With the services now available and the help of family members and physicians, it is usually possible to maintain these goals.

However, when the time comes that patients are no longer able to participate in such activities, we must all be sensible enough to ensure comfort by whatever methods we can. Even if mental ability has been compromised in order to relieve the pain, pain control should come first and remain all-important. *Comfort care* is the key phrase at this stage of life.

Treatment Follow-Up

People who have lung cancer have to be followed carefully by their physician, generally being examined every one to three months during the first two years, for that is when the risk of relapse is greatest.

• Chest CT scans every three to four months in the absence of symptoms
• Chest CT scans more often if symptoms occur
• Blood chemistry tests every three to four months
• Physical examination of the chest, lymph nodes, and abdomen
• Neurologic examination
• After two years, follow-up every six months with CT scans and blood surveillance

Patients should, of course, see their physician if any unusual symptoms occur.

Recurrent Cancer

See treatment for Stage IV disease.

The Most Important Questions You Can Ask

• What is the stage of my disease and what is my prognosis?
• What is the role of surgery and what is the chance of it curing me?
• What is the role of radiation therapy?
• How sick will I be on chemotherapy and can we control the sickness?
• If chemotherapy cannot cure my cancer, why should I expose myself to its side effects and toxicities?
• What is the chance that I will die from this tumor? How much time am I likely to have?

Lung: Small Cell

*Thierry M. Jahan, M.D., Sarita Dubey, M.D.,
Daphne A. Haas-Kogan, M.D., and David M. Jablons, M.D.*

■ ■ ■ ■

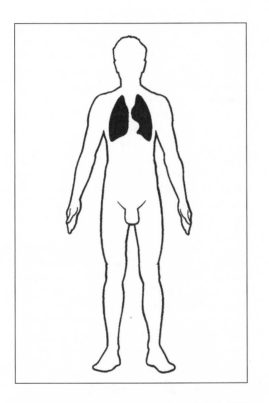

In 2007, there were an estimated 213,380 new cases of lung cancer in the United States. Small cell lung cancer accounts for about 20 percent of all lung cancer cases. Also called oat cell carcinoma of the lung, it has the most rapid clinical course of any type of lung cancer, with average survival of patients with extensive-stage disease from the time of diagnosis of only several months without treatment. Compared with other types of lung cancer, small cell carcinoma has a greater tendency to have spread widely by the time of diagnosis; although, because of its rapid growth, it tends to be more responsive to treatment with chemotherapy and radiation than are the other types of lung cancer.

The majority of patients with small cell carcinoma of the lung have distant metastases at the time of diagnosis. With modern staging procedures, the areas of spread can be discovered in two-thirds of these patients.

Small cell cancer is not always confined to the lung. Occasionally, it may occur in other organs such as the esophagus, prostate, and cervix, and sometimes it may occur without the primary site of origin being identified. The management of these tumors is addressed in the chapters concerning those organs; chemotherapy remains the fundamental basic treatment.

Types There are several types of small cell lung cancer, defined by the tumor's appearance under the microscope. These include small cell, mixed small cell/large cell, and combined small cell. It is unclear whether these types of tumors have different prognoses.

This tumor arises from what are called neuroendocrine cells and is known as an APUD (amine precursor uptake and decarboxylation) tumor. Under the electron microscope, hormone-producing (neurosecretory) granules can be seen. These tumors, therefore, can abnormally produce hormones and cause what have been known as paraneoplastic syndromes. For example, if the tumor produces too much cortisone, the condition is called Cushing's syndrome. If antidiuretic hormone (ADH) is produced, water is retained in the body and the apparent salt (sodium) level decreases. Each of these paraneoplastic syndromes produces its own signs and symptoms.

How It Spreads Small cell lung cancer can spread via lymphatic vessels to the lymph nodes in the center of the lung (hilar nodes), the center of the chest (mediastinal nodes), in the neck and above the collarbone (supraclavicular nodes), and in the abdominal cavity. It is likely to spread through the bloodstream to the liver, brain, and bone. Classically, small cell lung cancer presents with small primary tumors in the lung and large mediastinal lymph nodes.

What Causes It Cigarette smoking has been a major factor in the development of both small cell and nonsmall cell lung cancers. The increase in cigarette smoking by men in the 1920s was followed in the 1940s by a dramatic increase in the incidence of lung cancer in men. The marked increase in cigarette smoking by women in the 1940s was unfortunately followed twenty years later by a similar increase in the incidence of lung cancer among women. It has been estimated that if all tobacco disappeared from the earth, 17 percent of all cancers would also disappear. The attempt to discontinue cigarette smoking remains one of the most crucial medical issues in our society.

Lung cancer may predispose a person to a higher risk (ten- to twentyfold) of developing another lung cancer later.

Risk Factors

There is no specific environmental or genetic factor known except those discussed in the chapter on nonsmall cell lung cancer.

At Significantly Higher Risk
- Cigarette smokers
- Workers exposed to industrial substances such as asbestos, nickel, chromium compounds, chloromethyl ether, and/or air pollutants.

Screening

Lung cancer is very difficult to detect at an early stage. Tests such as the examination of sputum (phlegm) for malignant cells and regular chest X-rays have not proven to be beneficial. Chest X-rays can detect lung cancer in smokers, but it may not always be early enough to improve the survival of patients. A technique known as fluorescence bronchoscopy is in the process of being perfected, with a goal of detecting the cancer as early as possible. Recently, the use of spiral CT scanning in patients at high risk for developing lung cancer has shown promising preliminary results in detecting nonsmall cell lung cancer at a very early stage, when it may still be curable. Efforts are currently under way to confirm these promising results through a large national randomized clinical trial. These efforts may also lead to effective screening for small cell lung cancer, given that the risk factors and populations at risk overlap greatly with those of nonsmall cell lung cancer.

Common Signs and Symptoms

As with nonsmall cell cancer, a new or changing cough, sometimes containing blood, is a common symptom, along with hoarseness and shortness of breath or increased shortness of breath on exertion. There may also be an increase in the amount of sputum, recurrent episodes of lung infection (sometimes in the same lobe of the lung as the cancer), weight loss, fatigue, and swelling of the face or arms.

If the tumor has metastasized, the symptoms can include severe headaches, double vision, and pain in the bones, chest, abdomen, neck, and down the arms.

One point that needs to be emphasized is that this disease is usually widespread at the time of diagnosis.

Diagnosis

The diagnosis of small cell lung cancer is usually apparent by routine microscopy. Other techniques that may be useful in selected cases, particularly when the diagnosis is in doubt, include electron microscopy, which detects the small cell cancer's neuroendocrine granules, and immunohistochemical stains, which can detect certain markers characteristic for small cell cancer. Newer techniques, still investigational, include examining the tumor DNA for chromosome abnormalities, overexpression of oncogenes, and deletion of tumor suppressor genes.

Blood and Other Tests

- Chemistry profile.
- Sputum (phlegm) examination.
- Removal of fluid from the chest and examination of it for malignant cells.

Imaging

- Chest X-ray.
- CT scan of the chest and abdomen.
- MRI or CT scan of the brain.
- PET scans can be helpful in staging the mediastinum (the area between both lungs where a lot of the lymph nodes that drain the lungs are located) as well as in detecting metastases that have spread outside of the chest. A positive PET scan strongly suggests that cancer might be present.
- Bone scan.

Endoscopy and Biopsy

- Fiber-optic bronchoscopy with brushing or biopsy.
- Mediastinoscopy with biopsies. In this safe and outpatient procedure under general anesthesia, a small incision is made at the base of the neck and a long, thin tube called a mediastinoscope is inserted along the airway to assess the lymph nodes in the middle of the chest. Tissue can be removed through this instrument for analysis of tumor metastases to these lymph nodes.
- Needle aspiration through the chest wall (see the section on FNA biopsy in chapter 2, "How Cancer Is Diagnosed"), with a local anesthetic and often under CT guidance.
- Biopsies of the chest lining, lymph nodes, bone, and liver.

Staging

The detailed staging techniques and classifications used for nonsmall cell lung cancer are not commonly used for small cell lung cancer. Instead, the staging system focuses on whether disease is limited or extensive. The stage of the tumor (limited versus extensive) will determine the prognosis and may affect the choice of treatment.

The staging procedures commonly used to document distant metastases include CT scans of the brain and liver and radionuclide bone scans. MRI scans can also be used to evaluate the brain and bones. A bone marrow biopsy may be necessary to exclude the presence of metastatic disease if all of the other staging procedures prove to be negative.

Limited-stage disease means that the tumor is confined to the chest only, including the mediastinum and the supraclavicular nodes. This area can be encompassed within a tolerable radiotherapy field. *Extensive-stage disease* means that the tumor is too widespread to be included within the definition of limited-stage disease. Typically, these tumors involve multiple sites and therefore cannot be included in a single radiation field.

The definition of *limited stage* has changed somewhat over the years. In the past, patients with fluid around the lung (pleural effusion), massive or multiple pulmonary tumor masses on the same side, and enlarged supraclavicular nodes on the opposite side have been both included in and excluded from the "limited stage" by various treatment centers. At the present time, these patients would be considered to have "extensive-stage disease."

Treatment Overview

At the time of diagnosis, about one-third of patients with small cell lung carcinoma will have limited-stage disease. Most people who survive at least two years without a recurrence of the cancer come from this group. In limited-stage disease, average survival of ten to sixteen months is a reasonable expectation with current treatments. A few patients with limited stage are occasionally treated with surgery. These patients usually are at a very early stage (T1, N0, M0) and generally do well with surgery. Typically, they are initially thought to have nonsmall cell histology. The diagnosis of small cell or mixed histology is made from pathologic examination of the resected tumor.

With extensive-stage disease, the prognosis is worse. Average survival is six to twelve months with current treatments. There is long-term disease-free survival in some patients, so treatment is certainly recommended. Patients who achieve a complete response to treatment (the tumor appears to go away completely) have the best overall survival.

In small cell lung cancer, 10 to 20 percent of patients may achieve long-term remissions with aggressive combined radiation and chemotherapy. Most of the improvement in survival has been the result of treatments discovered by clinical trials.

Surgery Removing the primary tumor produces little benefit with this type of cancer, although a very small number of patients might possibly benefit from surgery followed by adjuvant chemotherapy or chemotherapy and radiotherapy. This is an option only for those patients who have small tumors limited to a single area of the lung and who possess adequate pulmonary function. Recent reports for T1 (less than $1\frac{1}{4}$ inches [3 cm]) small cell tumors treated with surgery, chemotherapy, and radiation have shown improved survival.

Chemotherapy Because of the frequent presence of hidden and undetectable spread to other parts of the body, chemotherapy is the cornerstone of treatment for small cell lung cancer, since it also treats tumors too small to detect. Once remission is achieved, there is no evidence that maintenance therapy is beneficial. There is no evidence that more than six months of treatment is of value.

Radiation Doses in the range of 4,000 to 5,000 cGy or more are needed to control chest tumors effectively. If radiation therapy is given with combination chemotherapy, there are higher response rates and better survival than when radiation therapy is given alone. Radiation therapy plus combination chemotherapy is also superior to chemotherapy alone for controlling the primary chest tumor. In a recently published randomized clinical trial, the combination of twice-per-day radiation ("hyper-fractionated" radiation) and chemotherapy was shown to provide better overall and disease-free survival than the control-arm treatment of once-daily radiation and chemotherapy. The study was criticized, however, in that the control dose of once-daily radiation was lower than what most radiation therapists would feel comfortable prescribing to patients with small cell lung cancer. Furthermore, hyperfractionated radiation does have significant drawbacks;

it is more toxic and it may not be the best choice for patients who start out debilitated. It should be considered only in patients who present with limited stage and excellent performance status, without additional underlying illnesses.

Studies have shown some survival benefit when combined therapy is given, especially in limited-stage disease, so long as radiation therapy does not result in a delay of the administration of proper doses of chemotherapy. There are increased side effects with combined programs and some treatment-related mortality because of lung and bone marrow toxicities.

Some patients have a tumor mass in the center of the chest that presses on the large vein draining blood from the head and arms (the superior vena cava). This pressure causes a fluid backup, resulting in swelling of the face and arms and sometimes even the brain. If this superior vena cava syndrome is present, combination chemotherapy alone can be given or radiation therapy given with it.

Because of the high frequency of brain metastases in small cell lung cancer, especially in patients with prolonged survival, many physicians use prophylactic radiation of the head. This reduces the frequency of subsequent brain metastases, especially in patients with complete responses to therapy, but has not been shown to influence survival. There may be late complications of this type of treatment, with neurological, mental, and thinking deficits in some long-term survivors who were given high-daily-dose fractionation. It may be preferable to give smaller doses each day.

There remains a certain amount of controversy regarding the use of prophylactic cranial irradiation (PCI). Until recently, there had not been a single strongly positive study to suggest that PCI increases survival, although a pooling of the results of the best studies did come up with a benefit in favor of PCI. Recently, a large Phase III study conducted in Europe demonstrated that the use of PCI in patients with extensive-stage small cell lung cancer who showed any degree of response after four to six cycles of chemotherapy did improve both disease-free and overall survival.

Treatment by Stage

■ *Limited Stage*

Standard Treatment Limited-stage small cell lung cancer is highly responsive to treatment with combination chemotherapy. Multiple drugs are clearly superior to single-agent treatment. Current programs give objective response rates (the tumor gets smaller) of 80 to 90 percent, with complete response rates (the tumor disappears) of 45 to 75 percent. Radiation therapy given at the same time as the chemotherapy improves the survival rate. Chemotherapy given twice daily, rather than the more conventional once daily, may improve survival over once-daily therapy. Twice-daily radiation and chemotherapy tends to be more toxic. When chemotherapy and radiation are given together, the radiation may be started as late as, but no later than, the second cycle of chemotherapy.

Efforts to increase the dose of chemotherapy to treat small cell lung cancer have included using stem cell transplants to rescue the heavily treated bone marrow. Unfortunately, the higher doses of chemotherapy did not prove more effective at increasing the survival of patients with limited-stage disease.

As noted, a small minority of very limited stage patients without evidence of tumor in the mediastinum might benefit from surgery followed by adjuvant chemotherapy.

Two-Year Survival 20 percent

■ *Extensive Stage*

Standard Treatment Extensive-stage small cell lung cancer patients are given chemotherapy in much the same fashion as those with limited-stage disease. Current programs result in objective response rates of 70 to 85 percent and complete response rates of 20 to 30 percent.

Commonly used combination chemotherapy regimens include PE (cisplatin [Platinol] + etoposide [Etopophos]), CE (carboplatin [Paraplatin] + etoposide), CAV (cyclophosphamide [Cytoxan] + doxorubicin [Adriamycin] + vincristine [Oncovin]), and CAVP-16 (cyclophosphamide + doxorubicin + etoposide). A randomized clinical trial in Japan showed that the combination of irinotecan (Camptosar, CPT-11) and cisplatin could be more effective in prolonging survival than the combination of cisplatin and etoposide. To date, these results have not been duplicated in Western populations. A cooperative group clinical trial headed by the Southwestern Oncology Group is currently under way to definitely prove whether the combination of irinotecan and cisplatin is superior to that of cisplatin and etoposide.

Unlike with limited-stage disease, there is no pressing need to include chest irradiation with combination chemotherapy. Radiotherapy may relieve symptoms caused by the primary tumor or metastatic disease. For example, symptoms from brain metastases and pain from bone metastases can be promptly relieved with radiation.

If the superior vena cava syndrome is present, chest irradiation may result in a very rapid initial response.

Two-Year Survival 5 percent

Supportive Therapy

The importance of supportive therapy in the treatment of lung cancer cannot be overemphasized.

• Quite clearly, malnutrition results in a bad outcome in patients with lung cancer. Patients must be served palatable meals and attempts must be made to work with patients to determine food preferences (see chapter 23, "Maintaining Good Nutrition").

• Pain control is of critical importance, and the tools to achieve control are available even for the most advanced cases. These include the use of pain-relieving (analgesic) drugs such as nonsteroidal anti-inflammatory agents, mild narcotics, strong narcotics, continuous narcotics, and narcotics delivered into the spinal canal (epidural). Pain control can generally be achieved without interfering with mental competence (see chapter 24, "Controlling Pain").

• Nausea can be controlled with a variety of drugs (see chapter 20, "Coping with the Side Effects of Chemotherapy").

• Physical therapy will help maintain muscle strength to keep life as normal as possible (see chapter 29, "Staying Physically Fit").

Maintaining the Quality of Life In the management of lung cancer (as well as all other malignancies), it is critical that patients maintain as high a quality of life as possible. Patients must feel that they are contributing members of society. Certainly, this keeps them in a happier mental frame.

Being with family and friends, going out to meals and movies, and participating in enjoyable recreational events are all important parts of maintaining lifestyle. With the services now available and the help of family members and physicians, it is usually possible to maintain these goals.

However, when the time comes that patients are no longer able to participate in such activities, we must all be sensible enough to ensure comfort by whatever methods we can. Even if mental ability has been compromised in order to relieve the pain, pain control should come first and remain all-important. *Comfort care* is the key phrase at this stage of life.

Treatment Follow-Up

After treatment is completed, patients should be seen every one or two months for at least two years. Visits can then be spread out, perhaps every four months for two years and every six months for another two years.

During the first two years, follow-up should include

- physical examination of the lungs, chest wall, lymph nodes, and abdomen;
- chest X-ray every three to four months or more frequently if required;
- blood chemistry tests every three to four months; and
- neurologic examination.

Recurrent Cancer

If small cell lung cancer recurs, the prognosis is determined in large part by how soon after the completion of chemotherapy the relapse occurred. If the cancer relapses less than three months after the completion of chemotherapy, patients have primary refractory disease. The prognosis is very poor regardless of stage or treatment. The expected average survival is two to three months, so a patient should be considered for either palliative therapy or participation in clinical trials.

- Palliative, or second-line, therapy could include chemotherapy agents that have not yet been used or radiation therapy for bone metastases or other metastases if appropriate. The drug topotecan (Hycamtin) has been approved especially for its use as a second-line treatment for relapsed small cell lung cancer. Other medications include paclitaxel (Taxol) and irinotecan (Camptosar, CPT-11). The likelihood of a response to a second type of chemotherapy for relapsed small cell lung cancer depends mostly on whether or not patients have primary refractory disease. The chance of a response from a second chemotherapy regime in patients with primary refractory disease is less than 10 percent. Patients whose disease returns between three months and one year after completing their initial treatment have a 50 percent chance of response to a second type of chemotherapy. Patients whose disease relapses over one year from the completion of their treatment have an 80 percent or better chance of response to second-line chemotherapy. So the decision to proceed with additional chemotherapy depends on the physical condition of the patient and the duration of the initial response to treatment.

- Other palliative treatments include measures for pain relief and orthopedic aids for patients with skeletal involvement and/or neurologic compromise.

The Most Important Questions You Can Ask

- What is the stage of my disease and what is my prognosis?
- How sick will I be on chemotherapy and what can be done to control the side effects?
- If chemotherapy cannot cure my cancer, why should I expose myself to its side effects and toxicities?
- What is the chance that I will die from this tumor? How much time am I likely to have?
- Are there investigational protocols for which I may be eligible?

Lymphoma: AIDS-Associated

Lawrence D. Kaplan, M.D., and Alexandra M. Levine, M.D.

■ ■ ■ ■

Lymphoma is not one disease, but rather consists of about twenty different types of tumors. In general, lymphoma is a cancer of a type of white blood cell called the lymphocyte, an extremely important cell in the immune system. In lymphoma, the lymphocytes start to grow for no known reason and continue to grow and expand, seemingly unable to stop. The result is enlargement of lymph glands or other organs in which lymphocytes normally grow and the development of "lumps and bumps" on the body. Dysfunction of various organs may also develop as the abnormal lymphocytes grow, taking up so much space that normal cells don't have room to function.

Types The lymphomas occurring in people infected with the human immunodeficiency virus (HIV) are high-grade B cell lymphomas. These are tumors that grow very rapidly. They usually consist of either small noncleaved lymphoma (also called Burkitt's lymphoma) or diffuse large B cell lymphoma. Other types of lymphoma are much less common and will not be discussed here.

What Causes It All people with HIV infection are at increased risk for developing lymphoma. The risk of developing lymphoma is significantly reduced by the use of anti-HIV medicines (highly active antiretroviral therapy [HAART]). The average number of new cases per year since the widespread use of HAART began is about six cases per 1,000 persons with AIDS.

Screening

There is no way to screen for this disease and no reason to do so, unless there are certain symptoms or findings that suggest lymphoma.

Common Signs and Symptoms

People with lymphoma usually develop abnormal lumps and bumps. This could be an enlarged lymph gland or an enlarged lump almost anywhere in the body, including the jaw, the stomach cavity, the skin, the liver, and elsewhere.

If lymphoma first starts in the stomach or intestines, the first symptom might be belly pain or bloating or enlargement of the abdominal area. If lymphoma first begins in the bone marrow (the factory where all blood cells are made), the initial symptom might be bone pain or anemia (lowering of the red blood cell count, causing weakness and fatigue).

Aside from tumor masses, "systemic B symptoms" may develop as the first manifestation of disease. These include persistent fever, drenching night sweats (so that the bed linens have to be changed several times each night), and the loss of more than 10 percent of the normal body weight.

Diagnosis

The diagnosis of lymphoma can be made only after biopsy. The biopsy is taken from the specific area of abnormality, such as an enlarged lymph gland or other mass.

Staging

Several tests are performed to determine the precise extent of lymphoma before starting treatment. This staging work-up usually includes a CT scan of the chest, abdomen, and pelvis; a bone marrow biopsy; and a spinal tap to see if there are lymphoma cells floating in the spinal fluid surrounding the brain and spinal cord. A PET scan may also be performed. If there are symptoms or other evidence suggesting involvement of the bone, stomach, or other specific areas, tests such as X-rays may be done. There are four disease stages. Stage I disease indicates that there is a single area of lymphoma. Stage IV refers to disease that is widespread.

Treatment Overview

Several factors affect the prognosis and, therefore, the decisions about treatment. Factors associated with a poorer prognosis include a history of AIDS before the diagnosis of lymphoma, CD4 cells less than 100, age over thirty-five years, a poor performance status (the patient is weak and debilitated instead of vigorous and strong), advanced disease (Stage III or IV), and the presence of primary central nervous system lymphoma, in which the only place the lymphoma is found is in the brain.

Having lymphoma in the body and also lymphoma cells in the spinal fluid is not a bad prognostic sign, provided that the spinal fluid is treated for involvement.

Before highly active antiretroviral therapy (HAART) became available for the treatment of HIV disease, the standard combinations of chemotherapy drugs required to treat and potentially cure lymphoma were difficult to administer to AIDS patients, were less effective than in non-AIDS patients, and often caused serious infections. As a result, most patients died within a year of diagnosis. The use of HAART has dramatically changed this for the better. It is now possible to treat most patients with AIDS-associated lymphoma the same way we treat non-AIDS lymphoma. With standard chemotherapy, similar outcomes can be expected and more than 50 percent of patients will be cured of their lymphoma.

Chemotherapy The most commonly used chemotherapy regimen for diffuse large cell lymphoma is CHOP, consisting of cyclophosphamide (Cytoxan), doxorubicin (hydrodoxorubicin [Adriamycin]), vincristine (Oncovin), and prednisone. These agents are given by vein during the first day of each three-week cycle. Usually about six of these treatment cycles are given (twelve weeks). Rituximab (Rituxan) is an antibody (a protein that attaches to a specific molecule on the surface of the lymphoma cell) that is commonly added to the chemotherapy (CHOP becomes R-CHOP). It improves the likelihood of cure in non-HIV patients and may do the same in HIV patients. It may not be used in some patients with very low CD4 counts (less than fifty) because of a possible increased risk of infection. To prevent relapse of lymphoma in the spinal fluid, spinal taps may be repeated weekly or on alternate weeks for four to six treatments. A specific chemotherapy drug such as cytosine arabinoside (Ara-C, cytarabin [Cytosar-U]), cytarabine liposomal (DepoCyt), or methotrexate (Mexate, Amethopterin, Folex) is injected directly into the spinal fluid during the procedure.

Other chemotherapy might be used instead of R-CHOP. Some of these other regimens may involve continuous intravenous infusion of several drugs over a four-day period of time. These regimens often require a hospital stay in order to receive the infusion. For Burkitt's lymphoma, more aggressive chemotherapy may be given, which would result in more time in the hospital. Burkitt's lymphoma is curable with these more intensive chemotherapy treatments.

Radiation Radiation therapy may be used in addition to chemotherapy in certain circumstances; mainly if the lymphoma is localized or if it involves the brain or spinal fluid. However, it is only rarely used alone without chemotherapy, since even when lymphoma appears to be localized, microscopic disease usually exists in other places.

Bone Marrow Transplant If lymphoma relapses after chemotherapy, high-dose chemotherapy and autologous (using the patient's own bone marrow) bone marrow or stem cell transplant may be recommended. This is an aggressive but often curative treatment for some individuals with relapse of their lymphoma. It has been used successfully in patients with AIDS-associated lymphoma. In this procedure, very high doses of chemotherapy are given, after which bone marrow stem cells are transfused by vein to rescue the bone marrow (where blood cells are made) from the effects of the chemotherapy.

Supportive Therapy

Many forms of supportive therapy can be given to someone with AIDS-associated lymphoma undergoing chemotherapy.

• Medicines to prevent nausea and vomiting should be given routinely. Ondansetion (Zofran) and granisetion (Kytril) are extremely effective antinausea medicines and are given by vein just before the chemotherapy, often combined with lorazepam (Ativan). Ondansetion, granisetion, prochlorperazine (Compazine), lorazepam, or other antinausea medications should also be given for use on an outpatient basis.

• G-CSF (filgrastim [Neupogen]) is an important medicine that can limit the decrease of normal white blood cells caused by chemotherapy. When the level of these normal white blood cells (granulocytes, neutrophils, or polys) is lowered by chemotherapy, patients are at an increased risk for developing serious, even life-threatening, infection. Patients can inject themselves with Neupogen under the skin, similar to an insulin injection.

The G-CSF is begun on the day following chemotherapy and is continued until the white blood cells have fully recovered (about ten days). G-CSF can prevent serious infection, decrease the number of days spent in the hospital for infections, and decrease the need for antibiotics, which can be very expensive. A newer drug called pegfilgrastim (Neulasta) is frequently used in place of filgrastim. It is a long-acting form of the drug. It is injected only once (usually the day after chemotherapy).

• If the red blood cell count becomes low because of the chemotherapy, erythropoietin (epoetin alfa [Procrit] or darbepoetin [Aranesp]) can be given once every two to three weeks by injection under the skin, similar to G-CSF. This will increase the bone marrow's production of red blood cells and improve or resolve the anemia possibly caused by the chemotherapy.

• Medication to prevent *Pneumocystis carinii* pneumonia (PCP) is mandatory during and for at least three months after chemotherapy, regardless of the CD4 count.

In addition, other antibiotics may be given during the period of low white blood cells to prevent other types of infections.

• Anti-HIV drugs (HAART) should be used along with chemotherapy. Although there is always some risk of interactions between antiretroviral medicines and chemotherapy, most of these drugs can be administered safely with chemotherapy and may reduce the risk of some chemotherapy-related side effects. The only anti-HIV drug that should not be used with chemotherapy is zidovudine (AZT, Retrovir) or any combination drug that contains AZT. There may be times when it is advisable to discontinue anti-HIV drugs and to restart them after chemotherapy is completed (for example, if nausea from chemotherapy makes it difficult to take the anti-HIV medicines). This should not have a negative effect on the curability of the disease or on the treatment of the HIV infection.

• Psychological support can be helpful for anyone receiving therapy for lymphoma and HIV. This may take on different forms for different people and might include meditation, prayer, participation in support groups, acupuncture, exercise, talking to a psychologist or psychiatrist, family members, or friends, and other such endeavors.

Treatment Follow-Up

A CT scan is repeated after two to four months of chemotherapy to be sure that all the sites of lymphoma have responded well to the chemotherapy. When complete remission is documented on the scan, an additional two cycles of chemotherapy will be given in an attempt to prevent the lymphoma from coming back.

When chemotherapy has been stopped, follow-up includes visits to the physician once each month or more frequently, depending on other illnesses or conditions.

• Routine blood tests are obtained, including a chemistry panel and a complete blood count (CBC).

• An elevation of the LDH is an important indication that the lymphoma might have relapsed, so this test should be routinely ordered during follow-up.

• A physical exam should be performed once each month and a careful history taken to see if any new symptoms have developed.

• CT scans may be repeated periodically to ensure that a patient is still in remission. They should also be repeated if any new symptoms or findings on physical exam develop or if the LDH becomes elevated.

The likelihood of relapse becomes smaller as time goes by after completion of chemotherapy. After two years, the risk of relapse is less than 10 percent.

The Most Important Questions You Can Ask

• Have you treated other patients with AIDS-associated lymphoma? With AIDS?

• What specific type of lymphoma do I have and what is its extent in my body?

• What regimen of chemotherapy will be used?

• Will I need to be hospitalized?

• Will you use Neupogen or Neulasta?

• Will I be able to continue (or start) anti-HIV drugs?

• Will you let me participate in my own care by sharing my lab values, test results, and so forth with me?

Lymphoma: Hodgkin's Disease

Sandra J. Horning, M.D., and Steven M. Horwitz, M.D.

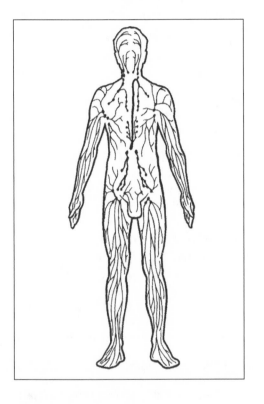

Hodgkin's disease—also called Hodgkin's lymphoma—is a cancer of the lymphoid system. It has special historical interest, because it was the first malignancy of the lymphoid system to be described. The first cases were reported in 1832 by British physician Thomas Hodgkin, who recognized that this disorder was distinct from other causes of enlarged lymph nodes, such as tuberculosis and other infectious diseases. Hodgkin's disease has characteristic features that distinguish it from all the other cancers of the lymphoid system, which have come to be collectively referred to as non-Hodgkin's lymphomas.

Hodgkin's disease (HD) is an uncommon malignancy. In 2007, an estimated 8,190 new cases of HD are expected in the United States out of over 1,400,000 new cases of cancer. Despite the relatively low incidence, HD is an important disease because it afflicts adolescents and young adults and because it has a substantial cure rate. Treatment is approached with great optimism.

The systematic approach to the pathologic diagnosis, staging, treatment strategies, and clinical trials that have been developed for Hodgkin's disease over the past thirty years serves as a model for all modern cancer therapy. These methods transformed an almost uniformly fatal disease into one of the most curable cancers. With so many cases being cured, attention has turned toward the complications of therapy and issues of "survivorship." Here again, Hodgkin's disease is leading the way in treatment design and evaluation.

Types The malignant cell characteristic of Hodgkin's disease is known as the Reed-Sternberg cell, named after the two pathologists who first described it. The Reed-Sternberg cell has been shown to originate from a B lymphocyte similar to most non-Hodgkin's lymphomas. One feature unique to Hodgkin's disease among other cancers is that the "tumors" contain few cancer cells. In most cases, the affected lymph nodes contain mixtures of mostly normal and less frequent malignant cells. It is believed that the collections of normal cells and scar tissue within affected lymph nodes represent a host response to the tumor cells. Occasionally, it can be very difficult or impossible to locate a single diagnostic Reed-Sternberg cell, but Reed-Sternberg "variants" or atypical large cells are regularly identified in HD tissues.

Like the non-Hodgkin's lymphomas, Hodgkin's disease is divided into subtypes according to the appearance of the affected lymph nodes under the microscope. The most recent World Health Organization classification system describes categories of Hodgkin's disease based on the types and arrangements of malignant and nonmalignant cells and on associated pathologic features. Nodular lymphocyte predominant Hodgkin's disease is separated from classical Hodgkin's disease because of its distinct pathology and clinical features. Each subtype of Hodgkin's disease is associated with characteristic age groups, sex, and stages of the disease, but because of the overall success of therapy, subtype generally has less prognostic importance in HD than in the non-Hodgkin's lymphomas.

World Health Organization Classification

Nodular Lymphocyte Predominance (NLP) This subtype can be difficult to distinguish from non-Hodgkin's lymphoma—a critical distinction when planning treatments or evaluating prognosis. The malignant cells are distinct from Reed-Sternberg cells and are called L&H (lymphocytic and histiocytic) or "popcorn" cells due to their appearance. The cells are typically arrayed in a nodular pattern. This subtype accounts for 5 to 10 percent of cases and affects men more frequently than women. It is typically diagnosed in early stage. Despite a greater tendency for relapse than classical Hodgkin's disease, the prognosis is excellent.

Classical Hodgkin's Disease

Nodular Sclerosis (NS) The affected lymph node has nodules of normal lymphocytes and other reactive cells, together with Reed-Sternberg cells, separated by bands of scarlike tissue. This is the most common type of Hodgkin's disease, making up 60 to 75 percent of cases. It is the only type that is more common in women than in men. It is often found as a limited-stage disease involving the lymph nodes of the lower neck, above the collarbone, and within the chest in adolescents and young adults. This type is unusual in people over age fifty.

Mixed Cellularity (MC) The affected lymph node contains a mixture of inflammatory cells in addition to abundant Reed-Sternberg cells. Adults with this type are often older and have widespread disease at the time of diagnosis. It is also seen in boys under the age of ten. MC accounts for 5 to 15 percent of cases of Hodgkin's disease.

Lymphocyte Depletion (LD) This is the least common variant of HD, occurring in less than 5 percent of cases. It is usually discovered in an advanced stage. Two forms have been described. One has abundant scarlike tissue (fibrosis) with sparse lymphocytes and Reed-Sternberg cells. The other has sheets of malignant cells of different sizes and shapes. It is important to distinguish this subtype from non-Hodgkin's lymphoma.

Lymphocyte Rich (LR) This is a newly proposed subtype of Hodgkin's disease that combines features of classical Hodgkin's disease and nodular lymphocyte predominance. It tends to be diagnosed at an early stage in somewhat older patients, usually men.

How It Spreads One of the unique features of Hodgkin's disease is its pattern of spread. As a rule, HD progresses in an orderly fashion from one lymph node group to the next group on the same side (ipsilateral) or the opposite side (contralateral). Non-Hodgkin's lymphomas, by contrast, are often widespread at diagnosis. The most characteristic pattern of HD spread is extension of the disease from the lymph nodes in the neck (cervical) to the nodes above the collarbone (supraclavicular), then to the nodes under the arms (axillary) and within the chest (mediastinal and hilar). Although there are different patterns, it is unusual to find areas that have been skipped, meaning that no apparent disease is found at a site where it would be expected by the rule of orderly progression. Hodgkin's disease often involves the spleen and may spread to the liver, bone, and bone marrow. Involvement of the central nervous system is extremely rare.

What Causes It Unknown. There is a theory that HD is the rare result, possibly

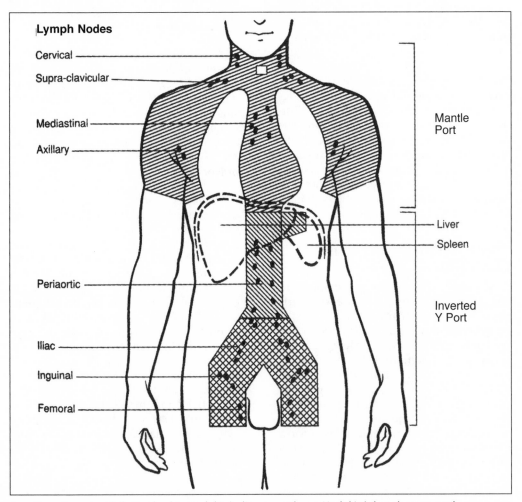

Lymph nodes potentially involved in Hodgkin's disease and non-Hodgkin's lymphomas, and radiotherapy ports

determined by genetics, of an infection acquired in late adolescence or early adulthood. Family clusters have been reported, and the Epstein-Barr virus has been suggested as the cause in about 40 percent of cases, but no genetic or infectious basis for the disease has been proven.

Risk Factors

In developed countries, there are two peaks of incidence of Hodgkin's disease, the first in young adults (ages fifteen to thirty-five), and the second after age fifty. Men are affected slightly more commonly than women. The frequency of the various subtypes depends on age. At the National Cancer Institute, where the majority of patients are young, nodular sclerosis accounts for 70 percent of cases and nodular lymphocyte predominance accounts for 15 percent. Mixed cellularity and lymphocyte depletion are more common in the elderly, in young children, in socioeconomically underdeveloped areas, and in people with AIDS.

There are no clearly established risk factors for Hodgkin's disease, although in the United States, there is some increased risk with small family size, higher education, and higher socioeconomic position. Brothers and sisters of people with Hodgkin's disease have an incidence seven times higher than in the general population. Sophisticated studies are in progress to explore the genetics of Hodgkin's disease.

Screening

There are no known effective ways to screen for Hodgkin's disease other than a physical examination and a chest X-ray when an enlarged lymph node is found.

Common Signs and Symptoms

People who develop Hodgkin's disease often see their physician because of the persistent swelling of painless lymph nodes in the neck or underarms. The swollen nodes may be the only sign of disease, or they may be accompanied by unexplained fevers, chills, drenching night sweats, weight loss, or itching. Young people with limited disease usually feel entirely well but occasionally have symptoms such as itching. Cough, shortness of breath, or chest discomfort can be the first symptom of Hodgkin's disease in the chest, although it is not unusual for a mass to be detected on a chest X-ray done for totally unrelated reasons. Less commonly, Hodgkin's disease in the abdomen may be signaled by an enlarged spleen or enlarged lymph nodes in the groin. These are much more likely to be signs of non-Hodgkin's lymphoma than of HD. Rarely, people will develop pain at lymph node sites immediately after ingesting alcohol. This peculiar phenomenon seems specific to Hodgkin's disease.

Diagnosis

Physical Examination

• Enlarged lymph nodes in the neck, above the clavicle, under the arms, or in the groin.

• Skin breakdown from scratching (excoriation) over most of the body because of itching.

• Fluid around the lungs (pleural effusion).

• Liver or spleen enlargement.

• Abdominal mass.

• Areas of bony tenderness.

Blood and Other Tests

• Complete blood count, including erythrocyte (red cell) sedimentation rate.

• Blood chemistries. These may be abnormal because of the tumor or because of the involvement of the bone, kidneys, or liver.

Imaging

• Chest X-ray may show masses within the chest, direct involvement of the lung, or a pleural effusion.

• CT scan of the chest, abdomen, and pelvis to look for enlarged lymph nodes or the involvement of the liver or spleen.

• Positron-emission tomography (PET) scan uses a radioisotope to highlight areas of increased metabolic activity such as sites of Hodgkin's disease. PET scans can be very effective in identifying sites of disease at diagnosis and in assessing residual masses after treatment. A negative, or normal, PET scan at the conclusion of treatment appears to portend a good prognosis in classical Hodgkin's disease.

• Bone X-rays and/or bone scan if there are any tender bony areas or there are areas of clarification required after PET scanning.

Biopsy

• Bone marrow biopsy to look for the presence of Hodgkin's disease for symptomatic and advanced-stage patients.

• Biopsy of an enlarged lymph node.

Staging

The stage is identified through a careful history, a physical exam, and laboratory and radiologic studies. The classification used for staging Hodgkin's disease is known as the Ann Arbor Staging System.

■ *Stage I*

Involvement of a single lymph node region (Stage I) or localized involvement of a single organ or site other than lymph nodes (extranodal; Stage IE).

■ *Stage II*

Involvement of two or more lymph node regions on the same side of the diaphragm (either above or below the breathing muscle separating the chest from the abdomen; Stage II) or localized involvement of a single associated organ or site other than lymph nodes and its nearby lymph nodes, with or without other lymph node regions on the same side of the diaphragm (IIE).

■ *Stage III*

Involvement of lymph node regions on both sides of the diaphragm (Stage III) that may also be accompanied by localized involvement of an extranodal organ or site (IIIE), involvement of the spleen (IIIS), or both (IIIS+E).

■ *Stage IV*

Widespread involvement of one or more sites other than lymph nodes, with or without associated lymph node involvement, or isolated extranodal organ involvement with distant lymph node involvement.

Each stage may be subdivided into A or B according to the presence or absence of general symptoms. "A" means the absence of "B" symptoms, which include any of the following: unexplained fevers over 100.4°F (38°C), drenching night sweats, and the unexplained loss of more than 10 percent of body weight.

Prognostic Factors Prognostic factors for early-stage Hodgkin's disease include the symptoms defined above, older age, male sex, abnormally elevated level of the erythrocyte sedimentation level, number of nodal sites, presence of extranodal sites, and size of mediastinal lymph nodes. In North America, patients with symptomatic or bulky mediastinal disease are treated for "unfavorable" disease. In Europe, about two-thirds of patients with early-stage Hodgkin's disease are considered "unfavorable" based on a list of the described prognostic factors. Because the cure rate for all patients with early-stage Hodgkin's disease is so high, this terminology is outdated but serves to select patients for treatment.

Different prognostic factors have been identified for advanced Hodgkin's disease. Adverse prognostic factors include Stage IV, male sex, age forty-five or older, and various laboratory tests that predict for poorer results of treatment (e.g., low hemoglobin [anemia], high white blood cell count, low lymphocyte count, and low albumin). Each additional factor confers a small increase in risk of relapse.

Treatment Overview

More than 80 percent of all newly diagnosed people with Hodgkin's disease can be cured with current combination chemotherapy and radiation therapy.

The most important factors for determining prognosis and outlining treatment plans are the stage of disease, the presence or absence of symptoms, the presence of large masses, and an assessment of prognostic factors.

 Radiation Historically, radiation therapy was the standard treatment for those with favorable localized disease—Stage I and Stage II—with no large masses and no symptoms. The recognition of the late effects associated with radiotherapy has led to the use of smaller fields and doses as a consolidation after chemotherapy. The exception, as described below, is nodular lymphocyte predominance.

Chemotherapy Chemotherapy is required for patients of any stage of classical Hodgkin's disease. Combined radiation and chemotherapy is commonly used for large individual tumor masses, so-called bulky disease. Patients with recurrent disease after chemotherapy have a less favorable prognosis, but long remissions have been reported after additional chemotherapy or intensive chemotherapy by

stem cell transplantation. Chemotherapy regimens include

- ABVD (doxorubicin [Adriamycin] + bleomycin [Blenoxane] + vinblastine [Velban] + dacarbazine [DTIC-Dome]),
- Stanford V (nitrogen mustard [mechlorethamine, Mustargen] + doxorubicin + vinblastine + vincristine [Oncovin] + bleomycin + etoposide [Etopophos] + prednisone + local radiation), and
- BEACOPP (bleomycin + etoposide + doxorubicin [Adriamycin] + cyclophosphamide [Cytoxan] + vincristine [Oncovin] + procarbazine + prednisone).

Combined Modality Therapy (Chemotherapy Plus Radiation) Clinical trials in early-stage Hodgkin's disease are designed to decrease the toxicity of treatment without reducing the overall excellent results. More effective therapy is sought for patients with high-risk and slowly responsive disease. Many newer regimens use combinations of chemotherapy and radiation. In early-stage Hodgkin's disease, combined modality therapy allows lower total doses of chemotherapy and less radiation to hopefully reduce late toxicities. In advanced stages, radiation may be used for bulky sites.

Treatment by Stage

■ Stages IA and IIA "Favorable"

The disease is classified as favorable if there are no large masses and no systemic symptoms. In Europe, only patients without risk factors (see above) are considered favorable.

Standard Treatment Combined modality therapy has become the standard treatment. Abbreviated forms of regimens such as ABVD and Stanford V are combined with limited radiation in lower dose, leading to a high rate of cure. Chemotherapy alone, given for a longer course, is an option to consider when avoiding radiation is an important goal.

There are different approaches to the treatment of nodular lymphocyte predominant Hodgkin's disease. Less extensive, regional, or involved field radiation may be used. Immunotherapy with rituximab (Rituxan) shows promise in early trials, but longer follow-up is needed. A watch-and-wait approach following complete surgical removal is being studied in children.

Five-Year Survival Above 90 percent

■ Stages IA, IIA, IB, and IIB "Unfavorable"

The disease is classified as unfavorable if there is a large mass or "B" symptoms.

Standard Treatment Combination chemotherapy regimens such ABVD and Stanford V are given with radiation therapy to the involved fields. If no bulky sites are present, chemotherapy alone is an option.

Five-Year Survival 85 to 95 percent

■ Stages IIIB and IV

Standard Treatment Combination chemotherapy with ABVD, which has the best efficacy and toxicity profile. Escalated BEACOPP may be particularly effective in high-risk disease (four or more adverse factors as described above). Ongoing studies will determine if newer regimens such as BEACOPP and Stanford V are superior to standard approaches.

The role of radiation therapy for advanced Hodgkin's disease is controversial. It may be helpful when added to standard chemotherapy for Stage III patients or when given to sites of bulky disease.

Five-Year Survival 65 to 85 percent, based on prognostic factors

Treatment Follow-Up

All patients must be followed up at regular intervals with a physical examination, blood counts, and radiological studies. This is particularly important because of the young age of the population and the ability to cure patients with secondary therapy.

• For patients treated with limited radiation after clinical staging alone, annual abdominal CT scans are recommended. Sites of previous bulky disease should receive particular attention.

• All patients receiving radiation therapy to the thyroid should have annual thyroid function tests. In a significant percentage of patients, thyroid function may become low (hypothyroid) because of radiation treatments, and thyroid hormone must be taken by mouth indefinitely.

• Surveillance is needed for secondary cancers, solid tumors in patients treated with irradiation, and acute leukemia in patients treated with BEACOPP (see "Complications of Therapy," below).

Complications of Therapy These may be divided into acute and chronic. Acute toxicities for the various chemotherapy drugs are well described and should be discussed before treatment. Acute toxicities of radiation therapy depend on which area of the body is irradiated.

Now that the cure rate for Hodgkin's disease is so high and so many patients are alive many years after treatment, the late complications of therapy are receiving more attention. These include the following:

• Nearly universal sterility in males and infertility and premature menopause in women over age twenty-five who receive BEACOPP. These effects appear to be largely irreversible. Fertility is usually preserved with the chemotherapy regimens ABVD and Stanford V. Children born to parents treated for Hodgkin's disease by any of the standard treatments have had normal birth weights and no increased incidence of birth defects.

• Intensive chemotherapy such as BEACOPP carries a leukemia risk, whereas there is much less risk of leukemia with ABVD.

• Non-Hodgkin's lymphomas are increased in HD patients treated by any method.

• Patients receiving radiotherapy are at increased risk of developing a second malignancy in the irradiated tissues, particularly skin cancer, breast cancer, stomach cancer, soft tissue and bone cancer, and lung cancer. Any patient who is irradiated would be very wise to stop smoking, since the incidence of lung cancer is strongly related to tobacco use. Mammograms are recommended for women who received chest or axillary irradiation before the age of thirty.

• There are concerns with the use of ABVD in that bleomycin may be toxic to the lungs and doxorubicin (Adriamycin) is associated with cardiac toxicity. Both of these effects depend on the dose used and are also affected by the combined use of radiotherapy.

Recurrent Cancer

Cancer that recurs more than one year after chemotherapy may be approached in a variety of ways, including an alternative drug combination, combined modality therapy, or, most commonly, high-dose chemotherapy or chemotherapy and radiation therapy followed by hematopoietic stem cell transplantation.

Progression on initial treatment with chemotherapy or relapse during the first year after chemotherapy should be approached with high-dose chemotherapy or chemotherapy and radiation therapy (depending on the earlier treatment) followed by hematopoietic stem cell transplantation.

Patients with a relapse after brief treatment for favorable early-stage disease may be secondarily cured in a variety of ways, including radiation alone, a more extended course of chemotherapy, combined modality treatment, or high-dose therapy and transplantation.

The Most Important Questions You Can Ask

• What is my stage? Is it a favorable or unfavorable presentation of that stage?

• What is my prognosis?

• Should I have treatment with chemotherapy and radiation, or chemotherapy alone? Why? What is the standard treatment and what clinical trials are being conducted for my stage and prognosis?

• Will this treatment make me sterile (or infertile)? If yes, what should I do to preserve fertility?

• What is my risk of a second malignancy or other complications of the recommended treatment?

• If the Hodgkin's disease recurs, what therapy will be required and what are my chances for cure? Should stem cell transplantation be considered?

• How should I be followed after treatment?

Lymphoma: Non-Hodgkin's

Steven M. Horwitz, M.D., and Sandra J. Horning, M.D.

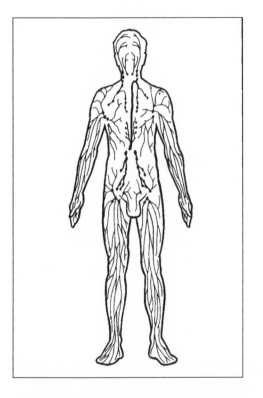

Malignant lymphomas are cancers that arise from the lymphoid system, the complex network of cells and channels that run throughout the body as a basic part of the immune system. Normally, the cells of the lymphoid system, known as lymphocytes, either are arranged in clusters—called lymph nodes or lymph glands—or circulate through the bloodstream and the lymphatic channels to all the tissues of the body. Cancers that develop within the lymphoid system—malignant lymphomas—may be found wherever normal lymphocytes go. They may occur in an isolated lymph node or a group of lymph nodes, in organs such as the stomach and intestine, in the sinuses, bone, or skin, or in any combination of these sites.

An estimated 63,190 new cases of non-Hodgkin's lymphoma are expected in the United States in the year 2007. Non-Hodgkin's lymphomas are the second leading cause of cancer deaths in patients ages fifteen to thirty-four and the third leading cause of cancer deaths in patients ages thirty-five to fifty-four. For unclear reasons, the incidence of non-Hodgkin's lymphomas has been increasing at about 3 percent each year for more than twenty years.

Although lymphoma refers to any cancer of the lymphoid system, malignant lymphomas actually represent a variety of cancers ranging from slow-growing chronic diseases to rapidly progressive acute diseases that may be life-threatening if appropriate therapy is not begun quickly. Cancer of the lymphoid system was first described by British physician Thomas Hodgkin in 1832. The form he described behaves in a very predictable way and has come to be called Hodgkin's disease. Despite their diversity, all of the other malignant lymphomas are referred to as non-Hodgkin's lymphomas (NHL).

Types There are two main types of cells in the normal lymphoid system: *B cells,* which make antibodies in response to infection, and *T cells,* which are responsible for the regulation of the immune system. Both B cell and T cell lymphomas occur, but the vast majority of lymphomas in the United States are of B cell

Table 1. International Working Formulation

LOW GRADE

Small lymphocytic, consistent with chronic
   lymphocytic leukemia
Follicular, predominantly small cleaved cell
Follicular mixed, small cleaved and large cell

INTERMEDIATE GRADE

Follicular, predominantly large cell
Diffuse, small cleaved cell
Diffuse mixed, small and large cell
Diffuse large cell (cleaved or noncleaved)

HIGH GRADE

Immunoblastic, diffuse large cell
Lymphoblastic (convoluted or
   nonconvoluted)
Small noncleaved cell, Burkitt's or non-
   Burkitt's lymphoma

Table 2. Lymphoid Neoplasms Recognized in the WHO Classification

B CELL NEOPLASMS

Precursor B Cell Neoplasm

   B lymphoblastic lymphoma/leukemia

Mature B Cell Neoplasms

   B cell chronic lymphocytic leukemia/small
      lymphocytic lymphoma
   B cell prolymphocytic leukemia
   Lymphoplasmacytoid lymphoma
   Splenic marginal-zone lymphoma
   Hairy cell leukemia
   Plasma cell myeloma/plasmacytoma
   Extranodal marginal-zone B cell
      lymphoma (MALT lymphoma)
   Nodal marginal-zone B cell lymphoma
   Mantle cell lymphoma
   Follicular lymphoma
   Diffuse large-cell lymphoma
   Burkitt's lymphoma

T CELL AND NATURAL KILLER (NK) CELL NEOPLASMS

Precursor T Cell Neoplasm

   T lymphoblastic lymphoma/leukemia

Peripheral T Cell and NK Cell Neoplasms

   T cell prolymphocytic leukemia
   T cell granular lymphocytic leukemia
   Aggressive NK cell leukemia
   Adult T cell lymphoma/leukemia
   Extranodal NK/T cell lymphoma, nasal
      type
   Enteropathy-type T cell lymphoma
   Hepatosplenic g/d T cell lymphoma
   Subcutaneous panniculitis-like T cell
      lymphoma
   Mycosis fungoides/Sezary syndrome
   Anaplastic large-cell lymphoma, primary
      systemic type
   Anaplastic large-cell lymphoma, primary
      cutaneous type
   Peripheral T cell lymphoma
   Angioimmunoblastic T cell lymphoma

origin. A variety of systems have been used to classify NHL subtypes according to their microscopic appearance and the behavior of the disease. In the 1980s, an international group of pathologists and clinicians published a working formulation that was developed to establish a common terminology. This defined ten major subtypes categorized as low, intermediate, or high grade (see Table 1). The current World Health Organization (WHO) classification now includes nearly thirty distinct subtypes of non-Hodgkin's lymphomas that can be distinguished on the basis of their microscopic appearance, cell surface markers, and clinical characteristics (see Table 2). As a result, the International Working Formulation is somewhat outdated, but it still provides a useful framework with which to conceptualize the various types of non-Hodgkin's lymphomas. The complex WHO system can be simplified for most patients by focusing on the behaviors of the major non-Hodgkin's lymphoma subtypes (see Table 3).

Table 3. **Major Subtypes of Non-Hodgkin's Lymphomas**

INDOLENT	% OF NHLS
Follicular	22%
Small lymphocytic	6%
Extranodal marginal zone	5%
Marginal zone	1%
Lymphoplasmacytoid	1%
MODERATELY AGGRESSIVE	
Mantle cell	6%
Diffuse large B cell	31%
Peripheral T cell	6%
Anaplastic large cell	2%
HIGHLY AGGRESSIVE	
Lymphoblastic	2%
Burkitt's	1%

How It Spreads Since lymphocytes normally travel throughout the body via the blood and lymphatic system, malignant lymphomas can either start in or spread to virtually any organ.

A lymphoma may arise in a single lymph node or organ and stay there even when a large mass is present, or many different sites may be involved at the time of diagnosis. Indolent lymphomas most often involve lymph nodes, the bone marrow, and the spleen when they are diagnosed. Aggressive lymphomas are most commonly found in lymph nodes, but a significant proportion of cases primarily involve organs separate from lymph nodes and are called extranodal.

What Causes It The immune system is so complex and dynamic that there are many opportunities for errors in regulation. Many lymphomas are thought to result from such errors or "accidents," which are statistically more probable when the immune system is continually stimulated.

Chronic disorders of the immune system or the chronic administration of drugs to suppress the immune system (such as those used after an organ transplant) predispose a person to lymphoma. Exposure to radiation increases the risk, too.

Several types of viruses have been linked. The Epstein-Barr virus, which causes infectious mononucleosis, is associated with African Burkitt's lymphoma. A T cell virus related to the HIV virus associated with AIDS has been linked to adult T cell lymphoma/leukemia, which is prominent in Japan, the Caribbean, and the southeastern United States. The mechanism common to each of these appears to be a significant alteration in the normal regulation of the immune system.

Risk Factors

At Significantly Higher Risk

• The incidence of lymphoma increases with age and is more common in men than in women. Most lymphomas occur in people who were previously healthy.

• Occupational exposure in the flour and agricultural industries has been reported to increase the risk of developing certain types of aggressive lymphomas.

• People with congenital or acquired abnormalities of their immune system or who take medicine to suppress their immune system have a higher incidence of lymphoma.

• There is an increased incidence of aggressive lymphomas in people infected with the HIV virus for four or more years.

• Exposure to radiation or chemotherapy is associated with increased risk.

Screening

There are no known effective ways to screen for lymphoma.

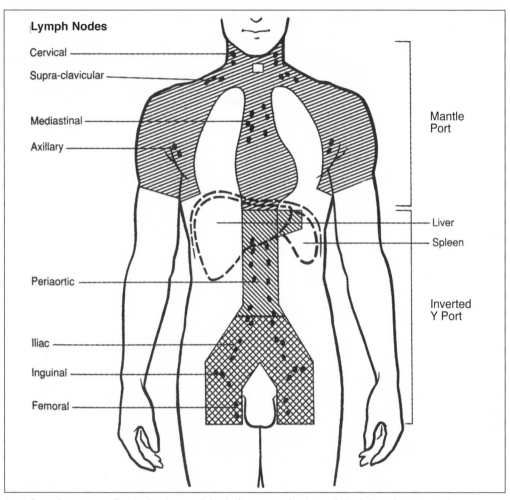

Lymph Nodes

Cervical

Supra-clavicular

Mediastinal

Axillary

Periaortic

Iliac

Inguinal

Femoral

Mantle Port

Liver

Spleen

Inverted Y Port

Lymph nodes potentially involved in Hodgkin's disease and non-Hodgkin's lymphomas, and radiotherapy ports

Common Signs and Symptoms

People with lymphoma most often seek medical attention because of one or more enlarged lymph nodes. Sometimes these have developed in association with a variety of nonspecific symptoms such as fatigue, fevers, chills, night sweats, decreased appetite, and weight loss.

But many people are found to have lymphoma when they see their doctor about a variety of symptoms related to the site and extent of tumor involvement.

They may develop shortness of breath or a cough because of chest disease; abdominal pain or fullness because of an abdominal mass; or ulcers, bleeding, or a change in bowel habits because of stomach or intestinal involvement. There can also be nasal stuffiness or sore throat or difficulty swallowing because of a lymphoma involving the sinus, upper airway, or throat. If the brain is involved, there may be headaches, changes in vision, or seizures. If the bone marrow is involved, there may be recurrent or persistent infections, bleeding, or profound fatigue.

Disease outside the lymphatic system is more common in intermediate- and high-grade lymphomas.

Diagnosis

Physical Examination

- Enlarged lymph nodes in the neck, under the arms, or in the groin.
- Swelling in the area of the tonsils, throat, or upper airway.
- Fluid around the lungs (pleural effusion).
- Liver or spleen enlargement.
- Abdominal mass.
- Soft-tissue swelling.
- Tenderness when pressure is applied to areas of the skeleton.
- Neurologic findings such as numbness and muscle weakness.

Blood and Other Tests

- A complete blood count may show circulating lymphoma cells or other blood abnormalities because of lymphoma in the bone marrow.
- Blood chemistries may be abnormal because of the tumor or because of the involvement of the bone, lung, liver, or kidneys.
- HIV test.

Imaging

- Chest X-ray may show masses within the center of the chest (mediastinum or hilum), involvement of the lungs, or fluid around the heart or lungs.
- CT scan of the chest, abdomen, and pelvis may show enlargement of the lymph nodes, spleen, or liver, or the involvement of the lungs or other organs.
- Positron-emission tomography (PET) may show "hot spots" in areas involved with lymphoma. PET scanning appears to be very effective in evaluating areas that are equivocal on CT scanning. It can also be helpful in assessing the completeness

of response at the conclusion of treatment. A negative, or normal, PET scan at the conclusion of treatment appears to portend a good prognosis in diffuse large B cell lymphoma, and PET scans are becoming a standard imaging test for other aggressive lymphomas.

- A CT or MRI scan of the brain may be done if central nervous system involvement is suspected. MRI may allow more accurate assessment of the tumor, particularly in the spinal cord and vertebrae.

Biopsy

- The diagnosis is usually made in a lymph node, but a biopsy of other involved tissues (extranodal) may be performed. In general, a surgical or core needle tissue biopsy provides more tissue and is more reliable for diagnosis than a fine needle aspiration (FNA).
- Bone marrow biopsy may detect the presence of lymphoma, in which case further studies will be done to identify the type.
- Lumbar puncture, sampling of spinal fluid by placing a small needle in the back, is necessary for certain patients with aggressive lymphomas who are at high risk of central nervous system involvement.

Staging

The staging system used for non-Hodgkin's lymphomas is the Ann Arbor convention developed for the staging and treatment (primarily with radiation) of Hodgkin's disease.

■ *Stage I*

Involvement of a single lymph node region (I) or localized involvement of a single organ or site other than lymph nodes (extranodal; Stage IE).

■ *Stage II*

Involvement of two or more lymph node regions on the same side of the diaphragm (either above or below the breathing muscle separating the chest from the abdomen; Stage II) or localized involvement of a single associated organ or site other than lymph nodes and its regional lymph nodes, with or without other lymph node regions on the same side of the diaphragm (IIE).

▓ Stage III

Involvement of lymph node regions on both sides of the diaphragm (Stage III) that may also be accompanied by localized involvement of an extranodal organ or site (IIIE), involvement of the spleen (IIIS), or both (IIIS+E).

▓ Stage IV

Widespread involvement of one or more extranodal sites, with or without associated lymph node involvement, or isolated extranodal organ involvement with distant lymph node involvement.

Each stage may be subdivided into A or B according to the presence or absence of general symptoms. "A" means the absence of "B" symptoms, which include any of the following: fevers over 100.4°F (38°C), drenching night sweats, and the unexplained loss of more than 10 percent of body weight.

Treatment Overview by Grade

The pathologic diagnosis and the clinical characteristics of the lymphoma are both important factors in determining the prognosis and the appropriate therapy. An international group has validated a number of prognostic factors for patients with diffuse large-cell lymphoma and developed the International Prognostic Factors Index. Good prognostic features include age under sixty years, a normal serum lactate dehydrogenase (LDH; a blood chemistry measurement), good ambulatory performance status, limited (Stages I and II) disease, and no or only one extranodal site of disease. These prognostic factors are most applicable to aggressive lymphomas, although similar prognostic models exist for indolent lymphomas.

With greater understanding of the biology of NHL, other factors have recently been recognized—for example, molecular features of the cells of the lymphoma—that can be related to the clinical outcome of the disease. It is expected that these will play a greater role in deciding on treatment in the future.

Indolent Lymphomas

Follicular, Grades 1 and 2, Small Lymphocytic; Extranodal Marginal Zone; Marginal Zone; Lymphoplasmacytoid Although the indolent lymphomas grow slowly and respond readily to chemotherapy, they almost invariably return and are generally regarded as incurable cancers.

It is usual for the indolent lymphomas to be widespread at the time of diagnosis, including involvement in the bone marrow. Despite this, the average survival of people with these lymphomas has been six to twelve years and appears to be improving with advances in therapy.

The long-term outcome of the disease has not been affected favorably by the use of immediate chemotherapy in selected patients who have no symptoms, so close observation alone may be the initial therapy of choice, particularly in older patients. Single-agent or combination chemotherapy, immunotherapy, or radiation therapy may be required when the disease progresses or begins to cause symptoms. Treatments targeted to the B cell (see below) are impacting both the timing and choice of therapy and may be improving the prognosis.

Following are exceptions to the general treatment guidelines:

• The extranodal marginal-zone lymphoma subtype, also called mucosa-associated lymphoid tissue (MALT) lymphoma, frequently arises in the stomach and, when so, is regularly associated with the bacterium *Helicobacter pylori*. Shrinkage of this lymphoma with antibiotics has now been reported in a significant number of patients and should be considered a standard therapy. However, close follow-up is required to detect early recurrences. When extranodal marginal-zone lymphomas occur at other sites such as the skin, salivary glands, and lungs, they are often managed as other low-grade lymphomas.

• The more aggressive subtype follicular lymphoma, Grade 3, is less common and less well characterized. There is controversy as to whether it should be treated more like the indolent lymphomas or an intermediate-grade lymphoma. Many experts approach this lymphoma as they would diffuse large B cell lymphoma.

Because of the apparent inability to cure indolent lymphoma patients, it is important that patients with this diagnosis are presented with the opportunity to participate in clinical trials designed to test new strategies or new agents with the goal of improving the prognosis for indolent lymphomas.

Patients with limited (Stages I and II) disease may provide the exception. They can enjoy prolonged responses to radiation therapy.

It is well known that indolent lymphomas may transform into more aggressive lymphomas. Therapy appropriate for the more aggressive cancer is required at that time.

Moderately Aggressive Lymphomas

Mantle Cell, Diffuse Large Cell, Peripheral T Cell, Anaplastic Large Cell These lymphomas are often curable. Combination chemotherapy is almost always necessary for successful treatment. Chemotherapy alone, chemotherapy plus irradiation, or abbreviated chemotherapy and irradiation cure nearly 80 percent of patients

with limited (Stages I and II) moderately aggressive lymphomas. Advanced (Stages II bulky, III, and IV) disease can be eradicated in 30 to 50 percent of patients. As stated above, a more precise assessment of prognosis can be made by the International Prognostic Factors Index.

Following are comments about specific subtypes:

• The addition of the B cell targeted antibody, rituximab (Rituxan), improves upon the results with combination chemotherapy and is now part of standard treatment for diffuse large B cell lymphoma.

• The behavior of mantle cell lymphoma is unique. Like indolent lymphomas, treatment is not considered to be curative, although the average survival time is shorter. However, like aggressive lymphomas, mantle cell lymphomas tend to grow more quickly and require treatment. There is no standard approach to mantle cell lymphoma. Investigational treatments, including combinations of chemotherapy, chemotherapy combined with immunotherapy, radioimmunotherapy (antibodies attached to radioisotopes), and high-dose chemotherapy with bone marrow or stem cell transplant, are being studied as ways to prolong remissions and survival.

• T cell lymphomas, particularly at advanced stage, are less favorable for cure.

• A subtype of anaplastic large T cell lymphoma that expresses a protein called ALK-1 has a more favorable prognosis than other moderately aggressive lymphomas, but the treatments are similar.

• Diffuse large-cell lymphoma and anaplastic large T cell lymphoma confined to the skin may have more favorable prognoses and behave more like indolent lymphomas than aggressive lymphomas. Certain patients may be effectively treated with radiation therapy alone.

Highly Aggressive Lymphomas

Burkitt's, Lymphoblastic For each of these highly aggressive malignancies, there is a 40 to 50 percent cure rate with conventional therapy. These lymphomas are potentially curable at any stage, with limited-stage patients having a high rate of cure. The prognosis is considerably worse for those with the greatest tumor burden.

Burkitt's lymphomas are exquisitely sensitive to chemotherapy. They should be approached with specialized treatments developed for childhood lymphoma. Lymphoblastic lymphomas are treated with an intensive drug program similar to that used for acute leukemia, including treatment of the central nervous system. Because of medical problems that may occur when treatment is started, patients with extensive lymphoblastic lymphoma or Burkitt's lymphoma should receive their initial chemotherapy treatment in the hospital.

Treatment by Grade and Stage

Indolent Lymphomas

■ Stages I and II

Standard Treatment True early-stage patients with indolent lymphomas are rare. Careful staging, including CT scanning, adequate bone marrow biopsy, and, in some cases, a PET scan, should be performed before assigning Stage I or II. Radiation therapy is the standard treatment, as some patients treated in this fashion will not relapse. While total lymphoid irradiation has been associated with longer disease-free survival, there is no overall survival benefit over regional or limited irradiation.

■ Stages III and IV

Standard Treatment The best treatment for advanced-stage disease remains controversial. Options are as follows:

• No initial treatment, with close observation for selected patients who have no symptoms.

• Rituximab (Rituxan) and chemotherapy improves the results of chemotherapy alone for patients with indications for immediate treatment. Combinations of chemotherapy and immunotherapy are the most commonly used regimens for initial treatment of indolent lymphomas. Whether it is best to give the rituximab with the chemotherapy or intermittently following the completion of the chemotherapy is an active area of study.

• Chemotherapy may be a single drug therapy such as oral chlorambucil (Leukeran) or cyclophosphamide (Cytoxan) but is more commonly given in combination. Combination regimens include CVP (cyclophosphamide + vincristine [Oncovin] + prednisone), CHOP (cyclophosphamide + doxorubicin [hydroxydoxorubicin, Adriamycin] + vincristine [Oncovin] + prednisone), FND (fludarabine [Fludara] + mitoxantrone [Novantrone] + dexamethasone [Decadron]), and CF (cyclophosphamide + fludarabine). No single combination is established to be superior to another.

• Rituximab as initial therapy alone is an active area of clinical investigation.

Five-Year Survival 90 percent for Stages I and II; 80 percent for Stages III and IV

Investigational

• Long-term, intermittent treatment with rituximab (Rituxan), also called maintenance therapy.

• Antibodies to CD20 tagged with a radioisotope (referred to as radioimmunotherapy, or RIT), either alone or in combination with chemotherapy, as initial treatment.

• Second-generation anti-CD20 antibodies engineered to be more effective.

• Phase III trials with tumor-specific vaccines administered after chemotherapy or rituximab are completed and the results are awaited.

• New chemotherapies, combinations of chemotherapies, numerous biological treatments, and combinations of these are under investigation.

• Allogeneic or donor stem cell transplantation for relapsed disease.

Therapy for Relapsed Disease The treatment used initially is often successful when used again after a relapse in the low-grade lymphomas. Rituximab (Rituxan) is effective for relapsed disease. Radioimmunotherapy is approved for relapsed disease. Fludarabine (Fludara) produces significant responses in previously treated patients. High-dose chemoradiotherapy and bone marrow transplantation have been associated with long remissions but carry a risk of secondary leukemia. Radiotherapy may be useful to reduce bulky or painful disease sites. Many of the investigational treatments may also be used.

Moderately Aggressive Lymphomas

■ Stages I and II

Standard Treatment

• A full course (usually six to eight cycles) of chemotherapy with R-CHOP (rituximab [Rituxan] added to cyclophosphamide [Cytoxan] + doxorubicin [hydroxyrubicin, Adriamycin] + vincristine [Oncovin] + prednisone). Results may be improved with the addition of limited radiation therapy to bulky sites.

• Abbreviated (three cycles) combination chemotherapy with R-CHOP plus limited radiation therapy is an alternative to a full course of chemotherapy for patients without bulky disease.

• Adding rituximab to chemotherapy for diffuse large B cell lymphoma significantly improves the cure rate.

Five-Year Survival 70 to 90 percent

Investigational Because initial therapy is so successful, the goals of investigational efforts are reducing the toxicity of treatment and trying to predict which patients are most likely to fail primary therapy and therefore need other treatment approaches.

■ Stages III and IV

Standard Treatment

• In a large multi-institutional trial, a number of chemotherapy regimens were found to be of equal efficacy for diffuse large B cell lymphoma. Because CHOP (cyclophosphamide [Cytoxan] + doxorubicin [hydroxyrubicin, Adriamycin] + vincristine [Oncovin] + prednisone) therapy is easy to administer and is relatively nontoxic, many physicians now consider it to be the treatment of choice.

• Several large randomized trials have shown that adding rituximab (Rituxan) to chemotherapy for diffuse large B cell lymphoma significantly improves the cure rate. R-CHOP is considered the standard treatment for diffuse large B cell lymphoma.

• The rates of cure for T cell lymphomas are poor with the above regimens, and often a more aggressive treatment such as intensive chemotherapy followed by bone marrow or stem cell transplantation or investigational therapies are considered.

• No standard treatment for mantle cell lymphoma has been defined. Choices for therapy include R-CHOP alone or consolidated with an autologous stem cell transplant or R-HyperCVAD (hyperfractionated cyclophosphamide [Cytoxan] + vincristin [Oncovin] + doxorubicin [Adriamycin] + dexamethasone [Decadron] alternating with cytosine arabinoside [Ara-C], and methotrexate). Clinical trials should be considered.

Five-Year Survival Ranging from 20 to 90 percent, with prognosis for patients varying according to the specific subtype of lymphoma and the International Prognostic Factors Index mentioned above

Investigational Because patients with multiple risk factors have a poor prognosis, participation in an investigational program should be considered. Current investigations include the earlier use of intensive chemotherapy followed by stem cell transplant; reducing the time interval between treatments; infusional chemotherapy; and the incorporation of radioimmunotherapy, new drugs, and new biologics in combination with chemotherapy.

Therapy for Relapsed Disease A number of chemotherapy combinations have demonstrated antitumor activity:

• CHAD/DHAP (cisplatin [Platinol] + cytosine arabinoside [Ara-C, cytarabine, Cytosar-U] + dexamethasone [Decadron]).
• ESHAP (etoposide [VP-16, Etopophos] + methylprednisolone [Solu-Medrol] + cytosine arabinoside [Ara-C] + cisplatin).
• ICE (ifosfamide [Ifex] + carboplatin [Paraplatin] + etoposide).
• EPOCH (etoposide + prednisone + vincristine [Oncovin] + cyclophosphamide [Cytoxan] + doxorubicine [hydroxydoxorubicin, Adriamycin]).
• CEPP (cyclophosphamide + etoposide + procarbazine [Matulane] + prednisone).
• For B cell lymphomas, rituximab (Rituxan) is often added to the above regimens.
• Because secondary chemotherapy alone generally fails to provide a cure, patients who are eligible are recommended to receive high-dose chemotherapy followed by stem cell transplanation. This approach has moderate success (40 to 50 percent long-term disease-free survival).

Highly Aggressive Lymphomas

Lymphoblastic Lymphoma

Standard Therapy Intensive multiagent chemotherapy, primarily with cyclophosphamide (Cytoxan), doxorubicin (Adriamycin), vincristine (Oncovin), and prednisone, is given together with central nervous system prophylactic therapy. Maintenance chemotherapy, including methotrexate (Mexate, Amethopterin, Folex), 6-mercaptopurine (Purinethol), and other agents, is often continued for up to six months after completion of standard treatment.

Patients with extensive disease—usually Stage IV on the basis of bone marrow and/or central nervous system involvement—and a high serum lactate dehydrogenase (LDH) have a higher risk for treatment failure.

Five-Year Survival 80 percent for limited disease; 20 percent for extensive disease with bone marrow and central nervous system involvement.

Investigational Intensified treatment for high-risk patients is being investigated. One strategy is early use of bone marrow transplantation.

Therapy for Relapsed Disease Secondary chemotherapy and bone marrow transplantation at relapse have some antitumor activity but have most often failed to cure this rapidly fatal condition.

Burkitt's Lymphoma

Standard Treatment The most successful therapies for this lymphoma are based on treatments for childhood lymphoma. Multiagent chemotherapy, based upon high-dose cyclophosphamide (Cytoxan), frequently incorporates methotrexate (Mexate, Amethopterin, Folex), cytosine arabinoside (Ara-C, cytarabine [Cytosar-U], vincristin (Oncovin), prednisone, doxorubicin (Adriamycin), and others together with central nervous system prophylactic therapy.

Patients with extensive disease—usually Stage IV on the basis of bone marrow and especially central nervous system involvement—and a high serum lactic dehydrogenase (LDH) require more intensive therapy.

Survival data, investigational approaches, and therapy for relapsed disease are essentially the same as for lymphoblastic lymphoma.

■ AIDS-Associated Lymphomas

The incidence of aggressive lymphomas frequently seen in HIV-infected patients has declined due to more effective antiretroviral therapies. These tumors can be highly aggressive. The management of these patients is often challenging because their immune system is already compromised by the HIV infection. These patients can be extremely sensitive to the bone marrow suppressive effects of chemotherapy and are more likely to develop infectious complications than other lymphoma patients. The "best" chemotherapeutic regimen has yet to be identified, but a number of centers are investigating modified versions of regimens similar to those used for the other intermediate- and high-grade lymphomas and infusional therapies. Infectious prophylaxis and hematopoietic growth factors are incorporated in the treatment regimen. HIV-related lymphomas more often primarily involve the central nervous system. In addition to the prognostic factors described above, immunocompetence as assessed by quantification of T cells, viral load, and previous manifestation of AIDS has prognostic significance. Rituximab (Rituxan) may be incorporated into primary therapy but is associated with an increased infection risk for patients with severe compromise of the immune system (see the chapter "Lymphoma: AIDS-Associated").

Treatment Follow-Up

Follow-up varies considerably, depending on the initial grade of lymphoma and the treatment.

• Patients with indolent lymphomas require lifelong follow-up because of the strong likelihood that the disease will recur and/or will transform into a more aggressive lymphoma.
• Recurrence of moderately aggressive and highly aggressive lymphomas usually occurs within one to three years after treatment. Relapse is rarely hard to find, given the rapid growth characteristics of these lymphomas. All patients should be seen at regular intervals for physical examination, complete blood counts, and radiologic studies. Newer biological markers of minimal disease may be used in the future.

The Most Important Questions You Can Ask

• What is my prognosis? What is the likelihood of cure?
• What is the standard treatment for my disease? What clinical trials are available to me?
• If the standard treatment won't cure me, are there any investigational treatments I should consider?
• What side effects can I expect from the treatment and how can they be minimized?
• If I have an indolent lymphoma, what are the risks and benefits of immediate treatment as opposed to no initial therapy?
• If I have recurrent (relapsed) lymphoma, should bone marrow or stem cell transplantation be considered?

Melanoma

Omid Hamid, M.D., Mohammed Kashani-Sabet, M.D.,
Malcolm S. Mitchell, M.D., and Jeffrey S. Weber, M.D., Ph.D.

■ ■ ■ ■

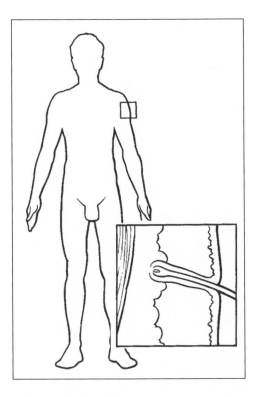

Most skin cancers are not generally considered very dangerous, since they are easily cured by surgery or medicines applied to the skin. The skin cancer called melanoma—which means black tumor—is a notable exception. Not only is melanoma the most malignant of all skin cancers, but it is among the most malignant of *all* cancers. Melanoma can spread to nearly every organ and tissue in the body and can lead to death within a year after it recurs in distant sites.

Yet amidst all these bleak aspects, there are some very encouraging ones. When melanoma first appears as a malignant mole on the skin or eye—and occasionally on the gums, in the vagina, or in the anus—it is often curable by limited surgery. In fact, at the current time, greater than 90 percent of patients are alive for five years or more following their melanoma diagnosis. This signifies the importance of recognizing the early signs of melanoma and bringing them to the attention of a physician, so that an experienced dermatologist, surgeon, or oncologist can become involved. In addition, several advances in biological treatment have prolonged useful survival, even at advanced stages of the disease.

Incidence The incidence of melanoma is rising faster worldwide than any other cancer. In the United States, melanoma is currently the fifth most common cancer, with almost 60,000 estimated cases in 2007. Over the past fifty years, the incidence of melanoma has risen 690 percent and is expected to continue to rise. However, the good news is that survival of patients with these tumors has increased due to growing public awareness and early detection leading to lower-stage, less aggressive tumors. Over 80 percent of melanomas diagnosed in the United States are diagnosed in a localized stage.

Melanomas can arise in somewhat unusual locations, such as under the nail of a finger or toe and on the mucosa lining the inside of the mouth, vagina, or anus. Primary melanomas have also been found on the pigmented tissue covering the brain (the meninges). It is important not to confuse melanomas under the nail with fungal infections, although that mistake is sometimes made at the beginning of the disease.

Melanomas are most commonly found on the skin, but 10 percent arise in the eye. The most common variants in the skin are called the superficial spreading melanoma and the nodular melanoma, terms that describe the pattern of enlargement.

Melanoma is most common in people in their forties to sixties and is rare before puberty. An increasing number of young adults with primary melanomas are being seen, however. A tumor known as clear cell sarcoma, arising in the soft tissues such as muscle and the tissue under the skin, is made up of the same type of malignant melanocytes as adult melanomas. Children and adults can have this form.

Types There is only one type of malignant cell composing all melanomas—the malignant pigment-producing cell called a melanocyte—but there are a few variants distinguished by their shape, such as cuboidal or spindle-shaped. The behavior of each is generally similar in skin melanomas, although in eye melanomas, the shape determines the behavior to a significant degree.

All melanocytes have pigment granules in them even when the cells are not black or dark brown. In all cases, they have the enzymes necessary to produce melanin, the black pigment. When melanomas spread, they often do not produce pigment and are said to be amelanotic, but the degree of malignancy of both amelanotic and melanotic melanomas seems to be the same.

How It Spreads There are two phases of growth of melanomas—the radial (outward on the surface of the skin) and the vertical (deeply into the layers of the skin). Sometimes, superficial spreading melanomas can remain in a radial growth phase

for a relatively long period of time. Nodular melanomas grow vertically soon after their appearance. Detection in a biologically early phase is, therefore, more likely with superficial spreading melanomas, but these latter tumors do eventually enter a vertical growth phase. When they do, they are as dangerous as nodular melanomas. Other less common types of melanomas include lentigo maligna melanoma, which describes a slowly expanding red or pigmented spot that usually occurs on sun-exposed areas (such as the face, scalp, and neck); acral lentiginous melanoma, which occurs on the palms or soles or underneath the fingernails; and desmoplastic melanoma, which can look like a cyst or a scar, frequently appearing on the head and neck.

Once the melanoma has penetrated deeply into the skin and has reached the lymphatic and blood vessels in the second level of the skin (the dermis), it is more difficult to cure, but a long period of quiescence may still be achieved by surgery. The melanoma can then utilize the lymphatics and bloodstream to spread to distant locations, including the lungs, liver, and brain (called metastasis).

What Causes It Caucasians living in tropical or subtropical climates, such as the American Southwest, equatorial Africa, Hawaii, and Australia, have the highest incidence. Obviously, exposure to ultraviolet light, particularly that leading to sunburn, is strongly suspected as a cause. Intermittent episodes of intense sun exposure causing sunburns have more commonly been associated with melanoma, although recent evidence is also pointing to the importance of chronic, cumulative exposure to sunlight generally associated with the development of more benign skin cancers. Typically, office workers and schoolchildren who spend hours on the beach on weekends, rather than farmers, dockworkers, and sailors who work in the sun daily, are liable to develop melanomas.

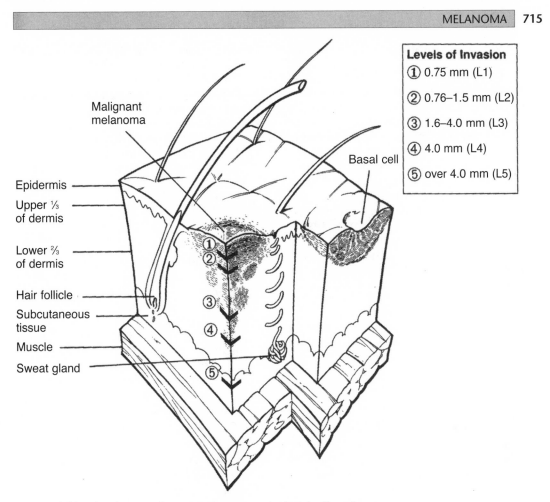

Levels of Invasion
① 0.75 mm (L1)
② 0.76–1.5 mm (L2)
③ 1.6–4.0 mm (L3)
④ 4.0 mm (L4)
⑤ over 4.0 mm (L5)

Malignant melanoma

Basal cell

Epidermis

Upper ⅓ of dermis

Lower ⅔ of dermis

Hair follicle

Subcutaneous tissue

Muscle

Sweat gland

Layers of skin, showing a malignant melanoma and a basal cell carcinoma

There is no conclusive evidence to support an association with hormones, although anecdotes continue to surface that suggest at least some women are highly susceptible to developing melanoma or recurrent melanoma when they are pregnant. Individual patients have had a striking history of recurrences and rapid progression of disease related to pregnancy. Recent evidence appears to suggest that taking oral contraceptives does not result in a significantly increased risk of developing melanoma.

Risk Factors

There are more than fifteen cases among each 100,000 Caucasians in California or Arizona, while more than sixty cases are found per 100,000 Caucasians in Australia, which is more tropical. African-Americans, Latinos, and Asians in the same regions have a much lower incidence.

• Among Caucasians, red-haired people with very fair complexions are at the highest risk, followed by blond, blue-eyed people.

• Primary melanomas can occur even in dark-skinned people on the palms and soles, under the skin, and in the membranes lining the mouth, rectum, and anus.

• Caucasian people with a large number of moles are at increased risk. Those with sporadic dysplastic nevi—unusual moles that under the microscope have features resembling melanoma—are at increased risk of developing melanoma, although their melanoma will not necessarily develop from one of those nevi. People with a strong family history (known as familial dysplastic nevus syndrome) can have a greatly increased tendency to develop melanoma.

Screening

There is no effective laboratory screening procedure, but because melanoma arises on the skin or in the eye, its presence is usually obvious to anyone aware of its features.

Common Signs and Symptoms

Cure requires early diagnosis and appropriate surgery. Family practitioners, internists, and patients themselves must recognize the early-warning signs, termed the ABCDEs of melanoma: A for *asymmetry,* B for *border irregularity* (jagged edges or borders), C for *color variation,* D for *diameter,* and E for *evolution,* or history of change. The often-quoted sign of bleeding is one of the later signs of the disease.

Further changes in the color of the mole, such as loss of pigmentation of a portion of it or a reddish or bluish tinge, may also occur. Bleeding usually occurs after some minor injury sometime after these changes become apparent. Itching can occur, as can scaling or crusting of the lesion. Occasionally, an entirely new pigmented spot appears.

It should be emphasized that most pigmented spots are not melanomas. Chronic inflammatory conditions, benign growth of skin cells (seborrheic keratoses), and basal cell carcinomas—one of the most common low-malignancy skin tumors—are sometimes pigmented. Benign tumors can also bleed after being irritated by underwear or after shaving. It is nevertheless better to bring any suspicious changes to the attention of a doctor. It is far better to risk being thought a hypochondriac than to run the risk of letting a melanoma get out of hand.

Diagnosis

Blood and Other Tests

• There are no blood tests available for screening or confirming the diagnosis of primary melanomas.

• Tumor-associated proteins (antigens) shed by the tumor are now being looked at as possible markers in the bloodstream, but results are inconclusive. Carcinoembryonic antigen (CEA), which is found in several cancers, is not found in melanomas.

Biopsy

• An adequate—in other words, an excisional—biopsy is preferred for diagnosis. Examination of the tumor under the microscope reveals characteristic melanoma cells, which are typically plump and usually contain dustlike grains of melanin pigment. The malignant melanocytes are seen to migrate into the dermis to various depths, where they are found singly, in small groups, or in large aggregations. Immunological staining procedures with special antibody-carrying dyes are now available to confirm the diagnosis in cases that do not appear typical.

• Shave biopsies that do not remove the entire melanoma are generally not recommended. They do not allow the depth of invasion into the skin to be determined, and this needs to be known to help predict the patient's risk of recurrence.

• Cauterization or freezing should never be done on a suspected melanoma. These procedures destroy the superficial part of the melanoma, making diagnosis and staging impossible. They also leave tumor cells in deeper locations at the site, which could later give rise to seeding of other parts of the body.

• Eye melanomas are not biopsied to avoid damage to sight. The appearance of eye melanomas is so characteristic that experienced ophthalmologists have no difficulty in making an accurate diagnosis in almost all cases.

Staging

The most commonly used staging system for cutaneous melanoma is that of the American Joint Committee on Cancer (AJCC), which lumps different tumor thickness levels and the presence or absence of ulceration into convenient smaller categories, called stages. The table on page 718 shows the stages, as modified and adopted in 2002. In this staging system, melanomas involving the skin only occupy Stages IA to IIC (with increasing thickness and presence of ulceration included). Melanomas involving the regional lymph nodes occupy Stages IIIA to IIIC, depending on the number of lymph nodes involved, whether the lymph node was microscopically or clinically involved, and whether ulceration was present in the original, primary melanoma. Stage IV melanomas comprise those melanomas with spread beyond the regional lymph nodes, including melanomas that show higher levels of the blood marker lactate dehydrogenase (LDH).

Several prognostic factors are used to stage skin melanomas. The factor with the best predictive ability measures the Breslow thickness, which is the exact measurement of the vertical thickness of the tumor under the microscope. Melanomas less than 1 mm are usually considered thin and highly curable by surgery alone (at least 95 percent five-year survival), although some people with such "thin" lesions have had recurrences. Tumors over 1 mm but less than 4 mm are considered to be in the intermediate range and are further subdivided into tumors less than or greater than 2 mm. Melanomas 4 mm or more are considered thick.

The depth of invasion is another well-known classification measurement, in which primary melanomas are categorized into five levels of invasion that a pathologist can easily recognize under the microscope (Clark's levels).

• Level I is melanoma at the place of origin, in the basal layer of the epidermis at the epidermal-dermal junction, the uppermost layer of the skin.

• Level II is extension to the top layer of the dermis, the papillary dermis.

• Level III melanoma extends to the border of the papillary and reticular dermis.

• Level IV involves the reticular dermis.

• Level V invades subcutaneous tissue, or the fatty layer.

Recently, a phenomenon called ulceration has also been included in the staging classification for melanoma. Ulceration is a break in the epidermis involving the melanoma and is measured by the pathologist by looking under the microscope. A bleeding tumor can sometimes alert the physician to the presence of ulceration, although this is a measurement that has to be made by the pathologist.

The presence of the tumor in regional lymph nodes draining the site of the primary tumor—such as the lymph nodes in the armpit draining a melanoma of the forearm—is another sign of a poor prognosis. Lymph nodes usually provide an immunological barrier against the tumor. When they are filled with tumor, they have obviously lost the battle, and cancer cells can pass beyond them into the bloodstream and travel to distant organs. The number of involved nodes has emerged as an important predictor of recurrence of the melanoma and is determined by analyzing a lymph node dissection specimen carefully under the microscope.

The Sentinel Node Biopsy Procedure A method of determining whether lymph nodes draining the primary melanoma site are involved with cancer, without doing an extensive surgical removal of all lymph nodes, is the sentinel node biopsy procedure. The sentinel node, or sometimes nodes, is the first lymph node that the tumor cells encounter as they travel along the lymphatic vessels from the tumor. If it is not involved with melanoma, it is unlikely that lymph nodes more distant from the primary tumor are involved.

A blue dye and usually a radioactive material are injected at the site of the tumor (or where the tumor used to be before its removal by biopsy) at the time of more complete surgery to remove all traces of the tumor. The surgeon sees where the blue dye and radioactivity have traveled—for example, into a lymph node in the armpit for a melanoma arising on the upper arm—removes that lymph node, and sends it to the pathologist to determine whether there are tumor cells in it. If not, only the remainder of the primary tumor is removed, and the other lymph nodes in the armpit are left alone. If the sentinel node has tumor cells in it ("positive" lymph node), the current practice is to remove other lymph nodes in the armpit, such as by removing the fat pad in which most of them reside. Some surgeons may remove only a few lymph nodes to sample them, and some may remove more than the fat pad, a radical resection.

Recent studies have shown that patients with a positive sentinel lymph node have a poorer outlook than those who have a negative sentinel node. Following the

American Joint Committee on Cancer Stage Grouping for Cutaneous Melanoma

STAGE	CRITERIA
IA	Localized melanomas $\leq$ 1 mm thick without ulceration or Clark level II/III (T1a, N0, M0)
IB	Localized melanomas $\leq$ 1 mm thick with ulceration or Clark level IV/V (T1b, N0, M0) *or* localized melanomas 1.01–2.0 mm thick without ulceration (T2a, N0, M0)
IIA	Localized melanomas 1.01–2.0 mm thick with ulceration (T2b, N0, M0) *or* localized melanomas 2.01–4.0 mm thick without ulceration (T3a, N0, M0)
IIB	Localized melanomas 2.01–4.0 mm thick with ulceration (T3b, N0, M0) *or* localized melanomas > 4 mm thick without ulceration (T4a, N0, M0)
IIC	Localized melanomas > 4 mm thick with ulceration (T4b, N0, M0)
IIIA–C	Nodal metastases depending on number of lymph nodes involved and presence of ulceration and/or in-transit metastases
IV	Any patient with distant metastases (any T, any N, any M1)

removal of any involved regional lymph nodes, many of these patients are receiving adjuvant therapy, such as with interferon-alpha or other experimental treatments. Another major benefit of the procedure is preventing extensive surgery on regional lymph nodes when the sentinel node is negative.

Treatment Overview

Sentinel Lymph Node Biopsy The removal of draining lymph nodes as a preventive measure in patients without clinically enlarged lymph nodes (sentinel lymph node biopsy) has not been definitely proven to improve the survival rate but has emerged as an important staging tool and an important predictor of further recurrence of the melanoma. Patients whose sentinel lymph node biopsy shows evidence of melanoma are clearly at higher risk for spread of their melanoma through the bloodstream and may be candidates for a systemic treatment termed adjuvant therapy to reduce the risk of melanoma recurrence.

Resected Melanoma

Adjuvant Therapy The only therapy for resected melanoma is interferon-alpha. Interferon-alpha (IFN-α, INTRONA) has been tested in three large trials. In the first trial, high-dose IFN-α given for one year improved disease-free survival and overall survival in patients with thick primary melanoma (defined as melanoma greater than 4 mm) and with positive lymph nodes compared with the no-treatment group. On the basis of this trial, IFN-α became approved by the FDA for use as adjuvant therapy for high-risk melanoma.

In the second trial, comparing no treatment, low-dose, and high-dose IFN-α, there was an improved disease-free survival in the high-dose group again, but overall survival was not improved. However, the additional treatments the patients received after relapse had improved between the time of the first trial and the second, so that the patients in the control group had a better overall survival than in the first trial. Thus, the second trial tended to confirm the better time to relapse found in the first trial, which was directly attributable to the interferon treatment.

In the third trial, high-dose IFN-α was compared with an experimental vaccine called GMK. This was the largest of all three interferon trials, and the trial was stopped early because the group receiving IFN-α treatment had a significantly improved survival (both disease-free and overall survival) compared with the GMK group.

While there has been suggestive evidence that some tumor vaccines can prolong disease-free survival when used after surgery for melanoma with positive lymph nodes, the recent completion of several trials including the vaccines known as GMK, CancerVax (or Canvaxin), and Melacine has not shown a significant benefit in survival when compared with IFN-α, placebo, or observation. At the current time, no vaccine has been approved by the FDA, and the use of vaccine remains experimental and should be undertaken only in a clinical trial setting.

Metastatic Melanoma

 Surgery The removal of the tumor, along with sufficient margins of normal skin, is the only curative treatment for all but the most advanced stages of disease. Nearby (i.e., sentinel) lymph nodes may also be removed depending on the thickness of the melanoma as well as other factors. Surgical removal of a single (or in special circumstances multiple) distant metastasis can also be very useful to control the tumor in a later stage.

Chemotherapy Single-drug chemotherapy is effective in no more than 20 percent of patients with advanced disease. Dacarbazine (DTIC-Dome) is the single-drug chemotherapy that is approved by the FDA, which is given by intravenous injections in an outpatient setting. Another reasonable choice for single-drug chemotherapy is temozolomide (Temodar), which is an oral drug that represents a natural metabolite of dacarbazine and has efficacy similar to dacarbazine. Temozolomide is approved for the treatment of brain tumors and may be reasonable to use in situations where the melanoma has spread to the brain.

At the current time, some physicians believe there is little rationale to pursue multidrug chemotherapy combinations. Combination chemotherapy drugs can cause higher responses, but an advantage in overall survival has not been borne out by larger studies.

Chemotherapy injected into the blood vessels of an arm or leg (known as isolated limb perfusion) has been effective in controlling disease in a particular region of the body. It is very useful for melanoma that has spread primarily or only to that region and has not shown up in many different parts of the body.

 Radiation Radiation therapy can help shrink isolated large lesions, particularly nodules under the skin, or relieve pain, but high individual doses of at least 500 cGy are usually required to overcome the resistance of melanoma cells to radiation. Somewhat lower daily radiation doses (300 to 400 cGy) are used for brain metastases. A newer method of focused radiation, stereotactic radiotherapy (CyberKnife or Gamma Knife), can be very effective for treatment of one or a low number of small brain metastases, sparing the patient the effects of whole brain radiation treatment.

Hyperthermia in conjunction with radiation may improve local control of large lesions.

 Biological Therapy Stimulating the immune system with biological response modifiers to reject the tumor has already shown some degree of success. It remains an option for therapy but is associated with significant toxicity. High doses of a biological substance called interleukin-2 (IL-2) have shown responses in approximately 20 percent of patients with advanced (usually Stage IV) melanoma. A major aspect of IL-2 treatment is the potential to achieve a complete response,

where all the patient's tumors are cleared by the treatment. A high percentage of patients who achieve complete responses with IL-2 can maintain those responses even two years later; this resulted in IL-2 being another drug approved by the FDA in 1998 for advanced melanoma. High-dose IL-2 is a very toxic treatment with many side effects, requiring intensive monitoring and treatment at experienced centers. So far, lower doses of IL-2 have not shown the same level of activity in melanoma. One recent modification of IL-2 treatment (done as part of an experimental clinical trial) is the addition of immune cells recognizing melanoma cells obtained from the patient's tumor.

Biochemotherapy is a combination treatment usually consisting of three chemotherapy drugs as well as IL-2 and interferon-alpha. Several studies have shown that biochemotherapy can result in responses in approximately 50 percent of patients, some with complete responses. However, at the current time, the question of whether biochemotherapy is superior to chemotherapy or high-dose IL-2 alone remains unanswered. Nevertheless, given the high proportion of responders, it remains a treatment option in many institutions. This is another intensive treatment that should be administered in experienced centers.

Treatment by Location
Skin Melanomas

■ *Stage I*
Standard Treatment Surgery with a wide excision around the tumor, usually with a margin of at least ½ inch (1 cm) in melanomas under ½ inch (1 cm). Sentinel lymph node biopsy is recommended for most cases of melanoma 1 mm in thickness or greater and selected cases under 1 mm.

Five-Year Survival 85 to 100 percent

Stage II

Standard Treatment Wide excision with ½ to ¾ inch (1 to 2 cm) margins in melanomas from 1 to 2 mm, and with ¾ inch (2 cm) margins (where possible) in melanomas greater than 2 mm thick. Sentinel lymph node biopsy is recommended for most cases of melanoma greater than 1 mm in thickness. Adjuvant therapy with Interferon-alpha may be considered in selected cases of melanoma over 4 mm.

Five-Year Survival 45 to 80 percent

Stage III

Standard Treatment Removal of the group of lymph nodes (lymph node dissection) that includes the ones that are felt by the doctor is the standard treatment. Patients with a sentinel lymph node biopsy showing melanoma also receive consideration for lymph node dissection. Interferon-alpha at high doses extended the average survival of patients with surgically removed Stage III melanoma by approximately a year more than surgery alone. Interferon-alpha, approved for use in the early phase of melanoma, is thus far the only treatment proven effective in preventing the recurrence of melanoma after surgery in a large-scale randomized trial. Patients with Stage III melanoma may be candidates for investigational therapies being compared with IFN-α or investigational therapies alone if they relapse following IFN-α or cannot undergo IFN-α treatment because of other medical problems.

Five-Year Survival 25 to 70 percent

Stage IV

Standard Treatment For metastasis involving distant skin, subcutaneous lesions, the lung, distant nodes, or viscera, treatment is either systemic therapy using immunological or chemotherapy agents or regional therapy with radiation (see "Treatment Overview" in this chapter).

Five-Year Survival Less than 20 percent

Other Types of Melanomas

Ocular Melanomas Melanomas of the eye occur in the colored regions at the front (the iris), just behind the iris in the structure controlling the shape of the lens (the ciliary body), and in the pigmented layer (the choroid) covering the eyeball behind the retina. Most eye melanomas grow very slowly. They may be observed with little increase in size.

Melanomas of the eye are classified by direct observation and ultrasound measurements into small, medium, and large tumors, based on their diameter and elevation. The appearance of eye melanoma cells under the microscope is also an indicator of outcome. Spindle-shaped cells are less malignant and patients almost always live fifteen years. Melanoma cells resembling skin cells (epithelioid) are more malignant, with 34 percent of patients living five years and 28 percent fifteen years. Survival is a little better for melanomas in which spindle cells are mixed with epithelioid cells (46 percent and 41 percent, five- and fifteen-year survivals, respectively).

Small tumors are usually followed closely by direct observation by an ophthalmologist, who uses a slit lamp and ultrasound or CT scanning to chart the exact diameter and height of the lesions. If they become large, they can be treated in the same way as medium and large melanomas. Such medium and large melanomas are treated either by removing the eye (enucleation) or increasingly by applying radioactive plaques.

If the melanoma extends outside the eye to the surrounding bone, the prognosis is very poor. Surgical treatment combined with radiation therapy is usually given, but there is no solid evidence that this intensive therapy alters the bad outcome.

Large melanomas of the epithelioid variety require treatment soon after discovery. Despite treatment, there is spread to a different part of the body—often the liver—in 65 percent of all patients.

Treatment of ocular melanomas that have spread depends on the site of metastasis. The most common site of metastasis is the liver, which may be treated with direct infusion of chemotherapy or immunotherapy into the liver. Other sites of disease can be treated with conventional therapeutic regimens, although controversy exists in regard to the efficacy of these regimens.

Mucosal Melanomas Mucosal melanomas arise in any area of the body that has mucous membranes, including the intestines, vagina, anus, nasal cavity, and oral cavity. Therapy is consistent with therapy for skin melanomas, although radiation is utilized in these cancers more frequently.

Brain Metastasis The most difficult challenge in melanoma is the treatment of brain metastasis. Unfortunately, there are few therapies for brain metastasis; dissemination of melanoma to the brain is associated with a poor prognosis. The most common therapy in these cases is radiation—whole brain or focused. Temozolomide (Temodar) is the only drug currently shown to cross the blood-brain barrier and is commonly used in these situations in concert with radiation. Additional studies with innovative therapeutics are in progress to improve this dismal situation.

Treatment Follow-Up

Resected Melanoma

Melanoma can involve so many parts of the body that any new symptom should be reported to the doctor. No surveillance program—including CT scans, chest X-rays, and blood tests—has been shown to provide a survival advantage.

• Since the liver and the lung are common sites for tumor cells to lodge and grow after traveling through the bloodstream, these organs should be watched carefully (at three- to six-month intervals) after removal of the primary melanoma and more often during treatment of disseminated disease.

• Chest X-rays and liver function tests (especially LDH) can be routinely done in patients with Stage IB melanoma or higher.

• In patients with Stage III melanoma, follow-up studies can be expanded to include the use of CT scans of the chest, abdomen, and pelvis, or, more recently, PET or even CT-PET fusion scans to detect melanoma relapse in various internal organs.

• Brain involvement causing neurologic symptoms is becoming more common as therapy improves for disease elsewhere in the body and patients live long enough to allow the slow-growing brain metastases to enlarge. Therefore MRI scans of the brain can be performed at the first sign of headaches or changes in mental ability, vision, muscle strength, sensation, or balance.

• Lumps under the skin, usually colorless or reddish-purple and occasionally black if in the skin, can be felt and seen by patients. Lymph nodes under the arms or in the groin can also be felt and/or seen. These can easily be diagnosed as melanoma using a technique called fine needle aspiration biopsy.

Metastatic Melanoma

In patients with metastatic melanoma, a baseline evaluation with a CT-PET fusion scan and MRI of the brain can accurately identify the site(s) of disease and should be routinely performed to assess the response to treatment.

Recurrent Cancer

Treatment is similar to that of Stage III and Stage IV. You may be eligible for re-treatment with your initial therapy, depending on the time interval and evidence of response that was observed with initial therapy. It is important that you obtain and keep all information in regard to your initial therapy to assist your physician in case of recurrent cancer.

Supportive Treatment

Melanoma usually has remarkably few debilitating effects on the system. Unless the tumor is in a place where it can cause symptoms because of its size—such as pressing on a nerve and causing pain, or causing headaches if it is in the brain—melanoma is not generally associated with severe symptoms. Patients feel and look good through most of their disease. This is in sharp contrast to cancers such as those of the head and neck or the bowel, where patients may lose their appetite and become thin fairly early in the course of their disease. Patients should do everything they feel like doing, without fear of adversely affecting their disease. Modern treatments are designed to permit and encourage a full and active life.

• Low- or nonimpact aerobic exercise, such as swimming or walking, can be pursued by all patients who feel good. More active exertion is often possible so long as there are no bad results, such as damage to the bones. Whether exercise itself has a beneficial effect on the course of the cancer is being studied actively at several university centers, but in any event it is not harmful unless overdone.

• Good, balanced nutrition is helpful, which means whole grains, lean meats, and complex carbohydrates. Fad diets should be avoided, as they often lack essential nutrients. Above all, enjoy the food that you eat.

• Review all additional "treatments" such as herbal medications, antioxidant medications, and "natural" medications with your oncologist, as they may have harmful effects when combined with your therapy. While it is true that some anticancer medications came from nat-ural beginnings, the majority of treatments took many years of testing. It is your right to refuse or accept any treatment; your physician serves as an advocate on your behalf to help you avoid unforeseen toxicities.

• As in any cancer, psychological support is essential to a good outcome. An upbeat attitude is an important element. Support groups emphasizing psychological adjustment and channeling of mental strength into overcoming the tumor, often with visualization techniques, are increasing in popularity and perform a valuable function. See the list of support groups in "Useful Readings and Resources," at the back of the book. While no one can yet explain it, there is little doubt that people who believe they will do well in fact do better than those who give up hope when they learn they have cancer. Mental attitude alone cannot do everything, but without a positive outlook, even an objective remission of disease cannot make a patient truly better.

• Your hospital and physician's office can offer additional support in the form of social workers and financial workers who are trained to assist patients in avoiding common issues during treatment.

Other Issues

Melanoma is such a variable disease that someone who is diagnosed should not feel totally disheartened. Long disease-free intervals are often achieved after the deep primary tumors are removed, and early melanomas are usually curable. If the disease comes back in a lymph node, it can be removed surgically. If it comes back elsewhere, such as in the lungs or liver, a variety of treatments are available. Some of the most exciting developments in immunotherapy are occurring in the treatment of melanoma, where prolonged survivals of several years are becoming fairly common.

It is important for all patients to know that there is now good news to replace the old bad news, when there was very little anyone could do about widespread disease. Check any information you may gain from reading about the disease with an oncologist who knows about melanoma. Look for information from trusted national sources and physicians, and not from individuals with anecdotal information. You will then have the opportunity to make an informed decision.

New Agents for Melanoma Therapy

Several new investigational treatment methods have shown some promise in treating melanoma. Newer strategies are being employed in order to improve the sensitivity of melanomas to chemotherapy.

CTLA4 Antibody Strategies to boost the immune response to melanoma continue to be an area of active investigation. One promising recent candidate is a monoclonal antibody targeting a protein called CTLA4. Cytotoxic T lymphocyte–associated antigen 4 (CTLA4) is an inhibitory receptor on immune cells (T cells) that dampens the body's immune response. Experiments in mice showed that removing CTLA4 in mice causes lethal immune proliferation, and genetic variations in human CTLA4 are associated with autoimmune disease. When given to patients with metastatic melanoma, CTLA4 antibody enhances the patient's immunity and has been associated with significant response. CTLA4 antibody's major side effects are diarrhea, rash, and inflammation. At the current time, the activity of anti-CTLA4 antibody is being investigated alone or in combination with other immune therapies in advanced melanoma, and early responses have been observed with anti-CTLA4 therapy.

Sorafenib (BAY 43-9006, Nexavar) Sorafenib is an orally taken medication that inhibits a defective signaling pathway in melanomas (the Raf kinase) leading to melanoma growth. More than 1,000 cancer patients have received sorafenib. Chronic administration is well tolerated. The most commonly observed toxicities are macular rash and hand-foot syndrome, which do not require discontinuation of the drug. Fatigue, anorexia, and diarrhea have also been observed in a minority of patients. Sorafenib is currently being evaluated in major clinical trials in combination with chemotherapy.

Dendritic Cells Dendritic cells (DC) are immune cells that form part of the mammalian immune system and are found throughout the body. They can also be found at an immature state in the blood. Once activated, they migrate to the lymphoid tissues, where they interact with T cells and B cells to initiate and shape the immune response.

Dendritic cells break the foreign proteins on the cancer cell surfaces into smaller pieces. The dendritic cells then display those pieces to the killer T cells. To make a dendritic cell vaccine, scientists extract some of the patient's dendritic cells and use immune cell stimulants to reproduce large amounts of dendritic cells in the lab. These dendritic cells are then exposed to antigens from the patient's cancer cells. This combination of dendritic cells and antigens is then injected into the patient, and the dendritic cells work to program the T cells.

Thalidomide (Thalomid) Investigators are studying agents that block angiogenesis, which is the formation of new blood vessels that feed tumors and help them to grow. Thalidomide is one of the anti-angiogenesis agents under investigation for melanoma, since recent studies have indicated that advanced melanoma may respond to thalidomide. The drug not only has antiangiogenic activity, but it also has other antitumor effects when given concurrently with chemotherapy.

The Most Important Questions You Can Ask

• What is the response rate and duration of response of the therapy you are proposing? Do you think they justify the side effects I may have?

• What are some of the difficulties and side effects that you have seen with this therapy?

• Are there other investigational treatments available anywhere in the country? Can you help me find out about them?

• What are the alternatives to the plan you are suggesting?

• What is your next choice for therapy if this one does not help me?

• Would a more (or less) aggressive treatment plan be more appropriate for me at this time?

• Can you arrange a second opinion about the treatment you are proposing?

• How many patients with melanoma do you treat annually?

Mesothelioma

Thierry M. Jahan, M.D., Sarita Dubey, M.D., Joycelyn L. Speight, M.D., Ph.D.,
Jasleen Kukreja, M.D., Malin Dollinger, M.D., and David M. Jablons, M.D.

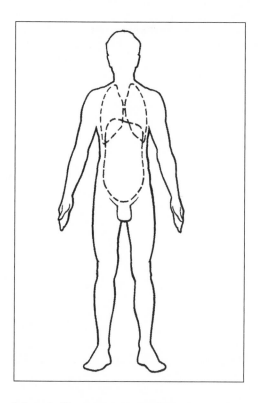

Mesothelioma is a malignant tumor in the lining of the chest and abdominal cavities. It is a rare form of cancer, with about 3,000 cases diagnosed in the United States each year. Most people who develop this cancer have a history of exposure to the widely found carcinogen asbestos.

Malignant mesothelioma is usually not curable, although some surgical cures have been reported in patients with very localized tumors. Most patients, however, have widespread disease at the time of diagnosis, with chest pain and a buildup of fluid within the cavity involved—chest or abdominal—that causes shortness of breath or abdominal swelling. Treatment at this stage, which may involve removing the fluid and the tumor, is usually directed toward relieving these symptoms.

Types Malignant mesothelioma is a tumor that can have both fibrous and epithelial elements. Epithelial cancers that develop in the tissues that cover the surface of or line internal organs are carcinomas, so the epithelial form of mesothelioma is sometimes confused with adenocarcinomas of the lung or with metastatic carcinomas. Epithelial mesotheliomas seem to have a better prognosis than other types.

How It Spreads Mesotheliomas start in the membranes lining the chest (pleural cavity) or in the membranes of the abdominal cavity (peritoneum). They can spread via the lymphatic channels to the lymph nodes of the middle of the chest. They can also spread via the bloodstream within and beyond the cavity of origin and metastasize to the chest wall and organs such as the lungs and bowel.

What Causes It Inhalation of asbestos fibers is a primary cause. Each year, about 70,000 tons of asbestos is used in the United States in cement, brake linings, roof shingles, insulation, flooring products, and packing materials. Asbestos has also been found as a contaminant in talc, which is also associated with ovarian cancer. Many urban water reservoirs contain asbestos-like fibers, and most public and private buildings contain asbestos. Only recently has the strong association between asbestos exposure and malignancy been recognized and appropriate industrial and health standards for exposure been put into effect.

There are also areas of the world where the soil contains asbestos-like fibers in very high concentration. People inhabiting these regions (including areas of Greece and Turkey) have an extremely high risk of developing mesothelioma. In addition, we expect to see a rise in the incidence of mesothelioma in the greater New York City area, due to the extensive exposure to debris from the 9/11 attacks and the collapse of the World Trade Center towers.

It is sometimes difficult to prove the relationship between asbestos exposure and the development of mesothelioma. The risk of developing the disease begins about fifteen years after the first exposure and increases each year up to forty to forty-five years after the first exposure. It is estimated that about 8 million people living in the United States have been occupationally exposed to asbestos over the last half century during the mining and milling of the mineral and during various manufacturing processes. It is believed that the incidence of mesothelioma will rise during the next ten to twenty years.

Risk Factors

At Significantly Higher Risk

Anyone exposed to asbestos fibers, even for a few months, particularly

- miners and millers in contact with asbestos;
- producers of asbestos products;
- laborers who install plumbing, boilers, and heating equipment in ships, factories, and homes;

- workers who are near the material but do not handle it directly (carpenters, electricians, and shipyard welders, for example);
- heating tradespeople and construction workers;
- firefighters and rescue personnel toiling in construction debris;
- people living near asbestos mines, who have an increased chance of developing asbestosis, an associated scarring of the lung, as well as mesothelioma; and
- inhabitants of the Anatoli region of Turkey, where zeolite is found in the soil and in homes.

At Somewhat Higher Risk

- Spouses and children of asbestos workers, presumably because of asbestos fibers brought home in the hair and on clothing.
- Demolition workers and workers who repair structures that contain asbestos.
- Although smoking greatly increases the risk of lung cancer in asbestos workers, it does not increase the risk of mesothelioma.

Screening

Regular chest X-rays are essential to follow the course of people with any significant asbestos exposure, although scar tissue and the shadows related to asbestosis that are seen on the X-rays will be chronic and may progress slowly over the years even without the development of malignant mesothelioma. Mesothelioma may also occur without asbestosis or scarring in the lungs. The tumor may not appear on a chest X-ray as a single mass with sharp edges, so rather than depending on X-rays as a screening method, the best procedure is to biopsy any suspicious area for a possible malignancy.

Common Signs and Symptoms

Patients with mesothelioma may have shadows on their chest X-rays related to

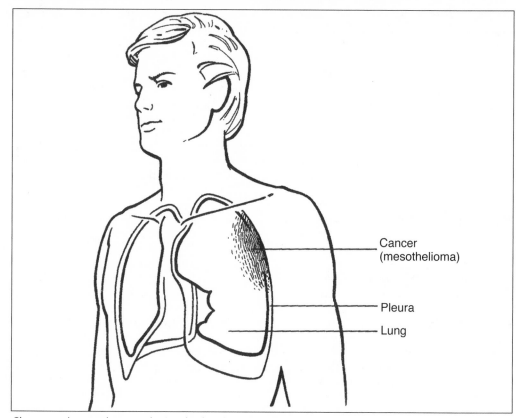

Cancer
(mesothelioma)

Pleura

Lung

Chest membranes that may be involved with mesothelioma

asbestosis, although the development of chest pain, significant shortness of breath, and especially fluid around one lung or in the abdomen should suggest a diagnosis of mesothelioma. People with peritoneal mesothelioma usually have signs of advanced disease, including an abdominal mass, pain, fluid in the abdomen (ascites), and weight loss.

If the tumor has extended to the ribs, bones, nerves, and the superior vena cava, common symptoms include pain, trouble swallowing, nerve compression syndromes, and swelling of the neck or face.

Involvement of the membrane around the heart (pericardium) may cause heart rhythm disturbances. Tumors in the lining of the abdominal cavity (peritoneum) may extend to produce bowel obstruction. Fever, clotting abnormalities, thrombophlebitis, and anemia have also been seen in a large number of patients with peritoneal mesothelioma.

Diagnosis

Careful questioning about the history of asbestos exposure should focus on the period twenty to fifty years before diagnosis and include possible exposure to household contacts. Because asbestos is so widespread, a brief exposure may have been forgotten.

Physical Examination

- Swelling of the neck and face.
- Abdominal mass.

Blood and Other Tests

- Lung function tests usually show a smaller amount of normal lung tissue available for breathing.
- A test for elevated levels of the carcinoembryonic antigen (CEA) in the blood may help distinguish an adenocarcinoma from mesothelioma, with a markedly elevated level suggesting an adenocarcinoma. This distinction may be important, for adenocarcinoma of the lung can be more treatable than mesothelioma.
- Patients with peritoneal mesothelioma may have elevated platelet counts and clotting abnormalities.
- Laboratory studies are not particularly helpful.

Imaging

- CT scans to assess the extent of disease and to assist decision making regarding therapy. Chest X-rays will often reveal thickening of the pleural membranes in half the patients with peritoneal mesothelioma.
- MRI scans can help define the relationships between the tumor mass(es) and anatomic structures of the chest or the abdomen more clearly. They can be useful to help decide whether or not surgery is possible.
- PET scans can provide information about the involvement of lymph nodes in the middle of the chest or the involvement of more distant structures, either of which will strongly influence the decision to operate.

Endoscopy and Biopsy

- If mesothelioma is suspected, attempts at a diagnostic biopsy should be made. Sometimes fluid removed during a chest "tap" (thoracentesis) may be examined for tumor cells in a way similar to a Pap test. A needle biopsy may also be done.
- Most cases require an open surgical biopsy, since needle biopsies seldom produce enough diagnostic material. Since a simple biopsy done with a surgical incision into the chest under general anesthesia (thoracotomy) may make it technically difficult to remove the tumor later, the surgeon doing the biopsy should be prepared to do the definitive surgical treatment if that seems appropriate.
- The usual examination of the biopsied tissue under the microscope will often prove that the tissue is malignant, but may not distinguish adenocarcinoma of the lung from mesothelioma. So a specimen is often processed by special methods—electron microscopy and special stains—to help document the type of tumor.
- Cytology of the sputum either coughed up by the patient or obtained through a bronchoscopy may document a lung cancer, an adenocarcinoma, which may not be visible on routine chest X-rays.
- Patients with peritoneal mesothelioma eventually have exploratory surgery of the abdomen (laparotomy), with an open directed biopsy. Sometimes a simpler procedure, peritoneoscopy, may yield enough tissue for diagnosis. An adequate biopsy is essential, since peritoneal mesothelioma can be confused with adenocarcinomas arising in other tissues, especially the ovary.

Staging

There are a number of different staging systems for malignant mesothelioma, including a TNM system. All list four stages of tumor from very localized to metastatic, but no one system is universally agreed upon. The PDQ classification into localized and advanced disease may be appropriate for decision making.

There is no satisfactory staging system for peritoneal mesothelioma, although the tumor is usually confined to the abdomen. Since metastasis is rare, extensive staging studies outside the abdomen may not be necessary. CT scans will usually adequately define the extent of tumor.

Treatment Overview

Surgery is the only treatment method that can lead to a cure, but only people with very early stage disease—a small minority of patients—will achieve long-term survival. Mesothelioma is usually incurable, so treatment efforts are designed to control the accumulation of fluids (effusion) as well as pain and other symptoms. Recently, new treatments have been implemented to help patients survive more comfortably for a longer time.

Despite its relative rarity, mesothelioma remains the subject of intense clinical trial investigation. These efforts are starting to yield positive results.

Chemotherapy Extensive attempts have been made to discover chemotherapeutic agents that have some effectiveness against this tumor. Many drugs have been tested, but only a few have modest activity. Doxorubicin (Adriamycin), cyclophosphamide (Cytoxan), and cisplatin (Platinol) are active, and so are 5-azacytidine (Vidaza), 5-fluorouracil, and high-dose methotrexate (Mexate, Amethopterin, Folex) with leucovorin (LV) rescue. The single agent vinorelbine (Navelbine) has also been reported to have some activity against epithelial mesothelioma. Recently, the drug pemetrexed (Alimta) has been shown to have excellent activity against mesothelioma, both as a single agent and as part of a combination. Pemetrexed was the first-ever chemotherapy drug approved by the FDA specifically for the treatment of this tumor.

Response rates to combinations of chemotherapy drugs usually tend to be higher. The use of pemetrexed in combination with cisplatin has been shown to be more effective than the use of cisplatin alone. The use of pemetrexed requires the use of both folic acid and vitamin B_{12} supplements in order to reduce the toxicity of the drug combination. The pemetrexed-cisplatin combination, while not a cure, has a good chance of improving the survival as well as the symptoms (chest pain, shortness of breath) of patients with advanced mesothelioma.

The combination of gemcitabine (Gemzar) and cisplatin has also been shown to have acceptable results in improving the symptoms of patients with mesothelioma. Finally, combinations with doxorubicin, which had been the standard for these patients previously, have activity but tend to be more toxic and therefore more difficult to administer than the more recent combinations mentioned above.

There has been a great deal of work in trying to understand microscopic and molecular events that control the development and the growth of mesothelioma. Some of these molecular events have been targeted through the use of newer therapies. As in many cancers, it appears that the growth of blood vessels is essential for the progression of mesothelioma. Consequently, recent clinical trials have attempted to target molecules involved in the development of blood vessels, a process known as angiogenesis. Clinical trials with agents specifically designed to interfere with angiogenesis continue to be carried out. A drug such as bevacizumab (Avastin) may prove to be effective when combined with chemotherapy. Other experimental molecules such as vatalanib (PTK/ZK) and ZD 6474, GW 70556, SAHA, tetrathiomolybdate, and ranpirnase (Onconase), to name a few, are being intensely studied for the treatment of malignant mesothelioma.

Results of these investigations should be available in the near future.

 Radiation The usefulness of radiation therapy is difficult to define. The natural history of these tumors varies and interpretation of the effects after treatment is difficult, both because of chronic shadows on the chest X-ray before and after treatment and because so few patients have been treated with this method. Early research did suggest some benefit from radiation therapy.

One problem is that usually one entire side of the chest is at risk for tumor and has to be treated. It may be difficult to administer a dose of radiation high enough to control tumor growth without risking toxic effects to adjacent structures, including the heart, stomach, intestines, liver, and kidneys. In addition, the pleura is a complex three-dimensional and superficial structure, which makes accurate and comprehensive radiation-treatment planning difficult.

The radiation oncologist must also be careful in giving radiation to the area of the heart. This is even more of a problem after surgery to remove the left lung, with the resulting shift of the heart toward the left side of the chest. Sophisticated radiation methods have to be used with this cancer, which may involve electron-beam treatments as well as the usual external radiation therapy. The use of radiation therapy at the time of surgery may help solve some of the technical difficulties in planning a treatment field. However, only a minority of patients will have surgery as part of their treatment.

Combined Therapy There has been a lot of interest in combining surgery with both chemotherapy and radiation as a comprehensive approach to the treatment of malignant mesothelioma. Clinical trials of surgery followed by radiation and chemotherapy reveal that the approach is feasible. In addition, for patients with limited disease, cures can be accomplished with this aggressive approach. Recently, the use of chemotherapy *before* surgery has been shown to be safe and feasible. It may prove to be useful in the management of mesothelioma patients.

Treatment by Stage
Malignant Mesothelioma
Localized
Localized mesotheliomas are either solitary tumors or tumors that have spread within the cavity involved (intracavitary) but are confined to the serosal surfaces where they started.

Standard Treatment Occasional patients with this stage of disease can be cured by aggressive surgery. A solitary tumor can be completely removed along with adjacent structures to ensure wide margins of cancer-free tissue.

Standard surgery for intracavitary mesothelioma will also involve the removal of portions of the lung and diaphragm in selected patients. Some surgeons favor more extensive operations to include whatever tissue is necessary to remove all visible tumor as long as this doesn't interfere with the functioning of the remaining organs.

To relieve the symptoms of disease, collections of fluid in the cavity (effusions) are drained. A chemical irritant can then be introduced into the chest to make the layers of the membranes adhere to one another. This may prevent further fluid accumulations.

Radiotherapy is also sometimes given to the lung involved in order to eliminate blood flow in the area and improve breathing.

Five-Year Survival Possible if patients undergo complete resection and if no lymph nodes are involved. Average survival for localized chest disease is about twenty months.

Investigational

- Chemotherapy within the chest cavity (intracavitary) after aggressive surgery
- Clinical trials of new chemotherapeutic agents and radiotherapy techniques
- Clinical trials of combined modality therapy with chemotherapy plus radiation (intraoperative and conventional)

Advanced

In this stage, the tumor has spread beyond the cavity of origin, with metastasis outside the serosal surface. This extension can include the lung and chest wall, as well as abdominal organs such as the intestines.

Standard Treatment In some patients, surgical removal of the tumor may be done as a palliative measure. Radiation therapy may also be given in an attempt to control the growth of the malignancy and reduce symptoms in the lung.

As for localized disease, chemical irritants are used to control collections of fluid caused by irritation from the tumor. The fluid is drained beforehand and the chemical irritants are introduced through a chest tube.

Five-Year Survival Less than 10 percent. The average survival is six to nine months.

Investigational New drugs and new combinations of standard chemotherapies with some of the newer agents are being actively tested as mentioned above. The results of these clinical trials should be available shortly.

Peritoneal Mesothelioma

Standard Treatment Therapy for peritoneal mesothelioma is difficult, especially as it is usually widespread by the time it is diagnosed. Removal of the tumors for cure is rarely possible, and the role of surgery is generally confined to relief of bowel obstruction, relief of ascites by placing shunts for drainage, or the palliative removal of large tumors.

Radiation therapy has often been used, but its role has not yet been defined. Since the entire abdomen is at risk, all of the abdominal organs will also be affected by radiation. To protect the liver, kidney, bowel, and spinal cord, the dose has to be lower than would be desirable for tumor control.

Although radiation may not be effective in most patients with large, bulky tumors due to the problems posed by an adequate dose, there may be some benefit from lower doses—in the range of 3,000 cGy—if most of the tumor has successfully been removed and only small amounts remain.

The use of chemotherapy for peritoneal mesothelioma has lately focused on the use of chemotherapy given via a catheter directly into the abdominal cavity (intraperitoneal). This permits a much higher concentration of drug to be delivered to the area of the tumor. Intraperitoneal cisplatin (Platinol), with special measures to neutralize the drug's toxic effects in the body, resulted in a significant complete response rate in one study, but unfortunately many of these patients relapsed after treatment. It appears also that the drug pemetrexed (Alimta) administered alone or in combination with cisplatin, may be effective in controlling the symptoms and the fluid accumulation seen in peritoneal mesothelioma.

Five-Year Survival Beyond one year is unusual.

Investigational

- Because present treatment programs for advanced mesothelioma usually do not have a major impact on the disease, we strongly recommend participation in clinical trials of new forms of therapy.
- Important studies are currently under way with combined treatment therapy, using, for example, surgery, and chemotherapy (pemetrexed [Alimta] + cisplatinum [Platinol]) in combination with abdominal radiotherapy.

• Another current trial involves the removal of larger tumor nodules, followed by intraperitoneal chemotherapy, then followed by a "second-look" operation to determine response. Radiotherapy is given if there has been complete control of the tumor, and more chemotherapy is given before the radiation treatment if there is any residual disease left. The preliminary results of this combined program suggest that significant response rate with acceptable toxicity is possible.

Treatment Follow-Up

Mesotheliomas usually progress rapidly and frequent follow-up evaluations are needed.

• A physical examination every six to twelve weeks
• Chest or abdominal X-rays or CT scans every three to six months
• Blood counts and chemistry panel every three to six months
• Lung function tests, depending on symptoms

The Most Important Questions You Can Ask

• Should I stop smoking?
• What can surgery accomplish?
• Should radiation be used?
• Is there any role for chemotherapy?
• How long can I live with this tumor?

Metastatic Cancer

Alan P. Venook, M.D.

■ ■ ■ ■

When a cancer spreads (metastasizes) from its original site to another area of the body, it is termed metastatic cancer. Virtually all cancers have the potential to spread this way. Whether metastases do develop depends on the complex interaction of many tumor cell factors, including the type of cancer, the degree of maturity (differentiation) of the tumor cells, the location, and how long the cancer has been present, as well as other incompletely understood factors.

The treatment of metastatic cancer depends on where the cancer started. When breast cancer spreads to the lungs, for example, it remains a breast cancer and the treatment is determined by the tumor's origin within the breast, not by the fact that it is now in the lung. About 5 percent of the time, metastases are discovered but the primary tumor cannot be identified. The treatment of these metastases is dictated by their location rather than their origin (see the chapter "Cancer of an Unknown Primary Site [CUPS]").

Although the presence of metastases generally implies a poor prognosis, some metastatic cancers can be cured with conventional therapy.

Types Virtually all cancers can develop metastases.

How It Spreads Metastases spread in three ways—by local extension from the tumor to the surrounding tissues, through the bloodstream to distant sites, and through the lymphatic system to neighboring or distant lymph nodes. Each kind of cancer may have a typical route of spread. The most likely sites of metastases for each tumor are listed in the individual tumor chapters.

What Causes It The characteristics of each tumor are different, and it is not known what factors make the metastases develop in particular places.

Common Signs and Symptoms

Many patients have no or minimal symptoms related to the tumor, and their metastases are found during a routine medical evaluation. If there are symptoms, they depend on the site involved.

• Brain metastases may cause headaches, dizziness, blurred vision, nausea, or other symptoms related to the nervous system.
• Bone metastases may be evident because of pain, although they frequently cause no symptoms. The first sign of a bone metastasis may be when the affected bone breaks, often after a minor injury or no injury at all.
• Lung metastases may cause a nonproductive cough or a cough producing bloody sputum, chest pain, or shortness of breath.
• Liver metastases may cause weight loss, fevers, nausea, loss of appetite, abdominal pain, fluid in the abdomen, or jaundice (the skin turning yellow).

Diagnosis

Physical Examination There are no specific findings for metastatic cancer on physical examination. But there may be

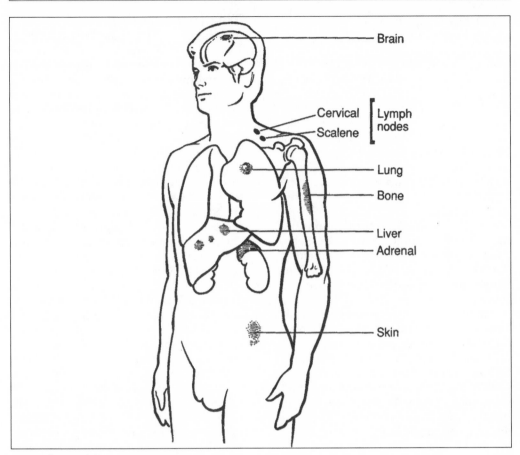

Areas of potential cancer metastases

- fever,
- tenderness of the bones,
- tumors under the skin,
- enlarged liver and spleen,
- enlarged, hard lymph nodes,
- fluid in the abdomen (ascites),
- jaundice (the skin turning yellow), or
- swelling of the legs (edema).

Blood and Other Tests

- Routine liver function studies—blood tests looking at serum bilirubin and liver enzymes—may be abnormal. They can, however, be completely normal even in advanced stages of metastatic cancer.

- There may be serum blood tests that are abnormal. Metastatic colon cancer, for example, may be associated with an elevated carcinoembryonic antigen (CEA), testicular cancer with a high alpha-fetoprotein (AFP) or human chorionic gonadotropin (HCG), pancreatic cancer with an elevated CA 19-9, and ovarian cancer with an elevated CA-125. But not all tumors have serum markers and not all markers are specific.

Imaging

- Abdominal ultrasound is one way to evaluate the abdomen if a mass is suspected.

It can reveal the presence of fluid in the abdomen and is particularly useful for distinguishing a solid mass from a noncancerous accumulation of fluid within the pelvis or liver (benign cyst).

• A bone scan will identify most tumor spread to the bones. It involves the injection of a special contrast agent into a vein, followed by whole body imaging by a special camera. But abnormal areas on a bone scan almost always have to be evaluated further with plain X-rays of the suspicious area.

• A CT scan is useful for determining the extent of a tumor within the head, chest, or abdomen and for evaluating the possible spread of tumor tissue into lymph nodes or other structures in the abdomen.

• Magnetic resonance imaging (MRI) may help determine if the cancer can be surgically removed, but it is usually not necessary except in specific situations such as tumors of the spinal cord.

• Positron-emission tomography (PET) scanning is a very popular new technique that distinguishes cancer areas from normal areas on the basis of metabolic activity. It can be a useful adjunctive test in determining the extent and distribution of cancer, but it is not indicated in many circumstances and is not particularly helpful in finding primary tumors that are otherwise not evident.

• If metastases have been found on biopsy, a chest X-ray should be done because the lungs are a very common site of metastases.

Biopsy A biopsy, with either a fine needle (FNA) or a regular needle, is often necessary. This procedure can be done through the skin without significant danger. The biopsy sample can be used to distinguish between types of malignancy because the tumor cells of different cancers have characteristic features under the microscope.

Treatment by Type
Treatment of metastatic cancer primarily depends on the original site of the cancer, so for specific treatment recommendations, refer to the chapters dealing with the primary cancers. In some clinical situations, however, metastases may be treated in specific ways.

Brain Metastases
Any cancer may spread to the brain, although the most common to do so are lung and breast cancers. The treatment of brain metastases depends on many factors, such as the tumor of origin, the number and location of lesions within the brain, and the extent of cancer in places other than the brain.

Standard Treatment Most patients are placed on steroids (dexamethasone [Decadron]) to relieve brain swelling that can cause severe symptoms. Many patients will also take an antiseizure medicine (phenytoin [Dilantin]), since seizures are a common complication.

Patients with brain metastases from lymphoma, leukemia, or small cell lung cancer should generally be given radiation therapy to the entire brain, although these tumors may also be treated with systemic chemotherapy.

The standard approach with brain metastases of any other origin is to decide if the tumor can be removed. A CT scan or an MRI should be done to discover whether there is more than one tumor and to define the specific site in the brain where the tumor or tumors are located.

• If there is only one tumor and the patient's overall condition is good, surgical removal of the metastasis may be attempted, although factors such as location within the brain, how long ago the primary cancer was treated, and the presence of metastases elsewhere in the body have to be considered. An alternative to conventional surgery on a single or a small number of brain metastases is the Gamma Knife. This is a type of radiation treatment delivered by a machine that focuses multiple radiation beams directly at the involved area. This technique is offered in certain centers in the United States. After the tumor is removed, radiation therapy is given to the entire brain.

• In patients with more than one brain metastasis, surgery is not usually an option and radiation is delivered to the entire brain.

Investigational A method of biopsying or removing tumors called stereotactic surgery is being studied. This allows for access to the brain tissue without causing extensive side effects (see the chapter "Brain").

Lung Metastases

Metastases to the lung are common for many types of cancer. Patients may have no symptoms or they may have symptoms such as shortness of breath and coughing up blood.

Standard Treatment Lung metastases are generally treated with chemotherapy directed against the primary tumor type. But occasionally tumors metastasize to form a single deposit in the lungs. The likeliest primary tumor to do this is a sarcoma, although it may occur with almost any primary cancer.

If the CT scan and MRI suggest that the tumor is isolated, it may be surgically removed without causing significant loss of lung function. In fact, some cancers like sarcomas and colorectal cancer may metastasize slowly enough that as many as three or four discrete tumors can be removed. This aggressive approach should be considered in any patient with a solitary lung metastasis, although most of the time the presence of other systemic tumors is likely to limit any gains from surgery.

One problem caused by metastases to the lung and the tissue lining the lung

(pleura) is the accumulation of fluid within the chest. This may make the lung collapse, creating breathing difficulties. The fluid can be removed through a needle or through a larger tube inserted through the skin into the chest cavity. After the fluid is removed, an irritant such as tetracycline, nitrogen mustard (Mustargen), or bleomycin (Blenoxane) may be injected into the cavity to cause scarring of the tissues and this may help to prevent the reaccumulation of fluid.

If a metastatic tumor causes bleeding into the lungs, a patient may begin coughing up blood. Radiation therapy directed precisely at the tumor may alleviate the problem. If that cannot be done, it may be possible to stop the bleeding by injecting a special material into a blood vessel in the lung. This requires a specific radiologic technique but occasionally is very effective.

Bone Metastases

The most common cancers to spread to the bones are prostate, lung, and breast cancers. Bone metastases may be discovered on a routine X-ray or bone scan or may be found because of pain, swelling, or a fracture of the weakened bone.

Standard Treatment Bone metastases that don't produce symptoms and involve bones that are not weight-bearing (weight-bearing bones include the hip, upper leg, and shoulder) may be treated with the chemotherapy appropriate for the primary tumor.

Bone metastases that cause symptoms can also be treated with systemic therapy, although to take this approach depends on the type of cancer and the likelihood of getting much benefit from the treatment. For example, a patient with prostate cancer involving the bones is likely to respond to hormonal therapy, but there is no such effective treatment for lung cancer that has spread to the bones. Other patients may benefit from the drug pamidronate (Aredia), which can diminish the progress of bone metastases in some diseases, including multiple myeloma and breast cancer.

If the tumor is not likely to respond to chemotherapy or if the bone involved is a weight-bearing one, the best option is to give radiation focused only on the involved area. The symptomatic relief is usually rapid and complete. Healing causes improvement in bone strength and makes the chance of a fracture less likely. Each bone can tolerate only a limited amount of radiation, although radiation can often be used to treat many different sites of tumor involvement.

If the bone metastases become apparent because of a fracture, the management issues are complicated. Surgery may be required to repair the bone and should be done if it is a weight-bearing bone. Fractured ribs, on the other hand, are not treated with a cast or immobilization. All such fractures should be treated with radiation therapy as well.

Bone metastases to the spine are a particular concern because a fractured vertebra can result in the loss of function of the limbs or bowel and bladder. Tumors in these bones, therefore, may need to be treated even though they are not weight-bearing bones and even when there are no symptoms.

Liver Metastases

Treatment of liver metastases depends on the organ where the cancer originated. The most common to metastasize to the liver are colon and other gastrointestinal cancers.

Standard Treatment For most metastatic tumors to the liver, systemic chemotherapy directed at the tumor type should be offered. But metastases from some cancers may be approached in a different way.

Occasionally, metastases to the liver are localized in one part of the liver or exist as solitary masses. Such tumors may be surgically removed with a possibility of achieving a cure, particularly with metastases from colon and kidney cancers or sarcoma. Generally, no more than four tumors should be removed from the liver, however. Removing more than four metastases rarely results in a cure and exposes the patient to significant surgical risks, although newer techniques are allowing for the liberalization of these parameters. Radiofrequency ablation in lieu of or in addition to surgical resection of liver metastases is gaining increasing popularity, especially in individuals with multiple areas of liver involvement (see chapter 13, "Radiofrequency-Generated Heat Treatment").

Liver metastases from colon cancer may be treated with systemic administration of combination chemotherapy and biological therapy—such as oxaliplatin (Eloxatin) + irinotecan (Camptosar) + 5-fluorouracil + leucovorin with bevacizumab (Avastin) and/or cetuximab (Erbitux)—but because of the particular biological properties of some colon cancers, patients may develop liver metastases without ever having other sites of tumor involvement. Patients with such limited cancer may benefit from chemotherapy infused directly into the liver. Delivered by an implanted pump connected to the hepatic artery, this therapy takes advantage of the liver's ability to metabolize some drugs, meaning that the tumor may be exposed to high concentrations of chemotherapy, while the rest of the body is spared the side effects.

This approach initially requires surgery to implant the pump and remove the gallbladder, but the rest of the therapy can be done on an outpatient basis. The treatment causes tumor regression more often than standard chemotherapy.

A treatment called chemoembolization involves administering a combination of chemotherapy and colloid particles directly into the liver tumor via the liver's main (hepatic) artery. The procedure is performed by a radiologist and does not require surgery or prolonged bed rest. It is very effective for primary tumors, but it is much less effective for metastases.

Investigational

• New combinations of chemotherapy drugs may improve results for patients with colon cancer metastases, both to the liver and elsewhere. Such combinations are being studied for systemic treatment as well as for treatment directly to the liver.

• Cryosurgery (cold surgery) has generally been supplanted by radiofrequency ablation (hot surgery) as a method of great promise allowing for the removal or destruction of some otherwise unresectable tumors. So far, this technique is performed only by a few specialized physicians.

• A liver transplant can be performed. But it should almost never be done for patients with metastatic tumors in the liver, for it can be assumed that the cancer will spread to other organs.

Supportive Therapy

• Pain relievers are sometimes called for in liberal doses. Narcotics may have excessive side effects, however, because they are metabolized by the liver, which may not be functioning properly.

• Nonsteroidal anti-inflammatory drugs may be effective even against the severe pain associated with metastatic cancer.

• The loss of appetite that often accompanies metastatic cancer may be relieved with megestrol acetate (Megace) or with medicinal marijuana.

• Water pills (diuretics) to alleviate fluid in the abdomen or legs may cause a significant imbalance in kidney function if their use is not carefully monitored.

• Nausea can be adequately treated with standard medications, including suppositories.

• Sleep disturbances are common, but sleeping pills (sedatives) should be used carefully, since most are metabolized by the liver.

Treatment Follow-Up

Careful follow-up is necessary after treatment of metastases. Depending upon the organs involved, diagnostic tests will be done to identify new areas of tumor involvement that may cause problems and to look for tumor recurrences.

The Most Important Questions You Can Ask

• Should any other tests be done to determine whether my cancer has metastasized?

• Should I see another physician to review the treatment of my metastatic tumor or to offer another viewpoint?

• If metastases are present, what effect do they have on the treatment plan and the curability of my cancer?

• Could I benefit from an investigational therapy available at another institution?

• How sick will the proposed chemotherapy make me relative to its potential benefit?

Multiple Myeloma

Robert A. Kyle, M.D., and S. Vincent Rajkumar, M.D.

■ ■ ■ ■

Multiple myeloma is a cancer of the plasma cell, a type of B lymphocyte responsible for producing antibodies that take part in the immune response. A treatable but rarely curable disease, multiple myeloma—also called plasma cell myeloma, myelomatosis, or Kahler's disease—is characterized by the overgrowth of malignant plasma cells, mostly in the bone marrow. Although multiple myeloma usually involves the bones, it must be distinguished from cancers that begin in another organ such as the breast or lung and then spread to the bones.

Multiple myeloma is an uncommon malignancy, making up only 1 percent of all cases of cancer. In a population of 1 million people, only forty cases would be found each year. There have been reports that the incidence of myeloma has increased two- to threefold during the past forty years, but careful studies from the United States and Europe suggest that the incidence has not truly changed. The apparent increase is most likely due to more and better medical facilities and diagnostic techniques.

Types Almost all cases of multiple myeloma involve the bone marrow. There are several types, each with its distinctive features and each producing a variety of diagnostic findings and symptoms:

• Patients with smoldering multiple myeloma (SMM) have enough myeloma cells in the bone marrow and/or a large amount of an abnormal protein (monoclonal protein, or M-protein) in the blood to indicate multiple myeloma, but

they do not have anemia, kidney failure, or skeletal lesions that are also characteristic of the disease. There are no symptoms. These patients should be followed closely and not treated until progression occurs.

• Patients with plasma cell leukemia have large numbers of plasma cells circulating in the blood. Plasma cell leukemia may be the first feature of multiple myeloma leading to a diagnosis or it may occur late in the myeloma's course after resistance to chemotherapy has developed.

• With nonsecretory myeloma, patients have abnormal plasma cells in the bone marrow and frequently have holes (lytic lesions) in the skeleton, but no abnormal protein is detectable in the blood or urine.

• Osteosclerotic myeloma ([POEMS syndrome), *endocrinopathy, monoclonal gammopathy*]) patients usually have pain, burning numbness, and weakness produced by the involvement of nerves by the disease (polyneuropathy). The liver and spleen are often enlarged (organomegaly); there may be a darkening of the skin and increased growth of body hair. The breasts may become enlarged and the testicles smaller. Bone X-rays usually reveal dense (sclerotic) areas in the bone. Anemia, kidney failure, and fractures are rare with this type of myeloma.

• Solitary plasmacytoma (solitary myeloma of bone) means there is a single plasma cell tumor in the bone. X-rays of the bones show no other lytic lesions, and the bone marrow is normal. Characteristically, the patients have no abnormal M-protein in the blood or urine. This tumor should be treated with high doses of radiation to the lesion, but about 60 percent of patients will develop multiple myeloma within ten years.

• Extramedullary plasmacytoma is a tumor consisting of myeloma cells but occurs outside the bone marrow. The most commonly involved area is the back of the nose and throat (nasopharynx), and the sinuses may also be involved. Eighty percent of cases involve the upper respiratory area. Extramedullary plasmacytomas may also involve the stomach, small bowel, colon, bladder, thyroid, breast, or brain. The bone marrow is normal, and the patients have no lytic bone lesions or M-protein in the blood or urine. If an abnormal protein is present, it should disappear after treatment. Diagnosis of a plasmacytoma is made after a biopsy of the tumor. It is treated with large doses of radiation. Most patients are cured, but the disease may recur in a nearby area. The development of typical multiple myeloma is uncommon.

What Causes It The cause is not known, although exposure to radiation may be a factor in some cases. Survivors of the atomic bomb explosions in Japan had an increased incidence of multiple myeloma.

There is little evidence that chemicals cause myeloma in humans, although some reports have linked multiple myeloma with benzene or other industrial toxins. An increased risk of multiple myeloma has been recognized in farmers in several countries and has been noted in rubber workers, furniture workers, and those exposed to pesticides. The number of cases is small, however, and more information is needed to confirm these associations.

There have been reports of two or more family members with multiple myeloma, but the genetic influence is minimal. There is no evidence that allergies, chronic infections, or other immune-stimulating conditions play a role.

Risk Factors

At Significantly Higher Risk

• Multiple myeloma occurs in older people. The average age is sixty-five to seventy years; 2 percent are under forty.

• Its incidence in African-Americans is twice that in Caucasians.

Screening

Screening is of no value in a healthy person because anyone with multiple myeloma should not be treated unless there are symptoms or serious laboratory abnormalities. Many patients are found to have an M-protein in their blood during a routine examination, but if there is no other evidence of multiple myeloma, these patients are considered to have a benign condition called monoclonal gammopathy of undetermined significance (MGUS).

Common Signs and Symptoms

At the time of diagnosis, more than two-thirds of people with multiple myeloma have bone pain, typically in the back or chest and less often in the arms and legs. The pain is usually made worse by movement and does not occur at night except after a change in position. Patients may lose several inches in height because of the collapse of vertebrae.

Weakness and fatigue are common and are often associated with anemia. Fever is rare, and when it occurs, it is usually from an infection. Occasionally, there may be bleeding from the nose and gums or easy bruising. The initial symptoms may be from an acute infection, most often pneumonia, although meningitis or bloodstream infections may also occur. There may also be symptoms of elevated serum calcium, which consist of loss of appetite, nausea, vomiting, constipation, excessive urination (polyuria), and stupor or coma.

Diagnosis

The criteria for diagnosis of multiple myeloma are listed below:

• There should be at least 10 percent abnormal plasma cells in the bone marrow or proof of an extramedullary plasmacytoma.
• An M-protein should be present in the serum or urine except in those patients considered to have nonsecretory myeloma.
• There should be evidence of end-organ damage: anemia, increased calcium, kidney failure, or bone lesions that are felt to be related to myeloma.

Connective tissue diseases (such as rheumatoid arthritis, polymyositis, and scleroderma), chronic infections, metastatic cancer, lymphoma, and leukemia may resemble some of the characteristics of multiple myeloma.

The diagnosis must differentiate those with true multiple myeloma from those with monoclonal gammopathy of undetermined significance (MGUS) and smoldering multiple myeloma (SMM), since people with these conditions should be observed indefinitely and not given therapy unless they develop features of multiple myeloma.

Physical Examination

• Physical findings are often general and nonspecific. Pallor (paleness) is the most common physical finding.
• The liver can be felt in less than 5 percent of patients; the spleen is rarely felt.
• There may be tumors outside the bone marrow (extramedullary plasmacytomas).

Blood and Other Tests

• A complete blood count (CBC) reveals anemia in two-thirds of patients.
• An increase in total serum protein may be one of the first clues to the presence of an M-protein. An elevated serum calcium occurs in 15 to 20 percent of patients. The level of serum creatinine (a measure of kidney function) is abnormal in one-fifth of patients at diagnosis. The serum beta-2 microglobulin level is helpful in prognosis.
• Serum protein electrophoresis (SPEP) shows an M-protein "spike" in 80 percent of patients. Immunofixation is necessary to determine the type of M-protein. The amount of M-protein is measured by SPEP or by the measurement of IgG or IgA, the two major types of M-protein found in multiple myeloma.
• Ninety-seven percent of patients with multiple myeloma will have an M-protein in the blood or in the urine. If the level of M-protein in the blood is high or if the patient has blurred vision or bleeding, determining the viscosity (thickness) of the serum is necessary. Measuring the M-protein in the serum and urine is a good way to determine whether the disease is getting worse or is responding to chemotherapy. The level of the M-protein is a direct measure of the tumor mass. If the patient has no spike by serum protein electrophoresis, the free light chain (FLC) should be measured.
• A twenty-four-hour urine specimen is essential. The total protein is determined and electrophoresis is performed, making it possible to measure the amount of monoclonal light chain (of kappa or lambda origin). This is called Bence Jones protein and should be detected by immunologic techniques (e.g., immunofixation).
• Bone marrow examination is essential for diagnosis, allowing the physician to determine the number of plasma cells (myeloma cells) in the marrow and their appearance. It also provides a measure of

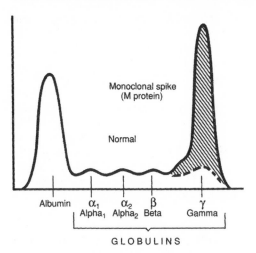

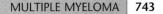

Serum protein electrophoresis (SPEP) patterns in multiple myeloma. Note the M-protein spike.

normal red cell, white cell, and platelet production.

Imaging

• X-rays of the skull, the entire spine, the pelvis, upper legs, and upper arms are necessary to detect lytic lesions, bone thinning (osteoporosis), or fractures. Skeletal abnormalities occur in 80 percent of patients at diagnosis.

• Bone scans with technetium-99 can be done but are not as effective as conventional X-rays for detecting lesions and are not recommended.

• CT or MRI scans are helpful when the patient has skeletal pain and negative X-rays or features of spinal nerve compression. PET scans may be helpful in determining the extent of disease.

Staging

A clinical staging system based on a combination of laboratory findings that correlate with the myeloma cell mass has often been used. Patients are generally separated into those with low-cell mass (Stage I), high-cell mass (Stage III),

and those whose cell mass is between Stages I and III (Stage II). A further classification divides patients according to whether they are "A" (kidney function test is normal or only slightly elevated, with a creatinine less than 2 mg/dl) or "B" (the serum creatinine is equal to or greater than 2 mg/dl). The International Staging System (ISS) utilizes only beta-2 microglobulin (β_2-M) and serum albumin values. The plasma cell labeling index (measure of the rate of growth of the myeloma cells) and the β_2-M level are more helpful prognostic factors than the staging system.

Treatment Overview

Multiple myeloma involves all of the red bone marrow and is usually widespread when the diagnosis is made.

Not all patients who meet the minimal criteria for diagnosis of multiple myeloma should be treated. Because the disease is not curable and therapy causes potential side effects and involves cost, treatment should be delayed in asymptomatic patients until there is evidence of progression, symptoms appear, or treatment is needed to prevent complications. There is no evidence that early treatment of multiple myeloma is advantageous.

Autologous Stem Cell Transplantation (ASCT) In patients with newly diagnosed multiple myeloma who are considered eligible for ASCT, it is important to avoid an alkylating agent such as melphalan (Alkeran) until stem cells can be collected, because such therapy can damage stem cells and interfere with their collection. Some patients older than seventy years are physiologically younger and can undergo a transplant, whereas some patients younger than seventy years may have medical problems and may not be suitable candidates for ASCT. Dexamethasone (Decadron) alone and thalidomide (Thalomid) + dexamethasone are two of the most commonly used induction regimens for patients who are candidates for ASCT. Patients receiving thalidomide + dexamethasone should be anticoagulated with warfarin (Coumadin) in therapeutic doses or with low-molecular-weight heparin. Aspirin may reduce the risk of blood clots and is an alternative. The old intravenous regimen of VAD (vincristine [Oncovin] + doxorubicin [Adriamycin] + dexamethasone) is infrequently used as induction therapy because of the increased risk of catheter-related sepsis and thrombosis. Bortezomib (Velcade) and lenalidomide (Revlimid) are currently being tested in clinical trials as initial therapy. Both produce a high response rate when combined with dexamethasone.

After stem cell collection, ASCT can proceed as soon as the patient has recovered, or transplant may be delayed and the patient treated with other agents with the transplant being reserved for relapsed disease.

Melphalan 200 mg/m^2 is the most widely used preparative regimen for ASCT. ASCT produces a longer progression-free survival and a median overall survival increase of approximately one year, when compared with chemotherapy. Approximately 60 percent of our patients receiving ASCT are treated as outpatients and the mortality is 1 to 2 percent.

With tandem (double) ASCT, patients receive a second planned ASCT after recovery from the first transplant. Benefit of a second ASCT is limited to patients in whom complete response or very good partial response (greater than 90 percent reduction in M–protein level) was not achieved with the first transplant.

Patients who are not candidates for ASCT on the basis of age, performance status, and comorbidity are treated with alkylating agent therapy. Melphalan (Alkeran) + prednisone, given orally, produces an objective response in 50 to 60 percent of patients. Leukocyte and platelet counts should be determined at three-week intervals after beginning therapy, because the melphalan dosage must be altered until midcycle neutropenia or thrombocytopenia occurs. Chemotherapy should be continued until the patient is in a plateau state with stable serum and urine M-protein and no evidence of progression. Patients should be followed closely during the plateau state and the same chemotherapy should be reinstituted if relapse occurs after six months.

Because of the shortcomings of melphalan + prednisone, new combinations of chemotherapy drugs have been used. Although a multivariate analysis comparing melphalan + prednisone with a variety of combinations of alkylating agents revealed higher response rates with the latter, there was no significant difference in overall survival. In addition, there was no evidence that high-risk patients benefited from these newer combinations of chemotherapy.

Two recent randomized trials have compared melphalan + prednisone with melphalan + prednisone + thalidomide (Thalomid), or MPT. These trials have showed superior response rates and event-free survival with MPT. Consequently, MPT is an additional option for patients with newly diagnosed myeloma who are not candidates for ASCT. However, MPT is associated with significantly greater toxicity, including thrombosis; therefore, care must be exercised in patient selection.

Maintenance Therapy Maintenance therapy with interferon-alpha$_2$ is of limited value and is seldom used. Prednisone 50 mg every other day may be useful, but experience is limited. Recently, results from a randomized trial from France have showed improvement in event-free and overall survival with maintenance thalidomide (Thalomid) + pamidronate

(Aredia) following autologous stem cell transplant.

Allogeneic Bone Marrow Transplantation
Allogeneic bone marrow transplantation is advantageous because the graft contains no tumor cells and there may be a graft-versus-tumor effect (see chapter 15, "Bone Marrow and Blood Stem Cell Transplantation"). However, there is a mortality rate of at least 25 percent. Furthermore, 90 to 95 percent of patients are ineligible because of their age, lack of an HLA-matched sibling donor, or inadequate renal, pulmonary, or cardiac function. Conventional allogeneic transplantation is associated with too high of a mortality rate and is not recommended. Nonmyeloablative ("mini allo") allogeneic studies are being pursued, but mortality is 10 to 15 percent, graft-versus-host disease is a potential problem, and many patients relapse. We feel that nonmyeloablative approaches should be limited to protocol studies.

Supportive Therapy

• *Radiation* The use of radiation therapy should be limited to those patients with disabling pain who have a local process that has not responded to chemotherapy. Tylenol with codeine or another narcotic can usually control the pain. This approach is preferred to local radiation because pain frequently recurs in another site and local radiation does not benefit anyone with generalized disease.

• *Hypercalcemia* Elevated blood calcium level occurs in 15 to 20 percent of patients and should be suspected if symptoms such as loss of appetite, nausea, vomiting, excessive thirst, increased urine output, constipation, weakness, change in mental alertness, and confusion develop. Treatment is urgent because kidney failure is common. Therapy with intravenous fluids and prednisone is usually effective,

but if it isn't, there are a variety of other effective agents such as zoledronic acid (Zometa) and pamidronate (Aredia).

• *Infections* Bacterial infections may occur and must be diagnosed and treated promptly with appropriate antibiotics. All patients should receive pneumococcal and influenza immunizations. Prophylactic penicillin or intravenous gamma globulin should be considered

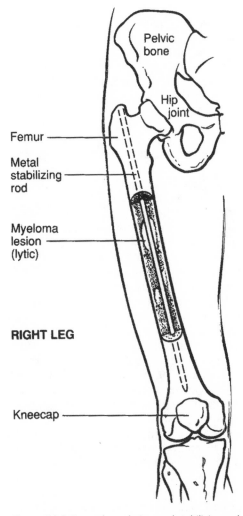

Bone with lytic myeloma lesion and stabilizing rod

for those with serious recurrent bacterial infections.

• *Skeletal Complications* Bone pain should be treated with analgesics or narcotics. People with multiple myeloma have to be as active as possible because confinement to bed increases bone loss. Patients must avoid falling because a fall can result in multiple fractures. Inserting an intramedullary rod into the long bone of the arm or leg should be considered when a large hole (lytic lesion) is seen on X-ray. The rod will stabilize the bone and prevent fractures. Radiation therapy to relieve pain may not be necessary for someone who is beginning chemotherapy. Intravenous bisphosphonates (zoledronic acid [Zometa] and pamidronate [Aredia]) help prevent fractures and reduce the number of skeletal lesions that need surgical or radiation intervention. They also improve quality of life and decrease the requirement for analgesics.

Patients with multiple myeloma who have lytic lesions or severe osteopenia (thinning of the bones) should be given intravenous bisphosphonates every four weeks. The dosage of bisphosphonates should be reduced in the presence of renal insufficiency. Serum creatinine and twenty-four-hour urine protein monitoring is necessary because renal insufficiency or nephrotic-range proteinuria may occur. One may consider stopping or reducing the intravenous bisphosphonate to every three months after two years of therapy unless there is evidence of progressive skeletal disease. Osteonecrosis of the jaw has been reported in patients receiving bisphosphonates. Consequently, it is essential to obtain a complete dental evaluation and perform preventive dental treatment prior to beginning bisphosphonates. Good oral hygiene should be practiced during therapy. Dental extractions or other invasive procedures should be avoided during bisphosphonate therapy.

Management of osteoporosis of the jaw should be conservative.

Both vertebroplasty (injection of methyl methacrylate [a cementlike substance] into a collapsed vertebral body) and kyphoplasty (introduction of an inflatable bone tamp into the vertebral body and after inflation the injection of methyl methacrylate into the vertebral cavity) have been used successfully to decrease pain and help restore height.

• *Kidney Failure* Increased fluid intake is necessary for patients with Bence Jones protein in the urine. They should drink enough fluids so that they produce approximately 3 quarts (3 l) of urine daily. Patients with acute kidney failure must be treated promptly with appropriate fluids and electrolytes. In some cases, removing large amounts of plasma from the blood (plasmapheresis) may be helpful in acute kidney failure. An artificial kidney (hemodialysis) may be necessary.

• *Anemia* Anemia occurs in almost all patients during the course of multiple myeloma. Symptomatic anemia requires therapy. Red cell transfusions are helpful. Erythropoietin may reduce or eliminate the need for transfusions. Erythropoietin improves the hemoglobin level and quality of life in about 60 percent of patients. Side effects are negligible and the major disadvantage is cost. The serum erythropoietin concentration is the most important factor predicting response, but some patients with normal levels will respond to the agent. Erythropoietin (epoetin alfa [Procrit, Epogen] or darbepoetin alfa [Aranesp], a long-acting erythropoietin), may be given. There is an increased risk of blood clots when erythropoietin therapy is combined with either thalidomide (Thalomid) or lenalidomide (Revlimid).

• *Hyperviscosity* This condition of "thick blood" is characterized by bleeding from the nose or gums, blurred vision, dizziness, shortness of breath, or mental confusion. It can be treated effectively with plasmapheresis.

• *Muscle Weakness* People with multiple myeloma may develop weakness or paralysis of their legs and have difficulty urinating or controlling their bowels. If this happens, a myeloma tumor pressing on the spinal cord is a possibility and can be diagnosed with an MRI or CT scan. The tumor can be treated effectively with radiation therapy.

• *Emotional Support* Anyone with multiple myeloma needs substantial and continuing emotional support. The approach must be positive, emphasizing the potential benefits of therapy. It is reassuring to know that some patients survive for ten years or more. It is vital that the physician caring for patients with multiple myeloma has the interest and capacity to deal with an incurable disease over a span of years with assurance, sympathy, and resourcefulness, and that patients can sense the doctor's confidence.

Treatment Follow-Up

• Complete blood count (CBC) every three weeks after each cycle of chemotherapy and before each treatment course
• Calcium and creatinine measured every six to twelve weeks
• Serum protein electrophoresis every six to twelve weeks
• Electrophoresis of a twenty-four-hour urine specimen every six to twelve weeks if an M-protein was found at the time of diagnosis
• Metastatic bone survey every six months or X-rays of bones in the event of new pain

• Bone marrow examination to confirm remission or relapse

Refractory Multiple Myeloma

Almost all patients who respond to chemotherapy or transplantation will eventually relapse. Until recently, the highest response rates in such patients have been with VAD given intravenously for ninety-six hours or as a bolus injection. Many physicians use dexamethasone (Decadron) as a single agent because it accounts for 80 percent of the effect of VAD.

New agents that have shown activity in relapsed myeloma in the past decade include thalidomide (Thalomid), lenalidomide (Revlimid), and the proteasome inhibitor bortezomib (Velcade). Thalidomide is usually given in a dosage of 50 to 200 mg daily with an objective response rate of 30 to 35 percent. Weakness, fatigue, constipation, somnolence, thrombotic events, skin rashes, and sensory-motor peripheral neuropathy are common side effects. Lenalidomide shows similar activity, but the side effects are much less troublesome. Bortezomib produces an objective response in about one-third of patients with relapsed, refractory disease. Fatigue, anorexia, nausea and vomiting, fever, diarrhea, constipation, anemia, neutropenia, thrombocytopenia, and peripheral neuropathy are adverse side effects.

The Most Important Questions You Can Ask

• Should I be treated now, or should therapy be delayed until I have symptoms?
• Should I receive an autologous or allogeneic bone marrow transplant?
• Should I get a second opinion?

Neuroendocrine (Islet Cell) Tumors of the Pancreas

Eric K. Nakakura, M.D., Ph.D., and Sean J. Mulvihill, M.D.

■ ■ ■ ■

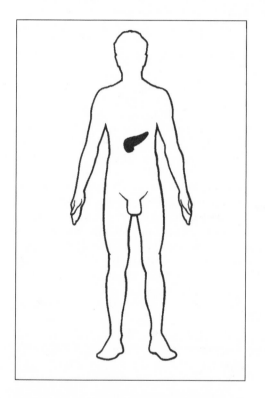

The pancreas is both an exocrine gland that produces enzymes to help digestion and an endocrine gland that produces insulin and other hormones to regulate the body's metabolism of glucose. Neuroendocrine tumors of the pancreas resemble the islet cells, the endocrine part of the gland; therefore, they are also commonly known as islet cell tumors. Neuroendocrine tumors of the pancreas are very uncommon, making up about 5 percent of all pancreatic cancers (about 1,300 cases each year). Pancreatic neuroendocrine tumors are much more curable than the more common exocrine pancreatic cancers.

These glandular tumors may be either functioning or nonfunctioning. Functioning tumors produce symptoms due to the secretion of one or more hormones normally produced by endocrine cells of the gut. These hormones include insulin, gastrin, glucagon, vasoactive intestinal polypeptide (VIP), somatostatin, pancreatic polypeptide (PP), and others.

Most functioning tumors producing insulin are benign, do not metastasize, and are classified as adenomas. Tumors producing gastrin, glucagon, or VIP are more likely to grow and spread to other organs, including the liver. About 90 percent of the nonfunctioning tumors are malignant.

Types The pancreatic islets are normally made up of four main cell types: alpha, beta, delta, and PP cells. These cells normally produce glucagon, insulin, somatostatin, and pancreatic polypeptide, respectively. Overproduction of a hormone or polypeptide by the tumor may produce symptoms. Pancreatic neuroendocrine tumors are named for the main type of hormone or polypeptide they produce—those that produce gastrin are called gastrinomas, those that produce insulin are insulinomas, and so on.

How It Spreads Spread may be by invasion of nearby tissues or metastases via the lymph system or bloodstream.

What Causes It The main underlying cause of these tumors remains unknown. In some tumors, genetic changes predisposing to cancer have been identified. In some cases, these genetic changes are familial—that is, they can be passed down from one generation to another.

Risk Factors

No special group is susceptible, but it is often found in those afflicted by the familial complex of tumors known as MEN (multiple endocrine neoplasia) type 1, a genetically transmitted group of endocrine abnormalities. These people develop several kinds of pancreatic neuroendocrine tumors—54 percent have multiple gastrinomas, 21 percent insulinomas, 3 percent glucagonomas, and 1 percent VIPomas. They also have a tendency to develop pituitary, parathyroid, and adrenal gland tumors.

Screening

When there is a family history of MEN-1, serum studies for calcium, gastrin, glucagon, insulin, and VIP may be useful. Genetic screening of patients from families at risk is becoming more common.

Common Signs and Symptoms

There is frequently a long delay between the initial symptoms and the diagnosis. The 90 percent of the nonfunctioning tumors that are malignant produce symptoms both by growing to a size where they put pressure on other tissues and by spreading to other organs.

The functioning, mainly benign pancreatic neuroendocrine tumors secrete active agents that have characteristic metabolic effects that create more symptoms than the tumor itself. When a functioning tumor becomes extremely large or metastatic, it will cause the same types of signs and symptoms as any other malignant tumor, as well as the hormonal symptoms.

• Gastrinomas (Zollinger-Ellison syndrome) produce an excess amount of gastrin, leading to increased production of stomach acid, severe peptic ulcer disease (multiple ulcers in an unusual location such as the jejunum), and often severe diarrhea. This syndrome accounts for less than 1 percent of all people with peptic ulcers. Other symptoms include abdominal pain and extreme weight loss.

• Insulinomas secrete excess insulin, leading to low blood sugar (hypoglycemia). Often, the symptoms of weight loss, fatigue, weakness, and hunger are attributed to psychological or neurologic disorders. Symptoms may be worse during fasting. In some patients, the low blood sugar is severe enough to cause fainting or loss of consciousness.

• The overproduction of glucagon by glucagonomas causes a characteristic skin rash (necrolytic migratory erythema) and a painful tongue (glossitis). Blood clots in the legs, which may travel to the lungs, have also been reported. Patients with glucagonoma often have unexpected weight loss.

• A pancreatic neuroendocrine tumor producing VIP results in a characteristic syndrome of massive, watery diarrhea and very low serum potassium. In addition, some patients have low serum chloride levels and high blood sugar (hyperglycemia) and calcium levels. The diarrhea in VIPomas is secretory (pancreatic cholera), in that it persists even when fasting. With severe diarrhea, up to $1\frac{1}{2}$ gallons (6 l) of small bowel fluid can be lost each day and patients can become dehydrated. Persistent diarrhea during fasting is very suspicious for VIPomas.

• Tumors that overproduce somatostatin cause electrolyte (mineral) abnormalities, diabetes mellitus, weight loss, malabsorption of food in the intestine (steatorrhea), loss of gastric acid (gastric achlorhydria), and occasionally gallstones.

Diagnosis

Blood and Other Tests

• Diagnosis of pancreatic neuroendocrine tumors can be confirmed with specific assays measuring the levels of gastrin, glucagon, insulin, VIP, somatostatin, or other hormones in the blood. Chromogranin A (CgA) levels may also be monitored, and elevated CgA levels may be found even in nonfunctioning pancreatic neuroendocrine tumors.

• An elevated serum gastrin level (often ten times normal) and an elevated stomach acid output raises suspicion of the Zollinger-Ellison syndrome and its associated gastrinoma.

• Measuring plasma proinsulin may help diagnose an insulinoma.

• Low serum potassium levels caused by secretory diarrhea may indicate a VIPoma.

• Elevated levels of serum somatostatin and diabetes with severe malabsorption should suggest a somatostatin-producing tumor.

Imaging

• Chest X-ray. This is done to check for spread of the tumor to the lungs.

• Abdominal CT or MRI scan. CT and MRI can show the main tumor if it is large enough (more than $\frac{1}{2}$ inch or 1 cm) and show spread to another organ such as the liver.

• Ultrasonography. This may be performed with a probe on the skin (transcutaneous), within the lumen of the stomach (endoscopic), or directly on the pancreas during surgery (intraoperative). Endoscopic or intraoperative ultrasound appears more sensitive than CT or MRI for finding very small tumors.

• Pancreatic arteriography can diagnose about 50 percent of cases, because some tumors—insulinoma, for example—are rich

in blood vessels and have a tumor "blush." This method is rarely used today, as it is more invasive than other techniques.

• Radioisotope scanning. It is possible to image most pancreatic neuroendocrine tumors with a scan using a specially labeled form of a peptidelike somatostatin (octreotide [Sandostatin]). This labeled peptide seeks out and binds to tumor cells, allowing them to be seen on the scan. The test is safe and painless but requires IV administration of the labeled compound.

Endoscopy and Biopsy Fine needle aspiration (FNA). This may be done to sample a tumor seen on CT or ultrasound, to confirm its nature. In most instances, a biopsy is not required; therefore, it is important to discuss this with a surgeon before it is done.

Staging/Classification

There is no universally accepted staging system for pancreatic neuroendocrine tumors. They can best be categorized as localized (in one site), regional (in the initial site and spread to lymph nodes), and metastatic to distant sites. In general, pancreatic neuroendocrine tumors are classified as well differentiated and poorly differentiated. The well-differentiated tumors are typically slow growing; however, there can be great variability in growth rate. The poorly differentiated tumors are highly aggressive and are typically treated with chemotherapy.

Treatment Overview

Surgery and chemotherapy are the two main treatment methods used, but only surgery can cure the disease. Careful observation may be an alternative approach for some pancreatic neuroendocrine tumors, especially those with few symptoms or slow-growing tumors. Radiotherapy is not effective.

Surgery Surgical removal of the tumor may lead to a cure. Depending on the location of the tumor, part of the pancreas may be removed (partial pancreatectomy) or the tumor mass may be excised—or "shelled out"—from the head of the pancreas (enucleation). When the tumor can't be completely removed, reducing its size (debulking) may still be a helpful palliative measure, given that these tumors are slow growing.

Chemotherapy When curative surgery is not possible, biotherapy and/or chemotherapy may be considered. Treatment with a somatostatin analogue called octreotide (Sandostatin; a form of biotherapy) is effective in controlling hormonally mediated symptoms and may stabilize tumor growth. Chemotherapy may be considered for patients with (1) symptoms due to pain, tumor bulk, or hormonal excess; (2) rapid disease progression; and (3) poorly differentiated pancreatic neuroendocrine tumors. Chemotherapy regimens containing streptozocin (Zanosar) are active against well-differentiated pancreatic neuroendocrine tumors. For poorly differentiated pancreatic neuroendocrine tumors, cisplatin (Platinol) and etoposide (Etopophos) are commonly used. Several biological and chemotherapy agents appear to be active against pancreatic neuroendocrine tumors. A technique called hepatic arterial chemoembolization delivers chemotherapy directly to the tumor via a catheter positioned in a suitable blood vessel. Currently this is useful for patients with tumor limited to the liver.

Treatment by Type

Gastrinoma

Sixty to 75 percent of gastrinomas are malignant and metastatic to lymph nodes or the liver at the time of diagnosis. Gastrinomas usually occur in the head of the pancreas, but up to one-third are found in the duodenum.

Standard Treatment The tumor should be removed if it can be precisely located by preoperative imaging studies or during surgery. Usually, small masses can be shelled out from the pancreas without the need for removing the whole organ. Removal of a localized tumor results in a high chance of cure.

Sometimes, the tumor cannot be found. In this case, the best approach is to block the acid production from the stomach with a proton-pump inhibitor. This prevents the two main symptoms of the tumor: ulcer pain and diarrhea.

Cutting the stomach nerves controlling acid secretion (vagotomy) and removing part of the stomach (partial gastrectomy) are old treatments not considered effective today. In rare cases in which medicines fail to control acid secretion and ulcerations recur or diarrhea persists, a total gastrectomy was once the treatment of choice; however, this has rarely been performed since the advent of proton-pump inhibitors.

In severe cases, primary management may include continuous stomach suction and intravenous replacement of sodium, potassium, and chloride to maintain electrolyte balance. Surgery can then remove a functioning tumor when the patient is stable. Postoperative gastrin levels are used for monitoring.

(For treatment for metastatic gastrinomas, see "Chemotherapy" in this chapter.)

Palliation Octreotide (Sandostatin) is a synthetic, long-acting somatostatin analogue that significantly decreases hormone secretion by tumor cells. It is useful for suppressing gastrin levels and inhibiting the hypersecretion of gastric acid characteristic of Zollinger-Ellison syndrome. This may be helpful if proton-pump inhibitor treatment fails.

Five-Year Survival 65 percent

Insulinomas

Insulinomas usually occur between ages forty and sixty. Ninety percent are benign and curable. Ninety percent occur within the pancreas.

Standard Treatment Removal of the pancreatic tumor is the basic approach. Most of these tumors can be enucleated (locally removed) and formal pancreatic resection is not required. Occasionally, patients benefit from surgical removal of metastases to help reduce symptoms from high levels of insulin and low blood sugar.

For pancreatic tumors that can't be removed or for widespread metastatic tumors, combination chemotherapy (streptozocin [Zanosar]–based), diazoxide (Proglycem), or somatostatin analogue (octreotide [Sandostatin]) can be given.

 Palliation Dietary changes, including frequent small meals and increased carbohydrates, may help reduce low blood sugar. An insulin-inhibiting drug such as diazoxide (Proglycem) may also help. Radiation therapy is not effective. Octreotide (Sandostatin) may be used to block insulin release from the tumor.

Five-Year Survival 80 percent

Glucagonomas

These tumors are often very large by the time they are discovered. They tend to be more aggressive than insulinomas.

Standard Treatment The tumor should be removed if possible. Because these tumors tend to be larger and more aggressive than insulinomas, removal of the portion of the pancreas around the tumor is usually necessary. If surgery is not possible because of widespread metastases or invasion into adjacent organs, palliation of symptoms is usually possible with octreotide (Sandostatin).

Chemotherapy with a streptozocin (Zanosar)–based regimen may be considered with advanced disease (see "Chemotherapy" in this chapter). Occasionally, partial surgical removal of the tumor (debulking) will relieve symptoms. Destruction of liver tumors through radiofrequency ablation (using heat to kill the tumor cells) can be helpful in reducing symptoms. (See chapter 13, "Radiofrequency-Generated Heat Treatment.")

VIPomas

Over 40 percent of these tumors are malignant. Most VIPomas occur in the pancreas, but some are associated with nerves in the back of the abdomen (retroperitoneum).

Standard Treatment Single lesions can be removed by a partial pancreatectomy. If the tumor has spread to the liver, it is sometimes helpful to remove both the primary tumor in the pancreas and as many liver lesions as possible. This debulking may reduce diarrhea. Radiofrequency ablation is also helpful for liver lesions that cannot be removed. Octreotide (Sandostatin) may also help relieve diarrhea.

Combination chemotherapy with a streptozocin (Zanosar)–based regimen may be given if the tumors cannot be removed (see "Chemotherapy" in this chapter).

 Palliation Octreotide (Sandostatin) is effective in reducing VIPoma symptoms, but it is not curative and often works for only a limited time. Fluids and electrolytes have to be replenished to avoid dehydration from the diarrhea.

Somatostatin-Producing Tumors

These are rare tumors, with fewer than 100 cases reported in the world medical literature. They are almost always malignant.

Standard Treatment Surgical removal of the tumor is the standard treatment for local disease. Combined chemotherapy with a streptozocin (Zanosar)–based regimen is used in patients with metastases (see "Chemotherapy" in this chapter). A few patients with liver metastases benefit from liver resection, radiofrequency ablation, or chemoembolization.

 Palliation Drugs used to relieve symptoms include the insulin-inhibiting drug diazoxide (Proglycem) and phenoxybenzamine (Dibenzyline), an alpha-adrenergic blocking agent.

Nonfunctioning Pancreatic Neuroendocrine Tumors

Nonfunctioning pancreatic neuroendocrine tumors do not produce clinical symptoms either because only a small amount of hormones are secreted or because a peptide without obvious activity, such as pancreatic polypeptide, is elaborated. In general, most nonfunctioning pancreatic neuroendocrine tumors are malignant, but they behave less aggressively than exocrine pancreatic cancer (cancer arising from the pancreatic duct cells).

Standard Treatment The only curative treatment is surgical resection. This is possible only in patients with tumor confined to the pancreas without invasion of adjacent organs or blood vessels. A radical pancreatic resection is often required. Radiation and chemotherapy are seldom effective against the main tumor.

 Palliation When the tumor has spread beyond the pancreas or invaded nearby organs or blood vessels, palliative therapy is considered (see "Chemotherapy" in this chapter).

Recurrent Cancer

Before deciding on further therapy for recurrences, the clinical situation will have to be reevaluated. Surgery or medical therapy for metastatic disease could be considered depending on the stage/classification, the site of recurrence, the presence of metastases, and individual factors. Participation in clinical trials should also be considered.

The Most Important Questions You Can Ask

• Will the removal of my tumor reduce or eliminate my symptoms?

• Can medical treatment control my cancer and reduce my symptoms?

• Are there any cancer centers where I could go for a second opinion?

Ovarian Germ Cell Tumors

Jeffrey L. Stern, M.D.

■ ■ ■ ■

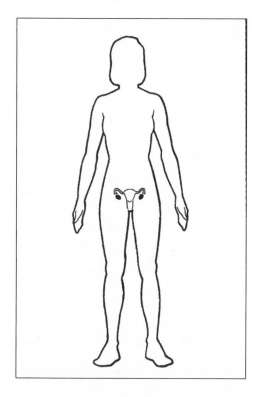

Germ cell tumors account for less than 5 percent of all ovarian malignancies. They almost always occur in women of reproductive age and are most frequently found in women in their teens or twenties. Many types of germ cell tumors are extremely aggressive, fast-growing malignancies. In the past, they were often fatal within two years even though frequently confined to one ovary at the time of diagnosis. With surgery and modern multiagent chemotherapy, the cure rate is excellent.

Types The main types of ovarian germ cell tumors include: dysgerminoma, endodermal sinus tumor, embryonal carcinoma, choriocarcinoma, immature teratoma, mixed germ cell tumor, and malignant transformation of a benign dermoid.

How It Spreads Ovarian germ cell tumors can spread directly to the adjacent pelvic organs and through the lymph system to the pelvic, aortic, chest (mediastinal), groin, and neck lymph nodes. They may also spread to the surfaces of the abdominal cavity and to distant organs such as the liver, lungs, and brain.

What Causes It The cause is not clear.

Risk Factors

At Significantly Higher Risk

- Premenopausal women
- Women with abnormal (dysgenetic) ovaries usually containing male chromosomes

Screening

No definitive screening method is available, except for a routine annual pelvic, abdominal, and rectal examination.

Common Signs and Symptoms

These tumors often do not cause any significant symptoms. Some women, however, will have a rapidly enlarging pelvic or abdominal mass and vague pain in the lower abdomen. Other women can experience abnormal vaginal bleeding or acute abdominal symptoms, including pain and shock.

Diagnosis

Physical Examination

- In addition to a careful pelvic exam, a general physical examination should pay particular attention to the lymph nodes in the neck above the collarbone, under the arms, and the groin.
- An abdominal examination may find an enlarged liver, a mass or masses, or excessive fluid (ascites).

Blood and Other Tests

- Serum beta human chorionic gonadotropin (HCG) is elevated in choriocarcinoma.
- Serum alpha-fetoprotein (AFP) is elevated in endodermal sinus tumors.
- Serum lactate dehydrogenase (LDH) is elevated in dysgerminoma.
- One or more of the tumor markers—serum HCG, AFP, and LDH—may be elevated in mixed germ cell tumors.
- Serum CA-125 may also be elevated.

Imaging

- Chest, abdominal, and pelvic PET/CT scan.
- Chest X-ray.

Endoscopy and Biopsy The definitive diagnosis is made on histologic evaluation of the removed ovary.

Staging

The International Federation of Gynecology and Obstetrics (FIGO) staging classification for malignant epithelial carcinomas of the ovaries is also used for staging malignant germ cell tumors of the ovary. Germ cell tumors of the ovary are surgically staged.

■ *Stage I* The cancer is confined to one or both ovaries.

- *IA* The cancer is limited to one ovary. There is no tumor on the surface of the ovary, the surface of the tumor is unruptured, and there is no ascites.
- *IB* Growth is limited to both ovaries. There is no tumor on the surface of either ovary, the surface of the tumors is unruptured, and there is no ascites.
- *IC* The tumor is either Stage IA or IB, but there is tumor on the surface of one or both ovaries, at least one of the tumors has ruptured, ascites is present, or the abdominal washings contain malignant cells.

■ *Stage II* The cancer involves one or both ovaries with extension to other pelvic structures.

- *IIA* There is extension of the tumor or metastases to the uterus and/or the fallopian tubes.
- *IIB* There is extension to other pelvic organs such as the bladder and rectum.
- *IIC* The cancer is either Stage IIA or IIB, but there is tumor on the surface of one or both ovaries, at least one of the tumors has ruptured, there is ascites with malignant cells, or the washings from the abdominal cavity contain malignant cells.

■ *Stage III* The tumor involves one or both ovaries with tumor present outside the pelvis or there is cancer in the abdominal or groin lymph nodes.

- *IIIA* The tumor is grossly limited to the pelvis, but there is microscopic cancer involving the abdominal cavity (peritoneal) surfaces. The lymph nodes are negative.
- *IIIB* The tumor involves one or both ovaries, and there are tumor implants on the peritoneal surfaces less than $\frac{3}{4}$ inch (2 cm) in diameter. The lymph nodes are negative.
- *IIIC* The tumor involves one or both ovaries, there are tumor implants on the

surface of the abdominal cavity greater than ¾ inch (2 cm) in diameter, or there is cancer in the pelvic, para-aortic, or groin lymph nodes.

■ *Stage IV* There are distant metastases to the liver or lungs or there are malignant cells present in the fluid accumulated in the chest cavity.

Treatment Overview

Surgery Surgical removal of the involved ovary or ovaries and removal of as much of the grossly visible tumor as possible is performed in all cases. If there is no spread beyond the ovaries, treatment will involve meticulous surgical staging, including removal of the pelvic and para-aortic lymph nodes, washings of the abdominal cavity to look for malignant cells, and careful inspection of the abdominal surfaces with multiple, random biopsies from the diaphragm and surfaces of the abdominal cavity. An omentectomy (removal of fatty tissue attached to the stomach and large intestine) will also be performed. Recently, laparoscopic minimally invasive surgery has been performed in selected cases with similar results.

The cell type of the tumor is an extremely important factor in determining the prognosis and the appropriate therapy after surgery.

Chemotherapy Women with a tumor confined to one ovary (Stage I) or with a well-differentiated (Grade 1) immature teratoma or dysgerminoma do not require postoperative chemotherapy. All others are usually treated with multidrug chemotherapy.

Until recently, external radiation therapy to the abdomen and pelvis with a boost to the para-aortic node region was standard therapy for dysgerminomas, but chemotherapy is now used more often to preserve fertility.

Women with other malignant germ cell tumors are treated with chemotherapy after surgery because radiation therapy is ineffective. The most commonly used chemotherapeutic drug regimen includes cisplatin (Platinol) and etoposide (Etopophos) with or without bleomycin (Blenoxane) given monthly for three or four courses.

Second-Look Surgery Occasionally, in women with Stage II, III, or sometimes IV disease who have no evidence of persistent cancer after chemotherapy, "second-look" exploratory abdominal surgery is performed to see if they are truly disease-free.

Second-look surgery is not usually performed on correctly staged women with well-differentiated immature teratomas, Stage IA and IB dysgerminomas, or other Stage I germ cell tumors who had elevated alpha-fetoprotein, HCG, or LDH levels before treatment that returned to normal with chemotherapy.

Women who have bulky disease after chemotherapy may occasionally benefit from tumor debulking at a second surgery.

Treatment by Stage and Cell Types
Dysgerminomas

■ *Stage IA*

Standard Treatment Removal of the involved ovary and fallopian tube as well as a wedge biopsy of the opposite, normal-appearing ovary and meticulous surgical staging is performed in women who want to preserve their fertility. For women who do not desire more children or who are approaching menopause, a hysterectomy and removal of both tubes and both ovaries may be performed. Women with Stage IA disease generally require no further treatment.

■ *Stage IB*

About 20 percent of women will have microscopic disease in the opposite, apparently normal ovary (Stage IB).

Standard Treatment Removal of both ovaries, tubes, and uterus and surgical staging. Women with this stage of disease are usually treated with three courses of cisplatin (Platinol) and etoposide (Etopophos) with or without bleomycin (Blenoxane).

Investigational

• Postoperative chemotherapy for women with microscopic disease in the opposite ovary, in an effort to preserve the ovary and fertility. Preserving the uterus in women who had both ovaries removed and who are desirous of having children.

• Combinations of chemotherapy, including varying doses and combinations of carboplatin (Paraplatin), cisplatin (Platinol), ifosfamide (Ifex), etoposide (Etopophos), vinblastine (Velban), paclitaxel (Taxol), docetaxel (Taxotere), and bleomycin (Blenoxane).

■ *Stage IC*

Standard Treatment After surgery, most gynecologic oncologists recommend three courses of cisplatin (Platinol) and etoposide (Etopophos) with or without bleomycin (Blenoxane).

■ *Stages II, III, and IV*

Standard Treatment Depending on the extent and location of disease, standard therapy includes a hysterectomy, removal of both tubes and both ovaries, aggressive tumor debulking to remove all grossly visible cancer, and at least three courses of cisplatin (Platinol) or carboplatin (Paraplatin), and etoposide (Etopophos) with or without bleomycin (Blenoxane). The opposite ovary and the uterus can be preserved, if normal, in women who want to maintain their reproductive capacity. Whole abdomen radiation may be given to those women who fail to respond to chemotherapy or who are not interested in preserving their reproductive function.

Investigational Same as for Stage IB.

Nondysgerminomatous Germ Cell Tumors

These include endodermal sinus tumors, embryonal carcinomas, choriocarcinomas, immature teratomas, and mixed germ cell tumors. Malignant transformation of a benign dermoid is its own unique entity that can result in a tumor of almost any histologic subtype, resembling tumors that arise from any other part of the body.

■ *Stage I*

Standard Treatment Removal of the affected tube and ovary and surgical staging are all that is required, since these tumors rarely occur in both ovaries. Postoperative chemotherapy, including cisplatin (Platinol) or carboplatin (Paraplatin), and etoposide (Etopophos) with or without bleomycin (Blenoxane), is given to all patients for three or four courses. Those with Grade 1 (well-differentiated) immature teratomas do not require chemotherapy.

Investigational Other chemotherapy drugs, including varying doses and combinations of carboplatin (Paraplatin), cisplatin (Platinol), platinum analogues, ifosfamide (Ifex), paclitaxel (Taxol), docetaxel (Taxotere), etoposide (Etopophos), and bleomycin (Blenoxane), are currently under investigation.

■ *Stages II, III, and IV*

Standard Treatment Depending on the extent and location of disease, a hysterectomy, bilateral removal of the tubes and ovaries, and aggressive tumor debulking is usually performed. If the opposite ovary and uterus are normal, they can be preserved in women who want to maintain their reproductive function. Four courses of chemotherapy, including cisplatin (Platinol), bleomycin (Blenoxane), and etoposide (Etopophos), are given after surgery.

Investigational

• Experimental therapy for advanced nondysgerminomatous germ cell tumors includes combinations of chemotherapeutic drugs such as carboplatin (Paraplatin), cisplatin (Platinol), bleomycin (Blenoxane), paclitaxel (Taxol), ifosfamide (Ifex), etoposide (Etopophos), and docetaxel (Taxotere). Dermoids that have transformed into malignancy are typically treated according to their dominant histologic appearance.

• High-dose chemotherapy and autologous bone marrow rescue.

Five-Year Survival Rates

The five-year survival rates for Stages IA and IB dysgerminomas and Grade 1 immature teratomas are over 95 percent. Even women with Stage III dysgerminomas have approximately an 80 percent survival rate.

Survival rates for women with Stages I and II nondysgerminomatous germ cell tumors are greater than 90 percent. Women with Stage III and IV disease have survival rates estimated to be greater than 75 percent.

Treatment Follow-Up

All women with germ cell tumors need careful follow-up every three months for the first two years after treatment.

• Follow-up should include a careful physical examination and serum HCG, alpha-fetoprotein, LDH, and CA-125 levels

(depending on which was elevated before therapy).

• Occasionally, radiologic studies such as an abdominal and pelvic PET/CT scan are performed as required.

Recurrent Cancer

Germ cell tumors may recur in the pelvis, abdominal cavity, liver, lungs, and lymph nodes. Symptoms may include pelvic or abdominal pain, bleeding, nausea, vomiting, abdominal swelling, weight loss, and chronic cough.

• Women with recurrent cancer in the pelvis and abdomen usually undergo an exploratory laparotomy with aggressive surgical debulking of the tumor.

• Women with recurrent dysgerminomas who did not receive chemotherapy or radiation therapy previously can be treated with combination chemotherapy or pelvic radiation up to a dose of 3,000 to 5,000 cGy over four to five weeks and whole abdomen radiation therapy up to 1,500 cGy, with a boost of up to 1,500 cGy to the para-aortic area, over several weeks.

• Women with recurrent nondysgerminomatous tumors are generally treated with chemotherapy after surgery, as radiation is not effective for these tumors. The chemotherapeutic drugs of choice typically include a combination of two or more of the following agents: cisplatin (Platinol), carboplatin (Paraplatin), ifosfamide (Ifex), bleomycin (Blenoxane), etoposide (Etopophos), vinblastine (Velban), vincristine (Oncovin), dactinomycin (Cosmegen), and cyclophosphamide (Cytoxan).

The Most Important Questions You Can Ask

• What qualifications do you have for treating cancer? Will a specialist in gynecologic oncology be involved in my care?

- What kind of germ cell tumor do I have?
- What stage is it?
- Will I still be able to have children?
- Will I need chemotherapy?
- Do I need a second-look operation?

Ovary

Jeffrey L. Stern, M.D.

■ ■ ■ ■

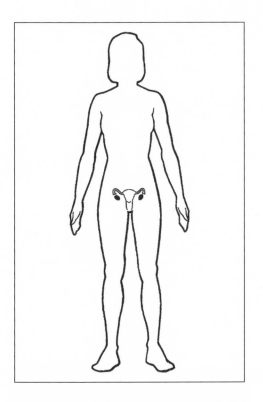

Carcinoma of the ovary is one of the most common gynecologic malignancies. In most cases, it is curable when found early, but because it may not cause any symptoms in its early stages, many women have widespread disease at the time of diagnosis. Partly because of this, the mortality rate from ovarian cancer exceeds that for all other gynecologic malignancies combined. It is the fourth most frequent cause of cancer death in women in the United States. About 1 in every 70 women will develop cancer of the ovary and 1 in every 100 women will die from it. The American Cancer Society estimates that there are 26,000 cases of ovarian cancer diagnosed each year with approximately 15,000 deaths.

Types The most common type of ovarian cancer arises from the cells covering the surface of the ovary and is known as epithelial carcinoma. There are five major cell types of this carcinoma—serous, mucinous, endometrioid, clear cell, and undifferentiated. Epithelial carcinomas are further divided into grades, according to how virulent they appear on microscopic examination.

Tumors of low malignant potential, also known as borderline tumors (Grade 0), are the slowest growing and account for 15 percent of all epithelial carcinomas of the ovary. The other three grades have progressively poorer prognoses: well differentiated (Grade 1), moderately differentiated (Grade 2), and poorly differentiated (Grade 3). Clear cell carcinomas and especially undifferentiated carcinomas have a poorer prognosis than the other cell types.

There are two other major types of ovarian cancers—germ cell tumors, which arise from the eggs, and ovarian stromal tumors, which arise from supportive tissue of the ovary. They are relatively uncommon and account for less than 10 percent of all ovarian malignancies (see the chapter "Ovarian Germ Cell Tumors").

How It Spreads Ovarian cancer spreads early by shedding malignant cells into the abdominal cavity. The cells implant on the lining of the abdominal cavity (peritoneum) and can grow on the surface of the liver, the fatty tissue attached to the stomach (omentum), the small and large intestines, the bladder, and the diaphragm.

Disease on the diaphragm may at times result in impaired drainage of fluid from the abdominal cavity, resulting, for some women, in a large collection of abdominal fluid known as ascites. The cancer cells spread to the surface of the lungs and chest cavity, resulting in a collection of fluid around the lungs known as a pleural effusion.

Ovarian cancer may also spread to the pelvic, aortic, groin, and neck lymph nodes.

What Causes It Unknown.

Risk Factors

There is a much higher incidence of ovarian cancer in industrialized countries. Some researchers have implicated talcum powder, which until recently contained asbestos, as a possible cause. Ovarian cancer can occur in any age group but is most common in postmenopausal women. Not ovulating—by having children, breast-feeding, using birth control pills, or having a condition that interferes with ovulation such as polycystic ovaries—has been shown to offer protection against developing cancer. There may also be a genetic predisposition to this cancer. There are families in which several members of the same or different generation develop ovarian cancer. This is known as hereditary ovarian cancer syndrome. Women with hereditary ovarian cancer syndrome are also at significant risk for the development of breast cancer, uterine cancer, and occasionally colon cancer. These individuals are often positive for the BRCA1 or BRCA2 gene, which can be detected in a blood test. There may be up to a 50 percent risk of

developing ovarian cancer in their lifetime. It can also be inherited through the male side of the family. This syndrome occurs in less than 3 percent of all women who have a positive family history of ovarian cancer. Approximately 7 percent of all women with ovarian cancer do not seem to have a genetic disposition but have a positive family history. Ninety percent of these women have only one other family member with ovarian cancer. Women who are positive for BRCA1 or BRCA2 generally develop cancer in their mid-forties.

Suggested management in women with a significant family history for ovarian cancer, or who are positive for the BRCA1 or BRCA2 gene, is as follows: removal of both ovaries and sometimes the uterus after childbearing, or very close follow-up with serum CA-125 and pelvic ultrasound every six months. In women who are BRCA1- or BRCA2-negative and who have only one relative with ovarian cancer, prophylactic removal of the ovaries is not recommended; while those women who have two to three close relatives with ovarian cancer, prophylactic removal of the ovaries is generally recommended by most gynecologic oncologists and geneticists.

Screening

There is no diagnostic method accurate enough to be used for routine screening of women without symptoms. Nonetheless, it is recommended that all women have an annual pelvic and rectal examination, since an ovarian mass can occasionally be detected. A Pap smear will detect ovarian cancer in only 10 percent of women. Studies have shown that a serum tumor marker known as CA-125 is elevated in 90 percent of women with advanced epithelial ovarian cancer and only 50 percent of women with cancer confined to the ovary (Stage I). Unfortunately, this test is not accurate enough for screening all women for ovarian cancer. Approximately 2 percent of normal women will have an elevated CA-125 (normal is less than 35). Approximately 1 percent of normal women will have a CA-125 greater than 65. Because of the small incidence of false positive tests, screening all women with CA-125 has not been recommended. A great deal of research is taking place exploring the use of CA-125 as well as other tumor markers for screening. Tumor markers are, however, very useful for assessing response to therapy.

A pelvic ultrasound (sonogram) examination can be used for screening and may become a part of the routine annual gynecologic examination in the future. At present, however, it is used for diagnosis and not as a screening test, except in women at high risk for ovarian cancer. It is performed using a minimally uncomfortable vaginal probe, as well as one through the abdominal wall, to examine the ovaries and the uterus. When used in combination with CA-125, it is fairly accurate in detecting ovarian neoplasms.

Common Signs and Symptoms

Often women with early stages of ovarian carcinoma have no symptoms. The unfortunate result is that two-thirds of all women with ovarian carcinoma have advanced disease at the time of diagnosis.

Many women have vague, nonspecific abdominal symptoms, including pain, pelvic pressure, low back discomfort, mild nausea, gas and bloating, feeling full early when eating, and constipation. Some women have abnormal uterine bleeding. Although some cases are diagnosed during a routine gynecologic examination, many women are diagnosed only when they have developed marked abdominal distention because of the accumulation of fluid called ascites.

Advanced ovarian cancer often results in blockage of the intestines, causing severe nausea, vomiting, crampy abdominal pain, and constipation. Shortness of breath can occur in women who also develop fluid around the lungs (known as a pleural effusion).

Diagnosis

Physical Examination

• A careful pelvic exam is performed with attention to the ovaries, uterus, bladder, and rectum.

• The neck, groin, and underarms (axillae) are examined for enlarged lymph nodes.

• The lungs are carefully examined for excess fluid.

• The abdomen is examined for the presence of a mass, ascites, or an enlarged liver.

Blood and Other Tests

• Complete blood count (CBC).

• Serum liver and kidney function tests.

• Serum CA-125.

Imaging

• Pelvic ultrasound (sonogram).

• Abdominal and pelvic CT or PET/ CT scans may be obtained in advanced cases.

• Chest X-ray or chest CT scan.

Endoscopy and Biopsy

• A definitive diagnosis requires microscopic examination of part or all of the involved ovary or any other suspicious abdominal mass. Cystic ovarian tumors that are less than $2\frac{1}{2}$ inches (6 cm) in diameter occurring in premenopausal women are usually benign cysts.

• Surgical evaluation is strongly recommended for any ovarian mass in a postmenopausal woman. In premenopausal women, masses that are larger than $2\frac{1}{2}$ inches (6 cm) in diameter, persist longer than one menstrual cycle, or are suspicious on imaging of the ovaries with or without an elevated CA-125 level should also undergo surgery.

Staging

Ovarian carcinoma is staged based on the findings found at surgery. Stages are defined according to the classification system devised by FIGO (International Federation of Gynecology and Obstetrics). The TNM system corresponds to the stages accepted by FIGO.

■ *Stage I* The cancer is confined to one or both ovaries.

• *IA* The cancer is limited to one ovary. There is no ascites (abdominal fluid) and no tumor on the surface of the ovary, and the surface of the tumor is unruptured.
• *IB* The cancer is limited to both ovaries. There is no ascites and no tumor on the surface of either ovary, and the surfaces of the tumors are unruptured.
• *IC* The cancer is either Stage IA or IB and one or more of the following applies: There is tumor on the surface of one or both ovaries, at least one of the tumors has ruptured, ascites is present, or the abdominal washings contain malignant cells.

Five-Year Survival 60 to 100 percent, depending on the substage, histologic type, and grade.

■ *Stage II* The tumor involves one or both ovaries with extension to other pelvic structures.

• *IIA* There is extension of the cancer or metastases to the uterus and/or fallopian tubes.
• *IIB* There is extension or metastases to the surface of the bladder or rectum or to other pelvic tissues.
• *IIC* The cancer is either Stage IIA or IIB and one or more of the following applies: There is tumor on the surface of one or both ovaries, at least one of the tumors has ruptured, the ascites contains malignant cells, or the washings from the abdominal cavity contain malignant cells.

Five-Year Survival 60 to 80 percent

■ *Stage III* The tumor involves one or both ovaries, with tumor implants confined to the abdominal cavity but outside the pelvis, or there is cancer in the pelvic, para-aortic, or groin nodes.

• *IIIA* The tumor is grossly limited to the pelvis, and the lymph nodes are negative, but there is biopsy-proven microscopic cancer on the upper intra-abdominal (peritoneal) surfaces.
• *IIIB* There are tumor implants on the upper abdominal surfaces less than $3/4$ inch (2 cm) in diameter. The lymph nodes are negative.
• *IIIC* There are tumor implants on the surface of the abdominal cavity greater than $3/4$ inch (2 cm) in diameter, or there is cancer in the pelvic, para-aortic, or groin lymph nodes.

Five-Year Survival 20 to 65 percent

■ *Stage IV* There are distant metastases in the liver, as opposed to on the surface of the liver; there are malignant cells in the fluid surrounding the lungs; or there are metastases to anywhere else in the body.

Five-Year Survival 10 to 40 percent

Treatment Overview

Surgery In women with early-stage cancer, one or both ovaries are usually removed (with or without removal of the uterus) and meticulous surgical staging is performed. This involves washings from the abdominal cavity to detect malignant cells, removal of the pelvic and aortic lymph nodes, careful inspection of the abdominal cavity surfaces with biopsy of any suspicious lesions, removal of the fatty tissue attached to the stomach and large intestine (omentectomy), and multiple random biopsies of the lining of the abdominal cavity, including the surfaces of the diaphragm.

In women with advanced cancer, surgical removal of as much tumor as possible, called tumor debulking, is standard therapy. If possible, the uterus, the omentum, and as much of the grossly visible cancer as is feasible is removed.

Recent studies have shown that 25 to 35 percent of women with ovarian carcinoma will require intestinal or urologic surgery to obtain optimal tumor debulking (defined as leaving behind no tumor implant greater than $\frac{3}{4}$ inch [2 cm] in diameter). An enormous effort is made by most gynecologic oncologists to leave no cancer at the end of surgery. A permanent colostomy may occasionally be necessary but is rare in women who have had a preoperative bowel prep—a cleansing of the intestines with enemas and laxatives and administration of antibiotics.

To decide if further treatment is required, second-look abdominal surgery may be performed after six cycles of chemotherapy in women without evidence of persistent cancer (see "Treatment Follow-Up" in this chapter).

In women with recurrent cancer, surgery is often required to relieve intestinal obstruction or to remove all visible cancer again if possible.

Complications of surgery can include infection; bleeding requiring transfusion; injury to the bladder, rectum, or ureter causing a leak (fistula); and injury to the blood vessels or nerves. There may be blood clots in the legs, which can occasionally dislodge and travel to the lungs (pulmonary embolism), pneumonia, wound infection, intestinal blockage, and hernia.

Minimally invasive surgery has become possible in women with undiagnosed ovarian tumors and occasionally in early ovarian cancer. Its use has primarily been in women who have ovarian tumors thought to be confined to the ovary. Laparoscopic removal of the ovary with a frozen section (intraoperative rapid histologic diagnosis) is performed, and if the specimen is cancerous, either a laparoscopic or an open traditional staging procedure can be performed.

Laparoscopy is actively being studied by the Gynecologic Oncology Group in the management of women who have had removal of one or both ovaries, as well as the uterus, for ovarian cancer, but who are incompletely staged. Within ten weeks of initial surgery, laparoscopic surgical staging can be performed.

In selected women, a second-look minimally invasive surgery can be performed in those women who are clinically free of disease and who are either thought to be at high risk for diffuse intra-abdominal small disease or thought to have no cancer.

Laparoscopy can also be performed to place an intra-abdominal catheter to administer chemotherapy (see below).

Chemotherapy In most cases, chemotherapy is begun within four weeks after surgery. The standard regimen includes carboplatin (Paraplatin) + paclitaxel (Taxol) or docetaxel (Taxotere) given intravenously every three weeks as tolerated for at least six cycles. Eighty percent of patients can be expected to respond. The response rate depends to a large degree on the amount of cancer remaining after surgery, with those who have no visible cancer after surgery having the best response rates.

Another technique, known as intraperitoneal (intra-abdominal) chemotherapy, may be used to deliver the chemotherapy directly into the abdominal cavity.

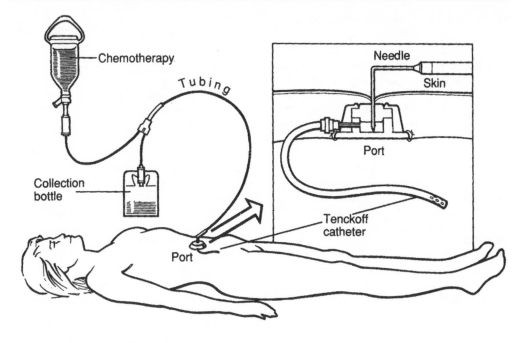

Intraperitoneal chemotherapy for ovarian cancer

This procedure requires surgery to place a plastic port and its attached catheter beneath the skin, usually on the upper abdomen. It is often placed at the time of the initial surgery, at the time of a second-look procedure, or with laparoscopy. The catheter is brought through the abdominal wall and placed directly in the abdominal cavity. The cancer drugs are then given via a needle directly into the port. The port requires periodic flushing with blood thinners to keep it open. Complications include infection, malfunction of the catheter, and occasionally intestinal blockage. Sometimes chemotherapy is given both intravenously and intra-abdominally.

Intraperitoneal chemotherapy is generally given monthly for six months. Recent trials have indicated a survival benefit for patients who receive both intravenous and intraperitoneal chemotherapy following surgery compared to those receiving intravenous chemotherapy alone following surgery.

Chemotherapy, depending on the drug, can cause hair loss; nausea and vomiting; infection or bleeding because of bone marrow toxicity; damage to the heart, kidneys, nerves, and liver; and numbness or tingling in the fingers and toes.

Preoperative Chemotherapy Chemotherapy is sometimes given prior to the initial surgery, especially in those women with advanced disease with a large amount of ascites (intra-abdominal fluid) and a pleural effusion (fluid around the lungs). It may also be given to patients who have surgical risks because of poor medical health. Many gynecologic oncologists also give preoperative chemotherapy (usually three to four courses over nine to twelve weeks) followed by surgery to almost all women with advanced disease.

The frequency of an optimal resection is significantly improved and the literature indicates that the morbidity, extent of surgery (i.e., the need for extensive intestinal surgery), and length of hospitalization are markedly lessened with preoperative chemotherapy. The survival rates appear to be equivalent to having surgery first.

 Radiation There is some evidence that external-beam radiation therapy is as effective as chemotherapy for patients with early stages of ovarian carcinoma who have no visible cancer remaining after their operation; however, it is rarely recommended because of its toxicity.

Sometimes radiation therapy is used to treat microscopic persistent ovarian cancer that has not responded well to chemotherapy. Radiation may be given to the pelvis or, more typically, to the entire abdomen (usually five days each week for four to five weeks), which results in a better survival rate. Complications and side effects can be considerable and include diarrhea, nausea and vomiting, bleeding from the bladder or rectum, vaginal scarring, intestinal obstruction, and leaks (fistulas) from the urinary or intestinal tract.

Treatment by Stage

■ Stage IA

Standard Treatment Therapy depends primarily on the age of the patient and the grade of the cancer.

For women who have a borderline or a well-differentiated tumor (Grade 1) and who want to preserve their reproductive function, standard therapy includes removal of the cancerous ovary and the adjacent fallopian tube (the other, apparently healthy ovary, however, should be biopsied), removal of the omentum, and removal of the pelvic and para-aortic lymph nodes.

For postmenopausal women and those who do not want to preserve their reproductive function, standard therapy includes a total hysterectomy, removal of both fallopian tubes and ovaries, and careful surgical staging. Women with Stage IA borderline or Grade 1 carcinoma are usually cured with surgery alone.

Standard therapy for Grade 2 (moderately differentiated) or 3 (poorly differentiated) tumors is total hysterectomy, removal of both tubes and ovaries, meticulous surgical staging, and six cycles of combination chemotherapy, usually with carboplatin (Paraplatin) + paclitaxel (Taxol) given every three weeks.

Investigational Intra-abdominal chemotherapy with agents such as cisplatin (Platinol) or carboplatin (Paraplatin).

■ Stage IB

Standard Treatment A total hysterectomy, removal of both fallopian tubes and ovaries, and meticulous surgical staging is performed. Women with tumors of low malignant potential or Grade 1 carcinoma do not require further treatment.

Women with Grade 2 or 3 cancers usually receive postoperative combination chemotherapy (usually carboplatin [Paraplatin] or cisplatin [Platinol] + paclitaxel [Taxol] given every three weeks for a total of six courses).

Investigational Same as for Stage IA.

■ Stage IC

Standard Treatment Hysterectomy, removal of both fallopian tubes and ovaries, partial omentectomy, and removal of the pelvic and para-aortic lymph nodes is done. Careful inspection of the remaining intra-abdominal surfaces is vital. Suspicious lesions should be biopsied, and washings of the abdominal cavity should be taken to check for malignant cells.

Standard therapy after surgery includes six courses of carboplatin (Paraplatin) or cisplatin (Platinol) + paclitaxel (Taxol).

Investigational

• Intra-abdominal cisplatin (Platinol) or carboplatin (Paraplatin) or etoposide (Etopophos) with or without other anti-cancer drugs
• Whole abdomen and pelvic radiation therapy

■ Stage IIA

Standard Treatment The surgical procedure is the same as for Stage IC, again with biopsy of any suspicious lesions, pelvic and aortic node dissection, and washings of the abdominal cavity to check for malignant cells. Standard therapy after surgery includes six courses of carboplatin (Paraplatin) and paclitaxel (Taxol).

Investigational Intra-abdominal carboplatin (Paraplatin) or cisplatin (Platinol) with or without other intravenous anti-cancer drugs

■ Stages IIB, IIC, IIIA, IIIB, IIIC, and IV

Standard Treatment In women with advanced ovarian carcinoma, standard therapy involves removing as much of the tumor as possible as well as the uterus, both fallopian tubes and ovaries, and the omentum. Removal of the pelvic and para-aortic nodes is also performed.

If disease is on the small or large intestine, removal of a segment of the bowel may be required, and sometimes a portion of the diaphragm, liver, or even the gallbladder or spleen is removed. Frequently, there are multiple tumor implants all over the intra-abdominal surfaces ranging in size from a few millimeters to several inches. A major effort is made to remove each one of them, as the size of the largest single tumor implant left behind correlates with survival. It has been shown that the prognosis worsens with the larger the size of the largest single residual cancer implant that remains after surgery. Although the definition of what is known as an optimal surgical resection is changing, many gynecologic oncologists believe that leaving no residual cancer is better than leaving 5 mm disease, which in turn is better than leaving disease greater than $\frac{1}{2}$ inch (1 cm) in diameter.

Combination chemotherapy, including intravenous cisplatin (Platinol) and carboplatin (Paraplatin) together with paclitaxel (Taxol), is given for six cycles (one course every three weeks). Intravenous paclitaxel plus intra-abdominal cisplatin and paclitaxel has been shown in a large randomized trial of patients with Stage III disease to produce better outcomes than intravenous cisplatin and paclitaxel alone. Many gynecologists and medical oncologists give a year of consolidation chemotherapy, as the disease-free and overall survival is improved by giving monthly paclitaxel for one year after an initial course of carboplatin and paclitaxel.

Investigational Many investigational protocols using different combinations of multiple drugs in varying doses and schedules are being conducted in the treatment of ovarian cancer:

• Different doses and schedules of intravenous carboplatin (Paraplatin) + paclitaxel (Taxol)
• Intravenous analogues of cisplatin (Platinol)—for example, oxaliplatin (Eloxatin)
• Intravenous paclitaxel with other drugs
• Intravenous topotecan (Hycamtin)
• Intravenous doxorubicin liposomal (Doxil)
• Docetaxel (Taxotere)
• Intravenous cisplatin + gemcitabine (Gemzar)
• Etoposide (Etopophos)
• Intravenous gemcitabine

• Topotecan + thalidomide (Thalomid)
• Intra-abdominal administration of single agents, such as interferon, cisplatin, carboplatin, 5-fluorouracil (5-FU), leucovorin (LV), and paclitaxel (Taxol)
• Vinorelbine (Navelbine)
• Intravenous carboplatin + ifosfamide (Ifex)
• Immunotherapy with interleukin-2 or interleukin-2–activated mononuclear cells
• Bevacizumab (Avastin)
• Tamoxifen (Nolvadex)
• Megastrol acetate (Megace)
• Oral altretamine (Hexalen) or etoposide
• Irinotecan (Camptosar, CPT11)

Treatment Follow-Up

Follow-up is generally performed every three months for the first two years after treatment.

• The lymph nodes in the neck, groin, lungs, abdomen, and pelvis are carefully examined at each visit.
• The serum CA-125 level is followed closely and is frequently the first indication of recurrent cancer.
• Abdominal and pelvic CT or PET/CT scans may be done, but their routine use has not been shown to be effective in the absence of symptoms.

Second-Look Surgery If after six cycles of chemotherapy or after consolidation chemotherapy, there is no evidence of persistent disease—as determined by physical examination, the serum CA-125 level, and pelvic and abdominal PET/CT scans—then second-look surgery may be performed. Although it is sometimes considered the standard of care, there has been no consistently proven survival benefit of this procedure. It is, however, the most reliable way of determining whether any cancer is left after treatment.

If no obvious cancer is found during the second-look operation, a thorough assessment looking for microscopic cancer requires taking peritoneal washings and biopsies from all adhesions or, if there are none, twenty to thirty random biopsies from the surfaces of the bladder, pelvis, pelvic sidewalls, and diaphragm and the removal of pelvic and aortic lymph nodes (if not removed previously). If some of the omentum is still present, it is also removed. An appendectomy is usually done as well. Traditionally, at the second-look operation, if all the biopsies are negative, no further treatment is required. If disease is found at second-look surgery, then an effort is made to remove all grossly visible disease.

In the hands of a gynecologic oncologist, 25 to 60 percent of the women who had sub-optimal disease (any tumor nodule greater than $1/2$ inch [1 cm]) after the initial surgery and were then given chemotherapy can have a subsequent optimal surgical debulking. This is known as a re-debulking procedure and not a second-look operation.

Prognosis

The prognosis primarily depends on the stage, grade, and type of carcinoma and especially the amount of residual disease after the initial surgery.

Women with Stage I disease, especially Grade I or II, have an excellent prognosis. Even those with Grade 3 do well with chemotherapy. Women who have Stage II, III, or IV, Grade 1, carcinoma and a negative second-look procedure have an excellent prognosis. Women with Grade 2 or 3 cancer and a negative second look also have a good prognosis but have a significant risk for developing recurrent disease. It is estimated that 30 to 50 percent of women with Grade 3 cancer will develop a recurrence within five years even after a negative second look.

Even those with Stage IIIC disease and a negative second-look procedure have a 40 percent chance of recurrence. For women who have microscopic disease at their second-look procedure, the prognosis is not as good and is partially dependent upon the grade of the cancer. These women are treated with more intravenous combination chemotherapy, intra-abdominal chemotherapy, or, occasionally, whole abdomen radiation.

Women with bulky residual cancer (implants greater than ½ inch [1 cm]) after a second-look procedure have a poor prognosis despite aggressive treatment with second-line chemotherapy.

Recurrent Cancer

Women whose cancer returns after initial therapy are candidates for exploratory surgery for further aggressive tumor debulking. The goal of surgery is to remove all visible disease. The prognosis is better the later the recurrence takes place after chemotherapy has ended. Postoperative therapy varies and may include intravenous chemotherapy and intra-abdominal chemotherapy. In many cases treatment may only be palliative.

Different regimens of chemotherapy have been used with some benefit, including various combinations and doses of carboplatin (Paraplatin), cisplatin (Platinol), oxaliplatin (Eloxatin), paclitaxel (Taxol), docetaxel (Taxotere), topotecan (Hycamtin), irinotecan (Camptosar, CPT11), doxorubicin liposomal (Doxil), cyclophosphamide (Cytoxan), gemcitabine (Gemzar), altretamine (Hexalen), 5-fluorouracil, ifosfamide (Ifex), doxorubicin (Adriamycin), etoposide (Etopophos), and melphalan (Alkeran) (see "Investigational" in this chapter).

The Most Important Questions You Can Ask

• What qualifications do you have for treating cancer? Will a gynecologic oncologist be involved in my care?

• Why will or will I not receive preoperative chemotherapy?

• What is the stage, cell type, and grade of my cancer?

• How much cancer remained after surgery?

• Should I receive intraperitoneal (intra-abdominal) chemotherapy?

• What is the reason for the type of therapy you recommended after surgery?

• What is the benefit of second-look surgery?

Pancreas

Andrew H. Ko, M.D., Margaret A. Tempero, M.D., and Sean J. Mulvihill, M.D.

■ ■ ■ ■

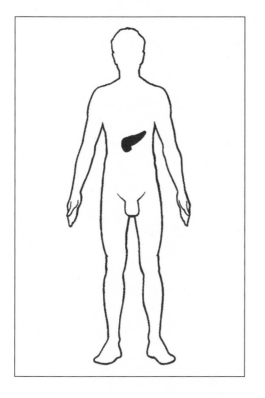

Pancreatic cancer is the fourth most common cause of cancer deaths in the United States. In 2007, there will be about 37,170 new cases and 33,370 deaths from the disease. For unknown reasons, the number of cases has been gradually increasing every year, especially in industrialized countries.

Types Ninety percent of pancreatic cancers are adenocarcinomas. These usually develop in the pancreatic ducts that carry enzymes made by the pancreas to the small intestine to aid digestion and are thus referred to as ductal adenocarcinomas. Other rare tumor types that can arise from the pancreas include adenosquamous, undifferentiated, small cell, and acinar cell carcinomas; cystadenocarcinomas; and lymphomas. An entirely different class of tumors that arise from the pancreas develop from the endocrine component of the organ known as the islets of Langerhans. These islets are normally responsible for the production of insulin and other hormones. Islet cell tumors of the pancreas, which are discussed in a separate chapter in this book, have very different prognostic and therapeutic implications from ductal adenocarcinomas (see "Neuroendocrine (Islet Cell) Tumors of the Pancreas").

How It Spreads Two-thirds of pancreatic cancers are located in the head of the organ (on the right side) and one-third arise in the body and tail (left side) of the gland (see the illustration of the gallbladder, liver, pancreas, and associated organs in the chapter "Gallbladder"). Tumor cells may spread by direct extension to adjacent

Pancreatic cancer is a common malignancy that is treatable if diagnosed early but is rarely curable. Diagnosis is usually not possible until symptoms appear, and by that time the cancer is often advanced. Because the pancreas resides deep in the abdomen close to the backbone near vital structures, and because tumors often produce few early symptoms, this cancer is not easily diagnosed at a possibly curable stage. Only about 10 percent of pancreatic cancers can be removed surgically.

structures such as the bile duct, duodenum, stomach, spleen, and colon. Tumor cells can also spread through lymphatic channels to regional lymph nodes. The most common sites for distant metastases are the liver, peritoneum, and lungs.

What Causes It It is not definitely known what causes pancreatic cancer, although age is a factor. There may also be racial or dietary factors. Smoking increases the risk of developing pancreatic cancer threefold. Concerns have been raised about the role of coffee, but there is no proof of an association.

Risk Factors

At Significantly Higher Risk

• Increasing age. Rare before age forty, the incidence peaks at around age sixty.

• Smokers of two packs a day. The incidence increases directly with the amount smoked and the number of years one smokes.

• Over ten years' exposure to chemicals, particularly petroleum compounds and solvents.

• Sufferers of chronic inflammation of the pancreas (chronic pancreatitis).

• Diet high in fat and red meat, low in fruits and vegetables.

At Slightly Higher Risk

• There is some association with alcohol consumption.

• History of diabetes or cirrhosis, particularly in women.

• Men outnumber women by a ratio of 3 to 1. African-Americans have a greater incidence than Caucasians.

• Prior gastrectomy. Decreased stomach acid leads to nitrates in foods becoming nitrosamines—carcinogens.

Screening

No effective screening methods are available for the general population. However, certain academic medical centers have developed programs to screen individuals who are at particularly high risk for developing pancreatic cancer, such as those with a strong family history.

Common Signs and Symptoms

There are no warning signs. The most common symptom is a vague upper abdominal or back pain. There may also be loss of appetite, nausea and vomiting, constipation (50 percent of patients), weight loss (early feeling of fullness is usual in 50 percent of cases), diarrhea, bloating, belching, and hiccups. Other symptoms include itching skin, swollen legs, sleeping problems, and fatigue. The cancer is often recognized late in its development, after spread to other organs has occurred.

Other symptoms vary according to the location of the cancer:

• Progressive jaundice, often painless, can be a sign of cancer in the head of the pancreas with bile duct obstruction. The whites of the eyes and the skin can turn yellowish. Often the urine is dark and cola colored and the stools are light and clay colored.

• Itching (pruritis) may occur due to bile duct obstruction.

• Diarrhea and swollen legs or mild diabetes may also develop.

There are few symptoms of cancer in the tail of the pancreas until the tumor is a large, often baseball-sized, mass.

Diagnosis

Physical Examination

• Jaundice.

• Abdominal masses.

• Enlarged gallbladder—50 percent of cases (carcinoma of head of pancreas).

• Enlarged liver (hepatomegaly).

- Abdominal fluid (ascites).
- Enlarged lymph nodes.
- Phlebitis (swollen legs).

Blood and Other Tests

- Complete blood count (CBC) and platelet count.
- The carcinoembryonic antigen (CEA), measured by a routine blood test, is elevated in 50 percent of cases.
- Carbohydrate antigen 19-9 (referred to commonly by its abbreviation, CA 19-9) is also measured in the blood. CA 19-9 levels are elevated in 70 to 80 percent of pancreatic cancer cases; testing for CA 19-9 is a better test than that for CEA because it is more specific. In many cases of pancreatic cancer, both the CEA and the CA 19-9 are elevated.
- Serum bilirubin is elevated in patients with bile duct obstruction.
- Serum alkaline phosphatase will be elevated if there are liver or bone metastases or if there is bile duct obstruction.

Imaging

- Abdominal ultrasound. Ultrasound may also be used at surgery to locate the exact borders of the tumor and to assess the liver for metastases.
- The single most important diagnostic test today is a high quality CT scan of the pancreas.
- CT scans may not detect small tumors but may identify pancreatic swelling, liver metastases, enlarged lymph nodes, dilated ducts, and fluid in the abdomen (ascites). It is hard to measure the size of a pancreatic mass by CT scan, as the edges of the tumor are often indistinct from the normal surrounding tissue.
- MRI may complement the CT scan.
- PET (positron-emission tomography) imaging is gaining acceptance as an aid to diagnosis and staging.

Endoscopy and Biopsy

- Endoscopic ultrasound (EUS) is a specialized technique available only at certain medical centers. It involves placing a telescope containing an ultrasound probe through the mouth into the stomach and duodenum. This allows good visualization of the pancreatic tumor in addition to any abnormal-appearing lymph nodes near the pancreas. An EUS-guided fine needle aspiration can be performed during the same procedure to obtain or confirm a tissue diagnosis.
- ERCP (endoscopic retrograde cholangiopancreatography) involves placing a telescope through the mouth into the duodenum and inserting a tube into the opening of the pancreatic duct. It can distinguish obstructive from nonobstructive jaundice and is very accurate.
- For a definite diagnosis, a biopsy is essential. Tissue can be drawn out with a fine needle (FNA) inserted into the tumor using CT guidance (diagnostic in 86 percent of cases). This will be necessary to differentiate pancreatic cancer from benign pancreatitis, a pancreatic pseudocyst, an islet cell carcinoma, or a lymphoma. FNA can also be done at the time of surgery. Brushings of cells from the lining of the bile duct can be obtained at ERCP.

Tests of Surrounding Organs

- Upper gastrointestinal tract X-rays (UGI series) may be done to examine the duodenum (the portion of the small intestine that surrounds the pancreas) to look for abnormalities.
- A needle may be inserted into the liver to discover obstructions in the bile duct (percutaneous transhepatic cholangiogram).
- Liver biopsy to confirm metastases, if indicated.

Staging

The staging system for pancreatic cancer is the TNM system. Knowing the location and extent of cancer in the head, body, or tail of the pancreas will help determine if surgery is feasible. Stage I cancers are localized to the pancreas without involvement of adjacent organs or lymph nodes. Stage II cancers are larger lesions that involve adjacent structures like the bile duct and duodenum. Stage III cancers include those with spread to regional lymph nodes. Stage IV, or the most advanced, pancreas cancers involve organs like the stomach and colon by direct extension or have metastasized to the liver or other organs via the bloodstream.

Treatment Overview

 Surgery Surgery is sometimes curative and is also used for palliation of certain symptoms, such as vomiting and jaundice. Surgery is, at present, the only potentially curative treatment. The extent and type of surgery depends on the location and stage of the tumor. Cancers in the head of the gland (the most common location) can be treated with pancreatico-duodenectomy (also known as a Whipple procedure) if they have not spread and do not involve or encase adjacent large blood vessels (such as the celiac trunk and the superior mesenteric artery, two main vessels that come off the aorta). In this operation, about 50 percent of the pancreas, the duodenum, the gallbladder, and the portion of the bile duct within the pancreas are removed. Small intestine is used to reconstruct the stomach, bile duct, and pancreatic duct so that normal digestion can occur. Cancers in the body and tail of the pancreas can be treated with distal pancreatectomy and splenectomy, in which about 80 percent of the pancreas and the spleen are removed. Rarely, total pancreatectomy is required for cancers that diffusely involve the pancreas. In all cases, the lymph nodes around the pancreas are removed en bloc with the main tumor, and the surgeon is careful to achieve a margin of normal tissue around the cancer. Radical surgery is more feasible when the tumor is small (less than 3/4 inch or 2 cm), no lymph nodes are involved, and there is no extension of the cancer beyond the "capsule" of the pancreas (a rare situation), although surgeons at specialized cancer centers will often attempt to fully resect pancreatic cancers that do not meet these criteria. Surgical removal of pancreatic cancer is unlikely to be beneficial if gross tumor is left behind. Five-year survival after complete surgical resection is about 20 percent.

Surgery may also be used to bypass an obstruction of the biliary or gastrointestinal tract. Alternatively, blockages of the bile duct can be opened with small tubes (stents) placed at the time of ERCP or by an interventional radiologist working with needles through the skin and into the liver.

Surgery for pancreatic cancer carries significant risk. It is clear that the chance of dying from a complication of the surgery is reduced in centers where the operations are performed frequently.

Radiation Radiation is used in several different settings in pancreatic cancer. It is routinely given in the postoperative setting, following a complete resection, to reduce the risk of the tumor recurring in or near the pancreas. Recently, however, large studies have called into question whether giving radiation to patients following resection of their pancreatic cancer really improves survival. Radiation is also frequently given in conjunction with chemotherapy (either at the same time or sequentially) for patients whose tumor cannot be removed surgically because of direct extension into, or involvement of, surrounding organs or vessels, known as locally advanced disease. Radiation can also be given for palliation of pain in patients who have metastatic disease; typically, such treatment is still directed toward the primary pancreatic tumor, which is the most common source of patients' pain. The risks of radiotherapy, such as damage to the kidneys, spleen, liver, spinal cord, and the bowel surrounding the pancreas, can be reduced with proper treatment planning. Radiation is typically administered together with low doses of chemotherapy—5-fluorouracil and capecitabine (Xeloda) being the most common chemotherapy agents used—which enhance the effectiveness of the radiation. Intraoperative radiotherapy (IORT) and interstitial I-125 radioactive implants have helped local tumor control but have not increased survival. Newer radiation techniques such as CyberKnife (stereotactic radiosurgery) are currently being explored.

 Chemotherapy Gemcitabine (Gemzar) represents the primary chemotherapy drug used for the treatment of pancreatic cancer. It was approved in 1996 based on an improvement in median survival by $1\frac{1}{2}$ months seen in patients with advanced stages of pancreatic cancer treated with gemcitabine compared to those treated with the previous standard of care, 5-fluorouracil (5-FU). The estimated one-year survival was also superior for gemcitabine compared to 5-FU (18 percent versus 2 percent). It also provides moderate palliation, with a 50 percent reduced need for analgesics for pain control.

Many clinical studies have been conducted over the past decade to try to improve on the outcomes seen with gemcitabine alone, most of them evaluating gemcitabine in combination with additional drugs. One recently reported large study demonstrated that the addition of erlotinib (Tarceva; a cancer drug used in lung cancer, taken in pill form) to gemcitabine resulted in a modest improvement in survival compared to gemcitabine alone. This led to the approval of Tarceva in 2005 for use in pancreatic cancer. Another study, conducted in Europe, showed that the combination of gemcitabine and capecitabine (Xeloda; also an oral drug) also resulted in longer survival times compared to gemcitabine by itself. Other combinations, including gemcitabine plus a platinum compound (cisplatin [Platinol] or oxaliplatin [Eloxatin]), have been evaluated extensively and show some evidence that they may also be more effective than gemcitabine alone.

Palliation Although treatment does not always improve the length of survival, it may improve the quality of life. Bypass of a blocked biliary tract or duodenum, or chemotherapy to shrink a tumor and relieve pain, can produce a dramatic effect on a patient's sense of well-being. This opportunity needs to be carefully weighed against the risks of treatment. Other palliative measures include pain control using analgesics, celiac and splanchnic (internal organ) nerve blocks, spinal morphine, antiemetics to control nausea or vomiting, and nutritional support with diets and replacement of pancreatic enzymes (see chapter 23, "Maintaining Good Nutrition"). Radiotherapy has been successfully used to control pain from bone metastases.

Treatment by Stage

▪ Stage I

TNM T1 or T2, N0, M0
In T1, the cancer is confined to the pancreas. T1A is less than $\frac{3}{4}$ inch (2 cm); T1B is larger. In T2, it has spread to involve the bile duct or duodenum.

Standard Treatment Stage I cancer is treatable by surgery and is occasionally curable. Radical surgery—the Whipple procedure—is the standard treatment for cancer of the head of the pancreas or the opening of the pancreatic duct. A hospital stay of ten to fourteen days is expected, and full recovery of appetite and strength may take three months. In the best centers, the risk of dying from a complication of surgery is 2 percent, although the average in all hospitals in the United States is about 10 percent. The main complications of Whipple resection include leakage from the place where the pancreatic remnant and intestine are sewn together, lung infections, and heart problems, including myocardial infarction. Transfusion is usually not required, unless unexpected problems are found during surgery. Surgery for cancer involving the body or tail of the pancreas is less common than the Whipple procedure, because tumors in the tail are usually large and far advanced before diagnosis.

Postsurgical (adjuvant) therapy consisting of chemotherapy and/or radiation is often used to try to reduce the risk of the cancer recurring. An early study published in 1985 suggested that the combination of radiotherapy and 5-FU may improve survival compared to no further treatment after surgery. In this study, about 40 percent of patients treated with such combined therapy were alive at two years, representing a twofold increase in survival compared to surgery by itself. As noted, however, more recent studies have called into question whether radiation is really an essential component of therapy after an operation or whether it should be considered only in select cases (such as for bulky tumors and for tumors that were removed with very close or microscopically positive surgical margins). On the other hand, evidence is mounting that chemotherapy does benefit individuals following pancreatic cancer surgery. A large German study demonstrated that six months of chemotherapy with gemcitabine (Gemzar) reduced the likelihood of disease recurrence compared to no further treatment after surgery.

Five-Year Survival 25 percent

Investigational
- The selection of chemotherapy and biological agents to use in addition to, or in lieu of, gemcitabine (Gemzar).
- Exciting work is ongoing evaluating administration of a pancreatic cancer vaccine following surgery, in conjunction with standard chemotherapy and/or radiation.
- The role and timing of radiation.
- At select institutions, chemotherapy and/or radiation are delivered prior to surgery. This should still be considered an investigational approach; the standard of care is to proceed immediately to surgery if the tumor appears resectable at the time of diagnosis.

Stage II
TNM T3, N0, M0
In T3 cancers, the tumor has directly spread to involve the bile duct or duodenum.

Standard Treatment The main treatment of Stage II patients is surgical resection, usually with the Whipple procedure. As with Stage I patients, postoperative adjuvant chemotherapy plus or minus radiation should be considered.

Five-Year Survival 15 percent

Investigational
- Same as for Stage I disease
- Standard versus extended lymph node dissection during Whipple resection

Stage III
TNM T1–3, N1, M0
In this stage, the cancer has spread to the regional lymph nodes. These nodes are the initial filters of lymph from around the pancreas. Involvement of these lymph nodes raises worries that tumor cells may have spread elsewhere, such as to the liver.

Standard Treatment Standard treatment for patients with Stage III pancreas cancer is surgical resection. All grossly enlarged lymph nodes in the region of the pancreas should be included in the resection specimen. Even if an apparently complete surgical resection can be achieved, the chance of recurrence is high, and patients should consider enrollment in a clinical trial or undergo postoperative adjuvant chemotherapy plus or minus radiation.

Five-Year Survival 5 percent

Investigational
- Same as for Stages I and II.
- Standard versus extended lymph node dissection during Whipple resection.

■ *Stage IV*
TNM T4, any N, M0 (Stage IVA); any T, any N, M1 (Stage IVB)
The cancer has spread to distant sites, most commonly the liver and lungs (Stage IVB), or involves adjacent organs such as the stomach, spleen, and colon, or large blood vessels (Stage IVA). For these patients, surgical resection is not possible and palliative treatment or investigational treatment is considered.

Standard Treatment Chemotherapy with gemcitabine (Gemzar)–based therapy is considered standard treatment. Multidrug regimens, such as gemcitabine in combination with erlotinib (Tarceva), capecitabine (Xeloda), or platinum compounds (carboplatin [Paraplatin], cisplatin [Platinol], oxaliplatin [Eloxatin]), should be offered to individuals who are still in relatively good shape. Palliative surgical, endoscopic, or transhepatic bypass may be necessary to relieve bile duct obstruction, as well as palliative gastrojejunostomy to relieve duodenal obstruction.

Five-Year Survival 1 to 2 percent

Investigational
Enrollment in clinical trials should be strongly considered. These trials may involve combinations of standard chemotherapy agents, evaluation of novel compounds (drugs that have shown promise in the laboratory but are not yet approved for widespread use), or some combination of both. Novel compounds include "targeted" agents often available in pill form, antibodies given intravenously, and vaccines.

Supportive Therapy
Nutrition Malnutrition is a common problem because of loss of appetite, diarrhea, poor fat absorption, and duodenal or bile duct obstruction. Fat-soluble vitamin deficiencies (A, D, E, and K) may also occur.

- Frequent feedings, digestive enzyme replacements (pancrelipase [Viokase]), and antinausea drugs will be needed.
- Low-fat food or supplements (medium-chain triglycerides) may help provide proteins and calories.
- Gastric and jejunal tube feeding can help supplement nutrition. Intravenous total parenteral nutrition does not appear to improve survival.

Pain Control Pain is often a major problem for Stage IV patients, but morphine or narcotics can help. If these are not effective, celiac nerve blocks or the infusion of morphine by vein or the spinal canal (typically administered by an anesthesiologist specializing in pain management) can help control pain in a majority of patients. Local radiotherapy has been used to control pain. Gemcitabine (Gemzar) has been shown to decrease pain in about 40 percent of patients.

Recurrent Cancer
For patients who have undergone surgical resection of their pancreatic cancer,

the cancer can recur either locally (in or around the surgical bed) or at distant sites throughout the body (most commonly the liver, lungs, and abdominal cavity). Locally recurrent pancreatic cancer can present with increased pain, jaundice, or symptoms of obstruction (food not being able to pass through, producing nausea, an early feeling of fullness, and vomiting). Recurrences either locally or distantly can produce weight loss, loss of appetite, and fluid buildup in the abdomen.

Recurrent cancer is rarely curable, although symptoms can often be effectively palliated by surgery or radiation therapy. Patients who remain in good physical condition can choose to receive chemotherapy (the choice of drugs dependent on what, if any, chemotherapy they have previously received) or participate in clinical trials.

The Most Important Questions You Can Ask

• What is the stage of my tumor and what treatment options are available?

• How experienced are my surgeon and hospital personnel in caring for patients undergoing surgery for pancreatic cancer?

• Do I qualify for any clinical trials testing new therapies?

Parathyroid

Orlo H. Clark, M.D., and Malin Dollinger, M.D.

■ ■ ■ ■

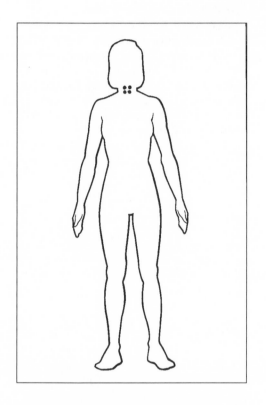

The parathyroid glands are usually located in the neck, two on each side of the thyroid gland (see the illustration of the thyroid and parathyroid glands in the chapter "Thyroid").

Parathyroid cancer is a rare and sometimes curable endocrine gland cancer. Though not all of these tumors are functioning, those that are produce increased amounts of parathyroid hormone (parathormone), which leads to a marked elevation in blood calcium level (hypercalcemia). It is usually the signs and symptoms of elevated calcium—painful bones, kidney stones, constipation, depression, and fatigue—that lead to the diagnosis.

Benign tumors of the parathyroid (adenomas) and an overgrowth of parathyroid tissue (hyperplasia) are much more common (99 percent) than malignant tumors (1 percent). Both benign and malignant parathyroid tumors produce parathyroid hormone that increases blood calcium levels, so it is sometimes difficult to know at surgery whether the tumor is benign or malignant. This distinction is extremely important because the treatment of a malignant parathyroid tumor requires not only removal of the tumor but often removal of the thyroid gland on that side. Muscles and tissues adjacent to the tumor are also removed when involved.

Recognition by the surgeon that the tumor is malignant rather than benign and performing the appropriate surgery (including removal of the lymph nodes) is important for good results. Malignancy is more likely if there is a very high serum calcium level, a palpable or hard mass in the neck, or hoarseness due to paralysis of the vocal cords on the same side.

Because this tumor usually grows slowly and because the main clinical problem is usually the effects of the elevated calcium level, palliative reduction or debulking of the primary tumor or metastases is recommended. This may lower the blood calcium level, which is difficult to treat any other way.

Types Parathyroid carcinomas are tumors with chief cell, oxyphil, clear cell, and mixed cell types.

How It Spreads Parathyroid tumors can spread directly to adjacent tissues, as well as through the lymphatic system to nearby lymph nodes and via the bloodstream to distant sites, usually the lung(s), liver, and bone.

What Causes It There is increased incidence following exposure to low-dose therapeutic radiation and in families with familial hyperparathyroidism or multiple endocrine neoplasia type 1 (MEN-1), especially with hyperparathyroidism–jaw tumor syndrome. The HRPT2 oncogene has been found in about 60 percent of patients with parathyroid cancer.

Risk Factors

There are no known environmental risk factors for parathyroid carcinoma, although benign tumors of the parathyroids (adenoma) occur more often if there has been radiation to the head and neck. Parathyroid tumors also occur in association with tumors of the adrenal and thyroid glands (MEN-1 and MEN-2A) and in patients with familial hyperparathyroidism–jaw tumor syndrome.

Screening

Because it is so rare, specific screening for this type of cancer is generally not done. Benign parathyroid disease is common, however, occurring in about 1 in 1,000 patients annually in the United States. Methods to search for parathyroid tumors, whether benign or malignant, include measuring the serum calcium level—commonly performed as part of a chemistry panel—and examining the thyroid region for suspicious masses during routine physical examinations.

Common Signs and Symptoms

Symptoms are due to the elevated calcium or parathyroid hormone level or rarely to the mass in the neck.

Clinical manifestations usually include fatigue, nausea and vomiting, muscle weakness, musculoskeletal aches and pains, depression, kidney stones or other kidney disease, osteoporosis, peptic ulcer, gout, inflammation of the pancreas (pancreatitis), and hoarseness.

Diagnosis

The diagnosis of overactive parathyroids is characterized by a combination of an elevated level of serum calcium plus an elevated level of serum parathyroid hormone in a patient without a low (less than 100 mg) twenty-four-hour urinary calcium level.

Diagnosis is usually made easily by documenting an increased two-site or intact parathyroid hormone (PTH) level in a patient with an elevated level of blood calcium. Only a very rare, nonparathyroid malignant tumor in such patients secretes pure parathyroid-hormone. Most nonparathyroid cancers secrete parathyroid-hormone-related peptide, and this substance does not cross-react with the new parathyroid hormone assays.

Physical Examination

• A mass in the neck is present in about 50 percent of cases. Benign parathyroid tumors rarely have a mass in the neck.

• Vocal cords may be paralyzed on one side, causing hoarseness.

Blood and Other Tests

• The normal serum calcium level is 8.5 to 10.5 mg/dl and the level in benign tumors averages 11 mg/dl, but most parathyroid cancers have levels over 14 mg/dl.

• Intact or two-site PTH levels are increased.

• Sometimes the presence and location of a primary parathyroid tumor can be confirmed in a patient with recurrent or persistent hyperparathyroidism by placing a catheter in the veins draining the parathyroids or metastatic deposits.

Blood samples are then taken from each site and serum parathyroid hormone levels are determined. This test is usually done only when imaging fails to localize the tumor.

Imaging

• Bone density studies documenting osteopenia or osteoporosis (loss of bone).

• Localization tests should be done before surgery. These include ultrasound, sestamibi, CT, and MRI scans of the neck and mediastinum.

• Localization tests are especially helpful in patients with persistent or recurrent disease, in patients who have had previous thyroid surgery, and in patients having a focused operation using intraoperative PTH assay.

Staging

There are only two stages of parathyroid cancer. One stage is localized, meaning that the disease is confined to the parathyroid with or without invasion of adjacent tissues. The other is metastatic, in which the cancer may have spread to regional lymph nodes and/or to distant sites such as the lung(s), liver, and bone.

Treatment Overview

The problem with these tumors is usually not the tumor itself, which grows rather slowly, but the marked elevation in calcium levels, which produces a condition (hypercalcemia) that is difficult to control medically and may eventually be fatal.

For this reason, aggressive surgical removal of bulk disease or metastatic disease is recommended. Unfortunately, this type of surgery is not always possible, because of widespread metastasis. Better results are obtained when a surgeon experienced with hyperparathyroidism is involved.

A variety of medical means can inhibit the action of parathyroid hormone and improve the hypercalcemia, including the use of calcimimetics such as cinacalcet (Sensipar), bisphosphonates, calcitonin (Miacalcin, Fortical), and plicamycin (Mithracin).

Treatment by Stage

■ Localized

Standard Treatment Localized parathyroid cancer is treated with removal of the tumor and the thyroid gland on the same side. Adjacent muscles and other tissues are removed if they appear to be involved. The laryngeal nerve must occasionally be removed, which may result in hoarseness. Local recurrence is common and may require repeat surgery.

Five-Year Survival About 50 percent

Investigational Clinical trials are evaluating combinations of surgery and radiation therapy, as well as radiation therapy alone.

■ Metastatic

Standard Treatment For metastatic parathyroid cancer, an operation is performed similar to that for localized cancer, with removal of adjacent, adherent, or involved neck muscles and regional lymph nodes.

An attempt is made to remove as much tumor as possible to eliminate the source of excess parathyroid hormone, hypercalcemia, and related metabolic problems.

Five-Year Survival 30 percent

Investigational

• As for localized cancer, clinical protocols are studying combinations of surgery and radiation therapy, as well as radiation therapy alone for metastatic parathyroid cancer.

• A few patients with metastatic parathyroid cancer have been treated with chemotherapy combinations, including the active agent dacarbazine (DTIC-Dome), as well as that agent combined with 5-fluorouracil and cyclophosphamide (Cytoxan). There are no current adjuvant treatment protocols for this tumor.

Treatment Follow-Up

Physical examination of the neck with ultrasound, sestamibi, CT, or MRI scanning and determinations of blood calcium and parathyroid hormone levels are the most appropriate methods of follow-up.

Recurrent Cancer

The treatment of recurrent parathyroid cancer is generally surgical removal of the primary tumor—with adjacent lymph nodes—or debulking the tumor to reduce the production of parathormone. Under investigation are the combination of surgery and radiation therapy, radiation therapy alone, and chemotherapy. Debulking the tumor or radiation often lowers the serum calcium level and provides palliation.

The Most Important Questions You Can Ask

• How does the surgeon decide whether a parathyroid tumor is benign or malignant?

• Is a frozen section reliable in helping to decide if the tumor is benign or malignant?

• Where does recurrent parathyroid cancer most often develop?

• Would radiation therapy be helpful along with surgery?

• What are the complication rates of the surgery?

Penis

Maxwell V. Meng, M.D., Norman R. Zinner, M.D., M.S., and Stanley A. Brosman, M.D.

■ ■ ■ ■

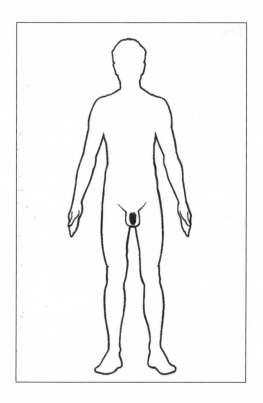

Cancer of the penis is rare in the United States, affecting fewer than 1,000 men each year. It most commonly arises from the head—or glans—of the penis or the foreskin but can arise from anywhere along the penile shaft. Removal of the foreskin before puberty nearly eliminates the occurrence of penile cancer, and good hygiene with prevention of chronic inflammation may also reduce the risk in those with the foreskin intact. The goals of therapy include cancer eradication with preservation of the penis and are often possible with early identification and treatment; unfortunately, many men do not seek medical attention until the cancer has become more advanced.

Types The most common type of penile cancer is known as squamous cell carcinoma, similar to that which occurs on the head and face. Melanoma may also develop on the penis, with the blue-brown, flat growths characteristic of melanomas elsewhere on the body; these tend to spread more rapidly and widely than squamous cell carcinoma. Rarely, cancers from other organs, such as the bladder and prostate, spread into the deep tissues of the penis. A superficial type of squamous cell carcinoma (carcinoma in situ) may occur on the penis as well as the rest of the genitalia and tends to be slow growing; however, some may progress to invasive squamous cell carcinoma, although metastasis rarely occurs.

How It Spreads These cancers begin on the surface and later grow into the deeper tissues of the penis. In addition to local growth, squamous cell carcinoma can spread through the lymph channels, and this is an orderly process sequentially involving the lymph nodes of the superficial groin, deep groin, and then the pelvis. Once the cancer has spread beyond the penis itself, more aggressive treatment is necessary, and if the cancer has moved beyond the groin lymph nodes, cure is usually not possible.

What Causes It Cancer of the penis is associated with several risk factors. These include lack of neonatal circumcision, inability to retract the foreskin (phimosis), infection with human papillomavirus (HPV), exposure to tobacco products, and possibly trauma and ultraviolet radiation. Thus, it appears that conditions that predispose to chronic irritation and inflammation may lead to the development of cancer over time. Among the numerous types of HPV, HPV 16 and 18 appear to be most frequently detected in men with penile squamous cell carcinoma, and these types are also implicated in the development of cancer of the cervix in women. Indeed, cervical cancer is more common in women whose sexual partners carry the HPV virus or have not been circumcised. Nevertheless, despite the elimination of penile squamous cell carcinoma by removing the foreskin, routine circumcision in the newborn remains a controversial subject.

Risk Factors

The cancer is usually diagnosed after the age of twenty-five, and typically men present after the age of fifty years. As mentioned, men with foreskins that cannot be retracted (phimosis) have poorer hygiene and chronic irritation and are therefore at greater risk. Other preventable causes of squamous cell carcinoma include tobacco and ultraviolet light exposure.

Screening

The only screening test is periodic self-examination or physical examination by a physician. One should routinely pull back the foreskin, permitting routine cleaning and inspection. There are no blood tests to detect this cancer. It is important to seek medical attention for any sores or lesions on the penis that do not heal and for pain or bleeding from the penis.

Common Signs and Symptoms

The most common finding is a surprisingly painless sore on the foreskin or a discolored area on the glans that does not heal or disappear. Phimosis may hide a lesion and allow it to grow to a large size, when it may protrude from beneath the foreskin or start bleeding. If untreated, these tumors become inflamed and infected, producing a foul odor, a discharge, and discomfort. An infected penile cancer can be associated with enlargement of the inguinal lymph nodes. As the cancer spreads into deeper tissues, the penis feels hard, but this type of cancer rarely presents with difficulty in urination.

Diagnosis

Physical Examination

- The primary physical finding is a painless sore on the foreskin or a discolored area on the head (glans) of the penis.
- The lymph nodes in the groin (inguinal) region may become enlarged from either infection or involvement with cancer.

Imaging CT or MRI scan, chest radiograph, and whole body bone scan may be helpful.

Biopsy

- Biopsy is the primary diagnostic test to confirm squamous cell carcinoma. All suspicious areas should be sampled and examined by a pathologist.
- Important pathologic factors include depth of invasion, grade, and status of vascular invasion.
- Biopsy or aspiration sampling of enlarged inguinal lymph nodes may be necessary.

Treatment by Stage

There is no universally accepted staging system for penile cancer. In general, outcome is determined by the penile structure invaded and whether the cancer has spread beyond the penis to lymph nodes or to distant sites.

■ Stage I

These cancers are confined to the skin or glans of the penis and do not invade the deeper layers beneath the skin. Usually the foreskin is involved, but the cancer can occur anywhere along the shaft of the penis.

Standard Treatment Cancers localized to the foreskin can be treated with circumcision. Small cancers on the glans or elsewhere on the shaft are treated by surgical removal, application of chemotherapy creams, or destruction using a laser. If the cancer is large or involves more than just the foreskin or glans, wider surgical removal is necessary and may require reconstructive methods or skin grafts.

Five-Year Survival Long-term survival approaches 100 percent.

■ Stage II

Stage II cancers have invaded below the skin and involve the underlying structures of the penis or have spread to only a single lymph node in the groin.

Standard Treatment Depending upon the depth and extent of the cancer, a partial or complete amputation of the penis may be necessary to completely remove the cancer. If the tumor involves only the end of the penis, a partial removal (penectomy) can be performed to preserve sexual and urinary function.

Cancers involving the base of the penis typically require more extensive surgery, which can mean total removal of the penis. The decision to remove the entire penis depends on whether the remaining penis is sufficient for sexual intercourse and urination while standing; techniques to reconstruct the penis

are available so that it is possible to create a new penis in some cases.

Many of these patients require sampling of groin lymph nodes to determine whether or not spread has occurred, the most important factor predicting survival in men with penile cancer. Removal of these lymph nodes not only provides staging information but can be curative if the extent of metastasis is limited. However, debate continues about who needs to undergo this surgery and how the surgery should be performed, since significant complications may occur.

Radiation therapy can be attempted in some situations, while in others a combination of surgery and radiation may be employed.

Five-Year Survival At least 75 percent

■ Stage III

In these cases, the cancer has spread to several lymph nodes of the superficial inguinal region, or the cancer has invaded the urethra or prostate gland. The ability to cure patients at this stage is limited.

Standard Treatment In patients with clear swelling of the inguinal lymph nodes, antibiotics are given to determine whether infection or cancer is the likely cause of enlargement. Most of these patients should undergo sampling of the lymph nodes in addition to treatment of the penile tumor itself. Chemotherapy is often added after surgery when there is evidence of metastasis beyond the inguinal lymph nodes.

Five-Year Survival Less than 50 percent

■ Stage IV

These patients have advanced cancers that have invaded adjacent structures other than the urethra or prostate, spread to deep inguinal or pelvic lymph nodes, or metastasized to distant sites.

Standard Treatment Treatment is primarily aimed at controlling any symptoms and preventing future complications. A combination of surgery, chemotherapy, and radiation therapy may slow the progression of cancer and prolong life.

Five-Year Survival Few patients are cured, but there is a five-year survival rate of 10 to 15 percent.

Treating Genital Warts

Genital warts (condylomata acuminata) are caused by HPV and may occur anywhere on the external genitalia, as well as the urethra and anus. Although the HPV types causing warts have low risk for conversion to squamous cell carcinoma, some lesions may become quite large and require treatment. Observation is an option, as genital warts may resolve with time, but patients should be informed that recurrence is common among sexually active individuals and that duration of infection and methods of prevention are not definitively known.

Treatment methods include

• application of topical chemical directly to the wart,
• freezing (cryotherapy) of the wart with liquid nitrogen,
• destruction of the wart using a laser, and
• surgical removal.

The Most Important Questions You Can Ask

• Is surgery necessary and how extensive will it be?
• Are lymph nodes going to be removed? If so, which ones?
• Is radiation and/or chemotherapy effective or necessary?
• What is the relationship between penile cancer and genital warts?
• Can the cancer by transmitted sexually?
• Should my sexual partner be tested for HPV?

Pituitary

Orlo H. Clark, M.D., and Malin Dollinger, M.D.

■ ■ ■ ■

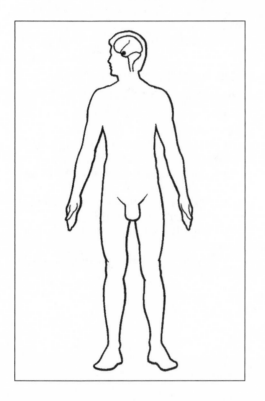

Tumors in the pituitary gland, which is located at the base of the brain (see the illustration of areas in the brain that develop brain tumors in the chapter "Brain"), are benign (adenomas) and curable over 90 percent of the time. But these tumors can become large enough to damage nearby nerves and brain tissue, sometimes permanently. By pressing on the nerves to the eyes, a pituitary tumor can cause progressive vision loss and even blindness. In some cases, the tumor compresses the pituitary gland, preventing it from producing the normal amount of hormones. Hypothyroidism, adrenal insufficiency, and a deficiency in growth hormone can result.

Types Many pituitary adenomas produce excess hormones, causing significant symptoms. The increased production of growth hormone can produce a disease called acromegaly. Excess prolactin can cause impotence in men and the loss of menstrual periods, infertility, and breast secretion in women. Excess ACTH (adrenocorticotropic hormone) can result in Cushing's disease. Some tumors, such as chromophobe adenomas, are nonfunctional but may lead to hormone deficiency by compressing the normal pituitary.

How It Spreads Since most pituitary tumors are benign, they do not spread like cancerous tumors. They may, however, cause erosion of the sella turcica, the bony structure surrounding the pituitary.

What Causes It There is no known cause, although the use of birth control pills may be a contributing factor in some cases. About 50 percent of patients with multiple endocrine neoplasia type I (MEN-1) have pituitary tumors.

Common Signs and Symptoms

Early symptoms depend on which hormone is involved. As the tumor grows, headaches may occur, and sight may deteriorate, starting with loss of lateral or peripheral vision.

Diagnosis

Blood and Other Tests Sensitive radioimmunoassays for any hormone suspected of overproduction

Imaging
• CT and MRI scans of the brain. MRI is the more sensitive study.
• X-rays of the skull may show destruction of the sella turcica.

Treatment Overview

Treatment depends on the type of tumor—whether it is functioning and whether it has grown beyond the area of the pituitary gland.

Prolactin-secreting tumors may stabilize and improve with time. People with these tumors usually benefit from treatment with bromocriptine (Parlodel).

Tumors that produce other hormones are treated with surgery or radiation, with the surgical approach—a transsphenoidal hypophysectomy (an operation that goes through the sinus cavities to remove the pituitary tumor)—usually the treatment chosen for tumors that have not grown outside the bony cavity. Larger tumors, usually nonfunctioning adenomas, need additional treatment with radiation.

Tumors that produce growth hormone and ACTH usually grow slowly. With any of the pituitary tumors, however, surgery is called for immediately if vision starts to deteriorate rapidly.

Treatment by Type

ACTH-Producing Pituitary Tumors (Cushing's disease)

Standard Treatment Treatment options include transsphenoidal resection of the tumor with or without radiation therapy, or radiation in combination with mitotane (Lysodren) or ketoconazole (Nizoral). Bilateral laparoscopic adrenalectomy is used for patients with recurrent or persistent disease. Posttreatment target hormone replacement therapy is administered if required.

Investigational Heavy-particle radiation

Prolactin-Producing Tumors

Standard Treatment Treatment options include surgical removal of the tumor, radiation, bromocriptine (Parlodel), or combinations of these treatments. Bromocriptine has been of considerable benefit in reducing symptoms. A new drug, CV 205-502 (quinagolide [Norprolac]), has been successful in patients who have failed to respond to bromocriptine.

Investigational Heavy-particle radiation

Growth Hormone–Producing Tumors

Standard Treatment Treatment options include transsphenoidal surgery with or without radiation therapy, and/or somatostatin (octreotide [Sandostatin]). Which treatment is chosen depends on the size and extent of the tumor and on how urgent it is to eliminate the excess hormone production. Posttreatment target hormone replacement therapy is administered if required.

Nonfunctioning Tumors

Standard Treatment These tumors, usually chromophobe adenomas, are treated with surgery and radiation. The choice depends on how big the tumor is, how fast it is growing, and its effect on adjacent pituitary tissue or other structures.

The surgical and radiotherapy techniques used to treat these tumors are very complex and sophisticated. Neurosurgeons, radiation oncologists, and endrocrinologists experienced in treating them are best able to judge which method is preferable and the posttreatment hormone therapy that is necessary.

Treatment Follow-Up

The intensity and schedule of follow-up depends on the amount of damage done to adjacent tissues before or during treatment and on whether the tumor was completely removed during surgery.

• An endocrinologist will usually be involved in follow-up after surgery, since hormone deficiency (ACTH, FSH, LH, TSH, sex hormones, and cortisol) may occur and replacement hormones may be essential.
• Follow-up CT or MRI scans may be useful.
• Hormone levels should be measured periodically if a hormone-producing tumor was treated.

The Most Important Questions You Can Ask

• Is my tumor producing extra hormones?
• Is surgery or radiation the best medical treatment for my type of tumor and why?
• What is the probability that the treatment will eliminate the tumor or make it decrease in size?
• What are the risks, complications, and side effects of treatment?
• Will I have to take hormones after surgery or other treatment and, if so, for how long?
• What are the chances that my vision will improve?

Prostate

Phillip L. Ross, M.D., Peter R. Carroll, M.D., Eric J. Small, M.D.,
Mack Roach III, M.D., Norman R. Zinner, M.D., M.S.,
and Stanley A. Brosman, M.D.

■ ■ ■ ■

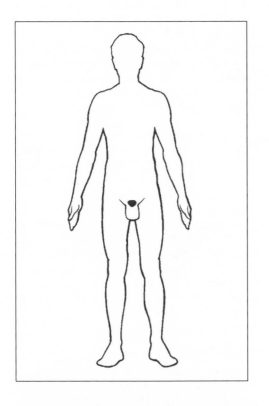

Aside from superficial skin cancers, prostate cancer is the most common form of cancer affecting men in the United States. The American Cancer Society[1] estimates 218,890 cases will be diagnosed in the United States in 2007 and 27,050 men will die from the disease. While there has been a slight decrease in the death rate since the mid-1990s, this still is the third leading cause of cancer death, behind lung cancer and colon cancer. That being said, prostate cancer represents an often curable and very treatable form of cancer. The vast majority of patients diagnosed with prostate cancer ultimately die from other causes.

Prostate cancer incidence rose sharply in the early 1990s with wider application of PSA (prostate-specific antigen) testing. While this sharp rise has since tapered off, the overall trend does continue to show an increasing incidence of prostate cancer over time in the United States. At the same time, clinicians who are involved in caring for patients with prostate cancer have noted a stage migration of the disease. That is, more and more patients are presenting at a younger age, with an earlier stage of the disease, and with lower PSA levels, and smaller less aggressive tumors. This trend is often attributed to the widespread use of PSA testing. Unlike with many cancers, the risk of a man developing prostate cancer continues to rise throughout his lifetime and is significantly affected by his age. For example, 1 in 10,000 men under forty will develop prostate cancer. For ages forty to fifty-nine, the odds are 1 in 103, and for men sixty to seventy-nine, the odds are 1 in 8. The risk of developing prostate cancer does appear to be slightly higher for African-American men. The risk of developing the disease is also higher for men with a primary relative affected by the disease. Recent data on this subject suggest that men with a primary relative (brother, father, or uncle) with prostate cancer have a higher likelihood of developing the disease, but once they are diagnosed, their disease does not appear to be any more aggressive than the average patient diagnosed with sporadic prostate cancer.[2]

Types Over 95 percent of prostate cancers are *adenocarcinomas,* which is the term for cancers arising from glands. Our discussion will focus on the treatment of adenocarcinomas. The remainder of prostate cancers consists primarily of transitional cell carcinomas (arising from the special lining cells of the urinary tract). Neuroendocrine (aka, small cell) carcinomas and sarcomas also exist but are extremely rare.

How It Spreads The chances of prostate cancer spreading are higher with increasing size and grade (determined by the Gleason score (see "Biopsy" and "Staging/Grading" in this chapter) of the primary tumor. The majority of prostate cancers detected today are localized to the prostate gland. When prostate cancers do spread, they first tend to penetrate the capsule of the prostate along the routes of the nerves. Prostate cancer can invade the seminal vesicles (a pair of accessory male sexual organs adjacent to the prostate) and when this occurs, there is an increased risk of the disease spreading both regionally and distantly. When the disease spreads locally, it can invade the part of the bladder where the ureters insert. The ureters transport urine from the kidneys to the bladder. When they are blocked by cancer or other processes, problems can occur, including an inability to urinate and the passage of blood in the urine. It should be noted that this is a rare cause of blood in the urine. The cancer also spreads via lymphatic drainage to the pelvic lymph nodes. The most common site of distant spread (metastasis) is bone, particularly the lumbar spine, femur, and pelvis. When prostate cancer

spreads to the bone, it is initially painless; however, if left untreated, these sites of bony metastasis may become painful and even brittle, putting the patient at risk for a pathologic fracture. This is when a fracture occurs because of a disease process in the bone (i.e., prostate cancer) rather than a traumatic injury. A particularly concerning situation in a patient with advanced, metastatic prostate cancer is known as cord compression. In this scenario, the cancer cells grow in or near the spine and compress the spinal cord and nerves, resulting in neurological symptoms. When this occurs, immediate medical attention is required. Prostate cancer can also spread to other organs, including the lung, liver, and adrenals.

What Causes It Prostate cancer researchers continue to work at uncovering the underlying cause(s) of this disease. There appear to be both genetic and environmental factors at play in the development of the disease. The role of genetics is an area of active investigation that will likely lead to significant advances in our ability to predict who will develop clinically significant prostate cancer. Such advances will lead to more sophisticated screening methods as well as molecular targeted therapies.

Risk Factors

The importance of the role of testosterone (the male sex hormone) in this disease is well established. The growth of both normal and cancerous prostate cells is dependent on testosterone. In fact, prostate cells contain a special compound (enzyme) that is able to convert regular testosterone into a much more potent form, known as dihydrotestosterone (DHT). It has been observed that men who are castrated before the onset of puberty do not develop prostate cancer.

Researchers and clinicians are well aware of evidence that prostate cancer

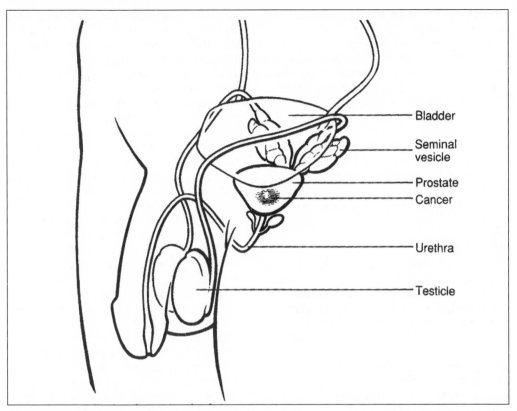

The prostate gland and associated pelvic organs

occurs at much lower rates in other parts of the world. They have also learned from studies that people who migrate from regions of low prostate cancer incidence (e.g., the Far East) to regions of higher incidence (e.g., North America) develop an increasing risk for prostate cancer, similar to men who have lived their entire lives in regions of higher incidence. Common factors of the lower incidence areas include a primarily low-fat, plant-based diet. Increased dietary amounts of animal fat in particular appear to be directly associated with prostate cancer. Other protective dietary components include lycopene (which is present in cooked tomatoes), selenium (a naturally occurring mineral), omega-3 fatty acids (present in fish), and vitamin E. Recently,

there has been increasing evidence suggesting that inflammation plays a role in the development of prostate cancer. Currently, however, there are no recommendations for men with a history of prostatitis (prostate infection/inflammation) to be more aggressively screened for prostate cancer.

Importantly, prostate cancer does not appear to be related to benign prostatic hyperplasia (BPH), which is a very common noncancerous condition affecting many men. BPH represents a noncancerous increase in the size of the prostate (specifically from the transition zone of the gland) that can result in a decreased urinary stream, a sense of urgency to void, and nocturia (waking up multiple times at night to void). There is no substantial evidence to suggest prostate cancer is related to having a vasectomy or to frequency of sexual activity. With rare exception, most patients in North America with prostate cancer have no symptoms at all when they are diagnosed. In fact, the symptoms that may actually lead to their doctor visit are often BPH symptoms or even something completely unrelated to the prostate. During the visit, a digital rectal exam is performed and/or the patient is recommended to have a PSA blood test, and this is what often leads to the diagnosis.

Screening

The most sensitive method for early detection of prostate cancer involves the combination of the PSA blood test along with the digital rectal exam (DRE). While the widespread use of PSA testing has led to a stage migration in the disease, the current (December 2002) finding of the Agency for Healthcare Research and Quality's U.S. Preventive Services Task Force is that there is not enough evidence to recommend for or against routinely screening patients for prostate cancer. Prostate cancer is often a slowly growing cancer, especially in its early stages, and therefore gathering clinical evidence that screening actually saves lives is a task that involves following the lives of thousands of patients over long periods of time. Further, while screening likely detects more cancers and at an earlier stage, we know that some of these cancers are not clinically significant (i.e., they would likely not affect the patient's quality or quantity of life had they never been detected). Therefore, the U.S. Preventive Services Task Force will not recommend prostate cancer screening until large randomized controlled studies have proven a beneficial effect. Such studies are currently under way and results should be expected within the next couple of years. Nonetheless, the American Urological Association (AUA) recommends offering PSA testing to patients fifty years of age or older who have at least a ten-year life expectancy. Men with risk factors such as a first-degree relative with prostate cancer or men of African-American race may be offered PSA testing at a younger age. The AUA encourages clinicians to discuss the option of PSA testing with the patient in light of the potential risks (morbidity of biopsy and possible treatment methods) and benefits (finding a potentially curable cancer), ultimately leaving the decision up to the patient.

The National Comprehensive Cancer Network (NCCN; information available on-line at *www.nccn.org*) has recently released guidelines for the early detection of prostate cancer. Given that the results of the large randomized studies on screening are still pending, the NCCN has assembled a panel of experts in the field to make use of the most up-to-date data to establish a set of guidelines that are reviewed on an annual basis. Following a baseline evaluation including a complete history (including a detailed history of prostate diseases, including prostate cancer) and physical examination, a discussion of the risks and benefits of screening should take place starting at age forty. Those patients who wish to pursue an early detection strategy should be offered a digital rectal exam (DRE) and PSA testing. At this age, if the PSA is less than 0.6, the panel recommends repeating the PSA at age forty-five. For patients in this age group with a PSA greater than or equal to 0.6, the panel recommends annual follow-up with DRE and PSA testing. Following this algorithm, as long as the DRE remains normal, the PSA remains less than 2.5 ng/ml, and the PSA velocity remains less than 0.5 ng/ml per year, the patient continues with annual DRE and PSA testing. If the DRE remains normal but the PSA is between 2.5 ng/ml and 4.0 ng/ml *or* the PSA velocity is greater than or equal to 0.5 ng/ml per year, a prostate biopsy should be considered (taking factors into account such as age, comorbid conditions, family history, and racial background). For patients with a negative DRE but a PSA in the 4 ng/ml to 10 ng/ml range, the panel recommends proceeding to biopsy or performing the free PSA test (see "Blood and Other Tests" in this chapter) in cases where the biopsy may present a risk to the patient or the patient has other comorbid conditions. Patients with a PSA greater than 10 ng/ml are encouraged to undergo prostate biopsy. A patient with a suspicious DRE should undergo biopsy regardless of the PSA level. The panel also gives recommendations on how to follow up on biopsies that do not indicate cancer. The full discussion of this topic is beyond the scope of this chapter.

Common Signs and Symptoms

As mentioned above, most patients with early-stage prostate cancer have no symptoms. Often, patients present to their urologist with voiding complaints that are related to BPH and not related to prostate cancer. In the more advanced stages of prostate cancer, voiding symptoms can occur that mimic the symptoms of BPH. Bone pain and pathological fractures are signs of advanced disease. Patients with cord compression note acute neurological changes such as altered levels of sensation in their arms and legs, weakness in their legs, and a change in their level of bowel or bladder control. Bulky involvement of the pelvic lymph nodes by regionally advanced prostate cancer can cause swelling in the legs as a result of poor lymph drainage (lymphedema).

Diagnosis

Physical Examination The key component of prostate cancer on physical exam is the presence of induration (firmness) on the digital rectal exam. It is possible for prostate cancer to be present in a prostate that feels completely normal to the clinician during the DRE. The availability of PSA testing should not be considered a substitute for a proper DRE.

Blood and Other Tests PSA is a substance produced by both normal and cancerous prostate cells. It exists in bound and unbound forms. Typically, normal PSA levels are considered less than or equal to 4 ng/ml; however, the rate of change from previous PSA levels can be very important, even if the total PSA remains below 4 ng/ml. An elevated or rising PSA may suggest the presence of prostate cancer. It is important to keep in mind that PSA will also go up with increasing prostate size (BPH), prostatitis, urinary tract infection, recent biopsy, and urethral instrumentation (e.g., cystoscopy)—potentially complicating the interpretation of an elevated PSA. Clinicians will often carefully examine the PSA velocity or doubling time to evaluate the rate of rise of the PSA. In cases of borderline elevated PSA levels, clinicians may also consider ordering a "free PSA," which is short for a "free to total PSA ratio." PSA circulates in the bloodstream in both free-form and bound to serum proteins. The ratio of the two is often a predictor for having prostate cancer. A patient with a PSA of 4 ng/ml and a high free PSA (greater than 25 percent) has a considerably lower likelihood of having prostate cancer than a patient with the same total PSA but a lower free PSA. Approximately 50 percent of men with a free PSA less than 10 percent will have prostate cancer. The free PSA result may allow a patient with a lower likelihood of disease to be spared the morbidity and inconvenience of undergoing a prostate biopsy.

PSA levels are also known to go up with age. For this reason, a normal PSA level for a patient in his forties or fifties may be considerably lower than the typical 4 ng/ml cutoff. Some have recommended lowering the cutoff for a normal PSA to 2.5 ng/ml. Others have recommended the use of age-adjusted PSA ranges whereby the upper limit of normal is 2.5 ng/ml for men in their forties, 3.5 ng/ml for men in their fifties, 4.5 ng/ml for men in their sixties, and 6.5 ng/ml for men in their seventies.

Imaging The first choice for imaging the prostate is the TRUS (transrectal ultrasound), which is often performed in conjunction with prostate biopsy. This study involves no radiation and can yield valuable information on prostate gland size and contour. The trained observer can get an impression of extracapsular disease and seminal vesicle involvement as well.

CT scans are often performed as part of the work-up for radiation therapy planning, where they are primarily used to exclude the presence of suspicious pelvic lymph nodes. MRI scans can also be used for this purpose. A further adaptation of MRI imaging of prostate cancer involves the use of an endorectal coil. In specialized centers, the endorectal coil–MRI images can be analyzed in combination with spectroscopy, which may improve the accuracy of imaging. The goal of the MRI-spectroscopic image is to determine the precise location(s) of the cancer.

Bone scans are performed to evaluate for the presence of bone metastases. Bone scans, while noninvasive, are typically reserved for patients with a clinical picture of more advanced disease—T3 and T4 tumors (see "Staging/Grading," below) and PSA greater than 15 ng/ml.

ProstaScint scans (monoclonal antibody imaging) look for the presence of prostate cancer cells in soft tissues. Due to relatively high false positive and false negative rates, this test is seldom used in clinical practice.

Biopsy Prostate biopsy is considered when there is reasonable clinical suspicion based on DRE and PSA results that prostate cancer exists, when the patient has at least a ten-year life expectancy, and when the patient feels he would consider a form of treatment if in fact prostate cancer were detected. Prostate biopsy is performed as a simple outpatient procedure with a local anesthetic under ultrasound guidance. Patients receive a short course of oral antibiotics and an enema prior to the procedure. A transrectal ultrasound (TRUS) probe is carefully inserted into the patient's rectum, allowing the clinician to visualize the prostate gland. Topical and local anesthetics may be used, making the procedure very tolerable for patients. The TRUS probe has an adaptor allowing the passage of a biopsy needle that takes a 15 mm–long core biopsy of prostate tissue. Typically, eight to sixteen cores are taken from specific anatomic areas within the prostate in order to sample those areas that are typically at the greatest risk of harboring cancer. The NCCN panel (see "Screening" in this chapter) recommends that an extended-pattern twelve-core biopsy be used.

Prostate biopsy is generally very well tolerated. Patients may notice a small amount of rectal bleeding and will typically notice blood-tinged or brownish-colored ejaculate for up to a couple of weeks following the biopsy; they may also notice blood in their urine. Those who experience persistent bleeding, pain, or fever following the procedure need to contact their physician.

Biopsy results are typically available in one to two weeks. The biopsy may show prostate cancer or other conditions that are not cancer but require close follow-up because they are associated with finding cancer on future biopsies. These conditions are known as atypical small acinar proliferation (ASAP) and high-grade prostatic intraepithelial neoplasia (PIN). Both of these findings should prompt the discussion of planning a repeat biopsy. Of the two conditions, ASAP carries a higher risk of finding cancer on the repeat biopsy.

Staging/Grading

Tumor grade describes the appearance of the prostate cancer cells under the microscope and is used to gauge the aggressiveness of the tumor. The most common grading system employed in prostate cancer is the Gleason grading system. In this system, the presence of prostate cancer cells is assigned a number from 1 to 5, where 1 represents the least-aggressive-appearing pattern and 5 represents the most-aggressive-appearing pattern. The pathologist reviews the specimen and assigns a primary Gleason grade to the most common pattern of cancer and a secondary Gleason grade to the second most common pattern. The Gleason score (or sum) is simply the sum of the primary and secondary Gleason grades. Clinicians will often quote the two grades (e.g., "Your biopsy shows Gleason three plus three") rather than simply stating the sum. The reason for this is that the primary Gleason has a very strong prognostic value, and therefore a Gleason 3 + 3 would be considerably more favorable than a Gleason 4 + 2. That being said, it should be noted that Gleason patterns 1 and 2 are very rarely found.

Tumor stage refers to the extent of cancer. Prostate cancer is included in the American Joint Committee on Cancer (AJCC) TNM (T = primary tumor, N = regional nodes, M = distant metastasis) staging system. The TNM staging system for prostate cancer was last revised in 2002. Importantly, the T stage for prostate cancer includes data from both the DRE and the TRUS. As long as the prostate is in the patient's body, clinicians are referring to the clinical T stage—that is, the best estimate of the stage of the tumor given all the clinical information available. Following radical prostatectomy, a pathological T stage is assigned, whereby the final assessment is made under the pathologist's microscope. The same staging system applies, but it is important to be aware of the difference between a clinical and pathological T stage.

The following is adapted from the *AJCC Cancer Staging Manual,* Sixth Edition:

T1 tumors are those tumors that are not clinically palpable on DRE or visible on TRUS.

T1a—Incidental finding of cancer in 5 percent or less of the tissue resected during a transurethral resection of the prostate.
T1b—Incidental finding of cancer in greater than 5 percent of the tissue resected during a transurethral resection of the prostate.
T1c—Tumor identified by needle biopsy (performed because of an elevated PSA).

T2 tumors are confined to the prostate, identified by DRE or TRUS.

T2a—Tumor involves one-half of one lobe or less.
T2b—Tumor involves more than one-half of one lobe, but not both lobes.
T2c—Tumor involves both lobes.

T3 tumors extend through the prostatic capsule.

T3a—Extracapsular extension (unilateral or bilateral).
T3b—Tumor invades the seminal vesicle(s).

T4 tumors are fixed or invade adjacent structures such as the bladder neck, external sphincter, rectum, levator muscles, and pelvic wall.
N1 refers to regional lymph node metastasis.
M1 refers to distant metastasis.

M1a—Nonregional lymph nodes.
M1b—Bones.
M1c—Other sites

Treatment Overview

There is great debate surrounding the optimal treatment of prostate cancer, and a focus of this debate is on the management of localized (T1 and T2) disease. The reason this debate exists is that there has been considerably successful outcomes with the various forms of treatment and it would be nearly impossible to devise a randomized, head-to-head study that would assign patients to various treatment modalities and determine which is the most effective. Treatment decisions are made by clinicians in conjunction with their patients, taking into consideration the grade and stage of disease, the life expectancy of the patient, and the anticipated side-effect profile of the various treatment modalities, as well as patient and clinician preferences. The goal is to maximize disease-free survival while optimizing quality of life. Treatment options include surgery (radical prostatectomy), radiation (external beam, brachytherapy with permanent implants, brachytherapy with temporary implants, cryotherapy, high-intensity focused ultrasound [HIFU], hormonal therapy, and active surveillance). These will be discussed below. Prediction tools (nomograms) are available to help predict patients' response to the various forms of treatment based on pretreatment parameters such as clinical stage, Gleason score determined from the prostate biopsy, and diagnostic PSA level.

Watchful Waiting or Active Surveillance

The risk of disease progression is low in patients with Gleason scores 2 to 6 (with no pattern 4 or 5 present), T1 or T2a disease, and serum PSAs that are low and stable. Men with these grade findings and well-characterized, early-stage prostate cancer can be followed carefully and treated at the first sign of progression. This should be performed in a structured way, where the clinician and patient are actively involved in a regular follow-up process. Such patients can be identified only after an extended core biopsy (i.e., more than ten or twelve cores obtained). Signs of progression are determined based on PSA trends, regular physical examination (DRE), and repeat prostatic biopsies. Although as many as 20 to 40 percent of men followed in such a way will ultimately be treated within a five-year period, treatment at the first sign of progression appears to be as effective as treatment at first diagnosis of cancer in this patient population. This modality may spare the patient (or at least defer) the side effects of definitive forms of treatment. It should be noted that the optimal follow-up strategies for patients on active surveillance are still in the process of being defined by researchers in this area.

Surgery Radical prostatectomy is a surgical procedure to remove the prostate and seminal vesicles. There are various surgical approaches to the prostate employed by urologists; these include radical perineal prostatectomy (midline incision between the scrotum and the anus), radical retropubic prostatectomy (midline incision from the waist level down to the pubic symphysis), and laparoscopic/robotic prostatectomy (involving five to six trocar incisions [5 to 15 mm each] across the abdominal wall). Surgery time is approximately two to four hours and the patient is typically hospitalized for two to four days. At the time of surgery, the surgeon may elect to remove the pelvic lymph nodes in higher-risk cases or if there is an intraoperative finding suggesting more advanced disease. This slightly increases the operative time and increases the risk of developing a lymphocele during the postoperative period. Regardless of the surgical approach, patients are typically eating a regular diet and walking around by one to two days after surgery and can be expected to return to full activity within $2\frac{1}{2}$ to 3 weeks.

While rare, complications do occur and may be attributed to the experience of the surgeon and the overall health status of the patient. Intraoperative complications include bleeding, rectal injury, and ureteral injury. Perioperative complications include deep venous thrombosis (blood clot), pulmonary embolism, lymphocele, and wound infection. Late complications include urinary incontinence and impotence. During surgery, the urethra is transected, allowing removal of the prostate, and then re-anastomosed (sewn back together) to the bladder neck. While this heals, a catheter is left in place. Most surgeons keep the catheter in place for one to two weeks. The patient can go home with the catheter and perform his regular activities of daily living. Many patients will regain continence within days to weeks after catheter removal. Total incontinence is rare; however, up to 20 percent of patients do experience stress incontinence (loss of urine with coughing, laughing, or strenuous activity). Preservation of potency is largely related to patient age, preoperative sexual function, and the ability of the surgeon to preserve the neurovascular bundles that course immediately alongside the prostate. In men under sixty with both neurovascular bundles preserved, postoperative potency rates are quoted from 40 to 82 percent. This figure drops to 20 to 60 percent if one bundle is preserved. It can take six to eighteen months to regain potency. Potency can be improved with the use of erectile medications such as sildenafil (Viagra), vardenafil (Levitra), and tadalfil (Cialis) in the early postoperative period. Potency can also be improved using injection therapy,

vacuum erection devices, or, more rarely, an implanted prosthesis.

Radiation

External-Beam Radiotherapy

The goal of radiation therapy in any form is to deliver a high enough dose of radiation to kill the cancerous tissue, while minimizing the radiation dose to the surrounding normal tissues. Higher-dose radiation not only carries a higher probability of killing the cancer cells, but also carries a higher risk of causing damaging side effects to the surrounding normal tissues. Traditional external-beam radiation uses bony landmarks or a single planning CT scan to define the target area. Improved imaging capabilities and novel treatment planning (three-dimensional conformal radiation therapy [3-D CRT] and intensity-modulated radiation therapy [IMRT]) allow radiation therapists to fine-tune the radiation dose to much more closely target the prostate. With these techniques, greater doses of radiation can be delivered, while minimizing the toxicity to the surrounding tissues. The application of 3-D CRT and IMRT has led to improved tumor control and decreased side effects. Proton-beam radiation is another modification. Proton-beams emit high-energy rays with special properties permitting the energy to be directed more precisely to the prostate compared to conventional radiation therapy. The ability to intensely focus the proton beam permits an effective dose of radiation to be given in fewer treatment sessions. Regardless of the specific technique used, doses greater than or equal to 7,200 cGy appear to be necessary to optimize treatment effect. Some believe there may be an added treatment benefit to radiating the pelvic lymph nodes; however, not all agree. There is evidence to suggest that daily variation in prostate and patient positioning can have a major impact on the effective dose of radiation delivered. For this reason, on-line daily portal imaging in the form of CT scans, ultrasound, endorectal balloon, and/or pretreatment placement of radio-opaque markers may be employed to optimize the dose of radiation delivered to the prostate.

In addition to dose escalation and improved tumor targeting, the results of radiation therapy may be improved with the use of neoadjuvant (prior to treatment), concurrent, and adjuvant androgen deprivation (see "Hormonal Therapy," in this chapter). Androgen deprivation has been proven to improve the outcome of radiation in patients with intermediate-risk (PSA 10 to 20 ng/ml, T2b, or Gleason score 7) or high-risk (PSA greater than 20 ng/ml, T3, or Gleason score 8, 9, or 10) disease. The use of short-term (three to four months) neoadjuvant and concurrent androgen deprivation is recommended for patients with intermediate-risk disease, whereas patients with high-risk disease appear to benefit from longer periods (twenty-four months) of androgen deprivation.

Like radical prostatectomy, men who receive radiation may experience side effects—typically related to urinary, bowel, and sexual function. Most such side effects are limited in extent. Whereas men who undergo surgery are more likely to suffer incontinence, men who undergo radiation are more likely to suffer obstructive or irritative voiding or bowel symptoms (diarrhea, rectal bleeding, or tenesmus—a painful spasm of the anal sphincter accompanied by an urgent desire to evacuate the bowel that results in the passing of little or no matter). Whereas the impact of surgery on sexual function occurs early and potency may improve with time, the impact of radiation on sexual function may not be seen for eighteen to twenty-four months, as the toxic side effects of the radiation on the nerves responsible for erectile function build up over time. The sexual side effects of radiation may be exacerbated with the concurrent use of androgen deprivation, especially if used long-term. However, most such men will respond to the use of medications or other maneuvers described above.

Brachytherapy and Permanent Implants Brachytherapy is a form of radiation whereby radioactive materials are placed in direct or close contact with the area being treated. Permanent implants in the form of iodine-125 or palladium-103 radioactive seeds may be used. Treatment planning involves integrating anatomical and radiopharmaceutical data to optimize the radiation dose delivered to the prostate. The procedure itself can be performed as a come-and-go, same day, outpatient procedure. No incisions are necessary. During the procedure, several needles loaded with the radioactive seeds are placed through the skin of the perineum and the seeds are delivered to their preplanned position within the prostate. The entire procedure can be performed in about one hour. Patients generally go home the same day and can resume their normal level of activity within a few days. The radioactivity of the seeds decays rather quickly, reaching half-strength in seventeen days (palladium) or sixty days (iodine).

Optimal patients for permanent-seed brachytherapy tend to be those with smaller prostates (less than 60 cc), no pubic arch interference (on TRUS imaging), minimal lower urinary tract symptoms, a PSA less than 10 ng/ml, and a Gleason score less than or equal to 6. Patients meeting these criteria tend to do well with brachytherapy as monotherapy and typically do not require additional radiation in the form of external-beam radiation or concurrent androgen deprivation. Patients with higher PSA levels and/or higher Gleason grade tumors may still be candidates for permanent implant brachytherapy; however, they will likely also be given external-beam radiation to the prostate and/or regional lymph nodes. They may also be given adjuvant androgen deprivation. When permanent-seed brachytherapy is employed as monotherapy, side effects are usually limited as described above and are generally related to irritative voiding symptoms (burning, frequency, and urgency), which tend to wane over time. There is minimal immediate effect on continence or potency. The cumulative effect of the radiation likely has a negative impact on erectile function over time.

High-Dose Rate Brachytherapy (Temporary Implants) Another form of brachytherapy is known as HDR (high-dose-rate) brachytherapy. With this modality, a series of approximately sixteen small hollow-bore catheters are passed through the perineum into the prostate gland under transrectal ultrasound guidance while the patient is sedated. These catheters are temporarily fixed in position and the patient is transferred to a CT scanner for treatment planning. Next, the hollow-bore catheters are filled with radioactive rods (iridium-192) that deliver a very high dose of radiation over a short period of time. Computer software customizes the amount of radiation delivered through each catheter. Typically, the patient receives two treatment sessions and is discharged home the following day. The patient can resume normal activities within a few days.

Since a very high dose of radiation is given, the placement of the catheters is a critical step in delivering effective radiation to the prostate and minimizing the side effects of the treatment. This modality is ideally suited for larger tumors and is typically employed in patients with higher-risk disease, where it is often combined with external-beam radiation and/or androgen deprivation. Researchers are currently investigating the role of HDR brachytherapy as monotherapy for patients with low-risk disease.

Based on contemporary information, radiation therapy delivered well, in appropriate doses by any means described above and when combined appropriately with androgen deprivation, appears to result in similar long-term, relapse-free outcomes as does surgery. Only well-designed randomized trials will determine whether or not there may be small to moderate differences in outcomes between these two forms of treatment.

 Cryosurgery Cryosurgery is an attempt at minimally invasive management of prostate cancer. Small cryoprobes are passed through the perineum under TRUS guidance. A freezing solution of argon gas or liquid nitrogen is used to cool the probes and freeze the prostate tissue. Typically, two freeze-thaw cycles are used, as both the freezing and thawing processes have their own properties that contribute to ablating tissue. Cancer cell destruction (the goal of the treatment modality) occurs when the prostate reaches –40°F (–40°C). Cryosurgery can result in negative posttreatment prostatic biopsies and low or undetectable serum PSA levels. However, the morbidity of cryosurgery is significant, including damage to the nerve bundles responsible for normal erectile function and sloughing of normal urethral tissue, causing significant and persistent urinary symptoms. Further, the long-term results are unknown. Some clinicians reserve the use of cryosurgery for cases of local recurrence involving a very specific location in the prostate. Others have advocated more focal cryosurgery as up-front treatment specifically directed to the site of presumed cancer in order to minimize side effects of treatment. Further refinements in imaging and tumor site identification are required before such treatment can be done with confidence in larger numbers of patients.

High-Intensity Focused Ultrasound (HIFU)
High-intensity focused ultrasound (HIFU) can be delivered to the prostate using a rectal probe. This technology kills normal and cancerous prostate tissue by heating the tissues to 185°F (85°C). Treatment sessions typically range from one to three hours and can be performed as an outpatient procedure. Clinical experience, largely from Europe and Japan, suggests that such treatment is associated with clinical outcomes similar to those seen with cryotherapy. Meanwhile, advocates of this procedure note that treatment failures may still be managed by surgery or radiation. A transurethral resection is typically planned in conjunction with the treatment to prevent the development of obstructive urinary symptoms. This form of treatment is not currently available in the United States outside of clinical trials.

Hormonal Therapy The goal of hormonal therapy is to prevent the delivery of androgens (primarily testosterone) to prostate cancer cells. Hormonal therapy may be used at all stages of the disease and can send prostate cancer cells into a prolonged state of hibernation and/or death. Ultimately, a population of prostate cancer cells adapt and learn how to survive and grow even if they are starved of androgens, and this modality becomes ineffective in controlling the disease—this is known as hormone-refractory prostate cancer (or androgen-independent disease).

Several medications are available that stop testosterone production and are generally referred to as LHRH (luteinizing hormone-releasing hormone) agonists. They manipulate a natural feedback system in the body that normally maintains a circulating level of testosterone, leading to a complete shutdown in testosterone production by the testes. This is termed medical castration. LHRH agonists are given by injection and are available in preparations that exert their effect for periods ranging from one to twelve months. When the testosterone level has been lowered, the PSA tends to drop quickly and the prostate shrinks. There are additional androgens produced in the adrenal glands. In some situations, the addition of oral medications called antiandrogens, which prevent androgens from entering the prostate cells, may be beneficial. The combination of these two types of hormonal medications is known as total androgen blockage or complete androgen deprivation.

While generally not thought of as a primary form of treatment, these medications are being used as primary treatment in many older patients with localized prostate cancer who do not undergo surgery or radiation. They are also used in combination with radiation to reduce the size of the prostate and decrease the number of cancer cells. Hormonal therapy has been shown to have a synergistic effect with radiation. The duration of therapy with these medications varies. They may be taken anywhere from three months to three years or indefinitely, depending upon the clinical indication.

A strategy known as intermittent androgen deprivation is used by some clinicians in an effort to minimize the side effects of the medications. Some clinicians believe the intermittent use of these medications may prolong their effectiveness, but this has not been proven. In this strategy, the therapy is administered for an initial period of six to twelve months, then stopped. Following withdrawal of the medication, PSA typically declines and then begins to rise at some point. When PSA begins to rise, hormonal therapy is resumed. The interval between these intermittent cycles can range from months to years.

An alternative to medical castration is high-dose antiandrogen therapy (bicalutamide [Casodex] 150 mg a day). This applies to men with locally advanced and metastatic disease who are interested in maintaining libido and erectile function.

An equally effective alternative to taking hormonal medications altogether is to stop the production of testosterone by having an orchiectomy (surgical removal of the testes). This eliminates the main source of testosterone.

As with any form of therapy for prostate cancer, side effects exist. Antiandrogen medications may produce gastrointestinal symptoms, breast tenderness, breast enlargement, and liver problems. There are remedies and alternative medications if these side effects occur. The absence of testosterone (caused by LHRH agonists or orchiectomy) can produce a loss in the desire for sex, weight gain, hot flashes, loss of muscle strength, fatigue, osteoporosis, cognitive delay, and sometimes mild depression. There are measures available to mitigate these potential side effects. Agents such as calcium and vitamin D supplements can be used to prevent bone loss; in more severe cases, bisphosphonates may be appropriate. Elderly patients, those on androgen deprivation for long periods of time, and those with a previous history of fractures should be screened for osteoporosis or osteopenia.

Treatment by Stage

The approach to treating patients with prostate cancer is generally based on determining the level of risk of the patient with regard to the ability of the various treatment modalities to maintain the patient in a disease-free state following treatment.

■ Stage T1

The finding of T1a disease prompts a discussion between the patient and his treating urologist. Typically, this is managed with close observation. The finding of T1b disease is quite rare in the PSA era.

T1c tumors prompt a significant discussion between the patient and his physician. Essentially, all treatment modalities are available to these patients, but it is very important to have a clear understanding of the risks and benefits of the various forms of treatment as well as the specific preferences of the patient. In the absence of any Gleason pattern 4 or 5, these patients tend to do well with surgery or brachytherapy (permanent-seed implant). Patients with a small volume of low-risk disease may consider active surveillance as a real option and appear not to jeopardize their treatment options by initially opting for a course of surveillance. Available studies suggest similar results with surgery and brachytherapy at six to eight years of follow-up. There is currently more long-term data available for surgery than for brachytherapy; this tends to make some clinicians more comfortable with surgery when dealing with younger patients. When Gleason pattern 4 or 5 is present, radiation therapy options will generally include a course of androgen deprivation. Treatment decisions at that point are largely impacted by the patient's feelings toward androgen deprivation.

In the absence of Gleason pattern 4 or 5, the five-year progression-free probability is greater than 90 percent regardless of treatment modality. In the presence of Gleason pattern 4 or 5, progression-free probability rates range from 80 to 90 percent.

■ Stage T2

T2a tumors generally have a very similar prognosis to T1c tumors, and essentially the same treatment options apply, including active surveillance when the patient presents with a low PSA and a small volume of low-grade disease.

Prognosis is quite similar to T1c disease.

T2b and T2c tumors represent more involvement of the prostate by the cancer

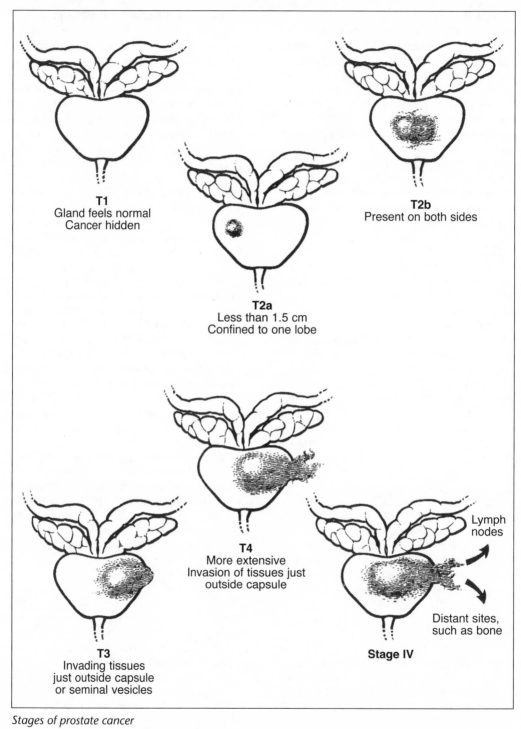

Stages of prostate cancer

and bump the patient into an intermediate or high-risk category depending on his PSA level and biopsy Gleason score. These patients tend to do well with surgery or radiation. Radiation may be of any of the various forms but will tend to include at least a short course of androgen deprivation and perhaps longer depending on the PSA level and biopsy Gleason score. Again, the patient's attitudes toward androgen deprivation will have a significant impact on treatment decision making.

Five-year progression-free probabilities range from 60 to 75 percent depending on the diagnostic PSA and biopsy Gleason score.

Stage T3

Patients with T3 disease may still be good candidates for surgery, particularly if their tumor appears to be bulging out in a very focal area, as the surgeon can tailor the approach to widely resect the affected area and remove the regional lymph nodes. More extensive disease with a large amount of Gleason pattern 4 and/or 5 or invasion of regional structures may have similar or better outcomes with radiation. Such cases would typically be treated with a protracted course (two to three years) of hormonal therapy, as well.

Five-year progression-free probabilities range from 15 to 60 percent and vary significantly depending on the diagnostic PSA and biopsy Gleason score. At this stage, the risk of regional lymph node involvement becomes considerable and treatment planning should address the possibility of finding cancer in the regional nodes.

Stage T4

The mainstay of treatment for T4 tumors is hormonal treatment. Radiation in conjunction with hormonal therapy may improve regional symptoms. There is generally a very limited role for radical surgery. Endoscopic procedures (transurethral resection of the prostate) may be employed to improve urinary symptoms.

N-positive and M-positive Disease

Some patients will be found to have tumors outside of the prostate at the time of their initial diagnosis of prostate cancer. A more likely scenario leading to the development of tumors outside the prostate gland is following a recurrence after surgery or radiation (see "Recurrent Cancer" in this chapter). The mainstay of treatment in these patients is hormonal treatment. There have been long debates on the optimal timing for initiating hormonal therapy in these patients, but we do know that patients who were found to have positive lymph nodes during radical prostatectomy and were given early hormonal therapy demonstrated a survival advantage compared to those given hormonal therapy at a later date.[3] There is some evidence to suggest that patients with metastatic disease who are treated with total androgen blockade demonstrate increased survival compared to patients treated with medical castration (LHRH agonist only). Other studies have failed to prove a survival advantage to either hormonal approach. In any event, patients with metastatic disease tend to demonstrate significant clinical improvement when given hormonal therapy. In the event a patient with metastatic disease is being treated with hormonal therapy and develops new bone pain, these lesions can be treated effectively (for palliation) with a short (three-day) course of radiation.

The development of a rising PSA despite hormonal therapy to suppress testosterone indicates the presence of what is called hormone refractory prostate cancer (HRPC) or androgen-independent prostate cancer. There are many treatment options in this situation and they include the use of further hormonal manipulations ("secondary" hormonal therapy), radiation, and chemotherapy, as well as bone-targeted therapy.

Secondary hormonal therapies usually consist of a drug called ketoconazole (Nizoral), which lowers the levels of testosterone-like hormones, or the use of another antiandrogen such as nilutamide (Nilandron) or flutamide (Drogenil). Steroid drugs like prednisone and dexamethasone (Decadron) are also used, as are estrogens such as diethylstilbestrol (DES) and estradiol.

Patients with cancer that has spread to the bones are susceptible to fractures and other complications in the bone. One drug, zoledronic acid (Zometa), has been shown to reduce the rate of complications in the bone and is in widespread use in this setting. It is administered intravenously approximately once per month.

Historically, chemotherapy for prostate cancer in the form of mitoxantrone (Novantrone) and prednisone was given for its palliative effects, as it demonstrated improved quality of life (primarily an improvement in pain) but failed to improve survival. Recently, docetaxel (Taxotere)–based chemotherapy regimens have for the first time proven to produce a survival advantage in patients with hormone refractory prostate cancer. These findings have prompted several ongoing studies to evaluate the role of docetaxel-based regimens at earlier stages of the disease.

In addition to novel hormonal and chemotherapeutic regimens, research into other new forms of therapy for men with advanced prostate cancer is currently under way. One approach now being studied in clinical trials is a form of active cellular immunotherapy known as dendritic cell–based therapy. A drug is designed to activate T cells against a particular prostate cancer cell target known as prostatic acid phosphatase. Another approach currently undergoing clinical trials involves targeting the androgen receptor of the prostate cancer cell through various mechanisms. Another

has been to target the blood supply to the tumor via an endothelin receptor antagonist. As our scientific understanding of the disease continues to grow, well-designed clinical trials will play an instrumental role in allowing new, molecular-based therapies to succeed.

Treatment Follow-Up

The primary follow-up of patients following definitive therapy consists of monitoring the PSA at regular intervals. Postsurgical patients look for an undetectable PSA. Patients who have had a form of radiation look for a low and nonrising PSA; attention is also paid to the time it takes for these patients to reach their nadir (lowest recorded) PSA. Patients treated with brachytherapy will often experience a PSA "bounce," a posttreatment PSA rise that is followed by a fall. This phenomenon can also occur in patients treated with external-beam radiation. This is not a cause for alarm or concern and does not represent a progression of their cancer. Patients with advanced disease are also monitored by their PSA. Hormonal medication can be manipulated in an effort to maximally control the disease (as represented by PSA level and findings on bone scans and CT scans). Patients on hormonal therapy for an extended period of time must be monitored for bone mineral density. Many of the side effects of hormonal therapy (such as anemia, bone loss, and hot flashes) can be mitigated with various medications. Patients should be forthcoming to their physician with any concerns they have.

Recurrent Cancer

Among surgically treated patients, recurrence is more common in those with positive surgical margins, established extracapsular extension, seminal vesicle invasion, and high-grade disease. For those patients in whom a detectable PSA level develops after radical prostatectomy, the site of recurrence (local versus distant) can be established with reasonable certainty based on the interval from surgery to the detectable PSA concentration, PSA doubling time, and selective use of imaging studies. Patients with persistently detectable serum PSA levels immediately after surgery, those with PSA levels that become detectable in the early postoperative period, and those with serum PSA levels that double rapidly are more likely to have systemic relapse. Those patients thought to have recurrent localized disease based on a long time from surgery to biochemical failure, prolonged PSA doubling times (greater than ten to twelve months), and the presence of positive surgical margins at the time of surgery are most likely to benefit from salvage radiation (in such cases, up to a 77 percent freedom from subsequent relapse may be achievable). Patients who have high-grade disease or seminal vesicle involvement at the time of surgery, who fail early, or who have rapid PSA kinetics after surgery are less likely to respond and should be considered for systemic therapy.

Among patients initially treated with radiation therapy, a rising PSA level following definitive radiotherapy is indicative of cancer recurrence. For those who undergo radiation and experience biochemical failure (persistently rising PSA), the site of recurrence may be identified using PSA kinetics, time to failure, prostate biopsies, and selective use of imaging studies. Most patients who fail radiation, irrespective of the site of recurrence, are managed with androgen deprivation (hormonal therapy). However, patients who are thought to have local recurrence only may be candidates for salvage local therapies in the form of brachytherapy, cryosurgery, or salvage prostatectomy. However, the morbidity of these salvage procedures is considerably higher than when they are used as primary treatment, and there is a significant risk of subsequent relapse.

Regardless of treatment course selected or the stage of disease, it is very important for the patient to feel he has the ability to have an open and honest discussion with his doctor. It is important to include the input of family and loved ones in treatment decision making, and patients should consider bringing these people with them to their appointments. There is an enormous amount of research going on in prostate cancer and our approach to the disease is continuously evolving. Patients may find great use in educational and supportive materials available in books and/or on the Internet. Patient support groups are an excellent avenue for discussing and sharing concerns and learning from the experiences of others.

The Most Important Questions You Can Ask

• Does my cancer appear to be confined to the prostate, and how can you tell?

• Does my cancer require treatment?

• Is there anything I can do to minimize my chances of being diagnosed with prostate cancer?

• Is there anything I can do to minimize the chances of this cancer progressing or recurring? Should I modify my diet or lifestyle in any way?

• Does my diagnosis have any impact on my brother's, son's, or grandson's risks of this disease?

• What is the difference in results between surgery and radiation for patients with tumors like mine? What are the major side effects of the various treatments? What are the outcomes? Are they the same? What is my likelihood of becoming impotent or incontinent as a result of the treatment? What is the risk of developing bowel problems? If I have these side effects, how would they be managed?

• How are most patients like me treated? What are their outcomes under your care?

• Are there any alternatives to the form of hormonal therapy that I am taking?

• How might I choose between surgery, radiation, androgen ablation, and watchful waiting? Why is one or the other treatment best for me? Should more than one be used? If so, is there a preferred sequence? If my cancer comes back after initial treatment, how will it be managed?

• Is my surgeon a board-certified urologist experienced in this kind of operation or technique? What is his or her experience with nerve-sparing procedures? Is he or she aware of its outcome in terms of cancer control, potency, and continence?

• Can you refer me to specialists who can give me additional opinions on forms of treatment for my disease?

• Are multiple treatment modalities offered at this medical center? Do the urologists, radiation oncologists, and medical oncologists act as a team and meet regularly to consult on and discuss patients? Should my case be discussed at a tumor board?

• Who will be following my prostate cancer after my initial treatment course?

• How can I get in contact with my provider if I have more questions or concerns or have any problems?

• Can you refer me to patients or support groups that can share their experiences with me?

• What are other sources of information?

Notes

1. Jemal et al., 2007.
2. Kupelian et al., 2006.
3. Messing et al., 1999.

Sarcomas of Bone and Soft Tissue

*Thierry M. Jahan, M.D., Richard J. O'Donnell, M.D., Eric K. Nakakura, M.D., Ph.D.,
Malin Dollinger, M.D., and Frederick Eilber, M.D.*

Sarcomas are uncommon malignant tumors that begin either in bones or in soft tissues such as muscles, cartilage, fat, and connective tissue. There are approximately 6,000 cases of soft-tissue sarcoma and 2,000 cases of bone sarcoma in the United States each year, making up about 1 percent of cancers in adults and 15 percent in children (see also the chapters "Childhood Cancers: Soft-Tissue and Bone Sarcomas," "Kaposi's Sarcoma," "Mesothelioma," and "Uterus: Uterine Sarcomas").

Sarcomas tend to affect certain age groups. Soft-tissue sarcomas most often occur in adults older than forty. Pediatric soft-tissue malignancies are exceedingly rare, with very young children being most frequently affected (specifically, by the rhabdomyosarcoma subtype). By contrast, bone sarcomas are more common in children than in adults. Osteosarcoma primarily affects teenagers. Ewing's sarcoma tends to affect children (ages five to nine) and young adults (ages twenty to thirty). Chondrosarcoma is the most common bone sarcoma affecting adults; it tends to affect the older age groups (fifty to sixty years).

Over the past forty years, there have been major advances in the diagnosis, treatment, and prognosis of these very rare tumors. Radiologic imaging—including computed tomography (CT), magnetic resonance (MR), technetium (bone), and positron-emission tomography (PET) scans—has served to promote early diagnosis and staging. Treatment has been enhanced by progress in the areas of radiation oncology and musculoskeletal

cancer surgery. Sarcomas in the extremities, for instance, can now be managed with limb-sparing techniques roughly 85 percent of the time. Dramatic improvements in overall survival, however, are attributed mainly to the establishment of effective chemotherapy guidelines. The overall survival for people with sarcomas, which had been on the order of 20 percent (bone) to 40 percent (soft tissue) in the late 1960s, has risen to approximately 70 percent in 2007.

Types Soft-tissue sarcomas are named according to the normal tissue from which the tumor is thought to have derived; more than fifty histologic subtypes are thought to exist. Many have characteristic patterns of growth and spread. Specialists use the specific type to help plan tests and treatment, but the likely behavior of the tumor is most closely related to three factors: *depth* (beneath the muscle fascia is worse), *size* (larger than 2 inches [5 cm] is concerning), and most especially *grade* (there are up to four grades, 1 through 4). Grade in turn is defined by *mitosis* (dividing cells), *necrosis* (cell death), *atypia* (tumor cells different from normal), and *pleomorphism* (tumor cells different from one another). Low-grade tumors have a chance to recur locally but generally do not spread; high-grade tumors (Grades 3 and 4) have the greatest propensity to metastasize.

Grade is also of great importance for bone sarcomas, which can also be subdivided according to Grades 1 through 4. By contrast, however, there are only three main subtypes of malignancies that arise in bone: osteosarcoma, Ewing's sarcoma, and chondrosarcoma.

How It Spreads Like other types of tumors, sarcomas are generally confined by a capsule, but "satellite" lesions can be present in surrounding soft tissues and "skip" metastases can sometimes occur in different parts of a bone affected by a tumor. However, by far the most common site for a sarcoma to spread is the lung. Other metastatic deposits can occur in nearby lymph nodes or in the liver.

What Causes It In most cases, the cause of sarcoma is unknown, although some tumors are related to certain diseases or exposure to specific agents. Soft-tissue sarcomas do not arise from benign tumors, but some apparently benign bone tumors—cartilage lesions, for example—can become malignant. Malignant bone tumors are more common in adolescents, supporting the theory that these tumors may occur because of rapid growth.

Risk Factors

• About 10 percent of people with von Recklinghausen's disease, a rare genetic abnormality affecting nerves, will develop malignant peripheral nerve sheath tumors.

• Other genetically linked diseases that have a slightly increased incidence of associated sarcomas include Werner's syndrome, tuberous sclerosis, intestinal polyposis, basal cell nevus syndrome, and Gardner's syndrome.

• Lymphangiosarcoma is associated with people who have chronic swelling of an arm or leg and can occur many years after a mastectomy, particularly when lymph nodes in the axilla have been resected and the area has been radiated.

• The risk of angiosarcoma of the liver increases with exposure to thorium dioxide (Thorotrast; an intravenous [radiographic] contrast agent no longer in use), arsenic, or vinyl chloride or in association with cirrhosis or hemochromatosis.

• Sarcomas of both bone and soft tissue can occur many years after radiotherapy, especially if it was given in childhood. Radiation exposure causes less than 5 percent of such tumors, however.

• Various causes of chronic irritation or stimulation to bones, including chronic bone infection, fibrous dysplasia, and Paget's disease, are risk factors for sarcoma development.

• Sarcomas have developed in old scars or areas of trauma or fracture, but a definite cause-and-effect relationship is very difficult to prove.

• Many types of bone and soft-tissue sarcomas have been found to be associated with characteristic chromosome abnormalities. Some families appear to have an increased incidence of sarcomas. Another inherited genetic abnormality —deletion of the retinoblastoma gene— also increases risk.

• Some chemotherapeutic agents, particularly "alkylating" agents, increase sarcoma risk.

Screening

Because these are rare tumors that can arise virtually anywhere in the body, there are no standard screening measures. Bone and soft-tissue sarcomas may appear silently, with an enlarging mass or swelling that may not be apparent until it causes pain or pressure symptoms. The masses evade discovery not only because these cancers grow without producing symptoms, but also because they often arise in inaccessible places.

Early detection requires that all unexplained masses arising in the bone and soft tissues be assessed by a physician. When appropriate, X-rays and scans (bone, CT, MRI, and PET) need to be ordered. Biopsy and surgical removal may be necessary.

Types of Sarcomas

TUMOR TYPE	TISSUE OF ORIGIN
Bone	
Chondrosarcoma	Cartilage
Osteosarcoma	Bone
Parosteal osteosarcoma	Bone surface
Ewing's sarcoma	Neural crest (primitive nerve)
Soft-Tissue	
Malignant fibrous histiocytoma	Primitive connective tissue
Liposarcoma	Fat
Rhabdomyosarcoma	Skeletal muscle
Leiomyosarcoma	Smooth muscle
Malignant peripheral nerve sheath tumor	Nerve structures
Angiosarcoma	Blood vessels
Lymphangiosarcoma	Lymph vessels
Fibrosarcoma	Connective (fibrous) tissue
Epithelioid sarcoma	Unknown
Clear cell sarcoma	Unknown
Synovial sarcoma	Unknown
Alveolar soft-part sarcoma	Unknown

Common Signs and Symptoms

The most common complaint is a swelling or a mass, which is most often painless. When pain occurs in the soft tissues or in an affected bone or joint, it is often worse at night. Very occasionally, there may be generalized symptoms such as fever, sweats, chills, weight loss, and fatigue.

Diagnosis

Blood and Other Tests Blood tests—including complete blood count, sedimentation rate, C-reactive protein level, electrolytes, liver function tests, and serum protein electrophoresis—aid in narrowing the differential diagnosis list. Unfortunately, blood results are neither sensitive nor specific for the detection of sarcoma.

Imaging

• X-rays will suggest a diagnosis of the most probable type of bone sarcomas, but soft-tissue sarcomas do not show up well on regular X-rays.

• For soft-tissue tumors, CT or MRI scans are useful for finding masses and determining their size and relationship to surrounding structures. CT scans are better for looking at cortical bone; MRI scans are better for soft tissues and bone marrow. A CT scan of the chest, abdomen, and pelvis is helpful in ruling out metastases.

• Bone scans add information about local and distant bone involvement (metastases).

• A PET or PET/CT scan can help to assess the grade of a particular tumor and to rule out hidden metastases. However, use of PET technology is not yet thought to be the "standard of care" for sarcomas.

Biopsy Biopsy of the suspected lesion is essential. The biopsy must be done carefully, under the direction of a physician skilled in minimally invasive (needle) and open (operative) techniques. The type of biopsy procedure used needs to take the ultimate surgical treatment into account, and complications such as bleeding and wound infection need to be avoided. Diagnosis of the biopsy material must be done by a pathologist familiar with musculoskeletal tumors.

Staging

Stage is determined by the tumor's size and grade and whether it has spread to nearby lymph nodes or distant sites. Several staging systems are used for adult soft-tissue sarcomas, pediatric sarcomas, and bone sarcomas.

The TNM classification system is useful to specialists, but a simplified staging system uses the grade of the tumor—the primary factor determining survival—to divide adult soft-tissue sarcomas into four stages (I through IV). Stages I, II, and III, none of which involve spread to nearby lymph nodes or distant sites, are also divided into substages A (tumors less than 2 inches [5 cm] in diameter) and B (tumors larger than that). Stage IV tumors have spread to regional lymph nodes (IVA) or to distant sites (IVB).

Grade is determined primarily by the percentage of dividing cells in the tumor. Grade 1 tumors are well differentiated and have only a small chance of spreading to another site. Grade 2 tumors are moderately differentiated and have a less than 20 percent chance of spreading. Grade 3 and 4 tumors are poorly differentiated, meaning that they contain immature cells that divide rapidly. They have a greater than 50 percent chance of metastasizing.

Five-year survival is usually better than 75 percent for low-grade tumors and less than 25 percent for high-grade tumors.

Adult Soft-Tissue Sarcomas: Treatment Overview

(For treatment of pediatric soft-tissue and bone sarcomas, see the chapter "Childhood Cancers: Soft-Tissue and Bone Sarcomas." Management of young adults and older individuals with bone tumors parallels that of children.)

Sarcomas are best treated by an experienced team of specialists in surgical oncology (often orthopedic oncologists in the case of bone tumors), radiation oncology, and medical oncology.

The initial biopsy must be carefully planned not only to ensure that enough tissue is available for diagnosis, but also to allow for subsequent surgery. This is especially important with sarcomas involving the arms or legs, where a poorly performed biopsy can decrease the likelihood of limb-sparing surgery.

Prognosis is affected by a patient's age; the size of the primary tumor; the grade and stage; the degree of lymphatic and blood vessel invasion; the duration of symptoms; and the location of the tumor on the arm, leg, or trunk. Unfavorable prognostic signs include age over sixty, a tumor larger than 2 inches (5 cm), a high-grade tumor, spread to lymph nodes or distant sites, a deep rather than a superficial malignancy, and symptoms lasting less than one year.

Low-grade tumors can usually be cured by surgery alone. High-grade sarcomas have a greater tendency to recur in the same area or to metastasize; thus, they are often treated with surgery, radiotherapy, and/or chemotherapy. A combination of these modalities is often used in order to improve the possibility of cure.

Surgery Surgery has been and remains the mainstay of treatment for sarcomas. Whether tumors involve the bone or soft tissue, limb-salvage procedures are now most commonly performed. Complete involvement of the blood vessels and nerves might well prompt an amputation, but otherwise there are few absolute contraindications to limb salvage. For sarcomas in the truncal region, surgical principles are the same, but particularly for retroperitoneal (back of the abdomen) tumors, local control by surgery is more difficult, and, of course, amputation is not an option.

In all cases of sarcoma, the goal is to achieve negative surgical margins. The definition of "wide" surgical margins is a matter of great debate, but at a minimum, "negative" margins (no microscopic cells at the edge of the resected tumor) are a desirable goal.

After tumor removal, some sort of simultaneous reconstructive process is often necessary. In the case of soft-tissue tumors, plastic surgical muscle flaps or skin grafts are sometimes needed. For bone defects, a wide variety of options are available, including bone grafts and metallic implants. Growing children are candidates for expandable devices that can be lengthened. Amputee patients have also benefited from tremendous advances in external prosthetic technology.

 Radiation Some sarcoma subtypes, such as osteosarcomas, are not sensitive to radiation therapy. However, for most sarcomas, the gold standard for tumor control has been surgery combined with radiation therapy. Radiation is thought to be necessary in most such cases in order to prevent local or regional recurrences from microscopic cells left behind after surgery or from adjacent "satellite" lesions that were not removed. Radiation therapy can be given before, during, or after surgery.

 Chemotherapy Several drugs have proven to be effective in treating bone and soft-tissue sarcomas. However, the dosages required to provide a good chance for cure often produce significant side effects. Chemotherapy is most effective for high-grade tumors and tends to be ineffective for low-grade tumors.

Effective single agents include doxorubicin (Adriamycin), cyclophosphamide (Cytoxan), high-dose methotrexate (Mexate, Amethopterin, Folex; with leucovorin [LV] rescue), ifosfamide (Ifex), dacarbazine (DTIC-Dome), vincristine (Oncovin), dactinomycin (actinomycin D, Cosmegen), and etoposide (Etopophos). Investigational agents also hold promise.

Commonly used combinations include

- mesna (Mesnex) + ifosfamide + doxorubicin (IA);
- mesna + doxorubicin + ifosfamide + dacarbazine (MAID);
- doxorubicin + cyclophosphamide + methotrexate;
- cyclophosphamide + vincristine + doxorubicin + dacarbazine (CyVADIC);
- ifosfamide + etoposide (IE);
- doxorubicin + cyclophosphamide; and
- doxorubicin + dacarbazine + cyclophosphamide.

Other combinations of these drugs have been used, but investigational agents have also been added.

Preoperative Chemotherapy Rhabdomyosarcoma, osteosarcoma, and Ewing's sarcoma are very rare malignancies that tend to occur in children and young adults. While rhabdomyosarcoma arises in the soft tissues and visceral organs, osteosarcoma and Ewing's sarcoma are generally found in bone, although soft-tissue variants do occur. Preoperative ("neoadjuvant") chemotherapy is part of the standard and optimal initial treatment for these three conditions in both children and adults. For Ewing's sarcoma and rhabdomyosarcoma, radiation therapy is generally added either before or after surgery, depending on the circumstances. Surgery is planned for all patients with osteosarcoma and for most patients with Ewing's sarcoma or rhabdomyosarcoma. Postoperative ("adjuvant") chemotherapy after surgery is mandatory for these diagnoses. In most centers, the resected tumor specimen is examined for significant tumor destruction to see if the same chemotherapeutic agents should be given again or if changes should be made.

In the past, adults with soft-tissue sarcoma were not treated with chemotherapy before surgery. Many studies failed to show a survival benefit for this treatment. However, great advances have been made in terms of supportive care for patients receiving chemotherapy, such that higher doses of drugs can be given in a safer (and more effective) manner. Therefore, most sarcoma centers will offer preoperative chemotherapy to otherwise healthy adult soft-tissue sarcoma patients, particularly when the tumor is high grade (3 or 4), deep (to the muscle fascia), and large (greater than 2 inches [5 cm]). Neoadjuvant chemotherapy is thought to be particularly effective against certain tumor types, including synovial sarcoma and malignant fibrous histiocytoma. After local control (surgery and radiation therapy) has occurred, the patient is still a candidate for additional postoperative chemotherapy.

Postoperative Chemotherapy Even if a bone or soft-tissue sarcoma was localized and entirely removed by surgery and radiation therapy, there is a significant risk (especially in high-grade, deep, and large lesions) that tumor cells have already spread to other places in the body. Postoperative treatment with chemotherapy attempts to eliminate these tumor deposits.

As mentioned above, adjuvant chemotherapy is commonly added to preoperative regimens for rhabdomyosarcoma, Ewing's sarcoma, and osteosarcoma, whether these tumors occur in children or adults. For adult soft-tissue sarcoma patients, postoperative chemotherapy is sometimes utilized even if preoperative chemotherapy has not been given. A recent study has indicated that adjuvant treatment of patients with high-grade soft-tissue sarcomas of the extremities using epirubicin (Ellence), ifosfamide (Ifex), and mesna (Mesnex) results in significant improvement in survival.

In Metastatic Disease The treatment of metastatic disease in both bone and soft-tissue sarcomas usually involves the use of chemotherapy. If metastases are confined to the lungs, an attempt may be made to surgically remove the deposits. Minimally invasive techniques for excision of lung lesions now exist, so that most often only a wedge of affected tissue needs to be sacrificed. Chemotherapy is sometimes used preoperatively in an attempt to shrink the metastases and to demonstrate that the tumor can be partially controlled with chemotherapy.

Investigational

• Adult soft-tissue sarcoma patients without metastases are the subject of investigational protocols utilizing preoperative chemotherapy. Treatment of patients with advanced disease is being studied with newly developed chemotherapy agents.

• There are investigational protocols for patients with high-risk Ewing's sarcoma (large tumors in the pelvis) who don't respond well to preoperative treatment. As well as the standard chemotherapy, radiation, and surgery, patients are now being entered into trials of high-dose chemotherapy and autologous bone marrow transplantation.

Adult Soft-Tissue Sarcomas: Treatment by Stage

■ *Stage I*

These are well-differentiated (low-grade) tumors that have not spread to nearby lymph nodes or other sites.

Standard Treatment The primary treatment is surgery, with margins free of tumor being essential. Radiotherapy is used for tumors that cannot be removed, when surgical margins are positive, or when wider resection would mean amputation or removal of a vital organ. Adjuvant therapy is generally used only in clinical trials.

Five-Year Survival Over 90 percent

■ *Stage II*

These are moderately well-differentiated (medium-grade) tumors that have not spread to nearby lymph nodes or to other sites. These lesions are highly treatable and curable, but they are more likely to spread than Stage I tumors.

Standard Treatment For sarcomas involving the arms or legs, limb-sparing surgery is often combined with preoperative or postoperative radiotherapy. In some centers, chemotherapy is given prior to and/or after surgery. Research is continuing on the best way to combine these treatments. In some cases involving limbs, amputation may still be necessary if conservative surgery combined with radiotherapy and/or chemotherapy is not possible.

Sarcomas of the head and neck, trunk, and abdomen are treated with surgery, often followed by high-dose radiotherapy. Preoperative radiotherapy sometimes permits more conservative surgery; radiotherapy is also given postoperatively. Some centers offer the use of radiation performed during the surgery (intraoperative radiotherapy) as a way to try to control the margins of resection. Again, the use of adjuvant chemotherapy is not fully established.

High-dose radiotherapy and chemotherapy are used for tumors that cannot be removed surgically (in the head and neck or abdomen, for example).

Five-Year Survival 70 percent

Investigational

- Preoperative and/or postoperative chemotherapy
- A variety of radiotherapy techniques

■ *Stage III*

These are poorly differentiated or undifferentiated (high-grade) tumors that have not spread to nearby lymph nodes or to distant sites. This stage is further divided into IIIA and IIIB according to the size of the primary tumor.

Standard Treatment Stage IIIA sarcomas are highly treatable and often curable but have an increased chance of metastatic spread. The standard treatment is surgery with radiotherapy, with or without chemotherapy.

Sarcomas of the arms or legs are treated in a similar way to Stage II tumors. Sarcomas of the head and neck, trunk, and abdomen are treated with surgery followed by high-dose radiation. Radiotherapy is also sometimes given before surgery. Furthermore, radiation is sometimes combined with chemotherapy if the tumor cannot be completely removed surgically. Some centers offer the use of radiation performed during the surgery (intraoperative radiotherapy) as a way to try to control the margins of resection.

Stage IIIB sarcomas are treated much like Stage II and IIIA tumors. Because these tumors are larger, however, amputation for extremity tumors will more often be necessary. In some cases, preoperative radiotherapy or combination chemotherapy may allow tumors to be surgically removed when it would not have been otherwise possible. Intraoperative radiation is also sometimes used.

Stage IIIB sarcomas of the head and neck, trunk, and abdomen are treated with surgery (with or without intraoperative radiation therapy), followed by high-dose radiotherapy and chemotherapy, depending upon the circumstances. If the tumor cannot be completely removed, high-dose radiotherapy combined with chemotherapy may relieve symptoms.

Five-Year Survival 20 to 50 percent

Investigational
• Investigational treatments similar to those for Stage II
• Intraoperative radiotherapy for Stage IIIA abdominal sarcomas

■ *Stage IV*
This stage is divided into two groups. Tumors of any grade or size that have spread to regional lymph nodes but not to distant sites are Stage IVA. Tumors that have spread to distant sites beyond the lymph nodes draining the area of the cancer (most commonly to the lung) are Stage IVB.

Standard Treatment In Stage IVA, local control of the primary tumor is best obtained with surgery (including removal of lymph nodes) followed by radiotherapy. In some centers, radiotherapy is given both pre- and postoperatively. If the tumor cannot be surgically removed, radiotherapy and chemotherapy are used.

In Stage IVB, if the lung is the only site of spread, cure may be possible in up to 30 percent of patients by aggressive treatment of the primary tumor similar to earlier stages and removal of the lung metastases, even if there are several.

If lung metastases are not removed or if there are other sites of metastasis, palliation may be provided by the administration of chemotherapy, generally including doxorubicin (Adriamycin) and ifosfamide (Ifex). Recently, the combination of docetaxel (Taxotere) and gemcitabine (Gemzar) has been shown to be effective in sarcomas that have been resistant to first-line therapy with doxorubicin (Adriamycin)–containing regimes.

Standard therapy is not curative, so patients should be considered candidates for clinical trials.

Five-Year Survival Up to 20 percent

Supportive Therapy

The resources of a multidisciplinary sarcoma team should be made available to all patients with these rare malignancies. Psychological and social support is invariably necessary. Physical therapy with active and passive range-of-motion and strengthening exercises for the arms and legs is extremely important for people with primary bone and soft-tissue tumors of the extremities. Exercise programs and elastic stockings can help to prevent stiffness and swelling of the extremities. For patients with very advanced disease, hospice care provides an invaluable resource.

Treatment Follow-Up

Patients with malignant bone and soft-tissue sarcomas must be followed on a regular basis by a team skilled in the management of these rare tumors.

• Routine physical examinations screen for pain or recurrence of a mass.
• Radiology surveillance studies must be done on a routine basis.
• Plain radiographs are needed for bone tumor follow-up.
• Chest imaging (chest X-rays alternating with chest CT scans) is required for the early detection of lung metastases, since, occasionally, removal can be curative.
• CT imaging of abdominopelvic and MRI scanning of extremity surgical sites is necessary to rule out local recurrence of the tumor.
• PET scans are helpful in some circumstances (for instance, to better define abnormalities noted on surveillance CT

or MRI scans), but they are not routinely used and cannot yet be considered the standard of care for sarcomas.

Recurrent Soft-Tissue Sarcomas

Treatment of sarcomas with local, regional, or distant recurrence depends upon many factors, including prior treatment. In general, recurrences often signal the need for more aggressive therapy in terms of surgery, radiation, and chemotherapy.

• Local recurrence in the extremities can occasionally be salvaged (with additional surgery, intraoperative radiation, and flap coverage), but amputation is often necessary.

• Regional (lymph node) recurrence can be treated with surgery and radiation; chemotherapy is often added.

• Distant (lung) metastasis is treated as outlined for Stage IV disease.

• If tumors recur after chemotherapy treatment, clinical trials using new agents are appropriate.

The Most Important Questions You Can Ask

• Am I being treated at a multidisciplinary sarcoma center, where I have access to physicians (including medical oncologists, radiation oncologists, surgical oncologists, orthopedic oncologists, musculoskeletal pathologists, and others) skilled in the diagnosis and management of these very rare but often aggressive tumors?

• What is my overall chance for survival?

• What is the chance for local control of my tumor?

• What are the side effects of surgery?

  • Can my limb be saved?

  • What will my function be like?

  • What activities will I be able to do?

• What are the side effects of radiation?

• Will my arm or leg be stiff, swollen, or weak?

  • Will my abdominal and pelvic organs be affected?

• What are the side effects of chemotherapy?

  • Will I become sick?

  • Will I lose my hair?

  • Will my fertility be affected?

Skin

Wendy Sara Long, M.D., and Kenneth A. Arndt, M.D.

Skin cancer is the most common form of cancer found in humans; one out of three cancers diagnosed in the United States is a skin cancer. Basal cell cancer (BCC) and squamous cell cancer (SCC) make up the majority of skin cancer diagnoses.

More than 800,000 cases of these non-melanoma skin cancers are diagnosed in the United States each year. This is up from 400,000 cases in 1980 and 600,000 in 1990. It is estimated that approximately 50 percent of fair-skinned people who live to be sixty-five years old will have at least one skin cancer.

Ten years ago, skin cancer was usually seen only in people over forty years old, but now it is commonly diagnosed in young adults. Both BCC and SCC are more common in men, but this is changing. BCC has disproportionately been increasing in women under the age of forty. This is likely due to the accepted practices of sunbathing and tanning-bed use more common among women to achieve a "healthy tan." There is no such thing as a "healthy tan." A tan, whether it is obtained by sunbathing or tanning-bed use, or simply during routine outdoor activities, is a sign of radiation damage.

Both BCC and SCC are almost always curable, especially when found and diagnosed early in their development. One cannot rely on symptoms of pain or itching to identify these tumors. Both BCC and SCC tend to be asymptomatic, perhaps with only slight tenderness or bleeding. This emphasizes the importance of knowing what to look for on a self-exam.

Below we will discuss the presentation, behavior, diagnosis, treatment, and prevention of basal and squamous cell skin cancers. Melanoma, another type of skin cancer, is significantly different from nonmelanomatous skin cancers. Please see the chapter "Melanoma" for a complete discussion of that tumor.

Types Basal cell cancer is the most common form of all skin cancers and accounts for 75 percent of all skin cancers diagnosed in the United States. One out of five fair-skinned Americans will have at least one BCC in his or her lifetime. BCC is not exclusively found in Caucasian people. It has been diagnosed in people with more pigmentation, including, but not exclusive to, those of Asian and Mediterranean descent.

BCC develops in the base (hence, *basal cell*) of the epidermis, the outermost layer of the skin. While it can develop on any hair-bearing skin on the body, greater than 90 percent are found on skin that has been chronically exposed to the sun, including the scalp. On the face, the most common area for a BCC to develop is the nose, although it can be found anywhere on the face, including the eyelids.

The appearance of BCC can vary considerably, and it is essential to be familiar with all the types of BCC in order to diagnose it early. All BCC can bleed or ulcerate if left untreated, but this frequently is a later development, so it should not be used as an initial diagnostic criterion.

The most common type is the nodular BCC, a flesh-colored to pink round or oval translucent papule with overlying small blood vessels and a pearly appearing rolled border. Frequently, people report that they thought it was a pimple or bug bite that just didn't go away. Nodular BCC may eventually ulcerate, form a crust, and/or bleed as it enlarges.

Another presentation of BCC is the pigmented form. This tumor appears darker than the nodular type, with blue, brown, or even black specks within a pink or flesh-colored papule. Occasionally, it can appear frighteningly similar to the very aggressive malignant melanoma tumor. Naturally, it is very important to distinguish between a malignant melanoma and a pigmented BCC, as the former is not uncommonly lethal, while the latter is a slow-growing tumor with little metastatic potential.

Another form of BCC that frequently poses a diagnostic challenge to those not trained in dermatology is the superficial type. It appears as a pink or red, often scaly, localized plaque, most often on the trunk. Superficial BCC can mimic the common skin disorders eczema and psoriasis. The main differentiating tool is that BCC is rarely, if ever, itchy, while these inflammatory disorders are frequently itchy. In addition, psoriasis almost never affects the face and eczema only rarely does.

The morpheaform or sclerosing BCC is frequently diagnosed later in its development because it often looks and feels like a scar and because it tends to ulcerate or bleed only after it has invaded the skin more deeply. It presents as a firm, ill-defined, slightly raised, or even depressed, lesion. It can be pink or even whitish in color.

Squamous cell carcinoma is the second most common form of skin cancer, affecting around 200,000 Americans each year. It arises from cells in the middle of the epidermis, the outermost layer of the skin. Squamous cells, under the microscope, resemble fish scales; the root word *squama-* is derived from the Latin word for "scale." These cells make keratin, the protective protein of the epidermis.

SCC usually occurs in areas of sun-damaged skin; at sites of previous burns, scars, or chronic ulcers; or on the mucous membranes of the mouth. SCC usually appears as a red, scaling, well-defined plaque and may gradually develop an ulcer, a scaly crust, or a wartlike surface. Eventually, it can spread into the deeper or surrounding tissues and has the potential to metastasize, or spread, to lymph nodes and internal organs.

SCC in situ, or superficial noninvasive SCC, consists of cancer cells that are only in the epidermis. The noninvasive SCCs are also known as Bowen's disease. A squamous cell carcinoma is considered superficially invasive when the cancer cells have invaded the upper part of the dermis, and infiltrative when the lower dermis and fat under the skin (subcutaneous tissue) are invaded. These cancers are also described based on how differentiated, or similar to normally behaving squamous cells, the cancer cells are, ranging from well to moderately to poorly differentiated. Tumors made up of poorly differentiated tumor cells tend to behave more aggressively.

Verrucous carcinoma is a cauliflower-like (fungating) type of SCC found on the mucosa of the mouth, on genital or perianal skin, or on the plantar surface of the foot. While this form of SCC can grow very large, it tends to be less likely to metastasize than other forms of SCC of equivalent size.

There are two lesions that are considered precancerous, with the potential to develop into SCC over years. Actinic keratoses are red, scaly, gritty-feeling, and frequently tender spots on sun-exposed areas of fair-skinned individuals. Cutaneous horns are hard, funnel-shaped lesions extending from a red base on the skin and can represent a precancerous actinic keratosis or a benign wart. Also, leukoplakia, a white patch on the oral or genital mucosa, can be a precursor to SCC.

How It Spreads Basal cell cancer usually remains unchanged for years or grows very slowly. It rarely metastasizes, or spreads, to lymph nodes or internal organs. One study reported less than 0.1 percent occurrence of metastatic disease from BCC. The lesions that metastasized were large, involved the head and neck with extensive local invasion, and had recurred after treatment. When metastatic disease occurs, it spreads to local lymph nodes and less often to the bone, lungs, and liver. Survival is less than one year once such spread has been discovered. A report of patients who had died from BCC found a mean age of eighty-five and documented refusal of surgical treatment in 40 percent of the cases.

SCC has a significantly higher rate of metastatic disease, with studies reporting a 3 percent rate of spread to distant sites. Squamous cell cancer spreads via the lymph system and can involve the bone, liver, and brain. The characteristics of both the tumor and the patient determine the potential for metastatic disease to develop.

Tumors with higher metastatic potential include, but are not limited to, tumors greater than $\frac{1}{10}$ inch (4 mm) in depth, tumors with an aggressive growth pattern (with many thin strands of tumor cells infiltrating the tissue), tumors with poorly differentiated cells, recurrent/previously treated tumors, tumors arising in a site of ionizing radiation exposure or thermal burn injury, and tumors on the central face and on the mucosal membranes of the mouth and genitalia. Metastases increase to a rate of 11 percent when SCC involves the oral and genital membranes and to 10 to 30 percent when the lesions are on areas of the skin previously injured from burns.

Patients who are at a higher risk of developing metastatic SCC include all patients with a weakened immune system. This includes patients with HIV or hematologic malignancies such as lymphoma, those undergoing chemotherapy, and those who are on chronic immunosuppression medication post–organ transplantation or to treat chronic autoimmune diseases.

What Causes It Most skin cancers are caused by excessive exposure to the ultraviolet radiation (UVR) in sunlight. Other forms of radiation—including X-ray radiation and radiation from exposure to an atomic bomb detonation or a nuclear power plant accident—can induce skin cancer, in addition to many other types of cancer. These forms of radiation can cause mutations in the skin cells, which can accumulate and develop into a skin cancer. Genetic background is also a factor, since light-skinned people suffer a more adverse reaction to the sun's ultraviolet radiation. Melanin, the pigment in the skin, serves as a shield to UVR. Therefore, people with less constitutive pigment in their skin are more likely to develop mutations in the skin cells exposed to UVR.

Risk Factors

The three major risk factors for developing skin cancer are the amount of exposure to UVR or other forms of ionizing radiation, the individual's genetic makeup, and the individual's immune status and general health.

At Significantly Higher Risk

• People who live in areas with high sun exposure and at high altitudes.

• People with fair skin (with less melanin in their skin).

• Males have a slightly higher incidence than females, although the incidence is beginning to equilibrate between the genders.

• Squamous cell carcinoma is most prevalent in people over fifty-five. Males predominate except on the lower leg, where women have a higher incidence.

• Individuals who spend significant amounts of time outdoors, while working or participating in recreational activities, such as golf and sailing.

• Individuals who have been exposed to ionizing radiation other than UVR, such as X-ray treatment of acne, or patients with wounds from thermal or chemical burns.

• People with medical conditions involving suppression of the immune system—those infected with HIV, people with any form of cancer, those who have undergone an organ transplant and are taking immunosuppressive drugs, those with debilitating chronic diseases, the malnourished, the elderly, and patients receiving chemotherapy drugs.

• Individuals with genetic skin disorders that predispose to skin cancer, including basal cell nevus syndrome, xeroderma pigmentosum, and albinism.

At Slightly Higher Risk

• Exposure to chemical carcinogens such as coal tar, arsenic in insecticides, and nitrogen mustard (chemotherapy) ointment (Mustargen).

• Some viral warts can be precursors to SCC depending on the type of virus implicated. This is especially true of genital warts.

• Individuals who have comorbid conditions resulting in chronic irritation and inflammation, such as nonhealing diabetic ulcers.

Prevention

People can protect themselves against the ultraviolet radiation damage leading to skin cancer by avoiding UVA/UVB light and taking sun-protective measures.

• *Using Sunscreens* Not all sunscreens are created equal. Until about five years ago, sunscreen protected only against UVB radiation. UVA radiation has also been linked to the development of skin cancer, especially melanoma. Now, most sunscreens are UVA/UVB blocking, or "broad spectrum." The SPF (sun protection factor) of a sunscreen indicates the sunscreen's ability to protect against UVB radiation only. The SPF number correlates with the amount of time one can spend in the sun before the skin becomes pink or red. For example, if an SPF 15 is worn, a person can remain exposed to the sun fifteen times longer without the skin becoming pink. A standardized rating system for UVA protection has yet to be developed. A sunscreen of at least SPF 15 is recommended, although the higher the better. The drawbacks to using sunscreens with high SPF is that they tend to be a bit more expensive, can be more irritating to the skin, and can give a false sense of security. The sunscreen preparation should be applied frequently, and more often with sweating and when swimming. While the lotion or gel may be sweatproof, waterproof, or rubproof, the active ingredients in the sunscreen that actually protect the skin start to degrade two to three hours after application. It is therefore essential to reapply every two to three hours.

As for UVA protection, there are several types of sunblocking ingredients that better protect against UVA-induced damage. Sunscreens containing micronized zinc oxide, titanium dioxide, or avobenzone are superior UVA blockers. Another fact about UVA is that it penetrates clouds and window glass and is therefore always present and causing radiation damage, even on a cold, cloudy winter day in the northern United States. Thus, it is advisable for those at higher risk of developing skin cancer to use a moisturizer or sunscreen with an SPF of 15 or greater on a daily basis, year-round.

Sunscreen use should begin in infancy. Regular use of sunscreens with an SPF of 15 during the first eighteen years of life can reduce the lifetime incidence of skin cancer by as much as 78 percent. One serious childhood or adolescent sunburn doubles the chances of developing skin cancer, especially malignant melanoma.

• *Wearing Protective Clothing* People who work outside should wear clothing that protects their skin, including long-sleeved shirts, hats, and pants. For people at particularly high risk of developing skin cancer, it is advisable to purchase a few pieces of UV-protective clothing to wear during periods of prolonged sun exposure. There are many companies that make UV-protective clothing. Outdoor recreational activities should be scheduled before 11:00 A.M. and after 2:30 P.M., when the concentration of ultraviolet light is decreased by 70 to 80 percent.

• *Avoiding Tanning Booths* Tanning booths have advertised that by using UVA (A-type ultraviolet light), a "safe"

tan is obtained. There is no such thing as a "safe" tan.

Tanning is a response of the skin to radiation injury. UVA does cause less redness than UVB, but, like UVB, it induces skin cancer and photoaging (drying, wrinkles, and pigment changes). UVA also reduces the immune system's ability to fight off precancerous lesions; therefore, it is not simply the ultraviolet radiation during youth that leads to skin cancer. UVA exposure in adulthood not only leads to more mutations, but allows previous radiation-induced precancers to flourish. UVA is actually used experimentally to produce skin cancer in mice. Since 1986, about 2 million people a year have visited tanning booths. This will contribute to an increase in the number of skin cancers we will see over the next ten to twenty years. A recent study investigating tanning-bed use by children found that 7 percent of fourteen-year-old females and 35 percent of eighteen-year-old females used tanning beds. This may be one factor contributing to why the rates of both melanoma and nonmelanoma skin cancers in females between twenty and forty years of age are exponentially increasing.

• *Being Aware of Skin Changes and Getting Early Treatment* In addition to avoiding ultraviolet light and taking sun-protective measures, decreasing the morbidity of skin cancer also relies on the early detection and swift removal of precancerous lesions and incipient cancers.

Screening

The best screening test is an extensive examination of the skin. Part of a yearly physical should be a thorough total body skin examination, including the mouth, ocular conjunctivae, along and behind the ears, around the nose, the scalp, the genitalia and perianal skin, the palms of the hands, and the soles of the feet.

Glasses, jewelry, hats, hair clips or bands, and hearing aids should be removed to facilitate a complete exam.

Everyone should be examined this way, especially fair-skinned, light-haired, blue-eyed individuals and people who have had previous skin cancers. Special attention should be given to areas where a previous skin cancer was removed. These people should also examine themselves often to assess any change or development of new lesions to bring to the attention of a physician. If a skin lesion is suspicious clinically or because of reported change by the patient, a dermatologist should be consulted.

Common Signs and Symptoms

The most common sign is simply a sore or mark on the skin that changes in size, color, or shape. Although skin cancers are usually asymptomatic, they may become itchy or painful, and the lesion may start to bleed or ulcerate. Frequently, patients report a pimple that just wouldn't resolve.

Diagnosis

During the initial doctor's appointment, a medical history will be obtained with particular attention given to previous skin lesions, genetic skin disorders, and exposure to chemical carcinogens or radiation. The history of the lesion in question should also be clarified—how long it has been present, how it has changed, and whether it has ever been treated.

Imaging No imaging studies—X-rays or CT, PET, or MRI scans—are necessary during an initial doctor visit. Imaging studies or blood tests are necessary only if there are signs or symptoms of metastatic disease from a previously diagnosed skin cancer that has the capability of metastasizing. These studies would be coordinated by an oncologist or dermatologist specializing in cutaneous oncology that has been following the patient's case.

Biopsy A biopsy should be performed on all suspicious lesions, and the specimen should be sent to a qualified pathologist, preferably a dermatopathologist. Biopsies are not usually designed to remove the entire lesion. They are performed to diagnose a lesion and to determine future treatment if needed.

Four biopsy techniques are employed for the diagnosis of suspicious skin lesions, with the type used depending on the size and location of the lesion, the equipment available, and the experience of the physician:

• A shave biopsy uses a scalpel to remove a thin slice of the suspicious lesion. This procedure is the most commonly used method of biopsy.

• Punch biopsy uses a cylindrical instrument that is rotated into the skin and removes a cylindrical specimen. The resulting skin defect is closed with sutures. This method of biopsy is used when tissue at a greater depth is required for diagnosis or when the cosmetic result of this method is vastly superior to that of a shave technique.

• Incisional biopsy removes a portion of the tumor with a scalpel. Sutures are commonly placed to repair the defect.

• Excisional biopsy removes the entire visible lesion. Sutures are commonly placed to repair the defect. It is important to understand, however, that an excisional biopsy removes only the clinically apparent lesion and does not ensure complete removal or sufficient treatment of the lesion.

Because of the ease and minimal complications of these procedures, they can all be performed in the office with a local anesthetic. The patient will have a scar from the biopsy, but it is usually minimal. Rare adverse effects include bleeding, irritant or allergic reaction to the tape adhesive of the bandage, allergic reaction to any topical antibiotic ointments applied, and infection. In fact, the use of topical antibiotic preparations is now discouraged among most dermatologists and dermatologic surgeons given the high rate of allergic reaction and the very low rate of infection from these types of procedures. A bland ointment is preferred, such as petrolatum.

Treatment Overview

There are several methods commonly used to treat skin cancer. In order to determine which method is ideal in any given case, the dermatologist must consider the characteristics of both the tumor and the patient. Tumor type, size, growth pattern, location, degree of differentiation, and history of previous treatment all need to be considered. The patient's age, health, immune status, access to medical facilities, and history of previous skin cancers are also considered.

All treatment methods have a cure rate of about 90 percent or more. Tumors that have less than a 90 percent cure rate with all methods, except Mohs micrographic surgery (see "Surgery" in this chapter), include sclerosing or morpheaform basal cell cancers, poorly differentiated squamous cell cancers, lesions around the eye, ear, nose, and forehead-temple region, tumors larger than $3/4$ inch (2 cm), older lesions, recurrent cancers, and cancers in severely immunosuppressed patients.

Basal cell and squamous cell cancers are treated using similar procedures. A larger amount of apparently normal tissue may have to be removed when surgically removing SCC, since there is a higher rate of metastasis than with BCC and SCC frequently has larger subclinical extension beyond the clinically apparent margins of the tumor.

Standard Treatments

The most appropriate method of treating skin cancer is the most effective treatment (i.e., the treatment modality with the lowest risk of recurrence), considering the characteristics of both the tumor and the patient. Other factors need to be considered, including patient age and comorbidities, potential adverse effects of treatment, and aesthetics, but complete removal of the tumor with the lowest risk of recurrence is the essential goal, the oncologic principle.

Curettage with (or without) Electrodessication (C&E) This is a two-step procedure in which a curette (sharp-tipped instrument) removes the more friable cancer tissue from normal tissue and bleeding is controlled by electrical current or by a chemical agent. This cycle is repeated two to four times. Nodular and superficial BCC and noninvasive SCC can usually be treated effectively with C&E.

C&E is ideal for small superficial primary tumors with distinct borders and well-differentiated histology. It is not recommended for large tumors; tumors invading dermis or fat; lesions with poorly defined borders; poorly differentiated squamous cell carcinomas; recurrent lesions; or lesions at certain anatomic sites that have lower cure rates (e.g., the central face and mucosal surfaces).

C&E is a low-risk procedure that can be performed on an outpatient basis. In contrast to surgical excision with sutured closure, an open wound is left that commonly requires one to three months of wound care and bandaging. C&E should be used with caution in patients with pacemakers, though the risk of pacemaker dysfunction is very small. Alternatives, such as thermal or chemical cautery, may be preferable.

 Cryosurgery This technique uses liquid nitrogen at very low temperatures to freeze the skin and induce necrosis of the skin in the treated area. The nitrogen is applied with an aerosol spray or cryoprobe to achieve tissue temperatures below –58°F (–50°C). The tissue is then allowed to thaw for about two minutes. This cycle is repeated two or three times.

Like C&E, cryosurgery is a low-risk procedure. It can therefore be used for people who refuse or cannot tolerate surgery.

Cryotherapy has been considered effective for treating primary superficial and nodular BCC, or superficial SCC. It is not useful for poorly defined lesions, poorly differentiated SCC, morpheaform BCC, recurrent lesions, or tumors that are in locations with higher recurrence rates; in patients with poor wound-healing potential; or on the extremities (arms and legs) where there is decreased blood flow.

Cryotherapy leaves an open wound that takes one to three months to heal. The wound may "weep" for two or three weeks after the procedure, and necrotic tissue can require debridement to facilitate healing. Topical antibiotic preparations are often used to prevent infection.

Nodular and superficial BCC and non-invasive SCC can usually be treated effectively with cryotherapy. This method of treatment has largely been abandoned, except for the treatment of very small lesions, given the postprocedure wound care required, the high recurrence rate, and the significant risk of excessive damage to surrounding healthy tissue because of the imprecise treatment margin.

 Radiation Treatment with radiation has a reported cure rate of 89 to 95 percent, depending on the tumor type, patient characteristics, and treatment regimen. Radiation is useful for older people who cannot tolerate surgery, for medium-sized tumors, and for lesions that are too inaccessible to be removed surgically. It is

particularly useful for lesions on or near the face. It can also be used as a palliative measure rather than for cure on excessively large cancers or as an adjuvant to surgical removal of aggressive SCC or SCC with growth along the nerves in the skin.

It should not be used for patients under fifty years old because of the high potential for recurrence and the possibility of inducing new cancers at the radiation site, and because the long-term cosmetic results are inferior to surgical removal. It is also less advantageous for lesions on the trunk and extremities because of a greater tendency to develop radiation side effects such as radiation dermatitis, skin atrophy, telangiectasia (superficial dilated blood vessels), and changes in the skin pigment.

For patients over fifty, radiation therapy can be used to treat nodular and superficial basal cell carcinomas and most squamous cell carcinomas.

Chemotherapy 5-Fluorouracil (5-FU) is a chemotherapeutic agent that blocks DNA synthesis, thereby preventing normal cell growth and ultimately causing cell death. Topical 5-FU is available in both cream and solution preparations. Topical 5-FU is most frequently applied directly to the skin twice a day for four weeks or more. It works by causing an inflammatory reaction, which heals after the treatment is stopped.

Advantages of 5-FU are that it is easy to use and does not require any procedures. Disadvantages are that it causes significant skin irritation and can result in skin pigmentation changes. In addition, 5-FU may treat only the superficial component of the skin cancer, leaving the deeper roots to continue growing underneath a clinically normal–appearing surface.

Imiquimod (Aldara) cream is a recent and scientifically elegant addition to the options for treating skin cancer and pre-cancerous lesions. This topical chemotherapeutic agent activates the specific arm of the cutaneous immune system that fights off cancerous and precancerous growths. It is applied three to seven days a week for four to six weeks. Like topical 5-FU, imiquimod causes significant irritation during treatment.

Both 5-FU and imiquimod creams can highlight skin lesions in or near the area of treatment that were not clinically obvious. Therefore, it is important to inform a person with a history of significant sun exposure that many inflamed lesions may develop in the treated areas as the creams activate a response against subclinical precancerous lesions.

It is essential that topical 5-FU and imiquimod, as is true of all topical chemotherapeutic agents for skin cancer, be used only in very specific cases and under the close supervision of a dermatologist, since recurrence rates are estimated to be up to 50 percent in some cases. Many dermatologists use topical chemotherapeutic agents only for the treatment of precancerous actinic keratoses, although their use in skin cancer is considered the standard of practice as long as specific patient and tumor parameters are met.

Surgery Excision is a surgical procedure that removes the entire lesion with an appropriate margin, usually 3 to 5 mm, of clinically normal tissue. The resulting defect is then repaired with sutures. This is a more invasive procedure than any of the previously mentioned treatment methods but has a much lower recurrence rate (3 to 5 percent). The wound closure results in more rapid healing and produces better cosmetic results than leaving an open wound, as from C&E, cryosurgery, or radiation. This procedure can be used effectively for all skin cancers in patients who can tolerate surgery.

Mohs Micrographic Surgery This technique was first described in 1936 by Dr. Frederick Mohs. It involves removing successive horizontal layers of the skin cancer and a small margin (1 to 2 mm) of surrounding tissue that may be involved. Each layer is mapped and microscopically examined. While only 2 to 3 percent of the margins are examined when a surgical excision specimen is sent for pathological examination, 100 percent of the Mohs layer is examined by the Mohs surgeon. If tumor extends to a margin, an additional layer is removed in the area that is still positive, sparing the normal tissue where the margins were clear. This layer is again examined microscopically until clear margins are attained both peripherally and at the deep margin of the tumor.

Mohs surgery has the highest cure rate of all treatment methods—97 to 99 percent. It is recommended for all tumors in the high-risk areas of the face (nose, eyelid, lip, temple, and ear); for very poorly differentiated tumors and tumors arising in patients with significant immuno-suppressed states or genetic cancer syndromes; for recurrent lesions and lesions with clinically indistinct borders; and for large tumors (greater than $\frac{3}{4}$ inch [2 cm]) in any location and tumors arising in areas of previous radiation or thermal burn damage. The disadvantages of Mohs surgery are that a great deal of expertise is required of the physician, the procedure is time-consuming, and more equipment is needed than in the other methods.

In addition to being experts in the surgical removal of skin cancers and the histopathologic examination of the Mohs layers, many Mohs micrographic surgeons have also trained extensively in the reconstructive methods resulting in the best cosmetic results possible. Well-trained Mohs surgeons, however, are very aware of when referral to a head and neck surgeon or an oculoplastic surgeon is indicated.

Laser Therapy The carbon dioxide laser may be used as a cutting instrument, much like a scalpel. It is useful for removing superficial basal and squamous cell carcinomas in patients who have tumors in locations that tend to be bloody, such as the scalp. It is also useful for patients who have a bleeding disorder or are taking anticoagulants, although at this point, most dermatologic surgeons agree that anticoagulants are not even a relative contraindication to the surgical removal of skin cancer. Most dermatologic surgeons, in fact, encourage their patients to remain on anticoagulant therapy regardless of a required surgery.

Laser resurfacing with the use of carbon dioxide and/or erbium:YAG lasers, which ablate the epidermis, effectively removes a large proportion of precancerous cells. It is the treatment of choice for actinic cheilitis, a precancerous condition that develops from extensive UVR damage to the lips. This should not be considered a routine treatment option for the sun-damaged, high-risk individual, but there is an advantage to having this procedure performed, even if it is primarily done for cosmetic improvement.

Investigational Although the treatments now most widely used have greater than a 90 percent cure rate, other therapies are being studied that may be more practical and effective.

Retinoids These are synthetic and natural derivatives of vitamin A. Patients with vitamin A deficiency may have an increased susceptibility to skin cancer. This deficiency causes a premalignant change of the skin that can be reversed by applying vitamin A.

Retinoids induce differentiation (maturing) of tumor cells derived from surface tissues (epithelium). Recent investigations have used the retinoids to treat premalignant and malignant skin cancers. Use of the locally applied (topical) form has shown some decrease in actinic keratoses of the face. Use of internal (systemic) retinoids has demonstrated a fair cure rate when treating basal cell carcinoma. Limited information exists for use in SCC, but one study reported a 70 percent response rate. Systemic retinoids have shown some success in high-risk patients who may develop numerous skin cancers, such as xeroderma pigmentosa and basal cell nevus syndrome, as well as in patients who are immunosuppressed. However, the long-term toxicity of these agents usually excludes them as the treatment of choice. Once the systemic retinoid is discontinued in the high-risk patient, the rate of carcinoma occurrence returns to the pretreatment rate.

Photodynamic Therapy (PDT) This treatment uses visible light in combination with a photosensitizer, a compound that attracts light. The photosensitizers include a hematoporphyrin derivative, HPD, given intravenously, and topical delta-aminolevulinic acid (ALA).

Approximately forty-eight to seventy-two hours after HPD is intravenously injected, most of the compound is cleared by the normal skin and selectively retained in the cancerous cells. Upon exposure to different wavelengths of light, HPD undergoes a photodynamic reaction that damages the tumor cells and spares the uninvolved tissue. In practice, HPD is given as an intravenous injection and is followed forty-eight to seventy-two hours later by irradiation with red or blue-green light. There are no well-controlled studies using HPD, but encouraging preliminary results have been reported in treating basal and squamous cell carcinomas.

A disadvantage of photodynamic therapy with HPD is that levels of HPD may stay in the normal skin for three to six weeks after the injection. During this time, patients need protection from all bright light, since exposure to light can result in severe redness and swelling of the skin. This adverse effect is eliminated by topical ALA, which is applied to the affected area of skin.

Twenty percent ALA emulsion is applied to the skin with or without a dressing for one to eight hours, depending on the regimen. The treated area is then irradiated with light from a variety of light sources, including intense pulsed-light and pulsed-dye laser emitting light at 595 nm wavelength. The treatment is administered daily until the redness and swelling clear up. This method appears to be most effective for superficial squamous cell carcinomas. It is also very useful in treating patients with excessive sun damage, as it can clear the treated area of a significant proportion of the precancerous lesions actinic keratoses.

Treatment Follow-Up

Twenty percent of people with a single basal cell cancer will develop a second one at another site within a year, 50 percent within three years. If there are two basal cell cancers at presentation, there is a 40 percent chance of developing a new one within a year. Patients should see their doctor twice a year for the first three years after treatment of a skin cancer, followed by yearly visits.

The Most Important Questions You Can Ask

• What risk factors do I have for developing skin cancer?

• Do I have a strong family history of skin cancer?

• What are the most important things I can do to lower my risk of getting skin cancer?

• Will you be carefully and regularly examining my entire skin surface to look for any premalignant and malignant lesions?

• Has the biopsy been reviewed by a pathologist with special training in skin tumors?

• What is the chance of recurrence or spread with this lesion and which method of treatment will give me the best cure rate?

Small Intestine

*Bert O'Neil, M.D., Andrew H. Ko, M.D., Ernest H. Rosenbaum, M.D.,
and Sean J. Mulvihill, M.D.*

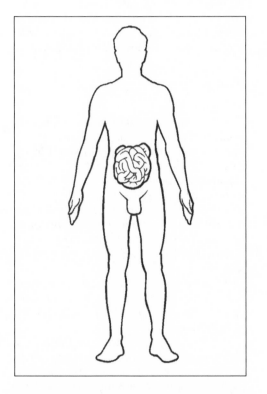

The small intestine is the longest segment of the gastrointestinal tract, making up three-quarters of its total length. Yet malignant tumors are much less common in this organ than they are in the esophagus, stomach, and large bowel. Of all the gastrointestinal tumors diagnosed, only 1.5 percent are found in the small intestine. About 4,600 new cases of and 1,140 deaths from cancer of the small intestine are seen annually. Most are patients over forty-five, and men account for 60 percent.

There are many reasons for the lower incidence. Cancer-causing agents have less contact with the surface membranes because of the rapid transit time of food through the small bowel compared with the colon. And since the stool is still liquid, there is less mechanical injury to the membranes.

The inner surface of the small intestine secretes a large amount of gamma globulin that protects the lining against disease. Benzpyrene hydrolase, which can detoxify carcinogens, is found in large amounts in the lining (mucosa) of the small intestine. Finally, the contents of the small bowel are alkaline, which reduces the production of carcinogens from bile and prevents the formation of nitrosamines, environmental carcinogens that are formed only under acidic conditions.

Malignancies of the small bowel are almost always treatable and some may be curable. Their prognosis and treatment depend on the cellular origin.

Types Small intestinal malignancies are most frequently adenocarcinomas. Other less common types include carcinoid tumors, sarcomas, gastrointestinal stromal tumors (GISTs), and lymphomas.

The most common of all—making up half of the small intestine tumors—are adenocarcinomas, which develop in glandular tissue, most frequently in the ileum. Most people with adenocarcinomas have metastases to the lymph nodes, liver, or peritoneum (abdominal lining) at the time of diagnosis.

Carcinoid tumors account for 20 percent of small bowel malignancies. They are often small (usually ½ to 1½ inches [1 to 5 cm] in diameter) and slow growing. There may be multiple lesions and they may be present for years (see the chapter "Carcinoids of the Gastrointestinal Tract").

Sarcomas are slow-growing tumors that account for 11 percent of small bowel cancers. Sarcomas can develop in any soft tissue such as fat cells (liposarcomas), blood vessels (angiosarcomas), or nerves (neural sarcomas, neurofibrosarcomas, or malignant schwannomas, which develop from the nerve sheath, most commonly in the ileum). But 75 percent of the sarcomas, called leiomyosarcomas, originate in the smooth muscles encircling the bowel. These malignancies may reach a large size before diagnosis (many are larger than 2 inches [5 cm]). Only a third of smooth-muscle tumors are malignant.

Gastrointestinal stromal tumors (GISTs) can occur anywhere in the GI tract (most frequently in the stomach), and under the microscope are often confused with sarcomas. GIST is defined by a particular gene mutation that can be identified with a simple test done by the pathologist (for more information, see the chapter "Gastrointestinal Stromal Tumor").

Lymphomas arising from lymphoid tissues in the wall of the small bowel make up 14 percent of small bowel tumors. They may occur in any part of the small intestine and 20 percent of them develop in multiple sites. Of all the lymphomas that start someplace other than in lymph nodes (extranodal lymphomas), 33 percent do so in the gastrointestinal tract, 10 percent in the small bowel. Most of these lesions are non-Hodgkin's lymphomas.

How It Spreads Small bowel cancers can spread directly through the bowel wall to adjacent tissues. Leiomyosarcomas grow in the muscle wall and extend to the surface (serosa). Sarcomas spread directly to the tissues supporting the bowel (mesentery), the retroperitoneum, or the adjacent bowel. These cancers also spread through the lymphatic system and bloodstream to regional lymph nodes or to the liver, lungs, or bone.

What Causes It There is an association with some inherited cancers and inflammatory bowel disease (Crohn's disease and celiac disease) and neurofibromatosis. Lymphomas are associated with immune deficiencies and celiac disease.

Risk Factors

At Higher Risk
• People older than sixty, especially those with a history of bowel disease.
• People with changes in small intestine acidity, rapid transit (food goes through the bowel quickly), and nitrosamine exposure.
• Those with inherited gastrointestinal disorders—Peutz-Jeghers syndrome, familial polyposis, inflammatory bowel disease, Crohn's disease, and neurofibromatosis.
• Those with increased lymphoid deposits in the ileum and immune deficiency diseases are at a higher risk for lymphomas.
• A history of or the presence of a *Helicobacter pylori* infection may lead to small bowel inflammation that may lead to the initiation of a lymphoma.

Screening

There are no general screening methods, but if a tumor is suspected because of abdominal pain, anemia, or some other symptom, a test for hidden blood in the stool is recommended.

Common Signs and Symptoms

Ten percent of people with small intestinal cancers have no symptoms. Most have abdominal pain or distension because of a partial or complete obstruction of the small bowel. There may also be weight loss, nausea and vomiting, fever, change in bowel habits, and a general malaise or weakness that may result from anemia caused by bleeding or malabsorption. The bowel may also become perforated, which can cause acute symptoms. With adenocarcinomas, jaundice may appear when the tumor is in the mid duodenum, blocking drainage of the common bile duct. Blockage of the bowel may also be caused by what is called pseudolymphoma, a benign overgrowth of the lymph nodes.

Diagnosis

Physical Examination
- Abdominal mass or painful distension.
- Rectal bleeding—possibly caused by ulcerations in the gastrointestinal tract—which may result in anemia.
- A partial or complete obstruction of the intestinal tract.
- Jaundice, which may be due to a tumor in the duodenum or to liver metastasis.
- Bowel kinking (intussusception).
- Often fatty fluid (chylous ascites) can collect in the abdomen.

Blood and Other Tests
- Blood counts usually show iron-deficiency anemia when bleeding occurs.
- The level of carcinoembryonic antigen (CEA) in the blood is often elevated with adenocarcinomas.

Imaging
- The most useful X-rays are an upper gastrointestinal and a small bowel series. These can detect a small cancer (often a "napkin ring" deformity) or a polyp.
- X-rays showing small bowel thickening with ulceration may indicate a lymphoma.

- An abdominal CT scan can help identify lesions outside the bowel, including metastases.
- Angiography is helpful for evaluating the abdominal tumor blood vessels, displaced vessels, and new blood vessels (neovascularization).
- A small bowel X-ray (enteroclysis) may locate a tumor. This procedure involves passing a small plastic tube through the nose to the duodenum and injecting barium and air to provide contrast.

Endoscopy and Biopsy
- A small part of the terminal ileum can be seen during a colonoscopic evaluation.
- Small bowel endoscopy is useful during surgery for additional evaluation.

Staging

Staging is similar to that of colon cancer. The tumor, or T, staging is based on the depth of invasion of the primary tumor, with T1 meaning superficial invasion only and T4 (the highest) meaning the tumor has grown into other organs or other loops of bowel. Lymph node involvement distinguishes Stage II from Stage III, and Stage IV is defined by metastatic disease.

Treatment Overview

As in other gastrointestinal cancers, the standard treatment is to remove the tumor surgically whenever possible.

 Surgery The best chance for cure is offered by the surgical removal of a part of the small bowel with a wide margin around the tumor, along with the attached tissues supporting the bowel (mesentery) and its lymphatic drainage. If this cannot be done, surgical bypass can be considered as a palliative measure for residual disease.

Radiation The small bowel is extremely sensitive to radiation, which limits the usefulness of this therapy. Radiation may be poorly tolerated and may result in weakness, nausea, vomiting, and diarrhea with small bowel inflammation. It may lead to occasional remissions for sarcomas but is usually used for relief of pain and symptoms of obstruction. Small bowel lymphomas are highly responsive to radiation at doses low enough to avoid some of the complications mentioned before.

Radiation can complement surgery and is often recommended in lymphomas. Intraoperative radiotherapy (IORT) to the tumor or the tumor bed and area at risk may be done, because normal tissues can be moved aside and protected.

 Chemotherapy Like radiotherapy, chemotherapy is a less effective therapy than surgery and is recommended only for disease that can't be surgically removed or for metastases. Chemotherapy is, however, instrumental in the treatment of lymphomas.

Treatment by Tumor Type

Small Intestine Adenocarcinoma

Standard Treatment If the tumor can be completely removed, radical surgery may lead to a cure. Simple excision of the tumor might be adequate for small malignancies, but for larger tumors, the recommended procedure requires the removal of a segment of the bowel with wide margins. If the cancer arises in the first part of the small bowel (duodenum), it should be noted that the duodenum is in a difficult location. It is behind the liver, pancreas, and stomach, and the Whipple surgical procedure—involving the removal of the pancreas and duodenum and the reconstruction of the bile duct drainage system—may be necessary.

Adjuvant Systemic Therapy 5-Fluorouracil (5-FU) + leucovorin is commonly used because of the rarity of the tumor. Clinical studies have not been done. Combination therapies used for colon cancer may be considered, although there are no studies to confirm that this helps.

Palliation If surgical removal of the tumor is impossible, the symptoms of the disease may be relieved by a surgical bypass or palliative radiation therapy. Chemotherapy used for colon cancer may be palliative in cases of advanced small bowel adenocarcinoma, although studies are small and few in number.

Five-Year Survival 20 percent (for resectable adenocarcinoma)

Investigational
- Radiation therapy with radiosensitizers, with or without chemotherapy.
- Various chemotherapy combinations have been tried, such as 5-FU + leucovorin, 5-FU + oxaliplatin (Eloxatin), and 5-FU + irinotecan (Camptosar).

Small Intestine Carcinoid
(See the chapter "Carcinoids of the Gastrointestinal Tract.")

Five-Year Survival 54 percent

Small Intestine Leiomyosarcoma

Standard Treatment If the primary tumor can be removed, radical surgery similar to that for adenocarcinomas may lead to a cure. Isolated metastases in the liver and lung can also be removed.

If the primary tumor cannot be removed, any tumor that is obstructing the bowel can be surgically bypassed. Tumors that can't be removed may also respond to high-dose radiation therapy, occasionally with long-term survival.

Palliation A combined approach using surgery and radiotherapy can help relieve pain and symptoms of obstruction in patients when metastases can't be removed.

Chemotherapy is also sometimes used for palliative purposes. Chemotherapy with doxorubicin (Adriamycin), cisplatin (Platinol), ifosfamide (Ifex), vincristine (Oncovin), or dacarbazine (DTIC-Dome) can have response rates of up to 65 percent. Adjuvant chemotherapy may also be given after surgery if the tumor is high grade, there is a high risk for local recurrence, or there is a significant risk of metastasis (lymphatic or blood vessel involvement), although there is not clear evidence that adjuvant chemotherapy improves the outcome of these cancers.

Five-Year Survival About 50 percent if the tumor can be removed surgically

Investigational

• Clinical trials are evaluating the use of new anticancer drugs and biologicals.

• Adjuvant radiotherapy in combination with chemotherapy is being studied.

Small Intestine Lymphoma

Standard Treatment It is unusual to find a single lymphoma as a primary small bowel tumor, so it is mandatory that the standard lymphoma staging work-up be done to look for evidence of other areas of disease. The work-up will include abdominal and pelvic CT scans, a chest X-ray, and bone marrow aspiration and biopsy. Depending on the stage and cell type, the standard treatment options include surgery, radiation, and combination chemotherapy, all of which may lead to a cure.

For disease that is localized to the bowel wall or has gone beyond the wall (local extension), surgical removal of the tumor alone may be adequate if twelve or more nearby lymph nodes are removed and show no evidence of disease (a 40 percent five-year survival). But the addition of combination chemotherapy or radiation should also be considered. Radiation may lead to a cure, control tumor growth, or relieve symptoms. For disease that extends into the regional lymph nodes, the tumor should be removed at the time of diagnosis. Combination chemotherapy is then the treatment of choice (see the chapter "Lymphomas: Non-Hodgkin's").

Combination chemotherapy is also the treatment of choice for disease that is extensive or cannot be removed surgically. Radiation therapy is often also used to eliminate any potential residual tumor cells, often in conjunction with chemotherapy.

Recent reports associate the infection *Helicobacter pylori* with small bowel lymphomas. Eradication of the bacteria with antibiotics may lead to a regression of lymphomas in some cases.

 Palliation Radiation therapy can relieve the symptoms associated with large lymphomas that cannot be removed, often in combination with chemotherapy. Single liver metastases may respond well to radiation (survival chances decrease as the number of metastases increases).

Five-Year Survival 25 percent for diffuse lymphoma, 50 percent or more for nodular lymphoma

Supportive Therapy

Nutritional support may be necessary after treatment of small intestinal cancers. This is especially so after a major portion of the small bowel has been removed or if the duodenum or terminal ileum has been removed or bypassed. These procedures result in poor absorption of iron, calcium, folate, vitamin B_{12}, fat and fat-soluble vitamins, and pancreatic/biliary digestive secretions, leading to deficiencies in essential nutrients. Nutritional replacement programs can correct these deficiencies (see chapter 23, "Maintaining Good Nutrition").

Recurrent or Metastatic Cancer

Tumors may come back in the small bowel after treatment or may metastasize from cancers arising elsewhere, especially cancers of the colon, kidney, pancreas, or stomach, which may extend directly into the small bowel. Symptoms include intestinal obstruction and bleeding from the tumor.

• If possible, surgery may be attempted for locally recurrent small intestine cancer, with removal of the lymph nodes if that is appropriate. Clinical trials are now evaluating ways of improving local control, such as the use of radiation therapy with radiosensitizers, with or without chemotherapy.

• There is no standard chemotherapy for recurrent metastatic adenocarcinoma or leiomyosarcoma of the small intestine. Patients may be considered candidates for standard combination chemotherapy programs, or for Phase I or Phase II clinical trials evaluating the use of new anticancer drugs or biologicals.

The Most Important Questions You Can Ask

• What is the role of surgery for small bowel tumors?

• How do you tell the difference between benign and malignant tumors of the small bowel?

• How are small bowel lymphomas evaluated?

• Is there a role for radiotherapy?

• How do you select a chemotherapy program for small bowel cancer?

• What is the role for supportive nutritional therapy?

Stomach

Bert O'Neil, M.D., Andrew H. Ko, M.D., Ernest H. Rosenbaum, M.D.,
Malin Dollinger, M.D., Sean J. Mulvihill, M.D., and David R. Byrd, M.D.

■ ■ ■ ■

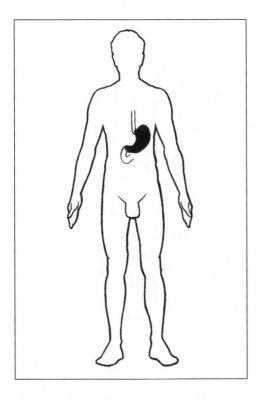

Cancer of the stomach—also called gastric cancer or gastric carcinoma—is a treatable disease that can often be cured when it is found and treated at a local stage. Unfortunately, the general outlook for this type of cancer is poor because 80 percent of the cases diagnosed in the United States are already at an advanced stage, having spread to nearby or distant organs. About 24,000 Americans are diagnosed yearly with gastric cancer, and 14,000 of them will die because of the disease.

A more encouraging fact about this cancer, however, is that the overall death rate has dramatically decreased, falling approximately 60 percent between 1930 and 1970. A more recent and disturbing trend, however, is that cancers of the part of the stomach nearest the esophagus have increased dramatically in recent years along with cancers of the gastroesophageal junction (where the esophagus meets the stomach). Stomach tumors in these locations are generally harder to cure than those arising in the distal (far) end of the stomach.

Stomach cancer was the leading cause of cancer deaths in the United States between 1900 and 1945 but is now the ninth most common cause in men and eleventh most common cause in women of cancer deaths. The exact reason for the decline—which is greatest among the elderly and whites—is not understood, although it is probably related to improved diets and the widespread use of refrigeration. Decreased use of food preservatives such as nitrates and salts are other possible factors. Differences in rates of stomach cancer between Asian immigrants (very high rate) who have moved to the United States and their descendants (lower incidence) strongly support the idea that dietary content is very important in the development of gastric cancer.

Types Stomach cancers are classified according to their tissue type. The most common type arises in the glandular tissue lining the stomach. These tumors are

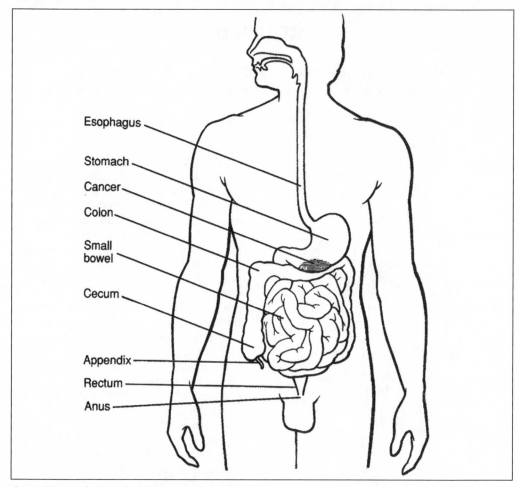

Esophagus

Stomach

Cancer

Colon

Small
bowel

Cecum

Appendix

Rectum

Anus

Gastrointestinal tract, showing stomach cancer

called adenocarcinomas and account for over 95 percent of all stomach tumors. One particular form of this cell type, unusual in the United States but more common in Japan, is the superficial spreading adenocarcinoma that essentially replaces the lining (mucosa) of the stomach with sheets of malignant cells. There is an increased rate in gastroesophageal junction adenocarcinoma. (Cancer right at the junction between the esophagus and the stomach.) These gastroesophageal junction cancers are sometimes treated as gastric cancers, and other times more like esophageal cancers (see the chapter "Esophagus"). A less common subtype is scirrhous carcinoma (linitis plastica), a poorly differentiated mixture of mucin-producing adenocarcinoma cells that infiltrates the muscle wall and turns it into rigid, leatherlike scar tissue that can't stretch or move during the normal digestive process (peristalsis).

Occasionally, a cancer may develop in lymph tissue (gastric lymphoma), from the smooth muscles of the stomach wall (leiomyosarcoma), or from stromal (supporting) cells (see the chapter "Gastrointestinal Stromal Tumor"). Carcinoids and plasmacytomas can also develop in the stomach.

How It Spreads The disease can spread directly through the stomach wall into adjacent organs and through the lymph system to nodes in the abdomen, the left side of the neck, and the left armpit. Metastases through the bloodstream can spread to the liver, lungs, bone, and brain. Metastases can also occur in the lining of the abdominal cavity (peritoneum) and in the pelvis around the rectum.

What Causes It The exact cause is unknown, but most gastric cancers are believed to be caused by carcinogens in the food we eat. Nitrites found in smoked meats, fish, and other foods, as well as the nitrates used as food preservatives, have been implicated, along with aflatoxin, a carcinogenic fungus contaminant that is present in some foodstuffs, such as peanuts. Smoking and excessive alcohol consumption may also be contributing factors.

Various medical conditions are also associated with the development of stomach cancer. A history of or the presence of *Helicobacter pylori* (a bacteria that causes most stomach ulcers) infection may lead to stomach inflammation that can induce mutations and DNA damage, leading to cancer. A lack of acid in stomach secretions (achlorhydria) allows growth of bacteria responsible for converting nitrates to carcinogenic nitrosamines. Five to 10 percent of people with pernicious anemia will develop gastric cancer. And the chronic backup, or reflux, of stomach acids into the esophagus can irritate the glandular tissue at the junction of the stomach and the esophagus, which may lead to cancer. Gastric polyps are another possibility, since they may become malignant.

Risk Factors
At Significantly Higher Risk
- Those aged between fifty and fifty-nine.
- Twice as frequent in lower socioeconomic groups in North America and western Europe.
- Workers in certain industries—coal mining, nickel refining (in Soviet Europe), rubber and timber processing.
- Workers exposed to asbestos fibers.
- People with pernicious anemia are 5 to 10 percent more likely to develop gastric cancer.
- People whose diet contains smoked, highly salted, and barbecued foods. Japanese immigrants have a decreased incidence of this cancer when they adopt an American diet and lifestyle, a tenfold drop after two generations.

At Slightly Higher Risk
- Tobacco use.
- People with type A blood and achlorhydria (lack of stomach acid).
- Males living in colder climates.
- Those who have had part of the stomach removed because of peptic ulcers, leading to a decrease in stomach acids. There is a 6.5 percent incidence of tumors in the remaining stomach (gastric remnant).
- Older people whose stomach lining produces less acid as it ages (atrophic gastritis).
- Peptic ulcer and atrophic gastritis associated with *Helicobacter pylori* infection (for carcinoma and lymphoma).
- Familial polyposis.
- HNPCC (hereditary nonpolyposis coli cancer) increases risk of familial genetic syndrome.

Screening

Screening can be helpful for finding early tumors that do not reach the outer wall of the stomach (serosa) or that penetrate the serosa but have not spread to lymph nodes. By looking at the stomach through a lighted tube (fiber-optic endoscopy) or by using X-rays of the upper gastrointestinal tract, smaller tumors can be detected. These tests are especially pertinent for people with gastric complaints.

Although screening programs are used in countries such as Japan with high gastric cancer rates, they are not common in the United States. Screening is not cost-effective, given the relatively low incidence of stomach cancer in the United States. Upper gastrointestinal X-rays, for example, discover cancer in only 0.15 percent (1 in 600) of apparently healthy people, in addition to often missing cancers that are present.

Common Signs and Symptoms

The symptoms of stomach cancer are similar to the symptoms of a hiatal hernia or peptic ulcer, namely a vague pain aggravated by food, nausea, heartburn, and indigestion. These symptoms are often thought to be due to stress and are treated with antacids or H-2 blockers. Unfortunately, the temporary relief this treatment brings often delays the tests that could diagnose cancer.

Loss of appetite, feelings of fullness after even a small meal, and weight loss are common (upper abdominal pain, vomiting after meals, and weight loss are seen in 80 to 90 percent of cases). There may also be mild anemia, weakness, gastrointestinal bleeding (40 percent of cases), and vomiting of blood. Both vomiting blood and rectal bleeding are seen in peptic ulcer disease, esophageal varices (varicose veins in the esophagus that grow and burst, a disease common in drinkers), and occasionally leiomyosarcomas.

Diagnosis

Gastric cancers often seem to be benign ulcers, which are like pits in the stomach lining. Larger ulcers—more than $\frac{3}{4}$ inch (2 cm) in diameter—that have borders raised above the level of the surrounding stomach are more likely to be malignant.

Physical Examination There are few specific findings on a physical examination, and they generally indicate an advanced tumor. Stomach tumors themselves can only rarely be felt.

- Enlarged lymph nodes above the left collarbone (supraclavicular node).
- Nodal masses around the rectum, inside the navel, or in the abdomen (involving the ovary).
- Enlarged liver (hepatomegaly).
- Increased fluid in the abdomen (ascites).

Blood and Other Tests

- Test for hidden blood in the stools.
- Complete blood count (CBC), which may indicate anemia from gastrointestinal bleeding.
- Serum chemistry profile to evaluate abnormal liver and bone chemistry enzymes, and levels of serum ferritin to indicate iron deficiency.

Imaging

- X-rays of the upper gastrointestinal tract (UGI series) by standard and double-contrast methods may find larger ulcer lesions (not considered as informative as endoscopy—see the following section).
- Chest X-rays.
- CT scan of the abdomen.
- Bone scan if the bone enzyme alkaline phosphatase is elevated in the serum or if there are symptoms such as new back or other bone pain.

Endoscopy and Biopsy

- Examination of the stomach through an endoscope (flexible fiber-optic camera) inserted through the esophagus may find ulcers and masses. It is the most definitive test for diagnosing stomach cancer.

Seventy percent of early malignant ulcers may look benign and even heal but are usually diagnosed on biopsy.

• A small piece of tissue may be removed from any suspicious area for biopsy analysis by a pathologist, or a brush can be passed through the endoscope to obtain cells in a way similar to a Pap smear. Tissue and brush biopsies can diagnose 98 percent of cases, although sometimes more than one attempt is necessary to make the diagnosis.

• Endoscopic ultrasound is a newer technique that uses a probe at the tip of an endoscope to get a good look at the lymph nodes near the stomach.

Staging

Stages are initially defined according to the findings of the diagnostic evaluation outlined above (clinical stage). After removal of the lesion, pathologic stage can be defined according to the TNM classification. For gastric cancer, the major factor in defining the T, or size of the primary tumor, is how deeply it invades into the stomach wall and whether it invades adjacent structures such as the spleen, small intestine, colon, liver, diaphragm, pancreas, kidney, and adrenal gland or the abdominal lining. Presence or absence of metastasis to local lymph nodes is also very important. The stage is important in determining the initial treatment options as well as the prognosis.

Treatment Overview

Stomach cancer can be treated, and over half the patients with early-stage disease are cured. Cancers arising in the lower part of the stomach (distal or antral cancers) have better cure rates than cancers rising in the upper stomach (proximal or cardial cancers). Unfortunately, early-stage disease accounts for only 10 to 20 percent of all cases diagnosed in the

United States. Five-year survival for more advanced cancers ranges from around 20 percent for those with regional disease (i.e., with extension to local lymph nodes or through the stomach wall) to almost nil for those with distant metastases. Treatment for metastatic cancer can relieve symptoms and sometimes prolong survival, but long remissions are not common. It is frustrating to medical oncologists that the results of treatment of metastatic disease are poor in spite of the fact that many drugs show activity against gastric cancer.

Radical surgery is the only treatment that by itself can lead to a cure, although lesser surgical procedures can play a significant role in therapy designed to relieve symptoms. Radiation and chemotherapy have recently been found to increase the chance of cure of gastric cancer when used in combination with surgery. This represents a major change in how resectable (surgically removable) gastric cancer is treated.

Surgery The best current treatment for gastric cancer is surgical resection (gastrectomy); however, this is not possible in all patients. If the tumor is localized and amenable to resection, surgeons term the condition operable, meaning an operation may lead to cure. If the tumor has spread beyond the stomach to the liver, lungs, or lining of the abdominal cavity, surgery has little, if any, benefit and the patient is considered "inoperable." Thus, before surgery is considered, a staging evaluation as outlined above is usually undertaken.

The extent of surgery depends on the extent of the tumor and the reason for the operation. Cancers confined to the distal stomach are usually treated with radical subtotal gastrectomy. In this operation, about 80 percent of the stomach, including the pylorus and first part of the duodenum, the adjacent lymph nodes, and

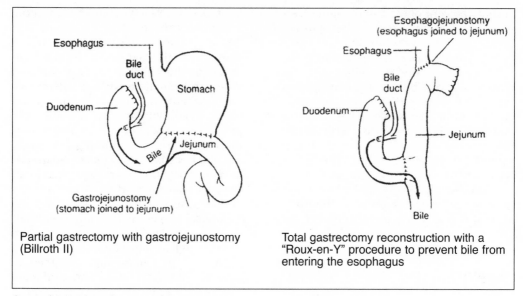

| Partial gastrectomy with gastrojejunostomy (Billroth II) | Total gastrectomy reconstruction with a "Roux-en-Y" procedure to prevent bile from entering the esophagus |

Surgical procedures for stomach cancer

the omentum (fatty tissue between the stomach and colon), is removed. Cancers arising in the proximal stomach are best treated with total gastrectomy, as well as lymph node dissection and omentectomy. There is controversy today regarding the value of more extensive surgery for gastric cancer, including removal of more lymph nodes, the spleen, and part of the pancreas. In Japan, these "super-radical" operations seem to lead to increased cure rates, but in Europe and the United States, no benefit has been found. It is generally agreed upon that more radical surgery is associated with increased complication rates.

If the tumor has spread to sites beyond the stomach, cure may not be possible, but some patients benefit from palliative surgery. Patients with large tumors causing pain or those with obstruction of the stomach may feel and eat better after gastrectomy. Sometimes, if gastrectomy is not possible due to tumor invasion into adjacent organs, a bypass procedure or placement of a feeding catheter can

help. Some patients have complications of their cancer, such as bleeding, obstruction, and perforation, in which case an emergency operation may be undertaken as an immediate lifesaving procedure, even in the presence of metastases.

Gastrectomy is a major operation performed under general anesthesia. A long incision from the breastbone down to or below the navel is usually required. A hospital stay of seven to ten days is expected for patients with an uncomplicated recovery, but it takes six to eight weeks before full strength returns. The chance of dying from a complication of surgery such as bleeding, infection, blood clots, heart attack, and the like is about 2 percent for distal gastrectomy but increases to 5 percent for total gastrectomy. After gastrectomy, patients can eat by mouth, as the GI tract is reconstructed with intestine. Most foods are tolerated well, although smaller, more frequent meals may be required. After total gastrectomy, vitamin B_{12} injections are given monthly to help prevent anemia.

Radiation Radiation is used either in combination with chemotherapy and surgery for cure, or for palliation of symptoms in cases where the tumor has spread such that surgery is not feasible. Doses between 4,000 and 4,500 cGy can help control tumors that can't be removed. Sometimes palliation is attempted over three to four weeks with 3,500 to 4,000 cGy, with infusions of 5-fluorouracil used as a radiation sensitizer during the first and fourth weeks, or continuously throughout radiation.

Intraoperative Radiation (IORT) Giving radiation therapy directly to the tumor area during surgery is sometimes done if there is an area that cannot be removed well enough to be certain that all cancer is gone (termed a positive margin).

Chemotherapy Gastric cancer is frequently affected by chemotherapy, with partial remissions (measurable tumors decreasing by half or more) occurring in as many as 40 to 50 percent of treated patients. Unfortunately, the beneficial effect of chemotherapy is usually relatively short-lived, as the cancer cells quickly develop resistance and regrow. True complete remissions are uncommon and, when they do occur, last on average only months. Chemotherapy *can* frequently improve cancer-related symptoms such as pain, difficulty eating, and ascites (fluid in the abdomen). Chemotherapy for advanced or metastatic disease can improve the duration of survival compared with supportive therapy alone, but the average benefit is measured only in months. An occasional patient may benefit dramatically from chemotherapy, although survival of more than two years from diagnosis of advanced stomach cancer remains unusual.

There is no agreed-upon "standard" chemotherapy for gastric cancer. Most oncologists use combination chemotherapy for this disease, which results in partial remissions more frequently than does single-drug chemotherapy. Regimens range from very toxic to relatively mild and the condition of the individual patient should be kept in mind when choosing a chemotherapy protocol. Most chemotherapy combinations include the drug 5-flourouracil. Among the more aggressive or potentially toxic regimens, comparative studies (primarily performed in Europe) have shown that the combinations ECF (epirubicin [Ellence] + cisplatin [Platinol] + 5-FU) and DCF (docetaxel [Taxotere] + cisplatin + 5-FU) may offer a survival advantage over other regimens, although the absolute degree of added benefit over less aggressive regimens is relatively small. Another recent study (also from Europe) showed that EOX (epirubicin [Ellence] + oxaliplatin [Eloxatin] + capecitabine [Xeloda]) may be an equivalent or better choice than ECF. Other chemotherapy combinations that have been extensively evaluated include FOLFIRI (5-FU + leucovorin [Wellcovorin] + irinotecan [Camptosar]), FAM (5-FU + doxorubicin [Adriamycin] + mitomycin [Mutamycin]), FAMtx (FAM + methotrexate [Mexate]), FLP (5-FU + leucovorin + cisplatin [Platinol]), FOLFOX (5-FU + leucovorin + oxaliplatin), ELF (etoposide [Etopophos] + leucovorin + 5-FU), EAP (etoposide + doxorubicin + cisplatin), and IC (irinotecan + cisplatin). These protocols again vary little in how often they induce a response, but may vary widely in how much toxicity they impart. For patients in whom one or more of the above combinations has stopped working or failed to work at all, or in whom combination chemotherapy may be too much to handle, single chemotherapy agents alone do have modest activity. These include drugs like paclitaxel (Taxol), docetaxel (Taxotere), irinotecan (Camptosar), and capecitabine (Xeloda).

The reasons for the poor outcomes of gastric cancer are poorly understood in spite of much research into mechanisms of resistance of the cancer to chemotherapy. Current studies include biologic agents in combination with chemotherapy (see chapter 44, "Investigational Anticancer Drugs").

Adjuvant Chemotherapy Many trials have been performed to examine whether the addition of chemotherapy either before or after surgical removal of stomach cancer can improve the chance of cure. The answer to this question until recently was unclear, with studies showing mixed results. However, a recent large trial done at many U.S. medical centers, both academic and private, has demonstrated that a combination of the drugs 5-flourouracil and leucovorin given along with radiation therapy to patients *after* complete removal of gastric cancers does indeed appear to improve the odds of cure. Another trial conducted in England utilized the ECF regimen before and after surgery (without radiation), and demonstrated improvement in the rate of cure compared with surgery alone. At present, it should be considered standard for patients with Stages II to IV gastric cancer that has been resected to undergo combined chemotherapy and radiation therapy if they have adequately recovered from surgery within four to eight weeks. Future studies will try to improve on the results of 5-FU and leucovorin alone using more aggressive chemotherapy protocols such as the ECF regimen.

Investigational and Biologic Agents Much effort is being put forth to define new kinds of treatment for all solid cancers, including gastric cancer. At present, there are a variety of new treatment strategies entering early clinical trials. Such strategies include (1) antiangiogenic agents (these are aimed at preventing tumor growth by targeting the blood vessels a tumor must create in order to survive and grow), (2) targeted molecular therapy (these are therapies, usually new kinds of drugs, aimed at specific genetic defects within tumors), (3) immunologic therapies (thus far, these have not shown significant promise in gastric cancers specifically, but research is ongoing to improve these therapies that help the immune system to fight cancers), and (4) gene therapy (this refers to strategies for replacing defective genes or removing errant genes that allow cancers to grow out of control; gene therapy remains in its infancy with significant technical hurdles yet to overcome).

Treatment by Stage

▪ Stage 0

TNM Tis, N0, M0

This is an in situ tumor that has not spread beyond the limiting membrane of the innermost level of the stomach lining (the mucosa).

Standard Treatment Experience in Japan, where this stage is diagnosed often, indicates that almost all patients who undergo a gastrectomy will survive beyond five years. An American series has recently confirmed these results. Certain patients can be treated with excision of the tumor with narrow margins of normal tissue, but without formal gastrectomy.

Five-Year Survival Over 90 percent

▪ Stage I

TNM T1, N0, M0 (Stage IA)
T1, N1, M0 or T2, N0, M0 (Stage IB)
The cancer is confined to the stomach wall and no lymph nodes are involved.

Standard Treatment Surgery is the treatment of choice, although how extensive the operation has to be depends on the tumor's location and how much of the stomach is involved.

For cancers arising in the lower (distal) part of the stomach, about 80 percent of the lower part of the stomach is removed, along with lymph nodes and the nearby connective tissue (a radical subtotal gastrectomy). This operation offers the best balance of high cure rates with low complication rates.

When the lesion involves the top, or proximal, part of the stomach (cardia), cure may be attempted by removing all of the stomach (total gastrectomy), along with lymph nodes, the omentum, and a sufficient length of the esophagus to obtain a clear margin. This operation is also the best choice for patients whose cancers diffusely involve the stomach (linitis plastica).

Because of the relatively good prognosis of Stage 1B tumors, it is unclear whether adding radiation and chemotherapy after surgery is of value, but it should be considered on an individual basis until more information is gathered. Stage 1A patients do not require additional therapy.

Five-Year Survival 52 to 85 percent for distal cancers; 10 to 15 percent for proximal cancers

Investigational

• Clinical trials of adjuvant combination chemotherapy and/or radiotherapy are appropriate whenever the tumor invades to the serosa or local lymph nodes either grossly or microscopically (Stage IB) to try to improve the survival.

• Neoadjuvant therapy is being evaluated for proximal cancers (stomach entry).

■ Stage II

TNM T1, N2, M0 or T2, N1, M0 or T3, N0, M0
The cancer is confined to the stomach wall and does not involve adjacent tissues. The lymph nodes very close to the

tumor or in the region around the stomach may be involved.

Standard Treatment This stage is sometimes curable with surgery. As in Stage I, the surgical procedure depends on the location and extent of the tumor. The procedures used are the same as for Stage I cancers. All visible tumor and grossly abnormal lymph nodes are removed.

Adjuvant postoperative chemotherapy and radiation therapy are warranted for this stage of disease and appear to improve the outcome by 30 to 40 percent. An acceptable alternative approach used more commonly in Europe is chemotherapy both pre- and postoperatively.

Five-Year Survival T1 or T2, N1 or N2, M0 over 20 percent; T3, N0, M0 about 20 percent

Investigational Same as for Stage I (adjuvant chemotherapy and/or radiotherapy).

■ *Stage III*

TNM T2, N2, M0 or T3, N1, M0 or T4, N0, M0 (Stage IIIA)
T3, N2, M0 or T4, N1, M0 (Stage IIIB)
The cancer involves tissues adjacent to the stomach and/or the lymph nodes very close to the tumor or in the region around the stomach.

Standard Treatment Cancer at this stage is treatable but not often curable. All patients whose tumors can be removed should have surgery, but radical surgery for cure is limited to those who do not have extensive lymph node involvement at the time of exploratory surgery. Up to 15 percent of selected patients can be cured by surgery alone if the lymph nodes involved are confined to the immediate vicinity of the tumor (N1).

Adjuvant postoperative chemotherapy and radiation therapy are warranted for this stage of disease and appear to improve the outcome by 30 to 40 percent.

An acceptable alternative approach used more commonly in Europe is chemotherapy both pre- and postoperatively.

Five-Year Survival 15 percent for distal cancers. Up to 15 percent can be cured if positive lymph nodes are confined to the immediate vicinity of the tumor.

Investigational Radiation therapy and/or adjuvant chemotherapy is being evaluated in patients with known residual disease.

■ *Stage IV*

TNM T4, N2, M0 (Stage IVA)
Any T, any N, M1 (Stage IVB)
The cancer has spread to adjacent tissues and to lymph nodes in the region around the stomach or has spread to distant sites, most commonly the liver or other organs.

Standard Treatment Because survival is so poor with all available single and combined treatment methods, no one approach can be considered state-of-the-art. Palliative surgery, combination chemotherapy, and occasionally radiotherapy are all options.

When it is possible to remove the primary tumor, palliative surgery will at least reduce the risk of bleeding or obstruction and may lead to a longer survival.

Chemotherapy can offer significant palliation to some patients, and long-term remissions are sometimes possible.

Stage IVA patients for whom complete resection of tumor is possible may benefit from adjuvant chemotherapy and radiation therapy.

Five-Year Survival Less than 5 percent

Investigational Neoadjuvant chemotherapy to shrink the tumor before surgery may make surgery possible. An occasional patient with Stage IV (T4, N3) cancer might be cured surgically. Investigational programs should be considered.

Treating Other Tumor Types

Gastric Lymphomas

These tumors, which may imitate primary adenocarcinomas of the stomach, are uncommon, making up only about 5 percent of gastric malignancies. These tumors are becoming more common, however.

A recent association has been shown between gastric lymphomas and ulcers and an infection with *Helicobacter pylori*. Eradication of the infection with antibiotics may lead to a regression of the lymphoma in some cases.

Patients with gastric lymphoma should have a general lymphoma evaluation, including a chest X-ray; chest, pelvic, and abdominal CT scans; and bone marrow biopsies.

Standard Treatment Removing part of the stomach, if possible, may be the ideal treatment. In one series of fifty consecutive cases, a survival of 90 percent was obtained when the tumor involved only the mucosa, 80 percent when it involved the submucosa. A study for Stages IE and IIE (local tumor extension) lymphomas showed that patients who had six courses of CHOP (cyclophosphamide [Cytoxan] + hydrodoxorubicin [Adriamycin] + vincristine [Oncovin] + prednisone) followed by radiation therapy and then additional chemotherapy did as well as patients who had surgery.

When the lymphoma fully penetrates the gastric wall and the lymph nodes in the region become involved, the survival is decreased to about 25 percent.

Radiation after surgery helps reduce the chance for local recurrences and is appropriate adjuvant therapy, especially for IE and IIE tumors. The radiation therapy port usually covers the upper abdomen as well as the regional lymph nodes, and radiation is given over several weeks. Combination chemotherapy following surgery is being studied and merits further investigation.

Leiomyosarcomas

If diagnosed with a sarcoma, it is important to discuss whether the diagnosis of gastrointestinal stromal tumor (GIST) has been definitively excluded. Treatment of GIST is very different and is discussed in a separate chapter (see the chapter "Gastrointestinal Stromal Tumor"). Leiomyosarcomas start in the smooth muscles of the stomach wall and account for only 1 to 3 percent of all gastric malignancies. Bleeding is common. Five-year survival is about 45 percent, but there are few long-term cures.

Standard Treatment The primary treatment is partial removal of the stomach, taking out just the area of the tumor and a rim of normal surrounding tissue. Radiation therapy and chemotherapy may be used after surgery or for metastatic disease. The most common chemotherapy combinations now used are doxorubicin (Adriamycin) + dacarbazine (DTIC-Dome) or doxorubicin + cisplatin (Platinol). High-dose ifosfamide (Ifex) is also used, although the role of chemotherapy in sarcomas remains unproven.

Supportive Care

Removing part or all of the stomach naturally produces many problems that require medical attention:

• Iron deficiency anemia often develops after a gastrectomy, since iron is absorbed mainly in the duodenum and stomach acids play a role in the process.
• Monthly doses of vitamin B_{12} should be given after a few years to prevent pernicious anemia.
• The dumping syndrome—with symptoms such as abdominal fullness, nausea, vomiting, a rapid heartbeat, weakness, and dizziness—is quite common after surgery because food passes through the system so quickly that there is little time for absorption. The dumping syndrome often resolves with time. Many treatments, including smaller meals, a lower-carbohydrate diet, and no chocolate or peppermint, can help. No food or fluid after 7:00 or 8:00 P.M. may help, too.
• Symptoms of upset stomach (gastritis) may be related to the alkaline backup, or reflux, of bile and intestinal secretions into the esophagus. Symptoms can be controlled by an antacid such as Maalox, Mylanta, or Riopan; by sucralfate (Carafate), which coats the stomach lining; or by a bile blocker such as cholestyramine (Questran).
• Walking or simply staying upright after meals as well as sleeping with the head elevated can help control reflux by improving the drainage of the gastric pouch and can also help reduce symptoms.
• If the antrum—the gastrin-producing part of the stomach—is removed, there will be little need for gastric acid blockers. But if acid is still being produced, an H-2 blocker such as Tagamet, Zantac, Pepsid, or Prilosec will help.
• Bacteria can grow in the loop of the duodenum bypassed by a connection of the stomach to the small bowel, producing what is called the blind loop syndrome. This bacteria breaks down bile and the acids pouring in from the pancreas, resulting in diarrhea and poor absorption of fats. The blind loop syndrome can be treated with oral antibiotics.

Recurrent Cancer

Survival is very poor with all available single and combined approaches to treatment, although an occasional patient might have a remission lasting several months or even a few years.

• All patients with recurrent stomach cancer should be considered candidates for Phase I and Phase II clinical trials testing anticancer drugs or biologicals.

• Standard treatment options are palliative chemotherapy with ECF, FAM, EAP, ELF, FAP (5-FU + doxorubicin [Adriamycin] + cisplatin [Platinol]), ELFI (etoposide [Etopophos] + leucovorin + 5-FU + interferon), and FAMtx.

• For the patient with either local disease that cannot be removed or local recurrent or residual disease after surgery, the use of radiation therapy in combination with chemotherapy has been considered effective palliative treatment (i.e., to prevent bleeding or obstruction of the stomach). This treatment has had no proven benefits for survival, however.

The Most Important Questions You Can Ask

• How do you tell a benign ulcer from a malignant one?

• What is the best way to cure my gastric cancer?

• How will the stage of my cancer be determined? Will I be a candidate for curative surgery?

• What disability might I have after surgery?

• Should I receive postoperative chemotherapy and radiation?

• What problems might I expect if I have all three treatments—surgery, chemotherapy, and radiation?

• What is a good program for palliation and support if that is needed?

• What clinical trials are available?

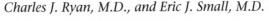

Testis

Charles J. Ryan, M.D., and Eric J. Small, M.D.

■ ■ ■ ■

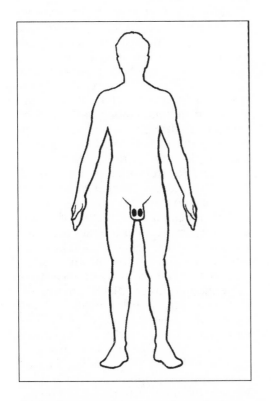

Testicular cancer accounts for only 1 percent of all male cancers, totaling about 7,400 annual cases in the United States. Fewer than 400 men will die of the disease each year because of its sensitivity to radiation therapy (seminoma) and chemotherapy (seminoma and nonseminoma). In the past thirty-five years, the five-year survival rate has increased from 63 percent to more than 91 percent. This improvement reflects not only advances in treatment (mostly chemotherapy), but also an increased awareness of the disease. Because of the young age of most patients with this disease, its high rate of curability translates into a substantial public health benefit. Currently, only 15 percent of patients have distant disease when they are diagnosed, while more than 60 percent have tumors confined to the testicle.

The vast majority of testis cancers are malignancies of the primordial germ cells—cells within the testicle that carry the genetic material required for the development of a fertilized egg. Although most germ cell tumors arise from the testicles, they can also develop in other locations that harbor germ cells (extragonadal germ cell tumors, or EGGCT), such as the chest, retroperitoneum, and brain. The testes, which are derived from the yolk sac early in the embryo's development, move from the center of a developing fetus to an area called the urogenital ridge. Since the embryonic germ cells from this ridge travel almost the whole length of the developing body to their destination in the scrotum, bits of primitive tissue called embryonic rests can be left behind during the migration. This explains why some germ cell tumors are found in nontesticular (extragonadal) sites in the chest or abdomen. Extragonadal germ cell tumors in general are very aggressive, carry a worse prognosis, and frequently require more intensive therapy.

Types Germ cell cancers are broadly divided into two types, based on their microscopic appearance—seminoma and nonseminoma. While both are initially treated with surgery to remove the testicle, the type of germ cell tumor may determine subsequent treatment: surgical removal of involved lymph nodes or chemotherapy for nonseminoma and radiation or chemotherapy for seminoma.

Seminoma Seminoma makes up approximately 40 percent of all testis tumors. A subtype is called spermatocytic seminoma, which is a rare variety occurring in elderly men. Spermatocytic seminoma almost never spreads. Seminoma is generally discovered in men in their thirties and forties. Seminoma is often confined to the testicles, and if it spreads, it tends to do so in an orderly fashion—first to lymph nodes and only later to the lungs. If there is any nonseminoma element present, or if one of the tumor markers (e.g., alpha-fetoprotein, or AFP) is elevated, by definition the tumor is considered to be a nonseminomatous germ cell tumor and the treatment may be different.

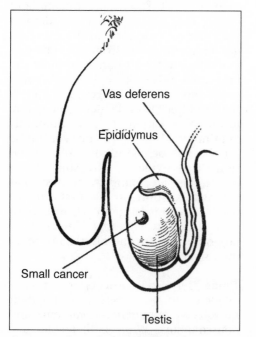

Cancer on the surface of testis

Nonseminoma Nonseminomatous germ cell tumors (NSGCT) most often occur in men in their twenties and early thirties. These tumors are composed of various cell types as seen under the microscope—embryonal carcinoma, teratoma, yolk-sac tumor (endodermal sinus carcinoma), and choriocarcinoma.

More than 90 percent of nonseminomatous germ cell tumors have more than one cell type in them, including seminoma cells. Pure embryonal carcinoma, pure teratoma, and pure yolk-sac tumor each account for 2 to 3 percent and pure choriocarcinoma for 0.03 percent of all germ cell tumors. Embryonal cell carcinoma is moderately aggressive. Its presence in the testicle predicts a higher likelihood of lymph node involvement. Pure choriocarcinoma is rare but is aggressive and has a higher frequency of metastases to the brain.

Teratocarcinoma is a mixture of embryonal cell carcinoma and teratoma, while so-called mature teratoma implies that embryonal cell carcinoma must have been present but has changed to a more mature (differentiated), more normal-appearing, and less malignant cell form either spontaneously or because of therapy. Patients with teratoma elements in their original tumor specimen are more likely to have residual masses, usually in the lymph nodes, made up of benign mature teratoma after chemotherapy. Mature teratoma in and of itself is unlikely to spread but can grow to a large size. Further, if teratoma tissue is not removed, it can (rarely) "transform" into a tumor type that is distinct from NSGCT, such as a lymphoma or a sarcoma. Pure yolk-sac tumors are extremely rare and more frequently observed in the chest (mediastinum), except in children under fifteen, where it accounts for 90 percent of testis cancers.

How It Spreads There is a difference in the way cancers of the testis spread.

Right-testis tumors spread by the spermatic cord and its associated blood and lymph vessels into lymph glands surrounding and between the large blood vessels, the aorta, and the inferior vena cava (the interaortocaval region).

Left-testis tumors drain via the spermatic cord vessels into the left kidney artery and venous lymphatic areas and to lymph nodes alongside the aorta (the para-aortic region). They are generally not found in the interaortocaval nodal system. Unless surgery has disturbed the scrotum—to remove the testis or repair an undescended testis through a scrotal incision—testis tumors always drain directly into the abdominal lymph nodes and not into the groin lymph nodes.

After spreading to lymph nodes, the most frequent site of organ metastases is the lungs, although in advanced cases the liver, bones, and brain can be involved, particularly in cases of choriocarcinoma and, to a lesser extent, embryonal cell carcinoma.

What Causes It Unknown. There is no firm evidence that heredity is a factor. There has been some association with a few uncommon genetic diseases such as hermaphroditism (mixture of male/female development) and Klinefelter's and Turner's syndromes. Failure of the testis to descend into the scrotum (cryptorchidism) accounts for 10 percent of testicular cancers. It is not known whether cryptorchidism is due to some underlying testicular abnormality that prevented the testicle's migration into the scrotum or to an anatomic abnormality that made an otherwise normal testis remain within the abdominal cavity, thereby leading to a cancerous change. Many patients with cryptorchid (undescended) testes never develop testicular cancer, and the majority of men who develop testicular cancer did not have cryptorchidism.

Risk Factors

At Significantly Higher Risk

- For men between twenty and thirty-four years old, testis tumors make up 22 percent of all cancers and rank first in cancer incidence. It is the second most common cancer for men ages thirty-five to thirty-nine years and third for those fifteen to nineteen.
- American white males have a rate four times that of black males.
- The incidence of this cancer among African-American men is increasing.

At Slightly Higher Risk Uncommonly, tumors are found in men with fertility problems. About 5 percent of men cured of testis cancer are at risk to develop another in the remaining testis within twenty-five years.

Screening

Testicular ultrasound is an accurate way to detect masses. However, the tumor is so uncommon that ultrasound screening is not generally done. The most cost-effective screening method is simple physical examination of the testicles. Although a program has been developed in the Scandinavian countries to educate men about self-examination (similar to that for breast cancer in women), it has not gained acceptance in the United States. At the very least, men who have already had a testis cancer and those who have had an undescended testicle should learn self-examination and intermittently undergo sonograms (ultrasound).

Common Signs and Symptoms

Swelling of the testicles, discomfort, or masses are present in over 90 percent of cases. Such symptoms are sometimes ignored or misdiagnosed as being caused by an injury, as an inflammation of the testis (orchitis) or spermatic cord (epididymitis) requiring only antibiotic therapy, or as enlarging veins of the spermatic cord. Sometimes testicular cancer occurs along with epididymitis, so that after the epididymitis resolves, testicular cancer should be ruled out. Frequently, the only symptom is a painless testicular mass.

In some situations, the cancer may spread outside the testicle before swelling in the testicle is large enough to be felt. Occasionally, the primary tumor (in the testicle) will shrink after this spread occurs. The testicle still needs to be removed in this situation.

In rare cases, breast tenderness or enlargement because of high levels of HCG (human chorionic gonadotropin) produced by the tumor, or abdominal pain or cough with or without blood-tinged sputum due to metastases, can be seen.

Testis Tumor Markers

Testis cancers produce proteins that can be measured in the blood. These measurements are extremely reliable tumor markers. The three main markers are human chorionic gonadotropin (HCG), lactate dehydrogenase (LDH), and alpha-fetoprotein (AFP). AFP and HCG are so dependable that any increase above normal blood levels almost always indicates a testis tumor recurrence. This is true even if there is no evidence of cancer by physical examination and X-ray examinations. Eighty percent of nonseminomas will have an elevated HCG or AFP or both. Seminomas never have an elevated AFP, and around 10 percent have an elevated HCG, which carries no prognostic significance. If there is an elevated AFP, by definition the tumor is considered a nonseminoma.

The Uses of Tumor Markers These markers are used to monitor the response to therapy. If the tumor markers decrease or return to normal levels after treatment, there is obviously a response. An increase

is a sign of disease progression or failure to respond.

If tumor marker levels do not normalize after surgical removal of the testicle, or normalize and then start climbing, chemotherapy or sometimes further surgery is needed. However, normal marker levels do not guarantee the complete absence of testis cancer, since microscopic deposits may still exist. This is why follow-up requires CT scans.

The rate of disappearance of a marker from the blood can also be predicted by its half-life, which is the time it takes for the amount of a marker in the bloodstream to be reduced by one-half. The half-life for HCG is about twenty-four to forty-eight hours, and for AFP five to seven days. Physicians using these formulas can determine to some degree whether the tumor is responding to treatment completely or partially.

Other Causes of Elevated Markers

HCG HCG is a rather specific testis tumor marker associated with breast enlargement and nipple tenderness in males when markedly increased. Some unusual lung, liver, bladder, and pancreatic cancers also can increase HCG levels, although these are uncommon. One caution in using this marker is that marijuana smokers may have increased HCG blood levels.

Rarely, patients can have a very slight false increase in the HCG after orchiectomy, which arises as a by-product of the low testosterone level following removal of the testicle.

LDH This hormone is increased frequently. While the level of LDH may be predictive of outcome, it is nonspecific and can be elevated with infections, and with using certain drugs, including filgrastim (G-CSF; Neupogen).

AFP AFP is elevated in 60 to 70 percent of testis tumor cases but never in seminoma. AFP can also be elevated in patients with a primary liver cancer (hepatoma) or with liver disease such as hepatitis or cirrhosis.

Diagnosis

Physical Examination

- A testicular mass that can be felt—particularly a painless mass or one that does not completely clear within two weeks of antibiotic therapy—requires further tests.
- Although many testicular cancers are painless, a painful testicular mass does not mean that cancer is not present.
- Enlarged lymph nodes in the abdomen and neck.

Blood and Other Tests

- Blood tests for LDH, AFP, and HCG.
- Blood counts, biochemical screening profile, serum magnesium, and a blood test (creatinine) to evaluate kidney function.
- If bleomycin (Blenoxane) is to be used, pulmonary function tests, including a DLCO (diffusing of the lung capacity), are performed as a baseline for future comparisons (bleomycin can cause lung scarring).
- Analysis of sperm and sperm banking should be considered in most patients, since treatment can result in infertility. This might be the result of chemotherapy-induced toxicity or of the loss of ejaculation if the surgical removal of lymph nodes requires cutting the nerves that control this function. However, it should be pointed out that about 40 percent of patients with testicular cancer are infertile *because* of their cancer. Testicular cancer and its treatment can result in infertility (inability to father a child) in about 35 percent of cases but not impotence (inability to have an erection).

Imaging

- Ultrasound is extremely accurate to evaluate the testicle, and any solid mass found on ultrasound should be considered cancerous until proven otherwise.
- Chest X-rays to evaluate lung metastases. Many oncologists advise obtaining a baseline CT of the chest, even with a normal chest X-ray, to aid in follow-up.
- CT or MRI scans of the abdomen and pelvis are part of the staging procedure to evaluate the abdominal (retroperitoneal) and pelvic lymph nodes.
- Lymphangiography may help in about 10 percent of cases, but it is no longer routinely used because CT scans are more accurate. Sometimes it is still used to plan radiation therapy ports.
- Radionuclide bone and brain CT scans have to be done only when there are symptoms, although some doctors routinely order these scans for men with pure choriocarcinoma.

Biopsy The removal of the testicle (orchiectomy) through an incision in the groin—never a scrotal incision or an aspiration biopsy—is required for diagnosis. Even when metastatic disease is found, the testis where the cancer started still has to be removed because the primary tumor does not always respond fully to chemotherapy, as it is located in a sheltered location, or "chemotherapy sanctuary."

Staging

Several staging divisions are used for testis cancer. The stage depends on whether the primary tumor involves the testis, epididymis, spermatic cord, and/or scrotum; whether a single node or multiple nodes are involved, and the size of those nodes; and whether there are distant metastases to other organs, the most common being the lungs or the lymph nodes above the diaphragm.

Treatment Overview

Surgery is necessary in all cases because the removal of the affected testicle is usually required for diagnosis. The use of further surgery, radiation, and chemotherapy depends on the stage of the disease as well as the components of the tumor (e.g., seminoma versus nonseminomatous germ cell tumors).

 Surgery For local tumors, the first step is to remove the testis, epididymis, and spermatic cord (radical orchiectomy). This is performed by an inguinal approach, meaning that it is removed through the groin. This is never done through an incision in the scrotum because that can open up new lymph drainage areas to the groin and alter the pattern of tumor spread.

For patients with nonseminomatous tumors confirmed by orchiectomy, if scans show no or limited lymph node involvement and no metastases, another operation is done to remove the lymph nodes in the back of the abdomen. This standard operation is known as a retroperitoneal lymph node dissection (RPLND). New surgical techniques have resolved many quality-of-life issues raised by this operation. The procedure is now much more acceptable, since the ability to have children is preserved in more than 60 percent of cases. There is usually no effect of surgery on potency (ability to have an erection).

Radiation For localized seminoma, radiation therapy to the pelvis and retroperitoneal lymph node areas can be used to prevent relapse.

Chemotherapy There are many commonly used chemotherapy regimens. Chemotherapy can be used as a preventive measure or as treatment for cancer that has spread. Each agent has been found to be active against testis tumors when given alone, but prolonged, complete disappearance of tumors is best when other drugs are combined with cisplatin (Platinol). The chemotherapy regimen used, and the number of times it is repeated, is determined by the extent and aggressiveness of the tumor.

In the United States, the most commonly used regimen is PEB (cisplatin [Platinol] + etoposide [Etopophos] + bleomycin [Blenoxane]). There is some controversy concerning the need for bleomycin, although it appears that it can be omitted in patients with good-risk tumors (see page 853).

How Standard Chemotherapy Is Administered PEB and PE (cisplatin [Platinol] + etoposide [Etopophos] without bleomycin [Blenoxane]) are given by vein, with the dosages of etoposide and cisplatin divided into five daily doses. When getting chemotherapy, the patient needs to be present for three to five consecutive days to get these divided doses. Bleomycin is given once a week, and every twenty-one days, this cycle of daily infusion is repeated. Most patients are treated with three (for PEB) or four (for PE) cycles.

Regimens containing ifosfamide (Ifex) are sometimes used as secondary therapy. Because ifosfamide is a bladder irritant that can produce blood in the urine, a

Chemotherapy Combinations Used for Testis Cancer	
PEB	Cisplatin (Platinol) + etoposide (Etopophos) + bleomycin (Blenoxane)
PE	Cisplatin + etoposide
VIP	Cisplatin + etoposide + ifosfamide (Ifex)
TIP	Paclitaxel (Taxol) + ifosfamide + cisplatin

protective drug such as mesna (Mesnex) is required to prevent this complication. Such drugs do not affect the antitumor activity of ifosfamide.

High-Dose Chemotherapy Another role for ifosfamide (Ifex), as well as for etoposide (Etopophos) and carboplatin (Paraplatin), is in high-dose regimens, in combination with autologous bone marrow or peripheral stem cell transplantation as salvage therapy for very poor risk cases. For some patients with relapsed germ cell tumors or very aggressive tumors, high-dose chemotherapy appears to offer the potential for cure. Since high-dose therapy usually damages the bone marrow, where red blood cells, white blood cells, and platelets are manufactured, a rescue, or transplant, of the patient's own bone marrow (bone marrow transplant) or, more commonly, of peripheral blood stem cells is required.

The use of high-dose chemotherapy as an initial treatment is no better than standard chemotherapy for patients with poor-risk disease.

Treatment by Stage

■ Stage I

TNM Tis–T3, N0, M0
The tumor is limited to the testis (Tis, T1) or the epididymis (T2). There are no lymph nodes involved or distant metastases. In the American Joint Committee on Cancer (AJCC) staging system, spermatic cord (T3) involvement is placed together with scrotal (T4) invasion in Stage II, although most oncologists would still consider this a Stage I tumor.

Standard Treatment Radical (inguinal) orchiectomy—removal of the testis, epididymis, and spermatic cord—is performed.

Seminoma Prophylactic radiation therapy is given to a total dose of 2,500 to 3,000 cGy to the pelvic and abdominal lymph node areas on the same side as the tumor. Prophylactic radiation will prevent virtually all relapses (98 percent). This is a very low dose of radiation and carries very little risk or side effects. Without radiation, only approximately 20 percent of seminomas will relapse. Thus, an investigational approach is simply to use surveillance or watchful waiting. However, since relapses can occur (in some cases, six to ten years later), long-term intensive surveillance is required for seminomas larger than $1\frac{1}{4}$ inches (3 cm) and those that have invaded the rete testis (a structure just outside the testicle but still within the scrotum).

It is also now apparent that either one or two doses of a single chemotherapy agent, carboplatin (Paraplatin), like radiation therapy, will prevent virtually all relapses. A recent large study suggests that this approach is a reasonable option for some patients with Stage I seminoma.

Nonseminomatous Germ Cell Tumors (NSGCT) After orchiectomy, patients with tumor confined to the testis (Stage I) can be treated with either RPLND (surgery to remove the abdominal lymph nodes that can be involved) or careful surveillance. Several important features are predictive of whether there will be microscopic involvement of the abdominal lymph nodes, even though the CT scan or MRI is negative. These adverse predictive features are (1) tumor type (the presence of a large proportion of embryonal carcinoma cells carries a worse prognosis); (2) involvement of blood vessels or lymphatic channels within the testicular mass; and (3) involvement of structures outside the testicle itself, like the spermatic cord, epididymis, or scrotum. For patients with one or more high-risk features, the risk of recurrence is in the 40 to 50 percent range, and RPLND is warranted. Node dissection becomes both a diagnostic and prophylactic measure. Removal of microscopically involved nodes (really a Stage II case) is not only diagnostic, but also therapeutic, for cure follows in almost all cases.

In situations where the serum tumor markers fail to normalize (after an appropriate waiting period), or rise after orchiectomy, chemotherapy should be utilized because ultimately all patients will develop metastatic tumors and are likely to do so even after RPLND. This situation is referred to as Stage IS because of the serum markers.

The concept of surveillance only—without lymph node surgery—has been investigated for nonseminomatous tumors because 60 to 80 percent of Stage I cases will never relapse and effective cisplatin (Platinol)–based chemotherapy will cure almost all early relapses. Good-risk patients (those with true T1 tumors, no or a small percentage of embryonal cells, normal markers, and no lymphatic or vascular invasion) are well suited for surveillance. For good-risk patients or those with a true T1, N0, M0 tumor, the relapse rate is 15 to 25 percent. In contrast, the relapse rate is over 50 percent for poor-risk Stage I cases having tumor invasion of the epididymis, spermatic cord, and lymphatic and/or blood vessels, particularly for the embryonal cell carcinoma variety. Surveillance should not be offered for such poor-risk cases.

If surveillance is the form of therapy chosen for good-risk cases, it should be realized that this demands very careful follow-up. For NSGCT, 80 percent of relapses that occur do so in the first year, and 95 percent occur within the first two years. Scans are obtained at least every three to four months for at least two years, and blood tests for tumor markers are obtained every six to eight weeks. Although almost all relapses will be found within the first twelve months, tumors have recurred as late as five years after diagnosis or beyond. With careful follow-up and by starting chemotherapy immediately after detection of a relapse, less than 1 to 2 percent

of men will die. For men with Stage I NSGCT who are not willing to make this type of follow-up commitment, the correct choice is surgery.

Five-Year Survival 95 to 100 percent

Investigational For patients with seminoma, although radiation therapy works well and generally has few side effects, options include surveillance and one or two doses of carboplatin (Paraplatin) chemotherapy. Chemotherapy for clinical Stage I NSGCT has been utilized and is being studied in patients, especially those with Stage I embryonal cell predominant disease. However, at this time, it is not a standard treatment and should be used only in certain circumstances.

■ *Stage II*
TNM Any T, N1–3, M0
The tumor involves the retroperitoneal lymph nodes either with a single node measuring $3/4$ inch (2 cm) or less (N1); with a single node $3/4$ to 2 inches (2 to 5 cm) or with multiple nodes all less than 2 inches (5 cm) (N2); or with any node larger than that (N3). An alternative staging system defines Stages IIA, IIIB, and IIC.

Stage IIA refers to minimally extensive disease. For seminoma, this generally refers to tumors greater than $3/4$ inch (2 cm) in size on CT, whereas for NSGCT, where RPLND is frequently undertaken, this also refers to tumors that have unexpected microscopic involvement of lymph nodes.

Stage IIB disease, or disease of intermediate extent, usually refers to tumors up to 2 inches (5 cm) in size, whereas Stage IIC refers to bulky disease, with tumors greater than 2 inches (5 cm) in size.

Standard Treatment
Seminoma Radical inguinal orchiectomy followed by therapeutic doses of radiation therapy (at least 4,000 cGy) to the abdominal lymph nodes will cure

more than 90 percent of nonbulky seminoma cases (Stage IIB or lower). Chemotherapy can be considered in situations where radiation would pose increased side effects or risk (e.g., inflammatory bowel disease or "horseshoe" kidney, a congenital abnormality in which the kidneys are fused together), or where the patient has previously received radiation.

For bulky Stage II seminoma (Stage IIC), chemotherapy is generally preferred, since older studies of radiation find the cure rate to be only about 70 percent, whereas chemotherapy will cure over 90 percent (see Stage III below).

NSGCT Patients with Stage IIA NSGCT who haven't already undergone surgery generally undergo RPLND. Stage IIB patients can be treated with RPLND or primary chemotherapy, whereas for Stage IIC NSGCT patients, chemotherapy is the preferred approach. After surgery, some patients with involved lymph nodes greater than or equal to $1\frac{1}{4}$ inches (3 cm) in size, with five or more lymph nodes involved, or with spread of cancer outside the capsule of the lymph node can receive adjuvant or prophylactic chemotherapy to reduce the risk of relapse. In that situation, generally two cycles of PE chemotherapy are given. Approximately half of the patients with no additional therapy relapse with tumor compared to less than 5 percent of those given two courses of prophylactic chemotherapy. However, almost all relapsing cases will subsequently respond when given standard chemotherapy. Clinical trials have indicated that if patients do not receive adjuvant chemotherapy, their overall survival is not affected, since chemotherapy is so effective if they relapse. However, careful surveillance is required, and upon relapse, three cycles of PEB are usually needed, so some patients prefer to receive adjuvant therapy, to try to get the treatment "over with."

Relapse rates are very low for Stage II cases in whom there are only a few positive lymph nodes found at surgery, provided none are larger than $3/4$ inch (2 cm). Consequently, chemotherapy can be withheld in such cases until relapse occurs.

Five-Year Survival 85 to 95 percent

▇ *Stage III*
TNM Any T, any N, M1
The tumor invades other organs, most commonly the lungs or lymph nodes above the diaphragm.

Standard Treatment Radical orchiectomy followed by chemotherapy for both seminoma and nonseminomatous tumors is the usual treatment. Patients with metastatic germ cell tumors can be classified into one of three categories: good risk, intermediate risk, and poor risk, based on the type of cancer, elevation of tumor markers, and site of disease.

For patients with good-risk tumors, the most frequently used drug combinations are cisplatin (Platinol) + etoposide (Etopophos), or PE, each day for five consecutive days repeated every three weeks for four doses or cycles, or cisplatin + etoposide + bleomycin (Blenoxane), or PEB, which uses the same doses and schedule of five days but adds bleomycin weekly for three cycles. Inadequate treatments include three cycles of PE (as opposed to four cycles) and the substitution of carboplatin (Paraplatin) for cisplatin in the PE regimen. For patients with high-risk tumors, four cycles of PEB or four cycles of etoposide (Etopophos) + ifosylamide (Ifex) + cisplatin, or VIP, are equivalent. Intermediate-risk patients, generally behave more like good-risk patients but are often treated as high-risk patients.

Fluids are given by vein to prevent cisplatin-induced kidney toxicity. Drugs are also given by vein to stop or minimize nausea and vomiting. A total of three to four cycles are given at no more than three- to four-week intervals, since it is

	NONSEMINOMA	SEMINOMA
Good risk	Arises in testicle *and* No disease outside nodes and lungs *and* Low tumor markers	Arises in testicle *and* No disease outside nodes and lungs
Intermediate risk	Arises in testicle *and* No disease outside nodes and lungs *and* Intermediate tumor markers	Disease outside nodes and lungs *or* Extragonadal germ cell tumors (EGGCT)
Poor risk	EGGCT *or* Disease outside nodes and lungs *or* High tumor markers	

harmful to space therapy at longer intervals. Only a complete response is acceptable, and surgery is required when CT scans of the chest, abdomen, and pelvis find any remaining disease, indicating a partial response.

For seminoma, if the remaining mass is less than 1¼ inches (3 cm), it is likely that only scar tissue will be found in the pathological specimen and no further surgery will be required. In seminoma, a PET scan can help discriminate between a residual mass that needs to be removed and one that is simply scar tissue. However, among nonseminoma patients with a remaining mass, 20 percent will have residual cancer, so surgery is required.

The relapse rate increases to 20 to 30 percent in men found to have viable (living) tumor (it is not unusual to find small areas of viable tumor in larger masses of dead tissue). In these cases, more chemotherapy, with a salvage regimen, must be given. Thereafter, careful follow-up is required.

Five-Year Survival Good risk, 80 to 90 percent; intermediate risk, 60 to 80 percent; poor risk, 40 to 60 percent.

Investigational For poor-risk patients not attaining a complete response and whose AFP and HCG markers are not decreasing at the normal half-life rate, consideration should be given to high-dose chemotherapy with peripheral stem cell transplant, which can cure at least 30 percent of heavily pretreated cases. The use of high-dose chemotherapy for high-risk patients as frontline therapy is no better than standard chemotherapy.

Treatment Follow-Up

Follow-up is an integral part of testis cancer therapy, particularly since most relapses occur quickly within the first year or two.

• Marker levels (some doctors also include a complete blood and platelet count) and chest X-rays should be taken every one to two months, with CT scans at three- to four-month intervals, during the first year.

• If abdominal or chest surgery has been performed, a repeat CT scan to serve as a new anatomic baseline can be done six weeks after the operation.

Similar tests are then repeated every three to four months during the second year. For NSGCT, since relapse is very uncommon after two years, the same tests can be done every four to six months for the third year and every six months thereafter. Seminoma tends to relapse later, so more intensive testing should be done for the first three to five years. Some doctors also do yearly examinations after that, but the value of such testing is uncertain.

• All men should be taught how to examine the remaining testicle and should have a sonogram when any change is found. The lifetime risk for a testicular cancer survivor to develop a tumor in the other testicle is 6 to 8 percent.

Long-Term Toxicity With many men being cured and having the expectation of a normal life span, therapy has been closely studied to evaluate any long-term toxicities.

• During therapy, nausea and vomiting can generally be prevented or minimized. Alopecia (hair loss) will occur, but hair will return—sometimes thicker, darker, and less wavy—within two to six months after chemotherapy is stopped.

• Low blood potassium, calcium, and magnesium levels may be found but can generally be easily corrected and disappear after therapy.

• Lung scarring can occur when bleomycin (Blenoxane) is used, so pulmonary function tests are used to monitor any change. It is recommended that these tests be obtained once every three to six weeks while on therapy. If lung function decreases, the drug must be stopped. Bleomycin is rarely fatal and rarely produces symptoms with current doses.

• Following some chemotherapy combinations, there have been reports of a chronic vascular disorder called Raynaud's phenomenon, in which fingers and toes are very sensitive to cold, turning red or blue, in 10 to 20 percent of cases.

• Sex drive (libido) is not changed by treatment and neither are erections. Chemotherapy may temporarily or permanently decrease the sperm count. Male hormone replacement is needed in men having orchiectomy for bilateral testicular cancers.

• Patients who have extensive surgery (RPLND) for large tumors may encounter irregularities in ejaculation, but erections are not changed.

• There is absolutely no evidence of any increased risk of abnormalities in children fathered by men who have had testis chemotherapy. Basically, either the sperm works or it doesn't. But it has been found that some men who have a testis cancer have low or zero sperm count before therapy, so a count should be done to document fertility *before* treatment is started and reevaluated thereafter.

• Chemotherapy can cause infertility in about 35 percent of patients.

• There is a very small (less than 2 percent) chance of developing other cancers, including leukemia, five to ten years after treatment. The risk of leukemia is due to one of the necessary chemotherapy drugs (etoposide [Etopophos]).

Recurrent or New Cancer

Since 6 to 8 percent of testis cancer patients will develop a second testis tumor in their remaining testicle, sequential self-examination and/or a baseline testicular sonography should always be done. A new testicular cancer is treated according to the stages listed earlier. A relapse indicated only by an increasing HCG or AFP marker requires a completely new work-up and is generally treated with chemotherapy.

• When the tumor is documented by CT scan, particularly in late relapsing cases, surgical debulking may be warranted to identify the type of tumor that has recurred, followed by salvage chemotherapy.

• When markers are positive yet cancer cannot be found by any diagnostic test (including MRI), salvage chemotherapy should be started, since it is generally successful in such cases.

• For metastases to the spinal cord and bone, radiation therapy is the treatment of choice to control local symptoms. Brain metastases may be removed surgically, if possible, and should be followed by therapeutic full-dose radiation therapy and chemotherapy.

The Most Important Questions You Can Ask

• What type of testis cancer do I have? What is the stage?

• Am I in the good-risk or poor-risk group?

• Will nerve-sparing surgery be possible?

• When should I sperm-bank?

• What are the toxic effects and risks of chemotherapy?

• What are the long-term toxic effects of radiation?

• What are my tumor markers? What other tests are needed for follow-up?

• What is my chance of cure?

Thymus

Tony Y. Eng, M.D., Malin Dollinger, M.D., and Ernest H. Rosenbaum, M.D.

■ ■ ■ ■

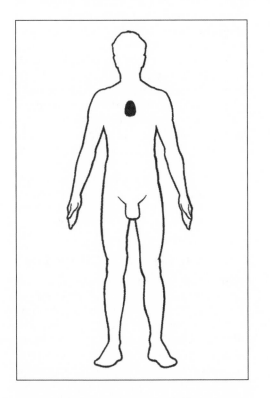

The thymus is a gland located in the upper front portion of the chest cavity (anterior mediastinum). It plays an important role in the production and maturation of T lymphocytes for the immune system. Most of these T lymphocytes, or thymus-derived lymphocytes, are formed before puberty as a major part of our immune system (cellular immunity) for our entire lives. Although these T lymphocytes look fairly similar under the microscope to the other major class of lymphocytes (B lymphocytes), they perform specialized immunologic functions to protect us from foreign organisms. The thymus gradually shrinks in size and function after puberty.

Types In general, thymus tumors are not common. But a variety of tumors can develop in the thymus. The most common thymus tumor is malignant thymoma. Five hundred to 700 people in the United States are diagnosed with thymoma each year. Thymoma originates in the lining, or epithelium, of the thymus gland. All other tumor types are uncommon. These include lymphomas, germ cell tumors, carcinoid tumors, carcinomas, and thymolipomas. This chapter will discuss only malignant thymoma.

Benign or Malignant? Some thymomas are noninvasive and appear to behave like benign tumors; others (malignant thymomas) have all of the invasive characteristics of malignancy. Although thymomas are usually encapsulated tumors, they can invade the capsule and infiltrate the surrounding tissues or even metastasize to regional and distant organs. Under the microscope, there are a number of cell subtypes of thymoma. Attempts have been made to correlate the different subtypes to clinical behavior and prognosis. However, it is difficult to consistently relate this microscopic appearance to how a tumor behaves. Sometimes, a malignant thymoma may be identified on body CT (computerized tomography) scan as showing invasion of adjacent tissues. So whether the tumors are called malignant depends not on their appearance but on their behavior (whether they have invasive characteristics). In the absence of invasion, the presence of a clearly defined covering, or "capsule," tends to classify the tumor as benign. But since all thymomas can become invasive and extend beyond the capsule, they should all be considered potentially malignant.

How It Spreads Most malignant thymomas grow slowly and do not usually spread outside of the thymus. However, they can eventually invade through the capsule into adjacent tissues and organs. Even after surgical removal, they have a tendency to recur in the chest at the site of origin. Although they seldom spread (metastasize) to elsewhere in the body, they can spread to the heart and lungs (especially the lining of the heart [pericardium] and lungs [pleura]) and to the liver.

What Causes It The true cause of thymoma is unknown. Epstein-Barr virus (EBV) infection, radiation exposure, and genetic abnormalities have been suggested as some of the potential causes. Also, there are several associated immune disorders linked to malignant thymomas, especially a type of muscle weakness called myasthenia gravis that may be present in 30 to 40 percent of the patients. Other associated immune disorders may be seen, including low red blood counts (pure red cell aplasia), low gamma globulins, connective tissue disorders, thyroiditis, ulcerative colitis, pernicious anemia, enteritis, and sarcoid. Various endocrine disorders can be associated with thymoma, such as hyperthyroidism, adrenal insufficiency (Addison's disease), Cushing's syndrome (adrenal overactivity), and hypopituitarism.

Risk Factors

Thymoma usually occurs in people between the ages of forty to sixty. It is slightly more common in males. However, there are no established risk factors identified for thymoma.

Screening

There are no general screening procedures for apparently healthy people. About a third of all thymoma cases are typically discovered during a routine or diagnostic chest X-ray. Myasthenia gravis, characterized by worsening muscle weakness and eye symptoms, is associated with a thymoma in up to 30 percent of cases. Therefore, patients who present with myasthenia gravis require a careful screening and evaluation for thymoma. Removing the tumor surgically will often produce a complete remission of the myasthenia gravis in about one-third of these patients, and at least half will improve. It is felt that the presence of myasthenia may be associated with a worse prognosis in some patients.

Common Signs and Symptoms

Most people with thymoma often have no symptoms initially, but as the tumor grows, they may have chest-related complaints such as a persistent cough, shortness of breath, difficulty swallowing, and chest pain or tightness due to tumor compression or invasion of surrounding organs. If the tumor is very large, the neck and face may be swollen because of an obstruction of the superior vena cava in the chest.

The associated diseases or syndromes can also produce a variety of symptoms. The predominant symptom of blurred or double vision, droopy eyelids, muscle weakness, and generalized fatigue may be found in patients with myasthenia gravis. Muscles that control breathing and movements of the arms and legs may also be affected. Severe depression of the red cells (pure red cell aplasia) in about 5 percent of patients with thymoma leads to severe anemia, and 5 to 10 percent have a low gamma globulin level.

Distinctive signs and symptoms of other autoimmune or endocrine disorders can lead to the diagnosis.

Diagnosis

A thymoma can be suspected in a patient with myasthenia gravis or one of the other autoimmune or endocrine disorders mentioned above. If a mass is seen on a chest X-ray in the location of the thymus in the chest, tumor samples may be obtained by needle biopsy, bronchoscopy, mediastinoscopy, video-assisted thoracoscopy, or open biopsy. Sometimes, when larger samples are required, definitive surgery may be done to get adequate tissue samples and to remove the tumor at the same time.

Definitive diagnosis is based on microscopic examination. Thymomas are classified based on predominant cell types (lymphocytic, epithelial, or spindle cell variants). As there is some association between histologic cell subtype and tumor invasiveness as well as prognosis, the World Health Organization classification groups thymomas based on cell type differences as types A, AB, B1, B2, B3, and C thymomas. Type C, or thymic carcinoma, is more aggressive and more likely than types A and AB thymomas to spread to other parts of the body and can also be more difficult to treat than other types of thymomas.

Imaging Imaging can determine if the cancer has spread to adjacent organs and other parts of the body. A chest X-ray can help determine the approximate size and location of the tumor and if it has spread to the lungs. A computerized tomography (CT) scan uses X-rays to create a three-dimensional picture of the inside of the body. It can show a detailed, cross-sectional view of the internal organs and identify any abnormalities or tumors. A magnetic resonance imaging (MRI) scan uses magnetic fields, not X-rays, to produce detailed images of the body. It may provide additional tumor information. Sometimes, a contrast substance (a special dye) is injected into a vein to provide a better picture. A positron-emission tomography (PET) scan uses radioactive sugar molecules as a tracer. When injected into the body, tumor cells absorb the radioactive sugar more quickly than normal cells and can be detected by the PET scan. Such information can help further delineate the extent of tumor spread even if it is not seen on X-rays or CT or MRI scan.

Prognostic Factors and Staging

The two major prognostic factors are invasiveness and completeness of surgical resection of the tumor. Long-term survival for patients with noninvasive thymoma is well over 90 percent after complete surgical resection. Patients who present with associated autoimmune diseases and those who are very young (children) may have a poorer prognosis, whereas young, healthy patients with no associated autoimmune diseases, ages thirty to forty, appear to have a better prognosis.

The Masaoka clinical staging system that is commonly used for thymoma is based on the extent of invasion into surrounding structures at the time of surgery. This staging system, which has important implications for prognosis, defines four stages according to whether the tumor has remained within the capsule (Stage I), broken through the capsule into adjacent fatty tissues (Stage II), invaded the surrounding structures within the mediastinum (Stage III), or spread beyond these areas and/or to distant sites (Stage IV).

Treatment Overview

Surgery An operation to remove a thymoma is called a thymectomy. The surgical approach typically involves a median sternotomy (incision through the breastbone), although sometimes a transcervical approach (horizontal incision across the lower portion of the neck) or, rarely, thoracotomy (incision through the lateral chest wall) are performed. If there is evidence of invasion by the tumor into adjacent tissues, such as adherent pericardium, pleura, or lung, these tissues should be resected along with the thymoma.

 Radiation The current state-of the-art-radiation therapy uses accurate CT treatment planning and advanced radiation delivery, targeting the tumor bed or residual tumor while sparing the surrounding critical organs. Some of these techniques include intensity-modulated radiation therapy (IMRT) and image-guided radiation therapy (IGRT) (see chapter 7, "What Happens in Radiation Therapy"). The

figure below shows a cross-sectional view of the chest. The tumor mass receives 100 percent of the radiation dose, while the surrounding organs receive substantially less radiation. Conventional doses, usually 4,500 to 5,400 cGy, can safely be given and are very effective. Treatment is given daily at 180 cGy to 200 cGy for five to six weeks. If there is visible disease left behind at the time of surgery, then higher doses (typically 6,000 cGy or more) will be required. Some long-term tumor control can be expected even for those patients with advanced tumors.

Patients receiving radiation treatment to the chest usually don't develop nausea and vomiting. The side effects of radiation therapy depend on the area treated and the total dose given. Fatigue during treatment is common in most patients. Some patients may also develop shortness of breath, skin irritation, chest tightness, fever, and coughing. Most of these

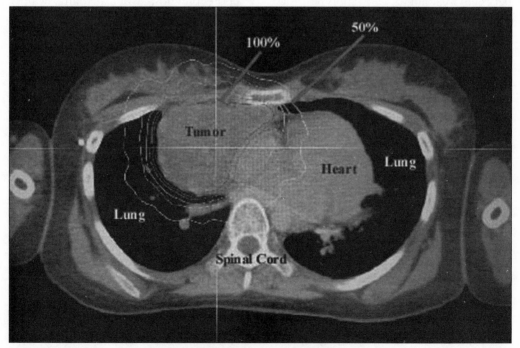

Intensity-modulated radiation therapy (IMRT) plan for thymoma

side effects will resolve after treatment is completed.

Chemotherapy Chemotherapy is constantly being evaluated in different combinations, and a variety of drugs have been found to be useful in patients who have advanced stages with residual or recurrent disease following surgery or radiation therapy. One study showed the combination of cisplatin (Platinol) + doxorubicin (Adriamycin) + vincristine (Onovin) + cyclophosphamide (Cytoxan) produced a 91 percent response rate (47 percent complete response). Similarly, in another trial, almost half of the patients treated with a four-drug combination of vincristine + cyclophosphamide + lomustine (CeeNU) + prednisone had complete responses. The three-drug combination of cisplatin + doxorubicin + cyclophosphamide has produced a 70 percent remission rate.

Depending on the chemotherapy regimen and the individual, side effects vary widely. Most patients may develop low blood cells, fatigue, or nausea and sometimes vomiting. Others may have hair loss, diarrhea, or secondary infection. A majority of these side effects usually go away once treatment is finished.

Treatment by Stage

Patients with thymoma should be managed by teams of oncologic surgeons, radiation oncologists, and medical oncologists. The treatment of thymoma depends on the size and location of the tumor, the stage, and the patient's overall health status.

▪ Stage I

The tumor is confined within the intact capsule (noninvasive thymoma).

Standard Treatment A noninvasive thymoma is treated by complete surgical removal of the tumor. Since the recurrence rate is very low (less than 5 percent), most patients don't need further treatment if the surgeon and the pathologist are certain that there is absolutely no evidence of spread through or beyond the capsule. In some circumstances, if follow-up cannot be done, radiation therapy may be considered after surgery to ensure the best chance for long-term tumor control.

For patients who present with myasthenia gravis, very specific and special precautions are needed before and after surgery because of the possibility of respiratory problems. Anesthesiologists experienced in this problem can dramatically reduce the rate of operative mortality; neurologists are also involved in the pre- and postoperative care of these patients.

▪ Stage II

The tumor penetrates the capsule into adjacent fatty tissues (invasive thymoma).

Standard Treatment When the tumor is discovered at surgery to have invaded the capsule and is completely removed, there is a difference of opinion about the role of adjuvant radiotherapy after surgery. Some physicians prefer to avoid the risks of additional radiation therapy. Others believe that radiation therapy is an essential part of treatment and can help prevent local recurrence, especially for tumors that are large or stuck to other organs. In general, most of these patients can achieve long-term tumor-free survival, especially when radiation therapy is used in addition to surgery.

▪ Stages III and IV

The tumor has penetrated the capsule and directly into surrounding organs (Stage III, or locally advanced invasive thymoma). The tumor has spread to elsewhere in the chest or body (Stage IV, or metastatic thymoma).

Advanced invasive malignant thymomas are also treated with surgical removal of the tumor if possible. Since the recurrence rate is very high, radiation therapy is given postoperatively whether or not the tumor has apparently been completely removed.

For locally advanced, invasive, or metastatic thymomas that are not resectable, radiation therapy alone or radiation therapy combined with chemotherapy may be considered. Other drug therapy includes the use of a steroid hormone such as prednisone or the somatostatin analogues octreotide (Sandostatin). These have caused regression of some thymomas that cannot be surgically removed and do not respond to radiation therapy.

Treatment Results

The approximate ten-year survival rates by stage are shown in the table below.

Overall Ten-Year Survival Rates for Patients with Thymoma

STAGE	TEN-YEAR SURVIVAL RATES
I	80–100%
II	50–90%
III	40–80%
IV	0–40%

Treatment Follow-Up

Follow-up care for thymoma depends on the stage of thymoma and the treatment received. Regular follow-up visits with the surgeon, radiation oncologist, and medical oncologist are required. Periodic physical examinations, blood tests, and CT scans are often needed, particularly for more advanced stages of thymoma— initially every two to three months during the first year and at longer intervals afterward—to detect recurrences. For those who have received radiation therapy, there may be a potential risk for a second cancer developing many years later in the treated area. Long-term follow up is important.

Recurrent Cancer

While the rate of recurrence is less than 5 percent for most noninvasive tumors, it is 20 to 50 percent for invasive malignancies. Local recurrences can be treated with repeat surgery, radiation therapy if not given previously, drug therapy with corticosteroids (e.g., prednisone), or chemotherapy. Chemotherapy regimens include the multiple drug combinations mentioned above. The five-year overall survival rate is reported to be 25 to 50 percent. However, long-term survival rates are typically poor.

The Most Important Questions You Can Ask

• How safe is surgery? Are there special precautions? What are the risks?
• Do I need radiation therapy? What are the side effects?
• Should chemotherapy be used? What are the side effects?
• If my tumor recurs, can I be treated again? Can I still be cured?

Reference

Huang A, Eng TY, Scarbrough TJ, Fuller CF, Thomas CR. "Mediastinal Tumors." In Perez and Brady's *Principles and Practice of Radiation Oncology,* 5th ed., edited by Edward C. Halperin, Carlos A. Perez, and Luthor W. Brady. Hagerstown, Md.: Lippincott Williams & Wilkins (November 2007).

Thyroid

Orlo H. Clark, M.D., Malin Dollinger, M.D., Thierry M. Jahan, M.D., and David M. Jablons, M.D.

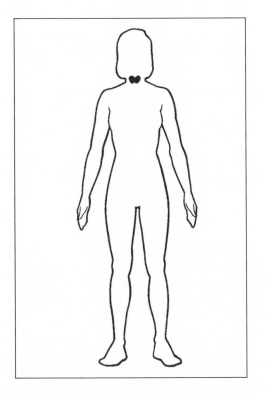

Cancer of the thyroid is the most common endocrine malignancy but is an uncommon cancer, making up only about 1 percent of invasive cancers. It is estimated that there will be about 25,000 new cases in the United States each year. It is the most rapidly increasing cancer in women. People with these malignancies are usually treated successfully.

Although invasive thyroid cancer is uncommon compared to benign thyroid nodules, doctors often have to diagnose and treat thyroid nodules, since about 4 percent of adults have clinically palpable thyroid nodules. Thyroid cancer commonly appears as a solitary nodule but can be present in multinodular goiters. Ultrasound examination and fine needle aspiration (FNA) biopsy have replaced radioiodine scanning for nodule evaluation.

Most cases occur between twenty-five and sixty-five years of age, and the age at diagnosis is one of the most important factors in predicting prognosis. Men under forty and women under fifty have significantly better survival rates than older patients.

Types About 80 percent of thyroid cancers are papillary, 10 percent follicular, 7 percent medullary, 3 percent Hurthle cell, and less than 1 percent anaplastic. About 5 percent of papillary thyroid cancers are familial, as are 2.5 percent of medullary thyroid cancers. Patients with well-differentiated tumors generally have a good prognosis. Those with undifferentiated or anaplastic tumors do not.

Papillary carcinomas are generally slow growing, with an 80 percent overall survival at fifteen years. Even when tumors spread to regional lymph nodes or the lungs, survival may be more than ten years. Tiny, clinically insignificant papillary carcinomas are found in about 10 percent of thyroid glands examined at routine autopsies.

Follicular carcinomas occur in patients who are about ten years older than those who get papillary carcinomas. Although these tumors are also usually slow growing, they behave somewhat more aggressively than papillary carcinomas and are more likely to spread to the lungs or bones. Hurthle cell cancers are generally included with follicular cancers but are more likely to be multifocal and involve regional lymph nodes. In contrast to follicular cancers, the metastases of Hurthle cell tumors also do not take up radioactive iodine.

Papillary, follicular, and Hurthle cell cancers make thyroglobulin, and medullary thyroid cancers make calcitonin. Undifferentiated (anaplastic) carcinomas usually occur in older patients, grow rapidly, behave aggressively, and respond poorly to treatment.

Medullary carcinomas secrete both calcitonin and carcinoembryonic antigen (CEA), which serve as tumor markers that help in diagnosis and follow-up. About 25 percent of patients with medullary thyroid cancer have familial disease. It occurs familially in multiple endocrine neoplasia (MEN) types 2A and 2B as well as in patients with only medullary thyroid cancers. Patients with MEN-2A have medullary thyroid cancer, hyperparathyroidism, and pheochromocytomas, whereas MEN-2B patients have a marfanoid habitus, mucosal neuromas, ganglioneuromatosis, and pheochromocytomas. Patients with familial disease can now be identified by testing for RET point mutations. All patients with medullary thyroid cancer should be tested for the RET proto-oncogene and if it is positive, a prophylactic total thyroidectomy is indicated before age six.

Unusual tumors that can arise in the thyroid gland include sarcomas, lymphomas, epidermoid carcinomas, and teratomas. The thyroid gland can also be a site of metastasis from other cancers, especially cancers of the lung, kidney, and breast and melanoma.

How It Spreads Papillary carcinomas spread to nearby lymph nodes and to adjacent tissues in the neck, with metastatic lesions to the lungs and bones. Follicular carcinomas invade locally but rarely invade lymph nodes. These tumors spread through the bloodstream, with metastasis occurring more often to lung and bone. Medullary carcinomas spread to lymph nodes and may invade blood vessels with metastases to the liver, lung, and bone. Anaplastic carcinomas usually extensively invade surrounding tissue, and distant metastases are present in about 50 percent at diagnosis.

What Causes It Papillary thyroid cancer is associated with radiation exposure and it is also slightly more common in areas of iodine excess. Follicular thyroid cancer, in contrast, occurs more frequently in areas of endemic goiter and iodine deficiency. Since the 1986 nuclear accident in Chernobyl, about 2,000 children have developed thyroid cancer.

Risk Factors

At Significantly Higher Risk

• Exposure to low-dose therapeutic radiation as used between 1920 and 1950 for enlarged lymph nodes in the neck, mastoiditis, tonsils, whooping cough, acne, enlarged thymus gland, keloids, and fungal infections dramatically increased the risk of thyroid cancer (as well as hyperparathyroidism, salivary tumors, and breast cancer). The incidence is directly related to the amount of radiation given and inversely related to the age of the person at the time of exposure. It generally takes ten to thirty years after radiation exposure for a thyroid tumor to develop, and about forty years for parathyroid tumors.

• Thyroid cancer will develop in about 13 percent of children treated with low-dose radiation to the head and neck. Four percent of thyroid cancer patients have a history of such radiation therapy. Factors for increasing the risk after radiation exposure include female sex, younger age at exposure, and a longer interval after radiation.

• Forty percent of patients with thyroid nodules and a history of exposure to external radiation have thyroid cancer.

• Papillary thyroid cancer is increased when other family members have thyroid cancer and in particular with familial polyposis and Cowden's disease.

• Risk for developing medullary carcinoma when a parent has familial disease (autosomal-dominant) is 50 percent.

At Slightly Higher Risk

• More follicular and anaplastic carcinomas develop in people from areas with endemic goiter. Eighty percent of patients with anaplastic carcinoma have a history of nodular goiter.

• Iodine deficiency is associated with follicular carcinoma, which is more common in iodine-deficient areas such as Germany.

• Iodine abundance is associated with papillary carcinoma, more common in areas using iodized salt (United States) or a high-iodine diet (Iceland and Japan).

• Patients with Hashimoto's thyroiditis have an increased incidence of thyroid lymphoma.

Screening

Physical examination is the best way to identify early-stage thyroid cancer. Two

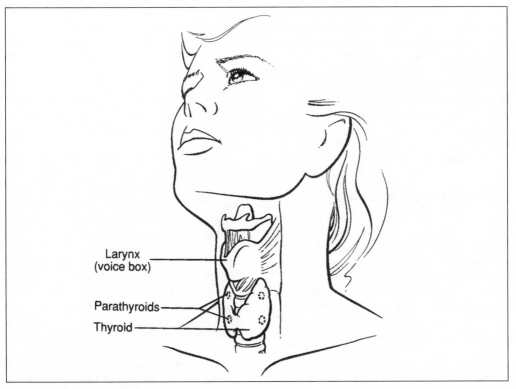

Thyroid and parathyroid glands

Larynx (voice box)

Parathyroids

Thyroid

groups of people need special screening procedures:

• Those with a family history of thyroid cancer or MEN-2. Serum thyroglobulin is useful in the former; RET point mutation testing, serum calcitonin, and CEA are important tumor marker in the latter.

• Those who have had radiation therapy to the neck who have no visible thyroid lumps should be examined at least every two years. A lump in the thyroid of these people generally suggests that the thyroid gland should be removed, since 40 percent will have cancer. To avoid surgery, small nodules are biopsied by FNA cytology under ultrasound guidance.

Patients with enlargement of the entire thyroid, without specific lumps or nodules, should have thyroid function tests and an ultrasound scan. If the thyroid is not overactive, thyroid hormone is given for six months. If a nodule grows, it is biopsied by FNA, and if suspicious or malignant, the thyroid lobe with the nodule is surgically removed. Otherwise, thyroid hormone treatment is continued. In general, the risk of cancer in an enlarged thyroid with many nodules is significantly lower than in a thyroid with a single nodule.

Common Signs and Symptoms

An enlargement of the entire thyroid or part of the thyroid or a lump or nodule is sometimes noticed while looking in the mirror while applying makeup or shaving. There may be enlarged lymph nodes in the neck that can be felt and there may be pain in the thyroid (especially with subacute thyroiditis or anaplastic carcinoma). Thyroid cancers also rarely occur at the base of the tongue in the pyramidal lobe or thyroglossal duct.

Pressure symptoms, including airway obstruction, hoarseness, and difficulty swallowing, develop in fewer than 5 percent of patients.

Diagnosis

The most cost-effective way to evaluate a patient with a thyroid nodule is to have a sensitive thyroid-stimulating hormone (TSH) blood test taken to document normal thyroid function and to perform a fine needle aspiration biopsy to determine whether the nodule is benign, suspicious, or malignant. Patients with benign nodules are sometimes treated with thyroid hormone to suppress TSH; about 50 percent of these nodules will shrink. Malignant and "suspicious" nodules should be removed, as should solitary "cold" nodules detected by radioactive iodine I-123 scanning. FNA is usually repeated after six months if the nodule has grown or has not decreased in size.

Physical Examination Careful examination of the thyroid gland and adjacent lymph nodes.

Blood and Other Tests Blood tests are not generally useful to determine if a thyroid nodule is benign or malignant.

• Serum thyroglobulin levels are elevated in most patients with well-differentiated thyroid cancers, but the level cannot indicate whether a lump is benign or malignant. The presence of thyroglobulin or an increasing thyroglobulin level after a total thyroidectomy (surgical removal of the thyroid gland) suggests recurrent or metastatic disease.

• An elevated serum calcitonin after total thyroidectomy, central neck node dissections, and a modified radical neck dissection for medullary carcinoma suggests persistent disease. Members of families of all patients with medullary carcinoma should also be screened for RET point mutations.

- CEA levels are useful in predicting prognosis in patients with medullary thyroid cancer.
- Blood tests, including serum alkaline phosphatase, are done to suggest metastatic disease in the liver or bone. An elevated alkaline phosphatase level when other liver function tests are normal could suggest either liver or bone metastasis, leading to liver and bone scans. Selective venous catheterization for serum calcitonin is sometimes helpful for locating metastatic tumors.

Imaging

- Images of the thyroid can be taken after injection of a radioactive iodine tracer or of technetium-99m. Because thyroid cancers do not generally take up as much iodine as normal thyroid tissue, a cancer appears as a cold area on a scan. Only 15 to 20 percent of cold, solitary nodules are cancer, however, and "warm" nodules are rarely malignant. Though used extensively in the past to classify nodules as hot or cold, thyroid scans are used less and less because more definitive information is provided by FNA and the greater sensitivity of ultrasound scanning.
- Ultrasound is a safe and simple way of determining if a mass is solid or filled with fluid (cystic). It can also detect multiple nodules where only one may be felt. High-resolution ultrasound can find nodules as small as 3 mm in diameter. It can suggest nodules that are more likely to be malignant with microcalcifications, small cysts, and irregular surfaces. Since it is noninvasive and sensitive, it is the most accurate way to measure and follow a suspicious nodule in a patient given thyroid hormone in an attempt to suppress the nodule. It may also be used to guide biopsy procedures and to identify regional lymphadenopathy.
- Standard X-rays, such as chest X-rays, to look for metastases. Spiral CT scans of the liver in patients with elevated calcitonin levels after total thyroidectomy.

- PET scanning is helpful for thyroglobulin-positive and radioiodine-negative patients and perhaps for patients with elevated calcitonin levels and negative scans.

Endoscopy and Biopsy

- Indirect or direct laryngoscopy if there is hoarseness, difficulty swallowing, coughing of blood (hemoptysis), or shortness of breath or if the patient has had a previous neck operation.
- Fine needle aspiration biopsy is the initial step in evaluating thyroid nodules in patients who do not have a history of exposure to low-dose radiation therapy, as it provides more information than any other diagnostic technique. It is over 95 percent accurate for benign lesions and about 99 percent accurate for malignancies. FNA is not recommended for those with a history of radiation therapy because 40 percent have cancer and most patients have multiple nodules, and the wrong nodule may be biopsied.

FNA helps select patients for surgery. Only about 3 percent of patients with benign findings on FNA will have thyroid cancer, so surgery can be postponed in these patients while the thyroid suppression trial is done. The TSH level must be mildly suppressed by the dosage of thyroid hormone. If the nodule decreases, thyroid hormone is continued. If the nodule does not change after six months, aspiration is often repeated. Malignant FNA results should lead to immediate surgery. About 20 percent of follicular or Hurthle cell neoplasms (suspicious biopsies) are cancer.

- Lesions larger than 2½ inches (6 cm), especially rapidly growing ones, are more likely to be lymphoma or anaplastic thyroid carcinoma. FNA may be satisfactory for diagnosis of anaplastic cancer, but the diagnosis of lymphoma of the thyroid usually requires a larger cutting needle or open biopsy.

Staging

The TNM staging system is useful but has not been uniformly accepted because it is more complex than other staging systems. Many clinicians use the DeGroot system, which classifies tumors according to Class 1 (confined to the thyroid), Class 2 (involving regional nodes), Class 3 (locally invasive), and Class 4 (distant metastases). Others use the AGES (age, grade, extent, and size) or AMES (age, metastases, extent, and size) classification to predict the tumor's aggressiveness. Staging systems have been designated for papillary and follicular carcinomas. Staging systems for medullary carcinoma and anaplastic carcinoma are now available. All patients with anaplastic cancer have Stage IV disease.

Treatment Overview

A number of factors affect the prognosis for papillary and follicular thyroid cancers. A better prognosis can be expected with a pure papillary carcinoma in younger patients (women under fifty and men under forty), a tumor smaller than $\frac{3}{4}$ inch (2 cm), small nodal metastases, female sex, and low-grade lesions.

A worse prognosis is related to age over forty, the degree of invasion (vascular and thyroid capsule) in follicular carcinoma, distant metastasis, a large tumor (especially over $1\frac{1}{2}$ inches [4 cm]), large nodular with extranodal invasion metastases, male sex, high-grade lesions (aneuploid), and tumors that cannot be completely resected.

Surgery The primary treatment of thyroid cancer is surgery, but there are some differences in opinion about the extent of thyroid resection required for the best prognosis. A near-total thyroidectomy—removing all thyroid tissue on one side and all but $\frac{1}{2}$ inch (1 cm) on the other—offers the best chance for cure, especially if the cancer is in several places within the gland. The removal of all functioning thyroid tissue also makes it possible to scan for metastatic disease with radioactive iodine and to use serum thyroglobulin values to detect persistent disease.

One of the risks of a total thyroidectomy is the inadvertent removal or devascularization of the parathyroid glands, which are situated, two on each side, at the edge of the thyroid. During thyroidectomy, an attempt is always made to leave all four parathyroid glands in place. At times, one cannot preserve a parathyroid gland and it should be auto-transplanted. The surgeon must maintain an adequate supply of blood to the parathyroid glands to prevent the symptoms and signs of hypoparathyroidism or parathyroid hormone deficiency. Thyroid operations also have some risk of damage to the nerves in the neck that supply the larynx (voice box).

Removing one side of the thyroid (called a lobectomy) has fewer complications because only one nerve and two parathyroids are at risk. It is the treatment of choice for all nodules that might be cancer and is useful in selected cases with small papillary cancers or follicular cancers with only minimal invasion.

The surgeon may select a procedure depending on the type of thyroid cancer as well as the size of the nodule and his or her own experience, but at least a total lobectomy on the side of the tumor is indicated. The National Cooperative Cancer Network has guidelines for treatment.

Radioactive Iodine Therapy It has been standard practice in many cancer treatment centers to give radioactive iodine after surgery. Such treatment generally requires that the patient has had a total or near-total thyroidectomy. When the thyroid scan demonstrates that the tumor takes up iodine, as occurs in about two-thirds of cases, there is general agreement that radioactive ablation therapy is useful. For low-risk patients with occult papillary thyroid cancers or minimally invasive follicular cancers, radioiodine ablation is not usually necessary.

Ablation therapy with I-131 has side effects, including temporary bone marrow suppression (at high doses), inflammation of salivary glands, nausea and vomiting, decreased sperm count, scarring of the lung when pulmonary metastases are present, pain in areas of metastasis, and, rarely, leukemia.

The radioactive iodine is given when the patient is hypothyroid in preparation for the scan and is receiving a low-iodine diet. A serum thyroglobulin level should also be obtained, since persistent disease is present when it is elevated. A pregnancy test should be done for all patients who are of childbearing potential. After scanning or treatment, patients are again placed on thyroid hormone in order to prevent hypothyroidism and to suppress the TSH levels, since high TSH levels might stimulate residual tumor cells to grow. Some patients will require re-treatment with radioactive iodine if the serum thyroglobulin level again becomes elevated or recurrent disease becomes evident. Ultrasound, MRI, or CT scanning is recommended after thyroidectomy for high-risk patients who are scan-negative and thyroglobulin-positive or -negative. Recombinant TSH is also used for scanning patients and monitoring blood thyroglobulin levels in patients with thyroid cancer after thyroidectomy. Although it is expensive, patients prefer recombinant TSH, since it avoids the symptoms of hypothyroidism.

Treatment by Type and Stage
Papillary Thyroid Carcinoma
■ Stage I
The tumor is confined to the thyroid gland. If it is on one side, it is considered Stage IA. If it is on both sides or there is more than one lump, it is Stage IB.

Standard Treatment The standard surgical procedure is removal of one side of the thyroid (lobectomy), but about 20 percent of patients will have a recurrence. Preoperative ultrasonography is encouraged and all enlarged or abnormal lymph nodes are also removed. Thyroid hormone is then given to suppress the thyroid-stimulating hormone (TSH) from the pituitary gland, which decreases the chance of recurrence.

Other options are a near-total or total thyroidectomy. The rationale for this is that there is an increased chance of multiple tumors in both lobes and any tumor left behind could grow, metastasize, or change into the highly malignant (anaplastic) form. More important, scanning for metastases is possible once the thyroid is removed, and thyroglobulin levels are more sensitive for detecting recurrent or persistent disease.

Five-Year Survival Over 95 percent

■ Stage II
Cancer has spread to lymph nodes (IIA if to nodes on one side, IIB if to both sides or to the mediastinal nodes—those in the center of the upper chest).

Standard Treatment The treatment is virtually identical to that for Stage I. The only difference between the two stages is the spread to lymph nodes. Removal of these metastases, usually by a functional or modified radical neck dissection preserving all motor nerves, reduces the chance of local recurrence and minimally improves survival. Total thyroidectomy allows persistent disease to be detected with radioiodine scanning and thyroglobulin monitoring and to be treated.

Five-Year Survival Over 95 percent

■ *Stage III*

The tumor has invaded the tissues of the neck.

Standard Treatment Total thyroidectomy, plus removal of all apparent areas of cancer that have spread to the neck (debulking). After surgery, radioactive iodine should be given if the tumor takes up this isotope. If the uptake is minimal or absent, external-beam radiation may be given, especially for high-risk patients.

Five-Year Survival 60 percent

■ *Stage IV*

There are distant metastases, usually to the lungs, bone, and distant lymph nodes.

Standard Treatment Patients who have small distant lymph node metastases are sometimes cured by radioactive iodine after a total thyroidectomy. Larger nodes should be removed surgically and then radioactive iodine used to treat micrometastases. Patients with radioiodine uptake in the lungs but no evidence of metastases in a chest X-ray can be "cured" in about 70 percent of cases, and about 95 percent are alive at ten years. Radioiodine scan–negative pulmonary metastases are more aggressive.

Solitary lung or bone metastases should be surgically removed, if possible. A therapeutic dose of radioactive iodine is then given; if there is no uptake, external-beam radiation therapy is given to the area involved. Patients with elevated thyroglobulin levels who are radioactive iodine scan–negative would probably benefit from a therapeutic dose of I-131, since in about 33 percent of such patients, thyroglobulin levels become undetectable. Taking thyroid hormone to suppress TSH appears to be effective in decreasing tumor recurrence.

Chemotherapy has produced occasional long-term remission. New trials with antiangiogenesis and anti–tyrosine kinase agents are available.

Ten-Year Survival Less than 20 percent

Follicular Thyroid Carcinoma

■ *Stage I*

The tumor is localized to the thyroid gland (IA if on one side, IB if on both sides or there are multiple lesions). Most follicular cancers are solitary.

Standard Treatment Patients are usually treated by a total thyroid lobectomy. When cancer is present, either a total or near-total thyroidectomy should be done. In patients with minimally invasive follicular cancers and only minimal invasion, lobectomy alone is usually sufficient. Follicular cancers are associated with a higher risk of metastasis to lung and bone. One disadvantage of leaving a remnant of thyroid is the difficulty in subsequent scanning with radioactive iodine (I-131). The residual thyroid rather than the metastasis will take up the isotope.

Sometimes, I-131 is used to eliminate any remaining normal thyroid tissue or thyroid tumor. Similarly, when therapeutic doses of I-131 are planned, all or almost all of the thyroid gland should be removed first.

Less extensive operations such as lobectomy have fewer complications, but about 10 percent of patients will develop a recurrence. Metastatic disease also cannot be treated with I-131 until the normal thyroid tissue has been removed.

As with papillary carcinoma, enlarged lymph nodes discovered at surgery, although less frequently involved, should be removed. In patients who have a limited surgical procedure (lobectomy), thyroid hormone is usually recommended postoperatively to suppress TSH and decrease the chance of recurrence.

Five-Year Survival 70 to 90 percent

Stage II

The tumor has spread to lymph nodes (IIA if to nodes on one side, IIB if to both sides or to the mediastinal nodes—those in the center of the chest).

Standard Treatment Treatment is similar to that for Stage I. The only difference is the involvement of nearby lymph nodes, which increases local recurrence but only minimally adversely influences survival.

Options include total or near-total thyroidectomy and lobectomy. The same considerations about hypoparathyroidism and distant metastases apply.

Five-Year Survival 50 to 70 percent

Stage III

The tumor invades the tissues of the neck (widely invasive follicular cancer).

Standard Treatment Total thyroidectomy and removal of local areas of tumor spread (debulking). If the tumor takes up radioactive iodine (I-131), the isotope is given in an attempt to treat all potential residual disease. When the I-131 uptake is low, external-beam radiotherapy is given to the neck.

Five-Year Survival 20 to 60 percent (worse if blood vessels are invaded)

Stage IV

There are distant metastases, usually to the lungs and bone.

Standard Treatment Treatment is usually not curative but may produce significant palliation.

The treatment options are similar to those for Stage IV papillary thyroid cancer and include therapeutic doses of radioactive iodine, after total or near-total thyroidectomy, if the metastases take up this isotope, and external-beam radiotherapy for localized lesions that do not respond to radioactive iodine. Tumors

in many patients can be suppressed with thyroid hormone. Investigative chemotherapy protocois are being developed for patients with metastatic disease that does not respond to these treatment programs.

Five-Year Survival 10 to 20 percent

Medullary Thyroid Carcinoma

In the sporadic form, the tumor is usually on only one side of the thyroid. In the inherited (familial) form, the tumor is almost always on both sides. It is usually a hard mass situated in the lateral portion of the thyroid lobe at the level of the cricoid cartilage.

Prognosis depends upon the size of the primary tumor, the involvement of nearby lymph nodes, whether the tumor can be completely removed, and whether there are distant metastases.

Standard Treatment A total thyroidectomy is done, with a thorough bilateral central neck clean out, meaning that all fibro-fatty and lymphoid tissue is removed between the carotid arteries. When the primary cancer is ½ inch (1.5 cm) or larger, an ipsilateral (same side) prophylactic modified neck dissection is recommended.

If the tumor is confined to the thyroid gland, almost all patients will be cured. If the blood calcitonin remains slightly increased after total thyroidectomy, central neck dissection, ipsilateral neck dissection, or a contralateral neck dissection should be done. In general, there is no benefit to radioactive iodine therapy, radiotherapy, or chemotherapy, although occasional responses to these treatments are seen in metastatic disease.

Treatment for metastatic disease has generally been unsatisfactory, pointing up the need for detection and diagnosis while the tumor is confined to the thyroid and can be cured surgically. Patients with metastatic disease benefit from palliative surgery. They may have significant symptoms, especially severe diarrhea and rarely Cushing's syndrome, related to the hormone produced by the tumor. Symptoms usually respond to treatment with somatostatin (octreotide [Sandostatin]) or nutmeg.

Five-Year Survival 40 to 95 percent. Survival is best in familial medullary thyroid cancer without other aspects of MEN, and intermediate for sporadic and for MEN-2A. It is worse for patients with MEN-2B—that is, in patients with a marfanoid habitus, mucosal neuromas, pheochromocytomas, and ganglioneuromatosis.

Anaplastic Thyroid Carcinoma

There are large cell spindle and small cell types. Both grow rapidly and often extend beyond the thyroid. Small cell tumors should be carefully analyzed to be sure they are not lymphomas or medullary thyroid cancers.

Standard Treatment Patients with this tumor have an extremely poor prognosis, most patients not surviving even six months after diagnosis.

After the diagnosis is established by FNA or a cutting needle biopsy, aggressive radiation therapy and chemotherapy is recommended for three weeks. No treatment is given for the following two weeks and then a thyroidectomy is performed. Radiation and chemotherapy are resumed two weeks after the operation. This treatment is usually not curative, but it appears to offer the best palliation and the best hope for survival.

Five-Year Survival About 2 percent, the average survival being less than six months

Primary Lymphoma of the Thyroid

Standard Treatment These patients have a rapidly enlarging thyroid mass, often with pressure symptoms. At least two-thirds have thyroiditis (Hashimoto's

thyroiditis). The prognosis depends on the lymphoma subtype as well as on the stage. Most are B cell lymphomas.

Treatment is similar to that for any B cell lymphoma arising outside lymph nodes. Since most patients have diffuse lymphomas, they tend to be treated after diagnosis by open biopsy with aggressive third-generation combination chemotherapy programs (see the chapter "Lymphomas: Non-Hodgkin's"). Radiation therapy is also used for recurrent or persistent disease.

Treatment Follow-Up

For well-differentiated thyroid cancers (papillary and follicular carcinomas):

• Periodic physical examination, especially of the thyroid and cervical lymph nodes
• Serologic marker (thyroglobulin)
• Scanning with radioactive iodine and treatment with 30 mCi (millicuries) for low-risk patients or 100 mCi for high-risk patients if they have had a total or near-total parathyroidectomy
• Periodic ultrasound, MRI, or CT examinations of the neck and mediastinum in high-risk patients to identify recurrence in the thyroid area or mediastinum or lymph node metastases
• Chest X-ray to detect metastases

For medullary thyroid cancer:

• Serum calcitonin level and CEA level every six months
• Physical examination, emphasizing the thyroid, although calcitonin level is more accurate than physical examination for following persistent disease
• Ultrasound of the neck, and CT or MRI scan of the neck and mediastinum
• Chest X-ray every six months until stable
• RET point mutation testing of all patients with medullary thyroid cancers

and of all first-degree (close) relatives of RET-positive patients

Recurrent and Metastatic Disease

When thyroid carcinoma is recurrent or metastatic and is also widespread or cannot be removed, it is treated with radioactive iodine. If it does not take up radioactive iodine, it should be treated with radiation therapy.

• For the papillary and follicular types, an effort is made to scan for metastatic disease with radioactive iodine. After the thyroid gland is removed and thyroid hormone is stopped for an appropriate time, a tracer dose of radioactive iodine is given. If hot spots appear at sites outside the thyroid area, suggesting metastases, a therapeutic dose of radioactive iodine is given. Radioactive iodine effectively irradiates microscopic metastases. Larger metastases should be removed surgically before radioactive iodine is given. If the thyroglobulin level is detectable or elevated after a total thyroidectomy, residual tumor is present.

• External-beam radiation is used in patients whose tumors do not take up radioactive iodine or are undifferentiated.

• Some patients respond to chemotherapy, with regimens containing doxorubicin (Adriamycin) having the highest response rate. The combination of cisplatin (Platinol) and doxorubicin may produce some complete and partial remissions in metastatic thyroid cancer. In a few cases, the complete responders survived more than two years. Another combination (doxorubicin + bleomycin [Blenoxane] + vincristine [Oncovin] + melphalan [Alkeran]) was reported to show responses in about one-third of patients. Paclitaxel (Taxol) has been used in some protocols.

• In patients with anaplastic thyroid cancer, chemotherapy is occasionally effective and is usually combined with external-beam radiation.

• Patients with metastatic thyroid carcinoma, especially those unsuitable for or unresponsive to radioactive iodine, should be considered for entry into clinical trials in the hope of finding a more effective chemotherapy program. New trials became available in 2006 for patients with various types of thyroid cancer.

The Most Important Questions You Can Ask

• How extensive should my surgery be?

• What is the chance of complications of surgery, especially damage to the parathyroid glands and the risk of nerve malfunction?

• Why do I need to take thyroid hormone after surgery?

• Will I need radioactive iodine?

• Should my family members be examined?

• What follow-up do I need?

• What is my chance of cure, and when can you be sure?

Trophoblastic Disease

Jeffrey L. Stern, M.D.

■ ■ ■ ■

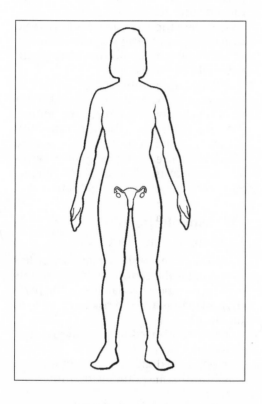

Gestational trophoblastic diseases (GTD) are disorders of abnormal growth of the placenta. They are always associated with a pregnancy. A key to understanding and managing patients with GTD is human chorionic gonadotropin (HCG), a protein hormone produced by the placenta. It can be detected in the blood and urine and is an extremely sensitive indicator for GTD. It is measured often during both therapy and follow-up to evaluate the response to treatment and to detect recurrent disease.

Types There are four types of gestational trophoblastic disease: hydatidiform mole (also called a molar pregnancy), invasive mole (chorioadenoma destruens), gestational choriocarcinoma, and placental site trophoblastic tumor. It is important to understand why the general term *gestational trophoblastic disease (GTD)* and the specific diseases hydatidiform mole, invasive mole, gestational choriocarcinoma, and placental site trophoblastic tumor (PST) coexist. The specific diagnosis requires biopsy material from the disease site for microscopic examination; however, the disease site(s) may be difficult to reach without risk (e.g., hemorrhage or loss of fertility). Furthermore, a biopsy is usually not required because human chorionic gonadotropin is a reliable indicator of disease presence and status. Lastly, management of the disease is based on the stage and not the histologic type.

Trophoblastic disease confined to the uterus regardless of cell type is known as nonmetastatic trophoblastic disease (NMTD).

• When there is evidence of metastatic disease, it is called metastatic trophoblastic disease (MTD).

• A hydatidiform mole results from an abnormal embryo. There are two types of hydatidiform moles, complete and incomplete (partial). A complete mole usually has little or no fetal development and a large overgrowth of the placenta in the form of cysts (hydatids). The diagnosis of a complete hydatidiform mole is usually made during the first half of a pregnancy. A variety of clinical conditions may be confused with a molar pregnancy, but these can usually be distinguished on the basis of medical history, a physical exam, and an ultrasound examination.

In contrast, a partial mole is associated with a fetus, placental tissue, umbilical cord, and membranes. It occurs much less frequently than a complete mole. The fetus usually dies within nine weeks after the last menstrual period, although occasionally it can survive to term.

Hydatidiform moles are sometimes associated with multiple ovarian cysts (theca-lutein cysts), high HCG titers, and pregnancy-induced hypertension. There is also the risk that the abnormal placental tissue will persist in the uterus or elsewhere in the body. These risks are greater for women with complete moles (10 to 20 percent) than for those with partial moles (5 to 10 percent).

• An invasive mole (chorioadenoma destruens) is defined as a hydatidiform mole that persists and invades the uterine wall. It develops in 10 to 20 percent of all molar pregnancies.

• Gestational choriocarcinoma (also known simply as choriocarcinoma) is a cancer composed of only the cells that cover the placenta (trophoblastic cells). It differs from an invasive mole, which is made up of all the placental tissues. Furthermore, choriocarcinoma can follow any type of pregnancy, but an invasive mole can only follow a hydatidiform mole. About 50 percent of all cases of gestational choriocarcinoma follow a hydatidiform mole, 25 percent follow a spontaneous abortion or tubal pregnancy, and 25 percent follow a normal term pregnancy. Choriocarcinoma follows a normal term pregnancy in 1 in 40,000 pregnancies. GTD after a normal pregnancy is always a choriocarcinoma, never a hydatidiform mole or an invasive mole.

• Prenatal-site trophoblastic tumor (PSTT) is a rare form of GTD that can develop after a normal pregnancy or an abortion. Some consider it a subtype of gestational choriocarcinoma. PSTT is found in the place where the placenta attaches to the uterus. It is generally more resistant to chemotherapy than are other types of GTD.

What Causes It A hydatidiform mole or an invasive mole occurs when a single sperm fertilizes an egg without a nucleus. The chromosomes from the sperm duplicate, resulting in an abnormal embryo that has only male genetic material. A mole can also occur when two sperm fertilize a single egg without a nucleus. A mole develops from the abnormally fertilized egg and is characterized by a lack of a normal fetus and by many small fluid-filled cysts.

The cause of gestational choriocarcinoma is uncertain. It can arise from a normal pregnancy, a miscarriage, or a tubal pregnancy, or from either type of mole.

How It Spreads Hydatidiform moles generally stay confined to the uterus. When they begin to invade the wall of the uterus, they are called invasive moles.

An invasive mole can penetrate the full thickness of the uterine wall and rupture, resulting in severe internal or vaginal bleeding. Invasive moles can also spread to other organs, most commonly to the vagina and the lung. This may be confusing, since women with proven invasive moles who have metastases may also have choriocarcinoma. Although an invasive mole is more locally aggressive than a noninvasive mole, it is no more likely to develop into choriocarcinoma.

Choriocarcinoma can spread virtually anywhere in the body but most commonly spreads to the lung, the lower genital tract (cervix, vagina, and vulva), the brain, liver, and kidney, and the gastrointestinal tract.

Risk Factors

Gestational trophoblastic disease occurs only in women of reproductive age. An invasive mole develops in 10 to 20 percent of all complete moles and 5 to 10 percent of all partial moles. Choriocarcinoma develops in 3 percent of complete moles but rarely in partial moles.

At Significantly Higher Risk Risks for the development of a hydatidiform mole, an invasive mole, or gestational choriocarcinoma include

- a prior mole (30 times the risk),
- maternal age greater than forty years (5 times) or less than twenty years (1.5 times), and
- a previous spontaneous abortion (twice the risk).

At Slightly Lower Risk Eating a diet high in vitamin A and having one or more children without having a previous spontaneous abortion is statistically correlated with a lower-than-average risk of developing a complete mole.

At Risk for Developing an Invasive Mole or Gestational Choriocarcinoma For women with a molar pregnancy, there are several risk factors associated with the subsequent development of an invasive mole or choriocarcinoma. These include delayed hemorrhage after removal of the mole by a D&C (dilation and curettage), large ovarian (theca-lutein) cysts, acute respiratory failure at the time of D&C, a large uterus before the D&C, a serum HCG level greater than 40,000 mIU/ml, a history of a previous mole, and maternal age over forty.

Screening

Gestational trophoblastic disease is not routinely screened for, since it is so rare. An ultrasound examination early in any subsequent pregnancy to document a normal pregnancy is usually performed for women with prior GTD.

Common Signs and Symptoms

A molar pregnancy is often associated with absence of menses, symptoms of pregnancy, bleeding in the first half of a pregnancy, pain in the lower abdomen, high blood pressure before twenty-four weeks of pregnancy (10 percent of all cases), excessive nausea or vomiting, a uterus larger than normal for gestational age (50 percent of all cases), an absent fetal heartbeat, and the expulsion of cysts.

Complications associated with a molar pregnancy include anemia because of blood loss, severe high blood pressure, symptoms similar to an overactive thyroid gland, heart failure, hemorrhage, infection, and acute respiratory failure.

Eighty to 90 percent of women with partial moles have abnormal uterine bleeding, the signs and symptoms of a spontaneous abortion, and a smaller than expected uterus for gestational age of the pregnancy.

The most common symptoms of choriocarcinoma are lack of menstrual period, symptoms of pregnancy, abnormal vaginal bleeding, and pelvic pain. Women with liver metastases may have bleeding within the abdomen because of a ruptured liver. Those with metastases to the lung may have a dry cough (occasionally with blood), chest pain, or shortness of breath. Spread to the intestinal tract may also be associated with chronic blood loss and anemia or with massive hemorrhage. Brain metastases are often associated with symptoms that suggest a brain tumor or stroke.

Diagnosis

The diagnosis of a mole is usually suspected after an ultrasound examination of the uterus, but absolute diagnosis is made by examining the cysts under a microscope. A serum HCG level far in excess of that of a normal pregnancy would support the diagnosis of a hydatidiform mole.

An invasive mole is seldom diagnosed definitively without a hysterectomy. The diagnosis is usually made after a hydatidiform mole is removed, the HCG titer remains persistently elevated, and there is no evidence of metastases. It is more properly referred to as nonmetastatic (confined to the uterus) trophoblastic disease (NMTD).

Confirmation of choriocarcinoma by removing cells for pathological analysis (biopsy) may be hazardous, since this tumor bleeds easily. Metastasis and an elevated HCG level in a recently pregnant woman indicate choriocarcinoma. Metastasis and an elevated HCG level following a hydatidiform mole can either be choriocarcinoma or an invasive mole. Since a biopsy is not usually done because of the risks, women with postmolar metastases are referred to as having metastatic trophoblastic disease (MTD).

Physical Examination Particular attention is given to the pelvis, the abdomen (specifically the liver), the lungs, and the brain.

Blood and Other Tests
- Complete blood count.
- Tests for liver and kidney function.
- Serum beta HCG.

Imaging Studies in the evaluation of a hydatidiform mole include

- pelvic ultrasound,
- chest X-ray, and
- tests for lung function (occasionally).

Imaging for persistent gestational trophoblastic disease or choriocarcinoma includes a CT scan of the head/chest/abdomen/pelvis or a PET scan.

Staging

Nonmetastatic trophoblastic disease is defined as having no disease outside the uterus and has a survival rate of 100 percent. Metastatic trophoblastic disease is further divided into low risk (good prognosis) and high risk (poor prognosis) based on several factors. Most physicians use the WHO (World Health Organization) scoring system of prognostic factors and not the FIGO (International Federation of Gynecology and Obstetrics) staging system to determine which combination chemotherapy protocol to use. A total score of less than 8 is defined as low risk, 8 to 12 is medium risk, and greater than 12 is high risk for treatment failure.

Treatment Overview

An important aspect of treating women with GTD is to start therapy as quickly as possible after the diagnosis is made. Chemotherapy is given until the serum HCG titer returns to normal.

Depending on the extent of the disease, most physicians give one to three cycles of chemotherapy following the first normal HCG level, then follow the titers monthly for six to twenty-four months after treatment. All women are advised to use oral contraceptives to prevent pregnancy for one to two years after therapy.

Treatment by Type and Stage

Hydatidiform Mole (Molar Pregnancy)

Standard Treatment As soon as the diagnosis is made, the molar tissue is removed from the uterus by a D&C in the operating room under anesthesia. For women who have completed childbearing, the removal of the uterus (hysterectomy) is also an option.

RH immune globulin is given to women with Rh-negative blood to prevent Rh sensitization. In about one-third

WHO Scoring System

PROGNOSTIC FACTOR	SCORE
Age	
Less than 39	0
Greater than 39	1
Antecedent Pregnancy	
Hydatidiform mole	0
Abortion	1
Term	2
Interval Between End of Antecedent Pregnancy and Start of Chemotherapy	
< 4 months	0
4–6 months	1
7–12 months	2
> 12 months	4
HCG (IU/ml)	
<1,000	0
1,000–10,000	1
10,000–100,000	2
>100,000	4
ABO Groups (Female x Male)	
O x A or A x O	1
B or AB	2
Largest Tumor, Including Uterine	
3.5 cm	1
>5 cm	2
Site of Metastases	
Spleen, kidney	1
Gastrointestinal tract or liver	2
Brain	4
Number of Metastases Identified	
1–4	1
4–8	2

of women with a molar pregnancy, there may be enlargement of one or both ovaries because of the high levels of HCG resulting in the development of multiple ovarian cysts (theca-lutein). Occasionally, the cysts can rupture, bleed, or become infected. In the vast majority of cases, these cysts do not need to be removed because they resolve with time, although sometimes it can take several weeks or months for them to disappear completely.

After the D&C, the HCG level is followed weekly until negative. Chemotherapy is usually given if (1) the serum HCG rises for two successive weeks or plateaus for three weeks (in the vast majority of women with persistent GTD, the HCG level plateaus or rises by seven weeks after the D&C), (2) the serum HCG rises again after reaching a normal level, or (3) there is a hemorrhage not related to an incomplete D&C.

Prior to giving chemotherapy, an evaluation for the presence of metastases is performed to determine whether or not it is NMTD or MTD.

Nonmetastatic Trophoblastic Disease

Nonmetastatic disease may be either an invasive mole or choriocarcinoma and is defined as having no disease outside the uterus with an abnormal HCG level.

Standard Treatment Chemotherapy for an invasive mole and non-metastatic choriocarcinoma is the same. All cases of NMTD are considered curable, even if there is extensive local disease. If chemotherapy fails, a hysterectomy may be recommended.

The HCG level is obtained weekly during and after treatment, until the titer is negative three weeks in a row.

The standard treatment is with a single chemotherapeutic drug. Most physicians use methotrexate (Mexate, Amethopterin, Folex) if the liver function tests are normal or dactinomycin (Actinomycin D, Cosmegen) if they are not. There are several different ways methotrexate may be used. Methotrexate may be given daily, either by injection into a muscle or intravenously, for five days. This schedule is repeated every fourteen days until the HCG level returns to normal. Three to four courses are usually required. Methotrexate may also be given on days 1, 3, 5, and 7, with leucovorin given on days 2, 4, 6, and 8. When used in this fashion, only one course of treatment is given (with a cure rate of around 80 percent). A second or third course is given only if the HCG titer does not return to normal.

Dactinomycin is usually given intravenously for five consecutive days and repeated every two weeks. Dactinomycin can also be given in various doses on a single day and be repeated every one or two weeks. Dactinomycin may also be given if treatment with methotrexate fails to bring about normalization of the HCG level (titer remission).

Women who fail to respond to methotrexate and dactinomycin are treated with multiple-agent chemotherapy as discussed below.

Five-Year Survival 100 percent for both invasive mole and nonmetastatic choriocarcinoma.

Low-Risk Metastatic Trophoblastic Disease

Metastatic trophoblastic disease is considered low risk when it is diagnosed less than four months after the onset of the pregnancy, when the HCG titer is less than 40,000 mIU/ml, when there are no liver or brain metastases, and when there has been no previous treatment with chemotherapy. A total WHO score of less than 8 is also considered low risk.

Standard Treatment Therapy for women with low-risk MTD may be with a single chemotherapeutic drug similar to treatment for nonmetastatic disease. However, most physicians use single-agent chemotherapy only for women who have an abnormal postmolar pregnancy HCG titer. All other cases with good prognostic features are treated with MAC or MA, a combination of methotrexate

(Mexate) + dactinomycin (Actinomycin D, Cosmegen) with or without cyclophosphamide (Cytoxan).

Those who fail chemotherapy with methotrexate alone (approximately 20 percent) are then treated with dactinomycin or with MAC. MAC is given intravenously for five consecutive days every two weeks until the HCG titer returns to normal. Often an additional course is given after the HCG titer reaches normal.

Five-Year Survival 97 to 100 percent

High-Risk Metastatic Trophoblastic Disease

Metastatic choriocarcinoma is considered high risk when it is diagnosed more than four months after the onset of pregnancy, when it is associated with a serum HCG titer greater than 40,000 mIU/ml, where there is liver or brain metastases, when there is a history of chemotherapy, when it occurs after a full-term pregnancy, or when the WHO score is greater than 8.

Standard Treatment High-risk metastatic disease should be treated as soon as possible with aggressive chemotherapy. Women with brain or liver metastases are usually treated immediately with radiation therapy to the brain or liver.

Standard chemotherapy includes the drugs etoposide (Etopophos), methotrexate (Mexate, Amethopterin, Folex), dactinomycin (Actinomycin D, Cosmegen), vincristine (Oncovin), and cyclophosphamide (Cytoxan). Another regimen, known as EMA-CE (cisplatin [Platinol] and etoposide are substituted for vincristine and cyclophosphamide), is also commonly used.

Five-Year Survival 80 percent

Treatment Follow-Up

A gynecologic examination and careful physical examination is done one week after the D&C for NMTD. Regular measurements of the serum HCG levels are the most important part of the follow-up surveillance for GTD. The levels are monitored weekly until normal. Usually, the level progressively declines to normal within fourteen weeks after the D&C for NMTD. After normalization of the titers, the HCG is followed monthly for six to twelve months for NMTD; for MTD, it is followed monthly for two to three years. Contraception (preferably oral contraceptives) should be used until pregnancy is permitted.

Pregnancy After Treatment for GTD Most physicians recommend avoiding pregnancy for the first year after GTD is treated. This will prevent any confusion about the interpretation of subsequent elevated HCG levels. Women with a history of GTD have a higher incidence of subsequent GTD. An ultrasound, an HCG titer, and a chest X-ray are usually obtained in subsequent pregnancies to check for GTD.

Side effects from chemotherapy for GTD may affect future pregnancies. There may be a slightly higher infertility rate, a lower chance for a successful term pregnancy, or a higher rate of spontaneous abortion. There does not appear to be an increased rate of birth defects in subsequent pregnancies.

Recurrent GTD

Recurrent GTD after therapy occurs in 2.5 percent of women with nonmetastatic disease, 3.7 percent of women with low-risk metastatic disease, and 13 percent of women with high-risk metastatic disease. Almost all recurrences take place within thirty-six months of remission, with 85 percent before eighteen months. Sometimes a recurrence can appear after an intervening normal pregnancy.

Recurrent disease is usually treated with chemotherapy or occasionally surgery if the metastases are isolated. Cure rates vary, depending on the site of metastases.

The Most Important Questions You Can Ask

• What type of gestational trophoblastic disease do I have, and what is its extent?

• What is the likelihood of cure?

• What type of chemotherapy is recommended?

• What are my prospects of having a normal pregnancy in the future?

• Will a specialist in gynecologic oncology be involved in my care?

Uterus: Endometrial Carcinoma

Jeffrey L. Stern, M.D.

■ ■ ■ ■

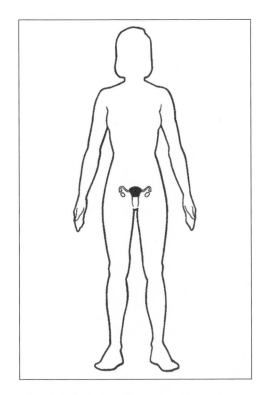

Endometrial cancer—carcinoma of the lining of the uterus—is the most common gynecologic malignancy and accounts for about 13 percent of all malignancies occurring in women. There are about 34,000 cases of endometrial cancer diagnosed in the United States each year, but encouragingly, there has been a significant decrease in the number of women who develop endometrial cancer each year since 1975.

Similarly, the death rate from endometrial cancer has steadily declined since 1950, falling more than 65 percent.

Since this cancer is usually diagnosed at an early stage, the cure rate is high, with an overall five-year survival rate of 85 percent.

Types All endometrial carcinomas arise from the glands of the lining of the uterus. Adenocarcinomas account for 75 percent of all endometrial carcinomas. Endometrial adenocarcinomas that contain benign or malignant squamous cells are known as adenocanthomas and adenosquamous carcinomas respectively and account for 30 percent of endometrial cancers.

The remaining types of endometrial carcinomas have a poorer prognosis. Three percent are clear cell carcinomas, and about 1 percent are papillary serous carcinomas.

Uterine sarcoma is another kind of uterine malignancy (see the chapter "Uterus: Uterine Sarcomas").

How It Spreads Endometrial carcinoma arises in the lining of the uterus and eventually invades the muscle wall of the uterus and may involve the cervix. With time, it can grow through the wall of the uterus into the surrounding tissues (the parametrium), the bladder, and the rectum.

It can also spread by the lymphatic system to the vagina, the fallopian tubes, the ovaries, the pelvic and aortic lymph nodes, and the lymph nodes in the groin and above the collarbone (supraclavicular). Like ovarian carcinoma, endometrial cancer can also spread throughout the pelvis and abdominal cavity, and occasionally through the bloodstream to the lung, liver, and brain. How rapidly it spreads depends on the histologic grade (virulence) and type of the cancer.

Endometrial cancer is often associated with a primary carcinoma of the ovary (see the chapter "Ovarian Germ Cell Tumors").

What Causes It Unknown.

Risk Factors

The use of birth control pills and postmenopausal hormone replacement therapy with estrogen and progesterone decreases the risk of developing endometrial cancer by half.

At Significantly Higher Risk

• Obesity greater than 50 pounds (23 kg) over ideal body weight (10 times as likely).

• Estrogen replacement therapy without supplemental progesterone (7 times as likely).

• Postmenopausal women.

• Menopause after age fifty-two (2.4 times as likely).

• Lack of children (twice as likely).

• Women with hypertension (twice as likely).

• Diabetics (2.8 times as likely). Probably related to obesity.

• Women who do not ovulate, those with polycystic ovaries (Stein-Leventhal syndrome).

• History of pelvic radiation therapy (8 times as likely).

• Family history of breast, ovarian, or, occasionally, colon cancer.

Screening

Screening for endometrial carcinoma is not as satisfactory as screening for cancer of the cervix because of the inaccessibility of the uterine cavity. Pap smears detect only a small percentage of endometrial cancers.

There have been a number of studies showing the benefit of endometrial biopsies to screen asymptomatic women at high risk. This procedure is associated with some discomfort, however, and may not be cost-effective in the absence of risk factors. A uterine sonogram (ultrasound) may be suggestive of cancer of the uterus, if the lining of the uterus cavity demonstrates increased thickness (greater than 5 mm thick). Routine annual screening for women without symptoms is not recommended by the American College of Obstetricians and Gynecologists.

Common Signs and Symptoms

In 90 percent of cases, there is abnormal uterine bleeding, ranging from insignificant staining to a hemorrhage. There may also be pain in the pelvis, back, or legs; bladder or rectal symptoms; weight loss; and general weakness. Five percent of women will have no symptoms.

Diagnosis

Physical Examination

• On a gynecologic examination, the external genitalia are usually normal. The cervix may be involved with cancer (Stage II), and the vagina may also be involved (Stage III).

• Occasionally, the uterus will be enlarged, hardened, or softened, and masses may be detected in the pelvis (a rectal examination is an important aspect of the pelvic examination).

• Enlarged lymph nodes in the neck and groin.

• Enlarged liver, an abdominal mass, or excessive abdominal fluid (ascites).

Blood and Other Tests

• Complete blood count.

• Serum liver and kidney function tests.

• Serum CA-125 is produced by a small percentage of women with early endometrial carcinoma, while advanced cancer is commonly associated with an elevation of CA-125. It is also useful in follow-up to detect recurrences.

Imaging

• A uterine sonogram with a thickened endometrial cavity (greater than 5 mm thick in postmenopausal women) may be suggestive of a uterine cancer.

• PET/CT scan of the chest, pelvis, and abdomen may be obtained for determining the extent of the cancer in the pelvis, the presence of ovarian disease, and the presence of pelvic and aortic lymph nodes and lung or liver metastases. It is performed for aggressive histologic cancer types, high-grade cancer, and suspected advanced cancer.

• Chest X-ray.

• MRI of the pelvis, in cases where the origin of the cancer is indeterminate (e.g., cervix versus uterine fundus).

Endoscopy and Biopsy The definitive diagnosis is made on an endometrial biopsy, which involves a small scraping of the uterus and is usually performed in the doctor's office. A dilation and curettage (D&C) is required for those women who have biopsy-proven endometrial hyperplasia (see "Endometrial Cancer Precursors," below), who have an insufficient specimen on an office biopsy, or who cannot tolerate an endometrial biopsy because of a small cervical opening or discomfort.

Staging

Cancer of the uterus is surgically staged. Between 70 and 80 percent of all endometrial cancers are Stage I. In 1988, the International Federation of Gynecology and Obstetrics (FIGO) staging system was revised to include the grade of the cancer (degree of virulence) as determined on microscopic examination. The cancers are divided into three grades, with Grade 1 (well differentiated) having the best prognosis and Grade 3 (poorly differentiated) having the poorest.

Endometrial Cancer Precursors

Endometrial hyperplasia, an overgrowth of the lining of the uterus, is a precursor to the development of cancer. Usually, hyperplasia is either a benign type without nuclear atypia, which has a very low risk of developing into cancer, or an intermediate-risk type (hyperplasia with atypia), which has a 50 percent chance of developing into cancer in four to ten years. On rare occasions, progression from a simple, benign hyperplasia confined to the lining of the uterus, to more severe atypical forms of hyperplasia, and eventually to an invasive malignancy, may occur. The risk factors for endometrial hyperplasia are similar to those of endometrial carcinoma.

Abnormal uterine bleeding is usually the first symptom. The diagnosis is made by evaluating the lining of the uterus by biopsy or D&C.

Treatment Overview

Treatment of endometrial carcinoma is based primarily on the stage and grade of the cancer.

Surgery The standard therapy is an abdominal hysterectomy with removal of both fallopian tubes and both ovaries, removal of pelvic and aortic lymph nodes, and washings from the abdominal cavity to look for malignant cells.

Most gynecologic oncologists recommend definitive surgery through a midline abdominal incision to gain access to the upper abdomen. Laparoscopic surgery (minimally invasive surgery) may be recommended in nonobese women, allowing a shorter hospital stay, a quicker recovery, and, where applicable, an earlier return to work.

Complications of surgery include infection, bleeding requiring transfusion, and injury to the bladder, rectum, or ureter causing a leak (rare). There may also be blood clots in the legs, occasionally dislodging and traveling to the lungs (pulmonary embolism); leg edema; and benign cysts around the blood vessels, secondary to the lymph node dissection, that occasionally require draining.

For women with advanced-stage disease, or very early stage, good-prognosis disease, many gynecologic oncologists recommend obtaining a specimen from the cancer for analysis of its estrogen- and progesterone-receptor content. The receptor content has prognostic value and may be useful in the selection of hormone therapy for recurrent or metastatic cancer, or for those women with severe menopausal symptoms such as hot flashes.

Radiation In the past, women with Stages IB, Grade 3, IC, or IIA uterine cancer were often treated two to six weeks after surgery with prophylactic radiation to the entire pelvis and upper vagina. External-beam radiation was given daily, five days a week, for four to five weeks. Although pelvic external-beam radiation therapy will decrease the frequency of recurrences in the pelvis and vagina, it does not statistically improve the five-year survival rate and as a result is recommended less often today. In some women with Stage II or Stage III disease, radiation therapy may be given preoperatively.

Intracavitary radiation (radioactive material temporarily placed directly in or near the tumor) may be used in select cases postoperatively, or occasionally prior to surgery, either alone or with external-beam radiation therapy. The radioactive material is of different types and left in place for different amounts of time, depending on a number of factors, including the size and location of the tumor and the type of radiation (i.e., low dose rate or high dose rate (see chapter 7, "What Happens in Radiation Therapy"). Side effects of radiation can include diarrhea, nausea and vomiting, bleeding from the bladder or rectum, vaginal scarring, intestinal obstruction, and leaks (fistulas) from the urinary or intestinal tract.

Chemotherapy Treatment with chemotherapy after surgery is used for later stages of the disease and recurrent cancer.

Treatment by Stage

Endometrial Hyperplasia

Total abdominal hysterectomy and removal of both tubes and both ovaries is the treatment of choice when fertility is no longer an issue or when progestational hormone therapy is contraindicated. For those women who desire more children or preservation of the uterus, a D&C, therapy with oral progestational agents, induction of ovulation, and avoidance of postmenopausal estrogen therapy without progesterone is frequently effective. Careful follow-up with an endometrial biopsy or a D&C is necessary every three to twelve months. Long-term treatment with progestational therapy is required because of recurrent hyperplasia.

Stage IA

The tumor is limited to the endometrium.

Standard Treatment Standard therapy is removal of the uterus, both tubes and both ovaries, and the pelvic and aortic lymph nodes. Unfortunately, the precise grade and depth of uterine wall invasion cannot be definitely determined at the time of surgery in women thought to be Stage I prior to surgery. As a result, the pelvic lymph nodes and aortic lymph nodes should be removed in all patients. Postoperative radiation therapy is not required.

Five-Year Survival 95 percent

Investigational Laparoscopic surgery

■ *Stage IB*

The tumor invades the uterine wall but through less than half of its thickness.

Standard Treatment The removal of the uterus, both tubes and both ovaries, and the pelvic and aortic lymph nodes and abdominal washings is all that is required.

Five-Year Survival Up to 90 percent

Investigational Laparoscopic surgery

■ *Stage IC*

The tumor invades the uterine wall by more than half of its thickness.

Standard Treatment Surgery is the same as for Stage IB. Usually, no further treatment is required. Some gynecologic oncologists and radiation therapists recommend whole pelvis radiation after surgery to decrease the frequency of recurrent disease in the vagina and pelvis. Although it does not statistically improve the five-year survival rate, it is effective in decreasing the incidence of local recurrences in the field of radiation.

Five-Year Survival 75 to 85 percent

■ *Stage IIA*

The glands that line the cervix are involved.

Standard Treatment This stage is generally treated like Stage IB.

Five-Year Survival Up to 90 percent

Investigational See Stage IB.

■ *Stage IIB*

The tumor cells invade the supporting tissue of the cervix.

Standard Treatment Before surgery, whole pelvis external-beam radiation therapy is given five days a week, over five weeks. After a two-week break, this is followed by a two- to three-day application of radioactive cesium to the upper vagina, the cervix, and the uterus or by high-dose-rate brachytherapy (see chapter 7, "What Happens in Radiation Therapy"). Six weeks later, an abdominal hysterectomy is performed, along with removal of both tubes and both ovaries, pelvic and aortic lymph node dissection, and cytological assessment of the abdominal cavity.

Alternative therapy for women in good medical condition is a radical abdominal hysterectomy (removal of the upper inch of the vagina and the tissue around the cervix and upper vagina), removal of the tubes and ovaries, and removal of all the pelvic and aortic lymph nodes.

Five-Year Survival 75 to 85 percent

Investigational High-dose rate brachytherapy in various doses, durations, and number of treatment sessions (see chapter 7, "What Happens in Radiation Therapy").

■ *Stage IIIA*

This stage is defined by involvement of the uterine surface and/or the tubes and ovaries and/or the presence of malignant cells in the abdominal fluid (positive peritoneal washings).

Standard Treatment After surgery, the type of additional treatment is controversial and should be considered investigational, as there is not enough information about the risk of recurrence, prognosis, and benefit of therapy. The chance of malignant cells being present within the abdominal cavity (Stage IIIA) increases with higher grades of cancer and with deeper invasion of the tumor into the uterine wall.

There is some controversy over the significance of malignant cells floating in the abdominal cavity. Many gynecologic oncologists recommend treatment with intravenous or intraperitoneal combination chemotherapy or with radiation therapy to the entire abdomen.

Five-Year Survival 60 to 70 percent; higher for those with only positive malignant cells in the washings

Investigational

• Pelvic and whole abdomen radiation
• Intravenous combination chemotherapy with cisplatin (Platinol) or carboplatin (Paraplatin), doxorubicin (Adriamycin), and paclitaxel (Taxol)
• Docetaxel (Taxotere), doxorubicin liposomal (Doxil), and topotecan (Hycamtin) in various doses and schedules
• Intra-abdominal chemotherapy (cisplatin or carboplatin)
• High-dose progestational hormones
• Intra-abdominal radiation (radioactive phosphorus)

■ *Stage IIIB*

Vaginal metastases or disease involving the tissue immediately around the uterus (the parametrium) or the tube and ovary.

Standard Treatment Women with vaginal metastases are usually treated by abdominal hysterectomy, removal of the tubes and ovaries, thorough staging with removal of the pelvic and aortic lymph nodes, and surgical excision of the vaginal metastases if possible.

Postoperatively, treatment with external-beam radiation therapy to the pelvis and vagina, five days a week for four to five weeks, is given, sometimes followed by either a temporary cesium insertion or the placement of radioactive iridium directly into and around the vaginal metastases (known as an interstitial implant). Alternatively, the radiation therapy precedes the definitive surgery by four to six weeks.

Endometrial cancer that extends locally outside the uterus is usually treated with radiation therapy—five days a week for five weeks of external-beam radiation therapy to the pelvis followed by two temporary cesium insertions two weeks apart or by a radioactive interstitial implant (low dose rate or high dose rate; see chapter 7, "What Happens in Radiation Therapy")—followed by surgery if possible.

Women with disease in the tubes or ovaries are treated with definitive surgery, including removal of the omentum (fatty tissue attached to the intestine and stomach). Chemotherapy is given postoperatively.

Five-Year Survival 40 to 75 percent

Investigational See Stage IIB.

■ *Stage IIIC*

Metastases to the pelvic and/or aortic lymph nodes.

Standard Treatment Most gynecologic oncologists recommend six courses of adjuvant chemotherapy such as carboplatin (Paraplatin) or cisplatin (Platinol), doxorubicin (Adriamycin), and paclitaxel (Taxol) or docetaxel (Taxotere), as well as external-beam radiation therapy over several weeks to the entire pelvis for those with positive pelvic nodes and to the entire pelvis and aortic nodes for those with positive pelvic and aortic nodes.

Five-Year Survival 60 to 80 percent

Investigational Chemotherapy (various drugs and doses) with or without pelvic and para-aortic radiation.

■ *Stage IVA*

The tumor invades the bladder or rectum.

Standard Treatment Treatment of cancer involving the bladder or rectum is usually with external-beam radiation therapy to the pelvis followed by two or more insertions of radioactive cesium or by interstitial radiation with iridium inserted directly into the tumor.

Another acceptable alternative is whole pelvis radiation therapy followed by the surgical removal of the uterus, vagina, bladder, and/or rectum (pelvic exenteration) and by pelvic and aortic lymph node dissection.

Five-Year Survival 10 to 50 percent

Investigational Studies are looking at the role of adjuvant chemotherapy with cisplatin (Platinol), carboplatin (Paraplatin), other platinum analogues, paclitaxel (Taxol), docetaxel (Taxotere), doxorubicin (Adriamycin), mitoxantrone (Novantrone), cyclophosphamide (Cytoxan), ifosfamide (Ifex), topotecan (Hycamtin), doxorubicin liposomal (Doxil), gemcitabine (Gemzar), or progestational hormones in various doses, combinations, and schedules prior to surgery. In those women with intra-abdominal spread of cancer, aggressive surgery is performed to remove all visible disease.

■ *Stage IVB*

Distant metastases (lung or liver the most common), intra-abdominal spread, or disease in the lymph nodes of the groin.

Standard Treatment Treatment is usually based on the location of the distant metastases. Surgery is performed whenever it can improve the survival rate (intra-abdominal disease, groin node metastases, isolated liver or lung metastases). Nowadays, chemotherapy and not progestational therapy is the preferred treatment. Chemotherapy with carboplatin (Paraplatin), cisplatin (Platinol), doxorubicin (Adriamycin), ifosfamide (Ifex), paclitaxel (Taxol), or docetaxel

(Taxotere) given every three to four weeks has been shown to be effective in some patients, with response rates in the range of 30 to 80 percent, depending on the site of disease. Women with microscopic or very small intra-abdominal metastases can be treated with intra-abdominal chemotherapy (cisplatin or carboplatin).

There is a 20 to 30 percent response rate to progestational hormones. If the metasteses or the initial uterine cancer is sensitive to progestational hormones, as shown by testing for progesterone receptors, the response rate to hormone therapy will be significantly higher. The most commonly used progestational agent is megestrol acetate (Megace). Similarly, if the tumor contains many estrogen receptors, then antiestrogen therapy with tamoxifen (Nolvadex) may be effective, with a response rate of 20 to 30 percent. Sometimes the two hormones are used together.

Occasionally, palliative radiation therapy may be given to a localized distant metastasis.

Five-Year Survival 5 to 40 percent

Investigational Chemotherapeutic drugs given in various doses and combinations are being studied. These include cisplatin (Platinol), carboplatin (Paraplatin), other platinum analogues, paclitaxel (Taxol), docetaxel (Taxotere), doxorubicin (Adriamycin), mitoxantrone (Novantrone), gemcitabine (Gemzar), cyclophosphamide (Cytoxan), ifosfamide (Ifex), 5-fluorouracil (5-FU), methotrexate (Mexate, Amethopterin, Folex), topotecan (Hycamtin), doxorubicin liposomal (Doxil), etoposide (Etopophos), and various types and doses of progestational hormones and antiestrogenic drugs.

Treatment Follow-Up

Most gynecologic oncologists recommend a general physical and pelvic examination with or without a Pap smear every three months for the first two years, then every six months for another three years.

• The serum CA-125 level can be monitored if it was elevated prior to therapy.

• CT scans or PET/CT scans are recommended whenever specific signs and symptoms warrant. Some physicians recommend imaging every six to twelve months for the first three years. Sometimes a baseline scan is performed six to eight weeks after surgery to compare with future studies.

Recurrent Cancer

Approximately 70 percent of recurrences take place within two to three years of the initial therapy. Symptoms of recurrent cancer may include vaginal bleeding or discharge; pain in the pelvis, abdomen, back, or legs; leg swelling (edema); chronic cough; urinary symptoms; constipation; and weight loss. Generally, the later the recurrence takes place after the initial treatment, the better the prognosis.

The pelvic wall, the vagina, and the tissue surrounding the cervix and uterus (parametrium) are the most common sites of local recurrences in women who have not previously received pelvic radiation. Distant metastases to the lung, liver, abdominal cavity, and distant lymph nodes may also occur.

Radiation therapy, if not given previously, may cure a high percentage of those women with only a vaginal or parametrial recurrence. Women who have a localized vaginal recurrence involving the bladder or rectum, especially if they have previously been treated with radiation therapy, are candidates for the removal of the bladder and/or rectum and vagina (pelvic exenteration). Cure is possible in 40 to 50 percent of women.

Unfortunately, most women with recurrent endometrial cancer outside the pelvis cannot be cured. Symptoms may be relieved and life prolonged with chemotherapy, progestational therapy, or antiestrogen therapy as noted above.

Estrogen Replacement Therapy

In the past, estrogen replacement therapy has been given to women with a low risk of recurrent cancer. Although giving women with uterine cancer estrogen replacement therapy is an absolute contraindication, it may be given on an individual basis for those with severe menopausal symptoms. Its use should be carefully considered, as estrogen may promote the growth of endometrial cancer.

The Most Important Questions You Can Ask

• What qualifications do you have for treating uterine cancer? Will a specialist in gynecologic oncology be involved in my case?

• Do I need radiation therapy?

• Is chemotherapy of any benefit?

• What symptoms of recurrent cancer should I be looking for after treatment?

• Can I use estrogen replacement therapy?

Uterus: Uterine Sarcomas

Jeffrey L. Stern, M.D.

■ ■ ■ ■

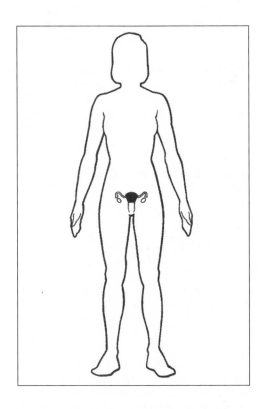

Uterine sarcomas are very rare. They are responsible for only 1 to 5 percent of all malignancies of the uterus (see the chapter "Uterus: Endometrial Carcinoma" for the much more common cancer of the uterus) and account for less than 1 percent of all gynecologic malignancies (see the chapter "Cervix").

Uterine sarcomas are treated like other uterine cancers; however, the rate of cure is less—50 to 70 percent for early-stage disease and less than 10 percent for advanced sarcomas.

Symptoms are similar to those of endometrial carcinoma, but some women are first diagnosed as having a common benign uterine tumor called a fibroid. After this occasionally rapidly growing, presumably benign fibroid is surgically removed, the pathologist finds that it is a cancerous tumor.

Types There are two general categories of sarcomas, pure and mixed. Those pure tumors arising from the smooth muscle of the uterine wall or from a benign fibroid are known as leiomyosarcomas and are considered benign if there are less than five dividing cells (mitoses) on microscopic examination and malignant if there are more than ten dividing cells. If there are between five to ten dividing cells, the tumor is considered a low-grade malignancy. Other histologic criteria, such as the degree of cellular nuclear atypia, are also factored into a diagnosis of benign versus malignant.

Another 15 percent of uterine sarcomas arise from the supporting (stromal) cells that surround the glands within the lining of the uterus (the endometrium) and are known as endometrial stromal sarcomas. They are classified according to grade, from the less virulent low-grade tumors to the extremely virulent high-grade tumors.

The most common type of uterine sarcomas—half of all cases—arise from both the endometrial glands *and* the supporting stromal cells of the endometrium. These are known as mixed mesodermal sarcomas and are further subdivided into homologous and heterologous tumors.

The homologous variety—also known as carcinosarcomas—contain malignant cells transformed from cells normally found in the uterus. The heterologous type contain cellular elements not normally found in the uterus, including malignant bone, fat, cartilage, and striated muscle.

Heterologous mixed mesodermal tumors are the most common type of uterine sarcoma and account for 1 to 3 percent of all uterine cancers. Homologous tumors are much less common.

How It Spreads Uterine sarcomas can grow locally to involve the cervix and the tissue surrounding the uterus and can spread to the rectum and bladder. They can also spread to the groin, the pelvic and aortic lymph nodes, the surfaces of the abdominal cavity, and distantly to the liver, lung, and brain.

Leiomyosarcomas spread by direct local extension, by abdominal implantation, or via the bloodstream. The lung is the most common site of metastases, followed by the liver, brain, and bone.

Low-grade stromal sarcomas are usually slow growing and tend to remain confined to the uterus in about 70 percent of cases. Spread beyond the uterus occurs via the lymph system or via the bloodstream. High-grade stromal sarcomas spread in a similar way, but they behave much more aggressively and are often advanced at the time of diagnosis.

What Causes It The exact cause is unknown; however, there is a significant association with previous pelvic radiation (10 to 30 percent of cases). The average time interval between pelvic radiation and development of the sarcoma is fifteen to twenty years.

Unlike other uterine sarcomas, leiomyosarcomas have no association with previous pelvic radiation.

Risk Factors

Heterologous mixed mesodermal tumors can occur in any age group, including infants, but they most commonly occur in postmenopausal women with a median age of sixty-five. Homologous mixed mesodermal tumors can also occur in all age groups, but the median age is fifty-seven years. The average age for leiomyosarcomas at diagnosis is fifty-three.

Low-grade stromal sarcomas occur much more frequently in premenopausal women, with 70 percent occurring in women under fifty. High-grade stromal sarcomas occur most commonly in postmenopausal women.

At Significantly Higher Risk Previous pelvic radiation.

Screening

Uterine sarcoma can occasionally be detected by a routine Pap smear; however, screening for any uterine cancer is not as satisfactory as that for cervical cancer because of the inaccessibility of the uterine cavity. There is no screening program routinely used for women without symptoms.

Although not as yet used for routine screening, sonography can detect uterine malignancies. The endometrial cavity is usually thicker than normal, indicating a growth within the endometrial cavity.

Common Signs and Symptoms

Usually, postmenopausal bleeding is the most common symptom in women with uterine sarcoma.

Most women with a leiomyosarcoma will have abnormal uterine bleeding, pressure or pain in the abdomen or pelvis, abnormal vaginal discharge, or a diagnosis of uterine fibroids. Many women will be asymptomatic.

Diagnosis

Physical Examination

- A careful pelvic examination.
- Examination of the lymph nodes in the groin and above the collarbone.
- Examination of the abdomen to detect an enlarged liver, abdominal masses, and excess fluid (ascites).

Blood and Other Tests Serum liver and kidney function tests, CA-125.

Imaging

- Chest X-ray.
- Pelvic, abdominal, and chest CT scans to detect pelvic extension of the tumor, pelvic and aortic lymph nodes, and liver and lung metastases.
- Pelvic MRI (on occasion).
- PET scan.

Endoscopy and Biopsy

- Cystoscopy and sigmoidoscopy (occasionally).
- The definitive diagnosis is made by a pathologist evaluating either an office endometrial biopsy, tissue removed during a D&C (dilation and curettage), or the tissue specimen after the uterus and cervix are removed (hysterectomy). While most endometrial stromal and mixed mesodermal tumors are diagnosed from an endometrial biopsy or D&C, most leiomyosarcomas are diagnosed after a hysterectomy for what are thought to be benign uterine fibroids. A preoperative diagnosis of leiomyosarcomas is uncommon.

Staging

The International Federation of Gynecology and Obstetrics (FIGO) staging classification for uterine sarcoma is the same as that for endometrial carcinoma. Uterine sarcomas are surgically staged.

Treatment Overview

Surgery is the primary treatment and can lead to a cure if the tumor is confined to the uterus. Radiation and chemotherapy may also be given after surgery for more advanced stages.

 Surgery Whenever possible, the uterus and cervix are removed (hysterectomy) along with the fallopian tubes and ovaries on both sides. The pelvic and aortic lymph nodes are also removed, and fluid from the pelvis and abdomen is taken for analysis (peritoneal cytologic washings), to look for cancer cells floating in the abdomen.

 Radiation External-beam radiation therapy is often given to the pelvis after surgery to decrease local recurrence in early-stage disease. This does not appear to improve survival, however. Side effects of radiation can include diarrhea, nausea and vomiting, bleeding from the bladder or rectum, vaginal scarring, intestinal obstruction, and leaks (fistulas) in the urinary or intestinal tract.

 Chemotherapy Although there is no definite proof of increased survival with adjuvant chemotherapy (treatment even if there is no obvious evidence of residual disease), many gynecologic oncologists and medical oncologists recommend its use even for early stages of disease. Metastatic sarcomas that have spread to distant organs are generally treated with chemotherapy.

Treatment by Cell Type
Mixed Mesodermal Sarcomas

The prognosis depends mainly on the stage of the cancer. There does not seem to be any difference in survival between homologous and heterologous mixed mesodermal tumors.

Generally, women with mixed mesodermal tumors are treated like women with high-grade endometrial cancer.

Standard Treatment Hysterectomy, removal of the tubes and ovaries on both sides, washings to check for malignant cells in the abdominal cavity, and removal of the pelvic and aortic lymph nodes on both sides is the usual treatment. Women at high risk for recurrent cancer, lymph node metastases, or metastatic disease to other organs are also treated with radiation therapy or chemotherapy or both.

Chemotherapy may be used as an adjuvant therapy, although there is no documented proof of its benefit. Chemotherapy is often recommended in women with documented metastases or node metastases.

Investigational

• Ifosfamide (Ifex), paclitaxel (Taxol) + carboplatin (Paraplatin).

• Doxorubicin (Adriamycin) + ifosfamide + dacarbazine (DTIC-Dome), ifosfamide + cisplatin (Platinol) or carboplatin.

• A clinical trial now being done by the Gynecologic Oncology Group is comparing ifosfamide and cisplatin with ifosfamide without cisplatin for the treatment of mixed mesodermal tumors. Thirty-five percent of women respond to intravenous ifosfamide alone.

• Doxorubicin in combination with dacarbazine or cyclophosphamide (Cytoxan) has been shown to be more effective than doxorubicin alone for advanced disease.

• Vincristine (Oncovin) and cyclophosphamide have also been used in combination with dactinomycin (actinomycin D, Cosmegen) or doxorubicin, with or without dacarbazine, with some effectiveness.

• Docetaxel (Taxotere), gemcitabine (Gemzar), topotecan (Hycamtin), and mitoxantrone (Novantrone).

Leiomyosarcoma

Good prognostic factors for this tumor type include the presence of a small tumor, a tumor arising from a benign uterine fibroid (5 to 10 percent of all cases), a low number of dividing cells, and being premenopausal.

Standard Treatment Abdominal hysterectomy, removal of both tubes and ovaries, washings to check for malignant cells in the abdominal cavity, and removal of the pelvic and aortic lymph nodes is the treatment of choice.

Additional treatment for women with early-stage disease and borderline tumors has not been shown to be beneficial.

Postoperative whole pelvis external-beam radiation therapy five days a week for five weeks is sometimes given to decrease the local recurrence rate in early-stage disease.

Although postoperative pelvic radiation and/or chemotherapy are often given to prevent recurrence, they have not been shown conclusively to increase survival. Commonly used chemotherapeutic drug regimens include doxorubicin (Adriamycin) + ifosfamide (Ifex) + dacarbazine (DTIC-Dome), and doxorubicin + cyclophosphamide (Cytoxan) + dacarbazine. Cisplatin (Platinol) alone has shown not to be of much benefit. Other agents such as docetaxel (Taxotere), paclitxel (Taxol), gemcitabine (Gemzar), and topotecan (Hycamtin) are also used in various combinations and doses.

Advanced leiomyosarcoma is treated with radiation therapy and/or chemotherapy.

Investigational

• Current studies are looking at postoperative pelvic radiation therapy versus no treatment and chemotherapy in various doses and schedules as prophylaxis.

• Docetaxel (Taxotere), gemcitabine (Gemzar), and topotecan (Hycamtin) in various combinations and doses.

• Mitoxantrone (Novantrone), a drug similar to doxorubicin (Adriamycin), and ifosfamide (Ifex) are also being studied.

Low-Grade Endometrial Stromal Sarcoma

Standard Treatment The standard treatment for these sarcomas usually includes a hysterectomy, removal of the tubes and ovaries on both sides, pelvic and aortic node dissection, and abdominal cytologic washings.

Early-stage disease can also be treated by a radical hysterectomy, removal of the pelvic and aortic lymph nodes, removal of the tubes and ovaries, and abdominal cytologic washings.

Postoperative radiation therapy to the pelvis (4,500 to 5,000 cGy given in divided doses, five days a week for five weeks) is sometimes given to decrease the chance of a pelvic recurrence. The frequency of recurrence depends primarily on the depth of uterine invasion.

Since these tumors frequently contain progesterone and/or estrogen receptors, hormone therapy with progestins or the antiestrogen tamoxifen (Nolvadex) is sometimes given.

Investigational Various types and doses of progestins and antiestrogens are being studied.

High-Grade Endometrial Stromal Sarcoma

Standard Treatment For high-grade stromal sarcomas, standard therapy is a hysterectomy, removal of the tubes and ovaries on both sides, removal of the pelvic and aortic nodes, and washings from the abdominal cavity to look for malignant cells.

For early-stage cancer, postoperative pelvic radiation therapy (4,000 to 5,000 cGy given in divided doses, five days a week for five weeks) is often recommended because it decreases the chance

of a pelvic recurrence. Radiation to the aortic nodes may be given as well.

Adjuvant chemotherapy is sometimes given, but it should be considered experimental.

Advanced cancers are treated like other high-grade endometrial cancers or like other sarcomas.

Investigational

• Since pelvic and distant recurrences are common and the prognosis of this malignancy is poor, many gynecologic oncologists and medical oncologists recommend adjuvant chemotherapy even though it has not yet been shown to be effective.

• Radiation therapy tailored to sites of disease.

• Doxorubicin (Adriamycin), ifosfamide (Ifex), and dacarbazine (DTIC-Dome), docetaxel (Taxotere), carboplatin (Paraplatin), gemcitabine (Gemzar), and topotecan (Hycamtin).

• Chemotherapy for advanced disease, such as doxorubicin (Adriamycin), ifosfamide (Ifex), and dacarbazine (DTIC-Dome); gemcitabine (Gemzar) with or withot docetaxel (Taxotere); carboplatin (Paraplatin) and paclitaxel (Taxol); or topotecan (Hycamtin).

Treatment by Stage

■ Stage I

Stage I cancer is further divided into Stages IA, IB, and IC. In Stage IA, the tumor is limited to the endometrium. In IB, it invades the wall of the uterus by less than half of the wall's thickness. In IC, it invades the wall by more than half of the thickness.

Standard Treatment Surgery should include a hysterectomy, removal of both fallopian tubes and both ovaries, washings from the abdominal cavity to look for malignant cells, and removal of the pelvic and aortic lymph nodes.

Postoperative radiation therapy is sometimes given prophylactically to the entire pelvis (4,000 to 5,000 cGy, given in divided doses, five days a week for five weeks).

Five-Year Survival 75 percent for Stage IA; 50 percent for Stages IB and IC

■ *Stage IIA*

The tumor involves the endocervical glands.

Standard Treatment Surgery as for Stage I and sometimes postoperative whole pelvis radiation therapy.

Five-Year Survival 50 percent

Investigational Same as for Stage I

■ *Stage IIB*

There is cervical stromal invasion.

Standard Treatment Surgery as for Stage I and postoperative radiation therapy is standard. An alternative is whole pelvis external-beam radiation therapy (4,000 to 5,000 cGy given in divided doses, five days a week for five weeks), followed two weeks later by the insertion of radioactive cesium into the uterus (intracavitary radiation) for one or two days. This will be followed six weeks later by a hysterectomy, removal of both tubes and both ovaries, cytologic washings of the abdominal cavity, and removal of the pelvic and aortic lymph nodes.

Equally effective for young women or those in good medical condition is a radical hysterectomy, removal of both tubes and both ovaries, removal of the pelvic and aortic lymph nodes, and meticulous staging.

Five-Year Survival 50 percent

Investigational See investigational adjuvant chemotherapies under "Treatment by Cell Type" in this chapter.

■ *Stage IIIA*

The surface of the uterus and/or the tubes and ovaries are involved and/or there are malignant cells in the abdominal fluid (positive peritoneal washings).

Standard Treatment Surgery as for Stage I. Postoperative pelvic radiation therapy (with or without whole abdomen radiation) therapy is given. Chemotherapy is also given sometimes.

Five-Year Survival Up to 20 percent

Investigational See investigational adjuvant chemotherapies under "Treatment by Cell Type" in this chapter.

■ *Stage IIIB*

There are vaginal metastases.

Standard Treatment For women with vaginal metastases, the standard treatment is surgery as for Stage I cancer and postoperative external-beam radiation therapy given to the whole pelvis and vagina. This is followed by vaginal brachytherapy (a radioactive substance is placed against the tumor) for one or two days or interstitial iridium (a radioactive substance is placed directly into the tumor) for one to three days. Multiple treatments are usually required.

Women with disease that extends locally outside the uterus are treated with whole pelvis radiation and one to three intracavitary cesium or interstitial iridium insertions, followed by surgery whenever possible.

Five-Year Survival Up to 10 percent

Investigational See investigational adjuvant chemotherapies under "Treatment by Cell Type" in this chapter.

• Interstitial radiation therapy with heat (hyperthermia) is being studied.

■ Stage IIIC

There are metastases to the pelvic and para-aortic lymph nodes.

Standard Treatment Surgery as for Stage I. Postoperative pelvic radiation therapy and radiation to the aortic lymph nodes (if they are involved) is usually given. Chemotherapy is often given as well.

Five-Year Survival Up to 10 percent

Investigational See investigational adjuvant chemotherapies under "Treatment by Cell Type" in this chapter.

■ Stage IVA

The tumor invades the bladder or rectum.

Standard Treatment Options include external-beam radiation therapy to the entire pelvis and intracavitary or interstitial radiation therapy (in one to three insertions). Occasionally, the uterus, vagina, bladder, and/or rectum are removed (pelvic exenteration).

Five-Year Survival Up to 5 percent

Investigational
- Adjuvant chemotherapy
- Interstitial radiation therapy

■ Stage IVB

There are distant metastases, with spread to organs within the abdomen and/or disease in the groin lymph nodes.

Standard Treatment Metastatic sarcomas are usually treated with chemotherapy. Commonly used drugs include doxorubicin (Adriamycin) and ifosfamide (Ifex), alone or together, and the combinations of gemcitabine (Gemzar) + paclitaxel (Taxol); doxorubicin + ifosfamide + dacarbazine (DTIC-Dome); vincristine (Oncovin) + dactinomycin (actinomycin D, Cosmegen); and doxorubin + cyclophosphamide (Cytoxan) + dacarbazine.

Five-Year Survival Up to 5 percent

Investigational
- Various doses and combinations of chemotherapy drugs are being evaluated.
- Doxorubicin (Adriamycin), ifosfamide (Ifex), carboplatin (Paraplatin), docetaxel (Taxotere), paclitaxel (Taxol), gemcitabine (Gemzar), topotecan (Hycamtin), and mitoxantrone (Novantrone).

Treatment Follow-Up

A general physical and pelvic examination is performed every three months for the first two years after treatment, then every six months for the next three years.

- A Pap smear may be performed at each visit.
- Diagnostic X-ray studies (CT/MRI/PET scan) are performed as specific signs and symptoms warrant.

Recurrent Cancer

Uterine sarcomas most often recur within three years of treatment and occur in the vagina, pelvis, lymph nodes, liver, and lungs. Recurrences of leiomyosarcomas are usually distant, with only 5 percent confined to the pelvis. Recurrences of low-grade stromal sarcomas can occur late, sometimes ten years after initial treatment. Although pelvic recurrences are the most common, these sarcomas can recur in the abdominal cavity or in the lungs.

Common symptoms of recurrent cancer include vaginal bleeding or discharge; pain in the pelvis, abdomen, back, or legs; swelling in the legs or abdomen; chronic cough; weight loss; change in bowel habits; and urinary symptoms.

There is no standard therapy for recurrent disease.

- The chemotherapy listed above in various combinations and doses has been used with variable effectiveness but rarely leads to a cure.

• Women with localized disease in the pelvis sometimes benefit from radiation therapy and occasionally from the removal of the pelvic organs (pelvic exenteration).

• Women with low-grade endometrial stromal sarcomas might benefit from progestational hormone or antiestrogen therapy.

The Most Important Questions You Can Ask

• What qualifications do you have for treating cancer? Are you a specialist in gynecologic oncology?

• What kind of sarcoma do I have?

• What is the stage?

• What benefit is there to having radiation therapy after surgery?

• Is there any benefit from chemotherapy?

Vagina

Jeffrey L. Stern, M.D.

■ ■ ■ ■

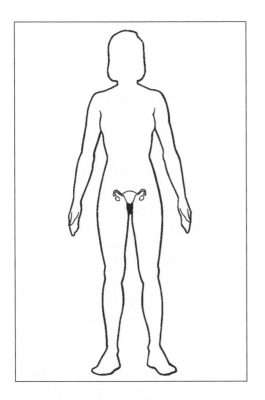

Carcinoma of the vagina is a relatively uncommon disease, affecting only about 2,000 women in the United States each year. It accounts for 1 to 2 percent of all gynecologic malignancies. Cancer arising in another organ that spreads to the vagina is much more common.

Types The most common type of vaginal cancer (85 percent) develops in the surface (squamous) cells lining the vagina (squamous cell carcinomas). About 5 percent develop in glandular tissues (adenocarcinomas). Other cell types include melanomas (3 percent), sarcomas (3 percent), and endodermal sinus tumors (1 percent).

Squamous cell carcinomas, leiomyosarcomas, and melanomas generally arise in older women. Adenocarcinomas usually occur in younger women. The very rare sarcoma botryoides and endodermal sinus tumors most frequently occur in infants.

How It Spreads Squamous cell carcinomas that originate in the skin that lines the vagina can remain confined to the lining for some time. At this stage, it is known as vaginal squamous intraepithelial lesion (SIL), vaginal intraepithelial neoplasia (VAIN), or vaginal dysplasia. Eventually, it will invade the vaginal wall and with time will extend directly into the tissue surrounding the vagina, the pelvic walls, the bladder, or the rectum.

Lymphatic invasion and metastases is another avenue of spread. Carcinomas arising in the upper vagina can spread to the pelvic and aortic lymph nodes, and those in the lower vagina to the lymph nodes in the groin.

Adenocarcinomas spread in a similar fashion, but they may have a higher incidence of metastases to the lymph nodes (see the chapter "Cervix").

What Causes It The human papillomavirus (HPV), a sexually transmitted virus responsible for genital warts, is believed to cause vaginal squamous intraepithelial lesion and invasive squamous cell carcinoma of the vagina. The time from infection to the development of an invasive cancer is thought to be from five to ten years.

Most cases of adenocarcinoma of the vagina used to be associated with exposure to diethylstilbestrol (DES) in embryonic life. DES was given in the 1950s to women who were thought to be at risk for miscarriage. The incidence of DES-related adenocarcinoma is highest for those women who were exposed during the first three months of their mother's pregnancy. The peak incidence is between ages seventeen and twenty-one. The incidence of this disease peaked in the early 1970s and is now rare, since DES use during pregnancy fell out of favor during the 1960s and was banned in the early 1970s.

In the future, vaccination against the human papillomavirus may prevent the squamous cell carcinomas and some of the adenocarcinomas of the vagina.

What causes the other vaginal tumors is not clear.

Risk Factors

Preinvasive and invasive squamous cell carcinomas of the vagina are associated with a previous history of genital warts or of intraepithelial or invasive carcinoma of the cervix or vulva. In 10 to 20 percent of women with squamous cell carcinoma of the vagina, there is a history of vaginal radiation therapy, usually for a cervical cancer.

Screening

Screening for malignancies of the vagina is similar to screening for cervical cancer. A careful annual pelvic examination and Pap smear is recommended. Women who have been exposed to DES are followed more carefully with twice-yearly pelvic examinations, Pap smears of the cervix and vaginal wall, and colposcopic (magnification) examination of the vagina.

Common Signs and Symptoms

The most common symptoms are abnormal vaginal bleeding, often painless and sometimes postcoital, and a foul-smelling vaginal discharge. There may be pain in the pelvis, back, or legs; leg swelling (edema); or urinary or lower-intestinal symptoms.

Diagnosis

Physical Examination

• A careful gynecologic, pelvic, and rectal examination is performed to assess the local spread of the cancer.

• Women with vaginal SIL are evaluated with a colposcope.

• Examination of the lymph nodes in the groin and neck and an abdominal examination are important to detect masses.

Blood and Other Tests

• Complete blood count (CBC).

• Serum carcinoembryonic antigen (CEA) and serum squamous cell carcinoma antigen.

• Serum alpha-fetoprotein (for an endodermal sinus tumor).

• Serum kidney and liver function tests.

Imaging

• Chest X-ray.

• CT or PET/CT scan of the chest, pelvis, and abdomen (for advanced cases).

• MRI of the pelvis (on occasion).

Endoscopy and Biopsy

• Cystourethroscopy for advanced cases.

• Proctosigmoidoscopy for advanced cases.

• The cancer is confirmed by a vaginal biopsy.

Staging

Vaginal carcinoma is staged by either the FIGO (International Federation of Gynecology and Obstetrics) system or the TNM classification. In the TNM system, N1 indicates pelvic lymph node metastases when the upper two-thirds of the vagina is involved or groin node metastases on one side when the lower two-thirds of the vagina is involved. N2 indicates groin node metastases on both sides.

Treatment Overview

Several factors are considered in choosing the most appropriate way to manage vaginal cancer, including the cell type, stage, size, location of the lesion, presence or absence of the uterus, and whether the woman has had previous radiation to the pelvis.

Early carcinomas are generally treated with either surgery or radiation therapy and concurrent chemotherapy. The radiation therapy involves radioactive material placed against the cancer (intracavitary radiation) or radioactive material temporarily placed directly in the cancer (interstitial radiation). External-beam radiation is given in divided doses to the pelvis five days a week for five weeks.

Locally advanced cancers are treated with radiation therapy with simultaneous administration of combination chemotherapy.

Treatment by Stage

■ Stage 0 (Squamous Cell Carcinoma)
TNM Tis, N0, M0
Carcinoma in situ or intraepithelial carcinoma.

Standard Treatment There are a number of effective treatments. Choice of treatment is based on whether there is only one lesion or multiple lesions, the size of the lesion(s), and the age and medical condition of the patient.

Partial vaginectomy has been the standard of treatment for decades, but today laser vaporization or topical 5-fluorouracil cream is used more frequently. Advanced cases on rare occasions require a total vaginectomy often with a skin graft. Radiation therapy is reserved for those in very poor medical condition.

Five-Year Survival 100 percent

■ Stage I (Squamous Cell Carcinoma or Adenocarcinoma)
TNM T1, N0, M0
The carcinoma is limited to the vaginal wall.

Standard Treatment Young women with lesions involving the upper third of the vagina can be treated by a radical partial vaginectomy, a radical hysterectomy, and removal of the pelvic and sometimes the aortic lymph nodes on both sides.

Equally effective for all Stage I tumors, regardless of age and site, is external-beam radiation therapy with concurrent chemotherapy and intracavitary or interstitial radiation therapy. Smaller lesions are sometimes treated with only intracavitary or interstitial radiation therapy.

Five-Year Survival 70 to 95 percent

Investigational
• Meticulous laparoscopic or conventional surgical staging before radiation therapy
• Various chemotherapeutic agents given simultaneously with radiation therapy
• High-dose-rate radiation therapy
• Radiation therapy with heat (hyperthermia)

■ Stage II (Squamous Cell Carcinoma and Adenocarcinoma)
TNM T2, N0, M0
The carcinoma involves the adjacent vaginal tissue but has not extended to the pelvic wall.

Standard Treatment External-beam radiation with concurrent chemotherapy and intracavitary or interstitial radiation.

Five-Year Survival 50 to 70 percent

Investigational Same as for Stage I.

■ *Stages III and IVA (Squamous Cell Carcinoma and Adenocarcinoma)*
TNM T3 (or less), N1, M0 or T3, N0, M0 (Stage III)
The carcinoma has extended to the pelvic wall.

TNM Any T, N2, M0 or T4, N0, M0 (Stage IVA)
The carcinoma has extended beyond the true pelvis or involves the lining of the bladder or rectum.

Standard Treatment Carcinomas in these stages are generally treated with external-beam radiation and with concurrent chemotherapy intracavitary or interstitial radiation. Radical surgery is an option in selected cases.

Five-Year Survival About 30 percent for Stage III; 10 to 20 percent for Stage IVA

Investigational Same as for Stage I.

■ *Stage IVB*
TNM Any T, any N, M1
There is spread to distant organs.

Standard Treatment Neither radiation nor surgery can cure women with distant metastases, but both are used for local relief of symptoms.
 A number of chemotherapy regimens that are effective in the treatment of metastatic cervical cancer are also used to treat metastatic vaginal cancers—various doses and combinations of cisplatin (Platinol), carboplatin (Paraplatin), paclitaxel (Taxol), cyclophosphamide (Cytoxan),

5-fluorouracil (5-FU), doxorubicin (Adriamycin), mitomycin (Mutamycin), vincristine (Oncovin), bleomycin (Blenoxane), ifosfamide (Ifex), and etoposide (Etopophos).

Five-Year Survival Less than 10 percent

Investigational Various doses and combinations of chemotherapeutic drugs are being evaluated, including cisplatin (Platinol), carboplatin (Paraplatin), ifosfamide (Ifex), etoposide (Etopophos), mitomycin (Mutamycin), 5-FU, vincristine (Oncovin), vinblastine (Velban), mitoxantrone (Novantrone), bleomycin (Blenoxane), and methotrexate (Mexate, Amethopterin, Folex).

Treating Other Cell Types

Endodermal Sinus Tumors These are extremely rare and are treated with surgery and a combination chemotherapy program such as cisplatin (Platinol) + bleomycin (Blenoxane) + etoposide (Etopophos).

Vaginal Sarcomas Sarcomas of the botryoid type are treated with combination chemotherapy, including vincristine (Oncovin), dactinomycin (actinomycin D, Cosmegen), cyclophosphamide (Cytoxan) and dacarbazine (DTIC-Dome), or mitomycin (Mutamycin), doxorubicin (Adriamycin), and ifosfamide (Ifex), followed by surgery or radiation therapy as indicated (see the chapters "Sarcomas of Bone and Soft Tissue" and "Uterus: Uterine Sarcomas").

Malignant Melanomas These tumors are generally treated by aggressive surgery, but the overall survival rate is extremely poor—less than 15 percent. Advanced melanomas are treated with chemotherapy regimens including dacarbazine (DTIC-Dome) + cisplatin (Platinol) + cyclophosphamide (Cytoxan) + tamoxifen (Nolvadex) (see the chapter "Melanoma").

Treatment Follow-Up

After therapy, women are followed every three months with a careful general physical examination and pelvic examination and a Pap smear.

- A chest X-ray or CT scan of the chest, abdomen, or pelvis or a PET/CT scan may be obtained if symptoms warrant.
- If the serum CEA, squamous cell carcinoma antigen, and/or alpha-fetoprotein were elevated before therapy, they can be followed to detect recurrent disease.

Recurrent Cancer

Vaginal cancer can recur in the vagina, pelvis, liver, lungs, and lymph nodes. Symptoms of recurrent disease include weight loss; vaginal or rectal bleeding; bleeding from the urinary tract; pain in the pelvis, back, or leg; leg swelling; and the development of a chronic cough.

- If previously treated with radiation therapy and the recurrent cancer is confined to the vagina, bladder, and/or rectum, surgical removal of the vagina, bladder, and/or rectum (pelvic exenteration) may be performed.
- Unresectable locally recurrent and/or metastatic disease is treated with a single chemotherapeutic drug such as cisplatin (Platinol) or carboplatin (Paraplatin), or combination chemotherapeutic drug regimens such as mitomycin (Mutamycin) + vincristine (Oncovin) + bleomycin (Blenoxane) + cisplatin, and carboplatin or cisplatin + ifosfamide (Ifex) + etoposide (Etopophos).

Investigational Various doses and combinations of the different chemotherapeutic drugs are being studied, including cisplatin (Platinol), carboplatin (Paraplatin), paclitaxel (Taxol), cyclophosphamide (Cytoxan), ifosfamide (Ifex), doxorubicin (Adriamycin), etoposide (Etopophos), mitomycin (Mutamycin), 5-FU, vincristine (Oncovin), vinblastine (Velban), mitoxantrone (Novantrone), bleomycin (Blenoxane), and methotrexate (Mexate, Amethopterin, Folex).

The Most Important Questions You Can Ask

- What qualifications do you have for treating cancer?
- Will a gynecologic oncologist be involved in my care?
- What stage of cancer do I have?
- What is the cell type?
- What signs and symptoms should I look for after I've been treated?

Vulva

Jeffrey L. Stern, M.D.

■ ■ ■ ■

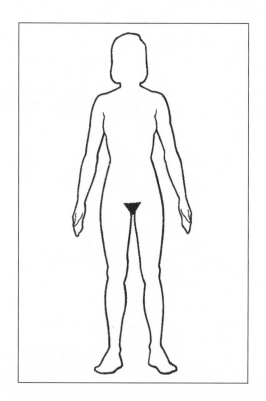

Malignant tumors of the vulva account for 3 to 5 percent of all cancers of the female genital tract and are usually cured when diagnosed at an early stage. Generally, because of better access to routine gynecologic care, these cancers are being diagnosed at an earlier stage.

Surgery has long been the mainstay of treatment, but views about the extent of surgery have changed over the years. In the 1940s, it was noted that the failure rate was much higher with conservative surgical measures. Since then, more radical operations have been performed with

a marked improvement in the survival rate. Now, however, as younger women with earlier disease are diagnosed with vulvar cancer, there has been a trend toward more conservative surgery with a greater emphasis on limiting the psychosexual consequences of therapy and preserving the normal female genital anatomy. Similarly, there has been a recent trend toward using local radiation therapy with chemotherapy in advanced cases either to reduce the amount of surgery needed or to improve the chance that the tumor can be surgically removed.

Types Squamous cell carcinomas account for about 86 percent of all vulvar malignancies. Melanomas account for another 6 percent, carcinomas of the Bartholin's gland for 4 percent, sarcomas for 2 percent, basal cell carcinomas for 2 percent, and Paget's disease for 0.5 percent of all vulvar cancers.

Some physicians believe that the grade of the tumor cells as seen under the microscope is also significant. Immature, or undifferentiated, cancers are more virulent and aggressive. Grade 1 (mature, or well-differentiated) cancers have a better prognosis than grade 3 (poorly differentiated) tumors.

How It Spreads Squamous cell carcinoma arises in the skin of the genitalia and stays confined to the skin for an estimated one to ten years. (At this stage, it is referred to as a carcinoma in situ, vulvar intraepithelial neoplasia [VIN], or vulvar squamous intraepithelial lesion [SIL]). Eventually, it becomes invasive. With time, it becomes locally destructive, growing to involve the urethra, vagina, and anus. It can also spread through the lymphatic system to the lymph nodes in the groin and then to the lymph nodes in the pelvis. Distant metastases, most frequently to the lungs and liver, are relatively rare (see the chapter "Cervix").

What Causes It Like carcinoma of the cervix, the risk factors for the development of vulvar cancer are primarily related to the likelihood of exposure to the sexually transmitted high-risk group of human papillomavirus (HPV). Both preinvasive and invasive vulvar cancers may be prevented in the future with a vaccination for HPV.

Risk Factors

• The majority of women with invasive vulvar carcinoma are postmenopausal. But there has been a definite trend over the past two decades of an increasing incidence of carcinoma in situ and cancer in younger women. Forty percent of women with carcinoma in situ are under forty years of age.

• Five to ten percent of women with invasive vulvar carcinoma have a history of genital warts, while 15 percent have a history of, or a subsequent diagnosis of, preinvasive (carcinoma in situ) or invasive carcinoma of the cervix.

• Over 90 percent of the invasive squamous lesions of the vulva are associated with the high-risk group of human papillomavirus (types 16 and 18).

• Other sexually transmitted diseases such as syphilis, lymphogranuloma vernerum, and herpes simplex virus II may also increase the risk for vulvar carcinoma.

• There is a higher incidence in women from lower socioeconomic groups, women with multiple partners, and women with a history of infectious vulvitis or a history of vulvar dystrophy (abnormal benign or premalignant skin changes).

Screening

Careful visual and manual inspection of the external genitalia during an annual gynecologic examination is important. Women with a diagnosis of an HPV-related infection of any portion of the lower genital tract should undergo a careful colposcopic (magnification) examination of the entire lower genital tract.

Common Signs and Symptoms

The most common signs and symptoms are a lump or an ulcer, itching, pain, burning, bleeding, discharge, and pain or burning with urination. Unfortunately, many women do not get early medical attention when these signs appear. At the time of the diagnosis, two out of three women with vulvar carcinoma have had symptoms for more than six months and one out of three has had symptoms for more than a year.

Diagnosis

Physical Examination

• Careful visual and manual inspection of the external genitalia, the anus, and the groin lymph nodes is crucial.

• Because of the association with precancerous and cancerous lesions of the cervix and vagina, a careful pelvic examination is also necessary.

• The majority of squamous cell carcinomas arise in the labia majora and minora. The clitoris, urethral opening, vulvar opening (introitus), outer vagina, and the skin between the vagina and the anus (perineum) may also be involved.

Endoscopy and Biopsy

• The definitive diagnosis is made on a biopsy, sometimes under colposcopic direction (magnification) for smaller lesions.

• Upon diagnosis, a metastatic work-up is done, including a chest X-ray, a complete blood count and serum and liver function tests, and CT scan of the pelvis and abdomen. Cystoscopy and proctoscopy, a PET/CT scan, or an MRI scan may also be recommended for advanced cancer. A serum CEA and squamous cell antigen may be elevated in some women.

Staging

Staging is based on physical findings, imaging, and pathology. Both the FIGO (International Federation of Gynecology and Obstetrics) and the TNM classifications are used to stage vulvar cancer.

Treatment Overview

The prognosis for vulvar cancer depends on several factors: (1) the extent of cancer (stage), (2) the size of the lesion, (3) the presence or absence of groin node metastases, (4) the depth of invasion, (5) whether the blood or lymphatic vessels are involved, and (6) the grade of the tumor and the pattern of invasion.

At diagnosis, about 35 percent of all vulvar carcinomas are Stage I, 30 percent of women have Stage II, 25 percent have Stage III, and 10 percent have Stage IV disease. The overall five-year survival rate for all women with invasive squamous cell carcinoma of the vulva is 70 percent.

Surgery The standard therapy for the past four decades has been radical surgical excision of the vulva and the removal of the lymph nodes in the groin and, occasionally, the pelvis. External-beam radiation therapy is frequently given to the groin and pelvis after surgery to women with positive groin and/or pelvic lymph nodes on one or both sides.

Over the past twenty years, less radical surgery and the removal of the groin nodes on one side has been shown to be equally effective in small, early-stage disease. Despite this trend toward conservative therapy, experience has taught that limiting surgery because of advanced age or frailty can result in overwhelming problems with locally advanced, persistent, or recurrent cancer in women who live longer than expected.

A radical vulvectomy and groin dissection is extraordinarily well tolerated and can be done in phases if the patient's medical condition warrants. Sexual function is also surprisingly more satisfactory than one would think and depends on the extent of surgery and the use of radiation therapy.

Complications of radical surgery for vulvar cancer include wound breakdown or infection, chronic leg swelling, collection of lymphatic fluid in the groin (lymphocyst), scarring of the vaginal opening, vaginal or uterine prolapse, loss of urine when coughing (stress incontinence), blood clots in the leg that can dislodge and go to the lung (pulmonary embolism, approximately 1 to 3 percent of women), and death (approximately 1 percent). Complications can be reduced with prophylactic antibiotics, compression stockings, wound drains, and early ambulation.

Chemotherapy and Radiotherapy In recent years, chemotherapy has been used in combination with local external-beam radiation therapy and occasionally with interstitial radiation, in which radioactive material is temporarily placed directly in the cancer. This treatment is reserved for women with advanced cancers. Occasionally, it may be given prior to surgical removal of the tumor, often allowing preservation of the bladder or anus.

Currently, there is no standard chemotherapy for advanced or recurrent cancer, but drugs that are sometimes effective for other squamous cell carcinomas of the genital tract—such as cisplatin (Platinol), mitomycin (Mutamycin), 5-fluorouracil (5-FU), carboplatin (Paraplatin), ifosfamide (Ifex), cyclophosphamide (Cytoxan), and bleomycin (Blenoxane)—have been used with some success.

Treatment by Stage

■ Stage 0
TNM Tis, N0, M0
Vulvar carcinoma in situ, also known as vulvar intraepithelial neoplasia III or high-grade SIL.

Standard Treatment Standard therapy has been either wide local excision, partial vulvectomy, or laser vaporization. Occasionally, a total vulvectomy is performed with or without skin grafting for very extensive disease. A topical cream containing 5 percent 5-fluorouracil is sometimes used as primary treatment or to prevent recurrences.

Five-Year Survival 100 percent

■ Stages IA and IB
TNM T1, N0, M0
(Stage IA)
The tumor is confined to the vulva or perineum, it is less than ¾ inch (2 cm) in diameter, and there is less than 1 mm invasion.

TNM T1, N0, M0
(Stage IB)
The tumor is confined to the vulva or perineum, it is less than ¾ inch (2 cm) in diameter, and there is stroma invasion greater than 1 mm. There are no nodal metastases.

Standard Treatment For Stage IA lesions with less than 1 mm of invasion and no vascular involvement, a wide local excision is adequate therapy.

For lesions with deeper invasion (Stage IB) that are clearly on one side of the vulva, a radical local excision (partial radical vulvectomy) with a complete groin node dissection on the same side is performed.

For other Stage I cancers involving the skin between the vaginal opening and the anus or clitoris, a radical vulvectomy and groin lymph node dissection on both sides may be performed.

Five-Year Survival Over 90 percent

Investigational
• Conservative surgery
• Treatment with radiation therapy with or without chemotherapy (5-FU + cisplatin [Platinol])
• Treatment with chemotherapy for high-risk factors: positive groin nodes, microscopic vessel involvement

■ Stage II
TNM T2, N0, M0
The tumor is confined to the vulva and/or perineum and is more than ¾ inch (2 cm) in diameter but has not spread to lymph nodes.

Standard Treatment Radical vulvectomy with removal of the groin lymph nodes on one or both sides depending on location.

Five-Year Survival 80 percent; up to 90 percent for those patients with surgically negative groin nodes

Investigational Same as for Stages IA and IB.

■ Stage III
TNM T3 (or less), N1 (or less), M0
The tumor may be of any size with either adjacent spread to the vagina, urethra, or anus or metastases to the groin lymph nodes on one side.

Standard Treatment Radical vulvectomy with groin lymph node dissection on both sides is the standard therapy. Sometimes, a pelvic lymph node dissection is done at the time of surgery if the groin lymph nodes are positive.

External-beam radiation therapy is frequently given postoperatively to the groin and pelvis if there are groin lymph node metastases. With two or more pathologically positive groin nodes, there has been a significantly better survival rate with pelvic radiation than with pelvic lymph node dissection in a study conducted by the Gynecologic Oncology Group.

Women with large vulvar lesions who have only a small margin of normal tissue around the tumor on microscopic examination of the surgical specimen may be treated with postoperative external-beam radiation therapy to the remaining genital skin.

Five-Year Survival About 50 percent

Investigational
• Radiation therapy given concurrently with chemotherapy has been used to improve resectability and to decrease the amount of surgery necessary in women with large cancers or cancers involving the urethra or anus.
• Preoperative external-beam and interstitial radiation therapy (radioactive substances inserted directly into the tumor for one to two days) with or without chemotherapy (cisplatin [Platinol], cisplatin + 5-FU).
• Treatment with cisplatin + 5-FU for high-risk factors: positive groin nodes, microscopic vessel involvement, close margins, large tumors.

■ *Stage IVA*
TNM Any T, N2, M0 or T4, N0, M0
The tumor may involve the upper urethra, the bladder mucosa, the rectal mucosa, or the pelvic bone, and/or there are bilateral groin node metastases.

Standard Treatment Options include

• radical vulvectomy, removal of the lymph nodes on both sides, and removal of the vagina, bladder, and/or rectum (pelvic exenteration);
• radical surgery followed by radiation therapy in those with close surgical margins; and
• radiation therapy with combination chemotherapy (5-FU + cisplatin [Platinol], 5-FU + mitomycin [Mutamycin] + cisplatin, cisplatin + ifosfamide [Ifex]) or cisplatin alone, followed by radical surgery.

Five-Year Survival About 15 percent

Investigational External-beam radiation therapy and interstitial radiation therapy with or without various doses of chemotherapeutic drugs are being evaluated.

■ *Stage IVB*
TNM Any T, any N, M1a or M1b
There are distant metastases to other organs, including pelvic lymph nodes.

Standard Treatment Vulvar cancer that has spread to distant sites is treated with chemotherapy, but at present there is no standard chemotherapeutic regimen. Cisplatin (Platinol), carboplatin (Paraplatin), paclitaxel (Taxol), ifosfamide (Ifex), doxorubicin (Adriamycin), cyclophosphamide (Cytoxan), 5-fluorouracil (5-FU), etoposide (Etopophos), methotrexate (Mexate, Amethopterin, Folex), vincristine (Oncovin), and bleomycin (Blenoxane) are commonly used in various doses and combinations.

Palliative local surgical removal or radiation therapy to the vulva may be performed for local symptom relief.

Women with metastases to the pelvic nodes are treated with pelvic external-beam radiation therapy and chemotherapy given concurrently.

Five-Year Survival From 5 percent (metastases to the lungs or liver) to 25 percent (metastases to the pelvic lymph nodes)

Investigational

• Cisplatin (Platinol), carboplatin (Paraplatin), other platinum analogues, ifosfamide (Ifex), doxorubicin (Adriamycin), 5-fluorouracil (5-FU), mitomycin (Mutamycin), methotrexate (Mexate, Amethopterin, Folex), vincristine (Oncovin), bleomycin (Blenoxane), paclitaxel (Taxol), and topotecan (Hycamtin), in various combinations and doses, are being investigated.

Treating Other Vulva Malignancies

Malignant Melanoma of the Vulva

Although relatively rare, this is the second most common type of vulvar cancer. It occurs most commonly in women around the age of menopause and in postmenopausal women.

More than 80 percent of melanomas arise from the labia minora and clitoris. Most women seek medical attention because of itching, bleeding, or a lump. Superficially spreading melanomas and mucocutaneous melanomas account for approximately 60 percent and 10 percent respectively of all vulvar melanomas and are somewhat slow growing until invasion occurs. Thirty percent are nodular melanomas, which behave much more aggressively.

Standard Treatment Radical vulvectomy and bilateral groin node dissection is the standard therapy, although over the past few years, there has been a trend toward more conservative surgery.

Melanomas that are less than 0.7 mm in thickness without vascular space involvement can be treated by a wide local excision with a ¾ inch (2 cm) skin margin, without a groin dissection.

The role of a pelvic lymph node dissection has not been determined, but if the groin nodes are involved, a pelvic lymph node dissection may be performed. The prognosis and survival is determined in large part by the depth of invasion and whether there are metastases.

Five-Year Survival 40 to 80 percent, depending on the stage and depth of invasion

Basal Cell Carcinoma

This type of vulvar cancer invades adjacent tissues but rarely metastasizes. It has an excellent cure rate and is managed with only a wide local excision.

Adenocarcinoma of the Vulva

This is a rare tumor and generally arises from the Bartholin's gland, located at the opening of the vagina. Survival is related to stage. Treatment is similar to that for squamous cell cancers of the vulva.

Paget's Disease

This occurs most commonly in postmenopausal Caucasian women. Intense itching is the most common symptom. They are frequently misdiagnosed as having a severe yeast infection.

About 30 percent of cases of Paget's disease are associated with an underlying invasive adenocarcinoma, and for these, the prognosis is quite poor. Paget's disease confined to the vulvar skin (Stage 0) has an excellent prognosis, with only rare instances of subsequent invasion or death.

If there is no underlying adenocarcinoma, a wide local excision or total vulvectomy is all that is required.

If there is an underlying adenocarcinoma, management is similar to that of other vulvar cancers.

Vulvar Sarcomas

This tumor accounts for only 1 to 2 percent of all vulvar malignancies. The majority of vulvar sarcomas arise from the smooth muscle and are known as leiomyosarcomas.

Treatment is usually radical surgery sometimes followed by radiation therapy.

Treatment Follow-Up

After therapy, most women are followed at three-month intervals with a careful physical examination, X-ray studies if symptoms warrant, and a serum CEA or squamous cell carcinoma antigen if elevated prior to treatment.

Recurrent Cancer

Recurrences are more common in women with large lesions or with positive nodes. They usually occur within the first three years after treatment. The recurrence may be anywhere on the remaining external genitalia (10 percent), in the groin or pelvic nodes, or at distant sites. Symptoms of recurrent cancer may include bleeding; discharge; pain in the genitals, groin, pelvis, or legs; leg swelling (edema); weight loss; chronic cough; and chest pain.

Treatment options include radical local excision (for a local recurrence), pelvic exenteration (removal of vulva, vagina, bladder, rectum), external-beam radiation therapy, interstitial radiation therapy, and chemotherapy.

The Most Important Questions You Can Ask

• What type of cancer do I have?

• Is a radical vulvectomy and removal of the groin lymph nodes on both sides necessary if I have Stage I disease?

• Is there a role for radiation therapy, with or without chemotherapy, for my cancer?

• What is my prognosis?

• What qualifications do you have for treating cancer? Will a gynecologic oncologist be involved in my care?

Glossary of Medical Terms

Malin Dollinger, M.D.

■ ■ ■ ■

A

Absolute neutrophil count (ANC) The actual count of the white blood cells (also called polys or granulocytes) that engulf and destroy bacteria. There is some concern about infection if the count is less than 1,000.

Acupressure The use of finger pressure over various points on the body (the same points used in acupuncture) to treat symptoms or disease.

Acupuncture A technique of inserting thin needles through the skin at specific points, to control pain and other symptoms.

Adenocarcinoma Cancer that arises from glandular tissues. Examples include cancers of the breast, lung, thyroid, colon, and pancreas.

Adenoma A benign (nonmalignant) tumor that arises from glandular tissues, such as the breast, lung, thyroid, colon, and pancreas.

Adjuvant chemotherapy Chemotherapy used along with surgery or radiation therapy. It is usually given after all visible and known cancer has been removed by surgery or radiotherapy. Adjuvant chemotherapy is usually used in cases where there is a high risk of hidden cancer cells remaining and may increase the likelihood of cure by destroying small amounts of undetectable cancer. Also see *Neoadjuvant chemotherapy.*

Agonists Drugs that cause a response in a cell or from another drug.

Alkaline phosphatase A blood enzyme commonly used in medical diagnosis. It is elevated in cases of bile obstruction (liver disease or cancer involving the liver) and in various bone diseases, including cancer involving bone. A variation of this test can distinguish between elevations due to bone and liver disease.

Alkylating agents A family of anticancer drugs that combine with a cancer cell's DNA to prevent normal cell division.

Allogeneic transplant A form of transplantation or transfer of a tissue—bone marrow, for example—from one individual to another. It is preferable that the tissue types match, but this is not always possible.

Allopurinol A drug that lowers the uric acid level to prevent gout and kidney damage resulting from tissue breakdown during chemotherapy (also called Zyloprim).

Alopecia Partial or complete loss of hair. This may result from radiotherapy to the head (hair may not completely return after therapy) or from certain chemotherapeutic agents (hair always returns).

Alpha-fetoprotein A protein that is elevated in the blood of patients with certain forms of cancer, such as liver and testis.

Alternative medicine Practices in addition to standard or conventional treatments, such as dietary supplements, herbs, megadose vitamins, enemas, special/unusual diets, spiritual healing, visualization, meditation, magnet therapy, and massage.

Ambulatory care The use of outpatient facilities—doctors' offices, home-care outpatient hospital clinics, and day-care facilities—to provide modern medical care without the need for hospitalization.

Ambulatory infusion The administration of chemotherapy by a small pump device usually worn under the clothes. The pump delivers anticancer drugs slowly and gradually. Since there is no need to remain in the hospital or even at home, this method allows patients to work and carry on with their normal activities.

Amenorrhea The temporary or permanent lack of menstrual periods. This may be a normal part of menopause or is sometimes brought on by severe physical or emotional stress. Some anticancer drugs can produce amenorrhea, especially if the woman is near the age when menopause would normally occur.

Amino acids The building blocks of proteins, analogous to the freight cars making up a train.

Analgesic A drug that relieves pain. Analgesics may be mild (aspirin or acetaminophen), stronger (codeine), or very strong (morphine). There are also a large number of mild, moderate, or strong synthetic analgesics.

Anaplastic A tumor that appears "wild" under a microscope, having no resemblance to the normal tissue of the organ involved. It is usually possible to tell where anaplastic tumors originate only by where the biopsy was taken or, knowing the area of involvement, by inference.

Anastomosis The point where two organs are joined together. In cancer therapy, it usually refers to joining two portions of the bowel after a segment containing cancer has been removed.

Androgens Male sex hormones. Testosterone is produced naturally, and several synthetic ones are used in treatment.

Anemia Having less than the normal amount of hemoglobin or red cells in the blood. This may be due to bleeding, to lack of blood production by the bone marrow, or to the brief survival of blood already manufactured. Symptoms include tiredness, shortness of breath, and weakness.

Aneuploid Tumor cells that do not have the normal number of chromosomes—forty-six—found in a human cell. Tumor cells that do have forty-six chromosomes are called euploid. Aneuploid tumors often have a worse prognosis.

Angiogenesis The growth of new blood vessels. This may be stimulated by certain chemicals produced by cancers and may be a requirement for cancers to spread. New treatments have been and are being developed to prevent this new blood vessel formation, such as the monoclonal antibody bevacizumab (Avastin).

Angiography The taking of X-ray pictures of blood vessels by injecting a radio-opaque contrast agent into the blood vessel. Angiograms may be taken to determine a tumor's blood supply before surgery, to place a catheter or infusion pump, or to determine the site for other intra-arterial procedures.

Anorexia Loss of appetite.

Antibody A protein made by white blood cells in response to a specific foreign protein, or antigen. The antigen may result from an infection, a cancer, or some other source. The antibody binds to the specific antigen to help destroy it. Antibodies against specific antigens are now being produced by companies for therapeutic purposes, including to treat certain types of cancers; examples of such antibodies include trastuzumab (Herceptin), cetuximab (Erbitux), and bevacizumab (Avastin).

Antiemetics Drugs given to prevent or minimize nausea and vomiting.

Antigens Substances that cause activation of the immune system.

Antimetabolites A family of antitumor drugs that resemble normal vitamins or building blocks of metabolism. They bind to the tumor's enzymes and chemical pathways. The tumor cells "think" they are getting the real vitamin or building block and starve to the point where they can't grow or multiply.

Apoptosis The programming of cells in the body to become old and die at the correct time. This vital feature of healthy human cells allows for replacement of tissues as needed. Cancer cells may persist because they may escape apoptosis. Some new methods of therapy are being studied to reprogram cancer cells to learn to die again.

Arteriogram An X-ray picture of arteries, especially inside a tumor, usually to facilitate surgery or to plan treatment involving injection of drugs or solid materials into the arteries.

Asbestosis Scarring of the lungs and the lining of the chest cavity from the inhalation of asbestos dust. This increases the risk of lung cancer and cancer of the chest cavity lining (mesothelioma).

Ascites An abnormal fluid collection in the abdomen from cancer or other causes.

Aspiration Removal of fluid or tissue, usually with a needle or tube, from a specific area of the body. This procedure may be done to obtain a diagnosis or to relieve symptoms.

Atrophy A withering or reduction in size of a tissue or a part of the body. This may result from lack of use during immobilization or prolonged bed rest or from pressure from an adjacent tumor.

Atypical Not usual or ordinary. For example, cancer is the result of atypical cell division.

Atypical hyperplasia A benign pattern of cells under the microscope, where the cells have abnormal features and are increased in number. It is not cancer.

Autoimmunity A condition in which the body's immune system fights and rejects its own tissues.

Autologous transplant Removal of a patient's own tissue, especially bone marrow, and its return to the same patient after chemotherapy. This might more correctly be called bone marrow reinfusion, or protection, rather than transplantation.

Autolymphocyte therapy A form of outpatient immunotherapy being tested, especially in kidney cancer, that involves readministering a patient's lymphocytes after they have been stimulated by a lymphokine (a substance that stimulates immunity) mixture. This is a form of "adoptive immunotherapy," in which the aim is to transfer to patients their own stimulated antitumor effector cells.

Autosomal A non-sex-linked method of inheritance. The inherited characteristic does not depend on whether the person is male or female, since the gene in question is not found on the sex (X or Y) chromosomes. A dominant gene requires that only one copy (allele) be present to be expressed (e.g., brown eyes). A recessive gene requires that two copies be present to be expressed (e.g., blue eyes).

Axilla The armpit. Lymph glands in the armpit are called the axillary nodes.

B

Barium enema An X-ray study of the colon (large bowel) in which the patient is given an enema of a liquid barium mixture before the X-rays are taken. Laxatives and/or regular enemas are usually required beforehand.

Barium swallow An X-ray study of the portion of the digestive canal between the throat and stomach (esophagus) in which the patient swallows a barium mixture while the radiologist watches for signs of narrowing, irregularity, or blockage. No preparation is required except fasting. Sometimes, in a procedure called an upper gastrointestinal (UGI) series, the barium is also observed after it enters the stomach to check for stomach problems or ulcers.

B cell Lymphocytes are the cells in the body that are intimately involved in the immune response. They occur in the blood, in lymph nodes, and in various organs. The two types of lymphocytes are B cells and T cells. Special techniques are needed to tell them apart because they look the same when viewed by ordinary methods under a microscope. It may be essential to make this distinction in cases of lymphomas, since the treatment and prognosis of B cell lymphomas may be very different from that of T cell lymphomas.

BCG A material prepared from killed bird tuberculosis bacteria. This has been widely used, especially in Europe, to vaccinate health care workers who work closely with tuberculosis patients and has been used in cancer treatment to stimulate the immune system.

Bench surgery Complete removal of a selected organ or tissue from the body during surgery in order to perform a separate, often delicate or complex, surgical procedure. The organ is then replaced in the body (usually in its original site, although sometimes the location is changed). Bench surgery can allow (1) better control for removal of a tumor, particularly in a vital organ that cannot or does not have to be totally sacrificed; (2) delicate surgery often requiring a microscope; (3) delineation of margins of resection to ensure a tumor is fully excised or to lessen spilling of cancer cells into the surrounding tissue or cavity, such as the peritoneum; and (4) cooling the organ to permit more time for surgery. A good example of bench surgery is in the treatment of kidney cancer, especially when it occurs in a patient with only one kidney or with borderline renal failure, and when the tumor is located in the center of the kidney. Blood vessels are disconnected temporarily, the kidney is completely removed to a separate operating table (bench), the tumor is removed with repair to the kidney, and then the kidney is replaced in the body.

Benign A tumor that has no tendency to grow into surrounding tissues or spread to other parts of the body. In other words, it is not malignant. Under a microscope, a benign tumor does not resemble cancer.

Benign prostatic hypertrophy (BPH) A very common benign overgrowth of prostate tissue, especially in older men, which may cause difficulty or blockage of urine flow. It is not a risk factor for prostate cancer but may cause mild elevations in PSA, which may require evaluation.

Bilateral Occurring on both sides of the body.

Biologic response modifiers Substances and agents that may have a direct antitumor effect and that also affect tumors indirectly by stimulating or triggering the immune system to fight cancer. Examples include interferon, IL-2, and LAK cells.

Biological therapy Certain complex substances produced within the body regulate cell growth and immunity. Biological therapy, which includes immunotherapy, is the use of these same substances to treat cancer. They may be produced in the laboratory or a production facility, or the person with cancer may be given drugs that stimulate the production of these substances.

Biopsy The surgical removal of a small portion of tissue for diagnosis. In almost all cases, a biopsy diagnosis of cancer is required before appropriate and correct treatment planning can take place. In some cases, a needle biopsy may be enough for diagnosis, but in others the removal of a pea-sized wedge of tissue is needed. In many cases, the biopsy may be the first step of the definitive surgical procedure that not only proves the diagnosis but attempts to cure the cancer by completely removing the tumor.

Blastic A bone lesion that appears on an X-ray to have more calcium (density) than normal.

Bleeding disorders Blood clotting is a complex process involving the interaction of many substances in the blood that promote coagulation. A deficiency of any of these substances results in a bleeding disorder. Some disorders are inherited (hemophilia, for example) and some are acquired (such as liver disease). A common disorder associated with cancer is a low platelet count (thrombocytopenia), which sometimes results from chemotherapy or radiotherapy and may make platelet transfusions necessary until the process subsides. Sophisticated tests are often needed to diagnose bleeding disorders.

Blood-brain barrier A microscopic structure in the brain that separates blood capillaries from nerve cells. This prevents some substances from entering the brain. Many cancer chemotherapeutic agents, for example, cannot be used to treat brain tumors because they cannot pass through the barrier. Some others (lomustine [CCNU], carmustine [BCNU]) are designed to penetrate it. There are techniques that can eliminate the barrier temporarily to allow the use of other antitumor drugs.

Blood cells The red cells, white cells, and platelets that make up the blood. They are made in the bone marrow.

Blood chemistry panel Multiple chemical analyses prepared by an automatic

apparatus from a single blood sample. These panels often include measurements of electrolytes (minerals) and proteins as well as tests of liver, kidney, and thyroid function. The advantages of panels include less cost and greater accuracy and speed, with results often available the same or the following day.

Bolus (or "push") chemotherapy Administration of intravenous chemotherapy over a short time, usually five minutes or less. The other method is called infusion chemotherapy, which may last from fifteen minutes to several hours or days.

Bone marrow A soft substance found within bone cavities. Marrow is composed of developing red cells, white cells, platelets, and fat. Some forms of cancer can be diagnosed by examining bone marrow.

Bone marrow examination The process of removing bone marrow by withdrawing it through a needle for pathological examination. It is usually withdrawn from the breastbone (sternum) or the hipbone. Both these bones are just under the skin, making the removal of marrow easy, safe, and only momentarily uncomfortable with a local anesthetic. The procedure takes about 10 minutes—9½ minutes for the anesthetic to take effect and 30 seconds for the actual procedure.

Bone marrow suppression A decrease in one or more of the blood counts. This condition can be caused by chemotherapy, radiation, disease, or various medications.

Bone marrow transplant Administration of bone marrow (one's own [autologous] or another person's [allogeneic]) into a patient who has been pretreated with high-dose chemotherapy and/or radiation therapy. Could also be termed *bone marrow protection*. (See also *stem cells/stem cell transplantation*.)

Bone scan A picture of all of the bones in the body taken about two hours after injection of a radioactive tracer. "Hot spots" indicate areas of bone abnormality that may indicate tumors, although they can also be due to another cause such as arthritis. No preparation is required and the test is easy. The main problem is lying still on a hard table for fifteen minutes. This test can help determine if cancer has spread to the bones, if therapy is working, and if damaged bony areas are healing.

Brachytherapy The use of a radioactive "seeds" implanted directly into a tumor. This allows a very high but sharply localized dose of radiation to be given to a tumor while sparing surrounding tissues from significant radiation exposure.

Brain scan (radionuclide) A picture of the brain taken after the intravenous injection of a radioactive tracer. CT and MRI scans have in most cases replaced such brain scans, since CT and MRI tend to discover smaller lesions and are more useful for following up the effects of therapy.

BRCA1; BRCA2 A gene that normally helps to suppress cell growth. If an altered version is inherited, there is an increased risk of breast, ovarian, or prostate cancer.

Bronchogenic carcinoma Carcinoma of the lung.

Bronchoscopy Inspection—and often biopsy—of the breathing tubes (bronchi) going to the lungs by means of a long tube inserted through the mouth or nose. The instrument usually used is a fiber-optic bronchoscope that is flexible and allows excellent visualization around corners. The procedure is often done on an outpatient basis after local anesthesia and sedation.

Bypass A surgical procedure to "go around" an organ or area affected by cancer and allow normal flow or drainage to continue. In cancer of the pancreas, for example, the bile ducts may be blocked. A bypass procedure will allow the bile to drain into the small bowel, as it should.

C

Cachexia The wasting away of the body, often due to malnutrition, disease, or cancer.

Calcium An important body mineral that is a vital component of bone. The calcium level may be elevated if tumors involve bone.

Cancer of an unknown primary site (CUPS) When cancer is found in a different place from where the cancer started, and the primary place or origin cannot be found.

Candidiasis; moniliasis A common fungal infection often seen as white patches on the tongue or the inside of the mouth.

Carcinogenesis The development or production of cancer.

Carcinoma A form of cancer that develops in the tissues covering or lining organs of the body such as the skin, uterus, lung, or breast (epithelial tissues). Eighty to 90 percent of all cancers are carcinomas.

Carcinoma in situ The earliest stage of cancer, in which the tumor is still confined to the local area, before it has grown to a significant size or has spread. In situ carcinomas are highly curable.

Cardiomyopathy A condition in which the heart muscle is diseased. It may develop because of the toxic effect of a few anticancer drugs.

CAT scan See *CT scan*.

Catheter A flexible tube made of rubber, plastic, or metal that can be inserted in a body cavity such as the bladder to drain fluid or to deliver fluids or medication.

Catheterization The process of introducing a catheter. The term is also used when a tube is placed in an artery or a vein to take X-rays.

CEA (carcinoembryonic antigen) A "tumor marker" in the blood that may indicate the presence of cancer. It may be elevated in some cancers, especially of the breast, bowel, and lung. By monitoring the amount of CEA, doctors can detect the presence of these cancers and assess the progress of treatment.

Cell cycle Each cell in the body, including a cancer cell, goes through several stages every time it divides. Various anticancer drugs affect the cell at certain stages of this cell cycle.

Cell cycle specific Chemotherapeutic drugs that kill only cells that are dividing rather than resting.

Cell surface markers Special proteins on the surface or edge of cells that can be used to identify them or their characteristics.

Cells The fundamental units, or building blocks, of human tissues.

Cellular immunity Immunity brought about by the action of immune cells such as lymphocytes.

Cellulitis Inflammation of the skin and underlying tissues.

Centigray (cGy) A unit of measurement of radiation therapy that is replacing the older term *rads*.

Central venous catheter (central line) A special IV tube surgically inserted into a large vein near the heart. It may exit through the skin or end in a reservoir under the skin. It is used to give chemotherapy, medication, fluids, and blood products (examples: Hickman, Broviac, Groshong). See also *Port*.

Central nervous system The brain and spinal cord.

Cerebrospinal fluid (CSF) The watery fluid around the brain and spinal cord. Samples may be removed by a "spinal tap" (lumbar puncture) to check for cancer cells, or anticancer drugs may be injected into the cerebrospinal fluid.

Cervical dysplasia The presence of abnormal—and possibly precancerous—cells in the mouth of the uterus (cervix).

Cervical (lymph) nodes The lymph nodes in the neck.

Cervix The lower portion of the uterus, which protrudes into the vagina and forms a portion of the birth canal during delivery. The Pap smear test is designed to check this area for cancer.

Chemoembolization Administration of anticancer drugs directly into the artery supplying a tumor. Usually the blood supply to the tumor is blocked. This concentrates the effect of the drug in the area of the tumor.

Chemoprevention Attempting to prevent cancer through drugs, chemicals, vitamins, or minerals.

Chemosensitivity assay Testing of tumor cells in the laboratory to see which chemotherapy drugs or combinations may be able to stop their growth.

Chemotherapy The treatment of cancer by chemicals (drugs) designed to kill cancer cells or stop them from growing.

Chromosomes The fundamental strands of genetic material (DNA) that carry all of our genes. There are twenty-three pairs in each cell. Tumor cells sometimes have more or fewer than twenty-three pairs. (See *Aneuploid*.)

Clinical Refers to the treatment of humans, as opposed to animals or laboratory studies. Also refers to the general use of a treatment by a practicing physician, as opposed to research done in cancer research centers ("preclinical").

Clinical trials The procedures in which new cancer treatments are tested in humans. Clinical trials are conducted after experiments in animals and preliminary studies in humans have shown that a new treatment method might be effective.

Clone A strain of cells—whether normal or malignant—derived from a single original cell.

Clonigenic assay A test done by growing tumor cells in the laboratory and identifying which chemotherapy agents will prevent their growth. This information is sometimes useful in deciding which drugs to use or not to use in treatment.

Cobalt; cobalt treatment A radiotherapy machine using gamma rays generated from the radioisotope cobalt 60.

Coin lesion A single "spot" on a chest X-ray that may be a tumor, infection, or other lesion. Given this name because it resembles the shadow of a coin.

Colonoscopy A procedure to inspect the rectum and colon by means of a long fiber-optic telescope that is lighted and flexible. Biopsy specimens of suspicious tissue can also be obtained. (See also *Sigmoidoscopy.*)

Colony-stimulating factor (CSF) A substance that stimulates the growth of bone marrow cells. Current clinical trials are using CSF to try to increase the dosage of chemotherapy that can be given safely.

Colostomy An artificial opening in the abdominal wall created so that feces drains from the colon into a bag. A colostomy is sometimes necessary after the removal of a diseased section of the large intestine, and can be either temporary or permanent. (See *Ostomy.*)

Colposcopy A way to detect small lesions by inspecting the cervix with special binocular magnifying instruments after applying a solution to stain cancer tissue.

Combination chemotherapy The use of several anticancer drugs at the same time. Most chemotherapy is now given this way, since it is a much more effective method.

Combined modality therapy Treatment with two or more types of therapy—surgery, radiotherapy, chemotherapy, and biological therapy. These may be used at the same time or one after the other. Surgery, for example, is often followed by chemotherapy to destroy random cancer cells that may have spread from the original site.

Computerized tomography See *CT scan.*

Cone biopsy Removal of a ring of tissue from the opening of the cervix.

Congestive heart failure Weakness of the heart muscle usually due to heart disease, but sometimes due to other causes, causing a buildup of fluid in body tissues.

Conscious sedation An altered state of consciousness, induced by certain pain relievers and sedatives, that minimizes pain and discomfort while usually still allowing the subject to speak and respond to questions during a procedure. Examples of such procedures include breast biopsy, upper gastrointestinal endoscopy, and colonoscopy. Patients usually cannot remember the procedure afterward.

Consolidation A second round of chemotherapy to further reduce the number of cancer cells.

Continuous infusion Administration of chemotherapy drugs (or other agents) by needle or catheter over a prolonged period of time.

Contralateral On the opposite side of the body. In cancer therapy, it refers to a tumor or a site of disease. (See also *Ipsilateral.*)

Control group The group of persons in the arm of a randomized clinical trial that receives the standard treatment or receives no treatment.

Cooperative group Clinical trials of new cancer treatments require many patients, generally more than any single physician or hospital can see. A number of physicians and/or hospitals form a cooperative group to treat a large number of patients in the same way so that the effectiveness of a new treatment can be evaluated quickly.

Core biopsy Removal of a small core of tissue, via a special needle, without surgery.

Cortisone A natural hormone produced by the adrenal glands. The term is also loosely used to designate synthetic forms of the hormone (for example, prednisone) that are used to treat inflammatory conditions and diseases, including certain cancers.

Cranial irradiation The delivery of radiation to the brain to treat brain tumors.

Creatinine clearance A sensitive test of kidney function that requires a twenty-four-hour urine sample and a blood sample. The test is often required to make sure it is safe to give anticancer drugs that may be toxic to the kidneys.

Cruciferous vegetables Vegetables such as cauliflower and brussels sprouts that are high in beta-carotene and are thought to help protect against colon cancer.

Cryotherapy; cryosurgery The use of an extremely cold probe as a surgical instrument to freeze areas of cancer, killing the cancer cells. The process usually involves several episodes of freezing and thawing, and is carefully controlled with temperature probes to avoid damage to surrounding healthy tissue.

CT scan A CT (computerized tomography) scan creates cross-sectional images of the body, which may show cancer or metastases earlier and more accurately than other imaging methods. This type of X-ray machine has revolutionized the diagnosis of cancer and other diseases.

Curettage Removal of tissue with a curette, a small "scraper" that looks like a spoon.

Cushing's syndrome A condition characterized by swelling of the face and back of the neck and purple lines over the abdomen. It results from an excess of cortisone or hydrocortisone caused either by disease or by the administration of these substances or their synthetic derivatives.

Cyst A fluid-filled sac of tissue that is usually benign but can be malignant. Cysts are sometimes removed just to be sure they are benign. Lumps in the breast are often found to be harmless cysts rather than cancer.

Cystitis An inflammation and irritation of the bladder caused by bacterial infection, chemotherapy, or radiation treatments. Symptoms include a burning sensation when urinating and a frequent urgent need to urinate.

Cystoscopy Inspection of the inside of the bladder by means of a telescope. During the procedure, a catheter may also be placed, biopsies taken, or tissue removed.

Cytogenetics Laboratory study or analysis of the chromosome pattern of a cell.

Cytokine A substance secreted by immune system cells, usually to send "messages" to other immune cells.

Cytology The study under a microscope of cells that have been cast off or scraped off organs such as the uterus, lungs, bladder, and stomach. Also called exfoliative cytology.

Cytomegalovirus A virus that is commonly carried without any medical problems. In patients whose immunity is suppressed, it can cause severe pneumonia (e.g., bone marrow transplant or leukemia or lymphoma patients).

D

Debulking A surgical procedure that removes a significant part or most of a tumor in cases where it is not possible to remove all of it. This may make subsequent radiotherapy or chemotherapy easier and more effective.

Deep venous thrombosis (DVT) A blood clot that forms in veins deep inside the body, commonly the lower leg and thigh. Many patients with cancer are at high risk for developing DVT.

DES Diethylstilbestrol. A synthetic hormone formerly used to treat complications of pregnancy. A rare type of vaginal cancer may occur in daughters of women who used DES during pregnancy. It has been used to treat prostate cancer.

Differentiation The process whereby immature (unspecialized) cells change to mature forms that have specific functions.

Diuretics Drugs that increase the elimination of water and salts in the urine.

DNA (deoxyribonucleic acid) The building block of our genetic material. DNA is responsible for passing on hereditary characteristics and information on cell growth, division, and function.

Dose limiting A side effect, complication, or risk that makes it impossible or unwise to exceed a specific dose of a chemotherapeutic agent. A total dosage of bleomycin of more than 400 units, for example, may produce severe lung scarring. Lung toxicity is, therefore, dose limiting.

Double-blinded A clinical trial in which there are several treatment choices and neither the patient nor the physician knows which treatment any person is receiving. The treatment is identified by a "code" that is deciphered only after the clinical trial is completed.

Drug resistance The development of resistance in cancer cells to a specific drug or drugs. If resistance develops, a patient in remission from chemotherapy may relapse despite continued administration of anticancer drugs.

Dysphagia Difficulty in swallowing; a sensation of food sticking in the throat.

Dysplasia Abnormal developments or changes in cells, which are sometimes an indication that cancer may develop.

Dyspnea Shortness of breath.

Dysuria Difficult or painful urination; burning on urination.

E

Edema The accumulation of fluid within tissues.

Effusion A collection of fluid inside a body cavity, such as around the lungs (pleural), intestines (peritoneal), or heart (pericardial). This can be caused by cancer invading the cavity.

EGD (esophagogastroduodenoscopy) Inspection of the esophagus and stomach with a flexible scope.

Electrolytes Certain chemicals—including sodium, potassium, chloride, and bicarbonate—found in the tissues and blood. They are often measured as an aid to patient care.

Electron beam A form of radiotherapy in which the beam does not penetrate completely through the body as ordinary X-rays do. It is used for treating the skin or lesions beneath the skin.

Electrophoresis See *Serum protein electrophoresis.*

Emboli Pieces of tissue, usually blood clots but sometimes tumor cells, that travel in the circulatory system until they lodge in a small artery or capillary, often in the lungs.

Embolization A method of treating tumors in a localized area by blocking the blood vessels to the area. This is done by inserting a thin tube (catheter) into an artery and injecting tiny pellets or other materials, which then travel "downstream" and block the smaller arteries. The pellets may also carry chemotherapeutic agents for release in the area ("chemoembolization").

Emesis A fancy word for vomiting.

Endemic Refers to a disease that is common in a particular community or population.

Endocrine glands Glands—such as the pituitary, thyroid, ovaries, and testes—that secrete hormones to control digestion, reproduction, growth, metabolism, or other body functions.

Endometrial carcinoma A cancer of the inner lining (endometrium) of the uterus.

Endoscope An instrument (telescope) for examining hollow organs or body cavities. There are many specialized types, such as the cystoscope for the bladder, colonoscope for the colon, gastroscope for the stomach, and bronchoscope for the lungs.

Endoscopy Examination of interior body structures with an endoscope. The physician is able to take photographs, obtain small samples of tissue, or remove small growths during the procedure.

Enteral feeding Administration of liquid food (nutrients) through a tube inserted into the stomach or intestine.

Enteroclysis A method of taking X-rays of the small bowel using a contrast agent administered through a tube inserted into the bowel.

Enterostomal therapist A medical professional specializing in the care of artificial openings in the abdominal wall and elsewhere—ileostomies, gastrostomies, or colostomies, for example.

Enterostomy The opening used for enteral feeding or for drainage if the bowel is obstructed.

Enzymes Proteins that play a part in specific chemical reactions. The level of enzymes in the blood is often measured

because abnormal levels may be a sign of various diseases.

Epidermal growth factor receptor (EGFR) A protein expressed on the surface of many tumor cells that is involved in cell division, growth, and survival. Several anticancer drugs targeting EGFR have now been approved, such as erlotinib (Tarceva) and cetuximab (Erbitux).

Epidermoid carcinoma A cancer arising from surface cells in an organ and resembling skin ("epidermis") when viewed under a microscope.

Epidural The space just outside the spinal cord. Plastic catheters may be inserted in the space to deliver anesthetics or morphine for pain control.

Epstein-Barr (EB) virus A virus known to cause infectious mononucleosis and associated with Burkitt's lymphoma and certain cancers of the head and neck.

ERCP (endoscopic retrograde cholangiopancreatography) A procedure in which a catheter is introduced through a gastroscope into the internal bile ducts.

Esophageal speech A way of speaking used by people who have had their larynges (voice boxes) removed. As air is expelled from the esophagus, the walls of the pharynx and esophagus vibrate to produce sound.

Esophagitis Soreness and inflammation of the esophagus due to infection, toxicity from radiotherapy or chemotherapy, or some physical injury.

Estrogen The female sex hormone produced by the ovaries. Estrogen controls the development of physical sexual characteristics, menstruation, and pregnancy. Synthetic forms are used in oral contraceptives and in various therapies.

Estrogen-receptor (ER) assay A test that determines whether the breast cancer in a particular patient is stimulated by estrogen.

Excision Surgical removal of tissue.

Extravasation Leakage into the surrounding tissues of intravenous fluids or drugs—especially cancer chemotherapeutic agents—from the vein being used for injection. Extravasation may damage tissues.

F

Familial adenomatous polyposis (FAP) A hereditary condition in which members of the same family develop intestinal polyps. It is considered a risk factor for colorectal cancer.

Fiber-optics Flexible tubes that transmit light by means of glass fibers. They are used to inspect and treat internal parts of the body. Various types of endoscopes use fiber-optic technology.

Fibrocystic breasts A condition, which may come and go in relation to the menstrual cycle, in which fluids normally absorbed by breast tissue become trapped and form cysts. There may be difficulty distinguishing between cysts and breast cancer.

Fine needle aspiration (FNA) A simple and painless way to obtain small bits of tissue for diagnosis. After local anesthesia, a small needle is inserted through the skin directly into a tumor and a sample of tissue is drawn up inside the needle. In some cases—thyroid cancer, for example—FNA has become an integral part of the early diagnostic process. But the amount of tissue obtained this way may not be enough to diagnose lymphomas and some other cancers.

Fissures Cracks or a splitting in the skin or an internal membrane.

Fistula An abnormal opening between the inside of the body and the skin or between two areas inside the body.

Frozen section A procedure done by the pathologist during surgery to give the surgeon an immediate answer as to whether a tissue is benign or malignant. Tissue is removed by biopsy, frozen, cut into thin slices, stained, and examined under a microscope. This information is vital in helping the surgeon decide the most appropriate course of action.

Fulguration Use of an electric current to destroy tissue.

G

Gamma globulins Proteins in the blood that contain antibodies, part of the body's defense against infection.

Gamma knife A special type of radiation therapy, used principally for tumors in the brain, in which many radiation sources are aimed from many angles toward a specific area of the brain containing the tumor. Other parts of the brain receive only a small amount of radiation, whereas the tumor area receives most of the radiation energy.

Gamma rays The form of electromagnetic radiation produced by certain radioactive sources. They are similar to X-rays but have a shorter wavelength.

Gene A biological unit of DNA capable of transmitting a single characteristic from parent to offspring.

Gleason score A system of grading the appearance of prostate cancer under the microscope. A low score usually means the cancer cells are very similar to normal prostate, and the cancer is likely to be indolent and grow slowly. A high score means the cells are very different from normal and more likely to grow, spread, and cause clinical problems.

Grade of tumor A way of describing tumors by their appearance under a microscope. Low-grade tumors are slow to grow and spread, whereas high-grade tumors grow and spread rapidly.

Graft-versus-host (GVH) disease After bone marrow transplantation, immune cells in the donated (grafted) material may identify the patient's tissues (the host) as foreign and try to destroy them. This can be a serious problem, and drugs are available to combat it. However, in some cases, a GVH reaction actually helps control the cancer. (See chapter 16.)

Granulocyte The most common type of white blood cell. Its function is to kill bacteria (also called neutrophil, poly, or PMN [polymorphonuclear leukocyte]).

Guaiac test A test to see if there is hidden blood in the stool. A positive result may be a sign of cancer, but many benign conditions also cause bleeding.

Gynecomastia Swelling of the breast tissues in men. Although this can be caused by medications and other diseases, in the cancer field it is caused by certain cancers of the testis or by female hormones used to treat prostate cancer.

H

Helicobacter pylori Previously, it was believed that peptic ulcers were caused by too much stomach acid and/or stress. A specific bacteria has now been found to be an important cause. This bacteria, *H. pylori,* can be cited as a cause of certain cancers of the stomach.

Hematocrit A way of measuring the red cell content of the blood. The normal level is about 40 to 45 in men and from 37 to 42 in women. A low hematocrit is a sign of anemia.

Hematologist A physician (internist) who specializes in blood diseases.

Hematoma A blood lump under the skin that appears like a "black and blue" mark.

Hematopoietic Pertaining to a blood-forming organ such as the bone marrow.

Hematuria Blood in the urine. This may be obvious (gross hematuria) or hidden (microscopic hematuria).

Hemoglobin A way of measuring the red cell content of the blood. The normal value in men is from 13 to 15 grams, in women from 12.5 to 14 grams.

Hemolytic anemia Anemia resulting from the breakdown of red blood cells in the bloodstream before the end of their usual life span of 120 days.

Hemorrhagic cystitis A bladder irritation, which may be caused by the anticancer drug cyclophosphamide (Cytoxan) or ifosfamide.

Hepatic Pertaining to the liver.

Hepatotoxicity Adverse effects of drugs on the liver indicated by abnormal blood tests of liver function. It is also sometimes associated with jaundice.

HER-2/*neu* (also called c-*erb*B-2) A gene that controls cell growth, involving human epidermal growth factor receptor 2. An antibody, Herceptin, is in clinical use.

Hereditary breast and ovarian cancer (HBOC) A syndrome predisposing women to the development of breast and ovarian cancers, among other malignancies. Commonly found in women of Ashkenazi Jewish ancestry. Usually caused by mutations in BRCA1 and BRCA2 genes.

Herpes simplex A common acute viral inflammation of the skin or mucous membranes characterized by the development of blisters. This infection around the mouth is commonly called a cold sore.

Herpes zoster; shingles A painful eruption in the skin caused by a virus infection that affects nerves. The same virus that causes shingles causes chicken pox.

Histology The appearance of tissues, including cancers, under a microscope.

HIV (human immunodeficiency virus) The virus that causes AIDS.

HLA (human leukocyte antigen) typing A blood test to match a potential donor for bone marrow transplantation.

Hormonal anticancer therapy A form of therapy that takes advantage of the tendency of some cancers—especially breast and prostate cancers—to stabilize or shrink if certain hormones are administered.

Hormonal replacement therapy A hormone (estrogen or progesterone) given to postmenopausal women or women who have had their ovaries removed, to replace the missing hormone.

Hormones Naturally occurring substances that are released by the endocrine organs and circulate in the blood. Hormones control growth, metabolism, reproduction, and other functions and can stimulate or turn off the growth or activity of specific target cells. Some hormones are used after surgery to treat breast, ovarian, prostate, uterine, and other cancers.

Hospice A facility and a philosophy of care that stress comfort, peace of mind, and the control of symptoms. Hospice care, provided on either an outpatient or inpatient basis, is generally invoked when no further anticancer therapy is available and life expectancy is six months or less. Hospice also helps family and friends to care for and cope with the loss of a dying loved one.

Humoral immunity Immunity mediated by substances such as proteins (gamma globulins) produced by the immune system.

Hyperalimentation Artificial feeding—temporary or permanent—by means of concentrated protein and fat solutions delivered intravenously. A special catheter is usually needed.

Hypercalcemia High levels of calcium in the blood. It is a sign of some forms of cancer or of cancer spreading to bone and also occurs in some benign conditions.

Hyperfractionation Radiation therapy given two or three times a day (usually in smaller doses) instead of once a day.

Hyperplasia The overgrowth of healthy cells; not a precursor of cancer.

Hyperthermia Increased body temperature. Generally used to mean the use of special devices to raise body temperature as a way of treating cancer. It is usually used along with radiation therapy.

Hypoechoic An ultrasound examination produces a picture of the area being examined. Hypoechoic areas "bounce" or echo the sound waves less than surrounding tissues (e.g., by a benign cyst in the breast).

Hypothermia Excessively low body temperature.

Hysterectomy Surgical removal of the uterus.

I

IL-2 See *Interleukins.*

Ileostomy An artificial opening in the skin of the abdomen, leading to the small bowel (ileum). (See *Ostomy.*)

Iliac The part of the lower abdomen just above the hipbone on each side of the body. Also refers to the iliac bone just above the hip joint.

Immune; immunity A state of adequate defense against infections or foreign substances. Some cancers are believed to produce immune responses.

Immune system The body mechanisms that resist and fight disease. The main defenders are white blood cells and antibodies, which, along with other specialized defenders, react to the presence of foreign substances in the body and try to destroy them.

Immunoelectrophoresis A way to separate serum gamma globulins—called IgA, IgG, and IgM—into groups according to their immunologic qualities.

Immunosuppression The state of having decreased immunity and thus being less able to fight infections and disease.

Immunosuppressive drug A drug that modifies the natural immune response so that it will not react to foreign substances. This type of drug is most commonly given after organ transplants so that the new organ will not be rejected.

Immunotherapy A method of cancer therapy that stimulates the body's defense mechanisms to attack cancer cells or combat a specific disease.

Incontinence Inability to control the flow of urine or stools.

Indirect laryngoscopy Inspection of the lower throat, pharynx, and larynx (voice box) by means of a small mirror placed in the back of the throat. (See *Laryngoscopy.*)

Induction The initial treatment—usually with chemotherapy—to eliminate or control cancer. Usually applied to leukemia or lymphoma.

Induration Firmness or hardness of tissues.

Inferior vena cava The large vein draining the blood from the legs and abdomen back into the heart.

Infiltration The leaking of fluid or medicines into tissues from a tube or needle. This can cause irritation or swelling. (See *Extravasation.*)

Inflammation The triggering of local body defenses causing defensive white blood cells (leukocytes) to pour into the tissues from the circulatory system. It is characterized by redness, heat, pain, and swelling.

Informed consent A legal standard defining how much a patient must know about the potential benefits and risks of therapy before agreeing to receive it.

Infusion Administration of fluids and/or medications into a vein or artery over a period of time.

Infusion pumps Small, preloaded mechanical devices used to continuously administer intravenous chemotherapy over a designated time.

Inguinal Pertaining to the groin, the common site for hernias and the location of the inguinal lymph nodes, an area where cancer may spread.

In situ A very early stage of cancer in which the tumor is localized to one area.

Interferons Natural substances produced in response to infections. They have been created artificially by recombinant DNA technology in an attempt to control cancer.

Interleukins A group of cytokines (chemicals) produced by body cells that convey molecular messages between cells of the immune system. Interleukin-2 (IL-2), the best known of these, acts primarily on T lymphocytes; it is being used in the treatment of cancer.

Intra-arterial Drugs directed into an artery through a catheter.

Intracavitary therapy Treatment directed into a body cavity via a catheter.

Intramuscular (IM) The injection of a drug into a muscle; from there it is absorbed into the circulation.

Intraperitoneal Delivery of drugs and fluids into the abdominal cavity.

Intrapleural Delivery of drugs and fluids into the space around the lung. Often employed when fluid collects there as a result of cancer.

Intrathecal Administration of drugs into the spinal fluid.

Intravenous (IV) Administration of drugs or fluids directly into a vein.

Intravenous pyelogram (IVP) An X-ray examination of the kidneys, ureters, and bladder.

Invasive cancer Cancer that spreads to the healthy tissue surrounding the original tumor site. This contrasts with in situ cancer, which has not yet begun to spread.

Ipsilateral On the same side of the body. (See also *Contralateral.*)

J

Jaundice The accumulation of bilirubin, a breakdown product of hemoglobin, which results in a yellow discoloration of the skin and the whites of the eyes. Jaundice is a sign of liver disease or blockage of the major bile ducts.

K

Kidney failure; renal failure Malfunction of the kidneys due to disease or the toxic effects of drugs or chemicals. Urine volume may or may not be diminished.

Killer cells (also called natural killer cells or NK cells) White blood cells that attack tumor cells and body cells that have been invaded by foreign substances.

L

Laparoscopy Insertion of a thin telescope (laparoscope) into the abdomen to inspect this area and remove tissue samples or biopsies.

Laparotomy An operation in which the abdominal cavity is opened.

Laryngectomy The surgical removal of the larynx (voice box) resulting in the loss of normal speech. A laryngectomee is someone who has undergone this operation.

Laryngoscopy Inspection of the lower throat, pharynx, and larynx by means of a small mirror placed in the back of the throat (indirect laryngoscopy) or by direct examination under anesthesia (direct laryngoscopy).

Leukocyte White blood cell.

Leukocytosis An increase in the number of leukocytes in the blood.

Leukopenia A decreased white blood cell count (below 5,000).

Leukopheresis A washing procedure that removes white blood cells from the blood.

Leukoplakia White plaque on the mucous membranes of the mouth and gums. This may be precancerous.

Ligation Tying off blood vessels to limit blood to a part of the body or a tumor.

Linear accelerator A radiation therapy machine that produces a high-energy beam.

Liver function tests A group—panel—of blood tests to check if the liver is healthy.

Liposomal An anticancer drug preparation in which the drug is attached to tiny fat particles. Absorption and distribution to the tumor may be improved.

Lobectomy Removal of one lobe of a lung; the right lung contains three lobes, the left lung contains two.

Localized A cancer confined to the site of origin without evidence of spread.

Lumbar puncture Removal of spinal fluid for examination. This simple procedure—also called a spinal tap—involves numbing the skin of the back with a local anesthetic and placing a needle in the numbed area to remove the spinal fluid.

Lumpectomy The removal of a breast cancer (lump) and the surrounding tissue without removing the entire breast. It is a less radical procedure than mastectomy and is usually followed by radiation treatment.

LVN Licensed vocational nurse. A nurse trained to do more limited tasks than a registered nurse (RN).

Lymph The watery fluid that circulates through the lymphatic system.

Lymph node mapping See *Sentinel node*.

Lymph nodes Oval-shaped organs, often the size of peas or beans, that are located throughout the body and contain clusters of cells called lymphocytes. They produce infection-fighting lymphocytes and also filter out and destroy bacteria, foreign substances, and cancer cells. They are connected by small vessels called lymphatics. Lymph nodes act as our first line of defense against infections and the spread of cancer.

Lymphadenectomy Removal of lymph nodes at surgery to see if they contain cancer and to improve the chance of cure in case they do.

Lymphangiogram An X-ray picture of the abdominal lymph nodes obtained by injecting a contrast substance under the skin on the feet. This test helps to determine if cancer has spread to the abdominal lymph nodes.

Lymphatic system The system of lymph nodes and the lymphatic vessels that connect them.

Lymphedema Swelling, usually of an arm or a leg, caused by obstructed lymphatic vessels. It can develop because of a tumor or as an unusual late effect of surgery or radiotherapy.

Lymphocytes A family of white blood cells responsible for the production of antibodies and for the direct destruction of invading organisms or cancer cells.

Lymphokine A specific protein (cytokine) created by lymphocytes.

Lymphokine-activated killer cells (LAK cells) White blood cells that are stimulated in the laboratory to kill tumor cells.

Lynch syndrome Also called hereditary nonpolyposis colon cancer (HNPCC). An inherited disorder in which affected people are at increased risk of developing colon cancer and certain other types of cancers, especially at a younger age than average.

Lytic A bone lesion that has less calcium than normal. On a scan, it may appear to be a "hole" in the bone.

M

Macrophages White blood cells that destroy invading organisms by ingesting them.

Malaise Tiredness or lack of "drive."

Malignant An adjective meaning cancerous. Two important qualities of malignancies are the tendency to sink roots into surrounding tissues and to break off and spread elsewhere ("metastasize").

MALT (mucosal-associated lymphoid tissue) lymphoma A type of lymphoma that arises in tissues lining the inside of organs, especially the gastrointestinal tract.

Markers; tumor markers Chemicals in the blood that are produced by certain cancers. Measuring the markers is useful for diagnosis but especially useful for following the course of treatment. (See *CEA [carcinoembryonic antigen]*.)

Median Most of the time when we talk about an "average," we add all the values together and divide by the number. Thus, adding up the ages of a group of people and then dividing by the number of people gives the average age. In the cancer field, particularly when talking about how long a response to treatment lasts or how long someone would be expected to live, a different kind of average is used, called the median. That is the middle value or the middle term, so half the values are higher and half are lower. If the median survival for a certain stage of cancer is eight years, that means that half the people live longer and half live shorter than eight years.

Mediastinum The central portion of the chest, comprising the heart, large blood vessels, esophagus, trachea, and surrounding tissues.

Metaplasia Cells that appear abnormal under a microscope and do not yet show signs of malignancy.

Metastasis The spread of cancer from one part of the body to another by way of the lymph system or bloodstream. Cells in the new cancer are like those in the original tumor.

Methadone A synthetic narcotic pain reliever related to morphine.

Micrometastases The presumed presence of tiny, as yet undetectable, deposits of cancer cells that have spread to other organs. A goal of adjuvant therapy is to attempt to eliminate these.

Milligrams/meter squared (mg/m²) A formula for calculating dosages of chemotherapy drugs according to the surface area of the body. Since the amount of skin is hard to determine exactly, it is closely estimated from height and weight. An average person might have 1.7 square meters of body surface area. If the standard drug dosage was 650 mg/m², then $650 \times 1.7 = 1105$ mg of drug would be given.

Mitosis The process of cell reproduction or division. Cancer cells usually have higher rates of mitosis than normal cells. The number of divisions seen under a microscope reflects how aggressive the cancer is.

Modality A general class or method of treatment. The basic modalities of cancer therapy include surgery, radiation therapy, chemotherapy, and immunotherapy.

Monoclonal antibodies (MAbs) Highly specific antibodies, usually manufactured in a laboratory, that react to a specific cancer antigen or are directed against a specific type of cancer. Current research is studying their role in therapy, and they are used in certain malignancies, such as non-Hodgkin's lymphoma. One potential use is to deliver chemotherapy and radiotherapy directly to a tumor, thus killing the cancer cells and sparing healthy tissue. Studies are also trying to find out if monoclonal antibodies can be produced to detect and diagnose cancer cells at a very early and curable stage.

Monoclonal gammopathy An elevation in gamma globulin in the blood caused by a single clone of plasma cells or lymphocytes. Such a protein pattern may be associated with multiple myeloma.

Morbidity Sickness; illness; symptoms and signs of disease. Not to be confused with mortality.

Mortality Death as a result of disease.

MRI (magnetic resonance imaging) A method of creating images of the body using a magnetic field and radio waves rather than X-rays. Although the images are similar to those of CT scans, they can be taken in all three directions (planes) rather than just in cross sections. There is no X-ray exposure.

Mucosa; mucous membrane The inner lining of the gastrointestinal tract or other structures such as the vagina and nose.

Mucositis Inflammation of the mucous membranes of the mouth or gastrointestinal tract. Soreness—like "cold sores"—

can develop in the mouth as a side effect of chemotherapy.

Multicentricity A tumor that appears to start growing in several places at once.

Multimodality Using a combination of two or more types of therapy—for example, radiotherapy plus chemotherapy, radiation plus surgery, or chemotherapy plus surgery.

Mutation A permanent change in a cell's DNA that alters its genetic potential. It may be a response to a chemical substance (mutagen) or result from a physical effect such as radiation. Sometimes the daughter cells may be cancerous.

Myeloid Pertaining to the bone marrow, where blood cells are made.

Myelogram An X-ray of the spinal cord after the introduction of radio-opaque dye into the sac surrounding it. Used to see if a tumor involves the spinal cord or nerve roots.

Myeloma A cancer of the protein-producing plasma cells of the bone marrow. Multiple bone lesions are common.

Myelosuppression A fall in the blood counts caused by therapy, especially chemotherapy and radiotherapy.

N

Nadir The lowest point to which white blood cell or platelet counts fall after chemotherapy.

Narcotics Pain-relieving (analgesic) substances whose use is closely regulated by government. There are natural and synthetic types.

Nasopharynx The part of the nasal cavity behind the nose and above the part of the throat that we can see.

National Cancer Institute A highly regarded research center in Bethesda, Maryland, that conducts basic and clinical research on new cancer treatments and supervises clinical trials of new treatments throughout the United States.

National Surgical Adjuvant Breast/Bowel Project (NSABP) A group of dedicated research and clinical physicians who have formed a large cooperative group to study new treatments. Many major advances in treatment are attributed to this group.

Natural killer (NK) cells Large, granular lymphocyte cells normally present in the body whose normal function is to kill virally infected cells. Some methods of cancer treatment take advantage of this ability of NK cells.

Neck dissection Surgery to remove groups of lymph nodes in the neck, to check for spread of cancer and to improve the chances of cure.

Necrosis The disintegration of tissues caused by some physical or chemical agent or by lack of blood supply. Cancers treated effectively by chemotherapy, radiotherapy, heat, or biological agents undergo necrosis.

Needle biopsy Removing a tiny bit of tissue for diagnosis by inserting a needle into a tumor. The procedure is usually done under local anesthesia. (See *Fine needle aspiration [FNA]*.)

Neoadjuvant chemotherapy Chemotherapy given *before* the primary treatment, either surgery or radiation therapy, to improve the effectiveness of treatment. (See *Adjuvant chemotherapy*.)

Neoplasm A new abnormal growth. Neoplasms may be benign or malignant.

Nephrotoxic Toxic to the kidneys. The term is generally used to refer to a drug's effect.

Nerve block Removing pain by numbing a nerve temporarily (with a local anesthetic) or permanently (with an alcohol injection).

Neuropathy Malfunction of a nerve, often causing numbness (sensory nerve) or weakness (motor nerve). It is sometimes a side effect of anticancer drugs.

Neurotoxicity Toxic effects (usually of drugs) on the nervous system.

Neutropenia An abnormally low number of neutrophils in the blood, often occurring as a result of chemotherapy. Neutropenia renders a person susceptible to bacterial infections.

Neutrophils One of the white blood cells that fight infection. Also called granulocytes, polys, or PMNs (polymorphonuclear leukocytes).

Nevus A benign growth on the skin, such as a mole.

Nitrosoureas A class of chemical compounds that can enter the brain through the blood-brain barrier. The anticancer drugs BCNU, CCNU, and methyl-CCNU are nitrosoureas. (See *Blood-brain barrier.*)

NK cells See *Natural killer (NK) cells.*

"No Code" An order, written in a hospital chart after careful and considered discussions, not to attempt to resuscitate a patient if breathing and/or the heartbeat should stop. This is usually considered if the patient, after all reasonable therapeutic efforts have been made and have failed, is suffering greatly and rapidly failing from a far-advanced malignancy. Also "Do Not Rescuscitate" (DNR).

Nodes See *Lymph nodes.*

Nodule A small lump or tumor that can be benign or malignant.

Non-cell-cycle specific Chemotherapeutic drugs capable of destroying cells that are not actively dividing.

NSAID Nonsteroidal anti-inflammatory drugs. A group of drugs used for pain, arthritis, and swelling.

Nuclear magnetic resonance (NMR) An old term for MRI.

O

OCN (oncology-certified nurse) A registered nurse who has passed an examination, following training and experience in oncology nursing practice.

Omentum A collection of fatty tissue inside the abdomen. It is often removed during cancer surgery, especially ovarian cancer, since it may collect cancer cells.

Ommaya reservoir A device consisting of a soft bulb implanted under the scalp, with a tube leading into a fluid compartment inside the brain. This is used to deliver anticancer drugs to the cerebrospinal fluid without the need for repeated spinal taps.

Oncogene A gene that normally directs cell growth. If altered or overexposed, it can facilitate the growth of cancer. It can be inherited or result from exposure to carcinogens.

Oncologist A physician who specializes in cancer therapy. There are surgical, radiation, pediatric, gynecologic, and medical oncologists. The term *oncologist* alone generally refers to medical oncologists, who are internists with expertise in chemotherapy and in handling the general medical problems that arise during the disease.

Oncology The medical specialty that deals with the diagnosis, treatment, and study of cancer.

Oophorectomy The surgical removal of one or both ovaries.

Opportunistic infections Many common fungi and bacteria and a few microscopic parasites do not ordinarily cause infections in healthy people. But such ordinarily harmless organisms can produce severe, life-threatening, and hard-to-control infections in cancer patients by taking advantage of the reduced immune response resulting from the disease or therapy.

Osteolytic Some tumors, if they spread to bones, cause the bone substance to break down and appear "thin" on X-ray. These areas may be more susceptible to fracture from even minor trauma ("pathologic fracture").

Ostomy A surgically created opening in the skin, leading to an internal organ, for purposes of drainage. (See *Colostomy; Ileostomy.*)

Ototoxicity Toxic effects on the ears, generally resulting in a ringing in the ears or hearing loss.

P

p-value A statistical term commonly used by scientists to express the probability that an observed difference between two groups or two treatments is really different, and not simply due to chance. The commonly used p-value of p = 0.05 means that there is only one chance in twenty that the observed difference is due only to chance.

p53 gene A tumor suppressor gene that usually inhibits tumor growth. It is altered in many forms of cancer.

Palate The roof of the mouth. The hard palate is in front, the soft palate just behind.

Palliative Treatment that aims to improve well-being, relieve symptoms, or control the growth of cancer, but not primarily intended or expected to produce a cure.

Palpation Examination by feeling an area of the body—such as the breast or prostate—with the fingers to detect abnormalities. A palpable mass is one that can be felt.

Paracentesis Removing fluid from the abdomen by inserting a small needle through the skin. This is usually done under local anesthesia.

Paraneoplastic syndromes Various symptoms and signs—changes in body minerals, nerve function, or water balance, for example—that indicate the presence of a tumor in the body but are not related to direct pressure by the tumor.

Parenteral nutrition Artificial feeding by the intravenous administration of concentrated amino acid, sugar, and fat solutions. (See *Hyperalimentation; TPN [total parenteral nutrition].*)

Partial remission Shrinkage but not complete disappearance of a tumor in response to therapy.

Pathologic fracture A fracture (break) in a bone through an area weakened by cancer. Usually little or no injury or trauma precedes the fracture, as is usually the case with the fracture of healthy bones.

Pathologist A physician skilled in the performance and interpretation of laboratory tests and in the examination of tissues to provide a diagnosis.

Pathology Study of disease through the examination of body tissues, organs, and materials. Any tumor suspected of being cancerous must be diagnosed by pathologic examination. The physician who does this is called a pathologist.

PCR (polymerase chain reaction) A technique to amplify short DNA or RNA sequences, from very small quantities. Used extensively in biology, medicine, and genetic research.

PDQ (Physician Data Query) A comprehensive, up-to-date information service on state-of-the-art cancer treatment, provided by the National Cancer Institute via computer and fax.

Percutaneous endoscopic gastrostomy Placement of a feeding tube through the skin directly into the stomach. This employs a technique of shining a light inside the stomach, by means of a gastroscope, to identify the exact location to safely pass the feeding tube through the skin, using a small incision under local anesthesia.

Performance status A score or scale to determine how a cancer patient is doing. The Karnofsky scale goes from 0 to 100 (100 being best). The Eastern Cooperative Oncology Group (ECOG) scale goes from 0 to 4, 0 being best.

Perfusion Administration of fluid, often containing chemotherapy drugs, to an organ or tissue, usually by the blood vessel supplying that area.

Pericardial effusion A fluid collection in the sac around the heart. Sometimes it needs to be drained if it causes pressure on the heart.

Perineum The part of the body between the anus and the genitals.

Perioperative Occurring at or around the time of surgery. Often used with reference to chemotherapy or radiotherapy treatments.

Peripheral stem cell transplantation Administration of immature blood cells, obtained either from the same person (autologous) or from another person (allogeneic), or from an identical twin (syngeneic). These cells help the bone marrow recover after high-dose chemotherapy. Also called peripheral stem cell support.

Peritoneal cavity The space inside the abdomen. It is enclosed by a membrane, the peritoneum, that also covers all the abdominal organs.

Peritonoscopy Inspection of the inside of the abdominal cavity by means of a telescope inserted under anesthesia through a tiny opening in the skin.

PET (positron-emission tomography) A type of scan that detects areas of cells that are living and growing more rapidly than others. It may thus find areas of cancer by detecting their growth, rather than the space they occupy, as in CT and MRI scans. It is becoming a vital tool for cancer staging and assessment.

Petechiae Tiny areas of bleeding under the skin usually caused by a low platelet count.

Phlebitis Inflammation of the veins, often causing pain and tenderness. (See *Pulmonary embolism; Thrombophlebitis.*)

Photodynamic therapy The injection of a light-sensitizing chemical or dye and the subsequent application of light, usually laser, to a tumor. The chemical improves the effect of the laser treatment and thus minimizes or prevents damage to normal tissues.

Photosensitivity Extreme sensitivity to the sun. Some medications—including a few anticancer drugs as well as tetracycline antibiotics—produce photosensitivity as a side effect, leaving the patient prone to sunburn.

Placebo An inactive substance, used in a research study or clinical trial, that looks like the medication. It is used to eliminate the improvement that may result from the belief that a medication is being given, rather than from the actual effect of a medication.

Plasma The clear yellow part of the blood, other than the blood cells.

Plasma cells A type of white blood cell, usually found only in the bone marrow, that produces antibodies. Cancer of this cell is called multiple myeloma.

Plasmapheresis The replacement or "washing" of a patient's plasma by donor plasma or saline.

Platelet One of the three kinds of circulating blood cells. The normal platelet count is about 150,000 to 300,000. Platelets are responsible for creating the first part of a blood clot. Platelet transfusions are used in cancer patients to prevent or control bleeding when the number of platelets has significantly decreased.

Plateletpheresis Collection of platelets in a machine for transfusion into another person.

Pleura The thin layer of tissue covering the lungs and the inside of the chest cavity. There is a small amount of fluid there normally. Sometimes if a cancer is present causing irritation, there may be a large fluid buildup, called pleural effusion.

Pneumonectomy Surgical removal of a lung.

Polycythemia An excessively high red blood cell count. This may be caused by a primary blood disease or be a response to another type of disease.

Polymerase chain reaction (PCR) A technique to amplify short DNA sequences from very small quantities. Used extensively in biology, medicine, and genetic research (e.g., to find occult cancer cells that have spread to lymph nodes).

Polyp A growth that protrudes from mucous membranes, often looking like a tiny mushroom. Polyps may be found in the nose, ears, mouth, lungs, vocal cords, uterus, cervix, rectum, bladder, and intestine. Some polyps occurring in the cervix, intestine, stomach, or colon can eventually become malignant and should be removed.

Poorly differentiated A tumor that under a microscope has little or only a slight resemblance to the normal tissue from the same organ. (See *Undifferentiated; Well differentiated.*)

Port (infusion) A small disk with a soft center (about the size of a quarter) that is surgically placed just below the skin in the chest or abdomen. A tube coming out of the side is connected to a large vein. By passing a small needle through the skin into the disk, fluids, drugs, or blood products can be delivered directly to the bloodstream without worrying about finding an adequate vein, making multiple venipunctures, or causing leakage of the fluids into surrounding tissues.

Port-a-Cath One type of infusion port, a venous access device that has nothing protruding from the skin. Injections are made into a chamber implanted just under the skin. (See *Port.*)

Potassium An important mineral in the body that is often lost during illness, especially with diarrhea. Low potassium levels can cause weakness.

Precancerous Abnormal cellular changes or conditions—intestinal polyps, for example—that tend to become malignant. Also called premalignant.

Primary tumor The place where a cancer first starts to grow. Even if it spreads elsewhere, it is still known by the place of origin. For example, breast cancer that has spread to the bone is still breast cancer, not bone cancer.

Proctoscopy See *Sigmoidoscopy.*

Progesterone One of the female hormones (the other is estrogen). It causes the buildup of the uterine lining in preparation for conception and performs other functions before and during pregnancy. Certain synthetic forms of the hormone are used in cancer treatment.

Progesterone-receptor (PR) assay A test that determines if breast cancer is stimulated by progesterone.

Prognosis A statement about the likely outcome of disease—the prospect of recovery—in a particular patient. In cancer, it is based on all available information about the type of tumor, staging, therapeutic possibilities, expected results, and other personal or medical factors. For example, breast cancer patients who are diagnosed early usually have a good prognosis.

Progression The growth or advancement of cancer, indicating a worsening of the disease.

Prophylactic Treatment designed to prevent a disease or complication that is likely to develop but has not yet appeared.

Prostate-specific antigen (PSA) A substance in the blood derived from the prostate gland. Its level may rise in prostatic cancer and it is useful as a marker to monitor the effects of treatment.

Prosthesis An artificial replacement or approximation of a body part—such as a leg, a breast, or an eye—that is missing because of disease or treatment.

Proteins The basic structures of our body, made up of a string of amino acids (like railroad cars coupled together). Some proteins are enzymes, cytokines, and antibodies.

Protocol A precisely written description of a research program to test a specific new treatment under controlled conditions.

Proto-oncogene A class of genes that encourage cell growth. Mutation of these genes produces a carcinogenic oncogene, one that can cause cancer.

Pulmonary embolism A life-threatening condition in which a blood clot travels to the lungs from veins in the legs or pelvis, often from thrombophlebitis. The clots are diagnosed with a lung scan and treated with anticoagulants.

R

Radiation fibrosis Scar tissue resulting from radiation therapy. This may be visible in the lung, for example, after radiation therapy treatment for lung cancer.

Radiation oncologist; radiotherapist A physician who specializes in the use of radiation to treat cancer.

Radiation therapy See *Radiotherapy*.

Radical mastectomy Removal of the entire breast along with the underlying muscle and the lymph nodes of the armpit (axilla). In a modified radical mastectomy, the underlying (pectoral) muscles are left in place.

Radical neck dissection An extensive surgical operation to remove all of the lymph glands on one side of the neck, usually in association with surgery to remove a primary tumor that may have spread to the lymph glands in the neck.

Radical surgery An extensive operation to remove the site of cancer and the adjacent structures and lymph nodes.

Radioactive implant A source of high-dose radiation that is placed directly in and around a cancer to kill the cancer cells.

Radioactive isotope A radioactive substance used for diagnosis (tracer dose used for scans) or treatment (therapeutic dose).

Radiofrequency ablation (RFA) A procedure that uses electrodes to generate heat and destroy abnormal tissue (e.g., primary or metastatic liver tumors).

Radiologist A doctor who specializes in the use of X-rays as well as other imaging techniques such as ultrasound, MRI, and radioactive tracers to diagnose and investigate disease. New radiology techniques are also used for treatment in some cases (interventional radiology).

Radiosensitive A cancer that usually responds to radiation therapy. The opposite is radioresistant.

Radiosensitizer A drug or biological agent that is given together with radiation therapy to increase its effect.

Radiotherapy The use of high-energy radiation from X-ray machines, cobalt, radium, or other sources for control or cure of cancer. It may reduce the size of a cancer before surgery or be used to destroy any remaining cancer cells after surgery. Radiotherapy can be helpful in treating recurrent cancers or relieving symptoms.

Rad An obsolete unit measuring radiation dosage, now replaced by the centigray (cGy).

Randomized clinical trial A scientific method of assigning subjects of a clinical trial to several groups at random. The results of the trial can be compared without bias and can be depended upon to reflect differences being studied instead of the results of accidental grouping.

Ras **gene** A gene that has been found to cause cancer if mutated or altered.

Recurrence The reappearance of a disease after treatment has caused it to apparently disappear.

Red blood cells Cells in the blood that bring oxygen to tissues and take carbon dioxide from them.

Refractory tumors Tumors that do not respond to chemotherapy.

Regional involvement The spread of cancer from its original site to nearby surrounding areas. Regional cancers are confined to one general location in the body.

Regression The shrinkage of a cancer usually as the result of therapy. In a complete regression, all tumors disappear. In a partial regression, some tumor remains.

Rehabilitation Programs that help patients adjust and return to a full productive life. Rehabilitation may involve physical measures such as physical therapy and prostheses, as well as counseling and emotional support.

Remission The partial or complete shrinkage of cancer usually occurring as the result of therapy. Also the period when the disease is under control. A remission is not necessarily a cure.

Renal Pertaining to the kidney.

Resection The surgical removal of tissue.

Residual disease; residual tumor Cancer left behind after surgery or other treatment.

Resistance Failure of a tumor to respond to radiotherapy or chemotherapy. The resistance may be evident during the first treatment (primary) or, after an initial response, during the subsequent treatment (secondary).

Response rate The percentage of patients whose cancer responds to treatment with shrinkage or disappearance.

Retroperitoneum The area of the abdomen near the back, behind all the organs, including the bowel.

Retrospective The use of medical records and interviews to study a disease, "looking backward."

Reverse isolation Isolation to prevent visitors or hospital staff from carrying an infection into a patient's room. This usually means that everyone must wear a gown, mask, and gloves.

Ribonucleic acid (RNA) A nucleic acid present in all cells and similar to DNA. It is the biochemical blueprint for the transfer of information from DNA to the formation of proteins by the cells.

Risk factors The habits or conditions that promote the development of many cancers. Cigarette smoking, for example, is the major risk factor for lung cancer. The major risk factor for skin cancer is overexposure to the sun.

Risk reduction Techniques used to reduce the chances of developing cancer. A high-fiber diet, for example, may help reduce the risk of colon cancer.

RNA See *Ribonucleic acid (RNA).*

S

Saline Saltwater solution resembling the amount of salt in the bloodstream.

Salvage The attempt to cure a patient by a second, third, or later alternative treatment program after the first-line treatment has failed to produce a cure.

Sampling Removal of a portion of a tissue for diagnostic tests.

Sarcoma A cancer of supporting or connective tissue such as cartilage, bone, muscle, or fat. Sarcomas are often highly malignant but account for only 2 percent of all human cancers.

Scans (radioisotope) Diagnostic procedures for assessing organs such as the liver, bone, and brain. Radioactive tracers are introduced intravenously and if a malignant tumor or other foreign material is present, pictures of the organ will show abnormalities that may indicate the presence of a tumor. There is no significant risk with this small, brief radiation exposure.

Screening The search for cancer in apparently healthy people who have no cancer symptoms. Screening may also refer to coordinated programs in large populations.

Second-look surgery Sometimes the only way to determine if aggressive therapy has worked is to explore the patient surgically sometime after initial therapy. Second-look surgery can discover if there is any residual or recurrent cancer, which may help decide whether treatment is complete or if more radiotherapy or chemotherapy is needed. Residual tumor may also be removed during the operation.

Segmentectomy Surgical removal of a portion (segment) of the breast or lung.

Seizure; convulsion Shaking of a part or all of the body, often with loss of consciousness. This can be caused by an injury, a benign condition (such as idiopathic epilepsy), or a brain tumor.

Selective angiography X-ray pictures of an organ taken after a catheter is passed through the artery to the organ and a dye, which shows on X-rays, is injected.

Sentinel node In the case of spread of cancers to nearby lymph nodes, there is usually a single lymph node (sometimes two) that first receives the cancer cells. This node can be identified by special dyes and/or radioisotopes. If only those nodes are removed, and examination shows no cancer, it is very unlikely that other lymph nodes contain cancer. This technique may eliminate extensive lymph node dissections, with their resulting possible problems, such as swelling. Most experience has been in melanoma and breast cancer, and the technique is now being developed in other forms of cancer.

Sepsis; septicemia; bacteremia Bacterial growth within the bloodstream. This very serious situation usually requires hospitalization for intravenous antibiotics.

Serum protein electrophoresis (SPEP) A laboratory testing method that separates serum proteins into different groups— albumin, alpha globulin, beta globulin, and gamma globulin. The different patterns produced are characteristic of various diseases.

Shingles See *Herpes zoster.*

Shunt A surgical path or diversion of fluid from one place to another, often used to relieve the effect of pressure from fluid.

Sigmoidoscopy An examination of the rectum and lower colon with a hollow lighted tube called a sigmoidoscope. It is used to detect colon polyps and cancer, to find the cause of bleeding, and to evaluate other bowel diseases. A newer instrument using fiber optics—the flexible sigmoidoscope—permits easier, safer, and more extensive examination. Also called proctoscopy. (See also *Colonoscopy.*)

Sodium An important mineral in the body that helps maintain fluid balance. It is measured as part of an electrolyte panel.

Soft tissue Refers to fat, muscle, fibrous tissue, or other supportive tissues. Soft-tissue sarcoma refers to cancers of these tissues.

Sonography The use of ultrasound pictures in diagnosis.

Speculum An instrument used to look inside an opening of the body.

Sphincter A circular muscle that tightens around an organ or cavity to close it and to regulate the flow of material. If the sphincter around the rectum and the mouth of the bladder aren't functioning properly, for example, urine and stool might be lost involuntarily.

Spinal tap Same as lumbar puncture. Insertion of a needle under local anesthesia, to remove spinal fluid for testing or treatment.

Spleen An organ adjacent to the stomach, composed mainly of lymphocytes, which removes worn-out blood cells and foreign materials from the bloodstream.

Sputum Material or secretions coughed up from the lungs. Also called phlegm.

Squamous cell (epidermoid) carcinoma Cancer arising from the skin or the surfaces of other structures, such as the mouth, cervix, and lungs.

Staging An organized process of determining how far a cancer has spread. Staging involves a physical exam, blood tests, X-rays, scans, and sometimes surgery. Knowing the stage helps determine the most appropriate treatment and the prognosis.

Stem cells/stem cell transplantation Primitive or early cells found in bone marrow and blood vessels that give rise to all of our blood cells. To protect patients from low blood counts and the resulting complications after high-dose chemotherapy, a complex device is used to remove stem cells from a vein in the arm and give them back intravenously a few days later. They find their way back into the bone marrow and replace the marrow that was depressed by chemotherapy. The use of peripheral stem cell transplants has made the need to collect bone marrow itself much less important. This procedure should really be called peripheral stem cell protection rather than transplantation, since patients get their own cells back.

Stent A tubular device placed inside a body structure to keep it open.

Stereotaxic needle biopsy A procedure often used in the diagnosis of brain tumors. A specialized frame is used to hold a patient's head or other body part stationary while the biopsy needle is directed to exactly the right spot. Usually a CT scanner or other computer-associated equipment is used to find the correct position. This method has also been applied to very small breast cancers.

Stereotaxic radiosurgery A technique of radiation to the brain using a rigid head frame, with administration of high-dose radiation through openings in the frame. The tumor receives the maximum dose and the normal brain a lesser dose.

Steroids A class of fat-soluble chemicals— including cortisone and male and female sex hormones—that are vital to many functions within the body. Some steroid derivatives are used in cancer treatment.

Stoma A surgically created opening in the skin for elimination of body wastes. A stoma is made in the abdominal wall for elimination of wastes, for example, when the colon and/or rectum can no longer perform this function. (See *Colostomy.*)

Stomatitis Inflammation and soreness of the mouth. This is sometimes a side effect of chemotherapy or radiotherapy.

Stool Feces or bowel movement.

Stool for occult blood A test to determine if bleeding has occurred. This may show signs of bleeding that are too mild to see with the naked eye. (See *Guaiac test.*)

Subcutaneous Beneath the skin, as in "subcutaneous injections."

Superior vena cava The large vein draining the blood from the head, neck, and arms back into the heart.

Supportive care Treatment given to prevent, control, or relieve symptoms, side effects, and complications, and to improve quality of life and comfort.

Suppository A way to administer medications by absorbing the drug into a wax preparation, then inserting it into the rectum or vagina. Suppositories are used to treat local conditions such as vaginitis and hemorrhoids and are also used when pills cannot be swallowed or kept down because of nausea, sore mouth, or narrowing of the esophagus. Antinausea suppositories such as Compazine and Tigan are often used to combat this side effect of chemotherapy.

Systemic Affecting the entire body.

T

T cell See *B cell.*

Targeted therapy A drug that targets a particular pathway or molecule that drives the growth, spread, survival, or maintenance of tumor cells specifically and preferentially while sparing normal cells. Many newer drugs in development in oncology are targeted therapies, as opposed to classic chemotherapy agents.

Telangiectasia Prominent or dilated small veins in the skin. This can occur without known cause, as part of certain medical conditions, and sometimes as a result of radiation therapy.

TENS (transcutaneous electrical nerve stimulation) The use of a small device that is connected to the skin and sends small, harmless amounts of electricity into the pain fibers so that they are "too busy" to recognize the real pain.

Teratogenic A drug or toxin that, if taken during pregnancy, can cause the fetus to be malformed.

Terminal This term has a number of definitions. Some people use it when cure is not possible, even if treatment can add years to the patient's life. Others say a patient is terminal when he or she has a specific short life expectancy, perhaps six months or one month. Still others mean that no other treatment can be given and that "nature will take its course." If this term comes up, discuss with your doctor exactly what is meant by it.

Thoracentesis Insertion of a needle or tube between the ribs and into the chest cavity to remove fluid. The procedure is done for diagnostic or treatment reasons and is performed under local anesthesia.

Thoracic Pertaining to the thorax or chest.

Thoracotomy A surgically created opening in the chest.

Thrombocytopenia An abnormally low number of platelets (thrombocytes)—fewer than 150,000—due to disease, reaction to a drug, or toxic reaction to treatments. Bleeding can occur if there are too few platelets, especially if the count falls to less than 20,000.

Thrombophlebitis Inflammation of veins with blood clots inside the veins. Usually associated with pain, swelling, and tenderness. (See also *Phlebitis; Pulmonary embolism.*)

Thrombopoietin A substance that stimulates the production of platelets. It is useful in improving low platelet counts after chemotherapy and thus reducing the risk of bleeding.

Thrombosis Formation of a blood clot within a blood vessel.

Tissue A collection of cells of the same type. There are four basic types of tissues in the body: epithelial, connective, muscle, and nerve.

TNM classification A complex and exact system for describing the stage of development of most kinds of cancer. This system is not used for lymphomas, leukemias, or Hodgkin's disease.

Topical On the surface of the body, usually the skin.

TPN (total parenteral nutrition) The use of complex protein and fat solutions to supply enough calories and nutrients to sustain life. The solutions are delivered intravenously.

Tracheostomy An artificial opening in the neck leading to the windpipe (trachea). The opening is created surgically to allow breathing when the trachea is blocked.

Tumor A lump, mass, or swelling. A tumor can be either benign or malignant.

Tumor debulking See *Debulking.*

Tumor necrosis factor A natural protein substance produced by the body that may make tumors shrink.

Tumor suppressor genes A class of genes that suppress cell growth.

Tyrosine kinase inhibitor (TKI) A new class of antitumor drugs that interfere with a particular enzymatic process important in cell communication and growth. Examples include imatinib (Gleevec) and erlotinib (Tarceva).

U

Ulcer A sore resulting from corrosion of normal tissue by some irritating process or substance such as stomach acid, chemicals, infections, impaired circulation, or cancerous involvement.

Ultrasound The use of high-frequency sound waves to create an image of the inside of the body. Also called ultrasonography.

Umbilical cord blood transplantation A new source of stem cells to be used to restore depleted bone marrow from high-dose chemotherapy. Active research is under way for cancer treatment.

Undifferentiated A tumor that appears "wild" under a microscope, not resembling the tissue of origin. These tumors tend to grow and spread faster than well-differentiated tumors, which do resemble the normal tissue they come from. (See *Anaplastic; Poorly differentiated; Well differentiated.*)

Unilateral On one side of the body.

Urethra The tube that leads from the bladder to the outside of the body to allow elimination of urine. Cancers rarely begin there.

Urostomy A surgical procedure in which the ureters, which carry urine from the kidneys to the bladder, are cut and connected to an opening in the skin outside the abdomen. This allows urine to flow into a collection bag. (See *Stoma.*)

Uterus The female reproductive organ, located in the pelvis; the womb in which an unborn child develops until birth.

V

Vaccine A substance that will stimulate an immune response to a tumor (or to microorganisms; for example, polio vaccine). Vaccines are being actively studied for treatment of cancer, especially melanoma.

Vascular endothelial growth factor (VEGF) A substance produced by certain cells that stimulates new blood vessel formation (angiogenesis). A number of anticancer drugs have been or are being developed that target VEGF and its receptor.

Venipuncture Inserting a needle into a vein in order to obtain blood samples, start an intravenous infusion, or give a medication.

Ventricles Four fluid-filled cavities in the brain all connected with each other. There are two lateral ventricles in the top part of the brain—one on each side—with the third and fourth ventricles in the center of the brain. Obstruction of the connections or the outflow tract leads to swelling (hydrocephalus). Also refers to the chambers in the heart.

Vesicant drugs Chemotherapeutic agents that can cause significant tissue irritation and soreness if they leak outside the vein after injection.

Video-assisted surgery Use of a video camera and TV screen to project an enlarged image of the inside of the body, to assist the surgery. For example, video-assisted thoracoscopy can perform surgery inside the chest through a relatively small incision.

Viral vector A virus used in cancer therapy, changed so it will not cause disease, and containing tumor antigens to stimulate an antitumor immune response in the body. Viral vectors may also carry genes that attempt to change cancer cells into normal cells.

Virus A tiny infectious agent that is smaller than bacteria. Many common infections such as colds and hepatitis are caused by viruses. Viruses invade cells, alter the cells' chemistry, and cause them to produce more viruses. Several viruses produce cancers in animals. Their role in the development of human cancers is now being studied.

W

Watchful waiting Close and careful monitoring of a person's cancer condition, without starting treatment until certain symptoms appear or change.

Well differentiated A tumor that under a microscope resembles normal tissue from the organ of origin. (See *Poorly differentiated; Undifferentiated.*)

White blood cells Cells in the blood that fight infection. These are composed of monocytes, lymphocytes, neutrophils, eosinophils, and basophils. The normal count is 5,000 to 10,000. It may be elevated or depressed in a wide variety of diseases. Chemotherapy and radiotherapy usually cause low white counts.

Z

Zoster See *Herpes zoster.*

Cancer Information Bibliography

Gail Sorrough, M.L.I.S., and Gloria Won, M.L.I.S.
H. M. Fishbon Memorial Library, UCSF Medical Center at Mount Zion

■ ■ ■ ■

A book about a topic as challenging as cancer becomes a helpful and at times comforting resource. You can read it anytime, anywhere, and easily share it with others.

Thousands of books about cancer have been published. Our goal with this bibliography is to present a short, representative selection of works for which we have found positive reviews from reliable resources (e.g., *Library Journal*) or that we have personally reviewed for integrity of data and credentials of authors, sponsors, and funding sources.

Testimonies about personal battles with cancer abound; many are beautifully written, inspirational, and filled with good advice. They have not been included in this list in part because there are so many, and it was decided that selection between them would be best left to the individual reader.

At the end of the bibliography is a list of books all beginning with the title "100 Questions & Answers." Jones and Bartlett, the publisher, works with the American Cancer Society and the National Comprehensive Cancer Network to produce this highly respected series.

The final section, "Web Resources," supplements the resources discussed in the chapter on cancer information.

■ General Textbooks

Abeloff, Martin D., James O. Armitage, John E. Niederhuber, et al., eds. 2004. *Clinical oncology*. 3rd ed. Elsevier Churchill Livingstone. 3205 pp.

American Joint Committee on Cancer. 2002. *AJCC cancer staging manual*. 6th ed. Springer. 421 pp.

DeVita, Vincent T., Samuel Hellman, and Steven A. Rosenberg, eds. 2005. *Cancer: principles and practice of oncology*. 7th ed. Lippincott Williams & Wilkins. 2 vols.

Hartmann, Lynn C., and Charles L. Loprinzi. 2005. *Mayo Clinic guide to women's cancers*. Mayo Clinic Health Information. 638 pp.

Kufe, Donald W., Robert C. Bast, and William N. Hait, eds. 2006. *Holland–Frei cancer medicine*. 7th ed. BC Decker. 2328 pp.

Volk, Ruti Malis. 2007. *The Medical Library Association guide to cancer information*. Neal-Schuman. 331 pp.

Yarbro, Connie Henke, Margaret Hansen Frogge, and Michelle Goodman. 2005. *Cancer nursing: principles and practice*. 6th ed. Jones and Bartlett. 1879 pp.

■ Diagnosis and Treatment

Adler, Elizabeth M. 2005. *Living with lymphoma: a patient's guide*. The Johns Hopkins University Press. 424 pp.

Boyd, D. Barry, and Marian Betancourt. 2005. *The Cancer recovery plan*. Avery. 256 pp.

Coleman, C. Norman. 2006. *Understanding cancer: a patient's guide to diagnosis, prognosis, and treatment*. 2nd ed. The Johns Hopkins University Press. 232 pp.

Cukier, Daniel, Frank Gingerelli, Grace Makari-Judson, and Virginia McCullough. 2005. *Coping with chemotherapy and radiation*. McGraw-Hill. 264 pp.

Dodd, Marylin J. 2001. *Managing the side effects of chemotherapy and radiation therapy*. UCSF Nursing Press. 324 pp.

Feuerstein, Michael, and Patricia Findley. 2006. *The cancer survivor's guide: the essential handbook to life after cancer*. Marlowe. 256 pp.

Figlin, Robert A. 2003. *Kidney cancer*. Kluwer. 256 pp.

Harpham, Wendy Schlessel. 2003. *Diagnosis, cancer: your guide to the first months of healthy survivorship*. Revised ed. W.W. Norton. 288 pp.

Levin, Bernard, Terri Ades, and Durado Brook. 2006. *American Cancer Society's complete guide to colorectal cancer*. American Cancer Society. 418 pp.

Link, John. 2007. *Breast cancer survival manual: a step-by-step guide for the woman with newly diagnosed breast cancer*. 4th ed. Henry Holt. 256 pp.

Lyss, Alan P., Humberto Fagundes, and Patricia Corrigan. 2005. *Chemotherapy and radiation for dummies*. Wiley. 380 pp.

Morra, Marion E., and Eve Potts. 2003. *Choices: the most complete sourcebook for cancer information*. 4th ed. HarperCollins. 1136 pp.

Rosenbaum, Ernest H., and Isadora Rosenbaum. 2005. *Everyone's guide to cancer supportive care: a comprehensive handbook for patients and their families*. Andrews McMeel. 579 pp.

Rosenbaum, Ernest H., David Spiegel, Patricia Fobair, and Holly Gautier. 2007. *Everyone's guide to cancer survivorship: a road map for better health*. Andrews McMeel. 349 pp.

Schofield, Jill R., and William A. Robinson. 2000. *What you really need to know about moles and melanoma*. The Johns Hopkins University Press. 248 pp.

Strum, Stephen, and Donna L. Pogliano. 2005. *A primer on prostate cancer: the empowered patient's guide*. 2nd ed. Life Extension Media. 368 pp.

Teeley, Peter, and Philip Bashe. 2005. *The complete cancer survival guide: the most comprehensive, up-to-date guide for patients and their families*. Broadway. 1008 pp.

Van Nostrand, Douglas, Gary Bloom, and Leonard Wartofsky, eds. 2004. *Thyroid cancer: a guide for patients*. Keystone Press. 336 pp.

Walsh, Patrick C., and Janet Farrar Worthington. 2002. *Dr. Patrick Walsh's guide to surviving prostate cancer*. Reprint ed. Warner Books. 480 pp.

Wilkes, Gail M. 2004. *American Cancer Society consumer's guide to cancer drugs*. 2nd ed. Jones and Bartlett. 535 pp.

■ Financial and Legal Matters

Doukas, David John, and William Reichel. 2007. *Planning for uncertainty: living wills and other advance directives for you and your family*. 2nd ed. The Johns Hopkins University Press. 160 pp.

Landay, David. 2000. *Be prepared: the complete financial, legal, and practical guide to living with cancer, HIV, and other life-challenging conditions*. St. Martin's Griffin. 480 pp.

National Cancer Institute. 2006. Financial resources for people with cancer. *FactSheet*, 10.

Shenkman, Martin M., and Patti S. Klein. 2004. *Living wills & health care proxies: assuring that your end-of-life decisions are respected*. Law Made Easy Press. 228 pp.

▓ Integrative Medicine

American Cancer Society's complete guide to complementary and alternative cancer methods. 2008. 2nd ed. American Cancer Society. 960 pp.

Cohen, Isaac, and Debu Tripathy. 2002. *Breast cancer: beyond convention; the world's foremost authorities on complementary and alternative medicine offer advice on healing.* Edited by M. Tagliaferri. Atria. 496 pp.

Gordon, James S., and Sharon Curtin. 2001. *Comprehensive cancer care: integrating alternative, complementary, and conventional therapies.* New ed. HarperCollins. 314 pp.

Halstead, Bruce, and Terry Halstead. 2006. *The scientific basis of Chinese integrative cancer therapy: including a color atlas of Chinese anticancer plants.* North Atlantic Books. 455 pp.

Kumar, Nagi B., Susan Moyers, Kathy Allen, Karen Besterman-Dahan, and Diane Riccardi. 2002. *Integrative nutritional therapies for cancer: a scientific guide to natural products used to treat and prevent cancer.* Facts and Comparisons Publishing Group. 165 pp.

Lerner, Michael. 1996. *Choices in healing: integrating the best of conventional and complementary approaches to cancer.* New ed. MIT Press. 696 pp.

Micozzi, Marc S. 2006. *Complementary and integrative medicine in cancer care and prevention: foundations and evidence-based interventions.* Springer. 600 pp.

Murray, Michael. 2003. *How to prevent and treat cancer with natural medicine.* Reprint ed. Riverhead Trade. 432 pp.

Tierra, Michael. 2003. *Treating cancer with herbs: an integrative approach.* Lotus Press. 528 pp.

▓ Nutrition and Fitness

Aker, Saundra N., and Polly Lenssen. 2000. *A guide to good nutrition during cancer treatment.* Fred Hutchinson Cancer Research Center. 147 pp.

Arnot, Bob. 1999. *The breast cancer prevention diet: the powerful foods, supplements, and drugs that can save your life.* Little, Brown. 304 pp.

Arnot, Bob. 2001. *The prostate cancer protection plan: the foods, supplements, and drugs that can combat prostate cancer.* Little, Brown. 352 pp.

Dalzell, Kim. 2002. *Challenge cancer and win! Step-by-step nutrition action plans for your specific cancer.* NutriQuest Press. 460 pp.

Elliott, Laura, Laura L. Molseed, and Paula Davis McCallum. 2006. *The clinical guide to oncology nutrition.* 2nd ed. American Dietetic Association. 270 pp.

Greenwood-Robinson, Maggie. 2006. *Foods that combat cancer: the nutritional way to wellness.* Avon. 240 pp.

Hickey, Steve, and Hilary Roberts. 2005. *Cancer: nutrition and survival.* Lulu.com. 300 pp.

Kaelin, Carolyn M., Francesca Coltera, Josie Gardiner, and Joy Prouty. 2007. *The breast cancer survivor's fitness plan: reclaim health, regain strength, live longer.* McGraw-Hill. 253 pp.

Keane, Maureen, and Daniella Chace. 2006. *What to eat if you have cancer: healing foods that boost your immune system.* Revised ed. McGraw-Hill. 288 pp.

Nixon, Daniel W. 1996. *The cancer recovery eating plan: the right foods to help fuel your recovery.* Reprint ed. Three Rivers Press. 464 pp.

Quillin, Patrick. 2005. *Beating cancer with nutrition: optimal nutrition can improve the outcome in medically-treated cancer patients*. Revised ed. Nutrition Times Press. 416 pp.

Simone, Charles B. 2004. *Cancer and nutrition: a ten point plan for prevention and cancer life extension*. Princeton Institute. 304 pp.

■ Supportive and Palliative Care

Berger, Ann, John L. Shuster, and Jamie H. Von Roenn. 2007. *Principles and practice of palliative care and supportive oncology*. 3rd ed. Lippincott Williams & Wilkins. 923 pp.

Brennan, James, and Clare Moynihan. 2004. *Cancer in context: a practical guide to supportive care*. Oxford University Press. 456 pp.

Harpham, Wendy Schlessel. 2004. *When a parent has cancer: a guide to caring for your children*. Revised, reprinted ed. HarperCollins. 240 pp.

Patt, Richard B., and Susan S. Lang. 2006. *The complete guide to relieving cancer pain and suffering*. New ed. Oxford University Press. 464 pp.

Rosenbaum, Ernest H., and Isadora Rosenbaum. 2005. *Everyone's guide to cancer supportive care: a comprehensive handbook for patients and their families*. Revised ed. Andrews McMeel. 600 pp.

SanKar, Andrea. 2000. *Dying at home: a family guide for caregiving*. 2nd ed. The Johns Hopkins University Press. 328 pp.

Silver, Julie K. 2006. *After cancer treatment: heal faster, better, stronger*. The Johns Hopkins University Press. 288 pp.

Waller, Diane, and Caryl Sibbett, eds. 2005. *Art therapy and cancer care*. Open University Press. 256 pp.

■ Jones and Bartlett Publishing

Abou-Alfa, Ghassan, and Ronald DeMatteo. 2006. *100 Questions & answers about liver cancer*. Jones and Bartlett. 126 pp.

Ball, Edward D., and Gregory Lelek. 2003. *100 Questions & answers about leukemia*. Jones and Bartlett. 133 pp.

Bashey, Asad, and James W. Huston. 2005. *100 Questions & answers about myeloma*. Jones and Bartlett. 143 pp.

Beck, Lindsay, Fertile Hope, and Kutluk H. Oktay. 2008. *100 Questions & answers about cancer & fertility*. Jones and Bartlett. 180 pp.

Brown, Zora K., Harold P. Freeman, and Elizabeth Platt. 2007. *100 Questions & answers about breast cancer*. 2nd ed. Jones and Bartlett. 263 pp.

Bub, David, Susannah Rose, and Douglas Wong. 2003. *100 Questions & answers about colorectal cancer*. Jones and Bartlett. 278 pp.

Carper, Elise, Kenneth Hu, and Elena Kuzin. 2007. *100 Questions & answers about head and neck cancer*. Jones and Bartlett. 160 pp.

Carrier, Ewa, and Gracy Ledingham. 2004. *100 Questions & answers about bone marrow and stem cell transplantation*. Jones and Bartlett. 130 pp.

Carroll, William L., and Jessica Reisman. 2005. *100 Questions & answers about your child's cancer*. Jones and Bartlett. 181 pp.

DeMatteo, Ronald, Marina Symcox, and George D. Demetri. 2007. *100 Questions & answers about gastrointestinal stromal tumor (GIST)*. Jones and Bartlett. 140 pp.

Dizon, Don S., and Nadeem R. Abu-Rustum. 2007. *100 Questions & answers about ovarian cancer*. 2nd ed. Jones and Bartlett. 165 pp.

Ellsworth, Pamela, and Brett Carswell. 2006. *100 Questions & answers about bladder cancer*. Jones and Bartlett. 155 pp.

Ellsworth, Pamela, John A. Heaney, and Oliver Gill. 2003. *100 Questions & answers about prostate cancer*. Jones and Bartlett. 238 pp.

Ginex, Pamela K., Manit S. Bains, Jacqueline Hanson, and Bart L. Frazzitta. 2005. *100 Questions & answers about esophageal cancer*. Jones and Bartlett. 160 pp.

Holman, Peter, Jodi Garrett, and William Jansen. 2004. *100 Questions & answers about lymphoma*. Jones and Bartlett. 180 pp.

Kelvin, Joanne Frankel, and Leslie Tyson. 2005. *100 Questions & answers about cancer symptoms and cancer treatment side effects*. Jones and Bartlett. 228 pp.

Krychman, Michael L. 2007. *100 Questions & answers for women living with cancer: a practical guide for survivorship*. Jones and Bartlett. 180 pp.

McClay, Edward F., Mary-Eileen T. McClay, and Jodie Smith. 2004. *100 Questions & answers about melanoma and other skin cancers*. Jones and Bartlett. 158 pp.

O'Reilly, Eileen, Joanne Kelvin, John R. Harty, and Joy McCully. 2003. *100 Questions & answers about pancreatic cancer*. Jones and Bartlett. 177 pp.

Parles, Karen, and Joan H. Schiller. 2006. *100 Questions & answers about lung cancer*. Updated ed. Jones and Bartlett. 208 pp.

Rose, Susannah, and Richard Hara. 2005. *100 Questions & answers about caring for family or friends with cancer*. Jones and Bartlett. 223 pp.

Stark-Vance, Virginia, and Mary Louise Dubay. 2004. *100 Questions & answers about brain tumors*. Jones and Bartlett. 239 pp.

■ Web Resources

American Academy of Dermatology: SkinCancerNet
Available at www.skincarephysicians.com/skincancernet

American Academy of Family Physicians: familydoctor.org
Available at familydoctor.org

American Lung Association
Available at www.lungusa.org

American Society of Clinical Oncology and the ASCO Foundation: People Living with Cancer (PLWC)
Available at www.plwc.org/portal/site/PLWC
PLWC provides timely, oncologist-approved information to help patients and families make informed health care decisions. All content is subject to a formal peer review process by the PLWC Editorial Board, composed of more than 150 medical, surgical, radiation, and pediatric oncologists, oncology nurses, social workers, and patient advocates. In addition, ASCO editorial staff reviews the content for easy readability.

The Brain Tumor Society
Available at www.tbts.org
The Brain Tumor Society was founded in 1989 as a national nonprofit organization to provide hope and comfort to patients, survivors, and families and to help them in their struggle against a brain tumor by offering concrete informational resources and supportive services. The society was also chartered with the goal to fund brain tumor research in order to find new treatments and, ultimately, a cure.

breastcancer.org
Available at www.breastcancer.org
All medical information on the breast-cancer.org Web site and in their printed materials is reviewed by members of their Professional Advisory Board, which includes more than sixty practicing medical professionals from around the world who are leaders in their fields.

CancerCare
Available at www.cancercare.org
CancerCare is a national nonprofit organization that provides free, professional support services to anyone affected by cancer: people with cancer, caregivers, children, loved ones, and the bereaved. CancerCare programs, including counseling, education, financial assistance, and practical help, are provided by trained oncology social workers and are completely free of charge. Founded in 1944, CancerCare now provides individual help to more than 91,000 people each year, in addition to the 1.6 million people who gain information and resources from its Web site.

Centers for Disease Control and Prevention Division of Cancer Prevention and Control: Cancer A to Z
Available at www.cdc.gov/cancer/az
The Division of Cancer Prevention and Control (DCPC) works with national organizations, state health agencies, and other key groups to develop, implement, and promote effective cancer prevention and control practices. A DCPC partner promotes DCPC's mission through programmatic implementation and outreach that puts research findings into action in order to achieve mutually beneficial goals.

Centers for Disease Control and Prevention: Cancer Survivorship
Available at www.cdc.gov/cancer/survivorship

Harvard School of Public Health. Harvard Center for Cancer Prevention
Available at www.hsph.harvard.edu/cancer/
Established in 1994, the Harvard Center for Cancer Prevention at the Harvard School of Public Health is dedicated to helping people learn about healthy behavior and decrease their risk of cancer and other chronic diseases. The center's communication, education, and research activities grow from collaborations with a variety of partners throughout Harvard University, local communities, and national and international organizations. The center takes a multidimensional approach to reaching diverse communities and motivating healthy behavior change.

The Leukemia & Lymphoma Society
Available at www.leukemia-lymphoma.org
The Leukemia & Lymphoma Society is the world's largest voluntary health organization dedicated to funding blood cancer research, education, and patient services. The society's mission is to cure leukemia, lymphoma, Hodgkin's disease, and myeloma and improve the quality of life of patients and their families. Since its founding in 1949, the society has invested more than $550.8 million for research specifically targeting blood cancers.

Lung Cancer Alliance
Available at www.lungcanceralliance.org
Lung Cancer Alliance is the only national nonprofit organization dedicated exclusively to patient support and advocacy for people living with lung cancer or those at risk for the disease. Their programs include the Lung Cancer Information Line, a toll-free information and referral service for people with lung cancer and their caregivers; the Phone Buddy program, a peer-to-peer support network; Lung Cancer Awareness Month, a national education and advocacy campaign; Spirit & Breath, their quarterly newsletter; and Advocacy Alert, where advocates can receive alerts to participate in or respond to important lung cancer issues.

National Cancer Institute
Available at www.cancer.gov

National Coalition for Cancer Survivorship
Available at www.canceradvocacy.org
The National Coalition for Cancer Survivorship (NCCS) is the oldest survivor-led cancer advocacy organization in the country and a highly respected voice

at the federal level, advocating high-quality cancer care for all Americans and empowering cancer survivors. NCCS believes in evidence-based advocacy for systemic changes at the federal level in how the nation researches, regulates, finances, and delivers cancer care. In 2004, NCCS launched Cancer Advocacy Now!™, a legislative advocacy network that seeks to involve constituents from across the country in federal cancer-related issues. Patient education is also a priority for NCCS. NCCS believes that access to credible and accurate patient information, such as NCCS's award-winning Cancer Survival Toolbox®, is key to demanding and receiving high-quality cancer care.

National Comprehensive Cancer Network (NCCN)
Available at www.nccn.org

National Library of Medicine and National Institutes of Health: MedlinePlus
Available at medlineplus.gov

Oncology Nursing Society: CancerSymptoms.org
Available at www.cancersymptoms.org
This Web site is designed to provide patients and caregivers with information on learning about and managing each of ten common cancer treatment–related symptoms: anorexia, cognitive dysfunction, depression, dyspnea, fatigue, hormonal disturbances, neutropenia, pain, peripheral neuropathy, and sexual dysfunction.

Prostate Cancer Foundation
Available at www.prostatecancerfoundation.org
Prostate Cancer Foundation (PCF) is the world's largest philanthropic source of support for prostate cancer research. The PCF has a single goal: to find better treatments and a cure for recurrent prostate cancer. The PCF, a 501(c)(3) organization, pursues its mission by reaching out to individuals, corporations, and others to harness society's resources, financial and human, to fight this deadly disease. Founded in 1993, the PCF has raised more than $300 million and provided funding to more than 1,400 researchers at 100 institutions worldwide.

U.S. Department of Health and Human Services: healthfinder.gov
Available at www.healthfinder.gov
Healthfinder.gov is an award-winning federal Web site for consumers, developed by the U.S. Department of Health and Human Services together with other federal agencies. Since 1997, healthfinder.gov has been recognized as a key resource for finding the best government and nonprofit health and human service information on the Internet. The site links to carefully selected information and Web sites from more than 1,500 health-related organizations.

U.S. Food and Drug Administration: Cancer Liaison Program
Available at www.fda.gov/oashi/cancer/cancer.html
The staff of the Cancer Liaison Program, located in the FDA's Office of Special Health Issues, work with the FDA's oncology staff to bring the patient advocate's perspective into the review of new drugs to treat cancer. The staff also meets with organized patient advocacy groups to listen to their concerns about drug development and to assist them in understanding the FDA drug regulatory process. Calls from cancer patients and their loved ones are routinely answered by the staff to help callers with questions about cancer clinical trials and cancer drug development.

Index

■ ■ ■ ■

■ P